Dr Ante Bilić
liječnik - stomatolog

Ante Bilić

06.09.1982

Periodontal Disease

Basic Phenomena, Clinical Management, and

Occlusal and Restorative Interrelationships

Periodontal Disease

Basic Phenomena, Clinical Management, and

Occlusal and Restorative Interrelationships

Saul Schluger, D.D.S.

Ralph A. Yuodelis, D.D.S., M.S.D.

Roy C. Page, D.D.S., M.S.D., Ph.D.

University of Washington School of Dentistry
Seattle, Washington

Periodontal Disease

Basic Phenomena, Clinical Management, and

Occlusal and Restorative Interrelationships

LEA & FEBIGER · PHILADELPHIA

Library of Congress Cataloging in Publication Data

Schluger, Saul.
    Periodontal disease.

    Includes index.
    1. Periodontia. I. Yuodelis, Ralph, joint
author. II. Page, Roy C., joint author. III.
Title. [DNLM: 1. Periodontal diseases. WU240
S346p]
RK361.S34   617.6'32   76-2591

ISBN 0-8121-0558-3

Published in Great Britain by Henry Kimpton Publishers, London

PRINTED IN THE UNITED STATES OF AMERICA
Print No.   3

Dedicated to

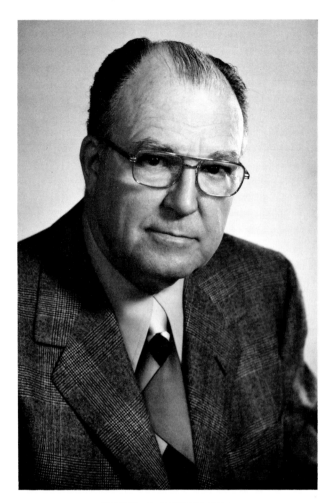

JOHN F. PRICHARD
Master Clinician and Student

Preface

PERIODONTICS has been called the "conscience of dentistry." This does not imply that this single area is the repository of all or much of the idealism, skill, and professionalism in dentistry. It is obvious that this is not the case, nor has it ever been so. What is meant, however, is that in clinical practice whatever derelictions may occur in treatment planning, standards, or skill, the results frequently become visible to the periodontist.

Periodontics is so pervasive throughout so many dental specialties that it almost seems to invade every area save full denture prosthesis. Restorative dentistry is particularly freighted with periodontal requirements and consequences. Approximately one third of this text is devoted to the subject.

We are addressing ourselves to a textbook on periodontics in the practice of dentistry. This is not a book on periodontics for the mythical general practitioner within the usual sense of that term. Such textbooks are sometimes watered down general treatises on periodontics deemed to be within the ability and interest of a dentist whose principal interest lies elsewhere. We hope this book will prove to be a complete and comprehensive text on periodontics. In addition it must, to fulfill our objectives, project periodontics against the variegated screen of the practice of dentistry in its most comprehensive sense.

Implicit in this objective is an authorship skilled in restorative dentistry and in its ancillary areas, knowledgeable in basic phenomena and in their clinical implications, and at the same time aware of the periodontal implications as only trained and practicing periodontists can be. Critical to such an effort is a more or less unified and consistent point of view.

The authors have been in close and intimate professional association for many years. That is not to say that the association has existed in harmonious agreement from the outset. Quite the contrary. Contention, discussion, and frank inquiry have been the rule. The resultant points of view are the product of lively and vigorous discussions until a common frame of reference emerged. It is from this frame of reference that this book is written.

Every book is written for a particular audience. This qualifies the level upon which the text is projected. It is our firm belief based upon many years of teaching periodontics on many levels and in all its ramifications that it is necessary only to be clear—not simple. This makes it possible to direct the book to the most sophisticated level of which we are capable, secure in the knowledge that the reader with a less than all-inclusive interest may profit from its use to the limit of his interest.

SAUL SCHLUGER
RALPH A. YUODELIS
ROY C. PAGE

Seattle

Acknowledgments

Dr. Robert Gottsegen of Columbia University was, in a real sense, the progenitor of this text. Even though his name does not appear as an author or contributor, he was the moving force behind this effort. To him belongs the credit for envisaging an encyclopedic book which would go beyond parochialism in periodontics. Sincere thanks are due and are freely given.

For contribution of material as well as critical review of portions of the manuscript, in addition to stimulating and valuable discussion, sincere thanks are due to Professor Jan Lindhe, Professor Hubert E. Schroeder, Dr. Earnest Newbrun, Dr. Robert Genco, Dr. Robin Davies, and Mr. Alan Saxton. Dr. Kenneth Morrison was an early supporter whose encouragement was most important to the projection of the restorative portions of the text. Dr. Robert H. Johnson and Dr. Val Jekkals were particularly helpful in literature search.

Virginia Brooks merits special mention for her outstanding effort with the illustrations. In working with three authors her task was a particularly difficult one. Alison Ross, too, rendered invaluable assistance in editorial labors to make the text clear as well as readable. Hers was no easy task. She was not alone, however, in her assistance to us. Ms. Judy Kotar also served ably and well in an editorial capacity.

We feel especially indebted to Ms. Gail Mathieson for her secretarial labors for all three of us. They were prodigious and indispensable to the project. Ms. Jan Dixon and Ms. Barbara Lorance also rendered valuable aid in this direction and their help is deeply appreciated.

Photographic reproduction, occupying as it does a critical position in the text, was the work of Mr. James Barrett, Mr. James Clark, and Mr. Clifford Freehe. In fact, all who helped—and they were many—did so in good spirit and humor, often when either or both qualities were in short supply and in great need.

The late Dean Maurice J. Hickey was a source of enormous strength and encouragement in every manner possible. We shall be eternally grateful for his efforts on our behalf. Dean Sheldon Rovin continued in the same manner and we thank him as well.

To that regiment of supporters and retainers must be added our wives, families, and dear friends who encouraged and endured.

Contributors

Neil Basaraba, D.D.S., M.S.D., F.A.C.D.
Private Practice
Vancouver, B.C. Canada

Gordon L. Douglass, D.D.S.
Private Practice
Sacramento, California

Walter B. Hall, A.B., D.D.S., M.S.D.
Professor and Chairman
Department of Periodontics
University of the Pacific
School of Dentistry
San Francisco, California

Elaine D. Henley, M.D., F.A.C.P.
Clinical Professor of Medicine
Division of Endocrinology and Metabolism
University of Washington
Seattle, Washington

Leonard Hirschfeld, A.B., D.D.S.
Clinical Professor
Department of Periodontics
Columbia University
New York, New York

Alfred L. Ogilvie, D.D.S., M.S.
Professor of Oral Medicine
Faculty of Dentistry
University of British Columbia
Vancouver, B.C. Canada

Gottfried A. Schmer, M.D.
Director, Coagulation Division
Department of Laboratory Medicine
Associate Professor of Laboratory Medicine
  and Biochemistry
University of Washington
Seattle, Washington

Hubert E. Schroeder, Dr. Med. Dent.
Professor of Oral Structural Biology
Dental Institute
University of Zurich
Zurich, Switzerland

Introduction to Periodontics

Contents

Introduction to Periodontics

Periodontal disease is one of the most ubiquitous diseases known to man. It is not only widely distributed throughout the world, but there is ample evidence reaching back to the border of prehistory that it has been an old and constant scourge of man. No race is immune; no region is free from the widespread incidence of chronic destructive periodontal disease.

The essential pathogenesis of the disease is not well understood, but the best available investigative minds are in the process of extending our areas of knowledge. At this time not enough has been revealed to permit a spectacular change in therapeutic approach. Therapy must still be administered primarily on a local basis. Within these limitations, however, advances have been made in both prevention and in treatment.

Central to the problem is prevention. In any disease such as chronic destructive periodontal disease in which the involved tissues are responsive to plaque and to other irritational factors, the key to prevention is plaque removal performed on a never-ending daily basis.

Dependence on the patient's effort is admittedly a variable and unreliable expedient. Public health measures such as a vaccine or another immunizing agent would be far more effective, but we have no such agent; we must be content with the less efficient and more personally demanding efforts with toothbrush, floss, and other debriding instruments.

Early recognition is, as in all preventable diseases, critical to optimal therapy. Here the responsibility is clearly that of the general practitioner of dentistry, the pedodontist, or the orthodontist. The old view that chronic destructive periodontal disease is essentially a disease of middle age has been successfully challenged again and again. Too many signs of early breakdown are being found in young patients and even in children. Knowledgeable observers no longer regard these signs as precocious periodontal disease. The pedodontist and the orthodontist should have wider diagnostic and therapeutic horizons than caries and malposition of teeth, and a steadily increasing number of these dental specialists are recognizing their responsibility in discovering periodontal disease.

OBJECTIVES OF PERIODONTAL THERAPY

The objectives of periodontal therapy can be consolidated into one great overriding aim: the survival of the dentition in relative health throughout the life of the individual. From this simple statement many complicated factors flow. For example, where in the therapeutic picture would one place pocket elimination? Is this not a reasonable objective of treatment?

1

In response, let us state that pocket elimination is one of the most important objectives in treatment. It is important insofar as it contributes to survival of the dentition. This in turn has implications of pocket elimination as an aid to plaque removal and maintenance by the patient. A good case can be made for the shallow sulcus as a basic aid to plaque control. Accessibility becomes the touchstone to the dedicated patient.

Since performance in the daily maintenance of the tissues is critical to survival of the dentition, what happens to the patient who does well in this direction but is not capable either psychologically or manually to do an outstanding job? Such a patient desperately needs a shallow sulcus for optimum results. The patient who is outstanding in his efforts may be able to overcome the handicaps of a sulcus somewhat deeper than normal.

Before making such demands upon the patient, searching evaluation of effort and effectiveness is in order. The safer situation by far is the shallow sulcus, but it is by no means the only acceptable one. The objective of therapy keeps intruding. In the multifaceted approach lies the basic attraction of periodontics to the most active and inquiring minds in dentistry.

In an area in dentistry so involved with variables and subject to so many influences as is the periodontium, therapy can become a complicated series of procedures. The search for simple methods is constant and must be continued. In the meantime, we must guard against simplistic thinking and action. It is easy and attractive to adopt a single method to apply to all cases of periodontal disease, no matter how complex. To do that, however, means the lowering of objectives and the acceptance of the loss of teeth that might otherwise have been restored to health.

In the horizons of therapy periodontists also establish their concepts of cure. The restoration of a diseased periodontium to health means a number of things that are definite and can by no means be equivocated.

1. There must be complete resolution of inflammation.
2. There may be no exudate of any kind.
3. There must be complete resolution of edema.
4. Normal probing must not elicit bleeding.
5. Gingival contours must be within normal range in color, texture, and form.
6. The foregoing criteria must describe the homeostasis, or steady state, of the gingiva and the attachment apparatus long enough to become the established state; this would be for a period of several years so that a reasonable judgment may be rendered.

Certain omissions in the foregoing criteria may be somewhat surprising. Elimination of mobility as an absolute requirement should be noted. This is particularly true if the mobility is slight and creates no great problems of retention and impaction of debris because of shifting contact relationships in function. It has been found that the dentition of patients who are heavy nocturnal or diurnal tooth grinders survives in health over extremely long time spans if the teeth are worn to accommodate to heavy use and thus do not make demands upon the supporting apparatus which it cannot meet. There are, however, many patients in which these special conditions do not obtain and who require extensive prosthetic stabilization. The lesson to be learned is that there is no substitute for diagnosis and treatment planning.

Pocket depth is another criterion which must be considered judgmentally on an individual basis. Some of the reasons for this have been given, but in essence we revert to time factors and careful periodic oral scrutiny for the patient who is responsive both in efficacy of effort and tissue quality. In short, we are attempting to use temporal factors instead of linear ones. Here, too, the rule is far from rigid. Most patients do better with shallow sulci to maintain, but not all. These exceptions make it necessary to remove complete pocket elimination from our list of indispensable requirements. In the final analysis, there is only one major and overriding objective of therapy and concept of cure—longevity of the dentition in health.

In establishing this objective, we must alter our conceptions of the importance of maintenance in therapy. A much more imaginative view of this aspect of treatment is required. It may no longer be regarded as ancillary and supportive to so-called active therapy. The entire procedural conglomerate of treatment planning, initial therapy, tooth movement, surgical methodology, restorative methods, and maintenance regimens becomes the single multifaceted assault on periodontal disease. Any and all methods may properly become an integral part of periodontal maintenance.

Two chapters, as well as Section IV, are devoted to techniques and administrative methods commonly ascribed to maintenance. If this is all there is to maintenance, then a larger number of cases will fail than should. Maintenance should properly be on-going therapy. In a certain sense, we as periodontists should regard maintenance much as a cardiologist does his specialty—as the very essence of therapy, with so-called active therapy being only one phase of treatment. This concept places therapy on a continuum throughout the rest of the patient's lifetime. It also means that *all* methods at our disposal will be brought to bear, when necessary, in the long-range management of the case. No longer may we segment treatment as we have in the past.

As for the large number of techniques available, it will be noted by the astute reader that none is universally applicable except, perhaps, subgingival curettage following coronal scaling. All the others have indications and contraindications as well as selective applicability. The student would be well-advised to look with suspicion on the protagonist of a single method as the one of choice.

The way of the periodontist is hard. As the watchdog and critic of others in dentistry, he should be above reproach himself. He rarely is. He is merely another soldier in the good fight.

Periodontics is rather young as specialties go. Using restorative dentistry as an example, with its long history of disagreement over principles of occlusion and restorative precepts, periodontics can look forward to a more universal approach to the periodontal problem. We must struggle against the effect of strong personalities on the acceptability and value of therapeutic alternatives. All methods must be tested in the arena of clinical experience. Individual testimony is useful only as clinical opinion with few, if any, objective criteria possible.

More than in most dental disciplines, time is the final arbiter. Because of the chronicity of the lesion and the variable factors involved—factors such as the patient's performance, resistance to breakdown, and age at onset—all conclusions must be tentative and all opinions, no matter how firmly held, must be subject to change.

TERMINOLOGY

Terminology and nomenclature in this text are that in common usage and in general acceptance by the last report of the Nomenclature Committee of the American Academy of Periodontology. This committee seems not to have met in over a decade. Having been a member of this committee for several years, one of us was engaged, without much success, in evaluating the then current nomenclature. Hope was entertained, forlorn as it proved, that some semblance of order could be achieved in the mixture of Latin and Greek roots in our terms. The answers were once again equivocal. We are precisely back where we were 25 years ago.

Serious attempts were made in this text to adhere to official Academy of Periodontology usage. In the absence of firm guidelines, some aberrations were inevitable, and for these the authors accept full responsibility. A term like *inverse bevel* was downgraded in favor of *internal bevel*. Both *intrabony* and *infrabony* were recognized as open to serious question as accurate terms. We did not, however, go so far as to offer *intra-alveolar* as a substitute even though a far better case can be made for it. We chose intrabony as the better term.

The term we prefer for the removal of material from the surfaces of the teeth or from the walls of a cavity with a curet is *curettage*. When a curet is used for a procedure, the text will generally refer to curettage rather than to scaling, scraping, or planing.

The reader may be struck with the enormous range covered by a text on periodontics and restorative dentistry and periodontal pathology. If there seems to be little in dentistry that has slipped through this net, it is because the material in this text *is* involved with almost all of dentistry.

Section I
Basic Phenomena

6

1

The Normal Periodontium

1

The
Normal
Periodontium

HUBERT E. SCHROEDER
AND ROY C. PAGE

Problems related to the structure of the periodontium are of more than academic interest: they pervade all of our concepts of normal function and pathogenesis, treatment, and prevention of disease. In recent years major advances have been made in our understanding of certain aspects of periodontal structure. Possibly the most significant of these has been resolution of the century-old controversy regarding the nature of the epithelial attachment.[137] In spite of these advances, our knowledge of periodontal structure is still inadequate in many respects, for example: (1) We know little about the comparative periodontal anatomy and histology of various mammalian species in spite of the fact that most experimental observations on the pathogenesis of disease are made in animals; (2) It is not yet possible to distinguish definitively between the normal periodontium and tissue that may have undergone early pathologic alteration; (3) Controversy persists with regard to whether passive eruption of the teeth and noninflammatory gingival recession are normal phenomena related to aging or are pathologic processes; (4) We have almost no information about the properties of the macromolecular components of the periodontal tissues, about how they are made, nor about their turnover rates in the normal state; (5) The normal defense mechanisms of the periodontium are only poorly understood.

It is our aim in this section to summarize the current knowledge of normal structure, physiology, and host defense and to point out areas of deficiency in our understanding. It is assumed that the reader has a prior grounding in oral embryology and histology.

The *dental unit* is an organ made up of the teeth and their supporting hard and soft tissues. The dental unit evolved primarily for the purpose of obtaining and processing food; however, it also plays a key role in deglutition, phonation, proprioception, support of the facial musculature and temporomandibular joint, and in the maintenance of a general sense of social well-being.

The supporting tissues of the teeth, known collectively as the periodontium (from the Greek *peri*, around and *odontos*, a tooth), are made up of gingiva, periodontal ligament, cementum, and alveolar and supporting bone. These tissues are uniquely organized to carry out the following functions:

1. *Attach* the tooth to its bony housing.
2. *Resist* and *resolve* the forces generated by mastication, speech, and deglutition.
3. *Maintain* the integrity of the body surface by separating the external and internal environment.
4. *Adjust* for structural changes associated with wear and aging through continuous remodeling and regeneration.

5. *Defend* against the noxious external environmental influences that are present in the oral cavity.

GENERAL FEATURES OF THE GINGIVA

The oral cavity is lined by a *mucous membrane* which is continous anteriorly with the skin of the lip and posteriorly with the mucosa of the soft palate and pharynx. The oral mucous membrane has three components: The _masticatory_ mucosa covers the hard palate and alveolar bone, a _specialized_ mucosa covers the dorsum of the tongue, and the _lining_ mucosa comprises the remaining oral mucous membrane. The portion of the oral mucous membrane covering and attached to the alveolar bone and cervical region of the teeth is known as the *gingiva*. Normal gingiva is salmon pink, lightly or heavily stippled, and exhibits no exudate and no plaque accumulation. The gingiva generally terminates coronally in a knife-edge relationship with the tooth surface. Histologically, the epithelium and the connective tissues are relatively free of migrating leukocytes, although in most instances a few neutrophilic granulocytes will be observed within the epithelium immediately adjacent to the tooth surface. Dense collagen bundles form the bulk of the underlying connective tissue and extend to and unite with the basement membrane.

The gingiva has three parts: the *free marginal gingiva* which extends from the most coronal soft-tissue margin to the gingival groove, the *interdental gingiva* which fills the interproximal space from the alveolar crest to the area of contact between the teeth, and the *attached gingiva* which extends from the gingival groove to the mucogingival line of the vestibular fornix and floor of the mouth (Figs. 1-1, 1-2). In the palatal region, there is no distinct line of demarcation between attached gingiva and the palatal mucous membrane.

The free marginal gingiva and the interdental gingiva are of special interest, since they make up the region of junction between the soft tissue and the surface of the crown or root, and they are the site of initiation of inflammatory gingival and periodontal disease. The *facial, palatal,* and *lingual* components of

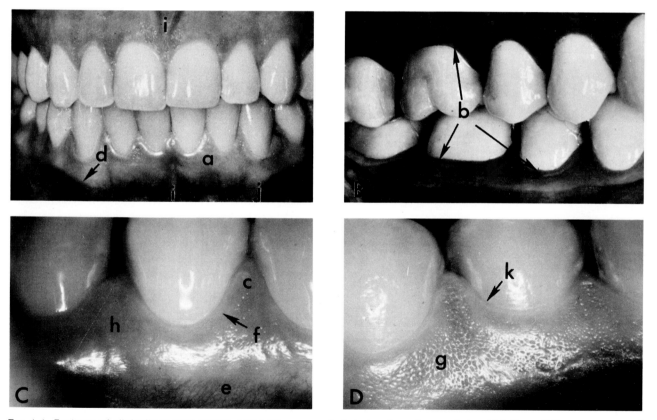

FIG. 1-1. *Features of clinically normal gingiva and oral mucosa. A. Anterior view of a mouth in which the soft tissues are normal except for the frena which are attached abnormally close to the free gingival margin. B. Clinically normal right posterior quadrants showing gingiva and oral mucosa. C and D. Normal gingiva and oral mucosa of the premolar region which are lightly (C) and heavily (D) stippled.*

Key to abbreviations: a. Attached gingiva; b. Buccal free marginal gingiva; c. Interdental papillae or interdental gingiva; d. Mucogingival line; e. Oral mucosa; f. Gingival groove; g. Heavily stippled attached gingiva; h. Attached gingiva relatively free of stippling; i. Labial frena; j. Vestibule; k. Gingival sulcus.

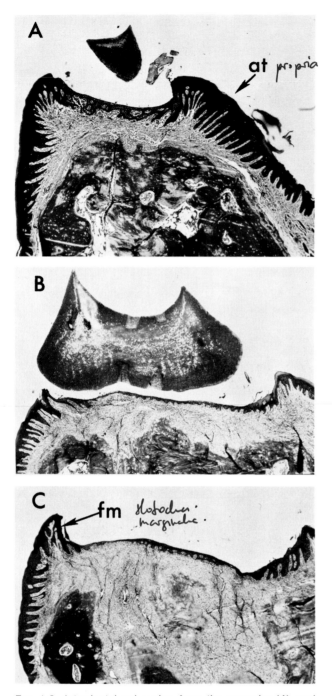

FIG. 1-2. *Interdental col region from the premolar (A) and molar (B and C) regions of a normal marmoset. The free marginal gingiva (fm) and attached gingiva (at) are indicated. Note the buccal and lingual papillae which are covered with keratinized oral epithelium and have typical rete pegs at the epithelial-connective tissue junction. (Trichrome stain, original magnification 32 ×.)*

contour of the teeth. The interdental gingiva is protected, and its shape and size are determined by the mesiobuccal, mesiolingual, distobuccal, and distolingual line angles and by the contact areas of the teeth. In the anterior segments of the dentition, depending upon the width of the interdental space, the interdental gingiva assumes a pyramidal or conical shape and is referred to as the *interdental papilla* (Fig. 1-1). Generally, the papillary surface is keratinized. In contrast, in the molar and premolar region the apex of the interdental gingiva is blunted buccolingually (Fig. 1-2). The extent of this blunting, which may assume the shape of *a col,* is determined by the breadth of the adjacent teeth and their contact relationships. Generally the width and depth of the col region become greater with increasing buccolingual and decreasing occlusal tooth dimension. The surface of the col area is not keratinized and may therefore be unusually susceptible to noxious influences such as plaque.

The free marginal gingiva adheres closely to the tooth surfaces, and its slightly rounded periphery forms the lateral or soft tissue wall of the gingival sulcus (Figs. 1-1, 1-3). The tissues that make up the free marginal gingiva include the oral epithelium coronal to the gingival groove, the oral sulcular epithelium (Fig. 1-3), the junctional epithelium referred to previously as attachment or crevicular epithelium,[137] and the subjacent connective tissues. The free marginal gingiva and the coronal portion of the interdental gingiva are not attached to bone, but they are united organically through the junctional epithelium to the tooth surface.

There is considerable confusion relating to the use of the terms *crevicular, sulcular, attachment,* and *junctional* epithelia. The terms *crevicular* and *sulcular epithelium* have been used to connote the cells extending from the crest of the free marginal and interdental gingiva to the most apical extent of epithelium in the region of the cementoenamel junction. The terms were especially used in relationship to the concept of Waerhaug that the gingival sulcus extends to the cementoenamel junction (see Fig. 1-12). The term *attachment epithelium* was defined by Gottlieb as the cells mediating the attachment of the soft tissues to the crown or root surface. More recently the terms *junctional epithelium,* and *oral sulcular epithelium* have come into widespread usage. The junctional epithelium is that layer of epithelial cells united to the surface of the crown or root by hemidesmosomes and a basal lamina and having as its sloughing surface the base of the gingival sulcus. The oral sulcular epithelium extends from the base of the gingival sulcus to the crest of the free marginal and interdental gingiva (see Figs. 1-3, 1-12).

The attached gingiva is bound firmly by the perios-

the free marginal gingiva vary in width from 0.5 to 2.0 mm and follow the scalloped pattern of contour of the cementoenamel junctions of the teeth (Fig. 1-1). The oral surface of the gingiva is keratinized, and it is protected by the buccal and lingual heights of the

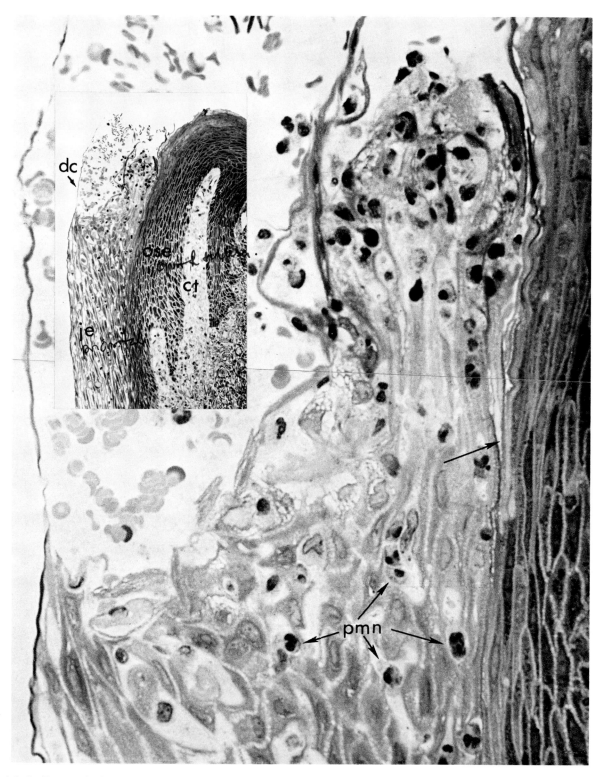

FIG. 1-3. *An Epon-embedded human biopsy specimen showing a relatively normal gingival sulcus. The soft tissue wall of the gingival sulcus is made up of the oral sulcular epithelium (ose) and its underlying connective tissue (ct), while the base of the gingival sulcus is formed by the sloughing surface of the junctional epithelium (je). The enamel space is delineated by a dense cuticular structure (dc). There is a relatively sharp line of demarcation between the je and the ose (arrow), and several polymorphonuclear leukocytes (pmn) can be seen traversing the je. The sulculus contains red blood cells resulting from the hemorrhage occurring at the time of biopsy. (Magnification 391 × and inset 55 ×).*

teum to the alveolar bone and by the gingival collagen fibers to the cementum, resulting in its characteristic immobility (Fig. 1-1). The tissue is subjected to the masticated food being shed from the sluiceways of the occlusal surfaces of the teeth. It is not protected by the anatomic contours of the teeth, and both the keratinized surface and the tightly woven dense collagenous corium reflect this stress-bearing function. Normal attached gingiva is salmon pink and may present a rough stippled texture (Fig. 1-1). It may vary in width from one individual to another and from one site to another.[1] The width of the attached gingiva may be as great as 9 mm or more on the facial aspect of the anterior maxillary and mandibular teeth and as little as 1 mm in the region of the premolars and canines. The width of the band of attached gingiva does not vary with age, but in the presence of pathologic alteration, it may become narrowed or it may disappear entirely.

At the *mucogingival line*, the attached gingiva merges with the *lining oral mucosa* (Fig. 1-1). The lining mucosa is freely movable, elastic, and bound only to the underlying muscle and fascia. It is covered with nonkeratinizing epithelium through which blood vessels can be seen. The corium is composed of loosely arranged collagen and elastic fibers. Because lining mucosa is not a stress-bearing tissue, it exhibits inflammatory and degenerative responses when subjected to stress.

THE GINGIVAL EPITHELIUM

A keratinizing stratified squamous epithelium covers the surface of the free and attached gingiva. This epithelium, which is separated from the underlying connective tissues by a basal lamina, is made up of basal, spinous, granular, and cornified layers (Fig. 1-4B). Nutritional support reaches the avascular epithelial tissues by diffusion or active transport from the connective tissue papillae that extend into the epithelium. The structure of the gingival epithelium has been studied recently by several investigators.[86,133,134,141]

The *basal layer* contains a heterogeneous population of cuboidal or low columnar cells which contact the basal lamina (Fig. 1-4B). Their long axes are more or less at right angles to the basal lamina. As they progress

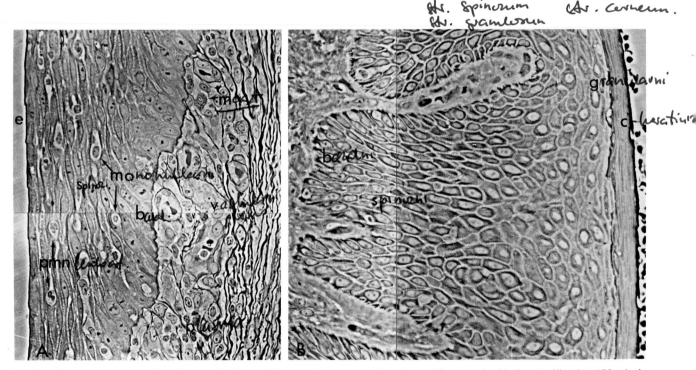

FIG. 1-4. *Features of oral and junctional epithelia and the underlying connective tissues (Epon-embedded, magnification 450 ×). A. Junctional epithelium. The cells of the junctional epithelium are in intimate contact with the enamel (e) and reproduce the surface indentations of the enamel. The epithelium has basal (b) and spinous (s) layers. There is no tendency toward keratinization. Numerous polymorphonuclear leukocytes (pmn) and mononuclear cells (mo) are present in both layers. In the connective tissue zone, portions of the gingival vascular plexus (v), mast cells, (m), and plasma cells (p) can be seen. There is a slight inflammatory cell infiltrate in the connective tissue. (Schroeder, H. E.: Struktur und ultrastruktur des normalen marginalen paradonts. Paradontologie, 23:159, 1969). B. Typical keratinizing oral epithelium. The epithelium is made up of basal (b), spinous (s), granular (g), and cornified (c) layers. (Schroeder, H. E.: Ultrastructure of the junctional epithelium of the human gingiva. Helv. Odontol., Acta, 13:65, 1969.)*

toward the surface, they become flattened and elongated with the long axis parallel to the tissue surface. The plasma membrane of the basal cells forms broad undulating microvilli that follow the contours of the basal lamina to which the cells are attached by *hemidesmosomes* (Fig. 1-4B, 1-5B, 1-5D). Frequently, small vesicles are seen opening onto the surface of the lamina from the basal cells between the hemidesmosomes (Fig. 1-5B). The lateral borders of the cells may exhibit extremely complex infoldings that result in a greatly augmented surface area and extensive interdigitation with the adjacent cells. The cells are attached laterally by desmosomes and by tight and gap junctions. The plasma membrane is coated on the external surface by a thin, electron-dense fuzzy material.

The cells destined to traverse the epithelium and keratinize are referred to as *keratinocytes*. They have a large round or oval nucleus with one or more prominent nucleoli. Their cytoplasm, which is palely basophilic in light-microscope preparations, is densely packed with organelles (Fig. 1-5A). The Golgi complex is prominent. Mitochondria are located preferentially in a perinuclear position in the basal part of the cell. Lamellae of rough endoplasmic reticulum are observed, but most of the ribosomes are present as free bodies or rosettes. Cytoplasmic filaments may be a prominent feature of the cells. They gather into fibrils, traverse the cell cytoplasm, and insert into attachment condensations at the sites of desmosome junctions (Fig. 1-5B). Cells of the basal layer exhibit two primary functions. They undergo self-replication, serving as a source of new cells for the constant renewal of the tissue, and they produce and secrete the materials that make up the basal lamina.

The cell turnover time in the attached gingival epithelium is similar to that observed for other surface epithelia. In both the rat and the marmoset, the time required for newly produced basal cells to reach the surface is about 10 to 12 days.[12,156,157]

Pigment-containing cells are present in the basal layer of the gingival epithelium of both light- and dark-skinned persons.[131,132] Dopa-positive cells occur with a frequency of about 7 percent throughout the basal layer of the free and attached gingival epithelium.[11] The stellate pigment cell, the *melanocyte,* contains granules called premelanosomes and melanosomes (Fig. 1-6A). The pigment-containing granules tend to accumulate in the terminal portions of the cytoplasmic processes. Melanocytes differ from the remaining basal cells, the keratinocytes, in that they do not exhibit attachments to neighboring cells or to the basal lamina and they are comparatively free of cytoplasmic filaments and fibrils. Melanin is transferred from the melanocytes to the nonpigment-producing

basal cells, the keratinocytes (Fig. 1-6B), and to cells within the connective tissues, presumably by phagocytosis.

The *spinous layer* located immediately peripheral to the basal layer derives its name from the characteristic bridges that appear to extend from one cell to another in fixed preparations (Figs. 1-4B, 1-5C). Relative to the basal layer, cells of the spinous zone exhibit features characteristic of increased specialization and maturation. The spinous cells have a decreased mitotic rate relative to the cells of the basal layer and they have lost, presumably, their ability to synthesize and secrete basal lamina material. There are a significant increase in the size of the cytoplasmic filament population and a concurrent decrease in the numbers of mitochondria. The filaments, which occupy about 37 percent of the cytoplasmic volume gather into bundles (Fig. 1-7). The remaining organelles are located in filament-free zones near the nucleus. Relative to the cells of the basal layer there are increased numbers of desmosomes and the tight or gap junctions may extend for several thousand angstroms. In the superficial regions of the layer, cells contain glycogen and dense peripheral cytoplasmic granules (Odland bodies or membrane-coating granules).

Cells of the *granular layer* are flattened in a direction parallel to tissue surface (Figs. 1-4B, 1-5D). The nuclei are elongated and exhibit an increase in density. Remnants of rough endoplasmic reticulum and free or aggregated ribosomes are still present. Electron-dense keratohyalin bodies and clusters of glycogen granules are present. Numerous small electron-dense granules, the membrane-coating granules or Odland bodies, which are considered to contain enzymes and a cementing substance, are lined up along the superficial borders of the cells. As cells traverse the granular layer toward the surface, the number of membrane-coating granules within the cell cytoplasm is reduced, and the intercellular space is occupied by dense material and empty microvesicles of approximately the same size as the intracellular dense granules. In the granular cells the desmosomes are more prevalent, the size of the intercellular space is reduced, and the cellular interdigitations are less prominent than in the deeper epithelial layers. As the zone of keratinization is approached, the desmosomal attachments are fortified to a great extent, but not completely, by long stretches of tight and gap junctions.

Generally, there is an abrupt transition from the granular layer to the *stratum corneum* reflecting keratinization of the cells and their conversion into thin parallel anucleate sheets (Figs. 1-4B, 1-5D). The process of keratinization is an intracellular single-cell phenomenon based on the prior accumulation of the ap-

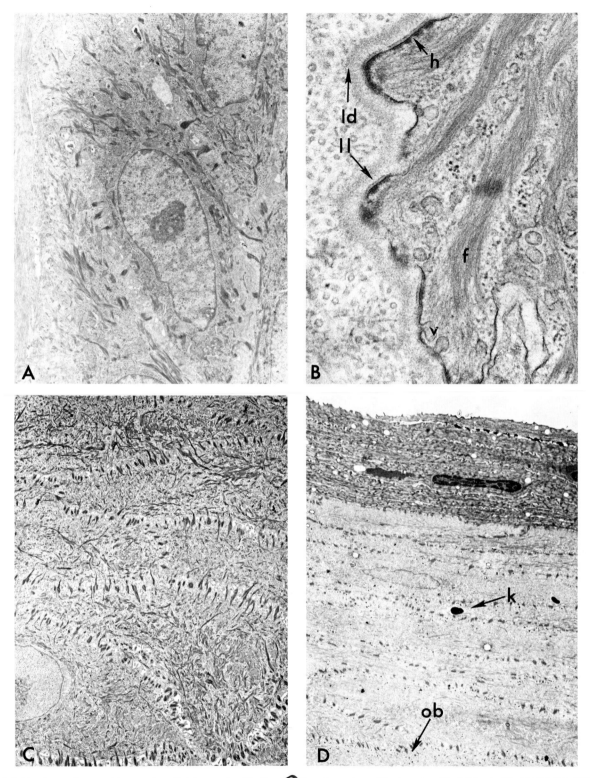

FIG. 1-5. *Sections of normal human keratinizing oral epithelium. (A) Keratinocytes of the basal epithelial layer along with the adjacent basal lamina and connective tissue. Note the large pale nucleus, extensive modification of the plasma membrane, nucleolus, rosettes of ribosomes, and lamellae of endoplasmic reticulum. Numerous mitochondria are present in a perinuclear position near the base of the cell. (Magnification approximately 5,500 ×). (B) Basal lamina with the adjacent connective tissue and basal cell. Note the lamina densa (ld) and lamina lucida (ll), anchoring fibers, hemidesmosomes (h) of the epithelial cell with inserting bundles of cytoplasmic filaments (f), vesicles (v) opening on to the lamina lucida, and adjacent connective tissue collagen fibers. (Magnification 34,200 ×). (C) Cells of the spinous layer of the gingival epithelium. Note the intercellular bridges, the extensive interdigitation of*

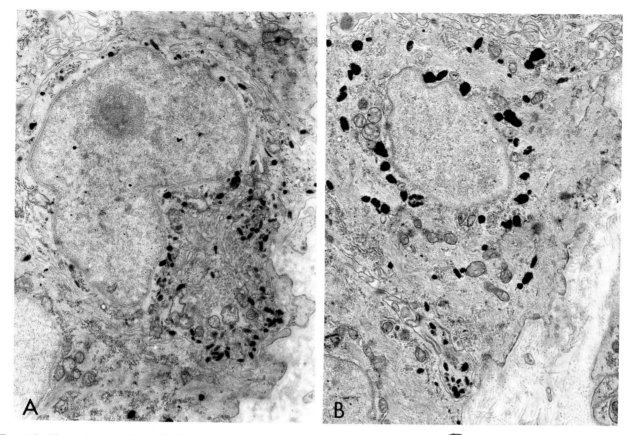

Fig. 1-6. *Pigment-containing cells located in the basal layer of the gingival epithelium. A. Melanocyte. Note the absence of hemidesmosome attachments to the basal lamina and adjacent cells, the large Golgi apparatus, absence of cytoplasmic filaments, and the presence of numerous melanin-containing granules (melanosomes) of variable density. B. Keratinocyte containing large dense phagocytosed granules of melanin and other cytoplasmic features characteristic of basal cells. There are desmosomal attachments to the basal lamina and adjacent cells, perinuclear mitochondria, and the cytoplasm is packed with filaments. (Magnification A, 4,950 ×; B, 5,700 ×.) (Schroeder, H. E.: Melanin containing organelles in cells of human gingiva. II. Melanocytes. J. Periodont. Res., 4:1, 1969. 4:235, 1969.*

propriate raw materials.[141] Several major cytologic events accompany this transition. The cells become densely packed with filament bundles that have undergone masking and keratohyalin granules. The entire synthetic and energy-producing apparatus, including the mitochondria, endoplasmic reticulum, Golgi apparatus, and nucleus, is removed from the cells probably by enzymatic breakdown. Individual filaments become coated and difficult to resolve morphologically. Changes in the cell membranes are also apparent. The outer leaflet becomes thin and difficult to resolve, while the inner leaflet thickens and acquires some condensed cytoplasm. In spite of the cytoplasmic and membrane changes, the cell junctions are maintained. There is no evidence of gradual degeneration of the junctional complexes as the cell approaches the surface; even sloughing cells are attached to the underlying adjacent layers by tight or gap junctions, and there is no direct communication between the exterior environment and the extracellular spaces.

Thus, as cells traverse the epithelium from the basal layer to the surface, they undergo continuous differentiation and specialization including (1) loss of the mitotic capacity and ability to synthesize and secrete basal lamina material, (2) enhanced protein production with accumulation of cytoplasmic filaments, amor-

Fig. 1-5. *Continued.*

the plasma membranes of the adjacent cells, the large amount of extracellular space, and cytoplasm densely packed with filaments and mitochondria and other cellular organelles. The nuclei are oval and frequently have nucleoli. (Approximate magnification 5,500 ×.) D. The granular and cornified layers of gingival epithelium. Cells of the granular layers contain elongated cells densely packed with cytoplasmic filaments. Few cytoplasmic organelles remain. Small dense cytoplasmic granules, the membrane-coating granules or the Odland Bodies (ob), are evident along the distal border of the cells. The remaining nuclei are dense and elongate. Keratohyalin (k) granules (arrow) are apparent. An abrupt transition between the two strata is demarcated by an increased density of the cell cytoplasm in the cornified layer. (Approximate magnification 4,500 ×.)

Volumetry of cytoplasm of various gingival epithelial cells

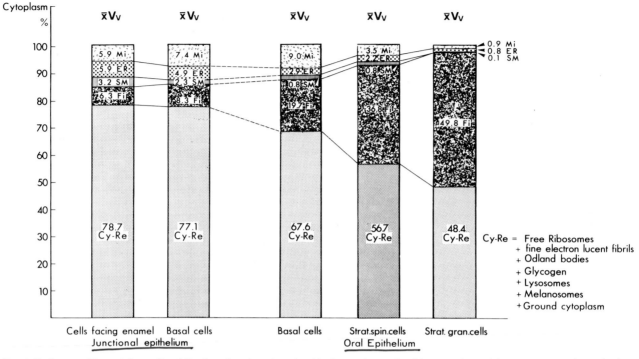

FIG. 1-7. Composition of the cells of the junctional and oral epithelia as determined by morphometric measurement on electron micrographs made from human biopsy specimens. The data are presented in units of $\bar{x}Vv$ which indicate the average portion of the total cytoplasmic volume occupied by various structures. The data permit comparison of the junctional with the oral epithelium and of the various layers of each epithelium with each other. Abbreviations used are Mi (mitochondria) ER (endoplasmic reticulum) SM (smooth membranes, including Golgi) Fi (fibrils in the cytoplasm), and Cy-Re (all remaining cytoplasmic consituents as indicated in the graph). As cells pass from the basal layer to the spinous and granular layers in the oral epithelium, they undergo maturation as demonstrated by the large increase in cytoplasmic fibrils and decrease in the volume occupied by mitochondria, endoplasmic reticulum, and smooth membranes. A maturation of this type is not seen in the junctional epithelium where the contents of the cells in the spinous layer do not differ significantly from those of the basal cells. (Based on Schroeder, H. E., and Münzel-Pedrazzoli, S.: Morphometric analysis comparing junctional and oral epithelium of normal human gingiva. Helv. Odontol. Acta, 14:53, 1970.)

phous matrix, and keratohyalin granules, (3) gradual breakdown of the energy-producing and synthesizing apparatus, (4) formation of a horny sheet by keratinization, (5) maintenance of lateral cell junctions, and (6) eventual loss of cell attachment leading to sloughing of cells from the surface.

Although keratinization is observed in the oral cavity at sites where the application of stress is greatest, such as the attached gingiva and hard palate, the association between stress application and keratinization is probably valid only from an evolutionary point of view. Any direct effect of stress in inducing keratinization is likely outweighed, by far, by epithelial-connective tissue interaction and other genetic factors involved in cell differentiation. While the application of unusual stress to normally nonkeratinized epithelial tissue surfaces, such as the oral mucosa, may induce the formation of an atypical stratum corneum, this is an abnormal pathologic event rather than a transforma-

tion of a normally nonkeratinizing to a normally keratinizing epithelium.

THE JUNCTIONAL EPITHELIUM

The term *junctional epithelium* denotes the tissue that is affixed to the tooth on the one side and to the oral sulcular epithelium or connective tissue on the other.[137] The junctional epithelium forms the base of the gingival sulcus (Figs. 1-3, 1-4A, 1-8). It has been examined in detail by several investigators.[88,90,134,137] Its structure and function differ significantly from those of gingival epithelium; indeed, in several respects the junctional epithelium appears to be a unique biologic system.

General structural features of the junctional epithelium are illustrated in Figures 1-2 and 1-4A. Thickness varies from about 15 to 18 cells at the base of the gingival sulcus to only 1 or 2 cells at the level of the

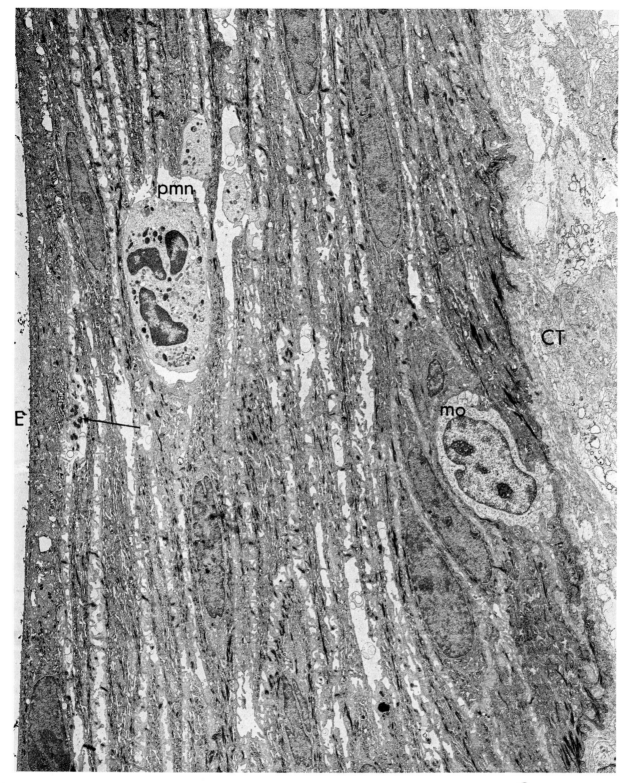

FIG. 1-8. *Electron micrograph of the junctional epithelium of a human biopsy specimen.* The enamel space (E) is on the left and the connective tissue (CT) on the right. At this level, a zone near the base of the gingival sulcus, the junctional epithelium is approximately 15 cells thick. One intact polymorphonuclear granulocyte (pmn) and cytoplasmic fragments of others are seen within the junctional epithelium. There is also a mononuclear cell (mo), probably a lymphocyte, among the basal cells. While desmosomes appear among all of the cells shown here (arrow), counts of these structures have shown that the total population in junctional epithelium is much lower than that of gingival epithelium. Note the relative absence of cytoplasmic filaments and fibrils, and the total absence of a granular layer. (Magnification 1,755 ×.) (Schroeder, H. E.: Ultrastructure of the junctional epithelium of the human gingiva. Helv. Odontol. Acta, 13:65, 1969.)

cementoenamel junction. The cells are arranged into basal and suprabasal layers only, and they exhibit no tendency toward maturation into granular or cornified layers. Cells originate from the basal layer, migrate in an oblique direction toward the tooth surface, and eventually reach the base of the gingival sulcus, where they are sloughed from the free surface (Fig. 1-3).

The cells of the junctional epithelium exhibit unusual cytologic features, differing significantly from other oral epithelia. The basal cells are cuboidal, or in some cases flattened, and relative to cells of the gingival epithelium, they contain slightly more rough endoplasmic reticulum and fewer cytoplasmic filaments (Figs. 1-7, 1-8). Upon leaving the basal layer, the cells become extremely flattened, and the nuclei elongate in a direction parallel to the long axis of the tooth surface. However, the cells do not undergo major cytologic modification upon leaving the basal layer, except that they alter in overall shape. Indeed, contrary to other epithelia, there is a slight increase in the amount of smooth and rough endoplasmic reticulum and a decrease in the content of cytoplasmic filaments of the cells as they migrate toward and along the tooth surface (Fig. 1-7).

The cells of the suprabasal layer, including those adjacent to the tooth surface, exhibit complex microvillus formation and interdigitation. The cell surfaces are covered with a fuzzy coat of polysaccharide material, which stains positively with ruthenium red (Fig. 1-9). The cells contain fewer cytoplasmic filaments, but more lamellae of rough endoplasmic reticulum and rosettes of ribosomes, than does gingival epithelium (Figs. 1-7, 1-8, 1-10). The Golgi complex is well developed and membrane-bound dense bodies, presumably lysosomes, are present (Fig. 1-10). Junctional epithelial cells, especially those near the base of the gingival sulcus, appear to have phagocytic capacity, and they stain intensely positively for lysosomal

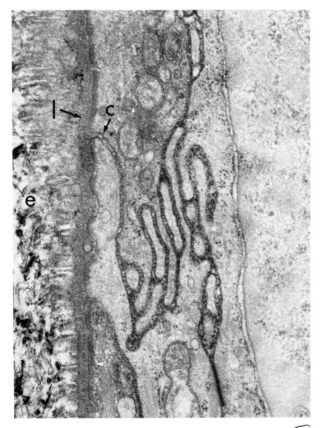

FIG. 1-9. *Features of junctional epithelial cells: enamel (e), epithelial attachment lamina (l), and communicating extracellular space from the junctional epithelium (c). A surface coating of ruthenium red-positive material can be seen in the intercellular space between the cell processes. (Magnification 27,700 ×.) (Schroeder, H. E.: Struktur und ultrastruktur des normalen marginalen paradonts. Paradontologie, 23:159, 1969.)*

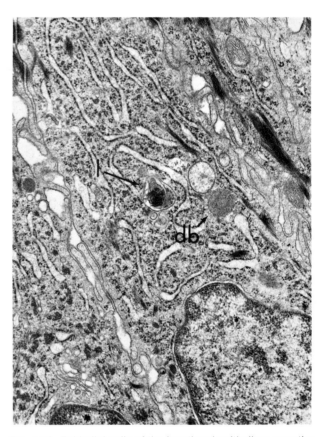

FIG. 1-10. *Epithelial cells of the junctional epithelium near the tooth surface. The cells exhibit extensive lamallae of rough endoplasmic reticulum, rosettes of ribosomes, dense bodies (db) which may be lysosomes, membrane-bound lipid-containing bodies which may be phagocytosed material (arrow). In many areas, the presence of an extracellular fuzzy coat can be seen. There are few desmosomes and cytoplasmic filaments. (Magnification 17,000 ×.)*

hydrolases.[75] The ruthenium red-positive material of the extracellular space appears to communicate with the epithelium-tooth interface (Fig. 1-9).

Leukocytes are seen within the junctional epithelium, even in clinically normal gingiva, and the presence of small numbers of these is considered to be normal (Fig. 1-8). Polymorphonuclear leukocytes enter the junctional epithelium from the vessels of the underlying connective tissue, migrate through the intercellular spaces, and enter the gingival sulcus. Large numbers of lymphoid cells, especially small lymphocytes, are also seen within the junctional epithelium of clinically normal gingiva along with a few cells exhibiting features of marcrophages. Although the function of the round cells is not clear at the present time, it has been speculated that they may be important in the host defense mechanism.[116,135,136]

THE EPITHELIUM-CONNECTIVE TISSUE INTERFACE

The morphology of the epithelium-connective tissue interface of the gingiva varies greatly in humans. In histologic sections, *rete pegs* of epithelial cells appear to project deeply into the connective tissues (Fig. 1-2). However, models constructed from serial sections show that the histologic observations may be misleading (Fig. 1-11). Ledges or conical connective tissue papillae project into a more or less uniform sheet of epithelium, resulting in the formation of a maze of interconnecting *epithelial ridges*. The zones of interconnection of these ridges are reflected as *stippling*, seen clinically on the epithelial surface (Fig. 1-1D). In the region of the junctional epithelium, the interface is more uniform and rete ridges are seen infrequently (Fig. 1-4A).

In the light microscope, a zone of specialization generally referred to as the *basement membrane* is seen. This structure measures 0.5 to 1.0 μ in thickness and stains positively for carbohydrates and for reticulin. It forms a continous sheet connecting epithelium and connective tissues. The electron microscope shows a faintly fibrillar, feltlike structure, referred to as the *basal lamina,* as part of the basement membrane (Fig. 1-5B). This structure can be resolved into a *lamina lucida* adjacent to the basal epithelial cells and joined to them through the hemidesmosomes and a *lamina densa.* The basal lamina usually forms a solid, intact sheet except in regions where mononuclear cells or polymorphonuclear leukocytes are in the process of moving from the connective tissues into the junctional epithelium. Fibrils measuring 200 to 400 angstroms in diameter appear to form loops extending from the hemidesmosomes of the basal cells through the basal lamina and into the underlying lamina propria of the

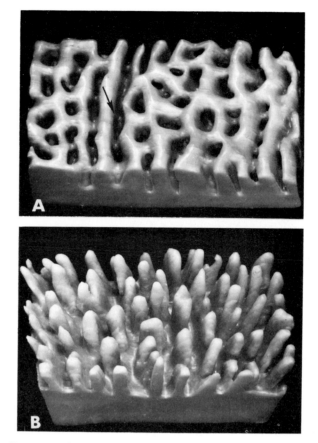

FIG. 1-11. *The anatomy of the epithelial-connective tissue interface.* Models of the oral aspect of the free and attached human gingiva adjacent to the buccal surface of the maxillary premolar of a 22-year-old female. A. Subsurface of the epithelium. B. Corresponding connective tissue surface. The specimen shows an even and regular distribution of tall conical connective tissue papillae, some of which have a common base. The subsurface of the epithelium is pitted, and some of the pits are connected by shallow grooves (arrows) (Magnification 160 ×). (Karring, T., and Löe, H.: The three-dimensional concept of the epithelium-connective tissue boundary of the gingiva. Acta Odontol. Scand., 28:917, 1970.)

connective tissues. These structures, which are presumed to bind the basal cells, basal lamina, and connective tissues together, have been seen subjacent to the oral,[166] sulcular, and junctional epithelium.[131,141]

Study of the structure of the gingival basal lamina is important for understanding of normal structure and pathologic alterations. Nutritional and gaseous exchange between the epithelial cells and connective tissues must occur across this membrane, and toxic substances must traverse it to reach the connective tissues and contact the structures involved in the inflammatory and immunologic responses. Important diseases such as desquamative gingivitis and several other bullous mucosal lesions appear to involve primary degenerative changes in the region of the basal lamina. Furthermore, the success of certain surgical procedures such as the survival of free gingival grafts is dependent upon diffusion across this membrane.

Although the basal lamina of the gingiva has not been studied chemically, currently available evidence supports the idea that its structure may be similar or indentical to that observed in other tissues. Extensive histochemical and biochemical studies have demonstrated numerous structural features held commonly by basal laminae of various organs, tissues, and species.[69,70,71,79,159] Basal lamina is produced by adjacent epithelial cells,[26,55,120] and it is made up predominantly of a collagenous protein and proteoglycans bonded covalently into a highly stable, totally insoluble complex. The collagenous protein differs chemically from that present in other connective tissues, especially in that many more of the lysyl residues have undergone hydroxylation and glycosylation.[159] This characteristic may lead to interference with fiber formation and a high state of hydration and thereby may account, at least in part, for the physical properties of the basal lamina.

THE EPITHELIUM-TOOTH INTERFACE

Knowledge of the details of structure of the soft tissue-tooth junction is of special interest. The initial stage of inflammatory gingival and periodontal disease involves pathologic alteration in the attachment apparatus, and most of the therapeutic methods currently available are directed toward restoration of a normal relationship. The nature of this structural relationship has been the subject of long-standing controversy. However, the disagreement has been resolved, at least to a large extent, by the studies of Schroeder and Listgarten.[137]

Prior to the time of Gottlieb, it was believed generally,[23,35] although not universally,[24] that the gingival soft tissues were closely apposed, but not organically united, to the surface of the enamel. However, experimental and clinical observations led Gottlieb to the concept that the soft tissues of the gingiva are organically united to the enamel surface (Fig. 1-12A).[47,48,107] He termed the epithelium contacting the tooth surface along with the interface substance the "epithelial attachment." According to this concept, a final act of the ameloblasts upon completion of the enamel matrix is the production of a primary enamel cuticle, which is continuous with the enamel matrix and attaches the cells of the reduced enamel epithelium to the calcified tooth surface. At the onset of tooth eruption, the cells of the reduced enamel epithelium unite with the proliferating oral epithelium. As eruption proceeds, the epithelial cells adjacent to the enamel surface produce

a cornified layer of material Gottlieb referred to as the secondary enamel cuticle and subsequently become separated from the enamel surface, leaving a small V-shaped groove, the gingival crevice.

Gottlieb's concept of the epithelial attachment dominated the thinking of oral structural biologists and clinicians for several decades. However, it did not go unchallenged. Weski provided histochemical evidence that dental cuticle was not a keratinous structure,[173] and Neuwirth[101] and Noyes[105] noted that the epithelial cells adjacent to the enamel surface were reduced ameloblasts rather than cornifying squamous epithelial cells. Other investigators noted that the cells adjacent to the enamel surface exhibited features similar to those of basal epithelial cells and suggested that the cells may have the capacity to produce a basement membrane.[53,80] There was also disagreement over Gottlieb's concept of the way the gingival crevice deepens. He felt that the epithelial cells cornify as they move near to the enamel surface and then separate from the surface, but Weski[173] and Skillen[155] suggested that the odontogenic epithelium gradually degenerates and is replaced by a lateral down-growth of oral epithelium. Gottlieb's concept was gradually modified by Orban and his colleagues. In 1944, Orban incorporated the views of Meyer,[94,95] Becks,[13,14,15] and Weski,[173] by stating that the separation of the epithelial-attachment cells from the tooth surface involved preparatory degenerative changes in the epithelium.[108] This was a sharp departure from Gottlieb's concept of production of a cornified cuticle. In 1953, the concept was modified even further when Orban stated that the ameloblasts shorten after enamel cuticle is formed and become part of the reduced enamel epithelium.[110]

In spite of objections, Gottlieb's concept of the epithelial attachment dominated thought until 1952, when Waerhaug presented the concept of the "epithelial cuff."[171] Waerhaug's concept was based on the observation that thin blades inserted between the surface of the tooth and the gingiva can be passed apically to the connective tissue attachment at the cementoenamel junction without resistance. On the basis of this and other observations with the light microscope, he concluded that the gingival tissues are closely apposed but not organically united to the tooth surface (Fig. 1-12B).

Resolution of the controversy regarding the nature of the epithelium-tooth interface was not possible until the increased resolving power of transmission electron microscopy became available. In 1962, Stern showed that in the rat incisor the epithelial cells are related to the tooth surface through hemidesmosomes.[163] The subsequent extensive studies of Schroeder and Listgarten illuminated the details of the structural rela-

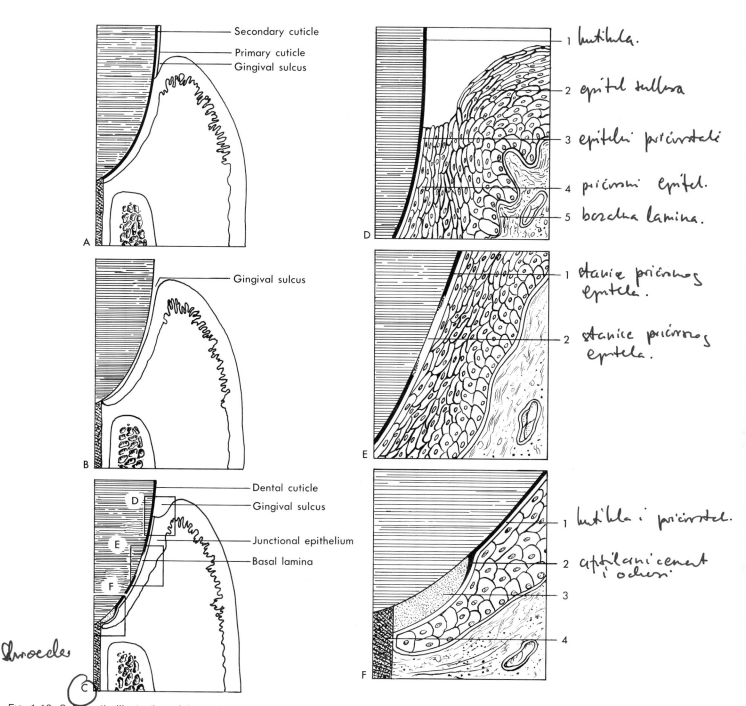

Secondary cuticle
Primary cuticle
Gingival sulcus

A

Gingival sulcus

B

Dental cuticle
Gingival sulcus
Junctional epithelium
Basal lamina

C

Shroeder

1 *cuticula.*

2 *epitel sulbu*

3 *epitelu pucinstali*

4 *pucinsni epitel.*

5 *bozelna lamina.*

D

1 *stanie pucinnos epitela.*

2 *stanice pucirrnos epitela.*

E

1 *cuticula i pucinstel.*

2 *aptilani cenent i ocren.*

3

4

F

FIG. 1-12. *Schematic illustration of the various concepts of the relationship of the gingival tissues to the calcified tooth surface. A. The epithelial attachment concept of Gottlieb. B. The epithelial cuff concept of Waerhaug. C. The basal lamina-hemidesmosome concept of Schroeder and Listgarten. D. Zone of the gingival sulcus: (1) dental cuticle; (2) oral sulcular epithelium; (3) epithelial attachment lamina; (4) junctional epithelium; (5) basal lamina. E. Zone apical to the base of the gingival sulcus: (1) junctional epithelial cells related to the enamel through the epithelial attachment lamina and the dental cuticle (compare to Fig. 1-14B); (2) Junctional epithelial cells related to the enamel through basal lamina only. F. Zone near the cementoenamel junction: (1) dental cuticle and epithelial attachment lamina interposed between the enamel and junctional epithelium (compare with Fig. 1-14B); (2) afibrillar cementum, dental cuticle, and epithelial attachment lamina interposed between enamel and junctional epithelium (compare with Fig. 1-14B); (3) afibrillar cementum and epithelial attachment lamina interposed between enamel and junctional epithelium (compare with Fig. 1-15A); (4) junctional epithelium united to root cementum through epithelial attachment lamina (compare with Fig. 1-16B).*

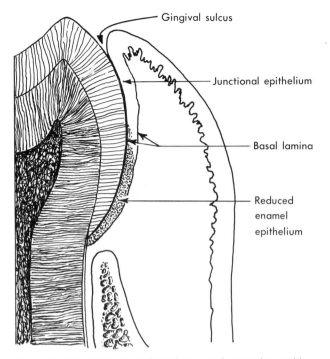

FIG. 1-13. *Development of the primary and secondary epithelial attachment.*

tionships in the human and monkey and served as the basis for a new system of terminology (Fig. 1-12C, 1-13).[137] The term *primary epithelial attachment* has been used to describe the relationship of the epithelium to the enamel of the unerupted tooth (Fig. 1-13). This relationship comes about as follows.[86,137] During maturation of the enamel, but prior to tooth eruption, the reduced ameloblasts elaborate a basal lamina referred to as the *epithelial attachment lamina.* This structure lies in direct contact with the enamel surface, and the epithelial cells are attached to it by hemidesmosomes; there is no evidence for the presence of a dental cuticle at this stage. As eruption proceeds, mitosis occurs in the basal layer of the oral epithelium and in the outer layer of the reduced enamel epithelium, but the ameloblasts no longer divide. The reduced ameloblasts and the other cells of the reduced enamel epithelium are transformed into junctional epithelial cells, and the primary epithelial attachment then becomes the *secondary epithelial attachment* (Fig. 1-13). The ameloblasts do not degenerate or cornify as was previously supposed; they undergo dramatic nuclear and cytoplasmic reorganization and transformation including development of cytoplasmic filaments, Golgi apparatus, and other features that make them indistinguishable from junctional epithelial cells.

The secondary epithelial attachment, in its simplest form, is made up of the epithelial attachment lamina and the hemidesmosomes (Fig. 1-12E, 1-14A). However, the interface structures at the secondary epithelial attachment are made more complex by the presence of dental cuticle and afibrillar cementum and by the fact that frequently the attachment zone may be located on the root surface instead of on the enamel.

At sites near the cementoenamel junction the completed enamel may become denuded of its epithelial covering and come to lie in direct contact with the connective tissues (Fig. 1-15B, C). When this occurs, a connective tissue product, *afibrillar cementum,* may be elaborated and deposited on the surface of the enamel (Figs. 1-12F, 14C). Afibrillar cementum resembles root cementum in that it undergoes calcification and exhibits incremental lines, but it does not contain a matrix of collagen fibrils. Generally, deposition of afibrillar cementum is confined to zones near the cementoenamel junction and later may become overlaid by junctional epithelium. Thus, in this region, in addition to the epithelial attachment lamina and desmosomes, afibrillar cementum may be interposed between enamel and the attachment lamina of the junctional epithelium (Figs. 1-12F, 1-14C).

The surface of enamel as well as afibrillar cementum may exhibit a layer of homogeneous, nonlaminated material that does not undergo calcification and differs morphologically from epithelial attachment lamina. This material, referred to as *dental cuticle,* occurs extremely irregularly, it stains intensely with uranyl acetate, and it may extend into the gingival sulcus and beyond. Presumably, dental cuticle is derived from epithelial cells, but this is by no means certain. Its composition is not known. When present, dental cuticle is interposed between the epithelial attachment lamina and the enamel or cemental surfaces (Figs. 1-12C, 1-14B, 1-15C, and 1-16A).

When the gingival margin is located on the root surface, the structure of the epithelial attachment resembles very closely that seen on enamel. As shown in Figure 1-16, the gingiva is attached to the root surface directly by the epithelial attachment lamina and hemidesmosomes, or it may be mediated by dental cuticle and afibrillar cementum.

While the junctional-epithelial cells arise initially by transformation of the reduced enamel epithelium, they can also be derived from other sources. Listgarten has shown that complete regeneration of an attachment apparatus which is normal in all respects follows surgical excision of the junctional epithelium.[87] Thus, the oral epithelium can give rise to de novo formation of junctional epithelial cells.

From the foregoing discussion it is apparent that the relationships of the junctional epithelial cells and the connective tissues to the calcified tooth surface are

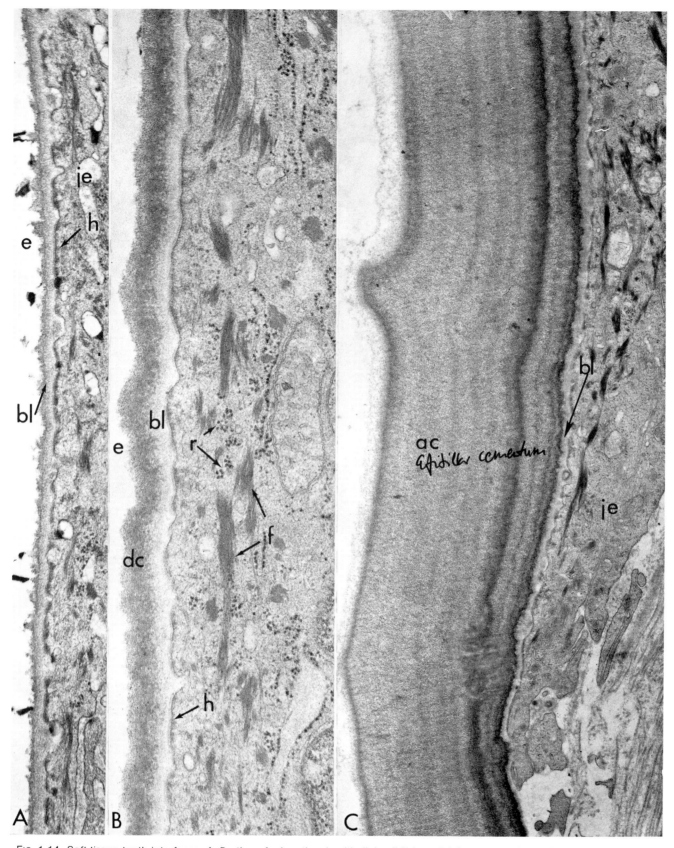

FIG. 1-14. *Soft tissue-tooth interfaces. A. Portion of a junctional epithelial cell (je) containing scattered cytoplasmic filaments and fibrils and exhibiting hemidesmosomes (h) separated from the enamel surface (e) by a basal lamina (bl). This is the most simple relationship observed between the epithelium and the enamel surface (Magnification 15,625 ×). B. A junctional epithelial cell exhibiting rosettes of ribosomes (r), aggregates of cytoplasmic fibrils (f), and hemidesmosomes (h) separated from the enamel surface (e) by a layer of dental cuticle (dc) and basal lamina (bl) (Magnification 21,250 ×). C. A portion of the most apical cells of the junctional epithelium (je) separated from the enamel surface by a thick layer of* afibrillar cementum (ac) *exhibiting incremental lines and basal lamina (bl). The presence of the afibrillar cementum indicates that the surface of the enamel in the region illustrated was at one time in contact with the connective tissues. The section was taken from the most apical zone of the junctional epithelium (magnification 9,375 ×).*

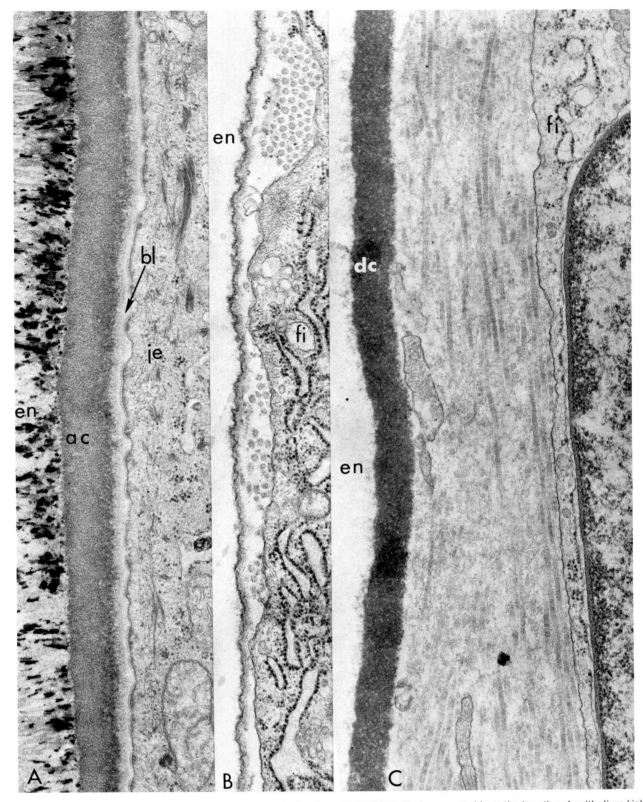

FIG. 1-15. *Soft tissue-tooth interfaces. A. Enamel surface (en) only partially decalcified, separated from the junctional epithelium (je) by a thick layer of afibrillar cementum (ac) and basal lamina (bl) (Magnification 21,250 ×). B. A connective tissue cell, probably a fibroblast (fi), with surrounding collagen fibers cut in cross section adjacent to the enamel surface (en) without distinctive interface material (Magnification 21,250 ×). C. A portion of a fibroblast (fi) and collagen fibers cut in long section separated from the enamel surface (en) by a thick layer of dental cuticle (dc) (Magnification 21,250 ×).*

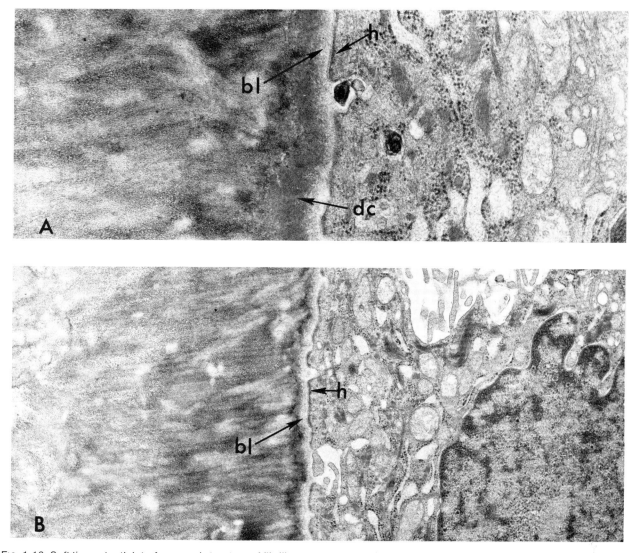

FIG. 1-16. *Soft tissue-tooth interfaces and structure of fibrillar cementum and junctional epithelial cells. A. A junctional epithelial cell related to root cementum by the epithelial attachment lamina (bl), hemidesmosomes (h), and dental cuticle (dc) (Magnification 20,250 ×). B. A junctional epithelial cell related to root cementum by the epithelial attachment lamina (bl) and hemidesmosomes (h) only. Typical fibrillar root cementum is seen (Magnification 12,375 ×).*

complex and may vary from one tooth to another and from one site on a single tooth to another. The relative prevalence of these various relationships has not been determined. In spite of the apparent complexity of the tooth-soft tissue relationships, one general principle emerges. A basal lamina is always interposed between epithelial cells and the crown or root surface, and the epithelial cells are united to the basal lamina by hemidesmosomes.

GINGIVAL CONNECTIVE TISSUES

The gingival connective tissues are highly organized into a characteristic architectural form, and they provide tone to the free and attached gingiva and tensile strength to the soft tissue-tooth interface.[6] The relative volumes occupied by the various constituents of the gingival connective tissues are illustrated in Figure 1-17. The major components are collagen fibers, vessels, and fibroblasts.

General Architecture

The gingiva is provided with blood from three sources (Fig. 1-18). The primary blood supply arises from the posterior superior alveolar and inferior alveolar arteries that supply the teeth. Branches of these vessels enter the interseptal bone near the tooth apices and pass coronally, exiting through numerous nutrient foramina in the cortical plate to supply the marginal and attached gingiva. Other vessels enter the marginal gingiva from the periodontal ligament. An additional blood supply, arising from the periosteal branches of the lingual, buccinator, mental, and palatine arteries, enters the gingiva from the vestibular fornix, floor of the mouth, and palate. This secondary blood supply is sufficiently rich to permit successful gingival flap surgery. There is a thorough anastomosis of the vessels from all of these sources. The veins and lymphatics run a course paralleling the arteries, and the lymphatic drainage from the gingiva is into the submental and cervical lymph nodes. The epithelial layer of the gingiva is innervated by nonmedullated sensory fibers

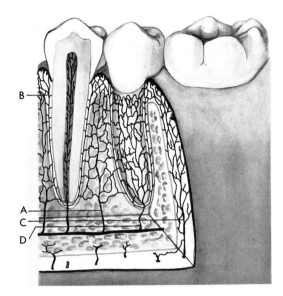

FIG. 1-18. *Schematic illustration of the blood supply of the periodontium. The alveolar arteries supplying the teeth give rise to branches (A) which pass coronally and exit into the gingiva through foramina in the crest of the interproximal bone. Vessels enter the free gingiva (B) from the periodontal ligament, and a further supply (C) derives from vessels entering the gingiva from the oral mucosa. Vessels from all three of these sources anastomose thoroughly. The tissues of the periodontal ligament are supplied primarily by branches of the alveolar vessels (D). These form a basketlike anastomosis throughout the periodontal ligament space. There is a rich anastomosis between these vessels and those in the alveolar bone through foramina in the cribriform plate (see Fig. 1-34).*

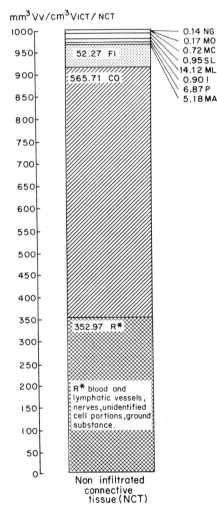

mm³Vv/cm³VICT/NCT

0.14 NG	
0.17 MO	
0.72 MC	
0.95 SL	
14.12 ML	
0.90 I	
6.87 P	
5.18 MA	

52.27 FI

565.71 CO

352.97 R*

R* blood and lymphatic vessels, nerves, unidentified cell portions, ground substance.

Non infiltrated connective tissue (NCT)

FIG. 1-17. *Relative volume occupied by various constituents of the gingival connective tissues as determined from light and electron micrographs of biopsies of normal human gingiva. Neutrophilic granulocytes (NG), monocytes (MO), macrophages (MC), small lymphocytes (SL), medium-sized lymphocytes (ML), immunoblasts (I), plasma cells (P), mast cells (MA), collagen (CO). (From Schroeder, H. E., Münzel-Pedrazzoli, S., and Page, R. C.: Correlated morphometric and biochemical analysis of gingival tissues. The early gingival lesion in man. Arch. Oral Biol., 18:899, 1973.)*

that extend from the connective tissues. Meissner and Krause corpuscles are present in the connective tissue layers.[18]

Immediately subjacent to the basal lamina of the junctional epithelium is a lamina propria-like zone of specialized connective tissue. This zone is rich in cells, poor in collagen bundles, and contains a rich anastomosis of blood vessels, which have been referred to as the *gingival plexus* (Fig. 1-4).[37] This zone, which has also been referred to as the *cell rich zone*, contains numerous macrophages and mononuclear cells and may be an important zone of host defense.[129]

Fiber Apparatus

The collagen of the gingival connective tissues is organized into groups of fiber bundles. These bundles have been described classically on the basis of their location, origin, and insertion as the dentogingival, dentoperiosteal, alveologingival, circular and transseptal fiber groups (Figs. 1-19, 1-20).[6,46]

The *dentogingival* fibers arise from the cementum of the root immediately apical to the base of the epithelial attachment, generally near the cementoenamel

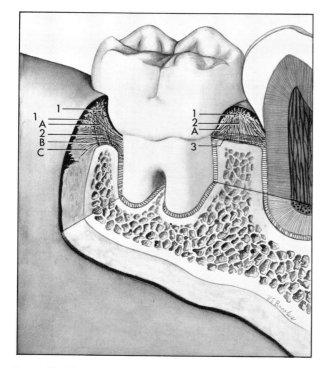

FIG. 1-19. *The gingival collagen fiber apparatus: the circular and semicircular fibers in cross section (1); the alveologingival fibers arising from the crest of the alveolar bone and extending into the free marginal gingiva (2); the transseptal fibers originating from the cementum of one tooth, traversing the interdental bone, and inserting into the cementum of the adjacent tooth (3); the dentogingival fibers that originate from the cementum and splay out into the gingiva in a coronal direction (A) and laterally (B); and the dentoperiosteal fibers (C) that insert into the periosteum on the surfaces of the alveolar bone.*

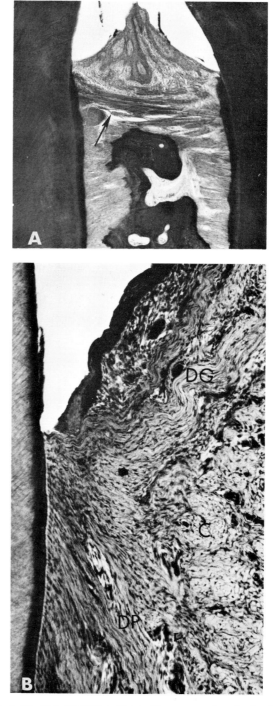

FIG. 1-20. *The gingival collagen fiber apparatus. A. Section from marmoset showing the transseptal gingival fibers (original magnification 37.5 ×). B. Section from human gingiva illustrating the dentogingival (DG), dentoperiosteal (DP) and circular (C) fibers (Magnification 153 ×).*

junction and splay out into the gingiva. One group of these fibers follows a coronal course subjacent to the junctional epithelium and terminates near the basal lamina of the free gingival margin. Another group courses laterally, and a third group, the *dentoperiosteal* fibers, bends apically over the alveolar crest and inserts into the buccal and lingual periostium (Fig. 1-20B). These three groups of fibers have been called groups A, B, and C by Goldman.[46] The *alveologingival* fibers arise from the crest of the alveolus and course coronally, terminating in the free and papillary gingiva. The *circular* fiber group passes circumferentially around the cervical region of the tooth in the free gingiva.[6] Additional fiber groups have been demonstrated recently in the marginal gingiva of the marmoset.[113] The *semicircular* fibers arise from the cementum of the proximal root surface just apical to the circular fiber group, extend into and traverse the facial or lingual free marginal gingiva, and insert into a comparable position on the opposite side of the same tooth (Fig. 1-21B,E). The *transgingival* fibers arise from the cementum in the region of the cementoenamel junction of one tooth and extend into the free marginal gingiva of an adjacent

tooth (Fig. 1-21A,D,E) while the *intergingival* fibers extend along the facial and lingual marginal gingiva from tooth to tooth (Fig. 1-21E). The transgingival fibers give rise to a crosshatching arrangement just lateral to the interdental bone crest (Fig. 1-21C). These

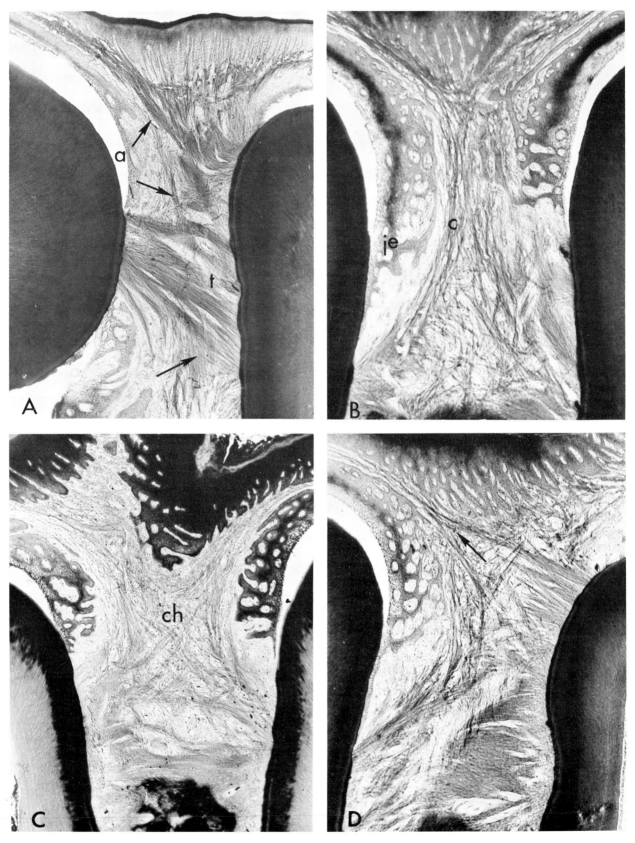

Fig. 1-21. *Legend on facing page.*

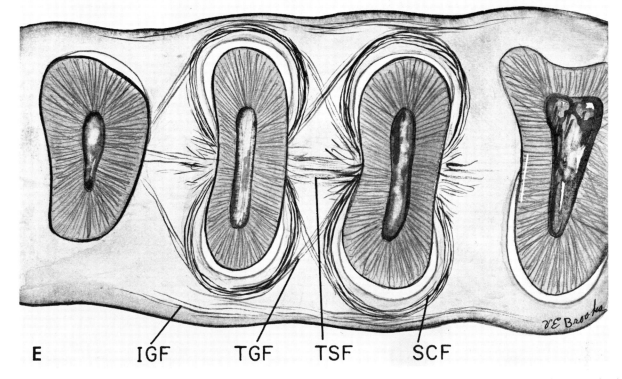

E   IGF   TGF   TSF   SCF

FIG. 1-21. *The gingival collagen fiber apparatus. Celloidin-embedded sections from the premolar region of the normal adult marmoset (Magnification 35 ×). A. Horizontal section coronal to the level of the interdental crest demonstrating the transseptal fibers (f) with branching or communicating fibers passing buccally and lingually (arrows). B. Horizontal section at the level of the interdental crest with semicircular fibers (c) arising from the cementum and bone and passing around the neck of the tooth subjacent to the junctional epithelium (je) to insert on the opposite side of the same tooth. C. Horizontal section illustrating the crosshatching fibers (ch) arising from the cementum of one tooth and traversing into the free marginal gingiva of the adjacent tooth. D. Horizontal section illustrating the intersection of semicircular fibers and transgingival fibers (arrow). E. Schematic illustration of the intergingival (IGF), transgingival (TGF) transseptal (TSF) and semicircular (SCF) fiber groups. (Page, R. C., et al.: Collagen fiber bundles of the normal gingiva. Arch. Oral. Biol., 19:1039, 1974.)*

fiber groups, which form the bulk of the free gingival connective tissue, may be considered collectively as the *gingival ligament*.

The *transseptal* fibers (Figs. 1-20A, 1-21A) arise from the cemental surface just apical to the base of the epithelial attachment, traverse the interdental bone, and insert into a comparable region of the adjacent tooth. The transseptal fibers collectively form an *interdental ligament* connecting all the teeth of the arch. This ligament appears to be uniquely important in maintaining the integrity of the dental apparatus. It is rapidly reformed after excision. When the transseptal fibers become involved in inflammatory disease, they usually reform at a more apical level, and shifting of the interdental ligament occurs in an apical direction. Residual portions of the transseptal fibers are seen even in advanced stages of periodontal disease.

The anatomic relationships of the fibers of the marginal gingiva may have an important bearing upon the behavior of the supporting structures in various disease states. There is a major degree of interdependence among the various segments of the gingiva. A large portion of the fibrillar structure of the facial and lingual marginal gingiva of a given tooth arises from the root surface or gingiva of the adjacent teeth (Fig. 1-21E). Therefore, the status of the marginal gingiva of one tooth may depend to a great extent upon the health of the supporting structures of the adjacent teeth. The presence of disease in the region of the gingival sulcus of one tooth may lead to disruption of the transgingival, intergingival, or transseptal fibers and thereby alter the tone and functional ability of the marginal gingiva of the neighboring teeth. In a similar manner, the extraction of one member of the arch may deleteriously affect the periodontal status of the remaining members. These anatomic features may aid in explaining the pattern of spread of inflammatory gingival and periodontal disease and the devastating effects of tooth extraction upon the periodontium of the remaining teeth.

Resident Cell Population

Cells make up 8.0 percent of the total volume of normal gingival connective tissues (Fig. 1-17). The cell population is heterogeneous and may vary from one site to another. Exclusive of the blood and lymphatic vessels, the cells present include fibroblasts, macrophages, mast cells, lymphoid cells, and blood leukocytes.

The *fibroblast* is the predominant cell, comprising 65 percent of the total cell population on a volume basis, and it is functionally the most important cell (Fig. 1-22A). Fibroblasts produce the connective tissue substances, including collagen, proteoglycans, and elastin, and thereby play a key role in maintaining the integrity of the gingival tissue. In the light microscope, fibroblasts are spindle-shaped with palely basophilic cytoplasm and large oval nuclei with one or more prominent nucleoli. When observed with the electron microscope, the cells exhibit all the features characteristic of actively synthesizing cells. These features include abundant mitochondria, a prominent Golgi apparatus, and densely packed lamellae of rough endoplasmic reticulum. Indeed, recent data indicate that they maintain a uniquely high level of activity, even in the adult.[29,111] At an early stage of inflammatory gingival disease, fibroblasts undergo severe cytopathic alterations.[115,140]

Large numbers of *mast cells* are present in normal human gingiva (Fig. 1-22C). Generally, these are located near the blood vessels and are characterized by the presence of large metachromatic or electron-dense granules containing heparin, histamine, and proteolytic enzymes. The cells undergo degranulation with tissue injury in certain pathologic conditions, but their function in the normal gingiva and in other connective tissues remains controversial. The release of histamine from these cells may contribute to acute gingival inflammation, and the release of heparin may be related to the bone loss associated with inflammatory periodontal disease.

A small population of *monocytes* and *macrophages* is present in normal noninflamed gingiva (Fig. 1-23). In the marmoset, this population is quite large, and a dense zone of macrophages is present immediately subjacent to the junctional epithelium.[129] Characteristic features of these cells include a relatively small oval or indented nucleus and abundant cytoplasm containing primary and secondary lysosomes, microfilaments, scattered lamellae of rough endoplasmic reticulum, and numerous small vessicles irregularly distributed throughout the cytoplasm. The cell periphery exhibits numerous microvilli varying in size. Macrophages, which have the capacity to produce large amounts of hydrolytic enzymes, may serve a scavenger and detoxification role in normal gingiva.[114]

Polymorphonuclear leukocytes are seen frequently within blood vessels and within the junctional epithelium in clinically normal human gingiva (Figs. 1-3, 1-4, 1-8, 1-23), but these cells are rarely present within the substance of noninflammed connective tissues. There is current evidence that granular leukocytes may emigrate from the vessels of the gingival plexus and rapidly enter the junctional epithelium, possibly in response to chemotactic substances released from plaque or saliva.

Lymphocytes and plasma cells are also prevalent in human gingival connective tissues that exhibit no other manifestations of pathologic alteration. The lymphocytes are generally located selectively in a zone immediately subjacent to the junctional epithelium, and plasma cells are present predominantly around the gingival vessels.[118] Whether the presence of these cells is indicative of an active pathologic process in the gingiva is not clear at the present time. Certainly, the lymphoid structures such as the tonsils, appendix, and Peyer's patches are seen at other sites in the gastrointestinal tract of otherwise normal individuals. Small lymphocytes are characterized cytologically by electron-dense nuclei and scanty cytoplasm relatively free of organelles (Fig. 1-24). Plasma cells exhibit clumped chromatin and their cytoplasm is packed with lamellae of rough endoplasmic reticulum. Lymphocytes and plasma cells are the predominant cells in inflammatory gingival lesions.

Macromolecular Components

The intercellular matrix of the gingival connective tissues is made up of the fibrous proteins, including collagen, reticulin, and elastin, and the ground substance. Ground substance is composed predominantly of proteoglycans, hyaluronic acid and serum-derived glycoproteins. Water, of course, is a major and important component. Characterization of the extracellular matrix components of the periodontal tissues has been of interest to oral morphologists and to investigators and clinicians interested in inflammatory gingival disease for several reasons. Collagen is the major structural component of the gingiva, alveolar bone, cementum, and periodontal ligament. In gingiva, the collagenous ligaments and their investing ground substance provide the tensile properties and tone that permit normal function of the supporting tissues. During the early stages of inflammatory gingival and periodontal disease, changes in the quality and quantity of the connective tissue components occur (see Chapter 7), and these changes appear to play a key role in

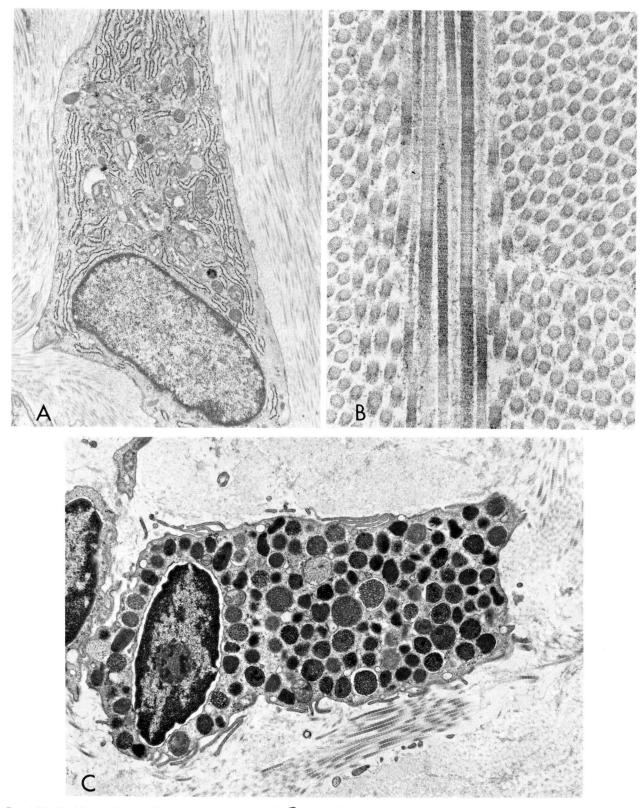

Fig. 1-22. *Resident cells and fibers of normal gingiva. A. A typical gingival fibroblast from the dog, containing lamellae of rough endoplasmic reticulum, dense bodies, Golgi apparatus, mitochondria, and a large palely staining nucleus. The cell is surrounded by bundles of collagen fibrils (Magnification 6,860 ×). B. Collagen bundles from dog gingiva. Note the 640 Å periodicity. See Fig. 1-25 for explanation of the mechanism of molecular aggravation. (Magnification 30,800 ×). C. Mast cell from gingival connective tissue of the marmoset. The cell cytoplasm contains abundant granules of varying density. (Magnification 7,700 ×). (Schectman, L. R., et al.: Host tissue response in chronic periodontal disease. J. Periodont. Res., 7:195, 1972.)*

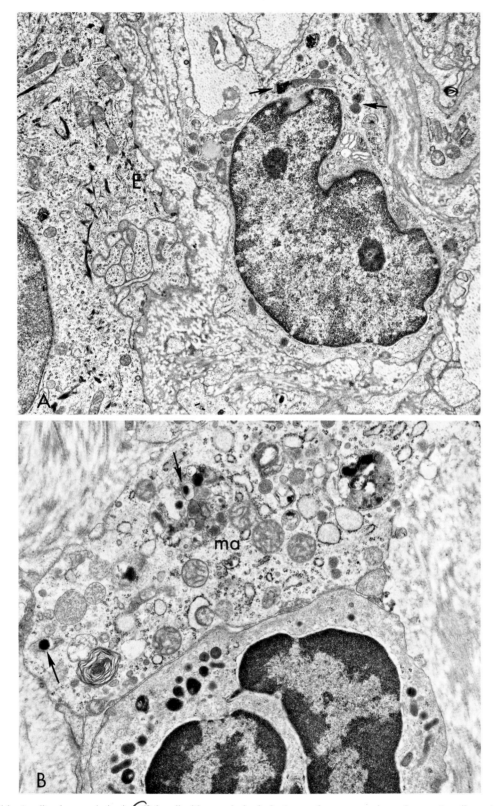

FIG. 1-23. *Resident cells of normal gingiva. A, A cell with morphologic features of a mononuclear phagocyte adjacent to the sulcular epithelium (E) of inflamed gingiva. Note the oval nucleus with dispersed chromatin and two nucleoli, small Golgi apparatus, and dense bodies (arrow) (Magnification 5,775 ×). B, Portions of a macrophage (ma) and a polymorphonuclear leukocyte from normal marmoset gingiva. The macrophage contains several dense granules similar in appearance to partially digested neutrophil granules (arrows) within phagocytic vacuoles (Magnification 8,250 ×). (Schectman, L. R., et al.: Host tissue response in chronic periodontal disease. J. Periodont. Res., 7:195, 1972.)*

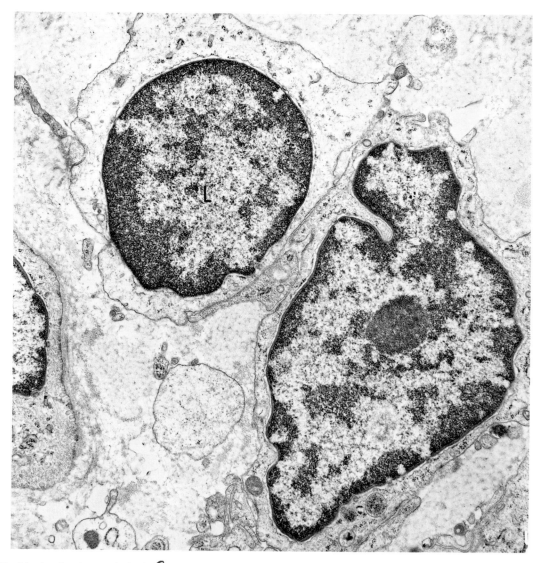

FIG. 1-24. *Resident cells of normal gingiva. A small lymphocyte (L) adjacent to a mononuclear leukocyte. Note the densely clumped nuclear chromatin and the paucity of cytoplasmic organelles in the lymphocyte (Magnification 7,425 ×). (Schectman, L. R., et al.: Host tissue response in chronic periodontal disease. J. Periodont. Res., 7:195, 1972.)*

the continuing loss of tissue integrity as the disease progresses.

MOLECULAR STRUCTURE OF THE FIBROUS PROTEINS AND THE GROUND SUBSTANCES

Important structural features of the intercellular matrix have been reviewed.[7,8,44,111,121,168] Collagen molecules are synthesized by resident fibroblasts and extruded into the extracellular compartment where they rapidly aggregate end to end and laterally to form collagen fibrils and bundles (Fig. 1-25).[33,58,106] Molecules are initially produced in a precursor form, which is converted into tropocollagen molecules of approximately 300,000 mw by cleavage of terminal peptides of approximately 30 amino acids each.[78] Each tropocollagen molecule is made up of three unbranched

parallel polypeptide chains of about 1,000 amino acids which run the entire length of the molecule. In most collagens, two of these chains, termed alpha-1, are identical in amino acid composition, and the third, the alpha-2 chain, has a different composition. Each chain is coiled into a left-hand helix, and all three chains have a gentle coil in the right-hand direction.

Collagen is subjected to the activity of several enzyme systems that modify the molecules during and after their synthesis. Hydroxylation of lysyl and prolyl residues is accomplished by specific enzyme systems located in the microsomes and using the polypeptide chain as substrate. Subsequent to hydroxylation, the chains are acted upon by a glycosyl transferase system that catalyzes glycosylation of certain hydroxylysyl side chains.[27] After extrusion to the extracellular space, tropocollagen molecules are acted upon by lysyl oxi-

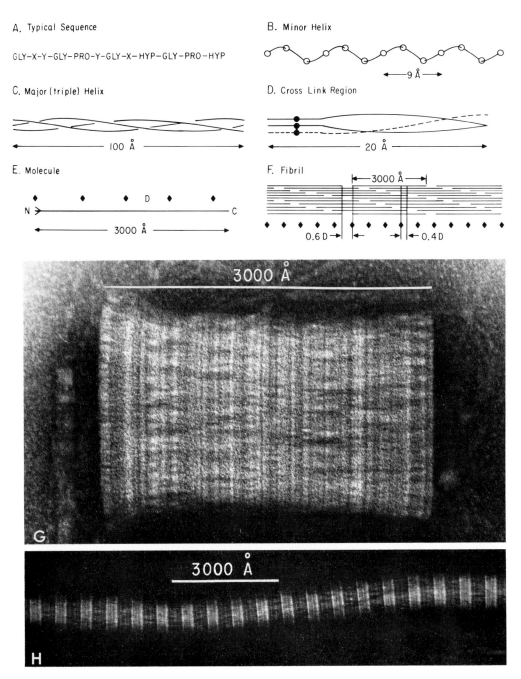

FIG. 1-25. *Illustration of the molecular structure of collagen and the mechanism of collagen fibril formation. A. Typical sequence. The polar and nonpolar amino acids are arranged in groups along the polypeptide chain. In the nonpolar regions, the typical sequences are made up of triplets of gly-x-y, gly-pro-y, gly-x-hy-, and gly-pro-hyp where x and y can be any amino acid. About half of the proline in collagen is converted enzymatically, after synthesis of the polypeptide chains, into hydroxyproline. Only proline residues in the number 3 position of the triplet can be hydroxylated. B. The minor helix. Each of the three polypeptide chains of collagen is approximately 1,000 amino acids in length and has a left-hand minor helix of the polyproline type. C. The major helix. The three polypeptide chains are intertwined about one another to form a right-hand major helix with a pitch of about 30°. The helical conformation results in the location of every third residue inside the molecule. Since glycine is the only amino acid without a side chain, it is the only residue that will fit into this position. Thus, all collagens contain 33 percent glycine. D. The cross-link region. The enclosed circles represent the lysyl and hydroxylysyl residue located near the N-terminus of each polypeptide chain which undergo oxidation enzymatically and condense to form the intramolecular cross-links. After fibril formation, other similar residues participate in intermolecular cross-linking. E, F, G, and H. Molecular aggregation. Each native collagen molecule is a stiff rod of approximately 3000 Å length. These molecules can be induced in vitro to relate to one another in register laterally to form segmented long-spaced aggregates as shown in G (Magnification 225,000 ×, negatively stained with phosphotungstic acid.) The resulting band pattern is a consequence of the grouping of amino acids with charged side chains in specific regions. Each molecule can be divided into regions of equal length, noted here as D, with an additional length of 0.4 D at the C-terminal end (E and F). Molecules aggregate laterally with an overlap of 0.4 D and end-to-end with a linear space interval of 0.6 D leading to fibrils with alternating regions of high and low density. These alternating zones are illustrated schematically in F and in a native fibril from rat tail tendon in H (negatively stained with phosphotungstic acid, magnification 225,000 ×). (Diagrams based on Piez, K. A.: Chemistry of collagen and elastin and biosynthesis of covalent cross-links. In Thule International Symposium Aging of Connective and Skeletal Tissues. 1969, p. 12.)*

dase, an enzyme that functions to initiate the maturation and stabilization process.[25,89,99,167]

The form of tropocollagen containing two α_1 and one α_2 chains per molecule is the major molecular species present in most connective tissues, but it is now apparent that other molecular types exist. A form of collagen with three α_1 chains which are homologous to, but not identical with, the α_1 chains described has been isolated from cartilage, and it now appears that additional molecular species may be present in basal lamina and, as a minor component, in other connective tissues.[44,96] The molecular form of collagen present in the periodontium is not known.

In addition to this biochemical heterogeneity in collagen, more than one kind of fibril can be demonstrated histochemically. With periodic acid Schiff reagent or silver staining techniques, reticulin fibrils can be demonstrated in most connective tissues, including the gingiva.[91,92] However, these fibrils are identical with small collagen fibers when viewed with the electron microscope and at the present time there is no evidence that they are composed of a protein other than collagen.

Elastin is the other major fibrous protein of connective tissue intercellular matrices. High concentrations of this protein are found in specialized structures such as the media of the aorta and large arteries, elastic cartilage, and elastic ligaments. In the periodontium, elastin is present in mucosa and attached gingiva and, to a limited extent, in the periodontal ligament. Soluble elastin, the precursor of elastin fibers and lamellae, has a molecular weight of approximately 74,000 daltons.[127] Soluble elastin molecules undergo aggregation, and the interchain covalent cross-linking system present in elastin is similar to that of collagen; all the cross-links so far demonstrated arise by condensation of lysyl side chains subsequent to oxidation by lysyl oxidase.[44,98]

Relative to the fibrous proteins, our knowledge of the components of the ground substance is scanty. While there is qualitative and quantitative variation from one connective tissue to another, in most tissues the ground substance is composed primarily of hyaluronic acid, proteoglycans, and glycoproteins. The details of structure of these substances have been reviewed.[9,10,64]

Hyaluronic acid is a linear polymer of alternating units of glucuronic acid and N-acetyl glucosamine with a molecular weight in the order of 10^6 daltons. In connective tissue matrix it likely exists as a randomly coiled hydrated globular structure. Hyaluronic acid is strongly affected by changes in ionic strength and pH. Whether hyaluronic acid forms noncovalent complexes with proteins of the matrix under condition of physiological pH and ionic strength is not known; however,

the material does exhibit a remarkable sieving effect on large globular molecules, and one of its major functions in connective tissues may be that of volume exclusion and sieving.[77]

Proteoglycans are made up of a protein core with covalently bonded glycosaminoglycan side chains. Proteoglycans exhibit immense variation. The protein core may be any one of a large family of related but different proteins, and the polysaccharide side chains may vary in their molecular size, composition, and degree of sulfation. Hybrids of chondroitin sulfates 4 and 6 have been found. Proteoglycans and hyaluronic acid form the bulk of the ground substance of most connective tissues and provide a gelatinous, highly hydrated matrix in which the fibers and cells are embedded.

PROPERTIES OF GINGIVAL COLLAGEN

On the basis of histologic and histochemical observations, the gingiva is usually considered to be a ligamentous tissue with a high collagen content. Extrapolation of data obtained from the chemical analysis of skin, tendon, and other connective tissues has led to the concept that the collagenous component is highly stable and turns over at a slow rate. However, it has recently been found that these concepts may not hold true for the gingival connective tissues.

The total collagen content of gingiva has been measured by several investigators.[4,139,143] Both in humans and in other primates, gingiva contains only about 60 percent as much collagen as the skin, while the collagen content of the adjacent palatal tissue is comparable to that of skin (Table 1-1). Furthermore,

TABLE 1-1. *Dry Weight and Collagen Content of Normal Adult Connective Tissues*

TISSUE	PERCENT DRY WEIGHT	HYDROXYPROLINE (MG/GM OF DRY TISSUE)
Human gingiva	26	60
Human skin	36	96
Marmoset gingiva	33	42
Marmoset palate	22	67
Marmoset skin	41	72
Marmoset tendon	36	103

From Page, R. C.: Macromolecular interactions in the connective tissue of the periodontium. *In* Developmental Aspects of Oral Biology. H. Slavkin and L. Bavetta, Eds. New York, Academic Press, 1972, p. 292.

the degree of interchain covalent cross-linking in gingiva may be much less than is seen in other mature connective tissues. Newly synthesized collagen molecules aggregate rapidly into fibrils, and within a matter of hours in most adult connective tissues undergo stabilization by covalent interchain cross-linking. Extraction of tissues with dilute saline solutions removes the newly synthesized noncross-linked collagen and serves as a simple way to measure the size of the unstabilized collagen compartment. Subsequent acid extraction of the tissue residue dissolves a partially stabilized form of collagen cross-linked by Schiff base. The most mature and highly cross-linked collagen is not solubilized by nondenaturing conditions. In both humans and marmosets, the size of the salt-soluble collagen component in clinically normal gingiva is several times larger than that of skin (Table 1-2), indicating that the gingiva may contain an unusually large pool of recently synthesized unstable collagen. The large size of the acid-soluble compartment in human gingiva indicates that Schiff base cross-links may be an important feature of this collagen.

Although the size of the various collagen compartments in connective tissues gives some indication of the degree of collagen stabilization, rates of production, maturation, and breakdown can best be measured by following the course of radioactively labeled precursor amino acid into and out of the connective tissues with time. This technique has been used to study collagen production and degradation in growing and mature animals, in inflammatory lesions, and in some forms of granulation tissue.[17,39,42,66,67,102,103,126,162] Generally, it has been found that in young growing animals and in granulating tissues the rates of collagen production and degradation are high, whereas in mature animals little label is incorporated and that which is used is retained. These observations have led to the concept that there is little or no turnover of normal mature collagenous structures. There is recent evidence that this may not be the case in the periodontium. For example, in rodents given radioactively labeled proline, large amounts of radioactivity can be detected by radioautography in the collagen of the gingiva and periodontal ligament.[29,31,34,158,161] More recently, the course of incorporation of ^{14}C-proline into collagen hydroxyproline of gingiva and several other mature connective tissues has been determined biochemically in normal mature marmosets.[112] In these experiments, prior to administration of the label, foam rubber sponges were implanted under the skin of the animals in order to have an internal control site of known rapid collagen production. Tendon was selected for analysis as a possible negative control site, since it is known to turn over in the mature animal at an exceptionally low rate. Palate, a contiguous oral collagenous tissue, and skin were also analyzed.

As seen in Table 1-3, the specific activity of hydroxyproline in the salt-soluble and acid-soluble collagens 6 days after administration of label is greater in the gingiva than in any of the other tissues analyzed except for sponge granulation tissue. The specific activities of hydroxyproline in insoluble collagen for all the time periods studied are shown in Figure 1-26. The counts in insoluble gingival collagen are several times greater than in any other tissue studied. Furthermore, the level of counts in insoluble collagen in gingiva is reduced

TABLE 1-2. *Extractability of Hydroxyproline in Normal Human and Marmoset Tissues Relative to Skin*[a]

	TOTAL HYDROXYPROLINE (MG/GM DRY WT)	SOLUBILITY	
		1 M NaCl	0.5 N HAc
Human gingiva	0.7	26.0	9.3
Human skin	1.0	1.0	1.0
Marmoset gingiva	0.6[b]	5.2	0.4
Marmoset palate	0.9	1.3	0.1
Marmoset tendon	1.4	0.3	1.0
Marmoset skin	1.0	1.0	1.0

From Page, R. C.: Macromolecular interactions in the connective tissue of the periodontium. *In* Developmental Aspects of Oral Biology. H. Slavkin and L. Bavetta, Eds. New York, Academic Press, 1972, p. 292.
  [a] Tissue of 10 animals, human gingival tissues from 8 subjects, and skin from 1 subject.
  [b] All data normalized to yield value of 1 for skin.

TABLE 1-3. *Incorporation of C[14]-Proline into Soluble Collagen Hydroxyproline Six Days After Administration of Label*[a]

TISSUE	SALT-SOLUBLE	ACID-SOLUBLE
Tendon	0	0
Aorta	ND[b]	524
Skin	11,921	1,310
Palate	ND[b]	2,620
Gingiva	21,091	7,598
Sponge	9,563	17,554

From Page, R. C.: Macromolecular interactions in the connective tissues of the periodontium. *In* Developmental Aspects of Oral Biology. H. Slavkin and L. Bavetta, Eds. New York, Academic Press, 1972, p. 292.

[a] Reported as DPM/μmole hydroxyproline.
[b] Not determined because of insufficient material.

with the passage of time, while the level in the other tissues is maintained near the maximum value. These observations support the concept that the collagenous component of the gingival connective tissues may be unusually labile and may turn over, even in the normal state, at an inordinately high rate. If this is the case, then several observations that have been poorly understood previously become clearer. The rapid turnover rate may help to explain the high potential for regen-

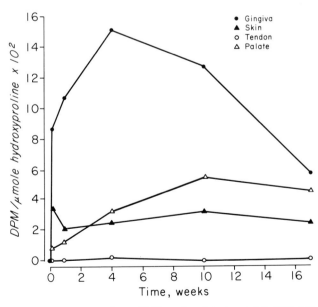

FIG. 1-26. *Incorporation of* [14]*C-proline into insoluble collagen hydroxyproline. (Page, R. C., and Ammons, W. F.: Collagen turnover in the gingiva and other connective tissues of the marmoset. Arch. Oral Biol., 19:1039, 1974.)*

eration and repair of the gingiva as well as the mechanism by which the general structural and architectural features of the gingiva and periodontium are maintained during tooth eruption, mesial drift, continuous eruption, and inflammatory disease. Furthermore, the rapid turnover rate hypothesis may help to explain the rapid loss of collagen observed in the early stages of inflammatory gingival disease,[139] since relatively minor alterations in collagen production or degradation can lead to dramatic changes in the collagen content.

THE GROUND SUBSTANCE OF GINGIVAL CONNECTIVE TISSUES

The ground substance of gingiva has been studied primarily from a histochemical point of view. Most of the data therefore are qualitative (see reviews by Balazs and Jeanloz, and Cabrini and Carranza.[10,28]) The matrix stains positively with periodic acid Schiff reagent, colloidal iron, and alcian blue, indicating the presence of both neutral and acidic mucopolysaccharides. Glycoproteins and hyaluronic acid can be extracted from normal human gingiva and the presence of both chondroitin sulfates 4 and 6 has been shown.[142]

ALVEOLAR BONE

The roots of the teeth are embedded in the *alveolar processes* of the maxillae and mandible. These processes are tooth-dependent structures. Their morphology is a function of tooth form and position. Furthermore, they develop as the teeth form and erupt, and they are resorbed, to a great extent, after the teeth have been lost. The alveolar bone anchors the teeth and their soft investing tissues and resolves the forces generated by intermittent tooth contact, mastication, deglutition, and phonation. The primary aim of preventive periodontics and of periodontal therapy is the preservation and maintenance of the alveolar bone. A thorough knowledge of alveolar bone structure, morphology, and physiology has become increasingly important to the periodontist in recent years as a result of the widespread use of advanced surgical techniques for bone in the treatment of periodontal disease.

Deposition

Mature alveolar bone is an unusually complex structure. The features of the mature structure can be explained best by beginning at an early stage of development while a measure of simplicity still exists. The initial stage in the formation of alveolar bone is characterized by the deposition of calcium salts in localized zones of connective tissue matrix near the developing tooth bud. This deposition results in the formation of zones or islands of immature bone separated from one another by uncalcified connective tissue matrix. Once established, these foci continue to enlarge, fuse, and undergo extensive remodeling. Active bone resorption and deposition go on concurrently. The external surface of the bone mass is covered by a thin layer of uncalcified bone matrix called *osteoid*, and this, in turn, is covered by a condensation of fine collagen fibers and cells referred to as the *periosteum* (Fig. 1-27). Cavities within the bone mass, or created there by resorption, are lined by the *endosteum* which is identical in structure with the periosteum. These layers contain *osteoblasts*, which have the capacity to deposit bone matrix and induce calcification, and *osteoclasts*, multinuclear cells participating in bone resorption. In addition, progenitor cells are also present. Under the influence of these cells, the alveolar bone undergoes appositional growth and remodeling to accommodate the demands

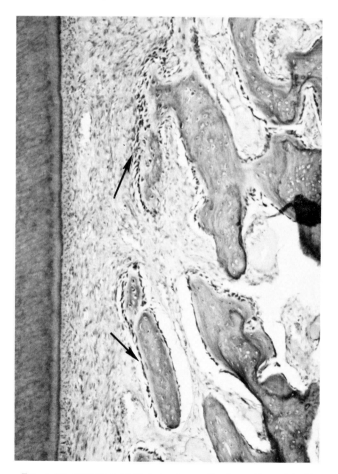

FIG. 1-27. *Features of alveolar bone. Region adjacent to the periodontal ligament in which the bony trabeculae contain lacunae with osteocytes and are covered by a periosteum made up of osteoblasts (arrows). (Magnification 200 ×.) (Courtesy Dr. B. Moffett.)*

of the developing and erupting teeth and evolves into a mature structure.

As growth continues, additional complexity is introduced. Cells present in the periosteum become embedded within the calcified matrix and are transformed into *osteocytes*. These cells reside in small cavities referred to as the *lacunae* (Fig. 1-28D), and extend processes through bony channels called *canaliculi*. The canaliculi become generally oriented in the direction of the blood supply, and osteocytes may communicate one with another through cytoplasmic processes in these channels. Blood vessels encountered by the enlarging bony mass are incorporated into the structure. The vessels become surrounded by concentric lamellae of bone referred to as *osteons* (Fig. 1-28C,D). The vessels course through channels in the osteons generally called *haversian canals*. Continuous peripheral appositional growth results in the formation of a dense surface layer of *cortical bone*, while internal resorption and remodeling give rise to the marrow spaces and the bony trabeculae characteristic of the *cancellous* or *spongy bone* (Fig. 1-28A). The trabeculae buttress the alveolus between the buccal and lingual cortical plates. The size, shape, and thickness of the bony trabeculae vary extensively from one individual to another and from one site to another in a given individual. Some trabeculae are uneven irregular sheets; others are cylindrical rods (Fig. 1-28A). All of the trabeculae are interconnected and join directly or indirectly with the cortical plates and the walls of the alveoli. No single trabecular bone pattern has been associated with specific disease states.[117] However, changes occur in the trabecular pattern from one time to another, and increases or decreases in the bone volume do indicate disease states.

As the teeth erupt and the roots form, a dense cortical layer of bone is laid down adjacent to the periodontal space. This layer is referred to as the *lamina dura* or *cribriform plate* (Figs. 1-28A, 1-29). This bony plate may be a sievelike structure, exhibiting numerous foramina through which blood vessels from the marrow spaces communicate with those of the periodontal ligament, or it may be a solid sheet of cortical bone (Fig. 1-29). The bone immediately adjacent to the root surface to which the fibers of the periodontal ligament attach has also been called the *alveolar bone proper* to contrast it to the *supporting bone* comprising the peripheral cortical plates and the cancellous bone.

Bone matrix is made up predominantly of collagen. Bone collagen molecules are made up of two alpha-1 and one alpha-2 chains and contain the lysyl family of cross-links.[97] Chemical and biologic properties of alveolar bone collagen have been studied.

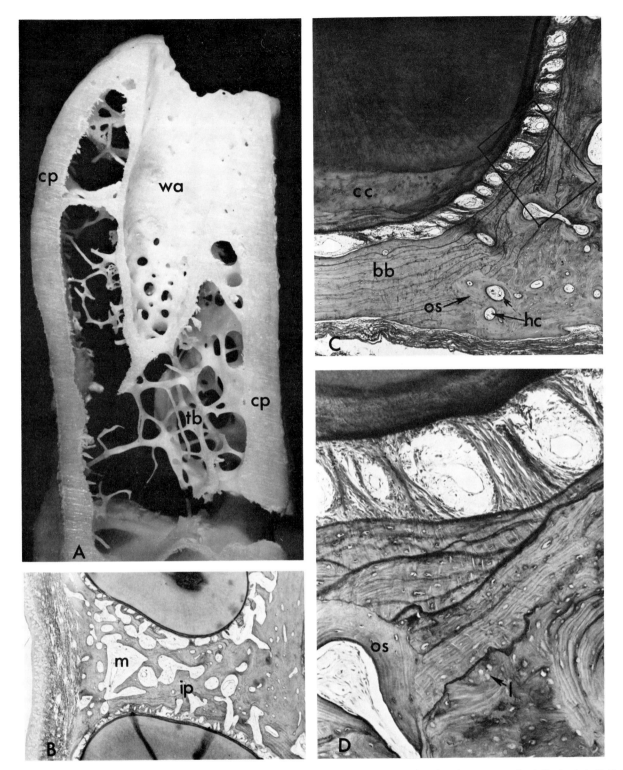

FIG. 1-28. *Structural features of alveolar bone. A. Section through the mandibular posterior alveolar process of a defleshed skull. Note the dense, thick buccal and lingual cortical plates (cp) and the thinner cortical bone forming the wall of the alveolus (wa), nutrient canals penetrating the cribriform plate in the apical one third of the alveolus, and spicules of trabecular bone (tb). B. Horizontal section near the middle third of the root in the mandibular premolar region. Note the buccal and lingual cortical bone and the trabecular interproximal bone (ip) with spaces filled with fatty marrow (m) (Magnification 30 ×). C. Horizontal section through the apical third of a premolar exhibiting features of bone, cementum, and periodontal ligament. Haversian canals (hc), fully developed osteons (os), and concentric layers of bundle bone (bb) exhibiting incremental lines are seen. A wide layer of cellular cementum (cc) on one surface of the root permits comparison of the histologic features of cementum and bone. (Magnification 60 ×). D. Higher magnification of area outlined in C. Note the osteon (os) and lacunae-containing osteocytes (l) (Magnification 120 ×). (Courtesy Dr. B. Moffett.)*

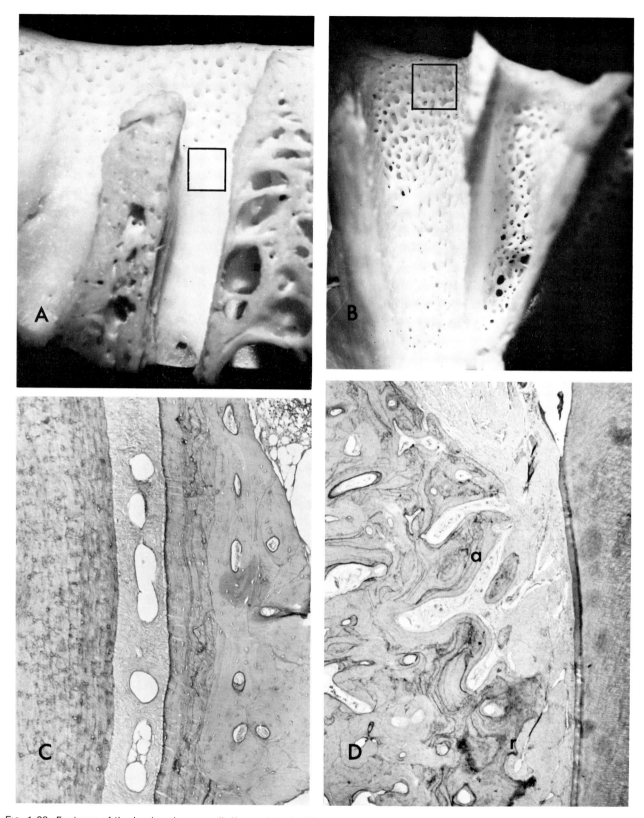

FIG. 1-29. *Features of the lamina dura or cribriform plate. A. Alveolus of a mandibular molar of Macacca mulatta from which the buccal aspect has been removed to illustrate regions where the cortical plates are uniform and free of nutrient canals in the apical region and a zone rich in canals in the gingival one third. B. Alveolus of a canine and lateral incisor from which the labial plate has been removed to show the dense population of nutrient canals that have given rise to the term cribriform plate. C. Histologic features of the alveolar wall from a region similar to that outlined in (A) are consistent with a surface resting or undergoing apposition and containing no nutrient canals (Magnification 120 ×). D. Histologic features of the alveolar wall from a zone similar to that outlined in (B). Areas of bone resorption (r) and bone apposition (a) are seen. The nutrient canals all slant in a coronal direction (Magnification 120 ×). (Courtesy Dr. B. Moffett.)*

Remodeling

One important functional characteristic of alveolar bone is its capacity to undergo continuous remodeling in response to functional demands. Under normal conditions, the teeth migrate mesially and erupt continuously to compensate for attritional reduction in the mesiodistal dimensions and in occlusal height. These movements induce renovation of the surrounding alveolar bone. Bone resorption is seen generally on the pressure side and bone deposition on the tension side of the moving tooth root. Surfaces undergoing remodeling exhibit characteristic anatomic and histologic features (Figs. 1-28C, 1-30). Zones of resorption exhibit rough uneven surfaces with numerous cavities and spicules. Histologically, the surfaces may appear moth-eaten and are covered with multinucleate osteoclasts. Surfaces upon which deposition is occurring exhibit layers of recently deposited *bundle bone* containing no marrow spaces or osteons. With the passage of time, bundle bone may undergo remodeling and become indistinguishable from the original alveolar bone. Bundle bone frequently contains embedded collagen fibers previously resident in the periodontal ligament and running at right angles to the bone surface. Apposition of bone is seen most often in the apical one third and on the distal aspect of the alveolus while bone resorption occurs most frequently on the mesial aspect.

Morphology

Alveolar structure varies greatly and an understanding of the range of variation is essential for diagnosis of bone defects. Generally, the form of the alveolar bone can be predicted on the basis of three general principles: (1) the position, state of eruption, size and shape of the teeth determine, to a great extent, the form of the alveolar bone,[57,125] (2) when subjected to forces within normal physiologic limits bone undergoes remodeling to form a structure that best resolves the forces applied, and (3) there is a finite thickness below which bone will not survive but will be resorbed.

The alveolar margin usually follows the contour of the cementoenamel line. Thus, scalloping of the bony margin is more prominent on the facial aspect of the anterior teeth than on the molars (Fig. 1-31A,B), and the interproximal bone between the anterior teeth is pyramidal, whereas that between the molars is flat buccolingually (Fig. 1-31C,D). The interproximal bone between adjacent teeth that are erupted to different planes of occlusion will be inclined toward the root of the less erupted tooth (Fig. 1-31G). Teeth that are rotated will exhibit a bone margin that is located more coronally and is less scalloped than that of adjacent normally positioned teeth (Fig. 1-31E). The size, position, and shape of the roots have a major influence upon bone form. Teeth in abnormal buccolingual position exhibit significant variation in bone form. On the prominent side the root surface may be covered by a thin layer of cortical bone with little or no spongiosa and with an apically positioned bone margin, dehiscence, or fenestration; on the contralateral surface the bone will be thick and will have a more coronally placed marginal ledge. Bone rarely exists as a paper-thin layer on the surface of roots. Instead, it is resorbed, giving rise to dehiscences and fenestrations (Fig. 1-31B,F). Most frequently dehiscences and fenestrations are variations of normal structure resulting from tooth position, and they are not necessarily a consequence of inflammatory periodontal disease.[38,76,160]

CEMENTUM

Cementum forms the interface between root dentin and the soft connective tissues of the periodontal ligament. It is a highly specialized form of calcified connective tissue, which resembles bone structurally but differs from bone in several important functional respects. Cementum has no innervation, no direct blood supply, and no lymph drainage. It covers the entire root surface and sometimes even portions of the crown of human teeth. Cementum undergoes only minor remodeling.[56,109,122,130]

Cementogenesis

The initial events in cementogenesis have been elucidated in young rats and mice by light and electron microscopy.[63,84,85,119,144,145,146,147,148,154,164] The formation of both dentin and cementum occurs in the presence of *Hertwig's epithelial root sheath*. This sheath is formed by an epithelial outgrowth, several layers thick, from the apical aspects of the *enamel organ*. As the cells of the sheath proliferate, a reduction in the thickness occurs in the more coronal portion of the structure. In zones where only one or two epithelial cell layers remain, the connective tissue cells on the pulpal side of the sheath differentiate into *odontoblasts* and begin to lay down *predentin*.[144,145]

When the layer of predentin reaches a thickness of from 3 to 5 microns, it becomes invested with an amorphous matrix substance and subsequently mineralizes. As mineralization progresses, the epithelial cells of the root sheath begin to separate from one another and from the dentin surface and migrate toward the periodontal connective tissue. Concurrently,

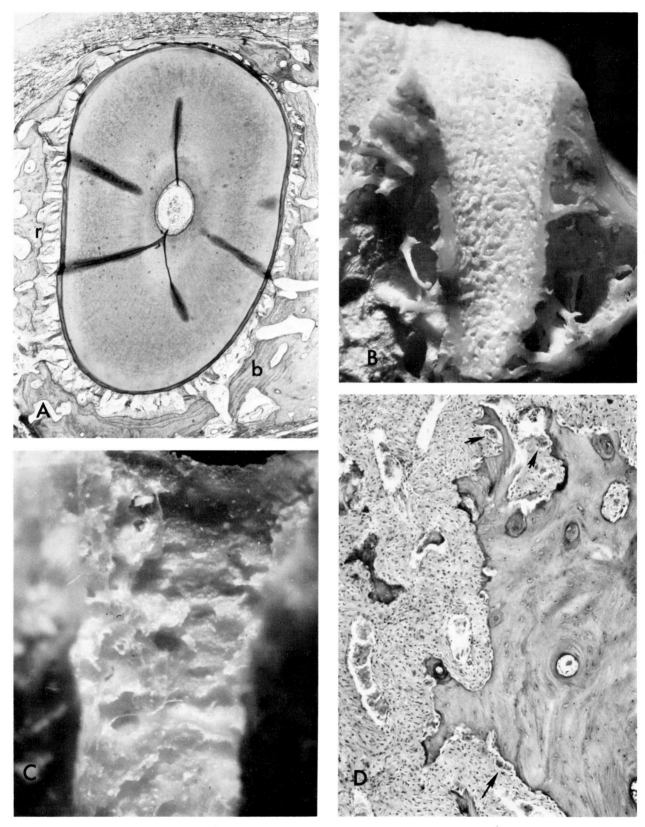

FIG. 1-30. *Features of remodeling alveolar bone. A. Horizontal section through a human premolar. The histologic pattern observed in the bone indicates that the tooth has moved in a mesiobuccal direction. Note the resorbing surface (r) on the mesial aspect and the layers of bundle bone (b) that have been laid down on the distolingual aspect. In some areas the bundle bone has undergone remodeling with the formation of nutrient canals (Magnification 30×). B. Alveolus of a molar from Macacca mulatta showing the rough uneven surface characteristics of a resorbing surface. C. Features of a resorbing surface. D. Histologic manifestations of resorbing alveolar bone and adjacent periodontal ligament. Note the moth-eaten surface and the replacement of the bone by fibrous connective tissue. The remaining fibers of the periodontal ligament exhibit little specific orientation. Multinuclear osteoclasts are present on the surface (arrows) (Magnification 150 ×). (Courtesy Dr. B. Moffett.)*

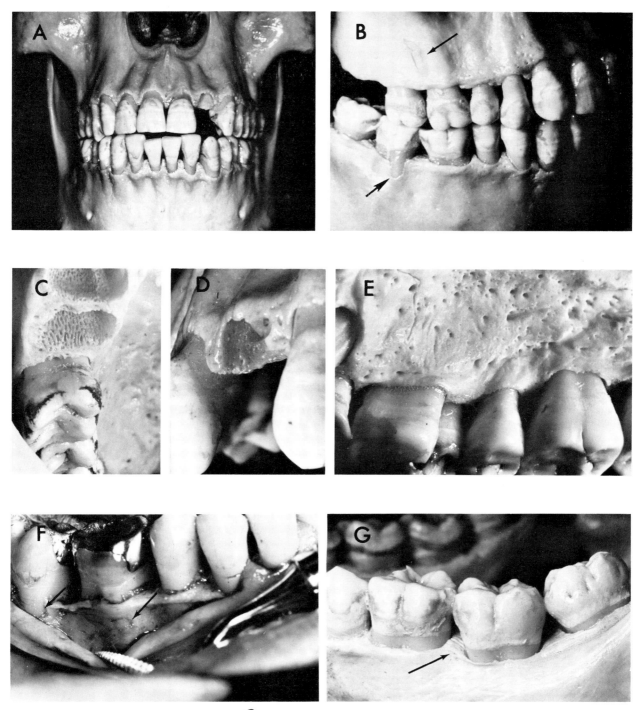

FIG. 1-31. *Anatomic features of the alveolar bone. A. Frontal view of the alveolar processes of a relatively normal human adult. The outlines of the root contours are evident in the labial plates. The bony margin follows the scalloped contours of the cementoenamel junction and terminates in a slightly rounded edge. In the mandibular region there is a slight bony ledge near the cervix of the teeth. B. Fenestration of the buccal plate over the distobuccal root of the maxillary first molar and an early dehiscence of the mesial root of the mandibular second molar. C. Bony housing of the maxillary left second and third molars illustrating the flatness of the interseptal bone in the molar region. The bony crest follows closely the cementoenamel junction. Also, note the porosity of the cribriform plates and the nutrient foramina in the interdental crests. D. Alveolus of a maxillary lateral incisor showing the conical shape of the interproximal bone and its parallelism with the cementoenamel junction. E. Palatal aspect of the maxillary right posterior quadrant. A slight fluting in the palatal root of the first molar is reproduced in the bone margin. The first premolar is in buccal version relative to the second premolar and exhibits a thicker and more coronally placed cortical plate than the second premolar. The adjacent tooth is rotated such that the mesial surface is placed palatally. Note the lack of scalloping relative to the second premolar and molar. F. Mandibular right posterior region prior to osseous surgery illustrating a fenestration on the mesial root of the first molar and an early dehiscense on the mesial root of the second molar (arrows). Note the pencil ledge of bone on the premolars. G. Buccal aspect of the mandibular left posterior quadrant. In spite of the fact that the second molar is buccally positioned and in a lower occlusal plane than the adjacent molars (arrow), the bony margin follows the contour of the cemento-enamel junction, and the interproximal bone slants toward the second molar. (Courtesy Dr. J. Easley.)*

the basal lamina separating the epithelial cells from the developing dentin becomes diffuse and is replaced by a layer of fine, randomly oriented collagen fibrils. These fibrils extend between the separating epithelial cells, but not into the developing dentin. This layer makes up the *cementoid* or *precementum.* It accumulates an amorphous matrix and calcifies at the same time. As calcification progresses, the *cementoblasts* move away from the surface and usually are not incorporated. Thus, the primary layer of cementum investing the newly formed root is usually acellular. However, both cementoblasts and epithelial cells from Hertwig's sheath may become trapped, giving rise to cellular cementum. The cementoblasts differ from the other connective tissue cells in that they are located near the cemental surface and are polarized in that they extend cytoplasmic processes among the collagen fibrils into the precementum. The cells are more electron-dense than are the surrounding fibroblasts; they contain dense material in dilated endoplasmic cisternae and exhibit features generally associated with actively synthesizing cells.[21]

The end result of cementogenesis is the formation of a thin layer of extracellular calcified material at the interface of the dentin and the noncalcified connective tissue that serves as the attachment site for collagen fibers of the periodontal connective tissue. Residual cells of the epithelial root sheath form a network within the periodontal ligament. These are referred to as the *cell rests.*[110]

Morphology

Cementum deposition does not cease when root formation is complete, nor when the tooth erupts; indeed, apposition may continue intermittently throughout life.[174] Furthermore, cementum formation is not confined to the root surface; it may be deposited also on enamel. The morphologic features of cementum may vary significantly with the time and site of deposition.

CELLULAR AND ACELLULAR CEMENTUM

Acellular cementum is usually the earliest layer deposited; it is therefore found immediately adjacent to the dentin (Fig. 1-32B). It is present predominantly in the cervical region but may invest the entire root.[119] Cellular cementum covers the middle and apical portions of the root surface. There is no clear dividing line between these types, however, and one form may be sandwiched between layers of the other. Both forms may exhibit a matrix of fine collagen fibrils embedded in a finely granular or amorphous matrix (Fig. 1-33). The structure of cellular cementum is similar to that of the acellular form, except for the presence of trapped

cementoblasts and root-sheath epithelial cells. These cells are located in lacunae, and they extend cytoplasmic processes through channels or canaliculi, usually oriented toward the blood supply of the periodontal connective tissues. After incorporation into the cementum, they are referred to as *cementocytes.* Cementocytes differ from cementoblasts in that they exhibit fewer cytoplasmic organelles such as rough endoplasmic reticulum, mitochondria, and Golgi apparatus and increased numbers of lysosomes.[63] Cementocytes are separated from the surrounding calcified cementum by a perilacunar space which may contain globular material. In this regard, they resemble osteocytes. Most of the cells remain viable, especially near the periodontal surface. However, cells located near the dentinal surface may degenerate.[63] Both cellular and acellular forms of cementum may exhibit incremental lines indicating intermittent periods of appositional growth and quiescence (Fig. 1-32C).

PRIMARY AND SECONDARY CEMENTUM

The term *primary cementum* is generally used to describe the acellular layer that was deposited immediately adjacent to the dentin during root formation and prior to tooth eruption. Primary cementum is made up of fine, randomly oriented collagen fibrils embedded in a granular matrix. *Secondary cementum* includes layers deposited after eruption, usually in response to functional demands. Secondary cementum is usually cellular and contains coarse collagen fibrils oriented parallel to the root surface and may exhibit Sharpey's fibers (Fig. 1-32E,F). Generally, primary cementum is more uniformly and more completely mineralized than is secondary cementum and has fewer developmental lines.[62]

FIBRILLAR AND AFIBRILLAR CEMENTUM

Variation in the extracellular matrix structure permits classification of cementum as fibrillar and afibrillar. When cementum is viewed with the electron microscope, numerous bundles of banded collagen fibrils, as well as amorphous and finely granular interfibrillar matrix material, are seen in fibrillar cementum (Fig. 1-33), but afibrillar cementum is free of collagen fibrils.[119,137,145,146,164] Afibrillar cementum is seen most frequently in the cervical region on the root or crown surface. It may be deposited in isolated areas on the enamel surface in regions where the reduced enamel organ has undergone degeneration and the connective tissues have come into contact with the enamel.[137] Both forms of cementum undergo mineralization, and both may have incremental lines.

Fibrillar cementum has a dual fiber system. The

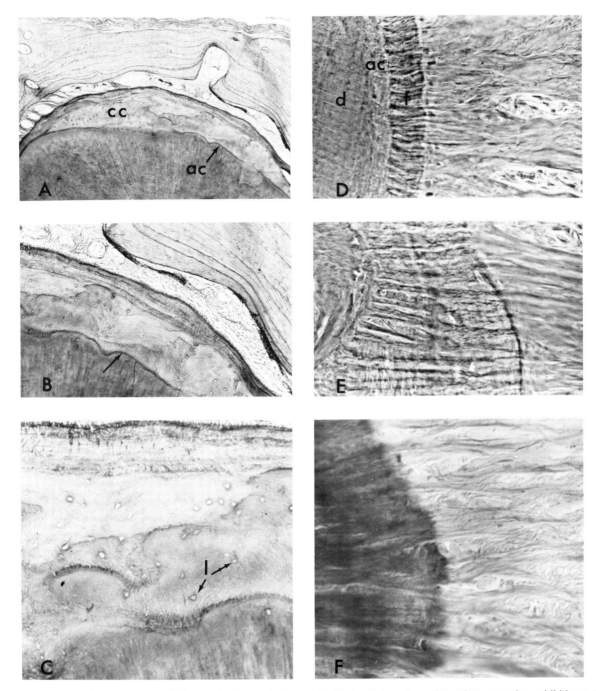

FIG. 1-32. Features of cementum and Sharpey's fibers. A, B, and C. Horizontal sections through a premolar exhibiting a thick cemental deposition. A thin layer of acellular cementum (ac) at the dentinal surface (arrow) is covered by a thicker layer of cellular cementum (cc) containing lacunae (l) and a surface layer of acellular fibrillar cementum exhibiting incremental lines. Note the wavy, irregular structure of the cellular cementum (original magnifications 50, 100, and 200 ×, respectively). D. Dentinal surface (d) covered by a layer of afibrillar cementum (ac) and fibrous cementum (f) into which the fibers of the periodontal ligament insert. E. Higher power view of acellular fibrous cementum with Sharpey's fibers traversing the entire thickness. F. The surface region of fibrous cementum illustrating the insertion of Sharpey's fibers. Note the irregularity of the surface.

collagen laid down by the cementoblasts and oriented either randomly or parallel to the root surface forms the intrinsic fiber system (Fig. 1-32). As the tooth erupts and reaches functional occlusion, cementum deposition continues and the ends of the principal fibers of the periodontal ligament become embedded at right angles to the root surface (Fig. 1-32F). These are referred to as *Sharpey's fibers* and they form an *extrinsic fiber system*. The extrinsic fibers are produced by fibroblasts of the periodontal ligament. Initially,

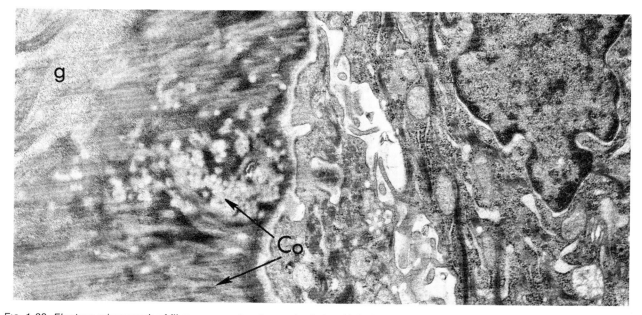

FIG. 1-33. *Electron micrograph of fibrous cementum from a tooth in which the epithelial attachment is located on the root surface. There is a granular matrix (g) between the collagen fibers (co). Fibers run parallel and at right angles to the plane of section. Note the similarity of the structure of the granular material with that of afibrillar cementum observed on the enamel surface (Fig. 1-14C). (Magnification 12,375 ×).*

Sharpey's fibers are inserted into the cementum at approximately right angles to the tooth surface; however, this angle may change greatly as tooth movement occurs. The number and diameter of Sharpey's fibers vary with the functional status and health of the tooth.[61] The density increases significantly after tooth eruption (Table 1-4). In humans, Sharpey's fibers are separated and surrounded by the intrinsic fiber system.[21] The average fiber diameter is about 4 microns.

There has been considerable controversy regarding the extent to which the various components of cementum mineralize. Some investigators support the idea that the matrix, but not the collagen fibers, calcify,[119,154] others have presented evidence that the intrinsic, but not the extrinsic, fibers mineralize; still others feel that the fibers as well as the matrix are involved in the calcification process.[144,145] Undoubtedly, some of this confusion stems from species variation. In the molars of the adult mice both the intrinsic and extrinsic fibers, as well as the interfibrillar matrix, mineralize.[145] However, in man the situation is more complex. There is a zone of from 10 to 50 microns near the dentinal surface where Sharpey's fibers are closely packed and calcification is usually complete; however, in cellular cementum where Sharpey's fibers may be separated from one another by intrinsic fibers located either randomly or parallel to the cemental surface, only the periphery of the fibers is calcified, leaving an uncalcified core.[145,146] It is also clear that although primary cementum is uniformly mineralized, cellular cementum is more laminated and less calcified.[62]

Composition and Properties

The chemical composition of cementum is similar to bone, but there are important differences. Of the normally mineralized connective tissues, cementum contains the least amount of inorganic salt. Of the total dry weight, inorganic salts make up about 70 percent of bone, but only 46 percent of cementum.[148] The inorganic salts are present in the form of hydroxyapatite crystals. The matrix is made up of collagen fibers, which apparently do not differ from those of other tissues, and a fairly dense amorphous and finely granular interfibrillar investing material, which appears to

TABLE 1-4. *Sharpey's Fibers*

FUNCTIONAL STAGE	DENSITY / 100 μ^2 (S.D.)	DIAMETER, μ (S.D.)
Pre-eruptive and eruptive	53.4 (13.5)	3.0 (0.02)
Normal function	28.0 (3.2)	4.0 (0.03)
Completely embedded	2.1 (5.3)	4.1 (0.03)
Fixed-bridge abutment	21.3 (5.2)	4.6 (0.06)

Adapted from Akiyoshi, M., and Inoue, M.: On the functional structure of cementum. Bull. Tokyo Med. Dent. Univ., *10*:41, 1963.

be the unique product of the cementoblasts (Fig. 1-33). Sasso,[128] and Paynter and Purdy,[119] have provided evidence that the investing substance is made up of proteoglycans and of neutral and acid mucopolysaccharides.

Cementum is a relatively brittle structure. Fractures may result from traumatic injury. The tissue is also permeable. Dyes and radioactive substances can diffuse from the pulp through the cementum into the surrounding connective tissues.[172]

Physiology

Cementum serves three major functions: it attaches the fibers of the periodontal ligament to the root surface, it helps to maintain and control the width of the periodontal ligament space, and it serves as the medium through which damage to the root surface is repaired.[65] Cementum deposition continues, at least intermittently, throughout life. On normal human teeth the thickness of cementum increases more or less linearly with increasing age, but on periodontally diseased teeth this incremental increase levels off.[60,174] In a study of 233 single-rooted teeth, it was noted that the thickness of cementum increased threefold between the ages of 11 and 76 years with the greatest increase occurring in the apical one third of the root.[174] The average cemental thickness at age 20 years is 95 microns; at age 60 it is about 215 microns.[60] The thickness varies from one location on the root surface to another. While the thickness in the cervical one third may be between 16 and 60 microns, a thickness of 150 to 200 microns has been noted in the apical third of the same teeth.[108] There is no clear-cut relationship between cemental thickness and functional stress. Thick layers of cementum have been observed on impacted and unerupted teeth.[50,74]

The continuous deposition of cementum is considered to be essential for normal mesial drift and compensatory eruption of the teeth, in that it permits rearrangement of the fibers of the periodontal ligament and maintains the attachment of the fibers during tooth movement. Gottlieb has suggested that continuous deposition of cementum is essential for the maintenance of a healthy periodontium and that defects in cementum deposition may underlie pocket formation.[49]

The principal functional difference between bone and cementum is that the latter does not undergo extensive physiologic resorption and remodeling.[109,122,130] Kerr has noted that cementum is resorbed less than bone,[72] and others have stated that resorption of cementum does not occur to any great extent under normal conditions.[56,74] However, the data indicate that some remodeling does occur. An examination of 261 human teeth revealed that 90.5 percent exhibited microscopic evidence of lacunar resorption. This was greatest in the apical third of the root and least in the cervical region.[54,56] Thus, lacunar resorption does not appear to be related to pocket formation or to inflammatory disease. The number and size of resorbed areas increased with increasing age. Resorption was more prevalent on the mesial and buccal surfaces than on the distal and lingual aspects of the roots. About 85 percent of the areas showed evidence of repair, and in most of these, repair was complete. Further evidence for cemental resorption and remodeling was presented by Bélanger[16]. Cementocytes have lytic capability as evidenced by the conversion of matrix component surrounding the lacunae into flocculent debris,[16,63,164] and this conversion is enhanced by the administration of parathyroid hormone.[16] Furthermore, radioactive substances are incorporated into cementum and have a high rate of turnover. Thus, current concepts regarding the inertness of cementum may require revision as more information is obtained.

THE PERIODONTAL LIGAMENT

The soft connective tissues enveloping the roots of the teeth and extending coronally to the crest of the alveolar bone are referred to as the *periodontal ligament*. The structural features of this tissue were accurately identified and described by Black and include resident cells, blood and lymphatic vessels, collagen bundles, and ground substance.[22] In recent years, only minor structural details have been added to his original description.

Formation

The periodontal ligament forms as the tooth develops and erupts into the oral cavity. The final structural form is not achieved until the tooth reaches occlusion, and functional force is applied. The ligament differentiates from the loose connective tissues investing the tooth bud.[3,40,43,144] Initially, this tissue is made up of undifferentiated or "resting" fibroblasts, containing a large amount of glycogen and few organelles and embedded in an amorphous argyrophilic matrix. The matrix contains a randomly oriented reticulum of branched, beaded microfibrils measuring 50 to 100 angstroms in diameter.[52] Subsequently, the fibroblasts develop into highly active cells rich in well-developed organelles and deposit collagen fibrils measuring 300 to 500 angstroms in diameter. These fibrils lack any specific orientation. As development proceeds, a fairly dense layer of connective tissue substance is laid down near the surface of the cementum, with an orientation generally paralleling the long axis of the tooth. Before eruption, cells near the cemental surface, especially in the coronal one third of the root, become oriented in an oblique direction, and a fibrillar matrix lying in a similar orientation is deposited.[82] As the tooth reaches its antagonist and functional force is applied, the periodontal tissues differentiate further and assume a definitive architectural form.

Structure

The collagenous component of the mature periodontal ligament is organized into the *principal fibers*, bundles that traverse the periodontal space obliquely, inserting into the cementum and alveolar bone as Sharpey's fibers, and the *secondary fibers*, bundles made up of more or less randomly oriented collagen fibrils located between the principal fiber bundles (Figs. 1-34, 1-35). In zones where there has been extensive mesiodistal tooth movement, Sharpey's fibers may be continuous through the interproximal bone from one tooth to another.[32,123]

The vascular supply to the periodontal ligament arises predominantly from three sources. Vessels enter the ligament from the alveolar bone through nutrient canals of the cribriform plate, from branches of the arteries supplying the teeth, and from the vessels of the free gingival margin (Figs. 1-18, 1-34). The blood vessels form a basketlike network throughout the periodontal ligament space.[41,73,81] Most of the vessels run between the principal fiber bundles in a direction paralleling the long axis of the root and have horizontal anastomoses.

Blind-end lymph vessels arise in the periodontal ligament and traverse one of three courses. They may pass over the alveolar crest and into the submucosa of the gingiva or palate, perforate the alveolar bone and pass into the spongiosa, or pass apically directly in the periodontal ligament.[83] The ligament around erupted teeth is innervated by fibers arising from the dental branches of the alveolar nerves and terminating as clublike free endings. In unerupted teeth, the periodontal ligament is supplied by fine nonmedullated fibers that are always associated with blood vessels and are considered to be autonomic.[20]

The structure of the principal fibers of the periodontal ligament has been the object of intensive investigation, and the nature of the mechanism by which these fibers are remodeled to accommodate eruption and physiologic tooth movement remains an enigma. Noyes noted that at least some of the fibers pass directly from cementum to alveolar bone.[104,105] However, observations on the structure of the periodontal ligament

around continuously erupting teeth in rodents led Sicher to postulate the existence of an intermediate zone, located approximately midway between the bone and the cementum in which the fibers intermesh.[149] This zone was presumed to be an area of high metabolic activity where the fibers could be spliced and unspliced with ease. Later, Sicher extended this concept to humans and he stated that the human periodontal ligament consists of alveolar fibers, dental fibers and an intermediate plexus.[150,151,152,153]

Support for the intermediate plexus concept was provided by several other investigators.[45,59] Eccles observed an intermediate plexus associated with erupting rat molars and noted morphologic differences between the fibers inserting into bone and those uniting with cementum.[36] However, he did not observe the intermediate zone around fully erupted teeth. Bernick also failed to demonstrate the presence of the three fiber zones around rat molars and fully erupted marmoset teeth, but did provide evidence for the presence of an intermediate plexus around erupting marmoset teeth.[19,20] Other investigators have been able to trace fibers from cementum to bone without interruption and on this basis have disputed the existence of an intermediate plexus.[30,169,175] Recent studies in which zones of high metabolic activity have been labeled with radioactive collagen precursors have also failed to demonstrate the presence of an intermediate plexus.[5,34,161] Indeed, most of the evidence currently available appears to support the idea that the collagenous component of the entire periodontal ligament may turn over at an unusually rapid rate, and this may account, at least in part, for the extensive remodeling that accompanies tooth movement.

THE DEFENSE MECHANISMS OF THE PERIODONTIUM

The teeth and gingiva exist in a septic environment containing innumerable different species and strains of microorganisms and masses of foreign and antigenic substances. Several lines of defense are present to protect the host from these potentially toxic substances. The first line of defense is the *surface barrier*, which has four components.

1. The soft tissues are covered by stratified squamous epithelium, a tissue which undergoes rapid regeneration and renewal (Figs. 1-4B, 1-5D). Cells produced in the basal layer traverse toward the surface and are shed, carrying with them toxic substances which may have penetrated the epithelial covering.
2. The gingival (Fig. 1-5) and in part the oral sulcu-

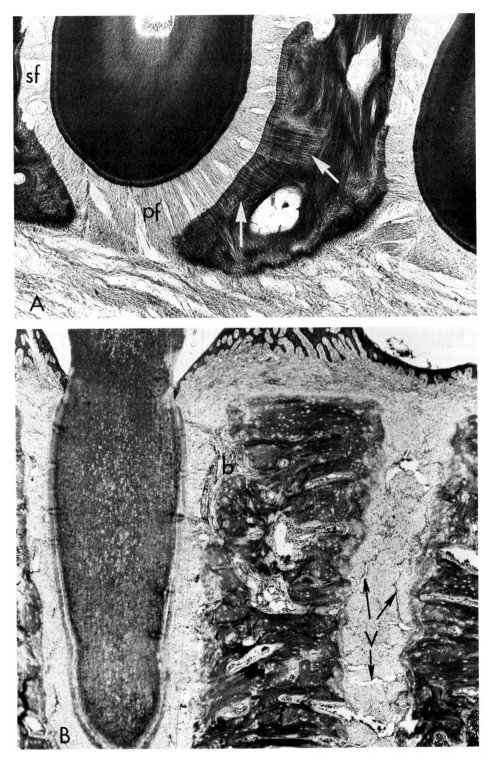

FIG. 1-34. *Structural features of the periodontal ligament and alveolar bone. A. Horizontal section from the mandibular premolar region of an adult marmoset. The principal fibers (pf) traverse the space between bone and cementum without interruption. They insert into the interdental bone as Sharpey's fibers. In one region these fibers traverse about halfway through the interproximal bone (arrow). The secondary fibers (sf) are less well developed and poorly oriented. (Van Gieson stain, magnification 27 ×). B. Vertical section from the buccal aspect of the mandibular premolars of a normal adult marmoset showing the very edge of the periodontal ligament. Note the vertical and horizontal blood vessels (V), and the passage of large vessels through the interseptal bone into the periodontal ligament (b). Compare the pattern observed here with the schematic illustration in Fig. 1-18. (Gomori's trichrome stain, magnification 27 ×).*

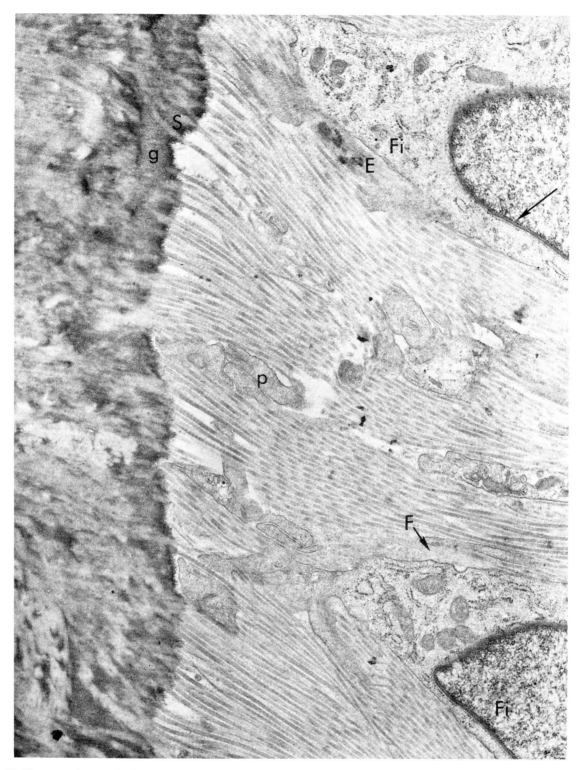

FIG. 1-35. *Electron micrograph of the periodontal ligament and root cementum. Portions of two fibroblasts (Fi) and processes from several others (p) are seen. The cells are rich in rough endoplasmic reticulum and mitochondria and exhibit the peripheral nuclear condensation of electron dense material which is characteristic of gingival fibroblasts (arrows). In addition, there is a network of fine fibrils throughout the cytoplasm. Fine, nonbanded fibrils are also present in the extracellular space (F), especially near the cell surfaces, but the predominant component is collagen fibrils of a rather uniform size and oriented obliquely. An immature elastin fibril (E) is also seen. Sharpey's fibers (S) inserting into fibrillar cementum are apparent. Also note the finely granular cementum (g) (Magnification 12,375 ×).*

lar (Fig. 1-3) epithelium undergo keratinization to produce a tough impenetrable surface layer.

3. The junctional epithelium (Fig. 1-3) in contact with calcified tooth surface elaborates a basal laminalike substance which effectively seals the soft tissue-tooth interface.

4. All the surface tissues, including the tooth, are covered by a glycoprotein coat.

Polymorphonuclear leukocytes migrate continuously from the vessels of the connective tissues into the junctional epithelium, the gingival sulcus, and the oral cavity. It has been estimated that under strictly normal conditions more than 500 polymorphonuclear leukocytes per second migrate through the junctional epithelium of a complete dentition and into the oral cavity.[124] The magnitude of this migration increases dramatically as the size of the microbial population near the gingiva increases. These cells have the capacity while in the tissues or in the gingival sulcus to phagocytose and kill microorganisms.

Macrophages are present within the gingival sulcus, the junctional epithelium, and the subjacent connective tissue. Unlike polymorphonuclear leukocytes, macrophages are long-lived. They have the capacity to serve as scavengers to kill, phagocytize, and digest microorganisms and foreign substances. In some animals such as the marmoset,[129] cells of this type are concentrated in a zone just deep to the junctional epithelium, where penetration of the surface barrier is most likely to occur.

Lymphoid cells, which have the capacity to trigger cellular and humoral immune responses, are also present in the junctional epithelium and the subjacent connective tissues. A continuing presence of microorganisms, such as that which occurs with plaque accumulation, results in sensitization of the host, with blast transformation of lymphocytes, the production of lymphokines, the differentiation of plasma cells, and the production of specific antibody.

The structure of the junctional epithelium allows the passage of *gingival fluid* into the sulcus. This fluid contains many of the constituents of blood, including specific antibody and nonspecific antimicrobial systems. A differentiation of lymphoid cells into plasma cells occurs within the gingival connective tissue with the synthesis and release of immunoglobulins.

The cells of the *junctional epithelium*, especially those located near the base of the gingival sulcus, constitute an important component of host defense. In many respects, the cells resemble epithelial cells migrating over an open wound. They contain primary and secondary lysosomes and have phagocytic capacity. Furthermore, the cells are continuously sloughed into the sulcus and replaced by cells moving coronally from the basal epithelial region.

References

1. Ainamo, J., and Löe, H.: Anatomical characteristics of gingiva. A clinical and microscopic study of the free and attached gingiva. J. Periodontol., 37:5, 1966.
2. Akiyoshi, M., and Inoue, M.: On the functional structure of cementum. Bull. Tokyo Med. Dent. Univ., 10:41, 1963.
3. Albright, J. T., and Flanagan, J. B.: Electron microscopy of cementum. IADR. Abs. of 40th General Meeting, 1962, p. 77.
4. Ammons, W. F.: Periodontal disease in the marmoset: A study of the nature of the collagenous component of the periodontium relative to that of man. M.S. Thesis in Dentistry, University of Washington, 1970.
5. Anderson, A. A.: The protein matrixes of the teeth and periodontium in hamsters: A tritiated proline study, J. Dent. Res., 46:67, 1967.
6. Arnim, S. S., and Hagerman, D. A.: The connective tissue fibers of the marginal gingiva. J. Am. Dent. Assoc., 47:271, 1953.
7. Bailey, A. J.: Comparative studies on the nature of the crosslinks in the collagen of various fish tissues. Biochim. Biophys. Acta, 221:652, 1970.
8. Bailey, A. J.: The nature of collagen. *In* Comprehensive Biochemistry. Eds. M. Florkin and E. H. Stotz. New York, Elsevier Publishing Co., 1968.
9. Balazs, E. A., ed.: Chemistry and Molecular Biology of the Intercellular Matrix. New York, Academic Press, 1970, Vols. I–III.
10. Balazs, E. A., and Jeanloz, R. W.: The amino sugar-containing compounds in bones and teeth. The Amino Sugars, vol. IIA. New York, Academic Press, 1965, 281.
11. Barker, S. D.: The dendritic cell system in human gingival epithelium. Arch. Oral Biol., 12:203, 1967.
12. Beagrie, G. S., and Skougaard, M. R.: Observations on the life cycle of the gingival epithelial cells of mice as revealed by autoradiography. Acta Odontol. Scand., 20:15, 1962.
13. Becks, H.: Mund- und Schmelzepithel in ihrem beiderseitigen Verhalten zur Zahnoberfläche. Paradentium, 3:51, 1931.
14. Becks, H.: Normal and pathologic pocket formation. J. Am. Dent. Assoc., 16:2167, 1929.
15. Becks, H.: Zur Frage der Taschenbildung. Paradentium, 2:137, 1930.
16. Bélanger, L. F.: Resorption of cementum by cementocyte activity (cementolysis). Calcif. Tissue Res., 2:229, 1968.
17. Bentley, J. P., and Jackson, D. S.: In vivo incorporation of labeled amino acids during early stages of collagen biosynthesis. Biochem. Biophys. Res. Commun., 10:271, 1963.

18. Bernick, S.: Innervation of teeth and periodontium after enzymatic removal of collagenous elements. Oral Surg., *10:*323, 1957.

19. Bernick, S.: Organization of the periodontal membrane fibers of the developing molars of rats. Arch. Oral Biol., *2:*57, 1960.

20. Bernick, S., and Levy, B. M.: Studies on the biology of the periodontium of marmosets: IV. Innervation of the periodontal ligament. J. Dent. Res., *47:*1158, 1968.

21. Bevelander, G., and Nakahara, H.: The fine structure of the human periodontal ligament. Anat. Rec., *162:*313, 1968.

22. Black, G. V.: A study of the histological characteristics of the periodontal ligament. Chicago, W. T. Keener, 1887, p. 138.

23. Black, G. V.: A Work on Special Dental Pathology. Chicago, Medico-Dental Publ. Co., 1915.

24. Bödecker, C. F. W.: The Anatomy and Pathology of the Teeth. Philadelphia, S. S. White Dental Mfg. Co., 1894, p. 41.

25. Bornstein, P., and Piez, K.: The nature of the intra-molecular crosslinks in collagen. Separation and characterization of peptides from the crosslink region of rat skin collagen. Biochemistry, *5:*3460, 1966.

26. Briggaman, R. A., Dalldorf, F. G., and Sheeler, C. E.: Formation and origin of basal lamina and anchoring fibrils in adult human skin. J. Cell. Biol., *51:*384, 1971.

27. Butler, W. T., and Cunningham, L. W.: Evidence for the linkage of a disaccharide to hydroxylysine in tropocollagen. J. Biol. Chem., *241:*3882, 1966.

28. Cabrini, R. L., and Carranza, F. A.: Histochemistry of periodontal tissues. A review of the literature. Int. Dent. J., *16:*466, 1966.

29. Carneiro, J.: Synthesis and turnover of collagen in periodontal tissues. Symp. of the Int. Soc. Cell Biol., *4:*247, 1965.

30. Ciancio, S. C., Neiders, M. E., and Hazen, S. P.: The principal fibers of the periodontal ligament. Periodontics, *5:*76, 1967.

31. Claycomb, C. K., Summers, G. W., and Dvorak, E. M.: Oral collagen biosynthesis in the guinea pig. J. Periodont. Res., *2:*115, 1967.

32. Cohn, S. A.: A new look at the orientation of cemento-alveolar fibers of the mouse periodontal ligament. Anat. Rec., *166:*292, 1970.

33. Cox, R. W., Grant, R. A., and Horne, R. W.: The structure and assembly of collagen fibrils. I. Native-collagen fibrils and their formation from tropocollagen. J. Roy. Microscop. Soc., *87:*123, 1967.

34. Crumley, P. J.: Collagen formation in the normal and stressed periodontium. Periodontics, *2:*53, 1964.

35. Ebner, V. von: Histologie der Zähne mit Einschluss der Histogenese. *In* Scheff, Handbuch der Zahnheilkunde. Wien, Holder, 1891, Vol. I., p. 236.

36. Eccles, J. D.: The effects of reducing function and stopping eruption on the periodontium of the rat incisor. J. Dent. Res., *44:*860, 1965.

37. Egelberg, J.: The blood vessels of the dento-gingival junction. J. Periodont. Res., *1:*163, 1966.

38. Elliott, J. R., and Bowers, G. M.: Alveolar dehiscence and fenestration. Periodontics, *1:*245, 1963.

39. Flieder, K. E., Sun, C. N., and Schneider, B. C.: Chemistry of normal and inflamed human gingival tissues. Periodontics, *4:*302, 1966.

40. Freeman, E., and Ten Cate, A. R.: Development of the periodontium: An electron microscopic study. J. Periodontol., *42:*387, 1971.

41. Fröhlich, E.: Die Bedeutung der peripheren Durchblutung des Parodontiums für die Entstehung und Therapie der Zahnbetterkrankungen. Dtsch. Zahnaertzl. Z., *19:*153, 1964.

42. From, S., and Schultz-Haudt, S.: Comparative histological and microchemical evaluations of the collagen content of human gingiva. J. Periodontol., *34:*216, 1963.

43. Furstman, L., and Bernick, S.: Early development of the periodontal membrane. Am. J. Orthod., *51:*482, 1965.

44. Gallop, P. M., Blumenfeld, O. O., and Seifter, S.: Structure and metabolism of connective tissue proteins. Ann. Rev. Biochem., *41:*617, 1972.

45. Goldman, H. M.: Discussion: A critique of normal connective tissues of the periodontium and some alterations with periodontal disease" by Harold M. Fuller. J. Dent. Res., *21:*223, 1962. J. Dent. Res., *41:*230, 1962.

46. Goldman, H. M.: The topography and role of the gingival fibers. J. Dent. Res., *30:*331, 1951.

47. Gottlieb, B.: Aetiologie und Prophylaxe der Zahnkaries. Z. Stomatol., *19:*129, 1921.

48. Gottlieb, B.: Der Epithenlansatz am Zahne. Dtsch. Mschr. Zahnheilk., *39:*142, 1921.

49. Gottlieb, B.: The new concept of periodontoclasia. J. Periodont., *17:*7, 1946.

50. Gottlieb, B., and Orban, B.: Biology and Pathology of the Tooth and Its Supporting Mechanism. Trans. by M. Diamond. New York, The Macmillan Co., 1938, p. 70.

51. Götze, W.: Über Altersveränderungen des Parodontiums (Volumenbestimmung der Gewebeanteile nach Henning). Forum Parodontologicum, *15:*17, May 1965, in Dtsch. Zahnaerztl. Z., *20:*465, 1965.

52. Griffin, C. J., and Harris, R.: The fine structure of the developing human periodontium. Arch. Oral Biol., *12:*971, 1967.

53. Gross, H.: Zur Genese der vertieften Zahnfleischtasche. Paradentium, *2:*70, 1930.

54. Harvey, B. L. C., and Zander, H. A.: Root surface resorption of periodontally diseased teeth. Oral Surg., *12:*1439, 1959.

55. Hay, E. D., and Revel, J. P.: Autoradiographic studies of the origin of basement lamella in Ambystoma. Dev. Biol., *7:*152, 1963.

56. Henry, J. L., and Weinmann, J. P.: The pattern of resorption and repair of human cementum. J. Am. Dent. Assoc., *42:*270, 1951.

57. Hirschfeld, I.: A study of skulls in the American Museum of Natural History in relation to periodontal disease. J. Dent. Res., *5:*241, 1923.

58. Hodge, A. J., and Schmitt, F. O.: The charge profile of the tropocollagen macromolecule and the packing arrangement in native-type collagen fibrils. Proc. Natl. Acad. Sci. (US), *46*:186, 1960.

59. Hunt, A. M.: A description of the molar teeth and investing tissues of normal guinea pigs. J. Dent. Res., *38*:216, 1959.

60. Hürzeler, B., and Zander, H. A.: Cementum apposition in periodontally diseased teeth. Helv. Odontol. Acta, *1*:1, 1957.

61. Inoue, M., and Akiyoshi, M.: Histological investigation on Sharpey's fibers in cementum of teeth in abnormal function. J. Dent. Res., *41*:503, 1962.

62. Ishikawa, G., et al.: Microradiographic study of cementum and alveolar bone. J. Dent. Res., *49*:936, 1964.

63. Jande, S. S., and Bélanger, L. F.: Fine structural study of rat molar cementum. Anat. Rec., *167*:439, 1970.

64. Jeanloz, R. W., and Balaz, E. A., Eds.: The Amino Sugars. New York, Academic Press, 1966, Vol. 2A, pp. 281–307.

65. Jepsen, A.: Root surface measurements and a method for X-ray determination of root surface area. Acta Odontol. Scand., *21*:35, 1963.

66. Kao, K-Y. T., Hilker, D. M., and McGavack, T. H.: Connective tissue. IV. Synthesis and turnover of proteins in tissues of rats. Proc. Soc. Exp. Med. Biol., *106*:121, 1961.

67. Kao, K-Y. T., Hilker, D. M., and McGavack, T. H.: Connective tissue. V. Comparison of synthesis and turnover of collagen and elastin in tissues of rat at several ages. Proc. Soc. Exp. Med. Biol., *106*:335, 1961.

68. Karring, T., and Löe, H.: The three-dimensional concept of the epithelium-connective tissue boundary of gingiva. Acta Odontol. Scand., *28*:917, 1970.

69. Kefalides, N. A.: Isolation and characterization of the collagen from glomerular basement membrane. Biochemistry, *7*:3103, 1968.

70. Kefalides, N. A.: Comparative biochemistry of mammalian basement membrane. *In* Chemistry and Molecular Biology of the Intercellular Matrix. *1*:536, 1970.

71. Kefalides, N. A., and Winzler, R. J.: The chemistry of glomerular basement membrane and its relation to collagen. Biochemistry, *5*:702, 1966.

72. Kerr, D. A.: The cementum: its role in periodontal health and disease. J. Periodontol., *32*:183, 1961.

73. Kindlova, M.: The blood supply in the marginal periodontium in *maccaca rhesus*. Arch. Oral Biol., *10*:869, 1965.

74. Kronfeld, R.: Biology of the cementum. J. Am. Dent. Assoc., *25*:1451, 1938.

75. Lange, D., and Schroeder, H. E.: Cytochemistry and ultrastructure of gingival sulcus cells. Helv. Odontol. Acta, *15*(Suppl. 4): 65, 1971.

76. Larato, D. C.: Alveolar plate fenestrations and dehiscences of the human skull. Oral Surg., *29*:816, 1970.

77. Laurent, T. C.: Structure of hyaluronic acid. *In* Chemistry and Molecular Biology of the Intercellular Matrix. E. A. Balaz, ed. *2*:703, 1970. New York, Academic Press.

78. Layman, D. L., McGoodwin, E. B., and Martin, G. R. The nature of the collagen synthesized by cultured human fibroblasts. Proc. Nat. Acad. Sci. (US), *68*:454, 1971.

79. Lazarow, A., and Speidel, E.: The chemical composition of the glomeruler basement membrane and its relationship to the production of diabetic complications. *In* Small Blood Vessel Involvement in Diabetes Mellitus. M. D. Siperstein, A. R. Colewell, Sr., and K. Meyer, eds. Washington, D.C., American Institute of Biological Science, 1964, p. 127.

80. Lehner, J.: Ein Beitrag zur Kenntniss vom Schmelzoberhäutchen. Z. Mikrosk. Anat. Forsch., *27*:613, 1931.

81. Lenz, P.: Zur Gefässtruktur des Parodontium. Untersuchungen an Korrosionspräparaten von Affenkiefern. Dtsch. Zahnaerztl. Z., *23*:357, 1968.

82. Levy, B., and Bernick, S.: Studies on the biology of the periodontium of marmosets: II. Development and organization of the periodontal ligament of decidous teeth in Marmosets (Callithrix jacchus). J. Dent. Res., *47*:27, 1968.

83. Levy, B. M., and Bernick, S.: Studies on the biology of the periodontium of marmosets: V. Lymphatic vessels of the periodontal ligament. J. Dent. Res., *47*:1166, 1968.

84. Lester, K. S.: The incorporation of epithelial cells by cementum. J. Ultrast. Res., *27*:63, 1969.

85. Lester, K. S.: The unusual nature of root formation in molar teeth of the laboratory rat. J. Ultrast. Res., *28*:481, 1969.

86. Listgarten, M. A.: Electron microscopic study of the gingivo-dental junction of man. Am. J. Anat., *119*:147, 1966.

87. Listgarten, M. A.: Electron microscopic study of the junction between surgically denuded root surfaces and regenerated periodontal tissues. J. Periodont. Res., *7*:68, 1972.

88. Löe, H.: The structure and physiology of the dento-gingival junction. *In* Structural and Chemical Organization of the Teeth. A. E. W. Miles, Ed. New York, Academic Press, 1967, Vol. II., p. 415.

89. Martin, G. R., Piez, K. A., and Lewis, M. S.: The incorporation of ^{14}C-glycine into the subunits of collagens from normal and lathyritic animals. Biochim. Biophys. Acta, *69*:472, 1963.

90. McHugh, W. D.: Some aspects of the development of gingival epithelium. Periodontics, *1*:239, 1963.

91. Melcher, A. H.: The architecture of human gingival reticulin. Arch. Oral Biol., *9*:111, 1964.

92. Melcher, A. H. Histological recognition of gingival reticulin. Arch. Oral Biol., *11*:219–224, 1966.

93. Melcher, A. H., and Eastoe, J. E.: The connective tissues of the periodontium. *In* Biology of the Periodontium, A. H. Melcher and W. H. Bowen, Eds. New York, Academic Press, 1969, p. 167.

94. Meyer, W.: Lehrbuch der normalen Histologie und Entwicklungsgeschichte der Zähne des Menschen. München, Lehmanns Verlag, 1932, p. 127.

95. Meyer, W.: Neue Befunde am Epithelansatz. Paradentium, *1*:22, 1929.

96. Miller, E. J.: The biochemical characterizations of various collagens. *In* Developmental Aspects of Oral Biology. H. C. Slavkin and L. A. Bavetta, Eds. New York, Academic Press, 1972, p. 275.

97. Miller, E. J., and Martin, G. R.: The collagen of bone. Clin. Orthop., *59*:195, 1968.

98. Miller, E. H., Martin, G. R., and Piez, K. A.: The utilization of lysine in the biosynthesis of elastin crosslinks. Biochem. Biophys. Res. Commun., *17*:248, 1964.

99. Narayanan, A. S., Siegel, R. C., and Martin, G. R.: On the inhibition of lysyl oxidase by beta-aminopropionitrile. Biochem. Biophys. Res. Commun., *46*:745, 1972.

100. Nasmyth, A.: On the structure, physiology and pathology of the persistent capsular investments and pulp of the tooth. Trans. Roy. Med. Chir. Soc., London. *22*:310, 1839.

101. Neuwirth, F.: Die Schmelzmembran und der Epithelansatz am Zahne. Z. Stomatol., *23*:318, 1925.

102. Nigra, T. R., Friedland, M., and Martin, G.: Controls of connective tissues synthesis: Collagen metabolism. J. Invest. Dermatol., *59*:44, 1972.

103. Nimni, M. E., de Guia, E., and Bavetta, L. A.: Synthesis and turnover of collagen precursors in rabbit skin. Biochem. J., *102*:143, 1967.

104. Noyes, F. B.: The structure of the periodontal membrane. Dent. Rev., *11*:448, 1897.

105. Noyes, F. B.: A Textbook of Dental Histology and Embryology Including Laboratory Directions. 5th ed., London, Kimpton, 1938, p. 81, 113.

106. Olsen, B. R.: Electron microscope studies on collagen II. Mechanism of linear polymerization of tropocollagen molecules. Z. Zellforsch., *59*:199, 1963.

107. Orban, B.: Zahnfleischtasche und Epithelansatz. Z. Stomatol., *29*:858, 1005, 1359, 1931.

108. Orban, B.: Oral Histology and Embryology. St. Louis, C. V. Mosby, 1944, p. 161.

109. Orban, B.: Oral Histology and Embryology, 2nd ed. St. Louis, C. V. Mosby, 1949.

110. Orban, B.: Oral Histology and Embryology, 3rd ed., St. Louis, C. V. Mosby, 1953, p. 227.

111. Page, R. C. Macromolecular interactions in the connective tissues of the periodontium. *In* Developmental Aspects of Oral Biology. H. Slavkin and L. Bavetta, Eds. New York, Academic Press, 1972, p. 292.

112. Page, R. C., and Ammons, W. F.: Collagen turnover in the gingiva and other connective tissues of the marmoset. Arch. Oral Biol., *19*:651, 1974.

113. Page, R. C., et al.: Collagen fiber bundles of the normal marginal gingiva. Arch. Oral Biol. *19*:1039, 1974.

114. Page, R. C., Davies, P., and Allison, A. C.: The role of macrophages in periodontal disease. *In* Host Resistance to Commensal Bacteria. T. MacPhee, Ed. Edinburgh, Churchill Livingstone, 1972, p. 195.

115. Page, R. C., and Schroeder, H. E.: Biochemical aspects of the connective tissue alterations in inflammatory gingival and periodontal disease. Int. Dent. J., *23*:455, 1973.

116. Page, R. C., et al.: Host tissue response in chronic periodontal disease. III. Clinical histologic and ultrastructural features of advanced disease in a colony-maintained marmoset. J. Periodont. Res., *7*:283, 1972.

117. Parfitt, G. J.: An investigation of the normal variations in alveolar bone trabeculation. Oral Surg., *15*:1453, 1962.

118. Payne, W. A., et al.: Histopathologic features of the initial and early stages of experimental gingivitis in man. J. Periodont. Res., *10*:51, 1975.

119. Paynter, K. J., and Purdy, G.: A study of the structure, chemical nature, and development of cementum in the rat. Anat. Rec., *131*:223, 1958.

120. Pierce, G. B., et al.: Basement membranes IV. Epithelial origin and immunological cross reactions. Am. J. Pathol., *45*:929, 1964.

121. Piez, K. A.: Chemistry of collagen and elastin and biosynthesis of covalent cross-links. *In* Thule International Symposium Aging of Connective and Skeletal Tissues. 1969, p. 12.

122. Provenza, V. D.: Oral Histology, Inheritance and Development. Philadelphia, J. B. Lippencott Co., 1964.

123. Quigley, M. B.: Perforating (Sharpy's) fibers of the periodontal ligament and bone. Alabama J. Med. Sci., *7*:336, 1970.

124. Rindom-Schiött, C., and Löe, H.: The origin and variation in number of leukocytes in the human saliva. J. Periodont. Res., *5*:36, 1970.

125. Ritchey, B., and Orban, B. The crests of the interdental alveolar septa. J. Periodontol., *24*:75, 1953.

126. Rysky, de S., Cattaneo, V., and Montanari, M. C.: Détermination quantitative des exosamines et de l'hydroxyproline dans les inflammations gingivales chroniques. Bull. Group. Int. Rech. Sci. Stomatol., *12*:359, 1969.

127. Sandberg, L. B., Weissman, N., and Smith, D. W.: The purification and partial characterization of a soluble elastin-like protein from copper-deficient porcine aorta. Biochemistry, *8*:2940, 1969.

128. Sasso, W.: Histochemical study of human dental cementum. Rev. Fac. Odont., *4*:189, 1966.

129. Schectman, L. R., et al.: Host tissue response in chronic periodontal disease II. Histologic features of the normal periodontium and histologic manifestations of disease in the marmoset. J. Periodont. Res., *7*:195, 1972.

130. Schour, I.: Noye's Oral Histology and Embryology, 8th ed. Philadelphia, Lea & Febiger, 1960.

131. Schroeder, H. E.: Melanin containing organelles in cells and human gingiva. J. Periodont. Res., *4*:1, 1969.

132. Schroeder, H. E.: Melanin containing organelles in cells of the human gingiva. II. Melanocytes. J. Periodont. Res., *4*:235, 1969.

133. Schroeder, H. E.: Struktur und Ultrastruktur des normalen marginalen Parodonts. Paradontologie, *23*:159, 1969.

134. Schroeder, H. E.: Ultrastructure of the junctional epithelium of the human gingiva. Helv. Odontol. Acta, *13*:65, 1969.

135. Schroeder, H. E.: Ultrastructure of the early gingival lesion. Rev. Fr. Odontostomatol. *20*:103, 1973.

136. Schroeder, H. E.: Transmigration and infiltration of leukocytes in human junctional epithelium. Helv. Odontol. Acta, *17:*16, 1973.

137. Schroeder, H. E., and Listgarten, M. A.: Fine Structure of the Developing Epithelial Attachment of Human Teeth. Monographs in Developmental Biology, Vol. II., Basel, S. Karger, 1971.

138. Schroeder, H. E., and Münzel-Pedrazzoli, S.: Morphometric analysis comparing junctional and oral epithelium of normal human gingiva. Helv. Odontol. Acta, *14:*53, 1970.

139. Schroeder, H. E., Münzel-Pedrazzoli, S., and Page, R. C.: Correlated morphometric and biochemical analysis of gingival tissues. The early gingival lesion in man. Arch. Oral Biol., *17:*899, 1973.

140. Schroeder, H. E., and Page, R. C.: Lymphocyte-fibroblast interaction in the pathogenesis of inflammatory gingival disease. Experientia, *28:*1228, 1972.

141. Schroeder, H. E., and Theilade, J.: Electron microscopy of normal human gingival epithelium. J. Periodont. Res., *1:*95, 1966.

142. Schultz-Haudt, S.: Observations on the acid mucopolysaccharides of human gingiva. Odont. Tidskr., *66:*1, 1958.

143. Schultz-Haudt, S. D., and Aas, E.: Observations on the status of collagen in human gingiva. Arch. Oral Biol., *2:*131, 1960.

144. Selvig, K. A.: Electron microscopy of Hertwig's epithelial sheath and of early dentin and cementum formation in the mouse incisor. Acta Odont. Scand., *21:*175, 1963.

145. Selvig, K. A.: An ultrastructural study of cementum formation. Acta Odont. Scand., *22:*105, 1964.

146. Selvig, K. A.: The fine structure of human cementum. Acta Odont. Scand., *23:*423, 1965.

147. Selvig, K. A.: Ultrastructural changes in cementum and adjacent connective tissue in periodontal disease. Acta Odont. Scand., *24:*459, 1966.

148. Selvig, K. A., and Selvig, S. K.: Mineral content of human and seal cementum. J. Dent. Res., *41:*624, 1962.

149. Sicher, H.: Bau und Funktion des Fixationsapparates der Meerschweinchenmolaren. Z. Stomatol., *21:*580, 1923.

150. Sicher, H.: Tooth eruption: The axial movement of continuously growing teeth. J. Dent. Res. *21:*201, 1942.

151. Sicher, H.: The principal fibers of the periodontal membrane. Bur, *55:*2, 1955.

152. Sicher, H.: Changing concepts of the supporting dental structure. Oral Surg., *12:*31, 1959.

153. Sicher, H.: Orban's Oral Histology and Embryology, 5th ed. St. Louis, C. V. Mosby, 1962.

154. Sicher, H., and Bhaskar, S. N., Eds: Orban's Oral Histology and Embryology, 7th ed. St. Louis, C. V. Mosby, 1972.

155. Skillen, W. G.: Normal characteristics of the gingiva and their relation to pathology. J. Am. Dent. Assoc., *17:*1088, 1930.

156. Skougaard, M. R.: Turnover of the gingival epithelium in marmosets. Acta Odont. Scand., *23:*623, 1965.

157. Skougaard, M. R., and Beagrie, G. S. The renewal of gingival epithelium in marmosets (Callithrix jacchus) as determined through autoradiography with thymidine-H^3. Acta Odont. Scand., *20:*467, 1962.

158. Skougaard, M. R., Levy, B. M., and Simpson, J.: Collagen metabolism in skin and periodontal membrane of the marmoset. J. Periodont. Res., Suppl., *4:*28, 1969.

159. Spiro, R. G.: Characterization and quantitative determination of the hydroxylysine-linked carbohydrate units of several collagens. J. Biol. Chem., *244:*602, 1969.

160. Stahl, S. S., Cantor, M., and Zwig, E.: Fenestrations of the labial alveolar plate in human skulls. Periodontics, *1:*99, 1963.

161. Stallard, R. E.: The utilization of H^3-proline by the connective tissue elements of the periodontium. Periodontics, *1:*185, 1963.

162. Stern, B. D.: Collagen solubility of normal and inflamed human gingiva. Periodontics, *5:*167, 1967.

163. Stern, I. B.: The fine structure of the ameloblast-enamel junction in rat incisors: epithelial attachment and cuticular membrane. *In* Breese Electron Microscopy, Vol. 2. New York, Academic Press, 1962.

164. Stern, I.: An electron microscopic study of the cementum, Sharpey's fibers and periodontal ligament in the rat incisor. Am. J. Anat., *115:*377, 1964.

165. Stern, I.: Electron microscopic observations of oral epithelium. I. Basal cells and basement membrane. Periodontics, *3:*224, 1965.

166. Susi, F. R., Belt, W. D., and Kelly, J. W.: Fine structure of fibrillar complexes associated with the basement membrane of human oral mucosa. J. Cell Biol., *34:*686, 1967.

167. Tanzer, M. L., Fairweather, R., and Gallop, P. M.: Collagen crosslinks: Isolation of reduced N-hexosylhydroxylysine from borohydride-reduced calf skin insoluble collagen. Arch. Biochem. Biophys., *151:*137, 1972.

168. Traub, W., and Piez, K. A.: The chemistry and structure of collagen. Adv. Protein Chem., *25:*243, 1971.

169. Trott, J. R.: The development of the periodontal attachment in the rat. Acta Anat., *51:*313, 1962.

170. Waerhaug, J.: Current concepts concerning gingival anatomy. The dynamic epithelial cuff. Dent. Clin. North Am., Nov. 1960, p. 715.

171. Waerhaug, J.: The gingival pocket. Odont. Tidskr. Suppl., 1, 1952.

172. Wasserman, F., et al.: Studies on the different pathways of exchange of minerals in teeth with the aid of radioactive phosphorus. J. Dent. Res., *20:*389, 1941.

173. Weski, O.: Röntgenographische-anatomische Studien aus dem Gebiete der Kieferpathologie II. Die chronischen marginalen Entzündungen des Alveolarfortsatzes mit besonderer Berücksichtigung der Alveolarpyorrhoe. Vjschr. Zahnheilk., *37:*1, 1921; *38:*1, 1922.

174. Zander, H. A., and Hürzeler, B.: Continuous cementum apposition. J. Dent. Res., *37:*1035, 1958.

175. Zwarych, P. D., and Quigley, M. B.: The intermediate plexus of the periodontal ligament: History and further observations. J. Dent. Res., *44:*383, 1965.

2

Diseases of the Periodontium

2

Diseases
of
the
Periodontium

A conceptual framework derived from the definition and classification of diseases affecting the periodontium strongly influences clinicians responsible for the diagnosis and treatment of individual patients, scientists investigating the nature of specific diseases, and public health workers, statisticians, and epidemiologists striving to improve the health of the entire population. The usefulness and accuracy of this conceptual framework are dependent upon the distinct, unequivocal identification and definition of the diseases affecting the periodontium. Although intensive efforts to identify, characterize, and classify these diseases extend back several decades, a universally accepted system of nomenclature and classification has not been devised. In this section we discuss the evolution of nomenclature and systems of classification and describe those currently used.

Every attempt to devise an acceptable system of classification has been plagued by major problems. Historically, a plethora of imprecise terms with vague definitions has been introduced and almost none of these has been discarded. Many terms such as *pyorrhea* were based on a single sign or symptom associated with only one stage of the disease; other terms have been all inclusive and have encompassed numerous different disease entities. Becks noted:

If we consider the difficulties which defy almost all attempts at classification, we are surprised at the frequency with which new names and definitions for the so-called "pyorrhea" appear in the literature, even before we have made a clear picture of the single factor which leads to its symptoms. The last few years of increased research in this special subject have resulted in nearly 350 theories of pyorrhea and an excessive nomenclature which has confused the clinical picture for the practitioner more and more.[3]

Further confusion in terminology and classification has resulted from our relatively poor understanding of the etiology and pathogenesis of the numerous diseases of the periodontium. Periodontal diseases are multifactorial and in general no single etiologic agent that totally accounts for the pathologic alterations can be found. Even in cases in which discrete clinical entities can be described, multiple causes may be at work and a complex picture may result.[14] Furthermore, what appear to be multiple distinct disease entities may in fact represent only different stages of the same malady modified in expression by time and by individual response.[11] Thus, we are faced with a cumbersome, vague terminology used to define a family of diseases which, in some cases, may involve common etiologies with different pathologic manifestations, and in others, may result from the action of differing etiologies producing common clinical and pathologic manifestations.

In distinguishing among and classifying the diseases of the periodontium several important factors must be taken into account. Among the more important of these are

1. Location, duration, history, and extent of the lesion
2. Clinical manifestations
3. Etiology
4. Pathologic characteristics
5. Biologic behavior of the lesion, especially rate and route of progress
6. Nature of response to treatment
7. Status of the host, especially age, sex, and physical and dental condition

Systems of nomenclature and classification taking all of these factors into account become too complex and cumbersome to be of general use, while those based on only one or two of these factors are equally unacceptable. The most useful systems, in general, have had the characteristics listed in Table 2-1.

HISTORICAL PERSPECTIVE

In order to grasp the full meaning of currently used terminology, it is important to understand how it evolved. Periodontal diseases have been a common affliction of man since he appeared on earth.

TABLE 2-1. *Characteristics of Useful Systems of Nomenclature and Classification*

Based on sound linguistic, scientific, and pathologic principles

Complete, although simple and free of excessive sub-classification

Emphasis on the commonly encountered diseases at the expense of the esoteric and the rare

Simple, unequivocal criteria that easily can be observed and measured

Easy modification of the system with the acquisition of new knowledge

Ancient Civilizations

A pattern of bone resorption characteristic of marginal periodontitis was noted in the fossil man of La Chapelle-aux-Saints who lived in the late paleolithic culture of Neanderthal man.[47] Among the ancient Egyptians some 4,000 years ago, a form of chronic suppurating periodontitis appears to have been one of the most common diseases. Jaws of mummies from this period exhibit both a generalized horizontal form of bone loss characteristic of marginal periodontitis and isolated vertical bone defects of the type usually associated with periodontosis (Fig. 2-1). Most of the ancient medical writings contain reference to disease of the gums and to loose teeth. The *Papyrus Ebers* (see Ebbell's translation, 1937)[41] contains a section on teeth in which remedies are given to "fasten loose teeth, to expel growth of purulency of the gums, to treat teeth which gnaw against an opening in the flesh, to treat the gums and to strengthen the gums." In the first century A.D., Celsus discussed diseases which "separate the gums from the teeth" and Hippocrates described diseases in which "the gums are detached from the teeth and smell bad."[52]

Knowledge of the diseases of the investing tissues of the teeth was not confined to the western civilizations. The oldest known Chinese medical work, that by Hwang-Fi written about 2500 B.C., classified oral disease into three types: Fong Ya, the inflammatory conditions; Ya Kon, the diseases of the soft investing tissues of the teeth; and Chong Ya, or dental caries.[52]

Possibly the most complete ancient account of diseases of the periodontium was that given by the early Arabian physician Rhazes (850–923) who devoted a great deal of time and care to study of the teeth. In his book *Al-Fakkir*, Rhazes includes chapters on Looseness of the Gums, Suppuration of the Gums, and Bleeding Gums. One of his contemporaries, Albucasis (963–1013) vividly describes the disease of the gums associated with the accumulation of tartar:

Sometimes on the surface of the teeth, both inside and outside, as well as under the gums, are deposited rough scales, of ugly appearance, and black, green or yellow in colour; thus corruption is communicated to the gums, and so the teeth are in the process of time denuded. It is necessary for thee to lay the patient's head upon thy lap and to scrape the teeth and molars, on which are observed these incrustations, or something similar to sand, and this until nothing more remains of such substance. . . .[52]

Fauchard, Hunter, and Fox

Almost all of the ancient medical works refer to the various maladies of the teeth and their investing tis-

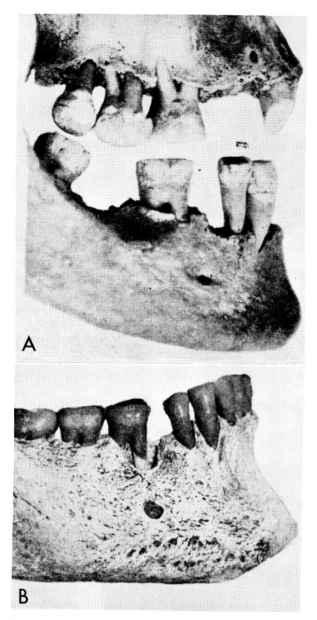

FIG. 2-1. *A. The jaw of a Gizeh pyramid-builder. In the lower jaw, the second molar had been lost during life and the alveolar socket healed. Severe marginal alveolar bone resorption is noted around the mesial root and in the bifurcation area of the first molar, and about two thirds of the total length of the roots of the mandibular canine and first premolar are exposed. In the maxillary arch, the surface of the remaining alveolar bone exhibits a moth-eaten appearance typical of that associated with perialveolar inflammation. Approximately one half of the alveolar bone has been resorbed, and there is furca involvement of all of the molars. These lesions are typical of those seen in chronic marginal periodontitis. B. The lower jaw from a person who lived during the XIIth-XVIth Dynasties in Egypt. Although the level of the alveolar bone around most of the teeth is located near the cementoenamel junction, a deep vertical defect is present around the mesial root of the first molar. The defect was considered to be a result of periodontal disease rather than a periapical abscess. (Ruffer, M. A.: Studies in Paleopathology of Egypt. Chicago, University of Chicago Press, 1921.)*

sues, but no specific terminology and no systematic body of knowledge evolved until the late eighteenth century. Descriptive terms such as "spongy gums," "inflamed gums," and "loosening of the teeth" were used. In the view of Weinberger, a detailed knowledge and appreciation of the conception and meaning of dentistry did not take place until about 1728.[52] The emergence of dentistry was in large part a consequence of the efforts of Pierre Fauchard and his contemporaries in France. Fauchard's book *Le Chirurgien Dentiste* (The Surgeon Dentist), written in 1723 and published in 1728, was the first compendium of knowledge on diagnosis and treatment of the diseases of the teeth and associated structures.[10] It remained the predominant textbook for over half a century. The first specific name for chronic marginal periodontitis, which Fauchard referred to as "scurvy of the gums" and the first accurate description of the disease, appeared in the second edition in 1746:

There is yet another, of which I think no other author has yet had occasion to speak, and which, without affecting the other parts of the body, attacks the gums, the alveoli and the teeth. Not only are softened, livid, prolonged and swollen gums affected by it but often those which are free from this vice are not exempt from the disease; it is to be recognized by rather white and sticky pus which can be made to come out of the gums by pressing the finger firmly above downwards upon those of the lower jaw, and from below upwards on those of the upper jaw.

. . . This pus often comes out from between the gums and the body of the alveoli, and sometimes from between the alveoli and the roots of the teeth; which happens more frequently on the external surface of the jaws than upon the internal, and rather around the incisors and canines of the lower jaw, than about those of the upper, which are, however, more ordinarily afflicted with this trouble than the molar teeth.[10]

The first important book in English was *Natural History of the Human Teeth* by John Hunter. Eleven editions of this work were published between 1771 and 1840. In Hunter's book,[26] and in a subsequent book by Joseph Fox,[12] we find the first system of classification of diseases of the periodontium. It is important to note that until the time of Weski,[53] the term *periodontium* was not defined, and both Hunter and Fox classified the diseases as those occurring in the alveolar bone and those of the gums. Under diseases affecting the gums, Hunter describes chronic marginal periodontitis thus:

The gums are extremely subject to diseases. . . . They swell, become extremely tender, and bleed upon every occasion, which circumstances being somewhat similar to those observable in the true scurvy, the disease has generally been called a scurvy of the gums . . . but as this seems to be the principal way in which the gums are affected, I suspect that the same symptoms may arise from various causes; as I have often seen the same appearances in children . . . and have also suspected them in grown people; they likewise frequently appear in persons, who are, in all other respects perfectly healthy.[26]

Hunter notes that when the gingiva becomes inflamed,

. . . it often happens, that the alveolar process disappears, after the manner described above, by taking part in the inflammation, or either from the same cause, or from sympathy. In such cases there is always a very considerable discharge of matter from inside of the gum, and alveolar process, which always takes the course of the tooth for its exit.[26]

Hunter also describes a form of gingival hyperplasia which he refers to as "excresences from the gums," although it seems unlikely that his description is directly relevant to our current concept of gingival hyperplasia. The soft tissue growths he describes are associated with large carious lesions or decayed root stumps which, because of therapeutic intervention, are rarely seen in most Western populations today. However, lesions of this sort are seen commonly in subhuman primates.[40] Although Hunter noted that the accumulation of tartar leads to swelling, ulceration, and bleeding of the gums and resorption of the alveolar process with exfoliation of the teeth, he does not appear to have associated the presence of tartar directly with scurvy of the gums.

The definition of terms and classification of various periodontal diseases evolved further with the publication in 1806 of Joseph Fox's book *Diseases of the Teeth, the Gums and the Alveolar Processes.* Fox described diseases of the gums, diseases of the alveolar bone, and disease resulting from the deposits of tartar on the teeth. He believed that diseases of three types affect the gums and the alveolar bone:

1. Those peculiar to the part
2. Those resulting from the presence of diseased teeth
3. Those deriving from "constitutional derangements"

Thus, the association of systemic factors with periodontal disease extends back nearly two centuries.

Diseases affecting the gums include gum boils and abscesses, hyperplastic growths (excrescences or preternatural growth of gums), and scurvy. Fox notes that scurvy is "the most common disease of the gums," and clearly he uses the term to denote chronic marginal periodontitis. In this disease, the tissue becomes red, is enlarged from turgescence of the vessels, and bleeds by the slightest cause. The gums become soft, spongy, and sore. This condition is followed by discharge of matter

from around the necks of the teeth and destruction of the interdental papillae. Subsequently, he notes, "the alveolar processes are resorbed and the teeth become loose and drop out" (Fig. 2-2).

Both Fox and Hunter consider the disease associated with the accumulation of tartar on the teeth to be separate from the other forms of periodontal disease.

. . . In addition to these various disease actions, there is an earthy deposit called tartar, which, in a greater or lesser degree accumulates about the teeth of most persons; this, if suffered to increase to any quantity, causes a separation of the gums from the necks of the teeth, and a consequent absorption of the alveolar process. . . . Excepting the disease of dental caries, nothing is so destructive of the healthy condition of the mouth or the duration of the teeth, as the accumulation of tartar.[12]

Thus by the end of the eighteenth century, a descriptive terminology and an elementary system of classification of diseases of the investing tissues had evolved. Distinction had been made between inflammatory lesions (scurvy of the gums) and atrophic or degenerative lesions (noninflammatory resorption of the alveolar processes), and a separate class of prolifer-

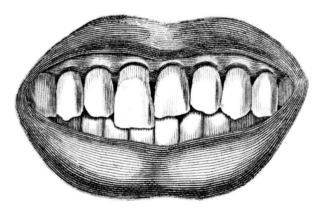

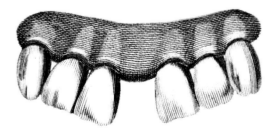

FIG. 2-2. *An illustration from Diseases of the Teeth, the Gums and the Alveolar Process by Joseph Fox depicting the manifestations of noninflammatory resorption of the alveolar process, a lesion subsequently referred to as "periodontosis." Note the typical diastema formation, drifting of the central and lateral incisors, and the extrusion of one of the maxillary teeth.*

ative or hyperplastic lesions (excrescences of the gums) had been described. The deleterious affects of tartar accumulation upon the health of the investing tissues was realized, although the possibility that deposits on the tooth surface could be the primary etiologic factor in "scurvy of the gums" had not been considered. Fox had classified the diseases of the gums and the alveolar bone on the basis of (1) those related to diseased teeth, (2) those deriving from constitutional or systemic causes, and (3) those peculiar to the gums or bone. However, little progress was made in nomenclature and terminology, and conception of the investing tissues of the teeth as a single functional and structural unit, or "periodontium," was to require the passage of another hundred years.

Riggs' Disease and Pyorrhoea Alveolaris

Between the time of Hunter and Fox in the late eighteenth and early nineteenth centuries and that of Riggs in the latter part of the nineteenth, most efforts were directed toward development of better means of treatment of diseases of the periodontium and very little advance was made in understanding their basic nature.[28] Black summarized the state of affairs thus: "Generally the entire subject was disposed of in a single paragraph, or at most in a page or two. This situation was changed radically through the efforts of Dr. J. M. Riggs who brought the subject prominently to the notice of the profession by clinics which he made before dental societies."[5] The term *Riggs' disease* came into use to denote inflammatory gingival and periodontal disease. Riggs' views of the disease were expressed in detail in a publication in 1877.[46] He considered the disease to exhibit four stages:

Stage I: *The margin of the gums shows decided inflammatory action, with some absorption of its substance, and bleeding at the slightest touch with a brush.*

Stage II. *The inflammation extends down over the thinner alveolar border, causing absorption of the bone as well as of the gum tissue, forming small pockets filled with pus beneath the gum.*

Stage III: *The disease action takes a deeper hold, involving the thicker portions of the alveolar process, absorbing it most rapidly nearest the tooth, causing the tooth to sway back and forth for lack of most of its bony support.*

Stage IV: *The disease has swept away all the alveoli and much of the gum, the tooth being held in place by the conversion of the periodontal membrane at the apex of the root into a tough ligamentous attachment.*

Some mouths present all four stages of the disease at the same time, while others, the younger patients, present only the first or second . . . . far from being a disease of old age,

cases are numerous at seventeen and even at fourteen years.[46]

Thus Riggs considered that a number of the inflammatory lesions of the periodontal tissues were simply different stages of single disease entities. Although he appears to have been an unusually astute and perceptive man whose ideas were considerably ahead of his time, his influence was not enduring. An intense opposition to him and to his views developed among his contemporaries. This dislike, which appears to have been rooted mostly in jealousy, resulted from Riggs' refusal to join certain dental organizations and from the naming of the disease after him.[5,45]

The term *pyorrhoea alveolaris* was first introduced by Rehnwinkel in a paper read before the American Dental Association in 1877. The term replaced Riggs' disease as the most popular name for the diseases of the tissues investing the teeth. Usage of the term by the professional and scientific communities continued until the 1950's,[11,25,27,56] and even today the term *pyorrhoea* is used frequently by laymen. Objection to the term was expressed at the time it was introduced and it has been repeated frequently since that time. One Dr. Judd, who was present in the audience when Rehnwinkel read his paper, was quoted as stating:

. . . he was befogged that he was listening to the description of a new disease when he heard about this "pyorrhoea alveolaris." He had analyzed the title to the paper, and asked the force of the adjective. It was probably intended to designate a flow of pus from the process; it would cover all flow of pus from these parts. There are cases where no pus is visible to the naked eye. . . . He thought we had better make use of the old terms; they are more definite and full as useful.[45]

In subsequent decades, Black,[5] Becks,[3] and others also expressed the view that the term *pyorrhoea alveolaris* which literally means "the running of pus from the alveoli," covers too much and does not properly describe the disease to which it is applied. Black thought that the term implied that the primary seat of the disease is in the margin of the alveolar process, when in fact the alveolar bone is the last of the investing tissues to become involved. He and his contemporaries introduced other terms such as *phagendenic pericementitis, suppurative pericementitis, alveolitis, dentoalveolar pyorrhea,* and *interstitial gingivitis,* although none of these terms was widely accepted.

Gottlieb and His Contemporaries

Modern concepts of nomenclature and classification of the diseases of the investing tissues are to a great extent an outgrowth of two developments occurring in the study of the normal structure of the periodontal tissues in the early 1920's. The first of these was the immensely important change in conceptual viewpoint expressed by Weski.[53] Until his time, each tissue around the tooth was viewed as an independent entity and as a primary seat of disease. Weski introduced the concept that the supporting tissues of the teeth comprise a single structural and functional unit to which he assigned the name *paradentium* (a term still sometimes used in European literature). As a consequence, for the first time it became possible to consider a single disease entity as affecting the entire tissue complex rather than separate diseases affecting each tissue independently. Thus terms such as *alveolitis* and *cementitis* gave way to terms such as *paradentitis* and *periodontitis*. A second major change was the partial elucidation, by Gottlieb, of the nature of the epithelial attachment and the subsequent focus on pocket formation as the cardinal manifestation of diseases of the periodontal tissues.[17,23] The importance of these two events on subsequent developments in periodontology and, indeed, on our current thinking cannot be overstressed.

The views of Gottlieb and those of Box[34] have had a major impact upon nomenclature and classification as well as upon our concepts of pathogenesis of the various periodontal diseases. Although distinction between diseases resulting predominantly from local causes such as accumulation of tartar and those arising from systemic factors or constitutional derangements can be traced back at least as far as the work of Joseph Fox,[12] Gottlieb is generally regarded as being the first writer to clearly distinguish between them.[29,37] He classified periodontal diseases into four types:[16,17,18,19,20,21,23]

Type I. Schmutz-Pyorrhöe *which results from an accumulation of deposits on the teeth and is characterized by hyperemia and inflammation of the gingiva with sulcular epithelial ulceration. In advanced stages, the disease may exhibit pus, shallow pockets, and resorption of the alveolar crest.*

Type II. Paradental-Pyorrhöe *a disease characterized by individual pockets irregularly distributed and of depths varying from shallow to extremely deep. This form of disease may begin as Schmutz-Pyorrhöe or as diffuse atrophy.*

Type III. Alveolar atrophy *or diffuse atrophy, a noninflammatory lesion exhibiting loosening, elongation and wandering of the teeth in individuals who are generally free of carious lesions and dental deposits. In this form of disease, pockets form only in the later stages.*

Type IV. Occlusal trauma *resulting in resorption of the alveolar bone and loosening of the teeth.*

The term *Schmutz-Pyorrhöe* came to be synonomous with a disease beginning primarily in the gingival tissues and resulting from local factors, whereas *alveolar atrophy* was considered to be seated predominantly in the alveolar bone and to result from systemic causes. *Paradental-Pyorrhöe* was regarded as either an advanced stage of Schmutz-Pyorrhöe or a form of diffuse atrophy, complicated by the presence of inflammation. This concept, or variations of it, were espoused by almost all of Gottlieb's contemporaries.

The classification of Box, presented about the same time as that of Gottlieb, was based upon the acuteness and extent of the lesion and the relative roles of local and systemic etiologic factors.[34] Box and his colleagues were strongly influenced by Weski's concept of the periodontium. They introduced the term *periodontitis* to denote those inflammatory diseases in which all three components of the periodontium, i.e., the gingiva, bone, and periodontal ligament are affected, in contrast to the lesions of occlusal traumatism and atrophic lesions in which only the bone and periodontal ligament may be involved. Box separated periodontitis into an *acute* form, subsequently to be known as acute necrotizing ulcerative gingivitis or Vincent's infection and a *chronic* form. On the basis of presumed etiologic factors, chronic periodontitis was subclassified into simplex and complex forms.

Simplex periodontitis, considered to result from local etiologic factors, was comparable to Gottlieb's Schmutz-Pyorrhöe. Its principal features included:

1. A local bacterial etiology with the relative absence of inflammation, pus formation, tartar accumulation, and tooth mobility
2. A slow progression without pocket formation or with the formation of shallow pockets
3. Progression through stages including chronic gingivitis, infective osteitis, and finally chronic pericementitis[34]

Complex periodontitis, a lesion caused predominantly by systemic etiologic factors, was described as the "typical lesion of so-called pyorrhea alveolaris" and did not have a direct counterpart in Gottlieb's classification. Its characteristics included:

1. The presence of deep pockets, pus formation, large amounts of tartar and varying degrees of tooth mobility
2. Occlusal traumatism as a consistently present feature, although occlusal trauma can occur without the development of complex periodontitis and factors other than occlusal traumatism and local bacterial factors are important

3. Evolution of lesions of two types as the disease progresses: a chronic pericementitis or conversion of a pocket on cementum to one extending into the pericementum, and an infective osteitis of the rarefying type[34]

The classification systems of Gottlieb and of Box, which comprise the foundation of our current terminology, were based upon (1) the clinical manifestations of the disease, (2) the putative role of local and systemic etiologic factors including occlusal traumatism, and (3) the presence of inflammatory or degenerative histopathologic alterations of tissue. The two concepts differed in important respects. In Gottlieb's view, systemic factors operate to produce a degenerative bone lesion referred to as alveolar atrophy or periodontosis which subsequently can be converted, at a late stage of evolution, into Paradental-Pyorrhöe, an inflammatory form of disease. Paradental-Pyorrhöe could also arise via Schmutz-Pyorrhöe from local causes. On the other hand, McCall and Box believed that systemic factors alone could lead directly to the formation of an inflammatory lesion which they called "periodontitis complex."[34] Their classification did not include a degenerative form of periodontal disease. At the time few data supported the contentions of either author. The criteria used to distinguish the complex and simplex forms of periodontitis were extremely vague, and most cases of disease could not be diagnosed definitively as either one or the other. Furthermore, there were, in fact, no data to show that a noninflammatory form of periodontal disease did indeed exist.

In spite of the problems, periodontal diseases for several decades were classified on the basis of presumed etiology and the presence or absence of inflammation. Numerous authors presented new classification systems and terms, although almost all of these were minor variations of the Gottlieb or Box concepts. For example, Simonton[48] and Becks[4] separated the disease of the investing tissues into *paradontitis*, the inflammatory disease, and *paradontosis*, the degenerative atrophic form of disease. Paradontitis was subclassified as (1) a chemicobacterial disease of completely local origin, comparable to Gottlieb's Schmutz-Pyorrhöe, which could be treated successfully by maintenance of a clean mouth, and (2) a form of disease beginning as gingivitis and extending into the pericementum or the alveolar bone, depending upon the relative resistance of the tissues encountered, and due predominantly to systemic causes. To the contrary, Häupl did not consider systemic factors to be of importance.[24] He referred to a superficial lesion (paradentitis marginalis superfacilis), comparable to Schmutz-Pyorrhöe or sim-

plex periodontitis, and a deep lesion (paradentitis marginalis profunda) exhibiting the same features as advanced periodontosis or periodontal atrophy described by Gottlieb. In his view, the latter is simply an advanced stage of the former.

Kronfeld modified Gottlieb's original classification in that he noted three classes of disease: gingivitis, paradental pyorrhea, and alveolar atrophy.[29] The term *gingivitis* was considered to be synonymous with Schmutz-Pyorrhöe or periodontitis simplex, and *alveolar atrophy* included both the traumatic occlusal lesions and diffuse atrophy of the type described by Gottlieb. Paradental pyorrhea was considered to serve as the link between gingivitis and alveolar atrophy, in that it could arise from either. Gingivitis was considered to rise from local factors, atrophy from systemic factors, and Paradental-Pyorrhöe from either or both. Thoma and Goldman used a similar approach, except that they re-defined gingivitis as an early stage of the inflammatory lesion, a definition still accepted today.[50]

In the 1940's, both Box and Gottlieb attempted to clarify further their systems of nomenclature and classification. Although Box retained his original definition and description of periodontitis simplex, he modified the definition of periodontitis complex to accommodate the concept of a degenerative lesion.[6,7] Gottlieb departed drastically from his earlier system of classification.[22] He suggested that all of the periodontal diseases, including gingival recession, pocket formation, and pathologic wandering of the teeth, result from a pathologic condition of the cementum he referred to as *cementopathia*. When the diseased cementum is located near the cervical region of the tooth in contact with the epithelial attachment *marginal cementopathia*, a lesion characterized by pocket formation and gingival recession, occurs; the lesion of *deep cementopathia*, a term used in lieu of diffuse atrophy or periodontosis, occurs when the diseased cementum is located more apically than the epithelial attachment. Marginal cementopathia may occur with or without inflammation and suppuration, and the resultant pockets may be confined to the soft tissues or they may extend into the bone.

Fish confused the issue even further in that his classification of the diseases of the periodontium reverted to use of the term pyorrhea. He states, "these diseases are generally classified together as "pyorrhea,' but there are three principal clinical types: *chronic marginal gingivitis, pyorrhoea simplex* and *pyorrhoea profunda*. These three conditions are really only different stages of the same malady, modified in expression as time goes on and as the disease affects different people."[11]

SUMMARY

Thus, by the 1950's, the nomenclature used for various periodontal lesions had become a morass of vague, ill-defined terms. Of the dozens of terms that had been introduced, only "scurvy of the gums" appears to have been dropped. Since the first system of classification by Fox one-and-one-half centuries earlier, literally dozens of systems of classification had been proposed, but none had become universally accepted, and many were, in fact, contradictory. Even though the etiology of various periodontal diseases remained essentially unknown, many of the systems of classification were devised on the basis of a presumed set of etiologic factors. For example, the distinction between periodontitis simplex and periodontitis complex rested predominantly upon the idea that the former was caused by "local" factors or deposits on the teeth, while the latter resulted from "systemic" or "constitutional" causes. The variety of possible causes was limited only by the imagination of the observer. Gottlieb's concept of cementopathia was based upon the assumption that all of the various periodontal diseases were caused by some undefined pathologic alteration in cementum, although evidence that cementum is indeed the primary seat of any of the diseases has never been shown. Distinction between periodontitis and periodontosis was based on the concept that the primary seat of the former is in the soft tissues and that of the latter is in the alveolar bone; the lesion was defined principally on evidence of degeneration of the connective tissue fibers and pocket formation in the absence of an inflammatory response. However, there has subsequently been no clear histopathologic evidence that such a lesion really occurs, and indeed, in light of current views on basic pathologic processes, it is unlikely to be the case. The distinction between periodontitis and gingivitis was defined on the basis of whether the inflammatory response extends beyond the confines of the marginal gingiva. Thus, even today, the definitive unequivocal distinction between these two entities would require procedures such as serial histopathologic sectioning and study which are impractical in most cases.

THE AMERICAN ACADEMY OF PERIODONTOLOGY TERMINOLOGY AND CLASSIFICATION SYSTEM

In order to resolve the nomenclature and classification problems, the American Academy of Periodontology formed a Committee on Nomenclature. The efforts of this Committee have resulted in clarification of many aspects of the nomenclature problem. The prefix *peri* (in lieu of *para* or *paro* was selected to designate the region immediately surrounding the tooth. Thus the term *periodontium* (peri-odontium, from the Greek, *odous, odontos,* a tooth) was accepted as the term designating the investing tissues, and *periodontitis* as the general name for the inflammatory diseases affecting the tissues.[1,34] A classification of periodontal diseases based upon the clinical manifestations, pathologic alterations, and etiology was devised (Table 2-2).[31,32,37,38] The diseases were designated as *inflammatory, degenerative, atrophic, hyperplastic,* and *traumatic.* Two inflammatory lesions were acknowledged. *Gingivitis* was defined as the inflammatory lesion confined to the tissues of the marginal gingiva (Fig. 2-3), and *periodontitis* was the term accepted to describe the inflammatory lesion extending into the deeper tissues (Fig. 2-4). It was noted that both inflammatory lesions could be described further on the basis of the character of the exudate as edematous, serous, purulent, or necrotic; on the basis of clinical manifestations as ulcerative, hemorrhagic, desquamative, or hypertrophic; on the basis of etiology as plaque-associated, nutrition-associated (scorbutic), endocrine-associated, as in adolescence or pregnancy, associated with generalized infection as in disseminated tuberculosis, or drug-induced as in Dilantin hyperplasia; and on the basis of duration as acute and chronic.

TABLE 2-2. *Periodontal Disturbances*

Inflammatory	Gingivitis (local origin, systemic origin) Periodontitis (simplex, complex)
Degenerative	Periodontosis (systemic, hereditary, idiopathic)
Atrophic	Periodontal atrophy (traumatic, presenile, senile, caused by disuse, idiopathic, inflammatory)
Hypertrophic	Gingival hyperplasia (chronic irritational, drug-induced, idiopathic)
Traumatic	Periodontal traumatism

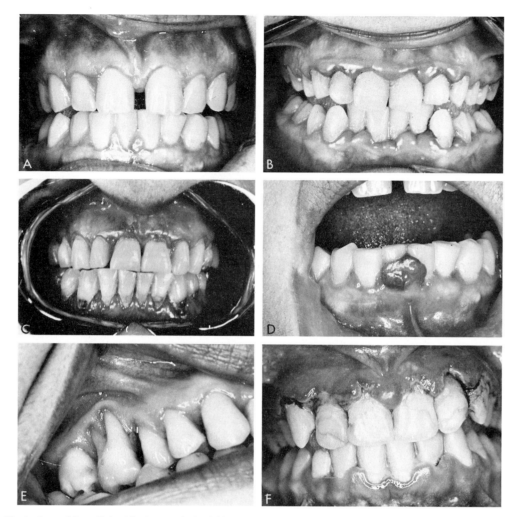

FIG. 2-3. *An illustration of the clinical features of gingivitis and the use of the system of nomenclature based upon the etiology, duration of the lesion, clinical features of the disease, character of the exudate, and combinations of these factors. A. A long-standing generalized inflammation of the papillary and marginal gingiva which later was alleviated completely by plaque removal. This lesion could be referred to as chronic plaque-associated or microbial gingivitis on the basis of duration and suspected etiology. B. A case of gingivitis, exhibiting plaque accumulation with thickened marginal gingiva and associated with mouth breathing, which on the basis of clinical features, duration, and suspected direct and indirect etiologic factors could be termed chronic fibrotic plaque-associated gingivitis, complicated by mouth breathing. C. Chronic idiopathic desquamative gingivitis, so named because of the clinical features, duration of the lesion, and unknown etiology. D. Gingivitis occurring during pregnancy in a relatively clean mouth. Note the generalized inflammation of the marginal and papillary gingiva and the hyperplastic lesions or "pregnancy tumor" between the incisor teeth. The disease could be referred to as chronic hyperplastic hormonal gingivitis. E. Chronic postsurgical gingivitis resulting from the inability of the patient to control plaque accumulation near the apically positioned gingival margins. F. Acute ulcerative necrotizing gingivitis. The nomenclature is based upon duration and clinical manifestations of the lesion. It may also be referred to as Vincent's infection or trench mouth.*

Gingivitis was subclassified on the basis of presumed etiology into local and systemic forms. Locally caused forms of gingivitis included those resulting from food impaction, calculus, irritating restorations, and drug reactions. Gingivitis with a systemic etiology included lesions seen in pregnant women or in individuals with various systemic diseases such as diabetes, endocrine dysfunctions, tuberculosis, syphilis, or leukemia. Additional systemic causes included drug reactions, allergies, and hereditary predisposition. Cases that could

not be resolved etiologically were classified as idiopathic. In general, this approach to classifying the various forms of gingivitis continues to be used.

Subdivision of periodontitis into simplex and complex forms as originally suggested by Box was accepted.[34] *Periodontitis simplex* was defined as the lesion evolving from gingivitis and resulting principally from local factors. It progresses relatively slowly, exhibiting shallow wide-mouthed pockets distributed throughout the mouth, with generalized bone loss. The pockets are

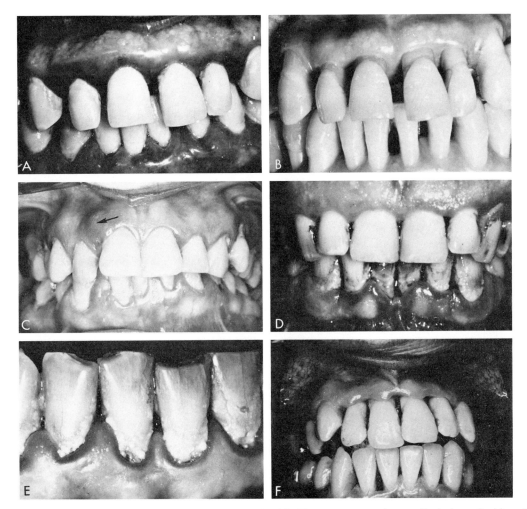

FIG. 2-4. *Clinical manifestations of adult chronic marginal periodontitis. The process may be manifested as a florid acute inflammatory phenomenon, a chronic inflammatory lesion dominated by gingival thickening and fibrosis, or as a mixture of these clinical features. A. Chronic marginal periodontitis in a 42-year-old woman resulting principally from the long-standing presence of debris on the teeth. Bone resorption was generalized with pocket depths in the range of 8 to 10 mm. The gingivae were fiery red and bled profusely upon probing. Calculus and plaque were present on all of the teeth. Fibrosis of the gingiva was not a major component. B. The same case shown in A, following treatment by root planing, curettage, and temporary stabilization, demonstrating a reasonably normal gingival contour gained through resolution of the acute inflammatory process. C. Chronic marginal periodontitis with an acute exacerbation. The disease is manifested clinically as erythema and swelling of the marginal gingiva with bleeding upon probing. However, there is an acute periodontal abscess associated with pocketing around the maxillary right central incisor (arrow). Fibrosis is not a feature in this case of periodontitis. D. Advanced chronic marginal periodontitis demonstrating areas of acute inflammation such as around the mandibular incisors where bleeding was profuse and areas of less acute response dominated by fibrosis, such as is evidenced around the maxillary incisors. Equally deep pockets were present around all teeth. E. Advanced chronic marginal periodontitis in which gingival fibrosis and thickening, along with massive deposits of plaque upon the teeth, are the major features. The tissues appear acutely inflamed only at the margin of the gingiva where the tissues are in actual contact with the microbial plaque. F. Very advanced marginal periodontitis which began as an acute necrotizing ulcerative gingivitis. Virtually all of the interdental soft and hard tissue has been lost, but the labial gingiva remains relatively intact.*

generally filled with plaque and debris, and there is an acute inflammatory reaction in the gingiva. The inflammatory reaction is most apparent in the perivascular areas, and it progresses into the alveolar bone and eventually into the periodontal membrane through the perivascular tissues. *Periodontitis complex* was considered to be caused predominantly by systemic disease or to be a periodontitis of local origin superimposed upon

a base of periodontosis. When the etiology is apparent, the disease is named accordingly as tubercular, diabetic, leukemic, or syphilitic. When the etiology is inapparent or not known, the disease is classified as idiopathic. The lesion can be further subclassified as acute, chronic, ulcerative, purulent, or suppurative.

Periodontosis was accepted as a general term and defined to include degenerative noninflammatory destruction of any one or more of the tissues of the periodontium. The characteristics of periodontosis include loosening and migration of the teeth in the presence or absence of secondary epithelial proliferation and pocket formation or secondary gingival disease. The disease was considered to have three pathologic stages: (1) the connective tissue fibers degenerate and the ligament space widens, (2) the epithelium near the sulcus proliferates and migrates apically to deepen the sulcus and convert it into a pocket, and (3) the attachment completely separates from the tooth leaving a deep pocket. Several features distinguishing periodontosis from periodontitis were noted:

1. In periodontitis, bone resorption begins at the alveolar crest and, as the disease progresses, extends into the central portion of the alveolar septum; in periodontosis, the bone is attacked from the periodontal ligament surface, leaving the remainder of the alveolar septum intact.
2. Periodontosis is predominantly a degenerative noninflammatory lesion; periodontitis is a destructive lesion resulting principally from inflammation.
3. Periodontosis most frequently affects young females and old males who frequently have caries-free teeth. The lesions are isolated and bone loss is vertical. Periodontitis, on the other hand, is seen most commonly in both males and females past the age of 30 years, the affected teeth may be carious, and the disease is usually generalized.[34]

Periodontal atrophy was accepted as an entity separate from periodontitis and defined as a decrease in the size of an organ or part by virtue of the loss of its cellular elements after it has attained mature size. Two forms of atrophy were distinguished. *Gingival recession* is the most commonly observed form of periodontal atrophy. In this condition, there is a noninflammatory loss of periodontal tissue, with concurrent apical movement of the soft tissue attachment to the tooth without pocket formation. The etiology may be traumatic, as for example, from the vigorous long-term use of a hard-bristled toothbrush, it may result from excessive occlusal forces, or it may occur spontaneously with aging. A second form is *atrophy of disuse* in which the functional forces have been removed from the tooth and in which there is a loss of alveolar bone and the principal fibers of the periodontal ligament without gingival recession; the alveolar bone proper persists, but the supporting bone trabeculae become thin and finally disappear as the marrow spaces increase in size.

The ligament space becomes narrowed and new cementum is deposited.

Hyperplastic lesions occur primarily in the gingiva (Fig. 2-5). Gingival hyperplasia is an overgrowth of tissue due to an increase in the number of its elements, and it serves no functional purpose. Gingival hyperplasia is generally subclassified on the basis of etiology. It may result from chronic irritation, from the endocrine imbalance of adolescence or pregnancy, from long-term use of certain drugs such as Dilantin sodium, or it may be hereditary as in cases of familial fibromatosis.

Periodontal traumatism was defined as a form of pressure necrosis characterized by thrombosis, hemorrhage, resorption of the bone and cementum resulting from mechanical trauma. The affected teeth may loosen, they may become sensitive to percussion, and they may contact prematurely in centric and excentric functional movements of the mandible. The term *primary occlusal traumatism* has been used when the affected teeth are otherwise healthy, the periodontium normal, and the force excessive; *secondary occlusal traumatism* is the term used for teeth around which the periodontium has been pathologically altered to the extent that otherwise normal occlusal forces cannot be tolerated.

CURRENT TERMINOLOGY AND CLASSIFICATION

Since publication of the initial recommendations of the American Academy of Periodontology, the accepted nomenclature and classification of the various periodontal diseases have undergone considerable change. In general, the changes have resulted from attempts to avoid vagueness in terminology and to attain simplification in classification.

The term *gingivitis* continues to be used to designate inflammatory lesions that are confined to the marginal gingiva, regardless of the etiology. The types most frequently encountered are *plaque-associated gingivitis, acute ulcerative necrotizing gingivitis, hormonal gingivitis* and *drug-induced gingivitis* (Fig. 2-5). Although these subclassifications are useful clinically, the need for a fresh view of the lesion of gingivitis is apparent. There is general agreement that periodontitis begins as gingivitis, although transient forms of gingivitis that may not progress to periodontitis appear to occur. Furthermore, there is no definite distinction between gingivitis and periodontitis on the basis of readily available clinical, radiologic, or histopathologic criteria. The ability to subclassify the lesion of gingivitis more accurately would be of immense importance

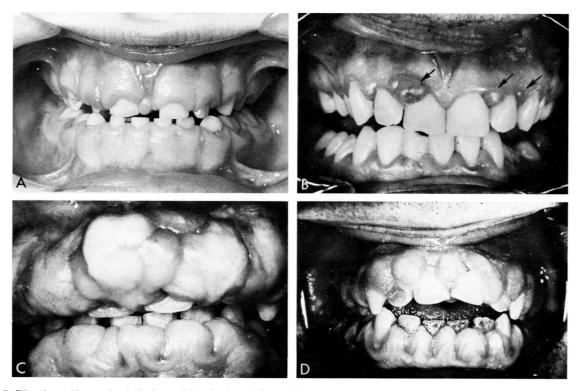

FIG. 2-5. *Fibrotic and hyperplastic lesions of the gingiva. A. Generalized fibrosis of the gingiva in a 5-year-old child. Note the extreme thickness of the attached gingiva. B. Nodular gingival fibromatosis. While there is a generalized thickening of the attached gingiva, several of the interdental papillae (arrows) are noticeably enlarged. C and D. Dilantin hyperplasia. Both patients had been on long-term Dilantin therapy for epilepsy. The overgrowth of tissue originates almost entirely from the interdental papillae and may be so extensive as to totally obscure the tooth. Barbiturates may induce a similar but less severe response in some patients.*

both in patient care and in research. It is hoped that laboratory tests or other procedures by which this can be accomplished can be devised in the future.

Although most investigators and clinicians agree that *marginal periodontitis* (Fig. 2-4) is not a homogeneous entity, it is no longer subclassified as periodontitis simplex and periodontitis complex. In spite of intensive efforts extending over several decades to refine the criteria, it has never been possible to diagnose definitively most cases of periodontitis as being of one type or the other. This is not to deny that cases differ greatly with regard to the extent and distribution of lesions, the amount of associated plaque and calculus, the rate of progression, the age of the individuals affected, and the characteristic bone and soft-tissue alterations. In addition, it is clear that while most cases respond well to therapeutic measures such as improved oral hygiene, root planing, and pocket elimination, directed toward control of the growth and accumulation of plaque significant numbers of cases do not respond to therapy, regardless of the aggressiveness with which it is applied. In spite of these differences, subclassification on the basis of the role of local etiologic factors versus systemic etiologic factors, or on the

basis of superimposition of an inflammatory lesion upon a previously existent degenerative lesion does not appear to be justified. The data now available appear to support subclassification of marginal periodontitis into *juvenile* and *adult* types.

The meaning and usage of the term *periodontosis* remain controversial. Indeed, a thorough reevaluation of all of the evidence leads us and many other writers to question whether or not a lesion exhibiting the clinical and pathologic features attributed to periodontosis actually exists.[24,31,33,35,42,43] Although the first description of periodontosis as a specific disease entity is generally attributed to Gottlieb,[2,4,9,29,33,39,44,49,50] the origin of the concept of a degenerative noninflammatory lesion leading to tooth mobility and exfoliation can be traced to much earlier literature. It appears to have originated before the evolution of the concept of the periodontium when diseases occurring around the teeth were considered to reside either in the gums or the alveolar bone, but not in both:

I come now to consider the diseases which take place primarily in the sockets, when the teeth are perfectly sound. The first effect, which takes place, is a wasting of the alveolar processes, which are in many people gradually absorbed, and taken into the system. This wasting begins first at the edge of the socket, and gradually goes on to the root bottom. The gum, which is supported by the alveolar process, loses its connection and recedes from the body of the tooth, in proportions as the socket is lost; in consequence of which, first the neck and then more or less the fang (root) itself becomes exposed.—John Hunter, 1839

The most common disease to which they (the alveolar processes) are subjected, is a gradual absorption of their substance, whereby the teeth lose their support, become weak, and at length are so loosened as to drop out. . . . As the disease progresses the gums partake. They lose their attachment to the teeth and recede in proportion to the wasting of the sockets. The gums may be completely free of inflammation and no cause may be apparent.—Joseph Fox, 1823.

Fox also notes that in the advanced stages of the disease, there may be massive inflammation and the oozing of pus. Thus, at least 100 years before the time of Gottlieb, a lesion distinct from scurvy of the gums and different from the disease associated with the accumulation of tartar on the teeth was known. The disease was considered to be a primary lesion of alveolar bone, to be noninflammatory in character except in the advanced stages, and to result from systemic or constitutional causes.

Periodontosis, as described by Gottlieb,[16] and subsequently by others,[3,15,29,39,49,51] was considered to be a noninflammatory degenerative lesion of the periodontium, occurring generally in the absence of debris or deposits on the teeth, and leading to migration, loosening, and exfoliation of the teeth. It was generally conceived that, in advanced stages, the lesion could become complicated by the presence of inflammation. Gottlieb considered the lesion to result from a pathologic alteration in cementum,[22] although other investigators believed that it could start as a noninflammatory degeneration of the principal fibers of the periodontal ligament.[13,31,39] Systemic factors were considered to be the principal cause of the disease.

When the published data are re-examined in the light of current knowledge, the validity of the conclusions drawn appears to be open to serious question. In several of the papers, the histopathologic specimens were from unknown sources or from individuals or animals on the brink of death from starvation or other causes, and in some instances illustrations of the same histopathologic section appeared repeatedly in publications.[13,16,39,51] The histologic features of all the illustrations of the periodontal pocket are characteristic of those seen in cases in which tooth movement has occurred either from excessive occlusal forces or from controlled orthodontic forces. Furthermore, in illustra-

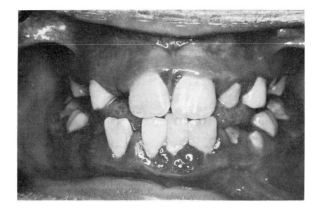

FIG. 2-6. *Clinical manifestations of juvenile periodontitis as seen in an 8-year-old child. Note the edema and other manifestations of florid acute inflammatory response of the marginal gingiva around the incisors. See Fig. 2-7 for radiographic manifestations.*

tions of sections taken from near the gingival sulcus or pocket, inflammatory cells are always present in the published material. The response generally given to the latter observation is that the pure noninflammatory phase of periodontosis exists for only a short time

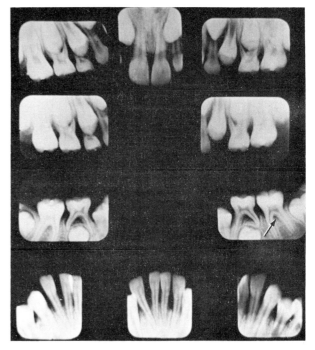

FIG. 2-7. *Radiographic manifestations of juvenile periodontitis as seen in an 8-year-old child. Note the loss of more than one half of the alveolar bone from the mandibular and maxillary incisors, as well as the significant bone loss around the posterior deciduous and permanent teeth. There is a bifurcation opening affecting the recently erupted left first molar (arrow). Refer to Fig. 2-6 for clinical manifestations.*

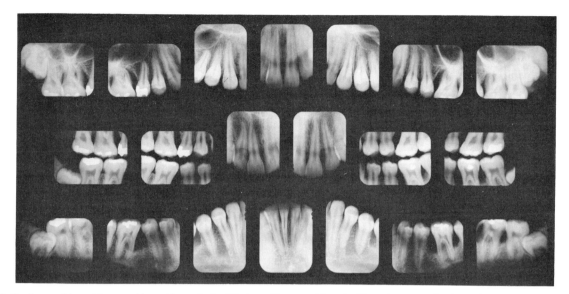

FIG. 2-8. *Radiographic evidence of juvenile periodontitis in a 16-year-old male. Note the extensive bone loss around all of the first molars.*

period and it is only in rare instances that the pure lesion can be found.[31,39]

The general conclusion is that periodontosis, as it is usually defined, does not exist as a specific disease entity,[31,55] but there seems little doubt that a form of periodontitis exhibiting features permitting definitive differentiation from the usual form does exist.[2,9,31,33,44,49] The disease occurs principally in young people, especially adolescent females, who are otherwise normal and healthy in all respects and who exhibit clean teeth; it appears to have a hereditary component. It has a predilection for the central incisors and first molars, but it is by no means confined to these teeth. The lesions, which may also affect the primary dentition, exhibit blatant inflammation; rapid progress; formation of isolated, deep, tortuous pockets; drifting and mobility of the teeth; and lack of response to standard therapeutic measures (Figs. 2-6, 2-7, 2-8).

Several investigators have suggested classification of the disease as *juvenile periodontitis* in contrast to *adult periodontitis*. This subclassification of periodontitis appears to have a firm scientific basis. In addition to the distinctive clinicopathologic manifestations noted, the immune response of persons exhibiting the juvenile lesion appears to differ both from that of normal persons and from persons with the adult form of the disease.[30,33] Furthermore, the adult and juvenile forms of periodontitis may differ with regard to the pocket flora. The flora of pockets of young people with rapidly progressing disease appears to contain about 60 percent gram-negative rods exhibiting a high pathogenic potential,[36] in contrast to the flora of pockets of adults with the slowly progressing form of the disease.[54]

References

1. Aiguier, J. E., McCall, J. O., and Merritt, A. H.: Report of the Committee on Nomenclature of the American Academy of Periodontology. J. Peridontol., *8:*88, 1937.
2. Baer, P. N., et al.: Advanced periodontal disease in an adolescent. J. Periodontol., *34:*533, 1963.
3. Becks, H.: General aspects of pyorrhea research. Pacific Dent. Gazette, *37:*259, 1929.
4. Becks, H.: What factors determine the early stage of paradontosis. J. Am. Dent. Assoc., *18:*922, 1931.
5. Black, G. V.: Special Dental Pathology. Chicago, Medicodental Publishing Co., 1915, p. 64.
6. Box, H. K.: Periodontal studies. Dent. Items Interest, *62:*915, 1940.
7. Box, H. K.: Twelve Periodontal Studies. Toronto, University of Toronto Press, 1940.
8. Box, H. K.: Oxygen Insufflation in Periodontal Disease. American Lectures in Dentistry, publication number 237. Springfield, Ill., Charles C Thomas, 1955.
9. Everett, F. G., and Baer, P. N.: A preliminary report on the treatment of the osseus defect in periodontosis. J. Periodontol., *35:*429, 1964.
10. Fauchard, P.: The Surgeon Dentist. Translated by L. Lindsay from the second edition, 1746. Pound Ridge, New York, 1969.
11. Fish, E. W.: Parodontal Disease. London, Eyre and Spottiswoode, 1952.
12. Fox, J.: Natural History and Diseases of the Human Teeth. Part II. Diseases of the Teeth the Gums and the Alveolar Processes. Third edition. London, E. Cox, 1823.
13. Goldman, H. M.: A similar condition to periodontosis found in two spider monkeys. Am. J. Ortho. and Oral Surg. *10:*749, 1947.

14. Goldman, H. M.: Periodontia, Third edition. St. Louis, C. V. Moshy Co., 1953.

15. Goldman, H. M.: Periodontosis in the spider monkey. A preliminary report. J. Periodontol., *18:*34, 1947.

16. Gottlieb, B.: Zur Aetiologie und Therapie der Alveolarpyorrhöe. Z. Stomatol., *18:*59, 1920.

17. Gottlieb, B.: Der Epithelansatz am Zahne. Dtsch. Mschr. Zahnheilk. *39:*142, 1921.

18. Gottlieb, B.: Die diffuse Atrophie des Alveolarknochens. Z. Stomatol., *31:*195, 1923.

19. Gottlieb, B.: Paradentalpyorrhöe und Alveolaratrophie. Munich, Verlag Urban und Schwarzenbaer, 1925.

20. Gottlieb, B.: Paradentalpyorrhöe und Alveolaratrophie. Mschr. Fortschr. Zahnheilk., *2:*363, 1926.

21. Gottlieb, B.: The formation of the pocket: Diffuse atrophy of the alveolar bone. J. Am. Dent. Assoc., *15:*462, 1928.

22. Gottlieb, B.: The new concept of periodontoclasia. J. Periodontol., *17:*7, 1946.

23. Gottlieb, B., and Orban, B.: Biology and Pathology of the Tooth and Its Supporting Mechanism. New York, The Macmillan Co., 1938.

24. Häupl, H.: Uber traumatisch verursachte Gewebsveränderungen im Paradentium. Z. Stomatol., *25:*307, 1927.

25. Hopewell-Smith, A.: Pyorrhea alveolaris, its pathohistology I. Preliminary note. II. Its interpretation. Dental Cosmos, *53:*397, 981, 1911.

26. Hunter, J.: A Practical Treatise on the Diseases of the Teeth. Supplement to Natural History of Human Teeth. Part II. London, 1835.

27. James, W. W., and Counsell, A.: A histological investigation into "so-called pyorrhoea alveolaris." Br. Dent. J., *48:*1253, 1927.

28. Koecker, L.: An essay on the devastation of the gums and the alveolar processes. Phila. J. Med. Phys. Sci., *2:*282, 1821.

29. Kronfeld, R., Histology of the Teeth and Their Surrounding Structures. Philadelphia, Lea & Febiger, 1933.

30. Lehner, T.: Immunological features of juvenile periodontitis (Periodontosis). Presented in the Symposium on Periodontosis, 52nd Gen. Meeting, IADR, Atlanta, Georgia, 1974.

31. Lyons, H., Bernier, H., and Goldman, H. M.: Report of the Nomenclature and Classification Committee. J. Periodontol., *30:*74, 1959.

32. Lyons, H., Kerr, D. M., and Hine, M. K.: Report from the 1949 Nomenclature Committee. J. Periodontol., *21:*40, 1950.

33. Manson, J. D., and Lehner, T.: Clinical features of juvenile periodontitis (Periodontosis). J. Periodontol., *45:*636, 1974.

34. McCall, J. O., and Box, H. K.: The pathology and diagnosis of the basic lesions of chronic periodontitis. J. Am. Dent. Assoc., *12:*1300, 1923.

35. Mezl, Z.: Contribution à l'histologie pathologique du paradentium. Paradentologie, *2:*60, 1948.

36. Newman, M. G., Socransky, S. S., and Listgarten, M. A.: Relationship of microorganisms to the etiology of periodontosis. Program and Abs. 52nd Gen. Session IADR, Atlanta, Georgia, 1974. Abs. #324.

37. Orban, B.: Classification and nomenclature of periodontal diseases. J. Periodontol., *13:*88, 1942.

38. Orban, B.: Classification of periodontal disease. Paradontologie, *3:*159, 1949.

39. Orban, B., and Weinmann, J. P.: A diffuse atrophy of the alveolar bone (Periodontosis). J. Periodontol., *13:*31, 1942.

40. Page, R. C., Simpson, D., and Ammons, W. F.: Host tissue response in chronic periodontal disease IV. The dental and periodontal status of a group of aged chimpanzees. J. Periodontol., *46:*144, 1975.

41. *Papyrus Ebers.* Translated by B. Ebbell. Copenhagen, Levin and Munksgaard, 1937.

42. Ramfjord, S.: Effects of acute febrile disease on the periodontium of monkeys with reference to poliomyelitis. J. Dent. Res., *30:*615, 1951.

43. Ramfjord, S.: Tuberculosis and periodontal disease, with special reference to collagen fibers. J. Dent. Res., *31:*5, 1952.

44. Rao, S. S., and Tewani, S. V.: Prevalence of periodontosis among Indians. J. Periodontol., *39:*27, 1968.

45. Rehnwinkel, F. H.: Pyorrhoea alveolaris. Dental Cosmos, *19:*572, 1877.

46. Riggs, J. W.: Suppurative inflammation of the gums, and absorption of the gums and alveolar process. Pa. J. Dent. Sci., *3:*99, 1876.

47. Ruffer, M. A.: Studies in the Paleopathology of Egypt. Chicago, University of Chicago Press, 1921.

48. Simonton, F. V.: Paradontoclasia. Pacific Dent. Gazette, *35:*251, 1927.

49. Tenenbaum, B., et al.: Clinical and microscopic study of gingivae in periodontosis. J. Am. Dent. Assoc., *40:*302, 1950.

50. Thoma, K. H., and Goldman, H. J.: Classification and histopathology of parodontal disease. J. Am. Dent. Assoc., *24:*1915, 1937.

51. Thomas, K. H., and Goldman, H. M.: Wandering and elongation of the teeth and pocket formation in periodontosis. J. Am. Dent. Assoc., *27:*335, 1940.

52. Weinberger, B. W.: Orthodontics: An Historical Review of its Origin and Evolution. St. Louis, C. V. Mosby Co., 1926.

53. Weski, O.: Röntgenologische-anatomische Studien aus dem Gebiete der Kieferpathologie. Vjschr. Zahnheilk., *37:*1, 1921.

54. Williams, B. L., and Sherris, J. C.: Studies on the predominant cultivatable subgingival microflora of patients with periodontitis. IADR Programs and Abstracts. 52nd Gen Meeting IADR, Atlanta, Georgia, 1974. Abs. #334.

55. World Workshop in Periodontics: S. P. Ramfjord, D. A., Kerr, and M. M. Ash Eds. Sponsored by the American Academy Periodontology and the University of Michigan, 1966.

56. Znamensky, N. N.: Alveolar pyorrhoea—its pathological anatomy and its radical treatment. J. Br. Dent. Assoc., *23:*39, 1902.

3

Epidemiology of Periodontal Diseases

The science of epidemiology is concerned with the discovery and measurement of factors related to health, disease, defects, disabilities and death in populations and aggregates of individuals.[2,3] In studies relating to a specific disease state, epidemiologists define and measure parameters considered to be important on the basis of data from other sources and strive to demonstrate interrelationships among these factors. The parameters of interest may vary from one disease state to another, but generally they include measurement of mortality and morbidity rates, the age distribution, the relationships to certain biologic and physiologic states, the role of various possible etiologic agents, and the efficacy of various therapeutic methods. When a sufficiently large body of information has been obtained, it may be assembled into an orderly array in an attempt to define and understand the chain of events that leads from the normal to the abnormal state. Once the chain of events has been established and understood, a means of alleviation or prevention of the abnormal state may emerge.

3

Epidemiology

of

Periodontal

Disease

EPIDEMIOLOGIC METHODS

Application of epidemiologic techniques to problems of gingival and periodontal disease has been a recent development. Early studies, using relatively crude methods of measurement and crudely defined criteria, were carried out by Marshall-Day and Shourie,[12] King,[9] and Schour and Massler.[21] The efforts of these investigators demonstrated the validity of the epidemiologic approach to the study of periodontal disease. Furthermore, they stimulated the subsequent development of several sophisticated techniques by which the prevalence and extent of periodontal disease and the level of oral cleanliness can be measured.[6,13,15,18,21] The information obtained by these techniques for the survey of large population groups throughout the world has had a major impact on our current concepts of the nature of gingival and periodontal disease. Using the epidemiologic approach, it has been shown that inflammatory disease of the supporting structures of the teeth comprises a worldwide public health problem of major proportions, and that the prevalence and extent of disease increase with increasing age and decreasing levels of oral cleanliness. (For reviews, see Scherp,[20] and Russell,[18]).

Problems

Application of epidemiologic methods to problems of gingival and periodontal disease is far more complex and difficult than is their use in the study of many other disease states such as dental caries or acute infectious disease. There are several important reasons for this. The long life span of man, the long-term chronic nature of periodontal disease, the need to measure prevalence and severity, the possible heterogeneity of the disease, and the lack of a pathognomonic manifestation or any simple test that is pathognomonic for chronic progressive periodontal disease have all seriously hampered development and application of epidemiologic methods.

CHRONICITY OF THE DISEASE STATE

Periodontal disease is a long-term chronic disorder of almost universal prevalence. The more widespread a condition or disease state, the more difficult it becomes to ferret out those environmental, societal, and cultural factors responsible or related to it. An example of this problem is the difficulty that has been encountered in the application of epidemiologic techniques to the study of atherosclerosis and heart disease.

EXTENDED LIFE SPAN OF MAN

Since the earliest manifestations of inflammatory gingival and periodontal disease may begin in childhood and extend throughout life, many important questions such as those relating to the natural history of the disease require the acquisition of longitudinal data. However, the unusually long life span of man relative to other animals precludes, to a great extent, the usefulness of longitudinal epidemiologic methods. For example, in most populations, studies of gingival and periodontal disease encompassing decades are interfered with severely by the mobility of the population, continually changing life styles, intermittent therapeutic intervention, and the periodic and unpredictable use of various preventive measures. As a consequence, questions posed are limited generally to those that can be answered by cross-sectional data.

PREVALENCE AND SEVERITY

Another equally difficult problem is the fact that while knowledge of the prevalence of the disease state may yield a reasonably clear insight into the magnitude of its effect on a population and may lead frequently to clarification of etiologic factors, measurement of prevalence alone is not sufficient in the study of gingival and periodontal disease. A knowledge of the severity or extent of the disease or lesion is of paramount importance. For example, consider two hypothetical populations, A and B. Assume that all members of group A exhibit a mild transient inflammatory response in the marginal gingiva, while all members of group B exhibit extensive gingival inflammation, pathologic pocket formation, and bone destruction. Measurements of prevalence alone would indicate that 100 percent of the individuals of both populations are affected by the disease state. The true periodontal status of the two populations would emerge only when techniques measuring both prevalence and severity were applied. Thus, it has been necessary to devise indices that take into account not only the presence or absence of pathologic alterations in the periodontium, but also the extent to which all the dentition is affected and the degree to which the lesions have progressed.

HETEROGENEITY OF PERIODONTAL DISEASE

Another factor that has hampered seriously the application of epidemiologic methods is the heterogeneity of gingival and periodontal diseases and the difficulty encountered by investigators in differentiating among them on a population-wide basis. Clearly, several forms of inflammatory disease which differ widely in their etiology, natural history, and clinical course exist. These include hormonal, drug-induced and nutritional gingivitis, acute ulcerative gingivitis, chronic progressive periodontal disease, and a host of other entities, limited only by one's taste for subclassification.[5,22] However, it has been necessary to consider all of these entities as a single disease process in order to formulate epidemiologic indices.

LACK OF A PATHOGNOMONIC FEATURE

A final factor complicating the use of epidemiologic techniques to study periodontal disease is that not only is it desirable that the disease under consideration be homogeneous, but also it is essential that the affected individuals exhibit pathognomonic features. For example, the application of epidemiologic techniques to the study of tuberculosis has been eminently successful because of the characteristic radiographic features observed in the lungs of affected individuals and the positive response to tuberculin skin tests. The cardinal clinical manifestations of chronic inflammatory periodontal disease include an inflammatory response in the gingival and periodontal tissues, various degrees of alteration in tissue form and texture, formation of periodontal pockets, loss of supporting alveolar bone, tooth mobility and drifting, and eventual tooth exfoliation. Unfortunately, no single pathologic alteration that can be measured conveniently in large populations reflects accurately the true periodontal status of a population.

Evaluation of the presence and extent of the inflammatory response is a major feature of most indices which purport to measure prevalence and extent of periodontal disease. However, the erythema, edema, ulceration, and hemorrhage upon which these judgments are based may frequently be more extensive in early mild gingivitis than in advanced disease states. Indeed, in the latter case the inflammatory response may be manifested only by alterations in texture and form. Likewise, measurements of sulcular depth alone may not reflect true periodontal status. Increased sulcular depth may be a consequence of enlargement of the marginal tissues rather than the apical migration of the junctional epithelium. Conversely, apical migration combined with resorption of the marginal tissues or recession may lead to normal sulcular depth even in the presence of advanced bone loss.

Measurement of alveolar bone loss is considered to be one of the best criteria for measuring periodontal status. However, this parameter cannot be measured by direct observation, and radiographic measurements on large populations are difficult and cumbersome. Furthermore, the irregular pattern of bone cratering and the poor definition of the relatively more important vertical defects on radiographs have seriously limited the use of bone loss as a pathognomonic feature in epidemiologic surveys. Within recent years, however, means have been devised to overcome many of these problems, and invaluable information has been obtained.

Techniques

The initial epidemiologic surveys of gingival and periodontal disease in large populations were directed simply toward segregation of individuals into subgroups on the basis of the clinical appearance of the tissues of the anterior teeth. These observations permitted evaluation of the relative proportions of the affected and unaffected individuals in the populations under consideration.[9,12,21] In 1944, Marshall-Day and Shourie devised a means for surveying the prevalence of alveolar bone loss. Subsequently, Russell and Ramfjord developed indices based on combinations of several pathologic manifestations and reflecting both prevalence and severity.[15,18] These indices permitted the periodontal status of a group of individuals to be resolved into a single reproducible numerical value. In 1960, Greene and Vermillion developed methods, later refined,[7] by which levels of oral cleanliness could be measured. During the past decade, these indices have been applied on a worldwide scale.

The Periodontal Index (PI) of Russell,[18] the Periodontal Disease Index (PDI) of Ramfjord,[15] and a simplified version of the Oral Hygiene Index (OHI-S) of Greene and Vermillion[7] are used extensively for the epidemiologic surveys of human and animal populations. Assessing PI is done by examining the tissues of each tooth and assigning a numerical value representative of the state of its attachment apparatus based on a set of rigid criteria (Table 3-1). The values for the individual teeth are summed and divided by the number of teeth examined to arrive at a final score. When there is doubt as to the correct value, the lower value is always chosen. This tends to give the Index a conservative feature. As seen in Table 3-1, the pathologic manifestations comprising the index include the presence and extent of inflammation, pocket formation, mobility, and loss of function. The index has a scale of values

TABLE 3-1. *Scoring and Criteria for the Periodontal Index*

SCORE	CRITERIA
0	*Negative.* There is neither overt inflammation in the investing tissues nor loss of function due to destruction of supporting tissues.
1	*Mild Gingivitis.* There is an overt area of inflammation in the free gingiva which does not circumscribe the tooth.
2	*Gingivitis.* Inflammation completely circumscribes the tooth, but there is no apparent break in the epithelial attachment.
6	*Gingivitis with Pocket Formation.* The epithelial attachment has been broken and there is a pocket (not merely a deepened gingival crevice due to swelling in the free gingivae). There is no interference with normal masticatory function; the tooth is firm in its socket and has not drifted.
8	*Advanced Destruction with Loss of Masticatory Function.* The tooth may be loose, may have drifted, may sound dull on percussion with a metallic instrument, or may be depressible in its socket.

Russell, A. L.: The Periodontal Index. *J. Periodontol.*, *38*(Part II):585, 1967.

TABLE 3-2. *Mouth Condition and Periodontal Index Scores*

SCORE	CLINICAL MANIFESTATIONS
0 –0.2	Clinically normal supportive tissues
0.3–0.9	Simple gingivitis
0.7–1.9	Beginning destructive periodontal disease
1.6–5.0	Established destructive periodontal disease
3.8–8.0	Terminal disease

Russell, A. L.: The Periodontal Index. *J. Periodontol., 38*(Part II):586, 1967.

which increases from 0 to 8 with increasing prevalence and severity of disease. The clinical conditions correlating to PI values are presented in Table 3-2. The method is highly reproducible for large populations, but it is of only limited value for individuals or small groups.

The PDI was devised for use in the characterization of the periodontal status of individuals and small groups, as well as of large populations. It is purported to be sufficiently accurate for use in longitudinal studies. The mesial and buccal aspects of only 6 teeth are examined. These include the right first molar, left central incisor, and left first premolar in the maxillary arch and the left first molar, right central incisor, and left first premolar in the mandibular arch. Gingivitis and pocket depth are scored separately. If a pocket is present, the gingivitis score is ignored. Gingivitis is scored on a scale of 0 to 3 on the basis of the extent of the inflammatory response. When the gingival pocket extends below the cementoenamel junction (CEJ), but not more than a distance of 3 mm, the tooth is given a score of 4. When the pocket extends 3 to 6 mm below the CEJ, the score is 5, and when the pocket extends more than 6 mm below the CEJ, the score is 6.

OBSERVATIONS

During the past two decades, epidemiologic surveys measuring the prevalence and severity of gingival and periodontal disease, the levels of oral cleanliness, and a large number of suspected correlative factors have been done throughout the world. These studies have been done on subjects with extremely divergent ethnic, cultural, and socioeconomic backgrounds who follow a wide range of oral hygiene practices. In spite of the diversity of the populations studied, the indices used, or the point of view and discipline of the observers, there has been an extraordinary uniformity in the results. The major contributions made by epidemiologists

to our concepts of periodontal disease will be discussed.

Prevalence and Extent in Human Populations

Gingival and periodontal disease appear to be universal human afflictions and comprise a worldwide public health problem of major proportions. Destructive inflammatory periodontal disease is the principal cause of tooth loss in all human adult populations studied. In a random sample representative of the entire United States male adult population for the period of 1960–1962, it was shown that 46 percent of the 55- to 64-year age group exhibited periodontal pockets, and the group as a whole had a PI score of 2.15 (Fig. 3-1).[8] PI values of this magnitude are considered to represent a significant deviation from the normal state (Table 3-2). The prevalence and extent of gingival and periodontal disease appear to become greater in poorly nourished populations and in groups of individuals such as refugees who are under long-term stress (Table 3-3).

Contrary to previously held opinion, gingivitis and periodontal disease are not confined to the adult population. In a survey by Russell of children in the United States, it was shown that over 3 percent of the group exhibited one or more obvious periodontal pockets by the age of 17 years (Fig. 3-2).[17] In many underdeveloped countries, gingivitis and destructive periodontal disease are even more prevalent and severe in the young.

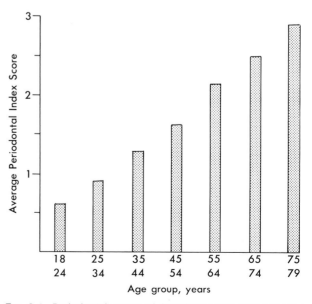

FIG. 3-1. *Periodontal status of American adult males for the years 1960–1962. (Adapted from data of Johnson, Kelly, and van Kirk. In Russell, A. L.: Epidemiology of periodontal disease. Int. Dent. J., 17:282, 1967.)*

TABLE 3-3. *Average Periodontal Index in Civilians of Both Sexes, Aged 44–49 Years*

POPULATION GROUP	AVERAGE PERIODONTAL INDEX
Baltimore, Maryland (White)	1.03
Colorado Springs, Colorado	1.04[a]
Alaska (Primitive Eskimos)	1.17[b]
Ecuador	1.85
Ethiopia	1.86
Baltimore, Maryland (Negro)	1.99
Vietnam (Vietnamese)	2.18
Colombia	2.21
Alaska (Urban Eskimos)	2.31[b]
Chile	2.74
Lebanon (Lebanese)	2.98
Thailand	3.30
Lebanon (Palestinian refugees)	3.52
Burma	3.58
Jordan (Jordanian civilians)	3.96
Vietnam (Hill tribesmen)	3.97
Trinidad	4.21
Jordan (Palestinian refugees)	4.41

The Epidemiology and Biometry Branch of the National Institute of Dental Research, U.S. Public Health Service.
[a]Ages 40–44 only.
[b]Males only.

Age Relationships

There is a positive correlation between the extent and prevalence of gingivitis and periodontal disease and increasing age. As seen in Figure 3-1, the PI scores of the population as a whole increase with increasing age. This increase in PI scores with increasing age reflects not only a worsening of a preexisting periodontal condition, but also an increase in the number of individuals affected. As illustrated in Figure 3-3, the portion of the population affected by the disease increased from about 10 percent in young adults to 60 percent in the 65- to 74-year age groups.

The relationship of PI score to age has been observed in all population groups studied. For example, note the similarity of the curve in Figure 3-1 and that in Figure 3-4, which is derived from a completely different population. The same result is observed, regardless of the index of measurement used. For exam-

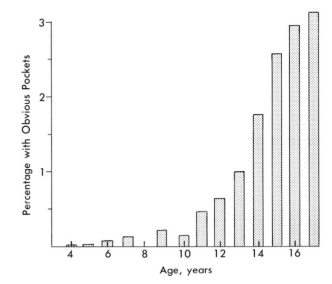

FIG. 3-2. *Percentage of children in the United States exhibiting one or more obvious periodontal pockets. (Adapted from data of Russell, A. L.: In Periodontal Therapy. H. M. Goldman and D. W. Cohn, Eds. St. Louis, C. V. Mosby, 1973, p. 69.)*

ple, Figure 3-5 presents data from a study in India where an index of bone loss measured radiographically was used and similar results are seen. The level of oral cleanliness is also related to age. As illustrated in Figures 3-6 and 3-7, both plaque and calculus scores increase with increasing age, and the portion of the population exhibiting poor oral hygiene also becomes larger. The true implication of these observations is not yet clear.

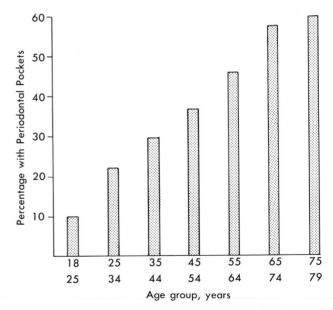

FIG. 3-3. *Periodontal status of American adult males for years 1960–1962. (Adapted from data of Johnson, Kelly, and van Kirk. In Russell, A. L.: Epidemiology of periodontal disease. Int. Dent. J., 17:282, 1967.)*

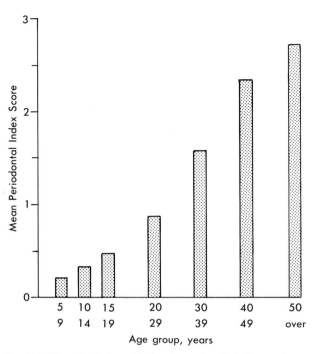

FIG. 3-4. *Mean Periodontal Index Score for all civilian males in Ecuador and Montana. (Adapted from Greene, J. C.: Oral hygiene and periodontal disease. Am. J. Public Health, 53:913, 1963.)*

Etiologic Factors

A strong positive correlation has been established between PI scores and the level of oral cleanliness. Indeed, as shown in Table 3-4, over 90 percent of the variance observed in populations with periodontal disease can be accounted for by the age and oral hygiene variables alone.

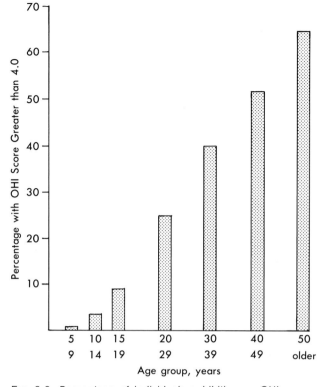

FIG. 3-6. *Percentage of individuals exhibiting an OHI score greater than 4.0. Combined data from Ecuador and Montana. (From Scherp, H.: Current concepts in periodontal disease research. J. Am. Dent. Assoc., 68:667, 1964. Copyright by the American Dental Association. Reprinted by permission.)*

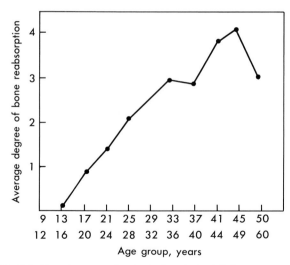

FIG. 3-5. *Prevalence and extent of periodontal disease vs age in population in India as measured by an index of bone resorption on radiographs. (Adapted from Marshall-Day, C. D., and Shourie, K. L.: The incidence of periodontal disease in the Punjab Indian. J. Am. Dent. Assoc., 39:572, 1944.)*

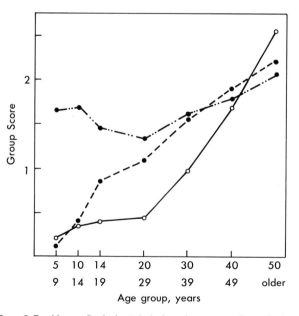

FIG. 3-7. *Mean Periodontal Index (—○———○—), calculus (--●---●--), and debris (—●— ·· —●—) scores for all individuals examined in Ecuador and Montana. Data for 5,685 persons including civilian and military personnel. (Adapted from Greene, J. C.: Oral hygiene and periodontal disease. Am. J. Public Health, 53:913, 1963.)*

TABLE 3-4. *Effects on Periodontal Index Scores of Age and Oral Hygiene Status Considered Simultaneously for Vietnamese and Lebanese Populations*

ITEM	SOUTH VIETNAM	LEBANON	BOTH COMBINED
Coefficient of multiple correlation	+0.96	+0.97	+0.95
Percentage of variance explained	91.7	93.3	90.3
Age	36.0	41.7	47.2
Hygiene	55.7	51.6	42.4

Data from Russell, A. L.: International nutrition surveys: A summary of preliminary dental findings. *J. Dent. Res.,* 42(suppl.):233, 1963.

Investigations aimed at demonstrating a relationship between PI scores and factors other than oral cleanliness have been generally unsuccessful. Russell failed to establish significant correlations between PI scores and each of the following: geography, fluoride content of the drinking water, ABO blood groups, serum protein levels, hemoglobin levels, socioeconomic status, or levels of vitamin A, ascorbic acid, thiamine, niacin, nicotinamide, or riboflavin.[17] Furthermore, with the exception of diabetes mellitus, various disease states do not appear to be associated specifically with gingival and periodontal status on an epidemiologic basis. Although early observations appeared to establish a greater prevalence of inflammatory gingival and periodontal disease in males than in females, this difference has been shown to disappear when the variables of age and oral hygiene status are taken into account.[5]

LIMITATIONS ON INTERPRETATION OF DATA

The Periodontal Index and the Periodontal Disease Index overcome many of the problems encountered in the application of epidemiologic methods to problems of gingival and periodontal disease. However, these indices and others in current use are based on assumptions and judgments that must be taken into account in the evaluation and interpretation of the resulting data.

Relative Values Upon Which the Indices are Based

The Periodontal Index and the Periodontal Disease Index were designed to reflect the true periodontal status of a population in order that differences among populations and within the same population at different times could be measured. Thus, it was essential to determine which manifestations of the disease are important and the relative values of these manifestations one to another. Furthermore, it was necessary that these relative values have validity in terms of the progress and eventual outcome of the disease. These judgments, of necessity, have been made on an empirical basis, since the natural history of gingivitis and periodontal disease is only poorly understood. Their absolute validity remains to be demonstrated.

Both the Periodontal Index and the Periodontal Disease Index are based on the presence and extent of soft-tissue inflammation and pathologic pocket formation. In addition, Russell included mobility and loss of function among his criteria. While both indices are based on similar pathologic manifestations of disease, they differ significantly in the relative values assigned to these manifestations and in the size of the scales used to measure them. In the PI, gingivitis may account for a score of 2 on a scale from 0 to 8; in the PDI it can account for a score of 3 on a scale from 0 to 6. Thus, the PDI would appear to be weighted more heavily in favor of the early manifestation of disease. In the PI, a tooth exhibiting early pocket formation merits a value three times as great as one with gingivitis alone; in the PDI, the score for early apical epithelial migration is 4 and for gingivitis is 3. Differences exist also in the upper ranges of the scales. In the PI, all teeth exhibiting stages of pocket formation from early to terminal disease, but still in functional occlusion, are assigned the same value of 6, but in the PDI no distinction is made among teeth with pocket depths greater than 6 mm. Thus, the PI appears to weigh early pocket formation as the most significant feature of the disease, and in the PDI, gingivitis is relatively the most important manifestation.

Assumption of Uniformity of the Disease State

Both the PI and the PDI are based on the assumption that all forms of inflammatory disease of the gingiva and other supporting tissues can be considered as a single entity. The term *periodontal disease* has been defined all-inclusively as "an inflammatory lesion affecting one or more of the supporting structures of the teeth. . . ."[16,20] This assumption may be partly justified on the basis that inflammatory disease resulting from plaque accumulation forms the great bulk of all gingival and periodontal disease. However, the essential corollary is the assumption that gingivitis is an early form of periodontal disease which, in the absence of therapeutic intervention, progresses to a chronic destructive lesion. While this assumption is a rational and safe therapeutic principle of long standing, the data available currently do not appear to justify its validity as a basis for epidemiologic investigations in man. Indeed, a form of gingivitis which is self-limiting and which does not usually progress to chronic inflammatory periodontal disease has been described in subhuman primates.[1,19] If a disease of this type also occurs in man, currently held views based on epidemiologic observations may require reconsideration.

CONCEPTS EMERGING FROM EPIDEMIOLOGIC CONSIDERATIONS

In spite of the limitations of the data, the epidemiologic studies have strongly influenced our views on prevention, diagnosis, and treatment of inflammatory gingival and periodontal disease.

Universality of Destructive Inflammatory Periodontal Disease

The view that periodontal disease is of almost universal prevalence in human populations is a widely held concept which influences both research and therapy in a major way. Support for this concept derives almost totally from the epidemiologic data. Careful scrutiny of the data demonstrates beyond doubt that gingivitis is indeed extremely widespread. However, extrapolation of the data to support the idea of the universal prevalence of inflammatory periodontal disease of a severity great enough to be clinically important appears to be open to serious question. As illustrated by the data presented in Figures 3-1, 3-4, and 3-7, Periodontal Index scores for adult males in the United States and indeed for most well-nourished population groups rarely exceed 3, even in the most advanced age groups. Since gingivitis alone can account for a score of 2, and the minimal value possible for pocket formation is 6, the data appear to suggest that it is gingivitis, not chronic periodontitis, that is present in most of the population studied. Thus, the whole concept of the universality of chronic destructive periodontal disease rests on the assumption that gingivitis is an early form of chronic periodontal disease. Although this assumption may be true, its validity remains to be proved.

Plaque and Calculus as the Primary Etiologic Agents

The major contribution of epidemiologists has been documentation of the concept that the presence of oral debris is related to the prevalence and extent of periodontal disease. It has been shown repeatedly that the correlation between these factors is positive and large. This observation has been interpreted generally to mean that the accumulation of microbial deposits on the teeth is related etiologically to gingivitis and periodontal disease. The conclusion has been justifiably criticized as an overextension of the data, and it has been pointed out that a positive correlation does not demonstrate a cause and effect relationship. Indeed, some investigators have suggested that tooth deposits may be a consequence rather than a cause of inflammatory disease resulting from the creation by the disease of a favorable milieu for the adherence and growth of microorganisms. There are compelling reasons for not accepting this view. Löe and his colleagues demonstrated that gingivitis can be induced in humans by allowing microbial colonization and growth on the teeth, and the manifestations of disease can be alleviated by reinstitution of plaque control measures.[10] Furthermore, Lövdal et al. reported a remarkable improvement in the periodontal status of a group of factory workers resulting from the institution of a program of controlled oral hygiene and professional care.[11] Thus, currently available evidence supports, but does not prove definitively, that the accumulation of microbial deposits is related in a determinative way to the induction and progress of inflammatory periodontal disease.

Debris-Time-Disease Relationships

Epidemiologic considerations have led Greene to formulate the whole problem of inflammatory periodontal disease in the following manner:[4,5]

$$\text{HEALTHY TISSUES} + \text{CALCULUS/DEBRIS} \xrightarrow{\text{Time}}$$

$$\text{INFLAMMATORY PERIODONTAL DISEASE}$$

This concept may be an oversimplification, since it tends to minimize the role of the host immunopathologic and other destructive inflammatory mechanisms in the tissue damage characteristic of the disease. Furthermore, it does not take into account the possibility that the presence of certain specific microorganisms, which may be absent from some plaques, may be essential for induction of the disease. The concept is supported by much of the epidemiologic data and it does serve to illustrate the interactions of the etiologic agent with time. The concept implies that a certain amount of gingival and periodontal disease may be an inevitable consequence of aging, since it is virtually impossible for the oral cavity to be free of debris continuously.

SUMMARY

Epidemiologic methods have been used to measure the extent and severity of inflammatory diseases of the periodontium in human populations on a worldwide scale. Indices devised for this purpose have been most useful in characterizing the relationships of microbiologic factors and age to the observed disease state. The indices are based on the assumption that gingivitis is an early form of destructive inflammatory periodontal disease and that inflammatory diseases of the periodontal tissues comprise a reasonably homogeneous group. These assumptions have not yet been shown to be entirely valid.

The data establish beyond reasonable doubt that plaque accumulation and increasing age of the host are intimately related to the induction and progress of gingivitis. The relationship of these factors to destructive inflammatory periodontal disease remains open for future investigation.

References

1. Ammons, W. F., Schectman, L. R., and Page, R. C.: Host tissue response in chronic periodontal disease. I. The normal periodontium and clinical manifestations of dental and periodontal disease in the marmoset. J. Periodont. Res., 7:131, 1972.
2. Clark, E. G.: Modern concepts of epidemiology. J. Chronic Dis., 2:593, 1955.
3. Fox, J. P., Hall, C. E., and Elveback, L. R.: Epidemiology, Man and Disease. New York, The Macmillan Co., 1970.
4. Greene, J. C.: Epidemiology and indexing of periodontal disease. J. Periodontol., 29:133, 1958.
5. Greene, J. C.: Oral hygiene and periodontal disease. Am. J. Public Health, 53:913, 1963.
6. Greene, J. C., and Vermillion, R. J.: Oral hygiene index: A method for classifying oral hygiene status. J. Am. Dent. Assoc., 61:172, 1960.
7. Greene, J. C., and Vermillion, R. J.: The simplified oral hygiene index. J. Am. Dent. Assoc., 68:7, 1964.
8. Johnson, E. S., Kelly, J. E., and Van Kirk, L. E.: Selected dental findings in adults by age, race and sex, U.S. 1960–1962. Vital Health Stat., 11:1, 1965.
9. King, J. D.: Gingival disease in Dundee. Dent. Rec., 65:9,32,38, 1945.
10. Löe, H., Theilade, E., and Jensen, S. B.: Experimental gingivitis in man. J. Periodont., 36:177, 1965.
11. Lövdal, A., et al.: Combined effect of subgingival scaling and controlled oral hygiene on the incidence of gingivitis. Acta Odont. Scand., 19:537, 1961.
12. Marshall-Day, C. D., and Shourie, K. L.: The incidence of periodontal disease in the Punjab Indian. J. Med. Res., 32:47, 1944.
13. Massler, M., Schour, I., and Chopra, B.: Occurrence of gingivitis in suburban Chicago school children. J. Periodontol., 21:146, 1950.
14. National Center for Health Statistics, Periodontal Disease and Oral Hygiene among Children. Series 11, #117, June 1972.
15. Ramfjord, S. P.: Indices for prevalence and incidence of periodontal disease. J. Periodontol., 30:51, 1959.
16. Rosebury, T.: Role of infection in periodontal disease. Oral Surg., 5:363, 1952.
17. Russell, A. L.: Epidemiology of periodontal disease. Int. Dent. J., 17:282, 1967.
18. Russell, A. L.: Systems of classification and scoring for prevalence surveys of periodontal disease. J. Dent. Res., 35:350, 1956.
19. Schectman, L. R., et al.: Host tissue response in chronic periodontal disease. II. Histologic features of the normal periodontium and histopathologic and ultrastructural manifestations of disease in the marmoset. J. Periodont. Res., 7:195, 1972.
20. Scherp, H.: Current concepts in periodontal disease research: Epidemiological contribution. J. Am. Dent. Assoc., 68:667, 1964.
21. Schour, I., and Massler, M.: Gingival disease in postwar Italy (1945). I. Prevalence of gingivitis in various age groups. J. Am. Dent. Assoc., 35:475, 1947.
22. World Health Organization. Periodontal disease: Report of an expert committee on dental health. (Members: Emslie, R. D., Held, A. M., Kostlan, J., Rice, F. B., Verhoestraete, L., Waerhaug, J.) Geneva, August, 1960. Int. Dent. J., 11:544, 1961.

4

Etiology of Periodontal Disease

It will not be necessary in this report to say anything of the etiology of the disease under discussion, beyond the expression of the belief that it is infectious, and that microorganisms are at least partially responsible for the disastrous results which are sure to follow if it is not checked before complete destruction of the alveoli.—A. W. Harlan, 1883

Etiology encompasses the sum of knowledge relating to the causes of a disease. Most of our presently held concepts of the etiology of inflammatory gingival and periodontal disease were originated over a century ago by individuals whose primary interest was in patient care, and these concepts were based predominantly upon clinical experience rather than upon scientific observation and experimentation. The picture generally presented of the etiology of inflammatory gingival and periodontal disease is one of an exceedingly complex interaction of local oral factors with systemic, emotional, and environmental conditions.[46,53,56] Historically, the relative importance placed on local and systemic factors has varied greatly from time to time. In order to grasp an understanding of the local and systemic concept of the etiology, it is important to examine its evolution.

Historical Perspective

In most ancient medical works, local tooth deposits were considered to be of utmost importance in causing chronic disease of the gums and alveolar bone, and removal of these deposits, along with tooth extraction, was the most commonly employed means of treatment (see Chapter 2). However, by the time the first books on dental pathology were published, systemic conditions were considered to be important.[35,38,76] For example, Koecker noted several "remote" causes,[89] and both Hunter and Fox discussed the role of "constitutional" factors.[38,76] Constitutional or remote causes noted by Koecker included irregularities in tooth position, the use of tobacco, neglect of cleanliness, injudiciously performed dental operations, excessive use of certain medicaments, application of irritating tooth powders, especially those containing charcoal, and systemic diseases including tuberculosis and scurvy. However, the bulk of opinion continued to espouse the idea that tooth deposits were the most important factor. Koecker and his contemporaries alike, felt that the remote causes or systemic factors were important primarily because they enhanced the accumulation of deposits on the teeth. Koecker stated "by the above causes, a collection of tartar, without which I have never seen this disease, is deposited upon particular parts of the teeth, and this becomes the immediate or exciting cause of the disease. . . ."[89]

4

Etiology

of

Periodontal

Disease

The key role of local factors or deposits in the induction of the disease pervaded thinking until the latter part of the nineteenth century. Hunter felt that "anything that occasions a considerable and long-contained inflammation" will induce the disease.[76] However, the importance of dental deposits and other local factors in the etiology of the disease was not universally accepted, and prior to the end of the nineteenth century, the pendulum began to swing more strongly toward the importance of systemic factors. In a paper presented before the meeting of the American Dental Association in Chicago in 1877, Rehnwinkel argued persuasively for the importance of hereditary and systemic factors.[149,151,184] Rawls wrote:

Local-cause theorists are at variance as to the cause, some claiming salivary calculus as its origin; a limited number sanguinary calculus; and still others that the affectation is resultant from a peculiar organism of fungus growth which always fills pockets.[149]

He refers somewhat caustically to Black's view of microbial plaque as an important factor thus:

This is one of the numerous germ theories, and is founded upon the fact of the presence in these cases of little hot-beds of peculiar organisms of fungi, which, according to supporters of the theory, cause melting away of the pericemental membrane, by what means is not definitely understood, but presumably the digestive fluids of the fungus growth causing a remolecularization of tissues exposed to their action.[149]

In light of this statement, it is interesting to note that the *Actinomyces*, an organism currently considered by many investigators to be an important etiologic agent, was classified until recently as a fungus.

The complexity of the etiologic problem resulting, at least in part, from the emphasis placed upon systemic factors and which remains to a great extent unresolved today, was heralded by Talbot who acknowledged no fewer than 22 causes of the disease:

We may consider, then, as predisposing and exciting causes a perverted condition of the secretions, low vitality, sanguinary calculus, and all diseases which affect the circulation, and as among the local causes catarrah, fistulae, salivary calculus, irritation from foreign substances such as detached bristles from the toothbrush, too great friction in brushing, injudicious use of the toothpick, the use of ligatures and regulating apparatus, application of the rubber dam and clamps, artificial dentures and regulating plates, accumulation and decomposition of food under artificial dentures and at the necks of the teeth, drugs which overstimulate the parts, the use of tobacco, fillings extending beyond the cervical margins, digestive derangements, contagion from unclean instruments, and improper mouthwashes and tooth powders, especially charcoal.[184]

Thus, by the turn of the nineteenth century, almost every facet of the human condition had been claimed as an etiologic factor in the disease. Talbot concluded that "in a word whatever irritates the peridental membrane is likely to produce the lesion under consideration."[184]

Current Views

While there seems little question that both local tooth deposits and constitutional or systemic factors are active in the disease, efforts to simplify the etiology problem and to evaluate the relative importance of various local and systemic factors by experimental observation have been fraught with difficulties, and these continue today to hamper progress. Inflammatory gingival and periodontal disease belongs to a family of long-term, chronic inflammatory diseases with immunopathologic aspects, including tuberculosis and rheumatoid arthritis. In diseases of this type, the initial inciting event, which may have occurred at some time in the distant past, may be obscured by subsequent developments to the extent that its recognition and definition may become impossible. In other words, it may not be possible to distinguish those features of the pathogenesis resulting from extrinsic factors such as microbial plaque or bacteria from those associated with exuberant or aberrant destructive host defense mechanisms. Furthermore, the natural history of the disease in humans is not understood, and observations have been severely limited by technical problems. In addition, until recently, satisfactory experimental animal models have not been available.[16]

In spite of the problems described, significant progress has been made in recent years. There is now overwhelming evidence that organisms present in microbial plaque and in the region of the gingival sulcus and pocket, or substances derived from them, constitute the primary and possibly the only extrinsic etiologic agent participating in the etiology of inflammatory gingival and periodontal disease.[31,40,177] However, it is also apparent that the disease is not an infection in the usual sense of the word in which bacteria invade the tissues and induce tissue destruction and necrosis. Except in specialized cases such as acute necrotizing gingivitis and acute periodontal abscess, microorganisms do not invade the tissues. Instead, they appear to participate by activation of destructive immunologic and other inflammatory reactions in the host and these lead, at least in major part, to the observed pathologic alterations in the tissues.[41,67,73,131,139] Thus, an understanding of the etiology of the disease requires consideration not only of (1) the role of microorganisms, but also of (2) conditions that may affect or enhance the accumulation and growth of plaque or preclude or interfere with its removal, (3) local and systemic or constitutional factors that may alter the resistance or susceptibility of the tissues of the periodontium to bacterial and other noxious substances, and (4) individual variation in the relative destructive and protective aspects of the host defense mechanisms.

MICROORGANISMS AS THE PRIMARY EXTRINSIC ETIOLOGIC AGENT

Although the mechanisms remain unclear, there now seems little doubt that microorganisms colonizing the tooth surface or residing within the gingival sulcus or periodontal pocket are the primary extrinsic etiologic agent causing inflammatory gingival and periodontal disease. The evidence supporting this contention derives from several different sources.

Population Studies

A positive correlation between the presence of microbial deposits on the teeth and the presence and extent of inflammatory disease of the periodontium has been shown repeatedly in human population studies.[57,165] However, since the presence of acute inflammation of the tissues may enhance bacterial colonization and plaque growth on the teeth,[164] it has not been possible to rule out unequivocally that the accumulation of deposits is a consequence rather than a cause of the disease, although the available evidence does not support this concept.[110] Although the association of deposits with gingivitis appears to be clear, problems inherent in the various epidemiologic indices (see Chapter 3), make a definitive association of microbial plaque per se with periodontitis more difficult.

Inducibility of Gingivitis and Periodontitis

Individuals previously exercising intensive plaque control measures, and free of gingivitis and periodontitis, develop gingivitis within 1 to 3 weeks after all means of plaque control are withdrawn.[79,108,142,188,196] A similar response occurs in beagle dogs,[64,100,103,163] and in subhuman primates.[91] In beagle dogs, continuation of conditions enhancing the growth of microbial plaque for months or years leads to the development of periodontitis with loss of the alveolar bone.[100] Whether a response of this type occurs in humans has not been proved definitively, although this appears likely to be the case. Accumulating plaque is made up almost totally of microorganisms.[182] Institution of measures to prevent the accumulation of microbial plaque, either by chemical means such as the use of chlorhexidine or antibiotics or mechanical means such as effective tooth brushing, results in the resolution of the disease and the restoration of gingival health.[79,107,109,124]

Effectiveness of Antibiotics

The use of antibiotics such as penicillin, kanamycin, vancomycin and others which act exclusively on microorganisms is effective in controlling some forms of gingival and periodontal disease in humans[79,124] and in preventing the periodontal syndrome in rats[25,59,126] and in hamsters.[82] These data indicate that microorganisms affected by antibiotics are related etiologically to the disease. More recently, Socransky and his colleagues have shown that broad-spectrum antibiotics such as chlortetracycline are effective adjuncts in treating rapidly progressing forms of periodontal disease.[128,129]

Ineffectiveness of Factors Other than Bacteria in Induction of the Disease

Local mechanical irritation and occlusal trauma have been proposed as important etiologic agents, but experimental observations do not support this concept. Rovin, Costich, and Gordon have shown that mechanical irritation induced in germ-free rats by the placement of silk ligatures around the necks of the teeth does not induce inflammatory changes, whereas this same procedure in conventional control animals results in plaque accumulation and gingival disease.[158] The placement of silk ligatures in beagle dogs[103] and subhuman primates leads to enhanced plaque accumulation and rapidly progressive periodontitis around teeth previously relatively free of the disease. Furthermore, in beagle dogs, experimentally induced occlusal trauma of teeth kept free of plaque fail to develop periodontitis, but similarly traumatized teeth in the same animal allowed to accumulate plaque exhibit periodontitis with rapid bone destruction.[102] A similar result from experimentally induced mechanical trauma was observed in subhuman primates.[144] While various systemic conditions including hormonal imbalance, protein-calorie malnutrition, vitamin and trace-mineral deficiency, and systemic diseases such as diabetes and various blood dyscrasias predispose to the development of inflammatory gingival and periodontal disease and aggravate previously existing disease, none of these conditions, in the absence of bacterial component, has the capacity to induce inflammatory periodontal disease.[46]

Nature of Effective Therapeutic Techniques

Techniques of treatment of gingivitis and chronic periodontal disease are directed almost totally toward debridement and control of the accumulation of bacterial plaque. In most individuals and animals, although not all,[65] these measures are effective.[110]

Transmissibility of the Disease in Animals

A form of gingival and periodontal disease can be induced in strains of hamsters which do not usually exhibit the disease by exposure to microorganisms obtained from susceptible hamsters which do exhibit the disease.[80,82,83] The agent responsible has been isolated and identified as *Actinomyces viscosus* (earlier classified as *Odontomyces viscosus*).[75] In addition, a penicillin-sensitive transmissible agent has also been shown to be responsible for the periodontal syndrome occurring in the rice rat.[25,59,126] The introduction of certain streptococci and gram-positive rods induces a transmissible form of gingival and periodontal disease in gnotobiotic rats and hamsters.[43] More recently, Socransky and his colleagues have demonstrated severe periodontal destruction in gnotobiotic rats monoinfected with various gram-negative microorganisms obtained from rapidly progressing human periodontitis.[77]

Pathogenicity of Plaque-Derived Microorganisms

Microorganisms present in plaque have considerable pathogenic potential when examined in various test systems. Rosebury and his colleagues showed that the injection of suspensions of viable plaque material into the skin of guinea pigs resulted in abscess formation, and that the lesion could be transmitted from one animal to another by use of the wound exudate, thereby demonstrating that these microorganisms can be pathogenic when they gain entrance to the connective tissues of skin.[37,111,155,156] In further experiments, attempts were made to differentiate between the potentially pathogenic and nonpathogenic flora. The observations indicated that spirochetes are necessary for abscess induction in the guinea pig system, and this observation gave rise to the concept, which was held for many years, that inflammatory gingival and periodontal disease may be a fusospirochetal infection.

The observations using the guinea pig system were extended by Macdonald and his colleagues.[110,112,113]

Pure cultures and various combinations of microorganisms were tested for their capacity to induce abscess formation. Generally, pure strains of these microorganisms were ineffective and, contrary to previous observations, spirochetes were not essential for positive results. Certain mixtures were able to induce abscess formation which could be transmitted from one animal to another. The mixture of microorganisms that was most effective in the guinea pig system consisted of two strains of *Bacteroides*, a motile gram-negative rod and a facultative diphtheroid. However, three of these four organisms could be replaced by substitution of other microorganisms or by specific nutrients, indicating that their role in the pathologic process was limited to that of providing favorable growth conditions for the remaining organisms. One microorganism, *Bacteroides melaninogenicus*, was essential for the induction of lesions. The pathogenicity of this microorganism was considered to be related to its unusual capacity to produce an enzyme that hydrolyzes native collagen.

The studies of Rosebury and Macdonald and their coworkers showed beyond doubt that the microorganisms present in dental plaque are potentially pathogenic, and that the pathogenicity of certain organisms may be enhanced by the presence of others in experimental lesions. The observations also highlighted the importance of the presence of viable, actively metabolizing microorganisms in lesion induction. These data, however, cannot be extrapolated to direct application to the problem of human gingival and periodontal disease. Since the assay system used was the induction of abscesses in guinea pig skin, lesions of this kind may bear little relationship to the long-term chronic inflammatory lesions seen in human periodontal disease. Furthermore, infectious microorganisms exhibit a considerable degree of species and tissue specificity. For example, bovine tubercle bacilli are not pathogenic in man, and the enteric microorganisms comprising the commensal flora of the gut are highly pathogenic when injected into the connective tissues. Thus, demonstration of the effectiveness of *Bacteroides melaninogenicus* and other microorganisms in the induction of abscesses in guinea pig skin indicates a measure of pathogenicity, but does not necessarily imply a comparable activity in the human gingival sulcus.

In addition to the demonstration of the capacity of plaque microorganisms to induce abscesses, there are other more compelling reasons to consider these microorganisms to be potential pathogens. Living, metabolizing plaque organisms elaborate a host of substances that may be noxious to viable tissues.[177] Among these are collagenase, hyaluronidase, fibrinolysin, chondroitin sulfatase, neuraminidase, DNAase and RNAase, several proteases, and numerous metabolites, including ammonia, urea, hydrogen sulfide, indole, toxic amines, and organic acids.

Nonviable plaque-derived microorganisms release cellular components that have the capacity to induce tissue damage. The injection of heat-killed human dental plaque into the skin of rabbits induces long-term chronic inflammatory lesions.[121,170] Gram-negative microorganisms, which make up a large portion of dental plaque, release endotoxin, a lipopolysaccharide-protein complex, upon death. The injection of this substance into gingival tissues of rabbits induces a reaction characterized by an acute inflammatory response that persists and leads to alveolar bone destruction.[152] Furthermore, a cell-wall component containing mucopeptide and polysaccharide can be obtained from *Actinomyces viscosus* and certain other gram-positive streptococci that are present in dental plaque. This substance induces chronic long-term inflammatory lesions in rabbits that exhibit many histopathologic features characteristic of chronic periodontal disease.[137] Thus, not only may actively metabolizing microorganisms be important in the pathogenesis of periodontal disease but also, upon death, the organisms present in plaque may induce a toxic effect upon the living gingival tissues.

Accessibility of Plaque-Derived Substances to the Connective Tissues

A large body of evidence indicates that substances from microbial plaque can gain entrance into the tissues of the inflamed periodontium and that these substances have the capacity to induce destructive inflammatory and immunopathologic reactions. Using standard immunofluorescence techniques, antigenic determinants of plaque microorganisms have been demonstrated in the connective-tissue portion of inflamed gingiva.[23,115,191] Similarly, Shapiro and his co-workers, using the limulus lysate assay procedure, demonstrated the presence of endotoxin both in the fluid exuding from the gingival sulcus of inflamed tissue and in the tissue itself.[172] The levels of endotoxin increased proportionately with the increasing severity of the inflammation. However, it should be pointed out that the dependability of the limulus lysate assay procedure has been recently questioned.

While there are considerable data to support the idea that plaque-derived substances can gain entrance into inflamed gingival tissues, transport or diffusion across the intact epithelial barrier appears to be essential for induction of the initial inflammatory lesion, and an important question remaining is whether this can occur. Although the pathway and mechanism of entrance remain unclear, the bulk of the evidence indicates that passage does occur. Over 20 years ago, Schultz-Haudt, Dewar, and Bibby and Schultz-Haudt, Bibby, and Bruce demonstrated that the application to the gingival sulcus of hydrolytic enzymes such as hyaluronidase, which can be elaborated by plaque microorganisms, results in alteration of the intercellular cementing substance between the epithelial cells adjacent to the tooth surface.[168,169] Test antigens such as albumin when applied repeatedly to the gingival sulcus region induce the differentiation of clones of plasma cells,[153] and a comparable application in monkeys leads to accumulation of plasma cells in the gingiva and development of an allergic form of gingival disease.[148] In normal beagle dogs, the application of radioactively labeled endotoxin to the gingival sulcus for a relatively short time interval resulted in the appearance of radioactivity within the connective tissues, especially around the blood vessels.[171]

Immunologic studies provide even more compelling evidence that plaque-derived substances can gain entrance to the gingival connective tissues. While the amount entering may be small and detection of the quantities present requires sophisticated techniques, the immune system can be considered to serve as an amplifier of the entrance of such substances, and demonstration of a humoral or cell-mediated immune response is proof tantamount to the presence of these substances. In both normal and periodontally diseased humans, circulating antibodies to oral microorganisms have been found,[34,122,181] and in some instances increased antibody titers have been recorded in humans with inflammatory periodontal disease.

The peripheral blood leukocytes of individuals with gingivitis and periodontitis, when maintained *in vitro* in the presence of plaque antigens or microorganisms, undergo blast transformation with lymphokine production.[74,78] This reaction is considered to be an *in vitro* correlate of cell-mediated hypersensitivity and serves to demonstrate the presence of sensitized lymphoid cells. In some individuals with periodontal disease, positive responses to skin tests indicative of humoral hypersensitivity reactions can be induced by using preparations of plaque microorganisms as antigens.[132] Diseased gingiva contains large amounts of immunoglobulin,[14,166] and a portion of this antibody is specific for antigens present in microbial plaque.[23,115,166,187] The application of test antigens such as horseradish peroxidase results in entrance of antigen into the tissues and to the differentiation of clones of plasma cells within the gingiva, producing antibody specific for the test antigen.[116,117,118] Thus, evidence from numerous sources supports the concept that antigenic and other noxious substances may cross the epithelial barrier in both normal and inflamed gingiva and gain access into the vascular and lymphoid systems.

Specific Microorganisms and Human Periodontitis

Although the case for a primary bacteriologic etiology for both gingivitis and periodontitis is well documented, the search for association of specific bacteria with the disease process has been unfruitful. Clearly this search comprises one of the most important quests in periodontal research today. If specific microorganisms or groups of microorganisms can be shown to be associated with the disease etiologically, then a means of controlling the disease by elimination or control of these specific microorganisms may emerge. This search is complicated by the fact that we do not yet know if actively metabolizing microorganisms, the products elaborated by these microorganisms, or the substances derived from them after death are the primary cause of the disease.

In order to associate specific bacteria or groups of microorganisms with gingivitis and periodontitis in a determinative way, the following criteria must be met. At the present time, no single microorganism, product or group of microorganisms has been shown to meet these criteria.

1. The presence of the organism (or group) or its products at the site of the gingival sulcus in quantities sufficiently large as to induce the observed disease state.
2. Demonstration that these organisms or products can gain access to the connective tissues of the periodontium across the intact epithelial barrier or can alter the intact epithelial barrier to the extent that subsequent passage is possible.
3. Demonstration of a capacity of the organism (or group) to induce progressive inflammatory disease in man or to induce the human form of the disease in experimental animal systems.

In spite of the dramatic successes in showing pathogenicity of oral microorganisms and inducing a form of periodontal disease in rodents, it has not yet been possible to associate definitively a specific microbiota with various forms of gingivitis and periodontitis in humans, although recently acquired data indicate that such a relationship may indeed exist.

One of the earliest attempts to demonstrate associa-

tion of a specific microbiota with human suppurative periodontitis was the study of Hemmens and Harrison.[68] These investigators found no major differences in the flora of normal and diseased human populations, although their negative result may have been due to technical problems. Using pooled samples of scrapings from the teeth and dark-field microscopy for analysis, Rosebury, Macdonald, and Clark found that certain organisms such as spirochetes, vibrios, and fusiform bacilli were present in material from diseased teeth in far greater numbers than in material from normal teeth, although qualitative differences were not demonstrated.[156] Subsequently, Schultz-Haudt, Bibby, and Bruce did a similar experiment using stained smears of scrapings from the teeth.[168] They, too, found no bacterial types in scrapings from patients with gingivitis and periodontitis that did not occur around normal teeth, although in most cases the total numbers of these organisms were considerably greater than normal.

Socransky et al.[178] and Gibbons et al.[44] thoroughly analyzed the cultivable microorganisms of pooled plaque from the region of the gingival sulcus of normal individuals and those with periodontal disease, using culture techniques, gross counts, and other means of analysis. They failed to find significant differences between normal and periodontally diseased individuals, except in the amount of gingival debris and therefore in the numbers of organisms present around the teeth. Salkind, Oshrain, and Mandel studied the populations of microorganisms accumulating on Mylar strips placed supragingivally and subgingivally in normal individuals with various states of gingival inflammation.[161] They found larger numbers of vibrios and fusobacteria in the subgingival than in the supragingival areas, and in a later study they found that the flora accumulating during the first 10 minutes on strips contained in a meticulously cleaned periodontal pocket was made up mostly of gram-positive cocci and rods with a few gram-negative rods and filaments.[136] Vibrios and fusobacteria were not seen.

Several recent studies have been done on specific types of pockets using sophisticated culture techniques for analysis of the microbiota. Dwyer and Socransky analyzed the microbiota of individual advanced periodontal pockets in 5 patients.[28] Streptococcus mitis was the most plentiful microorganism encountered, comprising 29.4 percent of the total flora, with Bacteroides melaninogenicus present in high numbers in 3 of 5 samples where it averaged 9.5 percent of the total flora. In a separate study Kelstrup was unable to correlate the presence of Bacteroides melaninogenicus with the inflammatory status.[81] Sabiston and Grigsby examined the flora of the roots of teeth around which 50 percent or more of the alveolar bone had been lost.[160]

They found low numbers of gram-negative organisms; of 50 strains studied, about half were facultative cocci and about half obligate anaerobes, mainly of the peptostreptococcal type.

Williams, Pantalone, and Sherris also studied the predominant cultivable subgingival flora of subjects with moderate periodontitis, using continuous anaerobic culture and sophisticated sampling techniques.[193] They found considerable variability in microbial populations at various sites in the same subjects. They detected no qualitative differences between the pathologically affected and the normal sites; however, they did find larger populations of facultative organisms of the *Actinomyces* type and other gram-positive rods in the pathologically affected sites than in the normal. Using material classified as mild periodontitis along with similar comprehensive sampling and culture techniques, Darwish, Hyppa, and Socransky studied pockets of four individual subjects.[24] As in the Williams, Pantalone, and Sherris study, they found considerable variation from one case to another. In two of the individuals where scaling had been done 2 weeks before sampling, the predominant cultivable flora was *Streptococcus sanguis* and *Actinomyces viscosus*, populations similar to those in supragingival plaque in the same individuals. However, in two other individuals in which no scaling had been done, predominantly anaerobic organisms with peptostreptococci predominating in one subject and *Bacteroides melaninogenicus* and *Actinomyces israelii* in the other were found. The microbiota differed from subject to subject, although the clinical conditions were seemingly similar.

Recently, Newman and Socransky studied the flora of pockets of individuals with rapidly progressing lesions classified as periodontosis as well as samples taken from clinically normal sites in the same individuals.[128] The flora from the control sites was predominantly gram-positive, comprising mostly *Streptococcus sanguis*, *Streptococcus mitis*, *Staphylococcus* and large numbers of gram-positive filamentous rods of the actinomyces type, and *Propionibacterium acnes*. On the other hand, the flora from the advancing front of the pockets was 43 to 78 percent gram-negative anaerobic rods, many of which had not been identified and characterized previously.

Currently there is no satisfactory explanation for the obvious variation and frequent outright contradiction in the data derived from studies of the flora of normal sulci and periodontal pockets. However, there are several possibilities. Techniques for sample collection, disaggregation, and culture have progressed remarkably in recent years, although serious problems remain. For example, it is still not possible to dissociate aggregates of microorganisms without loss of viability of some species. In addition, identification and cultural requirements of many pocket organisms remain unknown. Possibly the most important factor of all is the remarkable degree of organization and structure exhibited by the subgingival flora. This aspect has been investigated in humans by Listgarten, Mayo, and Tremblay[105] and in beagle dogs by Soames and Davies.[176] The composition and structure of subgingival flora appears to differ significantly, not only from one specific site to another within the pocket but also from one time to another. The surfaces of subgingivally placed epoxy crowns are first colonized by cocci which form microcolonies, multiply, coalesce, and form columns of microorganisms. Within one week, the surface of this coccoid plaque becomes colonized by filamentous microorganisms which, within 3 weeks, invade and replace the cocci. This structure remains attached to the crown or root surface in a manner similar to supragingival plaque. However, on the soft-tissue side or the advancing front of the sulcus or pocket, the flora is made up of freely floating unattached spirochetes, small unidentified cocci, gram-negative rods, many of which are motile, and unusual aggregates of microorganisms referred to as "corn cobs" and "test-tube brushes." The latter are seen only in subgingival plaque. In the pockets of humans as well as of beagle dogs, the composition of the flora differs as one progresses from the most coronal to the most apical portion. In beagle dogs, the most coronal region of the pocket is occupied by gram-negative rods and spirochetes, but the most apical regions contain only spirochetes. These observations are consistent with the idea that it will be necessary not only to determine the flora of single specific periodontal pockets of a carefully defined pathologic condition in lieu of pooled plaque samples but also to sample carefully various regions of the pocket at different times for an understanding of the floral relationships.

While the data now available are only preliminary and controversy remains, the facts appear to justify the claim that microorganisms constitute the principal and possibly the only extrinsic etiologic agent of significance in both gingivitis and periodontitis. Spontaneously accumulating plaque, regardless of its microbial composition, appears to have the capacity to induce gingivitis in humans and a number of animals. This material may or may not be able to induce periodontitis. The data indicate, but do not prove, that a specific microbiota consisting principally of gram-positive cocci and rods, particularly of the actinomyces type, is associated with slowly progressing forms of human periodontitis, and that a complex microbiota, exhibiting a highly organized plaque structure adherent to the tooth surface with freely floating predominately gram-negative anaerobic rods and populating sites near the soft tissue, is characteristic of rapidly progressing lesions. Whether it will be possible to prove that these organisms are the specific etiologic agent in periodontitis remains to be seen.

MICROBIAL PLAQUE GROWTH AND ITS RETENTION

Even though the key role of microorganisms in the etiology of inflammatory gingival and periodontal disease seems to be established clearly, there remains no doubt that numerous other secondary etiologic factors are involved. A large number of these appear to be important because they enhance the accumulation and growth of microbial plaque, interfere with plaque control measures, or lead to the establishment and growth within the dentogingival niche of pathogenic microorganisms not normally present. Since many of these factors and conditions are susceptible to therapeutic manipulation, awareness of their existence and an understanding of the pathways by which they may operate are essential for successful treatment and post-therapeutic maintenance of the periodontal patient.

Most of the factors leading to enhanced accumulation and growth of plaque or interfering with its removal are described and illustrated in Chapter 15; therefore, they will only be listed and alluded to briefly here.

Calcified Deposits (Calculus)

Microbial plaque allowed to remain without interference on the crown or root surfaces of the teeth undergoes mineralization and can no longer be removed by toothbrushing. While the mineralization process likely kills and inactivates some of the microorganisms and from that point of view may be beneficial, the resulting calcified deposit is deleterious for several reasons. The surface of calculus, even though recently polished with pumice, always contains large numbers of viable microorganisms of numerous species and gives rise to new plaque much more rapidly than do clean tooth surfaces. In addition, calculus may exert mechanical irritation upon the adjacent periodontal tissue;[85] it provides a rough surface and a favorable protected environment for rapid plaque growth, and its presence makes plaque removal and control difficult or impossible (Figs. 4-1A, 4-2A, 4-3A).

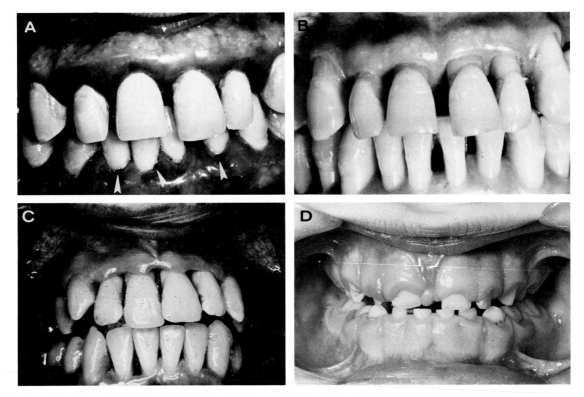

FIG. 4-1. *A and B. Advanced periodontal disease (A) before and (B) subsequent to treatment by root planing and curettage only. Note the location of subgingival calculi (arrows) and the intensely acute inflammatory reaction of the adjacent gingival tissues. C. Chronic ulcerative necrotizing periodontitis of long standing in which deep craters have formed between all the teeth. D. Gingival fibromatosis in which the gingival overgrowth almost covers the surfaces of the teeth. The soft tissues form thick fibrous ledges leading to plaque accumulation and interfering with application of the toothbrush.*

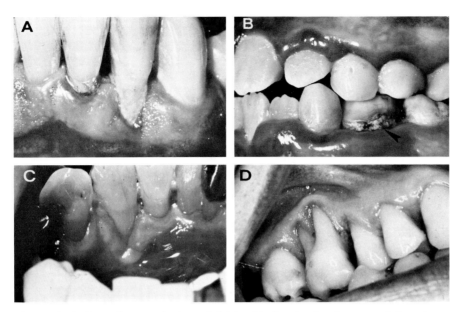

FIG. 4-2. *A. An inconsistent gingival margin around a lower left lateral incisor leading to accumulation of gross amounts of plaque and an associated inflammatory response. B. Inconsistent, acutely inflamed gingival margins associated with erupting permanent teeth. Note the presence of plaque on the buccal surfaces of the teeth, the acute marginal inflammation, and the mass of calculus and plaque on a lingually positioned tooth (arrow). C. Recession and thickening of the gingiva on the lingual aspect of a lower left canine. D. Apically positioned free marginal gingiva on the buccal aspect of a maxillary molar. Although the axial contour of the buccal surface is normal when the gingiva is normally positioned, it is excessive for the present apical position of the gingiva. This large area extending from the height of contour to the gingival margin is favorable for plaque accumulation and difficult to clean.*

Diet

The composition and consistency of the diet may be important determinants in the formation of microbial plaque on the teeth and in the development of inflammatory disease. Syrian hamsters[82,83,86,125] and rice rats[2,173] kept on soft, high carbohydrate diets exhibit extensive plaque accumulation and periodontal breakdown. In these animals, composition of the diet appears to be more important than its consistency; substitution of fat for the carbohydrate significantly reduces the degree of periodontal destruction.[173] Dietary composition also appears to be important in humans. Carlsson and Egelberg have shown that the teeth of humans consuming a diet either free of carbohydrate or containing only small amounts of this component develop within a few days a thin, structureless plaque that does not change significantly during a period of one week.[18] Supplementation with glucose does not alter this situation, although sucrose rinses cause the formation of remarkably larger amounts of microbial plaque.

In other species, consistency of the diet appears to be more important than composition. Contrary to the situation with hamsters and rats, beagle dogs kept on a soft protein-fat diet free of carbohydrates accumulate plaque and develop gingivitis.[19,29,30] In addition, the rate and amount of plaque accumulating in the beagle dog, as well as the presence and extent of periodontal inflammation, are all greatly increased by feeding a standard control diet which has previously been made into a mash by addition of water.[16,64] Likewise, ferrets fed meat scraps without bone and cartilage develop inflammatory disease, but feeding the same material attached to bone and cartilage alleviates the inflammatory lesion.[85]

Existing Pathologic Conditions

While there seems little doubt that accumulation of bacteria at the dentogingival junction leads to inflammation of the periodontal tissues, there is reason to believe that plaque accumulates more rapidly and to a greater extent on the surfaces of teeth invested with diseased tissues. For example, using the scanning electron microscope to study selective adherence, Saxton found that the rate of initial colonization of previously cleaned tooth surfaces is considerably greater when the surrounding gingiva is inflamed than when the teeth are invested by normal gingival tissue.[164] The reasons for this remain unclear, although the exudation of gingival fluid may enhance adherence and growth of microorganisms. Carious lesions, abnormally deep gingival sulci, or periodontal pockets provide niches in which growth conditions are highly favorable, especially of anaerobic microorganisms, and where their

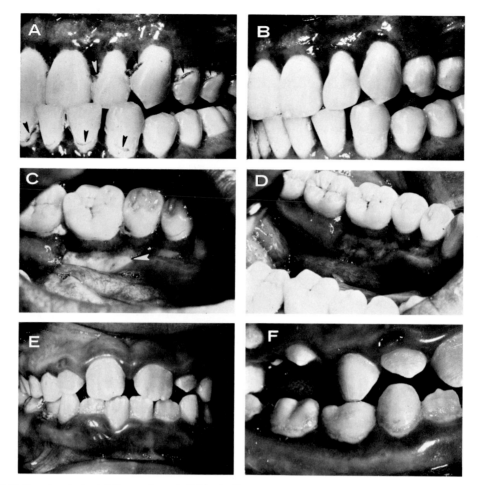

FIG. 4-3. *A–D. Gingival and periodontal disease in an individual with agranulocytosis resulting from drug hypersensitivity. A. Note the highly acute proliferative response especially apparent around the incisor teeth, and the presence of plaque-covered calculus (arrows). The deposits indicate the previous level of the gingival tissues. B. Following debridement and partial resolution of the disease. C. A large ulcer located lingually to the lower left first molar (arrow). D. Same as C but partially healed. (Courtesy Dr. T. Temple.) E–F. Periodontal condition of a child with neutropenia. Note the acute inflammation of the gingival tissues, the plaque covering the surfaces of all the teeth, and the thickened gingival margins resulting from edema. The mandibular lateral incisors have thick gingival margins and are covered with plaque, but the more prominent central incisor has a relatively normal gingiva and is relatively free of plaque. F. The teeth without antagonists tend to accumulate more plaque than teeth in normal occlusion. (Courtesy Dr. W. Lavine.)*

removal by tooth brushing or other mechanical means is virtually impossible (Fig. 4-1A,C).

Saliva

The consistency and composition of the saliva vary from one individual to another and from time to time, and it appears likely that salivary factors can affect the oral flora and the extent of plaque formation.[60] One important manifestation of the importance of saliva is the enhanced caries rate and the development of gingival and periodontal disease which almost always accompany pathologically decreased salivary flow. Saliva contains specific glycoproteins that enhance the capacity of organisms to colonize tooth surfaces and to aggregate with one another. In addition to certain antibacterial substances such as lysozyme, saliva also contains specific IgA antibody, which is capable of binding with certain oral microorganisms and thereby helping control the relative population sizes and adherence and aggregation properties.[42]

Abnormal Morphlology and Function

Anatomic and functional characteristics of the dentition and periodontal tissues are important in determining the propensity toward plaque accumulation and periodontal breakdown. They can operate along more than one pathway. In addition to affecting the rate and amount of plaque accumulation and the relative ease with which it can be removed, abnormal occlusal function, for example, can also alter the resistance of the periodontal tissues. Important anatomic and functional factors include the following:

1. Abnormal tooth position: prominent buccal or lingual position, tilting, tipping, rotation, or overlapping with adjacent teeth (Figs. 4-3E, 4-5B, 4-6A).
2. Abnormal tooth shape: unusually prominent buccal or lingual contours, abrasion, or tooth wear (Figs. 4-4D,E,F).
3. Functional status: teeth without antagonists (Figs. 4-3F, 4-4C).
4. Open contacts (Figs. 4-4B, 4-5A,B,D, 4-6B).
5. Gingival contour and position: the free marginal

gingiva may be thick from fibrosis or edema (Figs. 4-1D, 4-2B, 4-5C, 4-6A); it may be inconsistent in location relative to that of the adjacent teeth or located too far apically or coronally (Figs. 4-1D, 4-2D, 4-3E).

Iatrogenic Factors

Many of the secondary etiologic factors are the results of poorly executed therapeutic procedures. Among these are the following:

1. Open tooth contacts (Figs. 4-5A,B,D)
2. Improperly placed partial denture clasps and connectors and bars (Figs. 4-7B,C,E)
3. Improperly carved restorations, overhanging crown and filling margins (Figs. 4-5D, 4-7D,F)

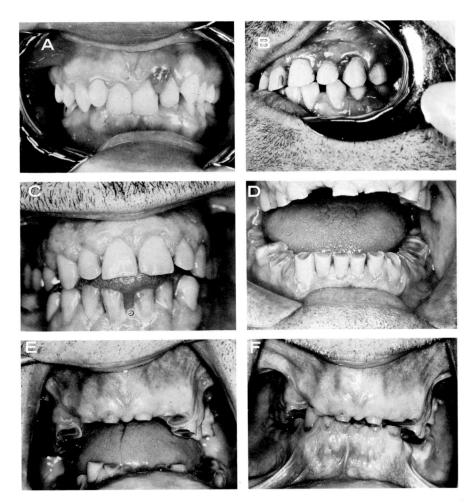

FIG. 4-4. *A. Dentition of a patient with a deep overbite whose maxillary incisor teeth contact the gingiva on the labial side of the mandibular incisor teeth, causing traumatic injury and predisposing the periodontium to breakdown. An open contact between the left central and lateral incisors with an associated pocket and hyperplastic inflamed gingival papilla is also apparent. B. Open contacts between most of the teeth shown with a plunger-cusp relationship between the maxillary canine, the maxillary lateral incisor, and the mandibular canine. Note the associated periodontal destruction. C. Dentition of a mouth breather, with open bite and tongue thrust. The anterior teeth have been driven apart, the gingiva is fibrotic and thick, and the mandibular incisors are covered with plaque. D, E, and F. Teeth severely worn from bruxism.*

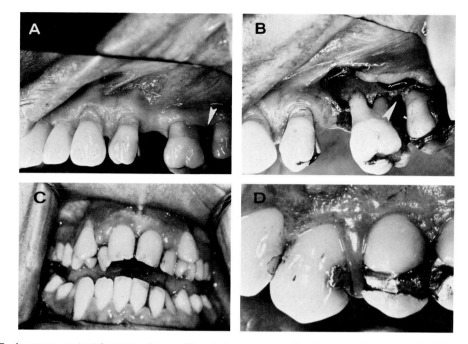

FIG. 4-5. *A and B. An open contact between the maxillary left molars resulting from drifting forward of the first molar into the endentulous space with formation of a bone crater (arrow). C. Severe malocclusion and poorly aligned teeth with attendant gingival and periodontal disease. Note the gingival recession on the labial aspect of the right maxillary and mandibular canines, the thick gingival ledges on the labial aspect of the lateral incisors, and the overlapping teeth. D. Proliferative response of the interdental tissue to an open contact between the maxillary canine and first premolars resulting from placement of undercontoured restorations. A deep bone crater was also present.*

Failure of the Patient to Maintain Plaque Control

Possibly the single most important factor contributing to the growth and accumulation of plaque is the failure or inability of the patient to maintain adequate daily mechanical plaque removal. Failure of plaque control measures may be a consequence of (1) lack of information and training in tooth brushing and other ancillary techniques; (2) presence of mouth conditions such as pockets, tissue ledges, defective restorations and appliances, open contacts, overlapping teeth, abnormal contours, open furcations and flutings, and exposed root surfaces, or (3) a lack of the required manual dexterity (see Chapter 15).

RESISTANCE OF THE PERIODONTAL TISSUES TO MICROBIAL CHALLENGE

Many secondary etiologic factors exert their effects by causing the periodontal tissues to be less resistant to

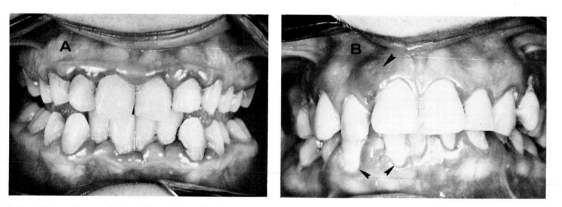

FIG. 4-6. *A. Dentition of a mouth breather with typically fibrotic labial gingiva, massive plaque accumulation, and malocclusion. B. Open contact between the maxillary right central and lateral incisors, with pocket formation and periodontal abscess (arrow). Also note the inconsistent gingival margins associated with the mandibular incisors and right canine (arrows).*

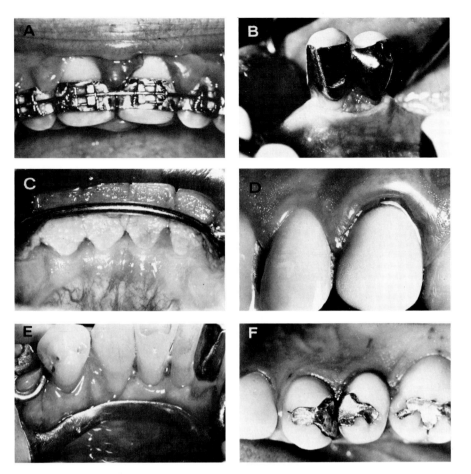

FIG. 4-7. *A. Hyperplastic, acutely inflamed gingival tissue associated with orthodontic bands. Appliances of this sort make adequate plaque control virtually impossible and may lead to periodontal destruction. B. Mandibular canine and premolar serving as abutments for a partial denture. The excessive force has predisposed this area to periodontal breakdown, as evidenced by the interdental formation of granulation tissue. C. Massive plaque accumulation associated with a bar located midway up the lingual surfaces of the lower incisors. D. A typical rolled, thickened free gingival margin associated with a poorly constructed jacket crown that has a rough, thick subgingival margin. E. Thickening and recession of the marginal gingiva on the lingual aspect of a lower left canine, resulting from impingement of the lingual bar of a partial denture. Recession and thickening has led to plaque accumulation and periodontal breakdown. F. Defective amalgam restorations in two adjacent premolars, with no marginal ridges or other proper occlusal anatomy, leading to food impaction, chronic inflammation, and pocket formation.*

the challenge posed by the presence of microorganisms. These factors are only poorly understood, and the pathways by which they operate remain largely unknown. In many instances, factors of this class are not amenable to therapeutic manipulation, although an appreciation of their existence is essential to the successful evaluation and treatment of the disease.

Aging

A strong and positive correlation between increasing age and the prevalence and severity of inflammatory periodontal disease has been shown repeatedly in human and animal populations.[57,65,93,110,165] The basis of this correlation is not understood, although it seems more likely to be related to time-dependent changes in the host than to alterations in the oral flora. The fact that certain other diseases exhibit a similar age relationship has led to the hypothesis that a decrease in the normal immunologic and other host defense systems may be important factors. The age dependency may also involve the general slowdown in cell replication and normal tissue-substance turnover that occurs with the passage of time.

Abnormal Morphology and Function

Mouth breathing,[87,106] the lack of normal lip seal, abnormal tooth position and functional occlusal problems associated with open bite and tongue thrust,[150] and abnormal habits including bruxism, clenching, and tapping the teeth[94,104,127,147,154,179,183] all create conditions leading to a decrease in the capacity of the periodontal tissues to withstand microbial insult (Figs. 4-4, 4-6A). Both hypo- and hyperfunction decrease resistance and enhance the likelihood of the development of inflammatory periodontal lesions.[102,144] The type, character, and amount of marginal gingival tissue are also important in determining the resistance properties of the periodontium. An abnormally narrow band of attached gingiva, or attached gingiva subjected to muscle pull through abnormal frenum attachment, is generally predisposed to periodontal breakdown in the presence of local irritation from plaque. In contrast to the keratinized attached gingiva, marginal tissues made up of oral mucosa are unable to withstand functional demands and become more susceptible to the deleterious effects of microorganisms than is attached gingiva. The basic mechanisms involving the enhancement of or predisposition to periodontal breakdown by these secondary etiologic factors are not understood.

Nutrition

The relationship between malnutrition and predisposition to inflammatory gingival and periodontal disease is not understood, although it has been studied by numerous investigators. All of the data available currently support the idea that deficiency or deprivation alone cannot cause inflammatory gingival and periodontal disease; however, these states aggravate and amplify the effects of local irritants and bacteria to make the disease more severe and more rapidly progressive.

There is little information regarding the effects of vitamin A deficiency on the periodontium of humans, although Radusch described periodontal disease associated with low daily intake of the vitamin.[145] Extensive studies have been done on experimental animals.[12,119,120] In vitamin A-deficient animals the gingiva becomes hyperkeratotic, and there is epithelial hyperplasia and proliferation of the junctional epithelium. Although gingival hyperplasia with inflammation and pocket formation occur in deficient animals also exposed to local irritation in the form of plaque, deficiency alone fails to induce these changes.[12,13,84,119]

Vitamin B complex deficiencies are manifested orally as glossitis, gingivitis, glossodynia, cheilosis, and stomatitis. However, the gingivitis is nonspecific, and its direct cause is bacterial rather than deficiency.[1]

Severe vitamin C deficiency causes scurvy, a disease manifested by abnormalities in the connective-tissue substance and in the small blood vessels. Scorbutic humans or animals may exhibit a florid gingivitis or periodontitis characterized by hemorrhagic, bluish-red, hyperplastic gingiva. However, not all deficient indi-

viduals exhibit this, and it is clear that the deficiency per se does not cause the periodontal problem. In experimental animals not allowed to accumulate microbial plaque, pockets do not form; instead, the state of deficiency alters the response of the supporting tissues to the extent that the destructive effects of the microbiota are accentuated.[45,72,134,192,195] Extensive efforts have been made to correlate the blood level of vitamin C with the periodontal status. However, results have been confusing,[189] with some investigators claiming a positive correlation and others finding no correlation.

Vitamin D deficiency and abnormal calcium metabolism result in rickets in young persons and osteomalacia and osteoporosis in adults. In experimental animals, deficiency leads to osteoclastic resorption of the alveolar bone, followed by formation of new but imperfect bone around the remnants of unresorbed bone.[7,26,70,135,175]

Protein deficiency and starvation accentuate the destructive effects of microbial plaque.[180] Experimental protein deficiency in animals causes changes in the oral tissues, including connective-tissue degeneration, osteoporosis of alveolar bone, retarded deposition of cementum, and delayed wound healing,[20,39,52] although deficiency alone does not cause gingival and periodontal disease.

Hormones

There is a predilection to inflammatory gingival and periodontal disease during periods of sex-hormone imbalance such as puberty, pregnancy, and menopause, and this tendency may be related to the effects these hormones have upon both normal and previously inflamed gingival and periodontal tissues. Young human females have considerably more gingival exudation at ovulation, a period when progesterone levels are high, than at menstruation when the levels are lower.[95] An increase in the amount of exudate obtainable on filter-paper strips placed in the gingival sulcus is greater in women regularly using oral contraceptives with specific progesterone effects than in comparable individuals not taking these drugs.[96] Knight and Wade found no increase in the levels of gingival inflammation, but there was increased periodontal breakdown in women taking hormonal oral contraceptives relative to a control group of comparable age.[88] A case of a plaque-dependent pregnancy tumor has been reported in a woman taking an oral contraceptive.[143]

The possible means by which the various sex hormones and contraceptives may affect the periodontal tissues have been examined in experimental animals. The administration of estrogens and gonadotropin to oophorectomized hamsters with microwounds in the cheek pouch had little effect; however, when progesterone was administered intramuscularly, acute inflammation developed within the wound area.[99] Elevated levels of progesterone result in vascular proliferation and inflammation of the venules and capillaries of slightly damaged tissues.[101] In rabbits, elevated levels of progesterone caused hypervascularization of granulation tissue along with inflammation and circulatory impairment.[98] In dogs relatively free of gingival inflammation, as well as in dogs with chronic gingivitis, administration of estrogen and progesterone increased the flow of exudate from the gingival sulcus, and this flow decreased remarkably at the termination of the hormone administration.[96,97] These observations have led to the concept that the use of contraceptives containing progestogens or other agents that may lead to the elevation in normal levels of progesterone may enhance normal levels of vascular permeability and exudation, predisposing to development of inflammatory lesions and aggravation of previously existing chronic inflammation of the periodontal tissues.

A variety of oral changes may be associated with diabetes mellitus, including dryness of the mouth, marginal indentations of the tongue with shedding of the papillae and inflammation, diffuse erythema of the oral mucosa, a tendency toward periodontal abscess formation, and increased prevalence of inflammatory periodontal disease with severe bone loss (see Chapter 10).[9,22,36,71,130,159,174,194] In general, it can be stated that individuals with diabetes are predisposed to gingivitis and periodontitis, that the disease is more severe and progresses more rapidly in those with the juvenile rather than in the adult form of the disease, that periodontal conditions may degenerate with dramatic rapidity in individuals in whom the diabetic problem is uncontrolled, and that, in general, response to the standard therapeutic measures is not as good in diabetic as in normal individuals (see Chapter 10). Although extensive research has been done and the relevant literature is massive, the above statements are based more upon clinical experience than upon experimentally derived observation. In fact, some investigators have failed to find an association between the diabetic state and periodontal breakdown.[133]

The association of hormonal abnormalities other than those discussed with predilection to inflammatory gingival and periodontal disease is not clearly established. Oral and dental changes in experimental animals in which abnormal levels of several hormones including thyroxin, parathyroid hormone, corticosteroids, and pituitary hormones have been studied.[5,6,33,47,48,49,51,61,157] Even though pathologic changes in the periodontal tissues, especially alveolar

bone, have been demonstrated, there is currently no definitive evidence to show that these conditions predispose in any specific way to inflammatory gingival and periodontal disease of microbial origin.

Debilitating Disease

Chronic debilitating diseases such as tuberculosis, leprosy, syphilis, scurvy, nephritis, and malignancy have long been suspected of predisposing to severe and rapid periodontal destruction. For example, Koecker listed both tuberculosis and syphilis among the constitutional causes of periodontal disease.[89] Although diseases of this type lead to cachexia, abnormally functioning homeostatic mechanisms, and a gradual failure of the normal host defense systems and individuals so affected are predisposed to infection in general, any specific relationship of these diseases to inflammatory periodontitis remains unclear.[162] For example, while an association between periodontal disease and tuberculosis has been reported,[17,146] it was not found by others.[58,185] Periodontitis has been described in lepers, although microorganisms characteristic of leprosy were not found in the periodontal tissues.[190]

Pathologic alterations of the periodontal tissues are frequently seen in anemic individuals,[92] although anemia is not a predisposing cause of inflammatory gingival and periodontal disease. Clotting defects and other blood dyscrasias causing an abnormal bleeding tendency lead to unusual hemorrhage from the gingiva.[27,32,90] Patients with one of the acute leukemias may have associated hyperplastic gingiva with inflammatory manifestations.[10,15,50] This is generally not seen in individuals with chronic leukemia. Oral lesions occur more frequently in monocytic than in lymphocytic and myelogenous leukemia. Individuals afflicted by agranulocytosis[4] or by neutropenia[21] may exhibit generalized ulcerative and necrotic changes of the oral mucous membranes, skin, and gastrointestinal tract, as well as of the attached gingiva (Fig. 4-3). Agranulocytosis is frequently a result of idiosyncratic or hypersensitive reactions to drugs.

Psychosomatic Disorders

Inflammatory gingival and periodontal diseases appear to be more prevalent and more severe in individuals with psychiatric and anxiety abnormalities than in psychologically normal individuals.[3,8,114,123] The mechanisms by which these disorders may be translated into a predilection to inflammatory periodontal disease are not understood, although it has been suggested that such individuals develop deleterious habits such as bruxism or that nutrition to the periodontal tissues or salivary flow may become altered.[11]

Heredity

There are several single mutant gene defects in which severe periodontal disease is a constant and striking component. These include cyclic neutropenia, acatalasia, and hypophosphatasia.[54,55] In addition to these diseases, severe periodontitis with remarkably early tooth loss is consistently present in humans and animals with the autosomal recessive trait, Chédiak-Higashi syndrome.[62,63,93,186] The manifestation of the disease in these cases is remarkably different from that seen in the common variety of plaque-associated periodontitis; the acute inflammatory component is much greater and necrosis of the gingiva and mucous membranes with ulceration is frequently observed. The effects of these genes are manifest in all oral environments, indicating that hereditary characteristics can be extremely potent in causing some forms of periodontal disease.

The association of hereditary factors with the commonly observed forms of inflammatory gingival and periodontal disease has not been clearly established, although the observations of most experienced clinicians indicate that such associations do indeed exist and that they are of considerable significance. The investigations done in this area have been reviewed.[55] It is clear that the clinical manifestations of inflammatory gingival and periodontal disease result from a confluence of numerous local, constitutional and environmental factors. Analysis of multifactorial inheritance patterns is extremely difficult, since the genetic tools that provide the most reliable and precise answers are those most easily applicable to clearly defined single-gene defects. In addition, most studies are based upon the use of index measurements of the periodontal status which are not dependable (see Chapter 3). In spite of these difficulties, pedigree analysis, the periodontal status of identical and fraternal twins, and the effects of age, sex, and race have been examined. Although the results of these studies remain generally inconclusive, major racial differences have been reported. For example, it has been reported that the incidence of periodontal disease is 50 to 60 percent in Persians, 20 to 40 percent in Kurds, and 15 to 20 percent in Armenians.

RESPONSIVENESS OF THE NORMAL HOST DEFENSE SYSTEMS

Normally functioning host defense systems are necessary for the maintenance of a healthy periodontium. These systems are consistently challenged by factors in the oral environment. This challenge is generally manifested by a low level of emigration of leukocytes through the gingival sulcus into the oral cavity and by the development of protective immune reactions to oral microorganisms and other antigens (see Chapter 1). Although these host defense systems have classically been considered to be defensive and protective, data now available indicate that they also have potent offensive and destructive capability as well (see Chapter 8).[69,138,140,141] The result of any challenge is a balance between the destructive and protective aspects of the systems activated. Indeed, in some diseases such as tuberculosis, it is clear that the causative microorganism is relatively innocuous in that it makes no exotoxins and does not contain endotoxin or other directly toxic substances; instead, it operates by activation of various host defense mechanisms, especially cell-mediated hypersensitivity and inflammation, and the destructive aspects of these produce the tissue damage observed. There is now a great deal of evidence that inflammatory gingival and periodontal disease belongs to this same family of diseases (see Chapter 8).[139,140] Therefore, hereditary factors or diseases such as the immunopathies and blood-cell defects of the type observed in the Chédiak-Higashi syndrome may predispose to periodontal disease through their capacity to amplify the destructive parts of the host defense systems relative to the protective parts.

SUMMARY

In 1885 Rawls posed these four questions that deserve investigation if we desire a correct knowledge of the etiology of periodontal disease:

First, do all persons who have deposits of salivary calculus about their teeth present the true characteristic signs and symptoms of this disease? If not, why?
Second, is the disease infectious? If so, why have so many of the human family escaped its ravages through the centuries of contact and exposure to its action; and why are not dentists, who daily and hourly stand almost mouth to mouth with patients, also infected?
Third, is the fact that this disease runs in families more an evidence of its infectious character than of its heredity?
Fourth, is it true that a peculiar and destructive fungus finds its habitat in the lesions of this malady, and cannot be found in mouths not so affected?[149]

Although none of the four questions originally posed by Rawls almost a century ago can be answered definitively, major insights have been achieved. The hypothesis that microorganisms are the principal extrinsic etiologic agent responsible for inflammatory gingival and periodontal disease is now widely accepted, and the disease can now be classified as infectious. However, it differs from classic infections in important ways: the microorganisms do not invade the tissues causing necrosis in the usual sense, and the disease is not transmissible, at least along the usual routes, explaining why the prevalence is not extremely high in dentists. It is clear that accumulating microbial plaque, regardless of its floral constituents, can cause gingivitis, although the question of whether "peculiar and destructive" microorganisms that cannot be found in normal mouths are associated with periodontitis remains unresolved. The work of Socransky and his colleagues and others indicates but does not prove that this may be the case. Although Rawls appears to have accepted the idea that inflammatory periodontal disease runs in families as fact, and clinical experience indicates that this is true, final proof has not yet been obtained; the influence of heredity and numerous other secondary etiologic factors remains undefined. Whether or not some humans are resistant to the disease in spite of the nature and magnitude of the microbial challenge is not known, although, in beagle dogs under experimental conditions, about 20 percent of the animals do not develop periodontitis even though plaque and calculus are allowed to accumulate. Consideration of the present rate of progress indicates that the answers to many of these important questions may be forthcoming in the near future.

References

1. Afonsky, D.: Oral lesions in niacin, riboflavine, pyridoxine, folic acid and pantothenic acid deficiencies in adult dogs. Oral Surg., 8:207, 315, 867, 1955.
2. Auskaps, A. M., Gupta, O. P., and Shaw, J. H.: Periodontal disease in the rice rat. III. Survey of dietary influences. J. Nutr., 63:325, 1957.
3. Baker, E. G., Crook, G. H., and Schwabacher, E. D.: Personality correlated to periodontal disease. J. Dent. Res., 40:396, 1961.
4. Bauer, W. H.: Agranulocytosis and the supporting dental tissues. J. Dent. Res., 25:501, 1946.
5. Baume, L. J., and Becks, H.: The effect of thyroid hormone in dental and paradental structures. Paradentologie, 6:89, 1952.
6. Bavetta, L. A., Bernick, S., and Ershoff, B.: The influence of dietary thyroid on the bones and periodontium of rats on total and partial tryptophane deficiencies. J. Dent. Res., 36:13, 1957.
7. Becks, H.: Dangerous effects of vitamin D overdosage on dental and paradental structure. J. Am. Dent. Assoc., 29:1947, 1942.
8. Belting, C. M., and Gupta, O. P.: The influence of psychiatric disturbances on the severity of periodontal disease. J. Periodontol., 32:219, 1961.
9. Belting, C. M., Hinicker, J. J., and Dummett, C. O.: Influence of diabetes mellitus on the severity of periodontal disease. J. Periodontol., 35:476, 1964.
10. Bender, I. B.: Bone changes in leukemia. Am. J. Orthodt. Oral Surg., 30:556, 1944.
11. Biber, O.: Autonomic symptoms in psychoneurotics. Psychosom. Med., 3:253, 1941.
12. Boyle, P. E.: Effect of vitamin A deficiency on the periodontal tissues. Am. J. Orthodt. Oral Surg., 33:744, 1947.
13. Boyle, P. E., and Bessey, O. A.: The effect of acute vitamin A deficiency on the molar teeth and periodontal tissues with a comment on deformed incisor teeth in this deficiency. J. Dent. Res., 20:236, 1941.
14. Brandtzaeg, P.: Local formation and transport of immunoglobulins related to the oral cavity. In Host Resistance to Commensal Bacteria. (T. MacPhee, Ed.). Edinburgh, Churchill Livingstone, 1972.
15. Burkett, L. W.: A histopathologic explanation for the oral lesions in the acute leukemias. Am. J. Orthodt. Oral Surg., 30:516, 1944.
16. Burwasser, P., and Hill, T. J.: The effect of hard and soft diets on the gingival tissues of dogs. J. Dent. Res., 18:389, 1939.
17. Cahn, L. R.: Observations in the effect of tuberculosis on the teeth, gums and jaws. Dental Cosmos, 67:479, 1925.
18. Carlsson, J., and Egelberg, J.: Effect of diet on early plaque formation in man. Odont. Rev. 16:112, 1965.
19. Carlsson, J., and Egelberg, J. Local effect of diet on plaque formation and development of gingivitis in dogs. II. Effect of high carbohydrate vs. high protein-fat diets. Odontol. Rev., 16:42, 1965.
20. Chawla, T. N., and Glickman, I.: Protein deprivation and the periodontal structures of the albino rat. Oral Surg., 4:578, 1951.
21. Cohen, D. W., and Morris, A. L.: Periodontal manifestations of cyclic neutropenia. J. Periodontol., 32:159, 1961.
22. Cohen, D. W., et al.: Studies on periodontal patterns in diabetes mellitus. J. Periodont. Res. Suppl., 4:35, 1969.
23. Courant, P. R., and Baeder, H.: Bacteroides melaninogenicus and its products in the gingiva of man. Periodontics, 4:131, 1966.
24. Darwish, S., Hyppa, T., and Socransky, S. S.: Predominant cultivable microorganisms in early periodontitis. J. Periodont. Res., in press.
25. Dick, D. S., and Shaw, J. H.: The infectious and transmissible nature of the periodontal syndrome of the rice rat. Arch. Oral Biol., 11:1095, 1966.
26. Dreizen, S., et al.: Studies on the biology of the periodontium of marmosets. III. Periodontal bone changes in marmosets with osteomalacia and hyperparathyroidism. Isr. J. Med. Sci., 3:731, 1967.
27. Durocher, R. T., Morris, A. L., and Burket, L. W.: Oral manifestations of hereditary hemorrhagic telangiectasia. Oral Surg., 14:550, 1961.
28. Dwyer, D. M., and Socransky, S. S.: Predominant cultivable microorganisms inhabiting periodontal pockets. Br. Dent. J., 124:560, 1968.
29. Egelberg, J.: The local effect of diet on plaque forma-

tion and development of gingivitis in dogs. I. Effect of soft and hard diets. Odontol. Rev., 16:31, 1965.

30. Egelberg, J.: Local effect of diet on plaque formation and development of gingivitis in dogs. III. Effect of frequency of means and tube feeding. Odontol. Rev., 16:50, 1965.

31. Ellison, S. A.: Oral bacteria in periodontal disease. J. Dent. Res., 49(supp. 2):198, 1970.

32. El Mostehy, M. R., and Stallard, R. E.: The Sturge-Weber syndrome: its periodontal significance. J. Periodontol., 40:243, 1969.

33. English, J. A.: Experimental effects of thiouracil and selenium on the teeth and jaws of dogs. J. Dent. Res., 28:172, 1949.

34. Evans, R. T., Spaeth, S., and Mergenhagen, S. E.: Bactericidal antibody in mammalian serum to obligatory anaerobic gram-negative bacteria. J. Immunol., 97:112, 1966.

35. Fauchard, P.: The Surgeon Dentist. Translated by L. Lindsay from the second edition, 1746. Pound Ridge, N.Y., 1969.

36. Fett, K. D., and Jutzi, E.: Die Bezahnung bei Diabetikern in Abhängigkeit vom Lebensalter und der Diabetesdauer. Dtsch. Zahnaerztl. Z., 20:121, 1965.

37. Foley, G., and Rosebury, T.: Comparative infectivity for guinea pigs of fusospirochetal exudates from different diseases. J. Dent. Res., 21:375, 1942.

38. Fox, J.: Natural History and Diseases of the Human Teeth. Part II. Diseases of the Teeth, the Gums and the Alveolar Processes. 3rd Ed., London, E. Cox, 1823.

39. Frandsen, A. M., et al.: The effects of various levels of dietary protein on the periodontal tissues of young rats. J. Periodontol., 24:135, 1953.

40. Genco, R. J., Evans, R. T., and Ellison, S. A.: Dental research in microbiology with emphasis on periodontal disease. J. Am. Dent. Assoc., 78:1016, 1969.

41. Genco, R. J., et al.: Antibody-mediated effects on the periodontium. J. Periodontol., 45:330, 1974.

42. Gibbons, R. J., and van Houte, J.: On the formation of dental plaque. J. Periodontol., 44:347, 1973.

43. Gibbons, R. J., et al.: Dental caries and alveolar bone loss in gnotobiotic rats infected with capsule forming streptococci of human origin. Arch. Oral Biol., 11:459, 1966.

44. Gibbons, R. J., et al.: The microbiota of the gingival crevice area of man. II. The predominant cultivable organisms. Arch. Oral Biol., 8:281, 1963.

45. Glickman, I.: Acute vitamin deficiency and periodontal disease. I. The periodontal tissues of the guinea pig in acute vitamin C deficiency. II. The effect of acute vitamin C deficiency upon the response of the periodontal tissues of the guinea pig to artificially induced inflammation. J. Dent. Res., 27:9, 201, 1948.

46. Glickman, I.: Clinical Periodontics. 4th Ed., Philadelphia, W. B. Saunders, 1972.

47. Glickman, I., and Pruzansy, S.: Propyl-thiouracil hypothyroidism in the ablino rat. J. Dent. Res., 26:471, 1947.

48. Glickman, I., and Shklar, G.: The steroid hormones and tissues of the periodontium. Oral Surg., 8:1179, 1955.

49. Glickman, I., Stone, I. C., and Chawla, T. N.: The effect of cortisone acetate upon the periodontium of white mice. J. Periodontol., 24:161, 1953.

50. Goldman, H. M.: Acute aleukemic leukemia. Am. J. Orthodt. Oral Surg., 26:89, 1940.

51. Goldman, H. M.: Experimental hyperthyroidism in guinea pigs. Am. J. Orthodt. Oral Surg., 29:665, 1943.

52. Goldman, H. M.: Protein deprivation in rats. J. Dent. Res., 39:690, 1960.

53. Goldman, H. M., and Cohen, W. D.: Periodontal Therapy. 4th Ed. St. Louis, C. V. Mosby Co., 1968.

54. Gorlin, R. J., and Pindborg, J. J.: Syndromes of the Head and Neck. New York, McGraw-Hill Book Co., 1964.

55. Gorlin, R. J., Stallard, R. E., and Shapiro, B. L.: Genetics and periodontal disease. J. Periodontol., 38:5, 1967.

56. Grant, D. A., Stern, I. B., and Everett, F. G.: Orban's Periodontics. 3rd Ed. St. Louis, C. V. Mosby, 1972.

57. Greene, J. C.: Oral hygiene and periodontal disease. Am. J. Public Health, 53:913, 1963.

58. Gruber, I. E.: The condition of the teeth and the attachment apparatus in tuberculosis. J. Dent. Res., 28:483, 1949.

59. Gupta, O. P., Auskaps, A. M., and Shaw, J. H.: Periodontal disease in the rice rat. IV. The effects of antibiotics on the incidence of periodontal lesions. Oral Surg., 10:1169, 1957.

60. Gupta, O. P., Blechman, H., and Stahl, S. S.: The effects of desalivation on periodontal tissues of the Syrian hamster. Oral Surg., 13:470, 1960.

61. Gupta, O. P., Blechman, H., and Stahl, S. S.: The effects of stress on the periodontal tissues of young adult male rats and hamsters. J. Periodontol. 31:413, 1960.

62. Gustafson, G. T.: Increased susceptibility to periodontitis in mink affected by a lysosomal disease. J. Periodont. Res., 4:259, 1969.

63. Hamilton, R. E., and Giansanti, J. S.: The Chediak-Highashi Syndrome. Report of a case and review of the literature. Oral Surg., 37:754, 1974.

64. Hamp, S.-E., Lindhe, J., and Heyden, G.: Experimental gingivitis in the dog. An enzyme histochemical study. Arch. Oral Biol., 17:329, 1972.

65. Hamp, S.-E., et al.: Prevalence of periodontal disease in dogs. I. Clinical and roentgenographical observations. Program and Abstracts, 53rd Gen. Session IADR, Abs. #L-19, 1975.

66. Harlan, A. W.: Treatment of pyorrhea alveolaris. Dental Cosmos, 25:517, 1883.

67. Hausmann, E.: Potential pathways for bone resorption in human periodontal disease. J. Periodontol., 45:338, 1974.

68. Hemmens, E. S., and Harrison, S. W.: Studies on the anaerobic bacterial flora of supprative periodontitis. J. Infect. Dis., 70:131, 1942.

69. Henson, P. M.: Interaction of cells with immune complexes: adherence, release of constituents and tissue injury. J. Exp. Med., *134*:114S, 1971.

70. Henrikson, P. A.: Periodontal disease and calcium deficiency. Acta Odont. Scand., *26* (suppl. 50) 1968.

71. Hirshfield, I.: Discussion of "the most significant findings of the California stomatological research group in the study of pyorrhea" by F. V. Simonton. J. Dent. Res., 8:261, 1928.

72. Hojer, J. A., and Westin, G.: Jaws and teeth in scorbutic guinea pig. Dental Cosmos, *67*:1, 1925.

73. Horton, J. E., Oppenheim, J. J., and Mergenhagen, S. E.: A role for cell-mediated immunity in the pathogenesis of periodontal disease. J. Periodontol., *45*:351, 1974.

74. Horton, J. E., et al.: Human lymphoproliferative reaction to saliva and dental plaque deposits: an in vitro correlation with periodontal disease. J. Periodontal., *43*:522, 1972.

75. Howell, A.: A filamentous microorganism isolated from periodontal plaque in hamsters. I. Isolation, morphology and general cultural characteristics. Sabouraudia, *4*:65, 1965.

76. Hunter, J.: A Practical Treatis on the Diseases of the Teeth. Supplement to Natural History of Human Teeth, Part II. London, 1835.

77. Irving, J. T., Socransky, S. S., and Heeley, J. D.: Histological changes in experimental periodontal disease in gnotobiotic rats and conventional hamsters. J. Periodont. Res., 9:73, 1974.

78. Iyanyi, L., and Lehner, T.: Stimulation of lymphocyte transformation by bacterial antigens in patients with periodontal disease. Arch. Oral Biol., *15*:1089, 1970.

79. Jensen, S. B., et al.: Experimental gingivitis in man. IV Vancomycin induced changes in bacterial plaque composition as related to development of gingival inflammation. J. Periodont. Res., 3:284, 1968.

80. Jordan, H. V., and Keyes, P. H.: Aerobic, gram-positive, filamentous bacteria as the agents of experimental periodontal disease in hamsters. Arch. Oral Biol., 9:401, 1964.

81. Kelstrup, J.: Bacteriodes melaninogenicus in human gingival sulci. Periodontics, 4:14, 1966.

82. Keyes, P. H., and Jordan, H. V.: Periodontal lesions in the syrian hamster. III. Findings related to an infectious and transmissible component. Arch. Oral Biol., 9:377, 1964.

83. Keyes, P. H., and Likin, R. C.: Plaque formation, periodontal disease, and dental caries in syrian hamsters. J. Dent. Res., 25:166, 1946.

84. King, J. D.: Abnormalities in the gingival and subgingival tissues due to diets deficient in vitamin A and carotene. Br. Dent. J., *68*:349, 1940.

85. King, J. D., and Glover, R. E.: The relative effects of dietary constituents and other factors upon calculus formation and gingival disease in the ferret. J. Pathol., *57*:353, 1945.

86. Klingsberg, J., and Butcher, E. W.: Aging, diet, and periodontal lesions in the hamster. J. Dent. Res., 38:421, 1959.

87. Klingsberg, J., Cancellaro, L. A., and Butcher, E. O.: Effects of air drying on rodent oral mucous membrane: A histologic study of simulated mouth breathing. J. Periodontol., 32:38, 1961.

88. Knight, G. M., and Wade, A. B.: The effects of hormonal contraceptives on the human periodontium. J. Periodont. Res., 9:18, 1974.

89. Koecker, L.: An essay on the devastation of the gums and the alveolar processes. Phila. J. Med. Phys. Sci., 2:282, 1821.

90. Kramer, G., and Grifel, A.: Christman Disease (Hemophilia B) in periodontal therapy. Oral Surg., *15*:1056, 1962.

91. Krygier, G., Genco, R. J. and Ellison, S. A.: Gingivitis in Macaca speciosa: Shifts in inflammatory cells and localization of immunoglobulins and complement (C3). Programs and Abstracts, 52nd Gen Session IADR. Abs. #503, 1974.

92. Lainson, P., Brady, P., and Fraleigh, C.: Anemia, a systemic cause of periodontal disease. J. Periodontol., *39*:35, 1968.

93. Lavine, W. S., Page, R. C., and Padgett, G. A.: Host response in chronic periodontal disease. The dental and periodontal status of mink and mice affected by Chediak-higashi Syndrome. J. Periodontol., in press.

94. Leof, M.: Clamping and grinding habits: their relation to periodontal disease. J. Am. Dent. Assoc., *31*:184, 1944.

95. Lindhe, J., and Attström, R.: Gingival exudation during the menstrual cycle. J. Periodont. Res., 2:194, 1967.

96. Lindhe, J., Attström, R., and Björn, A. L.: Influence of sex hormones on gingival exudation in gingivitis-free female dogs. J. Periodont. Res., 3:273, 1968.

97. Lindhe, J., Attström, R., and Björn, A. L.: Influence of sex hormones on gingival exudation in dogs with chronic gingivitis. J. Periodont. Res., 3:279, 1968.

98. Lindhe, J., Birch, J., and Branemark, P. I.: Wound healing in estrogen treated female rabbits. J. Periodont. Res., 3:21, 1968.

99. Lindhe, J., Branemark, P. I., and Birch, J.: Microvascular changes in cheek-pouch wounds of oophorectomized hamster following intramuscular injections of female sex hormones. J. Periodont. Res., 3:180, 1968.

100. Lindhe, J., Hamp, S.-E., and Löe, H.: Experimental periodontitis in the beagle dog. J. Periodont. Res., 8:1, 1973.

101. Lindhe, J., and Lundgren, D.: Influence of progesterone and estrogen on the permeability of crevicular vessels. *In* The Prevention of Periodontal Disease. J. Eastoe, D. C. A. Picton, and A. G. Alexander, Eds. London, Henry Kimpton, 1971.

102. Lindhe, J., and Svanberg, G.: Influence of trauma from occlusion on progression of experimental periodontitis in the beagle dog. J. Clin. Periodontol., *1*:3, 1974.

103. Lindhe, J., et al.: Clinical and steriologic analysis of the course of early gingivitis in dogs. J. Periodont. Res., in press.

104. Lipke, D., and Posselt, U.: Parafunctions of the masticatory system (bruxism): report of a panel discussion. J. West. Soc. Periodont., 8:133, 1960.

105. Listgarten, M. A., Mayo, H. E., and Tremblay, R.: Development of dental plaque on epoxy resin crowns in man. A light and electron microscopic study. J. Periodontol., 46:10, 1975.

106. Lite, T., DiMaio, D. J., and Burman, L. R.: Gingival pathosis in mouth breathers. A clinical and histopathologic study and a method of treatment. Oral Surg., 8:382, 1955.

107. Löe, H., and Rindom-Schiött, C.: The effect of mouth rinses and topical application of chlorhexidine on the development of dental plaque and gingivitis in man. J. Periodont. Res., 5:79, 1970.

108. Löe, H., Theilade, E. and Jensen, S. B.: Experimental gingivitis in man. J. Periodontol., 36:177, 1965.

109. Loesche, W. J., and Nafe, D.: Reduction of supragingival plaque accumulations in institutionalized Down's syndrome patients by periodic treatment with topical kanamycin. Arch. Oral Biol., 18:1131, 1973.

110. Lövdal, A., Arno, A., and Waerhaug, J.: Incidence of manifestations of periodontal disease in light of oral hygiens and calculus formation. Acta Odont. Scand., 14:21, 1958.

111. Macdonald, J. B.: The etiology of periodontal disease. Bacteria as part of a complex etiology. Dent. Clin. North Am., Nov:679, 1960.

112. Macdonald, J. B., Gibbons, R. J., and Socransky, S. S.: Bacterial mechanisms in periodontal disease. Ann. N.Y. Acad. Sci., 85:467, 1960.

113. Macdonald, J. B., Socransky, S. S., and Gibbons, R. J.: Aspects of the pathogenesis of mixed anaerobic infections of mucous membranes. J. Dent. Res., 42 (suppl 1):529, 1963.

114. Manhold, J. H.: Report of a study on the relationship of personality variables to periodontal conditions. J. Periodontal. 24:248, 1953.

115. Maryon, L. W., and Loiselle, R. J.: Bacterial antigens and antibodies in human periodontal tissue J. Periodontol., 44:164, 1973.

116. McDougall, W. A.: Penetration pathways of a topically applied foreign protein into rat gingiva. J. Periodont. Res., 6:89, 1971.

117. McDougall, W. A.: Ultrastructural localization of antibody to an antigen applied topically to rabbit gingiva. J. Periodont. Res., 7:304, 1972.

118. McDougall, W. A.: The effect of topical antigen on the gingiva of sensitized rabbits. J. Periodont. Res., 9:153, 1974.

119. Mellanby, M.: Diet and the teeth: An experimental study. Part I. Dental structures in dogs. Med. Res. Counc. Spec. Rep. Ser. London, 140, 1929.

120. Mellanby, M.: Dental research, with special reference to periodontal disease produced experimentally in animals. Dent. Record, 59:227, 1939.

121. Mergenhagen, S. E.: Endotoxic properties of oral bacteria as revealed by the local Shwartzman reaction. J. Dent. Res., 39:267, 1960.

122. Mergenhagen, S. E., DeAraujo, W. C., and Varah, E.: Antibody to leptotrichia buccalis in human sera. Arch. Oral Biol., 10:29, 1965.

123. Miller, S. C.: The use of the minnesota multiplastic personality inventory as a diagnostic aid in periodontal disease. A preliminary report. J. Periodontol., 27:248, 1953.

124. Mitchell, D. F., and Holmes, L. A.: Topical antibiotic control of dentogingival plaque. J. Periodontol., 36:303, 1965.

125. Mitchell, D. F., and Johnson, M.: The nature of the gingival plaque in the hamster. Production, prevention and removal. J. Dent. Res., 35:651, 1956.

126. Mulvihill, J. E., et al.: Histological studies of the periodontal syndrome in rice rats and the effects of penecillin. Arch. Oral Biol., 12:733, 1967.

127. Nadler, S. C.: The importance of bruxism. J. Oral Med., 23:124, 1968.

128. Newman, M. G., et al.: Studies of the microbiology of periodontosis. J. Periodontol., 47:373, 1976.

129. Newman, M. G., Socransky, S. S., and Listgarten, M. A.: Relationship of microorganisms to the etiology of periodontosis. Program and Abstracts, 52nd meeting, IADR., Abs #324, 1974.

130. Niles, J. G.: Early recognition of diabetes mellitus through interstitial alveolar resorption. Dental Cosmos, 74:161, 1932.

131. Nisengard, R. J.: Immediate hypersensitivity and periodontal disease. J. Periodontol., 45:344, 1974.

132. Nisengard, R. J., and Beutner, E. H.: Relation of immediate hypersensitivity to periodontitis in animals and man. J. Periodontol., 41:223, 1970.

133. O'Leary, T. J., Shannon, I., and Prigmore, J. R.: Clinical and systemic findings in periodontal disease. J. Periodontol., 33:243, 1962.

134. O'Leary, T. J., et al.: The effect of ascorbic acid supplementation on tooth mobility. J. Periodontol., 40:284, 1969.

135. Oliver, W. M.: The effect of deficiencies of calcium, vitamin D or calcium and vitamin D and of variations in the source of dietary protein on the supporting tissues of the rat molar. J. Periodont. Res., 4:56, 1969.

136. Oshrain, H. I., Salkind, A., and Mandel, I. D.: Bacteriologic studies of periodontal pockets 10 minutes after curettage. J. Periodontol., 43:685, 1972.

137. Page, R. C., Davies, P., and Allison, A. C.: Pathogenesis of the chronic inflammatory lesion induced by Group A streptococcal cell walls. Lab. Invest., 30:568, 1974.

138. Page, R. C., Davies, P., and Allison, A. C.: The role of the mononuclear phagocyte in chronic inflammatory disease. J. Reticuloendothel. Soc., 15:413, 1974.

139. Page, R. C., and Schroeder, H. E.: Biochemical aspects of the connective tissue alterations in inflammatory gingival and periodontal disease. Int. Dent. J., 23:455, 1973.

140. Page, R. C., and Schroeder, H. E.: The pathogenesis of inflammatory, periodontal disease. Lab. Invest., 33:235, 1976.

141. Pantalone, R. M., and Page, R. C.: Lymphokine induced production and release of acid hydrolases by macrophages. Proc. Nat. Acad. Sci., 72:2091, 1975.

142. Payne, W. A., et al.: Histopathologic features of the initial and early stages of experimental gingivitis in man. J. Periodont. Res., 10:51, 1975.

143. Pearlman, B. A.: An oral contraceptive drug and gingival enlargement: the relationship between local and systemic factors. J. Clin. Periodontol., 1:47, 1974.

144. Polson, A. M.: Trauma and progression of marginal periodontitis in squirrel monkeys. II. Co-destructive factors of periodontitis and mechanically produced injury. J. Periodont. Res., 9:108, 1974.

145. Radusch, D. F.: Nutritional aspects of periodontal disease. Ann. Dent., 7:169, 1940.

146. Ramfjord, S. P.: Tuberculosis and periodontal disease with special reference to the collagen fibers. J. Dent. Res., 31:5, 1952.

147. Ramfjord, S. P.: Bruxism, a clinical and electromyographic study. J. Am. Dent. Assoc., 62:21, 1961.

148. Ranny, R. R., and Zander, H. A.: Allergic periodontal disease in sensitized squirrel monkeys. J. Periodontol., 41:12, 1970.

149. Rawls, A. O.: Pyorrhea alveolaris. Dental Cosmos, 27:265, 1885.

150. Ray, H. G., and Santos, H. A.: Consideration of tongue-thrusting as a factor in periodontal disease. J. Periodontol., 25:250, 1954.

151. Rehnwinkel, F. H.: Pyorrhea alveolaris. Dental Cosmos, 19:572, 1877.

152. Rizzo, A. A., and Mergenhagen, S. E.: Local Shwartzman reaction in rabbit oral mucosa with endotoxin from oral bacteria. Proc. Soc. Exp. Biol. Med., 104:580, 1960.

153. Rizzo, A. A., and Mitchell, C. T.: Chronic allergic inflammation induced by repeated deposition of antigen in rabbit gingival pockets. Periodontics, 4:5, 1966.

154. Robinson, J., et al.: Nocturnal teeth-grinding: a reassessment for dentistry. J. Am. Dent. Assoc., 78:1308, 1969.

155. Rosebury, T.: The nature and significance of infection in periodontal disease. Am. J. Orthodt., 33:658, 1947.

156. Rosebury, T., Macdonald, J. B., and Clark, A. R.: A bacteriologic survey of gingival scrapings from periodontal infections by direct examination, guinea pig inoculation and anaerobic cultivation. J. Dent. Res., 29:718, 1950.

157. Rosenberg, M. M., Goldman, H. M., and Barger, E.: The effects of experimental thyrotoxicosis and myxedema in the periodontium of rabbits. J. Dent. Res., 40:807, 1961.

158. Rovin, S., Costich, E. R., and Gordon, H. A.: The influence of bacteria and initiation in the initiation of periodontal disease. J. Periodont. Res., 1:193, 1966.

159. Rutledge, C. E.: Oral and roentgenographic aspects of the teeth and jaws of juvenile diabetics. J. Am. Dent. Assoc., 27:1740, 1940.

160. Sabiston, C. B., and Grigsby, W. R.: Anaerobic bacteria from the advanced periodontal lesion. J. Periodontol., 43:199, 1972.

161. Salkind, A., Oshrain, H. I., and Mandel, I. D.: Bacterial aspects of developing supragingival and subgingival plaque. J. Periodontol., 42:706, 1971.

161a. Salton, M. R. J.: The Bacterial Cell Wall. New York, Elsevier Publishing Co., 1964, p. 252.

162. Sandler, H. C., and Stahl, S. S.: The influence of generalized diseases on clinical manifestations of periodontal disease. J. Am. Dent. Assoc., 49:656, 1954.

163. Saxe, S. R., et al.: Oral debris, calculus and periodontal disease in the beagle dog. Periodontics, 5:217, 1967.

164. Saxton, C. A.: Scanning electron microscopic study of the formation of dental plaque. Caries Res., 7:102, 1973.

165. Scherp, H. W.: Current concepts in periodontal disease research: Epidemiological contributions. J. Am. Dent. Assoc., 68:667, 1964.

166. Schneider, T. F., et al: Specific bacterial antibodies in the inflamed human gingiva. Periodontics, 4:53, 1966.

167. Schroeder, H. E., and Lindhe, J.: Conversion of a stable established gingivitis into destructive periodontitis. Arch. Oral Biol., in press.

168. Schultz-Haudt, S., Bibby, B. C., and Bruce, M. A.: Tissue destructive products of gingival bacteria from non-specific gingivitis. J. Dent. Res., 33:624, 1954.

169. Schultz-Haudt, S., Dewar, M., and Bibby, B. G.: Effects of hyaluronidase on human gingival epithelium. Science, 117:653, 1953.

170. Schuster, G. S., Hayashi, J. A., and Bahn, A. N.: Toxic properties of the cell wall of gram-positive bacteria. J. Bacteriol., 93:47, 1967.

171. Schwartz, J., Stinson, F. L., and Parker, R. B.: The passage of triated bacterial endotoxin across intact gingival crevicular epithelium. J. Periodontol., 43:270, 1972.

172. Shapiro, L., et al.: Endotoxin determinations in gingival inflammation. J. Periodontol., 43:591, 1972.

173. Shaw, J. H., and Griffith, D.: Relation of protein, carbohydrate and fat intake to the periodontal syndrome. J. Dent. Res., 40:614, 1961.

174. Sheppard, I. M.: Alveolar resorption in diabetes mellitus. Dental Cosmos, 78:1075, 1936.

175. Shoshan, S., Pisanti, S., and Sciaky, I.: The effect of hypervitaminosis D on the periodontal membrane collagen in lathyritic rats. J. Periodont. Res., 2:21, 1967.

176. Soames, J. V., and Davies, R. M.: The structure of subgingival plaque in a beagle dog. J. Periodont. Res., 9:333, 1974.

177. Socransky, S. S.: Relationship of bacteria to the etiology of periodontal disease. J. Dent. Res., 49(suppl 2):203, 1970.

178. Socransky, S. S., et al.: The microbiota of the gingival crevice area of man. I. Total microscopic and viable counts and counts of specific organisms. Arch. Oral Biol., 8:275, 1963.

179. Sorrin, S.: Habit: an etiologic factor of periodontal disease. Dent. Digest, 41:290, 1935.

180. Stahl, S. S., Sandler, H. C., and Cahn, L.: The effects of protein deprivation upon the oral tissues of the rat and

particularly upon the periodontal structure under irritation. Oral Surg., 8:760, 1955.

181. Steinberg, A. I.: Evidence for the presence of circulating antibodies to an oral spirochete in the sera of clinic patients. J. Periodontol., 41:312, 1970.

182. Stralfors, A.: Investigations into the bacterial chemistry of dental plaques. Odont. Tidskr. 58:151, 1950.

183. Takahama, Y.: Bruxism. J. Dent. Res., 40:227, 1961.

184. Talbot, E. S.: Pyorrhea alveolaris. Dental Cosmos, 28:689, 1886.

185. Tanchester, E. D., and Sorrin, S.: Dental lesions in relation to pulmonary tuberculosis. J. Dent. Res., 16:69, 1937.

186. Tempel, R. R., et al.: Host factors in periodontal disease: periodontal manifestations of Chediak-Higashi Syndrome. J. Periodont. Res. 7, Suppl., 10:26, 1973.

187. Terner, C.: Arthus reaction in the oral cavity of laboratory animals. Periodontics, 3:18, 1965.

188. Theilade, E., et al.: Experimental gingivitis in man II. A longitudinal clinical bacteriological investigation. J. Periodont. Ses., 1:1, 1966.

189. Thomas, A. E., et al.: Ascorbic acid and alveolar bone loss. Oral Surg., 15:555, 1962.

190. Torchichara, Y.: Pyorrhea alveolaris in leprosy. Nippar No Skikai, 13:165, 1933.

191. Tsutsui, M., Utsumi, N., and Tsubakimoto, K.: Cellular components of staphlococci and streptococci in inflamed human gingiva. J. Dent. Res., 47:663, 1968.

192. Weisberger, D., Young, A. P., and Morse, F. W.: Study of ascorbic acid blood levels in dental patients. J. Dent. Res., 17:101, 1938.

193. Williams, B. L., Pantalone, R. M., and Sherris, J. C.: Subgingival microflora and periodontitis. J. Periodont. Res., 11:1, 1976.

194. Williams, J. B.: Diabetic periodontoclasia. J. Am. Dent. Assoc., 15:523, 1928.

195. Wolbach, S. B., and Bessey, O. A.: Tissue changes in vitamin defficiencies. Physiol. Rev., 22:233, 1942.

196. Zachrisson, B. W.: A histological study of experimental gingivitis in man. J. Periodont. Res., 3:11, 1968.

5

Occlusal Traumatism as an Etiologic Factor

Other Predisposing Factors

    Loss of Teeth

    Faulty Restorative Dentistry

    Injudicious Periodontal Surgery

    Faulty Occlusal Adjustment

    Temporomandibular Joint Dysfunction

5

Occlusal Traumatism As An Etiologic Factor

For decades there has been disagreement about the role of abnormal occlusal stress in initiating periodontal disease. It is generally accepted that occlusal traumatism can be a distinct pathologic entity unassociated with periodontitis, and that related tissue changes are microscopic, noninflammatory, and limited to the attachment apparatus. When occlusal traumatism is associated with periodontitis, however, controversy arises. Can occlusal traumatism initiate gingivitis or periodontitis? Does it modify the response to local irritants that are the primary etiologic factors, or is the joint occurrence of occlusal traumatism and periodontitis merely coincidental? Many attempts, some excellent, have been made to resolve the controversy, yet much of the argument supporting the various hypotheses is still based on empiricism. Further study must be done to fill the serious gaps remaining in our knowledge of this relationship.

Occlusal traumatism is only one of the many terms used to denote injury to the periodontium by the forces of occlusion. Since there are several others, a review of the historical development of the terminology of occlusion and definitions of currently accepted terms will be helpful.

The term *traumatic occlusion*, introduced by Stillman, denoted abnormal stress capable of producing injury to the dental or periodontal tissues.[49] Box advocated use of the term *traumatogenic occlusion* for this stress and *traumatic occlusion* for the functional-contact relationship of occlusal surfaces that is the direct result of this trauma, for example, a disturbed occlusion resulting from tooth displacement in a jaw fracture.[5] Ramfjord and Ash, while admitting that *traumatic occlusion* is ambiguous, continued to use it merely as a matter of convenience, since it is so entrenched in the literature.[40]

Mühlemann and his associates pressed for a clearer distinction between *traumatogenic* and *traumatized* and suggested *traumatogenic occlusal situation* for factors initiating abnormal occlusal stress and *occlusal trauma* for the resulting microscopic lesion.[32] *Periodontal traumatism* was used by Orban[33] and also by Prichard[39] for the tissue injury caused by the occlusal forces and not for the occlusal forces themselves. Another term with the same meaning is *trauma from occlusion*.[15] Others have referred to *occlusal trauma* as the forces, resulting from mandibular movement, capable of producing periodontal disturbances.[7]

It is evident that disagreement in differentiation between causes and symptoms has contributed to the confusion. It may never be resolved. In this text the term *occlusal traumatism* is used for the sake of convenience to mean the effect and not the cause. When *occlusal trauma* is used, it refers to the stress created by the occlusal forces that leads to *occlusal traumatism*.

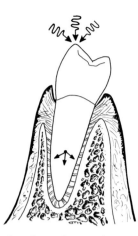

Fig. 5-1. *Effects of prolonged excessive occlusal force (wavy arrows) on tooth with relatively sound periodontal support, which can result in widening of the periodontal ligament space, yet cause no apical migration of the epithelial attachment, a condition often referred to as "primary occlusal traumatism."*

The division into primary and secondary occlusal traumatism has been attempted in much of the literature, but has led to much confusion. *Primary occlusal traumatism* is generally referred to as a condition resulting from abnormal occlusal forces on relatively sound periodontal structures. In effect, the traumatic forces acting on teeth with normal support are greater than can be withstood without injury to the periodontium. Those who adopt this definition imply that the forces are pathologic but that periodontal damage such as apical migration of the epithelial attachment resulting in bone loss is not appreciable (Fig. 5-1).

Secondary occlusal traumatism is applied to a condition resulting from physiologic or abnormal occlusal forces acting on a dentition that is seriously weakened by the loss of supporting alveolar bone. This lack of periodontal support may result not only from the effects of periodontal disease but also from injudicious osseous resection during periodontal therapy or oral surgery, from accidental trauma, or from excessive apical resorption associated with orthodontic or endodontic therapy. When one or more of these factors have caused a loss of periodontal support resulting in an apical shift in the fulcrum of the tooth within its alveolus, both functional and parafunctional occlusal loads may exceed the resistance and reparative capacity of the periodontium. Because of the increased crown-to-root ratio, the increased leverage applied to the teeth during even normal functions such as mastication may be intolerable and may lead to the condition termed secondary occlusal traumatism (Fig. 5-2).

The use of the terms *primary* and *secondary* as applied to occlusal traumatism is misleading. The confusion related to these definitions stems from the fact that primary occlusal traumatism refers to a histopathologic condition of the supporting structures, whereas secondary occlusal traumatism refers to the mechanical status of the tooth, for example, increase in crown-to-root ratio and an apically repositioned fulcrum. However, it is important to make it clear that all teeth categorized as suffering from secondary occlusal traumatism will also show histopathologic signs of primary occlusal traumatism of the supporting structures that remain attached to the tooth. Although secondary occlusal traumatism is never present without manifes-

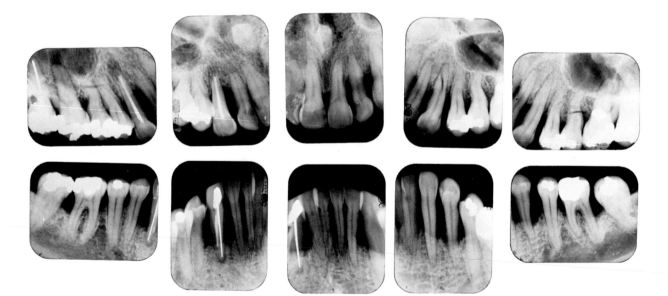

Fig. 5-2. *Example of so-called "secondary occlusal traumatism." Note the severe generalized loss of supporting bone.*

tations of primary occlusal traumatism, dentitions suffering from primary occlusal traumatism need not also be suffering from secondary occlusal traumatism.

In medical terms, *secondary* means that the condition is secondary to a separate disease or set of pathologic conditions. Unless the definition is revised and additional agents are identified as acting upon primary occlusal traumatism, the use of the terms, *secondary stage* or *secondary phase* would be more correct. However, this would imply that secondary occlusal traumatism is a progressive form or is the result of primary occlusal traumatism, which it has not as yet been demonstrated to be.

The clearest distinction between the two phases of occlusal traumatism can be derived from the definition of chronic destructive periodontal disease given by Ross.[42] He divides the factors causing chronic destructive periodontal disease into two groups: precipitating and predisposing. *Precipitating factors* are the irritants and the destructive occlusal forces that further destroy the tissues weakened by the predisposing factors. *Predisposing factors*, which take the place of those contributing to the histopathologic lesion, he lists as developmental factors, functional mechanisms, and the systemic component. These slowly and insidiously weaken the area. The terms *precipitating* and *predisposing* are equally applicable to the factors causing occlusal traumatism, and their adoption would rid the vocabulary of some imprecise terminology.

PRECIPITATING FACTOR IN OCCLUSAL TRAUMATISM

The precipitating factor in occlusal traumatism is *force*. All other factors are predisposing. Without force the classic histopathologic signs of occlusal traumatism would not appear. Force is applied to the teeth during both normal and abnormal functions. However, the reaction of teeth and their supporting structures to normal and abnormal functions can vary greatly.

Normal functions such as mastication, deglutition, and speech rarely, if ever, play a role in occlusal traumatism. Teeth seldom make functional contact during mastication, deglutition, and speech, and even when they do, the contact is of insufficient magnitude to be of much significance in occlusal traumatism. Even gross morphologic deformities can withstand the stresses of normal function, since the forces (for all practical purposes instantaneous) are usually well within the physiologic limits of the stress-absorbing system of the periodontium.

Of much greater significance are the effects of forces that result from parafunctions. The exertion of parafunctional force caused by the so-called occlusal neu-

roses such as grinding and clenching is of greatest significance as a precipitating factor in occlusal traumatism. Varying throughout life, parafunctional forces are of much greater intensity and longer duration than functional forces and are often exerted in a nonaxial direction. The periodontium can adapt to different functional forces, but traumatic lesions can appear if they exceed its physiologic limits, overcoming the adaptive capacity of the tissues by the intensity, duration, and frequency of application of forces. Repair cannot occur, especially if stress is combined with local or systemic factors inducing inflammation.

PREDISPOSING FACTORS

Predisposing factors can be divided into *intrinsic* and *extrinsic*.

Intrinsic Factors

Among the intrinsic factors are the following:

1. Morphologic characteristics of the roots. Factors such as their size, shape, and number are of prime importance. Teeth with short, conical, slender, or fused rather than divergent roots, are more predisposed to occlusal traumatism when subjected to prolonged excessive force (Figs. 5-3, 5-4) than are those with normal morphology.

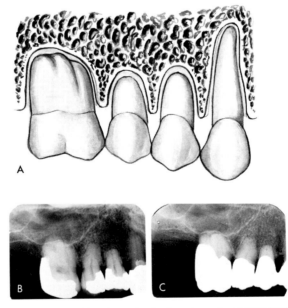

FIG. 5-3. *Teeth with extremely short roots, an important intrinsic factor that predisposes teeth towards occlusal traumatism. A. Schematic drawing of teeth seen in radiographs. Note fused roots of first molar, another predisposing intrinsic factor. B. Radiograph prior to stabilization. C. Radiograph after stabilization by fixed prosthesis.*

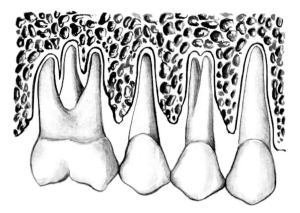

FIG. 5-4. *Schematic drawing of teeth with slender and conical roots, also an intrinsic predisposing factor.*

2. The manner in which occlusal surfaces and the roots are oriented in relation to the forces to which they are exposed. Axially inclined forces are more tolerable than are nonaxially inclined forces, which may be functional or parafunctional. If teeth are badly aligned, the effect of excessive force will be deleterious (Fig. 5-5).

3. Morphologic characteristics of the alveolar process. If the quantity or quality of alveolar bone is inherently lacking, the effects of prolonged parafunctional forces may result in rapid loss of the remaining support (Fig. 5-6).

Extrinsic Factors

Among the extrinsic factors that may seriously increase the rapidity of loss of supporting alveolar bone are the following:

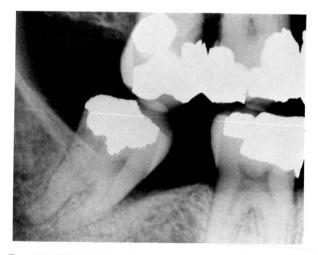

FIG. 5-5. *Tilted third molar, demonstrating effect of nonaxial forces, which may be functional or parafunctional. Note that the roots of the third molar are short and conical. This is another example of an intrinsic, predisposing factor. Note also the mesial osseous defect and the widened periodontal ligament space.*

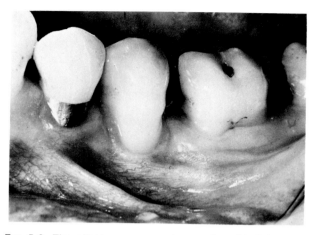

FIG. 5-6. *The effect, on a second premolar with little or no buccal supporting bone, of prolonged excessive occlusal force. This tooth had both centric and nonworking premature contacts. Note the gingival recession which followed the resorption of the buccal bone.*

1. Irritants. Microbial dental plaque is implicated as the most serious (Fig. 5-7). Other irritants that may have similar effects are food impaction that results in positive pressure on the tissues, overhanging fillings (Fig. 5-10B), poorly contoured crowns and bands, and ill-fitting partial denture clasps (Fig. 5-8).

2. Neuroses that result in parafunctional activities such as bruxism. These are the most prevalent and serious of all factors causing abnormal occlusal stresses (Figs. 5-2, 5-7, 5-20).

3. Loss of supporting bone (Fig. 5-9). Periodontitis, injudicious osseous resection (Figs. 5-22, 5-27), inadvertent trauma, and systemically related diseases are the chief causative factors.

4. Loss of teeth resulting in overloading of the remaining teeth, e.g., posterior-bite collapse (Fig. 5-23).

5. Iatrogenically created functional malocclusion (Figs. 5-10, 5-11).

STUDIES OF OCCLUSAL TRAUMATISM

Numerous reports describing the association of periodontal disease and occlusal traumatism have appeared in the literature. As early as 1901, Karolyi implied a cause-and-effect relationship, and since that time extensive investigations have been undertaken, using both experimental animals and humans to define the link between occlusal traumatism and periodontal disease.[23] Results from two studies supported Karolyi's hypothesis.[6,50] Box's study is unfortunately often quoted and has drawn much more attention than it deserves. He placed a gold crown, ended supragingivally, in supraocclusion on the lower incisor of a

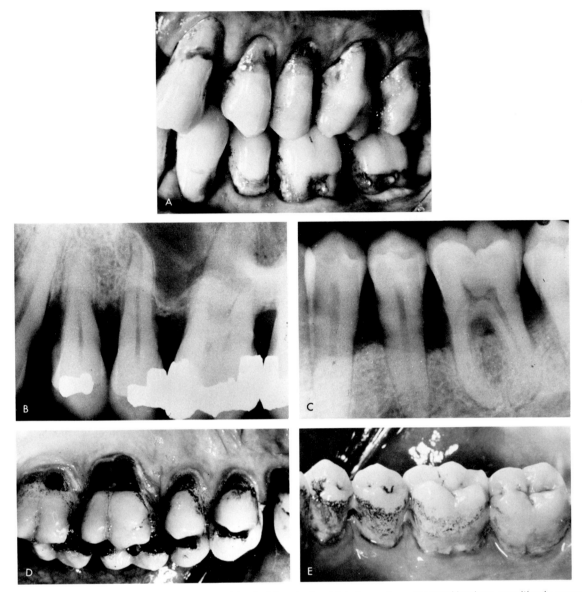

FIG. 5-7. *The co-destructive effects of a severe clenching habit and microbial plaque from poor oral hygiene, resulting in generalized loss of supporting bone and occlusal traumatism in the remaining attachment apparatus. Irritants such as microbial plaque also act as an important extrinsic predisposing factor in occlusal traumatism combined with periodontitis. A. Buccal view of teeth in occlusion. Note lack of cusp wear, which is symptomatic of clenching as distinct from grinding habits. B. Maxillary teeth of same patient. C. Mandibular teeth. C. Lingual view of maxillary teeth. E. Lingual view of mandibular teeth.*

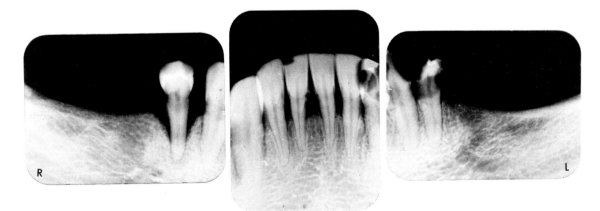

FIG. 5-8. *Mandibular teeth which helped support poorly designed removable partial denture. Right first premolar severely traumatized as a result of posterior settling and a poorly designed clasp. (The left premolar escaped occlusal traumatism only because extensive caries alleviated the deleterious force transmitted through a clasp of the same design.)*

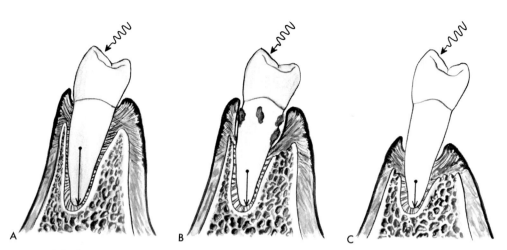

FIG. 5-9. *Force as a precipitating factor in occlusal traumatism. A. Effects of excessive and prolonged force (wavy arrow) on a tooth with normal support resulting in widening of the periodontal ligament space and increase in mobility. B. Effect of same forces on a tooth with moderate loss of periodontal support due to periodontitis. Because the fulcrum point (straight arrow) is more apically positioned there is an increased tendency toward occlusal traumatism, tooth mobility, and further breakdown of the remaining periodontal support. C. Severe loss of periodontal support where even masticatory forces cannot be tolerated, resulting in occlusal traumatism of the remaining periodontal support.*

sheep, thereby increasing the crown-root ratio and the labiolingual dimension of the tooth. After a little over 3 months, the crowned tooth demonstrated greater mobility and slightly increased pocket depth and had a greater accumulation of calculus than did the other three incisors. In addition, the pulp of the affected tooth showed subacute inflammation, and the surrounding tissues were edematous. The one tooth, one sheep study has since been widely criticized as not representing a scientific investigation. Regardless of Box's personal inferences, however, he never made a definite claim that a relationship exists between occlusal trauma and periodontal disease.

In a more sophisticated study, Stones demonstrated in monkeys what he felt was a causal relationship. He induced excessive occlusal stress by installing high occlusal restorations on adjacent teeth for up to 43 weeks.[50] After sacrifice, histopathologic changes similar to gingivitis and in some animals periodontitis were seen in the periodontium surrounding about 30 percent of the experimental teeth, being most pronounced in the tooth with the highest crown and its antagonist. Stones concluded that occlusal trauma led to periodontal disease and that the disease would increase in severity as long as the trauma was present.

Some felt that not all of Stones' conclusions had been correctly drawn. Among others, Bhaskar and Orban contended that apical migration of the epithelial attachment, observed previously by Stones in dogs, as well as in monkeys, was not pathologic but physiologic, representing nothing more than passive eruption.[4]

Most authors recognize the role of microbial plaque in producing gingival inflammation, which in turn is

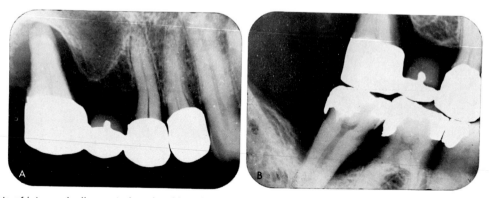

FIG. 5-10. *Effects of iatrogenically created occlusal interferences on the supporting structure. Examination revealed gross centric and nonworking interferences in the second molar region. In addition, poorly fitting restorations encouraged plaque retention—yet another destructive extrinsic factor;*

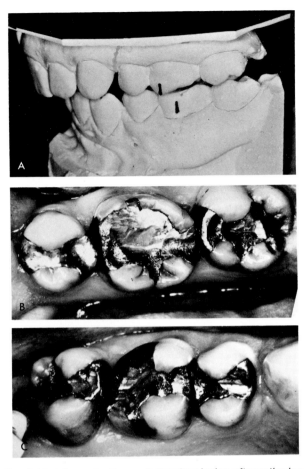

FIG. 5-11. *Iatrogenically created malocclusion after orthodontic therapy. Patient suffered from temporomandibular joint dysfunction. A. Articulated casts in centric relation occlusion. Vertical lines on the first molars indicate the discrepancy between the patient's centric relation occlusion and centric occlusion. B. Occlusal faceting, indicating attempt by the patient to function in a more retruded mandibular position. C. Occlusal faceting of the opposing maxillary teeth of the same patient. (Courtesy Dr. R. Fabrick.)*

essential to the development of periodontitis. Many believe that superimposed occlusal traumatism modifies or aggravates this response to local irritants such as plaque or faulty restorations, but the majority do not believe that occlusal trauma initiates gingivitis or periodontitis. Glickman and Weiss made it clear that inflammation is not caused by occlusal trauma, but that it is codestructive with it and cannot clinically be dissociated from it in periodontal disease.[14,20] The results of animal experiments and of observations on human surgical and autopsy material are reviewed.

Animal Experiments

Studies of animals generally consisted of creating overloading occlusal forces by placement of restorations in supraocclusion in dogs, monkeys, or occasion-

ally rats, followed by histologic examination of the teeth and surrounding tissues after varying time periods. Most of these experiments were designed so that the force employed eventually moved the tooth out of trauma. An analogous clinical situation would be a case in which anterior teeth move out in response to posterior prematurities.

The majority of the studies demonstrated early periodontal changes on both tension and pressure sides of the experimental teeth. The early changes on the tension side included widening of the ligament space, stretching or tearing of fibers, and thrombosis; on the pressure side, necrosis or disorientation of the ligament fibers, thrombosis and hemorrhage, and undermining bone resorption were seen. Signs of root resorption on both pressure and tension sides appeared later. After the tooth moved out of trauma a period of repair began. This was characterized by formation of new bone on the tension side and replacement of necrotic bone and connective tissue. The width of the ligament space returned to normal and the resorbed areas on the root underwent repair. The incidence and degree of gingivitis and periodontitis were not appreciably different in the experimental and control teeth in the majority of experiments. The characteristic destructive changes and subsequent repair were evident even if the induced occlusal overloads were repeated and prolonged. Damage to cementum, periodontal ligament, and alveolar bone was repaired when the tooth adjusted to its new position. Only under extremely "favorable" conditions could a deepening of the clinical pocket below the cementoenamel junction be produced, and this was considered the only evidence of permanent damage.[52]

Objections were raised regarding these studies in that the occlusal overloading did not represent the same type of jiggling trauma observed in humans, and experiments were designed to provide this.[54,57] Wentz and his colleagues fitted crowns to monkeys' teeth with lingual locks to force the experimental teeth buccally with each occlusal closure. An orthodontic appliance then pulled the teeth or tooth back lingually with disocclusion, thereby producing the buccolingual jiggling trauma. Thus, the experimental teeth could not escape the trauma by migration. The histologic evidence was the same except that pressure and tension areas occurred on both buccal and lingual sides, causing a widening of the periodontal ligament space and a lengthening of the fibers of the periodontal ligament. In no instance could recession of the epithelial attachment be seen. Inflammation was absent from the tissues after 3 months of the experiment, and in spite of a severe increase in mobility, new bone was being laid down simultaneously with alveolar bone resorption.

Animal studies, focused on the addition of further

stress, either mechanical, metabolic, or systemic, to occlusal overloading gave varying results. Protein deprivation further aggravated the effects of gingival injury and occlusal overloading in monkeys, causing exaggerated degenerative changes within the periodontium, with none of the signs of repair apparent in the control animals.[45] In other experiments systemic stress in addition to dental trauma, again in monkeys, produced reversible damage in the periodontal tissues, but not to any extent comparable to human periodontal disease.[57] Stahl, Miller, and Goldsmith were unable to induce migration of the epithelial attachment in rats by applying additional irritants that increased the inflammatory response and caused further alveolar bone resorption.[46,47]

Research findings from the majority of the animal studies gave the impression that excessive occlusal stress leading to occlusal traumatism was not necessarily of permanent importance in the diagnosis and treatment of periodontal disease. This separation of periodontitis and occlusal traumatism seriously influenced the method of treatment of periodontal disease by discounting the importance of occlusal adjustment by selective grinding. Since excessive occlusal forces apparently did not initiate apical migration of the epithelial attachment, the misconception arose that they would not aggravate existing periodontal pockets caused by other factors and since occlusal traumatism seemed to be reversible and capable of complete repair in animals, many believed that in humans repair would occur even if the excessive occlusal forces were persistent. The findings from these animal experiments, however, should not be extended to justify possibly erroneous conclusions about humans. The monkeys, dogs, and other animals used in many of these studies are not good experimental models. Even though the animal's mouth is constantly dirty, it is difficult, if not impossible, to produce periodontitis analogous to that in humans.[34]

The short duration of all these experiments is also significant. Even if jiggling forces are applied, they cannot possibly duplicate what years of excessive occlusal forces can do to a human dentition. Studies can only be satisfactorily made using human material.

Human Autopsy Material

Several investigations have been made using autopsy material to try to discover the relationship between histologic findings and the presence of forces causing occlusal traumatism in human jaws. Most of these jaws showed lesions that were similar to those described in animal experiments and which, provided that the reparative powers of the periodontium are not overtaxed by repeated insults, are reversible. Other jaws showed indications of prolonged and repeated insults that led to periodontal breakdown and loss of teeth. In such cases the areas of bone resorption had increased in number and size, and irreversible changes had occurred, making repair a disordered and irregular phenomenon. This stage is as a rule not reached in animal experiments.

Yet another phenomenon connected with increased functional occlusal forces has been described by Glickman.[18] A thickening of the cervical margin of the alveolar bone (buttressing) is seen in some human jaws that have been subjected to increased occlusal stress. He attributed this "seemingly paradoxical bulging bone contour" to an overcompensation by the forces of repair such as also occurs in the repair of alveolar bone elsewhere after injury.

Glickman and Smulow, describing the angular osseous defects that can be seen radiographically in cases showing microscopic evidence of occlusal traumatism, cautiously suggested the presence, following therapy, of osteoblastic activity within the osseous defects, especially those too small to be seen radiographically.[19] Their observations led them to associate occlusal traumatism with an alteration of the pathway of gingival inflammation, resulting in a modified pattern of tissue destruction and subsequently in intraosseous lesions. Their studies leading to this hypothesis are discussed later.

Histologic Changes in the Periodontium

Of particular interest was a statistical study made by Erausquin and Carranza of the histology of the periodontium when teeth are in normal occlusion and when they are subjected to trauma.[11] Their study showed that teeth in normal occlusion had the following characteristics: little or no apical migration of the epithelial attachment, physiologic gingival sulci or shallow supraalveolar pockets, scarcity of secondary cementum, a mean width of less than one-third a millimeter of the periodontal ligament space, scarcity of periodontal needles and nodules, intact cortical bone, and a few small-sized areas of alveolar resorption with compensatory reconstruction. In contrast, teeth that were subjected to trauma had the following characteristics: noticeable and very irregular apical migration of the gingival attachment, intraalveolar pockets, variable abundance of secondary cementum, a mean width of more than one-third a millimeter, an abundance of periodontal needles and nodules, osteoporotic cortical alveolar bone, and an abundance of large-sized areas of alveolar resorption with little or no compensatory reconstruction.

The periodontium is capable of adapting to either increased or decreased functional occlusal stress. Using block sections removed from patients scheduled for complete dentures, Ramfjord and Kohler observed that the midportion of the periodontal ligament and the crest of the alveolar bone are the structures most susceptible to increased pressure and that the Sharpey's fibers entering the cementum and the periodontal fibers coronal to them are the most stable.[41] Heavy stress was found to lead to extensive root (and even dentin) resorption and to changes in the cementoblasts such that they resembled odontoblasts and in the periodontal ligament such that it resembled periosteum. Teeth relieved of occlusal trauma from 2 weeks to 6 months before surgical removal showed rapid regeneration of bone along the alveolar crest and the surface of alveolar bone next to the periodontal ligament, and after 1 month deposition of precementum was evident on the root surfaces.

Clinical Studies

Epidemiologic studies on the relationship between occlusal traumatism and periodontal disease are limited in number and in most cases loosely controlled, presenting variables difficult to measure accurately. Several occlusal indices have been formulated, but all have some faults. Most investigators used an index that is morphologic rather than functional.[13,38] Interconnection between morphologic malocclusion and functional malocclusion has not stood the tests of research. Other criticisms are that oral hygiene practices and calculus deposition, very important factors, are not considered.

Beyron's long-term study of occlusal changes is a major contribution.[3] Although his study was not specifically designed to test a causal relationship between periodontal disease and occlusion, his results point to this. For up to 12 years he observed clinically healthy young adults requiring little or no restorative or periodontal care. By grouping their occlusions according to functional criteria (gliding patterns), he was able to note changes which characterized each category as follows (Fig. 5-12):

1. Dentitions with unrestricted multidirectional patterns of gliding movement. These developed more favorably than did other patterns, showing by the end of the study period uniform occlusion wear and no signs of undue stress on the periodontium.

2. Dentitions with predominantly bilateral movement but with somewhat restricted overbite. Predominating changes were attrition of the

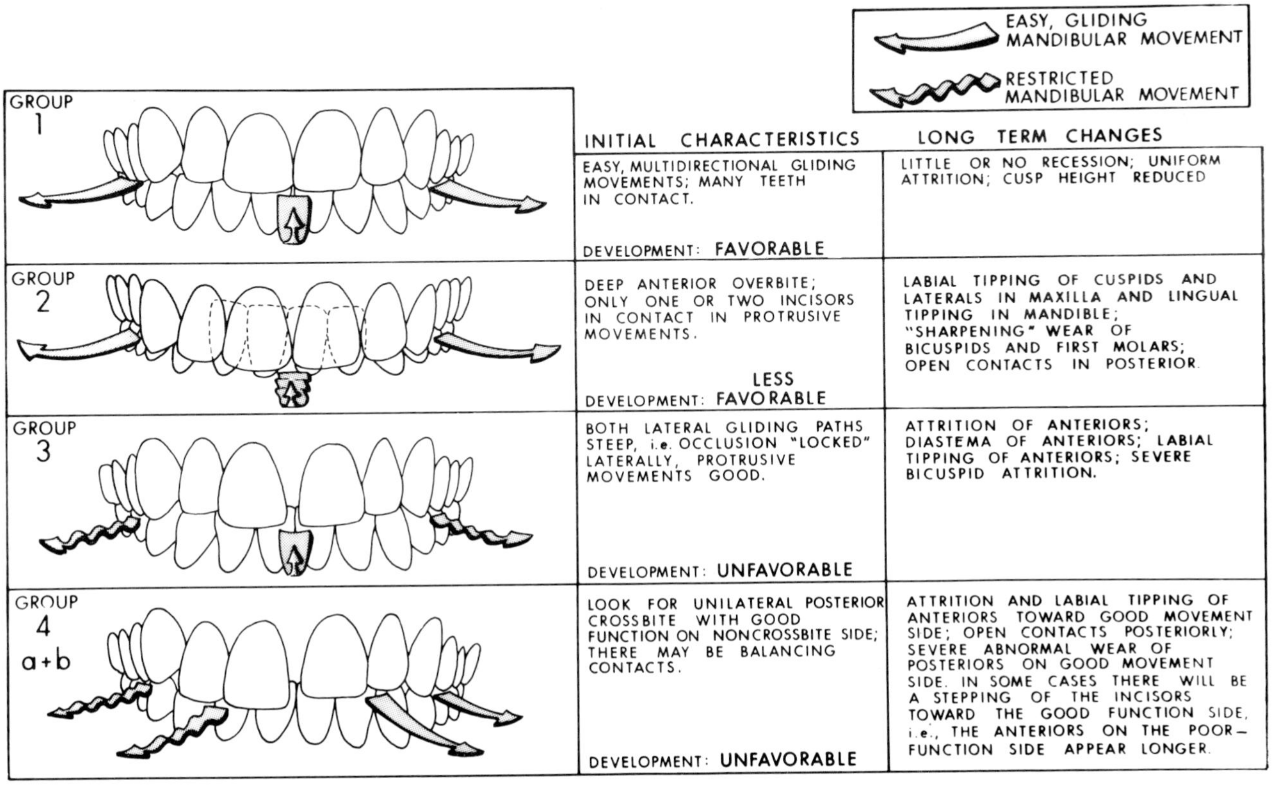

	EASY, GLIDING MANDIBULAR MOVEMENT
	RESTRICTED MANDIBULAR MOVEMENT

	INITIAL CHARACTERISTICS	LONG TERM CHANGES
GROUP 1	EASY, MULTIDIRECTIONAL GLIDING MOVEMENTS; MANY TEETH IN CONTACT. DEVELOPMENT: FAVORABLE	LITTLE OR NO RECESSION; UNIFORM ATTRITION; CUSP HEIGHT REDUCED
GROUP 2	DEEP ANTERIOR OVERBITE; ONLY ONE OR TWO INCISORS IN CONTACT IN PROTRUSIVE MOVEMENTS. LESS DEVELOPMENT: FAVORABLE	LABIAL TIPPING OF CUSPIDS AND LATERALS IN MAXILLA AND LINGUAL TIPPING IN MANDIBLE; "SHARPENING" WEAR OF BICUSPIDS AND FIRST MOLARS; OPEN CONTACTS IN POSTERIOR.
GROUP 3	BOTH LATERAL GLIDING PATHS STEEP, i.e. OCCLUSION "LOCKED" LATERALLY, PROTRUSIVE MOVEMENTS GOOD. DEVELOPMENT: UNFAVORABLE	ATTRITION OF ANTERIORS; DIASTEMA OF ANTERIORS; LABIAL TIPPING OF ANTERIORS; SEVERE BICUSPID ATTRITION.
GROUP 4 a+b	LOOK FOR UNILATERAL POSTERIOR CROSSBITE WITH GOOD FUNCTION ON NONCROSSBITE SIDE; THERE MAY BE BALANCING CONTACTS. DEVELOPMENT: UNFAVORABLE	ATTRITION AND LABIAL TIPPING OF ANTERIORS TOWARD GOOD MOVEMENT SIDE; OPEN CONTACTS POSTERIORLY; SEVERE ABNORMAL WEAR OF POSTERIORS ON GOOD MOVEMENT SIDE. IN SOME CASES THERE WILL BE A STEPPING OF THE INCISORS TOWARD THE GOOD FUNCTION SIDE, i.e., THE ANTERIORS ON THE POOR-FUNCTION SIDE APPEAR LONGER.

FIG. 5-12. *Long-term occlusal changes in the permanent dentition (after Beyron[3]). (Courtesy Dr. C. Castaldi.)*

posterior teeth and slight labial tipping of the maxillary cuspids and lateral incisors.

3. Dentitions demonstrating predominantly sagittal movements. These generally developed attrition and labial tipping of the anterior segments and diastemata between the maxillary teeth. Because of the tipping the occlusal stresses were less favorable. The type of wear exposed some teeth to a rocking and jarring action.

4. Dentitions featuring predominantly unilateral gliding movements.

   a. With a major difference in inclination between right and left lateral gliding paths; also such irregularities as crossbites, nonworking contacts, and irregular contacts on the working side. The predominant occlusal changes observed were some attrition and labial tipping of the maxillary anterior teeth on the functioning side and loss of interstitial contact in some cases due to direct damage of the periodontium through food impaction.

   b. With anterior components. The occlusal changes by the end of the study were pronounced attrition and slight labial tipping of the maxillary anterior teeth on the functioning side with no attrition on the opposite side.

Beyron's study showed that under a given set of conditions, with time, predictable occlusal and periodontal changes could occur which depended greatly on the functional pattern of the occlusion and to a lesser degree on the morphology.

Ramfjord and Kohler observed periodontal changes in response to known functional increase or decrease in occlusal stress and concluded that disuse atrophy of functionally oriented periodontal fibers was a slow process in adults.[41] They also stated that loss of posterior teeth may lead to occlusal traumatism with such sequelae as root resorption and resorption of the alveolar cortical plate with perforations causing dehiscences and fenestrations. The validity of these findings is questionable since there was an uncontrolled variable: labial mucoperiosteal flaps overlying the experimental teeth had been reflected as part of another experiment.

Another clinical investigation was conducted by Yuodelis and Mann in an attempt to determine the prevalence and possible role of nonworking (balancing) contacts in periodontal disease.[56] Statistical results showed that teeth with nonworking contacts were associated with significantly greater mobility, pocket depth, and interproximal bone loss than were those without such contacts. Although the findings did not indicate that nonworking contacts are the primary cause of periodontal breakdown, they suggest that they may play a modifying or aggravating role.

A Modifying Role

The majority of investigators on humans and animals seemed to dismiss abnormal occlusal stress as a primary etiologic factor in the initiation of periodontal disease, but an undercurrent was detected, implicating occlusal trauma as playing a modifying or aggravating role. Further studies on animals and humans led Glickman and Smulow to suggest that occlusal trauma alters the pathways of gingival inflammation into the deeper supporting structures, a theory currently accepted by several authorities.[17] A review of these studies will help explain this theory.

The major blood supply to the gingiva arises from vessels that parallel the ligament and exit into the gingiva. Weinmann's classic study led him to believe that the progress of chronic and acute gingival inflammation is related to the distribution and direction of these blood vessels.[55] Histologic evidence from human jaws demonstrated that gingival inflammation progressed into the alveolar bone marrow by following the course of the perivascular channels and penetrated directly into the periodontal ligament. This evidence suggested that perivascular channels offered a path of lesser resistance to the inflammation than did the ligament. Resorption of the alveolar crest from the gingival side led to destruction first of the supporting alveolar bone and then of the interseptal bone.

In a later study, Macapanpan and Weinmann observed the progress of gingival inflammation of local origin into ligaments previously damaged by tooth movement.[28] Rather than following the same course as that observed in Weinmann's earlier study, the gingival inflammation (as demonstrated by leukocytic infiltration) spread from the gingival papillae directly into the periodontal ligament.

Glickman and Smulow set themselves to discovering the factor responsible for the change of pathway and identified it as excessive force damaging the ligament on the tension side and allowing direct infiltration by inflammatory cells.[17]

Goldman studied the response of gingival tissue to induced occlusal traumatism.[21] He surmised that any undue pressure against the tooth would occlude the blood supply to the marginal gingiva from the periodontal ligament. Using india-ink perfusion, he demonstrated that in spite of obliteration of this route, the gingival blood supply was not embarrassed. In a similar study, Cohen et al. demonstrated changes typical of occlusal traumatism in the attachment apparatus, but the gingival blood supply was not affected.[8] Kennedy induced ischemia of the gingival circulation of squirrel monkeys and showed that the epithelial attachment is supplied collaterally by vasculature from the gingiva and from the periodontal ligament and that either one alone is sufficient to maintain it.[24] The lesions produced by gingival ischemia in no way resembled periodontal disease. Clinically, it is improbable that the blood supply to both gingiva and periodontal ligament can be cut off simultaneously. Thus, it is reasonable to deduce that necrosis of the epithelial attachment must be attributable to some other cause.

Glickman and Smulow demonstrated in a similar study (up to $4\frac{1}{2}$ months) on adult monkeys that excessive occlusal stress from experimentally induced abnormal functional relationships in the presence of gingival inflammation could produce the signs and symptoms of occlusal traumatism and noted the following:[17]

1. Alteration in the orientation of the periodontal fibers opened up a direct pathway for inflammation into the ligament.
2. Increased pressure on the crestal areas of the periodontal ligament caused osteoclastic resorption of alveolar bone.
3. Degeneration of the periodontal ligament eliminated the natural barrier provided by healthy fibers.
4. Formation of a funnel-shaped widening of the periodontal ligament by osteoclastic resorption at the crestal margins channeled the inflammation directly into the altered periodontal ligament.
5. Pressure sufficient to cause localized necrosis in the periodontal ligament set up a barrier to the direct extension of inflammation, and in these instances inflammation followed the usual course described in Weinmann's study.[55]
6. Changes on the tension side were not extensive enough to affect the pathway of inflammation in these experiments.
7. Evidence of repair could be seen in osseous lesions after 3 to 4 months.

Ewen and Stahl reported a similar investigation with somewhat different results: gingival inflammation spread primarily into the crestal alveolar zone and into the tension side of the periodontal ligament.[12] The combination of tilting forces and gingival irritation induced an intraosteal lesion with topography similar to that described in humans. The results were not, however, contradictory. The trauma was much more severe (tilting was induced by removal of an incisor and tying together of the two adjacent teeth across the gap) and the experiments lasted up to 1 year.

Glickman and Smulow subsequently proposed rec-

ognition of two disease zones, the zone of irritation and the zone of codestruction.[17] The *zone of irritation* consists of the marginal and interdental gingiva apically bounded by the gingival fibers; inflammation confined to this region is unaffected by occlusal forces. The *zone of co-destruction* includes the periodontal ligament, cementum, and surrounding alveolar bone and is coronally bounded by the transseptal fibers interproximally and the alveolar crest fibers facially and lingually. These fibers are disrupted by occlusal traumatism and gingival inflammation, thus allowing inflammation to spread directly into the periodontal ligament and its approximating base. This pattern of progression of inflammation leads to vertical or intraosteal defects pathognomonic of occlusal traumatism. Glickman and Smulow attempted to demonstrate the same disease zones, using human material.[19] They proposed that angular-bone defects specifically are strongly suggestive of occlusal traumatism. However, the modifying role concept was not freed from controversy, since only autopsy material was used and there were no results of occlusal examination to relate the signs of traumatism to the defects.

Stahl presented histologic data from the resected jaws of 4 patients treated for oral malignancies who were examined for occlusal discrepancies before surgery.[44] He observed a great variety of tissue responses, among them the limited degree of inflammatory infiltration into the crestal periodontal ligament when pressure had altered the ligament. It is difficult to draw conclusions from the study of these 4 patients because of the possibility that some tissue changes may have resulted from hypofunction.

Because of these inconsistencies, Comar and his colleagues conducted yet another study using monkeys.[9] Gold crowns with gross marginal discrepancies and open contacts were constructed and placed in supraocclusion to provide co-destructive factors, intensifying the already active gingivitis. However, animals sacrificed at varying intervals failed to show any apical migration of the epithelial attachment. In failing to confirm Glickman's co-destruction hypothesis, Comar and his associates admitted that although the trauma in their experiments was in excess of that found in humans, the degree of inflammation required to duplicate Glickman's results may not have been reached. It appeared as though additional factors such as bacterial or other systemic irritants are needed if the integrity of the dentogingival complex is to be altered.

Present Status

Data from studies using animals such as monkeys and dogs as the experimental subjects are of limited value, since inferences drawn cannot be reliably applied to humans. Although the animals' mouths may be dirty, it is difficult, if not impossible, to produce true periodontal disease in monkeys. In addition, no experiments have been extended for sufficient time to duplicate the effect of years of occlusal traumatism in humans. Therefore, negation of traumatic occlusion as either a primary etiologic factor or a modifying factor now would be premature.

The controversy remains incompletely resolved. Nonetheless, investigators agree that certain relationships exist between occlusal traumatism and periodontal disease.

We know that just as the periodontium exists to support the functional demands of the teeth, stimulation from normal functional occlusion is required to keep the periodontium healthy. We also know that in many cases it can accommodate increased functional demands, as evidenced by a thickening of the lamina dura and reinforcement of the bony trabeculae. If accommodation does not take place, injury may result even without local factors of sufficient intensity to cause inflammation. In such cases excessive occlusal stress can alter the attachment apparatus of the periodontium without producing an increase in pocket depth, for example, in occlusal traumatism unassociated with periodontitis, where histopathologic changes of the attachment apparatus are reversible only if the tooth can move away from the traumatic forces or if the trauma is eliminated. If the noxious force is chronic, the effect is a widening of the periodontal ligament thought to cushion the impact. Widening is due to bone resorption and results in excessive tooth mobility which becomes especially significant in the presence of gingival inflammation or systemic factors.

Inflammation is recognized as the principal factor responsible for tissue destruction in periodontal disease. Since inflammation occurs at least to some degree in most mouths, a tooth already weakened by occlusal traumatism offers less resistance to its spread, resulting in bone loss (Fig. 5-7). Occlusal traumatism does not initiate gingivitis or periodontitis, but probably modifies or intensifies the inflammation to result in its more rapid extension and in pocket formation (Fig. 5-9B,C). How this happens and at what stage in periodontal disease occlusal stresses become operant has not been conclusively demonstrated.

Systemic factors can modify the resistive capacity of the host to both abnormal occlusal stress and local gingival irritants and can exert an important influence.

There is no scientific evidence to support the thesis that occlusal traumatism is associated with gingival changes such as Stillman's clefts or McCall's festoons, described as manifestations of traumatic occlusion.

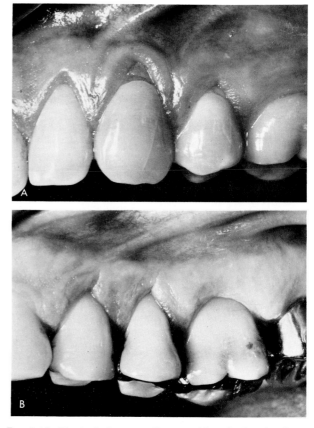

FIG. 5-13. *Gingival changes often considered related to bruxism. A. McCall's festoons. B. Stillman's clefts. There is no scientific evidence that such changes are related to occlusal stress, and they may be only coincidental.*

Occasionally, clinical cases demonstrating noninflammatory gingival changes may seem to be associated with occlusal traumatism (Fig. 5-13). These are, however, exceptions, and their relationship is biologically unexplainable, since no such changes have been produced by experimental occlusal traumatism in animals.

Regardless of its role in periodontal disease, occlusal traumatism is nevertheless a serious pathologic state of the periodontium and should therefore be regarded as pathognomonic of periodontal disease. It is often associated with periodontitis and its distressful symptoms must be treated.

ETIOLOGY OF OCCLUSAL TRAUMATISM

It has been stated earlier in the chapter that force is the precipitating factor in occlusal traumatism. In an intact dentition with normal or adequate periodontium, occlusal traumatism is rarely if ever the result of functional forces. Chiefly, it is associated with excessive occlusal forces, with those of a parafunctional nature, or with compulsive habits such as grinding, clenching, and other occlusal neuroses. The potentially damaging influence of these parafunctional forces to the attachment apparatus, teeth, and temporomandibular joint has been referred to earlier as a major factor in the etiology of certain degenerative forms of periodontal disease because the forces resulting from neuroses are applied more frequently and are of considerably longer duration than those resulting from normal function.

Function versus Parafunction

There are two major categories of activity performed by the stomatognathic system: normal function and parafunction. Mastication, occasional light contact during speech, swallowing, coughing, and yawning are all regarded as normal function; all other forms of pressure contact of the teeth are parafunctional.

With adequate periodontal support, normal functions are homeostatic, often under even the most unfavorable conditions of occlusal morphology. Normal functional stresses are injurious only when the dentition has suffered from excessive alveolar bone loss or apical resorption. Parafunctions are not homeostatic, since they are performed on a subconscious, reflex-controlled level and have a tendency to be prolonged for many hours during sleep or even during waking hours when the conscious attention of the patient is directed elsewhere. Thus, they are often injurious even under normal occlusal and periodontal conditions.

Parafunctional Activity (Bruxism)

Five categories of parafunctional activity have been identified:[10]

1. *Psychically motivated*, meaning that the parafunctions are of a neurotic nature, e.g., bruxism.
2. *Stress-motivated*, representing exaggerated response to stress, of a concentration often seen during athletic activities or some types of work.
3. *Habitual*, associated with one's trade or profession.
4. *Endogenous*, arising from systemic diseases such as epilepsy, tetanus, meningitis, and other infections.
5. *Excessively compensating*, and involuntary and unconsciously exaggerated, representing reactions to occlusal interferences and to disturbances of various kinds.

All these categories overlap and have a common psychic component. The terms *parafunctional activity* and *bruxism* are now often used interchangeably, but there is a trend toward grouping the various patterns of parafunctional clenching and grinding in centric and eccentric positions under the general term *bruxism*.[25,40] Since the specific distinctions in the neuromuscular basis of the different patterns cannot be established, use of the single term would seem justified. A slight distinction should be made between grinding habits and clenching habits. Although intimately related, they may be of dissimilar significance to the teeth and periodontium and often require different therapy, primarily because of the difference of degree and duration of the force applied. During episodes of grinding, the muscle contraction is isotonic, whereas during clenching isometric contraction prevails. Of the two, prolonged isometric contraction is considered more noxious, since it exerts as much as 200 to 300 pounds of pressure per square millimeter.[1] The different pathologic manifestations of the two habits will be discussed later in the chapter.

Other common parafunctions such as biting the tongue, cheek, lip, fingernails, pencils, bobby pins, and pipe stems have a definite psychogenic basis. They are clearly related to bruxism but should be classified as occlusal habits rather than bruxism per se. Their pathologic sequelae are usually localized, whereas more general damage may result from clenching or grinding.

PREVALENCE OF BRUXISM

Surveys of the prevalence of bruxism are unreliable for several reasons. Since bruxism is performed on a subconscious, reflex-controlled level, the habit is commonly unrecognized by the patient unless it has been called to his attention. Also, variations in concept as to what constitutes bruxism undoubtedly account for the large discrepancies in the incidence (20 to 88 percent) in the adult population reported.[30,36] If it is agreed that parafunctional movements, at least at some time in one's life, constitute bruxism, then the incidence might well approach 100 percent. However, the transient tendency to clench or grind briefly associated with anger, remorse, or physical exertion is not damaging and is considered normal. It is only when the need for bracing by clenching or grinding is persistent and prolonged that this parafunctional movement should be termed bruxism.

ETIOLOGY OF BRUXISM

Two major factors are intimately related to the mechanism of bruxism: the emotional or psychologic factor and the occlusal factor. The emotional factors implicated range from repressed aggression, emotional tension, anxiety, anger, and fear to oral dependency as the central life problem.[31] Occlusal factors include centric prematurities and cuspal interferences within excursive border movements. Bruxism is related to the state of hypertonicity of the masticatory muscles, which is in turn affected interdependently or independently by occlusion, emotion, pain, or discomfort. Damage results from the excessive forces of bruxism. Since the source of force is the jaw muscles, neuromuscular disturbances resulting in hypertonicity are considered important factors, either in initiating the compulsion or as a sequela of it.

It has not yet been possible to evaluate the relative significance of the emotional and occlusal factors in clenching, although electromyographic and clinical studies have revealed that there is often an interplay between them.

Bruxism resulting in occlusal traumatism may arise from severe functional disharmony and minimal psychic tension as well as from severe psychic tension and insignificant functional occlusal factors.[40] Here again, it is unclear how the interplay operates. According to one theory, the occlusal factor is more important, acting as a trigger mechanism to incite nervous tension. The most common occlusal factors are discrepancies between centric relation occlusion and centric occlusion and balancing (non-working) interferences.[40] This assertion is based on clinical electromyographic observation of severe bruxism where the imbalance in muscular activity could be eliminated by proper occlusal adjustment.

A different theory implicates emotional factors as being more important from the fact that emotional stress causes an increase in skeletal-muscle tension, initiating bruxism.[43] In one study, temporomandibular-joint dysfunction closely associated with bruxism was effectively treated without occlusal therapy by alleviating anxiety only.[26]

RELATIONSHIP OF BRUXISM TO PERIODONTAL DISEASE

The significance of bruxism as an etiologic factor in periodontitis depends on whether bruxism results in occlusal traumatism. If it does, it will play the same role as occlusal traumatism. However, occlusal traumatism is only one of several manifestations of bruxism; other major ones are occlusal attrition and dysfunction of the temporomandibular joint and associated musculature. Because of the high incidence of bruxism, it should be suspected in most cases of periodontal disease. The periodontal significance of bruxism increases with a decrease in periodontal support, resulting from either chronic destructive periodontitis or the loss of posterior teeth from caries or severe root resorption. In such cases the condition may precipitate occlusal traumatism.

MANIFESTATIONS OF BRUXISM

Manifestations of bruxism differ with the type of habit. *Clenching*, also referred to as *centric bruxism*,[40] is a repetitive, prolonged, forceful contact of the teeth with no or extremely minimal mandibular movement. Because of the lack of movement, clenching results in isometric muscle contraction (as distinct from isotonic contraction during grinding). The most serious results of clenching are primarily pathologic changes of the periodontal supporting structures and secondary disturbances of the temporomandibular joint.

The pathologic sequelae of clenching are usually greater, more generalized, and more serious than those resulting from grinding. Histologic evidence of crushing injury such as hemorrhage and necrosis is present. Clinically, the incidence of severe tooth mobility is higher and more generalized than results from grinding, and thus mobility contributes to food impaction (Fig. 5-2). Clenchers rarely show excessive occlusal attrition or faceting typical of grinders, and any tooth wear is slight and in the immediate vicinity of the centric holding areas.

Radiographically, the teeth show little wear if hypermobility is generalized, but instead manifest generalized widening of the ligament space, which is often accompanied by selective destruction of the alveolar bone. Root resorption (Fig. 5-14) and in more severe instances apical radiolucencies, indicating pulpal death, may be seen.

Disturbances of the temporomandibular joint and associated musculature typical of clenching commonly accompany periodontal manifestations and result from prolonged isometric muscle contraction. These in turn lead to progressive local decrease in blood circulation, accumulation of metabolic end products, and fatigue of the involved muscles.

Grinding, also referred to as *eccentric bruxism*,[40] may be limited to a single pair of teeth or involve segments of the dentition (Fig. 5-15). Because of mandibular movement, the muscle contraction is isotonic. Manifestations of grinding are (1) attrition of the occlusal surfaces, (2) injury to the periodontium, and (3) disturbances of the temporomandibular joint and associated musculature. The pathologic sequelae depend greatly on the ability of the periodontium to compensate for the increased stress. If stress is compensated for by an increased trabecular pattern of the bone, alveolar exostoses, or buttressing, the damage is greatest on the occlusal surfaces, which in such a case form the weakest link (Fig. 5-16). Damage to the supporting structures may be seen if the periodontium cannot accommodate the increased stress or if periodontal bone destruction is already present. It is not uncommon to find disturbances of varying degree in all

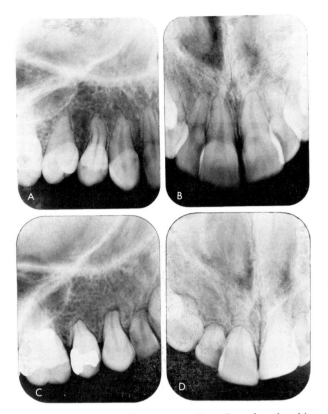

FIG. 5-14. *Root resorption as a manifestation of a clenching habit. A and B. Teeth of 14-year-old patient. C and D. Same teeth 10 years later.*

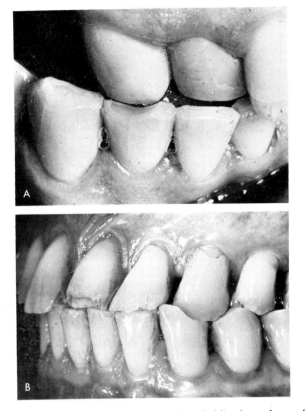

FIG. 5-15. *Faceting related to grinding habit, also a form of bruxism. A. Incisal wear on the mandibular lateral incisors is the result of atypical grinding in a lateral protrusive position, whereas the wear on the mandibular cuspid is due to grinding in a lateral functional position. B. Wear resulting from grinding, limited to a segment of the dentition.*

three areas: teeth, periodontium, and temporomandibular joint and associated musculature.

When grinding affects only one or two teeth, the pathologic sequelae may be isolated and irregular wear patterns, mobility, pain, pulpal death, and periodontal or apical abscess formation (Fig. 5-17). Radiographically and micrographically, signs of injury to the attachment apparatus are widening of the ligament space, cemental tears, root resorption, hypercementosis and, in more severe instances, root fracture with apical radiolucencies indicating pulpal death (Figs. 5-18, 5-19).

When large segments of the occlusion are involved, the manifestations are the same, but on a broader scale. The occlusal surfaces may show extensive nonfunctional patterns of attrition and no pathologic tooth mobility, but instead a compensatory alveolar nodular exostosis may be evident (Fig. 5-16). Attrition may result in variations in occlusal curvatures, highly polished matched facets (Fig. 5-20), sharp or ragged incisal edges (Fig. 5-15), and loss of clinical crown height. The wear and excessive stress may result in the fracture of teeth and restorations.

MISCELLANEOUS ORAL HABITS

Many oral habits, some closely related to bruxism, may be categorized as either nonspecific or occupational.

Nonspecific habits, such as lip, tongue, and cheek biting, or clamping of jaws in eccentric positions, all

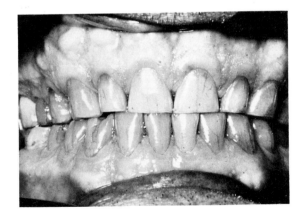

FIG. 5-16. *Generalized tooth wear as a manifestation of a grinding habit. Note the enamel crazing and fracturing as well as compensatory alveolar nodular exostoses.*

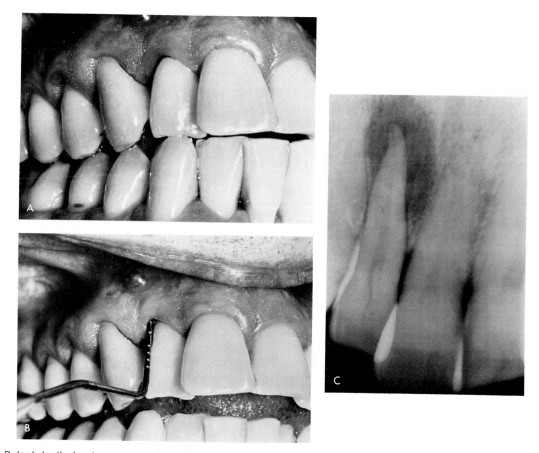

FIG. 5-17. *Pulpal death due to a severe atypical grinding habit involving the maxillary lateral incisor and the mandibular cuspid. A. Position of teeth during grinding. Note incisal faceting of the lateral incisor. B. Probing to indicate lack of apical migration of the epithelial attachment (pocket depth 3 mm). Note fistula above the lateral incisor. C. Radiograph showing apical radiolucency. (Courtesy Dr. R. L. Johnson.)*

serve, like bruxism, as outlets for emotional and psychic tension. Occlusal interferences may not be involved initially. Effects of such habits are dependent on their frequency and duration and the ability of the dentition to resist the consequent stress. Pathologic sequelae are usually more localized than are those of bruxism.

Cheek and lip biting usually cause excessive scarring of mucosal surfaces and, occasionally, malpositioning of the teeth involved. Localized malpositioning may in turn result in functional occlusal interferences and associated occlusal traumatism.

Faulty tongue posture or abnormal tongue habit in swallowing presents a perplexing problem for both the patient and the dentist who must treat it. This type of habit may be endogenous or acquired and usually results in both morphologic and functional malocclusion. Because the abnormal postures or excursions of the tongue are performed unconsciously, they are difficult to overcome. If the habit is a lateral thrusting of the tongue, a posterior open bite will develop (Fig.

5-21). A generalized anterior open bite with a poor occlusal relationship of the posterior teeth results from an anterior tongue thrust during swallowing.

Patients with an anterior open bite find it most difficult to incise, to masticate properly, and to swallow food. In an effort to perform these normal functions, much stress is exerted on the few posterior teeth remaining in occlusion. To protect the posterior teeth, a normal overjet-overbite relationship of the anterior teeth is important because it permits disclusion of the posterior teeth during lateral and protrusive movement. This is not possible with an anterior open bite, since every mandibular movement is met with deflective occlusal interferences during mastication. In order to close off the space during swallowing, great pressures are exerted on the anterior teeth by the tongue and by the mentalis, circumoral, and masseter muscles.

Such patients often show periodontal breakdown around the teeth remaining in occlusion, since they are the teeth subjected to abnormal stress. Generally, the

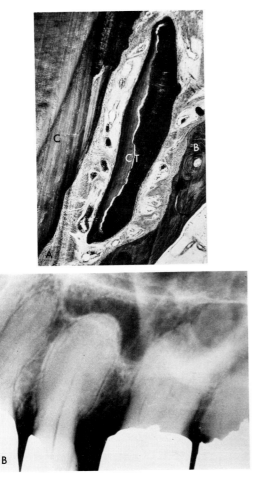

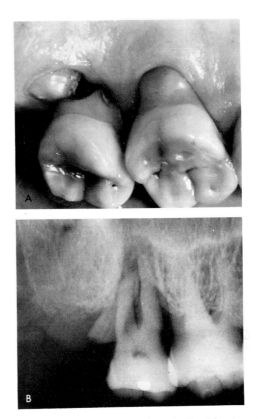

Fig. 5-19. *Manifestations of bruxism. A. Root fracture. Note occlusal wear and fractured palatal root of the second molar. B. Radiograph of A. (Courtesy Dr. G. Douglass.)*

Fig. 5-18. *Manifestations of bruxism. A. Micrograph of cemental tear: C, cementum; CT, cemental tear; B, bone. Note the fibrous attachment on each side of the tear. (Courtesy Dr. D. Grant.) B. Hypercementosis.*

periodontium surrounding the most distal molars shows signs of breakdown first. Teeth not in occlusion may show signs of greater plaque and calculus retention, which also results in periodontal disturbance.

Occupational habits may require or allow use of the teeth and mouth either actively or passively, and it is not uncommon to see localized effects from such habits as holding nails between the teeth, biting thread, and pressing mouthpieces of brass musical instruments tightly against the lips. Closely related habits are holding a pipe stem between the teeth for long periods, opening bobby pins, biting pencils, and prying open bottle caps. Such habits are not always psychically or occlusally induced. If damage to the periodontium results, it is usually localized. Occasionally such habits, if prolonged, can alter occlusal function and precipitate more occlusal disturbances that in turn lead to generalized occlusal traumatism. Even though such habits are not as common as bruxism, their recognition

is important because treatment of the effects and not the cause would result in only temporary improvement.

THE SIGNIFICANCE OF PARAFUNCTION

Parafunctional forces have been stressed as the major etiological factors in occlusal traumatism, with the psychic factor and occlusal disharmony implicated as initiating factors necessary in most cases to precipitate the various parafunctions, especially bruxism. However, the relative significance of the two initiating factors varies. For example, occlusal traumatism may be the result of moderate psychic tension and gross occlusal disharmony or of severe psychic disturbance with only minor occlusal discrepancies. Therefore, one must not rigidly prescribe the same therapeutic measures for all patients suffering from manifestations of occlusal traumatism. The help of a psychiatrist or psychologist is often necessary to overcome the psychic factor. In some cases this may be needed much more than complex occlusal therapy.

The significance of parafunction becomes increasingly greater in mouths already showing signs of alveolar bone loss, as is found in certain metabolic disturb-

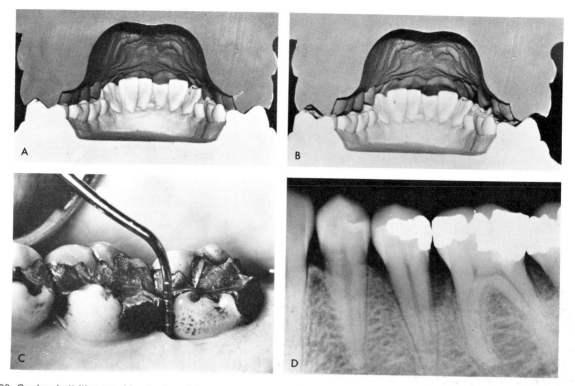

FIG. 5-20. *Occlusal attrition resulting in deep intercuspation of the posterior teeth and in periodontal pathology. A. Ground casts in centric occlusion, illustrating deep intercuspation of the posterior teeth. B. Same casts illustrating cross-arch and cross-tooth nonworking contacts during lateral excursion. C. Probing to illustrate loss of attachment. Note occlusal wear facets, especially on the molar marginal ridges, which were caused by plunger-cusp action and gave rise to interproximal food compaction. D. Radiograph of same region as in C, showing bone loss in premolar and molar regions and poor interproximal contact between premolar and molar.*

ances such as diabetes. Dentitions with moderate to severe loss of periodontal support are incapable of adequately resisting parafunctional forces. Alveolar support rapidly deteriorates unless proper therapeutic measures, including splinting and elimination of osseous craters and local factors, are undertaken. Here periodontal prosthetic measures are essential if an

environment for sufficient normal function is to be provided. They are necessary for good mastication and (often more important) in protecting the dentition from damage resulting from continued bruxism. Therefore, one must often reconstruct a dentition so that the patient can more safely grind or clench and more efficiently masticate. Too often periodontal ther-

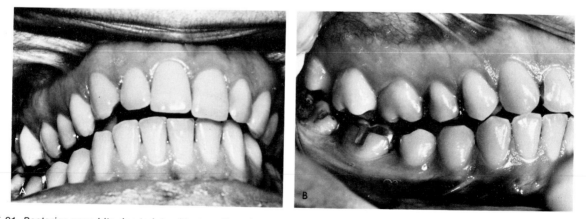

FIG. 5-21. *Posterior open bite due to lateral tongue-thrusting habit. A. Anterior view in centric occlusion. B. Lateral view of affected side in centric occlusion. The characteristics of this occlusion prevented normal disclusion of the posterior teeth by the cuspid during function and gave rise to contacts on the nonfunctioning side.*

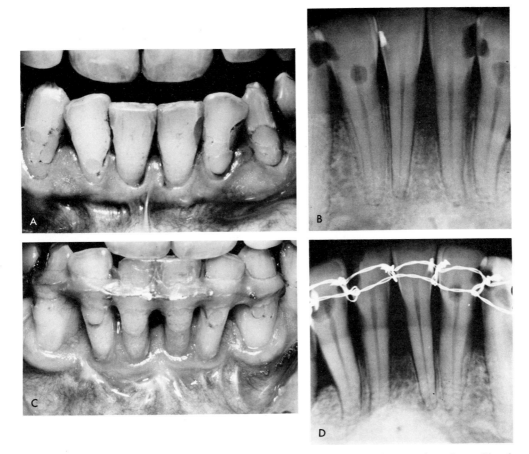

FIG. 5-22. *Permanent pathologic tooth mobility and occlusal traumatism of the remaining attachment, resulting from injudicious osseous resection to gain positive architecture in the incisor region. A. Presurgical view. B. Presurgical radiographs showing osseous involvement between central incisors. C. Postsurgical result. Mandibular incisors required temporary stabilization because of severe mobility. D. Postsurgical radiograph showing level of supporting bone. Incisors required extraction and replacement by a fixed bridge.*

apy ends with the elimination of pockets, leaving the patient a dental cripple, with many teeth that are sensitive and mobile and that have long clinical crowns. Such dentitions are incapable of proper function and could very well have been much more comfortable and capable of longer survival had they remained untreated (Figs. 5-22, 5-27). It is important to remember that pocket elimination is not the only goal in periodontics. Our knowledge of therapy must not be so narrow as to exclude the benefits of other disciplines. This subject will be discussed in Section III of the text.

Other Predisposing Factors

Although most important, parafunctions and microbial plaque are not the only extrinsic predisposing factors involved in occlusal traumatism. Several others predispose to this condition. However, occlusal traumatism does not result unless the adaptive capacity or resistance of the periodontium is overcome by the precipitating factor, which is force. In bruxism the protective response of the neuromuscular system is often seriously hampered, but this is not usually the case with tissue insult not initiated by neuromuscular disturbances. Here protective reflexes are normal and for this reason predisposing factors are considered less significant and are more easily eliminated or controlled.

Examples of predisposing factors are tooth loss, faulty restorations, periodontal, occlusal, or orthodontic therapy, and temporomandibular-joint dysfunction. Certain intrinsic anatomic abnormalities such as short, tapered roots provide less resistance to occlusal stress and also predispose toward occlusal traumatism.

LOSS OF TEETH

The early loss of teeth from caries or accident is common and predisposes toward occlusal traumatism. A classic example is posterior-bite collapse resulting from premature loss of the first permanent molar. It has been stated that the premature loss of the first permanent molar is the cause of almost all posterior-bite collapse.[2] Treatment of this type of case often taxes dentists' ability and patients' means and patience. Yet it is ironic that the unfortunate sequela of tooth loss, so universally understood and predictable, cannot be prevented more often, especially since its prevention is so easy. With all the modern restorative techniques available there is little reason to condemn grossly carious first molars. If they must be extracted the dentist should promptly preserve the space, either by means of a space maintainer if the patient is young, or preferably with a fixed bridge if the patient's age permits. This will prevent drifting and space closure leading to posterior-bite collapse.

The effects of tooth loss are not always restricted to the immediate vicinity of the loss. Changes often take place some distance from lost teeth. Classic examples are the occlusal changes from loss of the mandibular first permanent molar, including mesial and lingual tilting of the approximating molars and extrusion of the unopposed maxillary first molar, resulting in marginal-ridge discrepancies and inadequate or open-contact relationships of many posterior teeth (Fig. 5-23). This in turn contributes to food impaction, interproximal caries, and functional occlusal discrepancies. The discrepancies often cause an increased slide from centric relation occlusion to centric occlusion, the anterior teeth hitting each other with greater force during mastication. This functional disharmony causes the anterior teeth to drift labially, resulting in an open-contact relationship of the anterior segment. The next phase is usually further bite collapse and alveolar bone loss.

Another example is extrusion of an unopposed mandibular third molar (Fig. 5-24), resulting in a condition classically described by Thielemann.[51] This is referred to as Thielemann's Diagonal Law, which states that if an interference, such as an extruded or tipped tooth or third-molar gingival flaps, restricts the functional gliding movement of the mandible, extrusion of the anterior teeth will occur, and often periodontal disease will develop in the anterior region diagonally opposite to the interference.[40]

FAULTY RESTORATIVE DENTISTRY

Faulty restorative dentistry commonly predisposes toward acute occlusal traumatism. The traumatism may be transient if the tooth or teeth are able to drift or rotate into a harmonious occlusal relationship, but if not, the traumatic situation may become chronic. It is therefore imperative that principles of good functional occlusion be followed during restorative procedures.

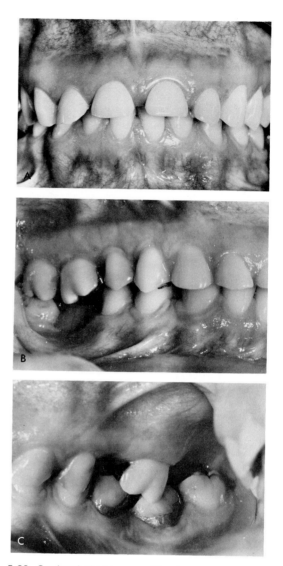

FIG. 5-23. *Occlusal changes resulting from premature loss of several posterior teeth and from superimposed bruxism. A. Anterior view, showing increased overjet, labial drifting, of incisors, and diastema formation. B. Right lateral view, showing extrusion of unopposed maxillary first molar. C. Left lateral view, showing mesial and lingual tilting of the second and third mandibular molars and distal tilting of the second mandibular premolar, obliterating the entire space of the missing first molar.*

Such mistakes as undercarving (Fig. 5-25) or overcarving occlusal anatomy (Fig. 17-19) or failure to restore proximal contacts may result in progressive detrimental occlusal change. A tooth with a high filling may become so painful that the patient is forced to acquire a different relationship of the mandible to the maxillae in order to avoid the imporperly restored tooth. This often puts many other teeth into traumatic functional relationship and may also lead to temporomandibular-joint dysfunction. Overcarving the occlusal anatomy so that centric holding areas are removed is a serious mistake, as it may allow teeth to erupt into a

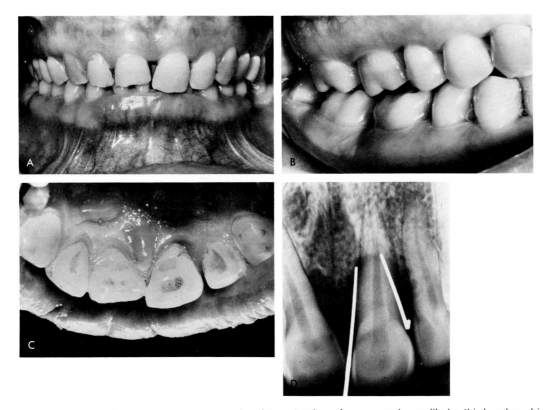

FIG. 5-24. *Condition resulting from occlusal changes related to extrusion of unopposed mandibular third molar which restricts function to one side of the mouth. A. Anterior view to show extruded and unworn side. B. Unopposed and extruded third molar diagonally opposite to affected anterior teeth. C. Lingual view of affected teeth to show migration to form diastema. D. Radiograph with silver points in place to indicate periodontal involvement. (Courtesy Dr. E. Sturdevant.)*

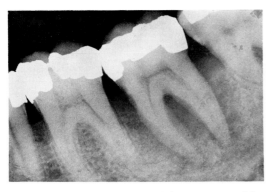

FIG. 5-25. *Severe acute periodontal damage around the second molar associated with undercarved amalgam restoration placed in supraocclusion. Note radiolucent area surrounding the roots.*

new occlusal relationship that may be traumatic to the periodontium during functional or parafunctional excursive movements of the mandible (Fig. 17-16).

INJUDICIOUS PERIODONTAL SURGERY

When periodontal disease is complicated by intraosseous defects or anatomic bone aberrations such as exostoses or tori, osseous resection has long been rec-

ognized as an effective remedy. As with any surgical resective procedure, there is a price to pay. In this case, further loss of supporting alveolar bone is often concomitant with the elimination of bone craters and results in a decrease in total alveolar support. Loss of alveolar support caused by either periodontal disease or corrective procedures may seriously aggravate occlusal traumatism. Therefore, in many severe cases the value of pocket elimination by osseous resection must be weighed carefully against this decrease in support. In such circumstances, functional forces previously within a physiologic range may become excessive, and irreversible breakdown may occur (Fig. 5-22).

Alternative therapeutic measures must be evaluated carefully. If total pocket elimination is imperative in severely involved dentitions, the patient must be informed that the therapy may embarrass total alveolar support to such an extent that complex and expensive long-term splinting will be necessary. Since many patients cannot afford the expense, a compromise treatment consisting of regular and definitive curettage, root planing, and oral physiotherapeutic procedures must be substituted.

Whether osseous resection will predispose toward occlusal traumatism depends on several factors. The

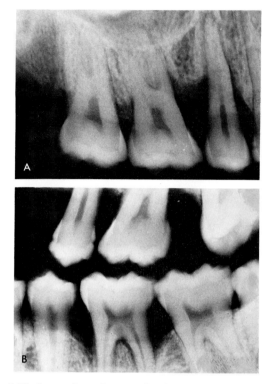

FIG. 5-26. *Severe loss of supporting bone and widening of the remaining ligament space due to occlusal stress. A. Attempts to eliminate the osseous defect around the second premolar by resection would seriously compromise the support of the first premolar and first molar. Extraction of the involved premolar is indicated. B. Pattern of bone loss surrounding the first molar warrants extraction of this tooth also.*

most significant are the amount and location of bone loss around the tooth prior to surgery (Fig. 5-26). One must relate the degree of loss to the tooth mobility and determine whether mobility is primarily the result of excessive force or is mainly caused by excessive bone loss.

Significant intrinsic predisposing factors to consider are the size, shape, number, and position of roots relative to the alveolar process. For example, a maxillary first molar with long, divergent roots and demonstrating no mobility can withstand removal of much more supporting bone in eliminating an intraosseous defect than one with short, spindly or closely grouped roots. Despite pocket elimination, the remaining bone around short, spindly or tapered roots will continue to resorb if the mobility patterns of these teeth are mainly attributable to loss of supporting bone. Osseous resection in such cases may cause teeth to topple over, evoking severe occlusal traumatism. It would often be better either to maintain the osseous defects with conservative therapy or to extract the teeth if they jeopardize the less involved adjacent teeth.

When severe bone involvement is localized on one or a few teeth, selective extraction of these teeth is often the wisest choice of therapy. It is not always possible or even advisable to save every tooth in every mouth. It is, however, our duty to save the mouth, and if the extraction of a few severely involved teeth makes this possible it should be done. Preservation of selectively involved teeth would necessitate gross removal of alveolar supporting bone from the adjacent teeth (Fig. 5-27). Inevitably this loss of tissue and support would result in increased sensitivity, difficulty in oral hygenic measures, and, most importantly, an increase in mobility, whereas extraction would preserve the support of adjacent prospective abutment teeth.

FAULTY OCCLUSAL ADJUSTMENT

Ironically, a therapeutic measure to correct faulty functional occlusion can result in further aggravation if used indiscriminately. Most rules for occlusal adjustment are flexible, but there are a few inviolate princi-

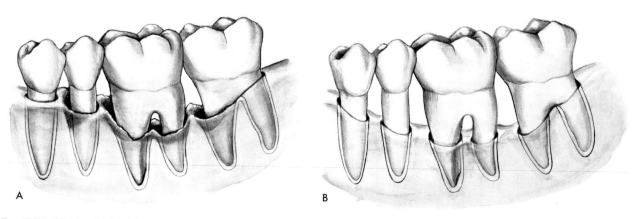

FIG. 5-27. *Effects of injudicious osseous resection. A. Characteristic bifurcation involvement, cratering, and hemiseptal osseous defects. B. Severe reduction of bone after injudicious attempt to create positive architecture.*

ples. Occlusal adjustment procedures resulting in occlusal contact relationships with forces not directed axially cause further trauma. This will be discussed in Chapter 17.

TEMPOROMANDIBULAR JOINT DYSFUNCTION

Temporomandibular joint dysfunction can result from minor functional occlusal discrepancies coupled with psychoneurotic habits, as well as from major dysfunctional occlusal relationships alone. Often patients demonstrate mandibular deviations resulting in bizarre occlusal relationships. Prior to any occlusal adjustment one must determine how much of the faulty occlusal relationship is due to mandibular deviation resulting from muscular spasm. Occlusal correction should not be done during the acute stages of temporomandibular-joint dysfunction. Muscle spasms should be alleviated first; if they are not, occlusal relationships might be "corrected" from an inaccurate centric relation position. Then, after the spasms have subsided, it would become apparent that occlusal relationships normal to the patient prior to temporomandibular-joint dysfunction had been permanently destroyed. This could result in a generalized occlusal traumatism.

References

1. Anderson, D. J.: Measurements of stress in mastication. J. Dent. Res., 35:671, 1956.
2. Amsterdam, M., and Abrams, L.: Periodontal prosthesis. *In* Periodontal Therapy, 5th ed. H. M. Goldman and D. W. Cohen, Eds. St. Louis, C. V. Mosby, 1973.
3. Beyron, H. L.: Occlusal changes in adult dentitions. J. Am. Dent. Assoc., 48:674, 1954.
4. Bhaskar, S. N., and Orban, B.: Experimental occlusal Trauma. J. Periodontol., 26:270, 1955.
5. Box, H. K.: Traumatic occlusion and traumatogenic occlusion. Oral Health, 20:642, 1930.
6. Box, H. K.: Experimental traumatogenic occlusion in sheep. Oral Health, 25:9, 1935.
7. Chacker, F. M.: Etiology. *In* Periodontal Therapy, 4th ed. H. M. Goldman and D. W. Cohen, Eds. St. Louis, C. V. Mosby, 1968.
8. Cohen, D. W., et al.: Effects of excessive occlusal forces on the gingival blood supply. J. Dent. Res., 39:677, 1960.
9. Comar, M. D., Kollar, J. A., and Gargiulo, A. W.: Local irritation and occlusal trauma as co-factors in the periodontal disease process. J. Periodontol., 40:193, 1969.
10. Drum, W.: *In* Parafunctions of the masticatory system (bruxism). D. Lipke and U. Posselt, Eds. J. West. Soc. Periodont., 8:133, 1960.
11. Erausquin, R., and Carranza, F. A.: Primeros hallazgos paradentosicos. Rev. Asoc. Odontol. Argentina (Buenos Aires), 27:486, 1939.
12. Ewen, S. J., and Stahl, S. S.: The response of the periodontium to chronic gingival irritation and long-term tilting forces in adult dogs. Oral Surg., 15:1426, 1962.
13. Geiger, A. M.: Occlusal studies in 188 consecutive cases of periodontal disease. Am. J. Orthod., 48:330, 1962.
14. Glickman, I.: Inflammation and trauma from occlusion, co-destructive factors in chronic periodontal disease. J. Periodontol., 34:5, 1963.
15. Glickman, I.: Clinical Periodontology, 4th ed. Philadelphia, W. B. Saunders Co., 1974, Chapter 24.
16. Glickman, I.: Clinical significance of trauma from occlusion. J. Am. Dent. Assoc., 70:607, 1965.
17. Glickman, I., and Smulow, J. B.: Alterations in the pathway of gingival inflammation into underlying tissues induced by excessive occlusal forces. J. Periodontol., 33:7, 1962.
18. Glickman, I., and Smulow, J. B.: Effect of excessive occlusal forces upon the pathway of gingival inflammation in humans. J. Periodontol., 36:51, 1965.
19. Glickman, I., and Smulow, J. B.: Further observations on the effects of trauma from occlusion in humans. J. Periodontol., 38:280, 1967.
20. Glickman, I., and Weiss, L.: Role of trauma from occlusion in initiation of periodontal pocket formation in experimental animals. J. Periodontol., 26:14, 1955.
21. Goldman, H. M.: Gingival vascular supply in induced occlusal traumatism. Oral Surg., 9:939, 1956.
22. Goldman, H. M., and C. W. Cohen: Periodontal Therapy, 4th ed. St. Louis, C. V. Mosby, 1968.
23. Karolyi, M.: Beobachtungen über Pyorrhea alveolaris. Oesterr-ungar. Vrtlschr. Zahnheilk., 17:279, 1901.
24. Kennedy, J.: Experimental ischemia in monkeys, I. Effect of ischemia on gingival epithelia. J. Dent. Res., 48:696, 1969.
25. Krogh-Poulsen, W. G., and Olsson, A.: Occlusal disharmonies and dysfunction of the stomatognathic system. Dent. Clin. North Am., November, 1966, p. 627.
26. Kydd, W. L.: Psychosomatic aspects of temporomandibular joint dysfunction. J. Am. Dent. Assoc., 59:31, 1959.
27. Lipke, D., and Posselt, U. (Eds.): Parafunctions of the masticatory system (bruxism). J. West. Soc. Periodont., 8:133, 1960.
28. Macapanpan, L. C., and Weinmann, J. P.: The influence of injury to the periodontal membrane on spread of gingival inflammation. J. Dent. Res., 33:263, 1954.
29. Maddick, I. H.: On occlusal stress—a discussion. Dent. Pract., 15:171, 1965.
30. Moore, D. S.: Bruxism: diagnosis and treatment. J. Periodontol., 27:[277], 1956.
31. Moulton, R., et al.: Emotional factors in periodontal disease. Oral Surg., 5:833, 1952.
32. Mühlemann, H. R., Herzog, H., and Vogel, A.: Occlusal trauma and tooth mobility. Schweiz. Mschr. Zahnheilk., 66:527, 1956.
33. Orban, B.: Periodontics: A Concept—Theory and Practice, St. Louis, C. V. Mosby, 1958.

34. Page, R., Ammons, W., and Schectman, L.: Personal communication, 1970.

35. Parfitt, G. J.: Dynamics of a tooth in function. J. Periodontol., 32:102, 1961.

36. Posselt, U.: *In* Parafunctions of the masticatory system (bruxism). D. Lipke and U. Posselt, Eds. J. West. Soc. Periodont., 8:133, 1960.

37. Posselt, U.: The Physiology of Occlusion and Rehabilitation, 2nd ed. Philadelphia, F. A. Davis, 1968.

38. Poulton, D. R., and Aaronson, S. A.: The relationship between occlusion and periodontal status. Am. J. Orthod., 47:690, 1961.

39. Prichard, J. R.: Advanced Periodontal Disease: Surgical and Prosthetic Management. Philadelphia, W. B. Saunders Co., 1965.

40. Ramfjord, S. P., and M. M. Ash: Occlusion, 2nd ed. Philadelphia, W. B. Saunders Co., 1972.

41. Ramfjord, S. P., and Kohler, C. A.: Periodontal reaction to functional occlusal stress. J. Periodontol., 30:95, 1959.

42. Ross, I. F.: Occlusion. St. Louis, C. V. Mosby, 1970.

43. Schwartz, L.: Disorders of the Temporomandibular Joint. Philadelphia, W. B. Saunders Co., 1959.

44. Stahl, S. S.: The response of the periodontium to combined gingival inflammation and occluso-functional stresses in four human surgical specimens. Periodontics, 6:14, 1968.

45. Stahl, S. S., Joly, O., and Goldsmith, E. D.: Adaptation of periodontal tissue to combined insults. Dent. Prog., 1:121, 1961.

46. Stahl, S. S., Miller, S. C., and Goldsmith, E. D.: The effects of vertical occlusal trauma on the periodontium of protein deprived young adult rats. J. Periodontol., 28:87, 1957.

47. Stahl, S. S., Miller, S. C., and Goldsmith, E. D.: The influence of occlusal trauma and protein deprivation on the response of periapical tissues following pulpal exposure in rats. Oral Surg., 11:536, 1958.

48. Stallard, R. E.: Occlusion: a factor in periodontal disease. Int. Dent. J., 18:121, 1968.

49. Stillman, P. R.: The management of pyorrhea. Dental Cosmos, 59:405, 1917.

50. Stones, H. H.: An experimental investigation into the association of traumatic occlusion with periodontal disease. Proc. Roy. Soc. Med. (Sec. Odont), 31:479, 1938.

51. Thielemann, K.: Biomechanik der Paradentose insbesondere Articulations ausgleich durch Einschleifen. Leipzig, Meusser, 1938.

52. Waerhaug, J.: Pathogenesis of pocket formation in traumatic occlusion. J. Periodontol., 26:107, 1955.

53. Weiss, M.: Bruxism: etiology and clinical significance. Ariz. Dent. J., 11:141, 1965.

54. Wentz, F. M., Jarabak, J., and Orban, B.: Experimental occlusal trauma imitating cuspal interferences. J. Periodont., 29:117, 1958.

55. Weinmann, J. P.: Progress of gingival inflammation into the supporting structures of the teeth. J. Periodontol., 12:71, 1941.

56. Yuodelis, R. A., and Mann, W. V., Jr.: The prevalence and possible role of nonworking contacts in periodontal disease. Periodontics, 3:219, 1965.

57. Zander, H. A., and Mühlemann, H. R.: Effect of stresses on the periodontal structures. Oral Surg., 9:380, 1956.

6

Dental Deposits

Microbiology of Plaque

Pathogenic Constituents of Plaque

Inflammation-Inducing Substances

Bacterial Products Inducing Direct Tissue
Damage

Substances Inducing Indirect Tissue
Damage

Control of Dental Plaque

Alteration of Interactions at the Tooth
Surface

Disaggregation of Plaque Matrix

Suppression of Plaque Flora

Mechanical Disruption of Plaque

After eruption, several organic deposits may form on the surfaces of the teeth. These include pellicle, materia alba and food debris, microbial plaque, and calculus. Since the presence of some of these substances, especially plaque, is intimately related to the induction and progress of dental caries and inflammatory gingival and periodontal disease, their source, structure, and nature have been the object of intensive investigation.

GENERAL BACKGROUND AND HISTORIC PERSPECTIVE

The disease association of dental deposits makes them of common interest to clinicians and investigators in all branches of dentistry, and the contributions from the clinical and basic sciences have led to the availability of a broad spectrum of information. While major discrepancies and missing links in our knowledge of dental deposits continue to exist and there are numerous unsolved problems, the general nature of these substances, their source, and their relationship to disease are beginning to become apparent. Most of this information has been obtained during the past decade, and it has led to important changes in our views of the nature of oral and dental disease. Although some of the recent information has been presented in monographs and symposia,[28,38,183] most of the recent advances have not been reported previously in a thorough, yet concise form that is readily available to students and to practitioners. It is our aim in this section to summarize this information and to present general concepts that emerge from the new data.

A relationship between the soft deposits on teeth and dental disease has been suspected since ancient times; such an association was recognized by Aristotle,[9] and the microbial nature of the deposits was described by van Leeuwenhoek almost three centuries ago.[30] Investigators of the late nineteenth century acknowledged the role of these deposits in the initiation and progress of diseases of the teeth and the soft supporting tissues and exhibited an intense interest in the pathogenic mechanisms involved.[11,150,151,213] However, early in the present century, interest shifted from the structure and pathogenic consequences of the soft deposits to mechanisms of calcification and calculus formation. The bulk of the research effort centered until recently upon calculus. As a consequence, little new information relating to plaque became available. However, during the past decade renewed interest in plaque was stimulated by the realization that microorganisms play a major role in the pathogenesis of both caries and periodontal disease and that both disease states can, in all probability, be prevented by effective plaque control measures.[48]

6

Dental

Deposits

DEFINITION OF TERMS

Dental deposits have been classified and defined as follows:[26,27,134,157,183,190]

ACQUIRED PELLICLE. Acquired pellicle is a homogeneous, membranous, acellular film covering most of the tooth surface and frequently forming the interface between the tooth surface and the dental plaque and calculus. It is composed of glycoproteins derived from saliva.

MATERIA ALBA. Materia alba is a deposit composed of aggregates of microorganisms, leukocytes, and dead exfoliated epithelial cells, randomly organized and loosely adherent to the surfaces of the teeth, plaque, and gingiva. Materia alba is a product of accumulation rather than of bacterial growth, and it can be removed either by vigorous rinsing or with a water spray. Many investigators have expressed doubt that materia alba exists as a specific entity, since all grossly visible dental deposits contain microorganisms and exhibit some degree of organization. Food debris may be present transiently on the surfaces of the teeth, or interdentally, especially after eating.

MICROBIAL PLAQUE. While there is general agreement today as to the meaning of the terms *microbial plaque* and *dental plaque*, formulation of an exact formal definition is still difficult and controversial.[183] Major handicaps have been the multiplicity of terms used to describe the soft deposits on the tooth surfaces and the general confusion over the specificity and structure of these deposits. In the English literature, literally dozens of terms have been used to describe the soft dental deposits. Among the more colorful of these are scum, filth, debris, slime, gelatinous plaque, and zoogloea plaque.[200] The descriptive term *gelatinous microbial plaque* was first introduced by Black in 1898 to describe microbial colonies on tooth surfaces.[11] However, Black's term was not understood by his contemporaries, who subsequently used it to denote loose accumulations of food debris, sloughed epithelial cells and leukocytes, and deposits of salivary mucin, as well as bacterial masses and colonies. More recently, Black's terminology has been shortened to the term *plaque*, and its usage has been restricted to denote only those deposits that are predominantly microbial in nature.

All recently published definitions of plaque are inadequate,[123,154,184,190,200] since none of them take into account the living, ever-changing nature of plaque structure and its variability with time and site.[194] Thus we have chosen to present a description of plaque rather than a formal definition. Plaque is a specific but highly variable structural entity resulting from colonization and growth of microorganisms on the surfaces of teeth, soft tissues, restorations, and oral appliances. Plaque exhibits structural and morphologic features sufficiently characteristic to distinguish it from other forms of dental deposits. It is a living, organized community of microorganisms, usually consisting of numerous species and strains embedded in an extracellular matrix made up of products of bacterial metabolism and substances from the serum, saliva, and diet. Plaque is predominantly, therefore, a product of bacterial growth rather than of accumulation. Although particles of food debris are not constituents of plaque on smooth surfaces, they may be present, at least initially, in plaque in pits and fissures.

Plaque originates by the colonization of surfaces, apparently by selective adherence of single microorganisms or clumps of microorganisms, especially in the cervical and interproximal locations of the teeth. It undergoes growth and maturation with the passage of time, by cumulative additions of gram-negative, anaerobic, and filamentous microorganisms. In the absence of interference, plaque gradually covers the entire tooth surface. It may undergo intermittent periods of active growth and quiescence.

DENTAL CALCULUS. Dental calculus is tightly adherent plaque that has undergone mineralization. Matrix and microorganisms calcify, but the free surface of calculus is usually covered by living microorganisms.

TECHNIQUES FOR PLAQUE ANALYSIS

A broad spectrum of techniques and methods of varying degrees of sophistication have been used for the observation and study of dental plaque. These include direct observation, metabolic measurements *in situ*, biochemical analysis of cellular and extracellular components, and various systems for the assay of toxicity and pathogenicity.

Direct Observation

The development of simple clinical index systems for use with or without disclosing solutions for the measurement of plaque accumulation on the teeth of individuals or large populations has served as the basis for most of the recent clinical observations.[5,65,126] These methods have resulted in demonstration of a relationship between plaque accumulation and the prevalence and extent of inflammatory disease. They have permitted investigation of the efficacy of various plaque control agents,[24,100,122,154] the role of dietary constituents in plaque formation,[17,18,34] and many other clinical parameters.

Morphologic Analysis

Stereomicroscopy and scanning electron microscopy have been used to study the initial events in bacterial colonization of the tooth surfaces, plaque growth, and plaque morphology.[10,91,92,158,176,185] The structure of plaque has been investigated by light and transmission electron microscopy. Several investigators have studied sections from extracted teeth with plaque of unknown age,[45,112,150,151,213] and others have examined plaque accumulating on enamel fragments and other materials inserted into prosthetic appliances.[113,114,145] Plaque of known age, grown on tooth surfaces *in situ*, has been studied by McDougall, Schroeder and De Boever, and Frank and Houver,[46,142,143,184] A significant technical advance was made by Mandel and his colleagues, who introduced the use of plastic strips as a surface upon which to collect plaque of known age and history.[135] Localization of specific substances and microorganisms in plaque has been achieved by histochemical methods and immunofluorescence.[135,167, 168,169,183,184,207] Radioautography has been used to study the salivary glycoprotein[8] and the dietary (Saxton, 1972 unpublished) contribution to plaque matrix.

Metabolic Studies In Situ

Microelectrodes inserted into plaque and radiotelemetry built into prosthetic appliances have been used to study pH changes associated with the metabolism of plaque.[75,99,155]

Biochemical Analysis

Classic biochemical techniques for extraction, purification, and characterization of unknown substances have been applied to the problems of matrix structure. These studies have been reviewed by Mandel, Leach, Guggenheim, and Hotz and co-workers.[66,85,109,133] High-molecular-weight polymers of glucose and other sugars,[22,23,49,53,85,175,210] altered salivary glycoprotein,[25,109,110,111,147,148] proteases,[196] and various chemotactic and inflammation-inducing substances[99,117,203] have been detected and partially characterized.

Microbiologic Techniques

Microorganisms are the predominant component of dental plaque, and there is a massive literature relating to them.[15,39,43,66,68,104,192,193] Classic techniques for sampling, isolation, enumeration, identification, and study of metabolism have been used. More recently special anaerobic techniques have been devised.[136,178] Generally these studies have been directed toward the following problems:

1. Determination of the number, viability, and identity of microorganisms
2. Changes in the microflora with plaque age, maturation, and pathogenicity
3. Utilization of metabolites such as sucrose and elaboration of extracellular materials, including the glucans and various toxic substances
4. Aggregation and adherence of microorganisms to tooth surfaces
5. Identification of odontopathic and periodontopathic microorganisms

Assays of Plaque Toxicity

One of the most important aspects of plaque research is detection and characterization of substances in plaque that have the capacity to induce disease. Investigations of this kind have been hampered by a lack of methods for detecting and assaying these substances. One of the earliest assay systems was assessment of lesions induced in skin or oral tissues by the injection of whole plaque, specific microorganisms,[44,132] or substances derived from plaque.[132, 146,170,171,172,188] Intraoral monoinfection of gnotobiotic animals has been used to identify suspected odontopathic and periodontopathic microorganisms.[29,41]

Recently, cell- and organ-culture systems have been devised to assess the toxicity of plaque substances. Page and his co-workers have assayed the capacity of plaque to induce synthesis and release of acid hydrolases from cultures of macrophages.[162] Lehner and his colleagues and Horton and his colleagues have shown that suspensions of sonicates of several plaque bacteria have the capacity to induce blast transformation of sensitized human lymphocytes in culture.[83,86,87] Furthermore, these cells release substances that are effective in inducing bone resorption.[84] Another valuable technique has been the use of the Boyden chamber to study leukocyte chemotaxis in response to the plaque-derived substances.[203] Thus, it is apparent that many of the methods of modern cellular and molecular biology are being applied to study plaque constituents and periodontal pathogenesis.

PELLICLE DEPOSITION

In 1943, Manly noted that individuals routinely using a nonabrasive dentifrice accumulated a brownish structureless film on the surfaces of the teeth, referred to as "acquired pellicle."[137] This film, which can be removed by polishing with an abrasive compound, re-forms soon after removal. More recent observations have revealed that this film forms on teeth as well as on other nonsloughing surfaces exposed to the oral environment, regardless of the dentifrice used. The film is probably a specialized form of the glycoprotein coat deposited on tissue surfaces throughout the gastrointestinal tract.

Morphology

Acquired pellicle exhibits histochemical and ultrastructural features that distinguish it from plaque and other exogenous dental deposits and provide evidence that it is composed of salivary glycoprotein.[135,142,143,145,197,198,205,207] In general, the staining properties of pellicle are quite similar to those of dried salivary films. It stains positively for sugars and proteins, but does not bind dyes that are specific for collagen or keratin. It does not contain heme or melanin; the brownish color results from the presence of tannins. When viewed with the electron microscope, pellicle is an acellular, afibrillar, faintly granular homogeneous material of variable thickness, in intimate contact with its supporting surface (Fig. 6-1).

The age and method of preparation of pellicle appear to affect the observed structure. Material forming for short time periods on previously polished tooth surfaces or on intraoral plastic strips exhibits a smooth even surface (Fig. 6-1A,B), but pellicle of unknown age and history, present on extracted teeth from which plaque has been removed by brushing under running tap water, may exhibit a honeycombed structure with a scalloped surface.[1,183] The cells of the honeycombed structure are approximately the size of individual microorganisms and frequently contain bacterial cell ghosts and debris.[1] Recent observations on plaque structure support the idea that the honeycombed material may not be pellicle in the usual sense of the word; it can be described more accurately as plaque interface material which may be made up of pellicle, cuticle, or some other material from which the microorganisms have been removed during preparation (Figs. 6-9, 6-11).[184]

Formation

Pellicle deposition has been studied by following the course of events on the surfaces of teeth polished previously with a rubber cup and pumice—a procedure that removes all uncalcified surface deposits except those present in the surface defects, pits, and fissures (Fig. 6-2A,B). Within minutes after exposure of the cleaned tooth surface to saliva, pellicle is reformed.[10,113,176,197,205] This film, which is essentially free of microorganisms, covers the tooth surface completely, filling pits, fissures, and enamel surface defects (Fig. 6-2C). A fully established pellicle can be seen

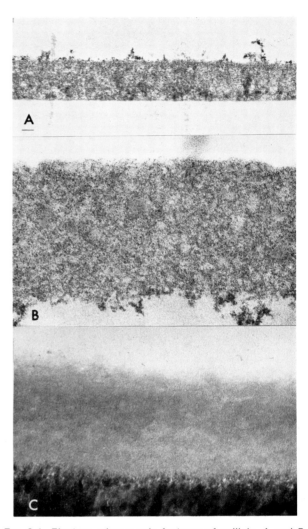

FIG. 6-1. *Electron microscopic features of pellicle. A and B. Sections from acquired pellicle deposited on intraoral Mylar strips during a time period of 30 minutes. The material appears to contain two morphologic components, a granular one of high electron density and a second of somewhat lower density comprising the bulk of the material (magnification 24,650 and 80,750 ×, respectively). (Courtesy Dr. J. Theilade.) C. Natural pellicle deposited on a tooth surface (magnification 65,960 ×). (Courtesy Dr. R. Frank.)*

within 30 minutes (Fig. 6-1A), and within 24 hours it may be faintly erythrosin dye-positive and 0.1 to 0.8 microns in thickness.[10]

Hypotheses that have been put forward to account for pellicle formation include acid precipitation, enzymatic enhancement, and selective adsorption.

ACID PRECIPITATION

Kirk first suggested that acid produced by oral microorganisms colonizing the surfaces of the teeth leads to precipitation of salivary glycoproteins and forma-

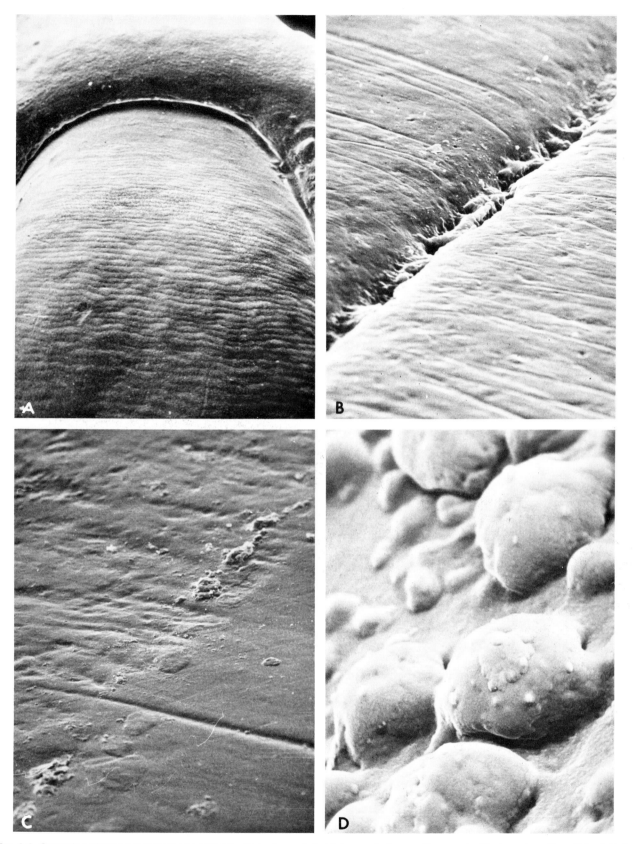

FIG. 6-2. *Scanning electron micrographs of the tooth surface. A. Labial aspect of a maxillary central incisor recently polished. Note the surface (magnification 18 ×). B. An enamel crack in the surface of a recently polished tooth surface containing residual organic material (magnification 1100 ×). C. Recently polished tooth surface to which Scotch tape was applied (lower right side of the illustration) to prevent pellicle accumulation. Initial pellicle deposit seen in the upper left area of the illustration. Bacterial colonization has not yet occurred (magnification 225 ×). D. Bacterial colonization of the tooth surface by aggregates of microorganisms and single microorganisms (magnification 2000 ×). (Saxton, C. A.: Scanning electron microscopic study of formation of dental plaque. Caries Res., 7:102, 1973. S. Karger AG, Basel.)*

tion of a layer of glycoprotein on the teeth.[98] This hypothesis appears to be unlikely for several reasons. Pellicle formation generally occurs prior to bacterial colonization, and it can occur both *in vivo* and *in vitro* in the absence of microorganisms. Furthermore, Dawes has shown that glycoprotein precipitation does not occur at pH levels observed at the tooth surfaces.[25]

ENZYMATIC ENHANCEMENT

Sialic acid (N-acetyl neuraminic acid) is a 9-carbon amino sugar found terminally on the carbohydrate prosthetic group of many salivary glycoproteins. Its presence enhances protein solubility at neutral pH by lowering the isoelectric point. Several investigators have shown that oral microorganisms produce an enzyme, neuramidinase, which has the capacity to cleave the sialic acid bond and enhance the tendency toward precipitation of glycoproteins at neutral pH.[47,109,110,148] Leach has suggested that neuramidinase activity may play a role in pellicle formation; however, definitive evidence to support this contention has not yet appeared.[66]

SELECTIVE ADSORPTION

Ericson has shown that salivary glycoproteins that are rich in sialic acid are selectively adsorbed to hydroxyapatite crystals,[36] and Hay has established electrophoretic identity between these glycoproteins and the constituents of pellicle.[77] Thus, it appears likely that pellicle is made up of a particular fraction of salivary glycoprotein which is selectively adsorbed to the surface of the hydroxyapatite crystals of the tooth surface. If this is the case, pellicle collected on Mylar strips and other artificial surfaces may differ significantly in composition from that present on natural teeth.

Classification

Three separate types of acquired pellicle, based on location, have been observed on human teeth.[145] The first, a *subsurface* type, which has also been referred to as "dendritic pellicle,"[112] is characterized by the presence of processes that extend 1 to 3 microns into defects in the enamel surface. Pellicle of this type is frequently observed interproximally. *Surface* pellicle is about 0.2 microns thick and covers most of the labial, buccal, and palatal surfaces of the teeth. Surface pellicle on the lingual and palatal aspects of the teeth is almost always calcified and only rarely has associated microorganisms. *Stained* pellicle is 1 to 10 microns or more in thickness and may be observed with the naked eye.

Composition and Source

Although the morphologic and chemical data support the idea that pellicle is composed of glycoprotein, there has been considerable disagreement with regard to the relative contributions of the saliva and of oral microorganisms to its composition. The lack of agreement among investigators who have analyzed pellicle biochemically is not surprising. Materials of unknown age and history have been used frequently. The isolation and collection procedures are empirical, and they cannot be monitored adequately. Generally, pellicle is collected from extracted teeth, from which the plaque has been removed following vigorous brushing under running tap water, by treatment with 2 percent hydrochloric acid. Acid treatment decalcifies the enamel surface, leading to possible contamination by enamel matrix protein, and leaches out soluble materials that are usually discarded prior to analysis.[138]

The data presented in Tables 6-1 and 6-2 permit comparison of several different pellicle preparations with mixed saliva and with salivary glycoprotein. Pellicle formed from bacteria-free saliva on the enamel surfaces *in vitro* exhibits a composition similar to pellicle accumulating on natural teeth intraorally during short time periods. Thus bacterial participation does not appear to be necessary for pellicle formation. Generally, amino acids make up only about 45 percent of the dry weight of pellicle. The amino acid composition of whole pellicle and insoluble pellicle is similar to that of mixed saliva and salivary glycoprotein, but important differences are apparent. Pellicle contains relatively more glucose and less nitrogen, and there are major differences in the content of tyrosine, glycine, serine, and alanine. The high content of glutamic acid and aspartic acid is characteristic of glycoproteins. There are also many similarities between the amino acid composition of insoluble pellicle and bacterial cell walls. It has been pointed out that the composition of insoluble pellicle is intermediate between those of salivary mucin and bacterial cell walls.[1,4]

Most of the evidence indicates that the principal component of pellicle is a select or altered fraction of saliva. Pellicle has been analyzed specifically for sialic acid and fucose, sugars present in salivary glycoprotein but absent from bacteria, and for rhamnose, muramic acid, and diaminopimelic acid, constituents of bacterial cell walls that are absent from saliva. The ratio of various hexoses present has also been of interest in determining whether or not the constituent glycoproteins have been altered, since unaltered mixed salivary glycoproteins contain about three times as much galactose as glucose. Leach and his associates and Mayhall have shown that while fucose is present in relatively large amounts in pellicle hydrolysates, only trace

TABLE 6-1. *Relative Amino Acid Compositions of Pellicle, Saliva, Bacterial Cell Walls*[1]

AMINO ACID	PELLICLE[a] INSOLUBLE	PELLICLE[b] MATURE TOTAL	PELLICLE[b] IN VIVO	PELLICLE[b] IN VITRO	SALIVA[b] MIXED	SALIVARY[c] MUCIN	BACTERIAL CELL[d] WALLS
Proline	44.51	61.9	136.2	148.8	270.3	55.19	23.60
Aspartic acid	71.26	89.0	71.4	61.6	76.8	83.61	67.62
Glutamic acid	133.32	132.7	196.8	209.1	185.5	126.69	139.32
Threonine	43.41	47.4	30.6	29.3	10.7	57.29	31.31
Serine	45.61	147.1	91.9	83.7	50.0	76.85	29.72
Alanine	145.84	79.9	38.4	31.3	23.6	75.92	301.79
Glycine	81.21	151.7	137.9	137.3	169.9	96.41	40.16
Valine	53.17	36.7	32.6	30.8	21.3	51.47	20.37
Isoleucine	30.49	26.5	22.9	22.2	15.5	38.66	14.98
Leucine	63.96	56.1	49.6	52.7	25.6	85.47	39.71
Tyrosine	14.05	28.2	51.5	63.5	19.2	26.55	14.07
Phenylalanine	28.96	30.5	37.6	42.1	16.6	32.60	13.16
Lysine	50.60	37.6	31.8	26.4	46.3	61.71	103.47
Histidine	18.72	28.1	19.1	11.2	18.8	19.10	—
Arginine	42.44	28.9	42.3	42.7	43.8	45.18	23.14
Ornithine	26.13					6.75	—
Cystine	12.69	12.1	5.5	4.7	5.0	10.12	—
Methionine	11.78	6.1	4.1	3.3	1.5	12.78	6.81

[1]Reported as residues/1000.
[a]Armstrong, W. G., and Hayward, A. F.: Acquired organic integuments of human enamel. Caries Res., *2*:294, 1968.
[b]Mayhall, C. W.: Concerning the composition and source of the acquired enamel pellicle of human teeth. Arch. Oral Biol., *15*:1237, 1970.
[c]Armstrong, W. G.: Amino acid composition of the acquired pellicle of tooth enamels. Nature (London), *210*:197, 1966.
[d]Salton, M. R. J.: The Bacterial Cell Wall. New York, Elsevier, 1964, p. 252.

TABLE 6-2. *Pellicle Composition*

SAMPLE	GLUCOSE[a]	NITROGEN[a]
Total natural pellicle	5.6 (1.2)	9.8 (1.7)
In vivo pellicle	3.1 (1.1)	9.3 (0.4)
In vitro pellicle	3.0 (0.9)	12.2 (0.8)
Mixed saliva	2.7 (0.4)	14.5 (0.6)

[a]Reported as mg/100 mg of ash-free sample from Mayhall, C. W.: Concerning the composition and source of the acquired enamel pellicle of human teeth. Arch. Oral Biol., *15*:1327, 1970.

quantities of rhamnose, muramic acid, and diamino-pimelic acid are present and the ratio of galactose to glucose is approximately 1:1.[111,138] On the basis of these observations it has been suggested that pellicle is essentially free of microbiologic products. On the other hand, preparations analyzed by others contained rhamnose, muramic acid, and diaminopimelic acid in quantities sufficiently large to indicate that bacterial substances may account for 30 to 60 percent of the total substance.[1,2,3,4] These differences may result from a variable amount of bacterial contamination because of various methods of preparation of the material.[1]

Function

Several features of pellicle structure have been clarified, but the relationship of pellicle deposition to normal oral homeostasis and to pathologic alterations remains unclear. Enamel coated with pellicle is unusually resistant to acid decalcification,[145] and pellicle may participate in the repair of early carious lesions by filling in surface defects.[113,114] On the other hand, many investigators consider pellicle formation to be an initial step in the formation of microbial plaque.[10,98,133,142,143,176]

PLAQUE INITIATION
AND MATURATION

Plaque formation occurs in two steps: (1) bacterial colonization of the tooth surface and (2) bacterial growth and maturation. Although many unsolved problems remain, the general features of plaque formation are now reasonably clear.

Colonization

Generally, pellicle deposition occurs prior to or concurrently with bacterial colonization and may facilitate plaque formation.[10,142,143,176] This idea is supported by several observations: (1) glycoproteins in saliva that are similar to or identical with those of pellicle enhance aggregation of plaque-forming bacteria;[57,78] (2) colonizing microorganisms alter the appearance of pellicle with which they make contact, possibly by using its components as substrate; (3) the pellicle subjacent to plaque exhibits features indicative of partial digestion (Fig. 6-9).[1] On the other hand, it is clear that pellicle deposition occurs frequently without subsequent colonization, and colonization may occur under some conditions without prior pellicle deposition.[12,39] Thus, the exact relationship between pellicle deposition and plaque formation, if any, remains unclear.

Colonization of the tooth surface occurs by either of two mechanisms: (1) single microorganisms or clumps of microorganisms become attached to the surface by selective adherence (Figs. 6-2D, 6-3) and multiply to produce discrete plaque colonies (Fig. 6-4); or (2) mixed cultures of microorganisms grow out from viable precursors remaining in pits, fissures, and cracks in the tooth surface (Fig. 6-4C).

COLONIZATION BY SELECTIVE ADHERENCE

The existence of intraoral ecologic niches exhibiting remarkably differing microbial populations is a well-established observation.[16,55,105,194] For example, *Streptoccocus salivarius* makes up about 45 percent of the total facultative streptococci in the saliva and 41 percent of those present on the tongue, while this organism comprises only 3.4 percent of the facultative

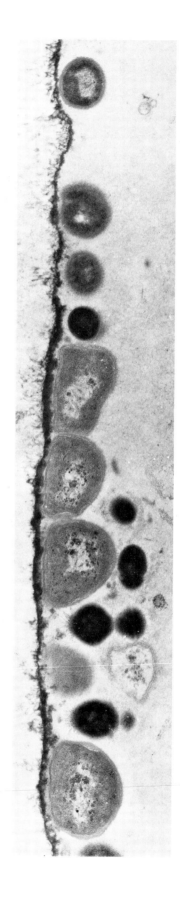

FIG. 6-3. *Early colonization of the tooth surface by cocci. Note the single layer of microorganisms adherent to an electron-dense interface material of unknown composition (magnification 13,400 ×). (Courtesy Dr. H. E. Schroeder.)*

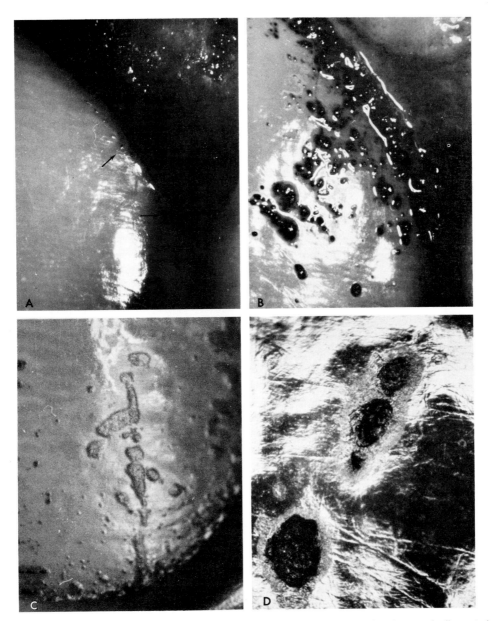

FIG. 6-4. *Early plaque formation on human teeth observed by stereomicroscopy. A. The labial surface and adjacent gingival papilla of a maxillary canine 24 hours after cleansing. Note the tiny plaque colonies near the free gingival margin (arrows) (magnification 17 ×). B. Tooth surface 68 hours after polishing, showing multiple colonies of microorganisms, colony enlargement, and coalescense, and the formation of halos of extracellular material (magnification 17 ×). C. Surface of a mandibular canine showing plaque growing from a surface enamel crack (magnification 21 ×). (Björn, H., and Carlsson, J.: Observations on a dental plaque morphogenesis. Odontol. Revy., 15:23, 1964.) D. Enlarged view of plaque colonies showing colonial morphology and surrounding extracellular material. Scratches in the enamel surface result from previous polishing (magnification approximately 35 ×). (Courtesy Dr. H. Björn.)*

streptococci on the tooth surface.[208] On the other hand, zooglea-producing streptococci other than *Streptococcus salivarius* account for 55.6 percent of the total facultative streptococci on the tooth surface but only 10.9 and 16.5 percent, respectively, of those on the tongue and in saliva.[208]

Factors relating to the initial colonization of the intraoral surfaces and those regulating subsequent growth may differ. Populations of 10^6 microorganisms per cm^2 of tooth surface have been detected within 5 minutes after thorough cleansing.[195] Thus, while factors enhancing or suppressing microbial replication and metabolism are undoubtedly important in determining the composition of the mature flora, it is likely that adherence mechanisms are dominant in the initial colonization.[164,169,177] Adherence mechanisms appear to

TABLE 6-3. *Relative Adherence of Bacteria to Human Cheek Epithelial Cells*

ORGANISM	RELATIVE ADHERENCE[a]
Streptococcus salivarius 9GS2	100
Streptococcus strain 26	33
Streptococcus strain B1	55
Fusobacterium strain F7	13
Streptococcus faecalis	0
A. naeslundii strain 1	49

Gibbons, R. J., and van Houte, J.: Selective bacterial adherence to oral epithelial surfaces and its role as an ecological determinant. Infect. Immun., 3:567, 1971.

[a]Relative adherence = 100 × average number of bacteria per cell/ average number of Streptococcus salivarius 9GS2 per cell.

be selective. Since the microorganisms involved in colonization are likely to come directly from the saliva bathing the teeth, random adsorption would be expected to result in the presence on the tooth surface of a population closely resembling that of saliva. This is, in fact, not the case. *Streptococcus sanguis* and pleomorphic rods are the principal organisms involved in colonization of the teeth,[195] whereas other types predominate in the saliva. These observations have led to the hypothesis that mechanisms of nonrandom adherence are operative in colonization of the tooth and soft tissue surfaces in the oral cavity and to intensive investigation of the relative adherence properties of oral microorganisms.[35,50,52,57,59,60,208]

The ability of various species of oral microorganisms to adhere to epithelial cells and to tooth surfaces varies widely.[58,82,209] However, it has been found that gener-

ally the selective adherence properties exhibited by microorganisms *in vitro* correlate well with the observed localization at various sites within the oral cavity.[58,116] For example, relative to other oral and nonoral microorganisms, *Streptococcus salivarius* exhibits a tendency to adhere to oral epithelial cells (Table 6-3), and it has a tendency to populate epithelial sites *in vivo*. *Streptococcus salivarius* becomes implanted in the oral cavity shortly following birth,[19] and it constitutes a high percentage of the total facultative streptococci in samples from the tongue and cheek mucosa of adults.[16,60,105] On the other hand, *Streptococcus sanguis* exhibits a far greater propensity than *Streptococcus salivarius* to adhere to tooth surfaces and to enamel powder. In experiments in which mixtures of the two microorganisms were held in the mouths of human volunteers for various time periods, ten to one hundred fold more *Streptococcus sanguis* than *Streptococcus salivarius* adhered to the teeth during a 45-minute test period (Table 6-4).

Several substances related to selective bacterial adherence have been identified. These include salivary glycoprotein, bacterial extracellular coat material, and dextran polymers.[79] Gibbons and Spinell showed that 28 of 46 strains of freshly isolated human plaque microorganisms exhibited agglutination in the presence of saliva.[57] Although both *Streptococcus sanguis* and *Streptococcus salivarius* have the capacity to adhere to enamel powder, the adherence of *Streptococcus sanguis*, the organism participating in colonization of the tooth surfaces, is greatly enhanced by pretreatment of the particles with saliva.[82] The active factor in saliva is a high-molecular-weight glycoprotein, which not only aggregates plaque-forming microorganisms in the presence of divalent cations but also adsorbs selectively to hydroxyapatite.[78] Thus, substances present in saliva,

TABLE 6-4. *Percentage of Streptomycin-Resistant S. salivarius and S. sanguis Adhering to Cleaned Tooth Surfaces*

SUBJECT	STRAINS	MIXTURE	SALIVA		TOOTH SURFACE[a]		
			15 min.	45 min.	1	2	3
1	S. salivarius Di-R	43.3[b]	46.6	21.1	2.3	1.0	1.2
	S. sanguis H7P-R	56.7	53.4	78.9	97.7	99.0	98.8
2	S. salivarius Di-R	40.2	71.2	36.2	0.5	3.9	1.9
	S. sanguis A12-R	59.8	28.8	63.8	99.5	96.1	98.1

[a]Lingual surfaces of upper central and/or lateral incisors.
[b]Expressed as percentage of the total of labeled cells of both species.
Van Houte, J., Gibbons, R. J., and Pulkinnen, A. V.: Adherence as an ecological determinant for streptococci in the human mouth. Arch. Oral Biol., 16:1131, 1971.

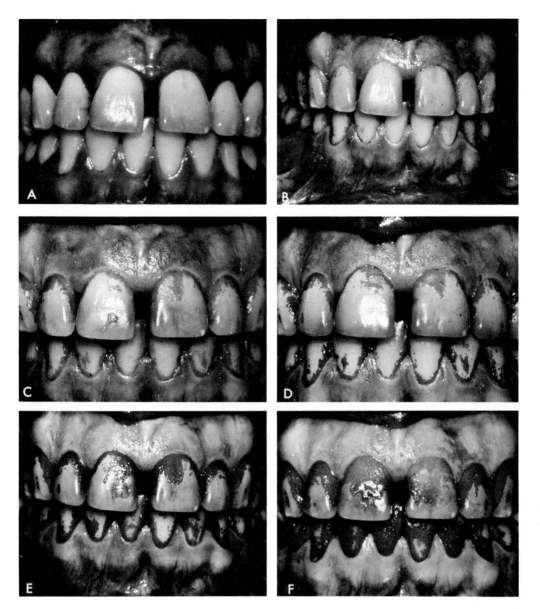

FIG. 6-5. *Plaque accumulation over a period of 10 days in an individual refraining from all oral hygiene procedures but consuming his regular diet. The teeth were stained with erythrocin dye and photographed daily. A. Day 0. There is a very faint dye binding indicating that pellicle is present. This is particularly apparent in the small labial depression of the left central incisor. The teeth were not polished prior to the experiment. B. Day 3. Discrete plaque colonies (maxillary lateral incisors), as well as a continuous layer of plaque (mesial right canine), can be seen. Growth is more prominent in the sheltered and protected areas of the surface. C. Day 4. The plaque is thicker and its coverage extended to form a continuous band apical to the height of contour of all of the teeth. Growth is apparent even on surfaces coronal to the height of contour on smooth surfaces in contact with the lips (maxillary right incisor). D. Day 5. The pattern of growth is now well established, and the plaque has become more luxuriant than on day 4. Note the slight change in the pattern on the right central incisor as compared with day 4. E. Day 7. An increase in thickness and extent of coverage is apparent. F. Day 10. The labial surfaces of the mandibular teeth are essentially completely covered as are all other surfaces which are protected from mechanical interference. The surface of the attached gingiva is relatively free of plaque except in the region of the left lateral incisor on the maxillary arch.*

and probably in pellicle, may play a critical role in selective colonization.

Cell wall determinants and extracellular substances produced by oral microorganisms may also be important in adherence phenomena. The oral streptococci selectively adhering to epithelial cells exhibit an extracellular fuzzy coat that may serve as a mediator of the attachment. Enzymatic removal of this coat interferes with subsequent adherence.[35,59] One component of the extracellular coat is M-protein. There is a positive correlation between the presence of this antigenic determinant and adherence properties.[35] Specific adherence can be inhibited by prior treatment of the bacterial cells with secretory immunoglobulin A, an indication that the immunologic system may also participate in the selectivity observed in colonization of the surfaces in the oral cavity.[214] The extracellular glucan polymers elaborated by certain streptococci involved in plaque formation enhance bacterial aggregation and adherence to the tooth surface.[49,50,173]

COLONIZATION BY OUTGROWTH FROM PITS, FISSURES, AND CRACKS

Selective adherence colonization is undoubtedly important, but the tooth surface can be colonized by a separate and independent means. While ordinary prophylactic measures remove all surface deposits, pellicle and viable microorganisms remain in the depths of fissures and cracks in the enamel surface (Fig. 6-2B), and these organisms can proliferate and give rise to plaque without the participation of specific adherence phenomena (Fig. 6-4C).[10,142,143] This outgrowth proceeds more slowly than does smooth-surface colonization by adherence, usually requiring 24 hours or more, but a mixed flora appears much sooner.[142,143] Furthermore, bacterial adherence probably contributes to the increasing mass.

Growth and Maturation

The events occurring in plaque growth and maturation have been followed closely during the initial 2 to 3 weeks, but events occurring beyond this time are poorly understood.[10,135,142,143,169] The process of maturation includes (1) growth and coalescence of the original discrete plaque colonies, (2) continued appositional growth by adherence to the tooth and plaque surface of additional organisms and clumps of organisms, (3) increasing complexity of the plaque flora, and (4) accumulation of inorganic salts with conversion of plaque to calculus.

Many important clinical features of plaque growth and maturation are shown in Figure 6-5 which illustrates the events occurring in an individual who refrained from all oral hygiene measures for a period of 10 days. The teeth, which were not polished before beginning the experiment, were stained daily with erythrosin dye and photographed. Although individual subjects may vary significantly with regard to the time required for plaque to form and the extent to which plaque accumulates, plaque growth can be seen generally within 2 days, and most of the interproximal surfaces of the teeth and areas apical to the heights of

contour become covered by day 3. The thickness of the plaque and the area of tooth coverage appear to increase throughout the 10-day observation period except in areas of mechanical interference. New areas of plaque colonization and growth appear throughout the period, demonstrating continued bacterial adherence. Growth was observed on the gingiva as well as on the teeth. Plaque levels on gingiva appear to increase for the first 3 to 4 days and then decrease noticeably. The decrease probably results from the sloughing of the surface epithelial cells.

There is a gradual and continual change in plaque structure during the first 1 or 2 weeks. The single microorganisms and discrete colonies (Fig. 6-4A) consisting mostly of streptococci evolve into more mature, highly complex structures covering a large portion of the tooth surface (Fig. 6-5). During this maturation, there is a shift from a predominantly gram-positive, aerobic coccal flora to a mixed flora with a preponderance of rodlike, filamentous, and spiral microorganisms. The relative populations of gram-negative and anaerobic microorganisms increase dramatically.[127,135,206,207] As maturation progresses, calcium phosphate salts are deposited in varying degrees, and at some sites conversion of plaque to calculus is seen. Plaque maturation may undergo intermittent phases of activity and quiescence.

Several lines of evidence support the idea that plaque growth and maturation may be more a result of microbial apposition by continued adherence than of microbial replication and colony enlargement. Plaque formation may be extremely rapid. For example, a large portion of the tooth surface may become covered by plaque within a period of 2 or 3 days (Fig. 6-6). The structure extends over the tooth surface to an extent and with a rapidity unlikely to result simply from bacterial replications (Fig. 6-5E,F). The increasing

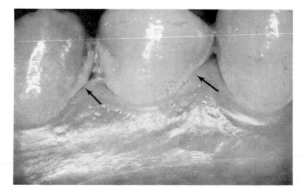

FIG. 6-6. A 2-day accumulation of plaque in a subject exhibiting rapid plaque formation. The structure is white, glistening, and lumpy. It is located below the heights of contour of the teeth in contact with the marginal gingival tissues (arrows). (Courtesy Dr. W. Payne.)

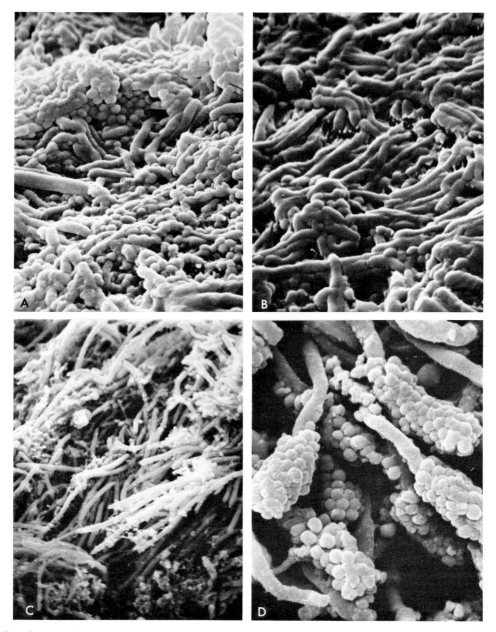

FIG. 6-7. *Scanning electron micrographs of the surface of mature dental plaque from human teeth. A. A mixed flora of intertwined filaments, cocci, and rods. The surface is free of food debris, epithelial cells, and leukocytes (magnification 4,500 ×). B. A predominantly filamentous flora with few intermixed cocci (magnification 4,500 ×). C. Filamentous flora with adhering material of unknown composition and relatively free of cocci (magnification 1,500 ×). D. Filamentous microorganisms with adhering cocci illustrating the selective adherence of organisms of different species which contributes to appositional growth (magnification 5,250 ×). (Courtesy C. A. Saxton.)*

complexity of the flora can only come about by the adherence of additional microbial species. Examination of plaque surfaces by scanning electron microscopy has provided direct evidence supporting the concept of continued adherence. As seen in Figure 6-7D, a highly specific form of intermicrobial adherence does occur in which cocci adhere to filamentous organisms[91,92,183]

Furthermore, Gibbons and Nygaard have shown that numerous microbiologic species from plaque aggregate in the presence of other unlike microorganisms.[52] Therefore, although replication and colony enlargement are important factors in plaque growth and maturation, specific adherence also continues to play a major role.

PLAQUE STRUCTURE

Since plaque is a living, continuously changing structure with the capacity to adapt to everchanging mechanical, physical, and chemical conditions, it presents exceptionally varied morphologic features. These features may vary with age, extent of maturation, location on the tooth surface, diet,[17,18,34] and many other currently unrecognized conditions. Most of the structural studies have dealt with relatively young plaque, and our knowledge of older structures is meager. Thus, only the general overall features seen in most plaques of 1 to 2 weeks of age will be described.

General Architectural Features

When observed clinically, unstained plaque is a yellowish-white, glistening, sometimes lumpy material of variable thickness covering portions of the tooth surface (Fig. 6-6). At higher magnification (Fig. 6-8), the dense microbial nature of the structure becomes apparent. The microbial component is made up of numerous different species and strains, which appear frequently to be mixed in a random fashion. The filamentous organisms radiate out from the tooth surface at approximately right angles to create a "palisade" (Figs. 6-8, 6-9). Large zones relatively free of viable microorganisms and containing cell ghosts, bacterial membranes, dead cell debris, and globular insoluble material can be seen (Fig. 6-10B). A matrix material that may be granular, globular, or fibrillar is present in regions between the bacteria (Figs. 6-11, 6-12). An electron-dense material, probably derived from salivary glycoprotein or elaborated by bacteria, forms the interface between the plaque and the tooth surface (Fig. 6-11). Although sloughed epithelial cells, leukocytes, and food debris are generally not components of smooth-surface plaque, these substances may be ob-

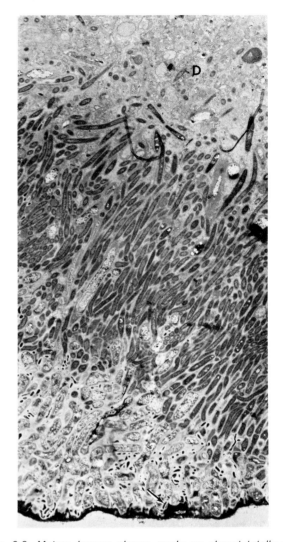

FIG. 6-9. *Mature human plaque made up almost totally of filamentous microorganisms arranged in a characteristic palisade. Note the presence of a scalloped layer of electron-dense material at the enamel-plaque interface (arrow) and the presence of dead cell debris (D) near the surface (magnification 4,160 ×). (Courtesy Dr. H. E. Schroeder.)*

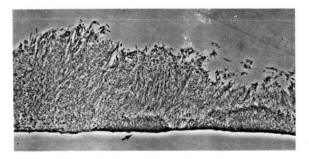

FIG. 6-8. *An Epon-embedded section of mature human dental plaque. Note the palisading of the filamentous microorganisms and the presence of more dense plaque colonies at the tooth-plaque interface (magnification 300 ×). (Courtesy Dr. H. E. Schroeder.)*

served on the plaque surface (Fig. 6-9), and residual food debris may be present in fissure plaque. At calculus-forming sites, especially on the lingual surfaces of the mandibular incisors and the buccal surfaces of the maxillary molars, plaque may be converted rapidly to calculus by acquisition of mineral salts.

Tooth-Plaque Interface

The relationship of the microorganisms to the calcified tooth surface varies greatly. Since bacterial colonization occurs usually after pellicle deposition, it is likely that salivary glycoproteins of pellicle form the tooth-plaque interface in most immature plaques. The

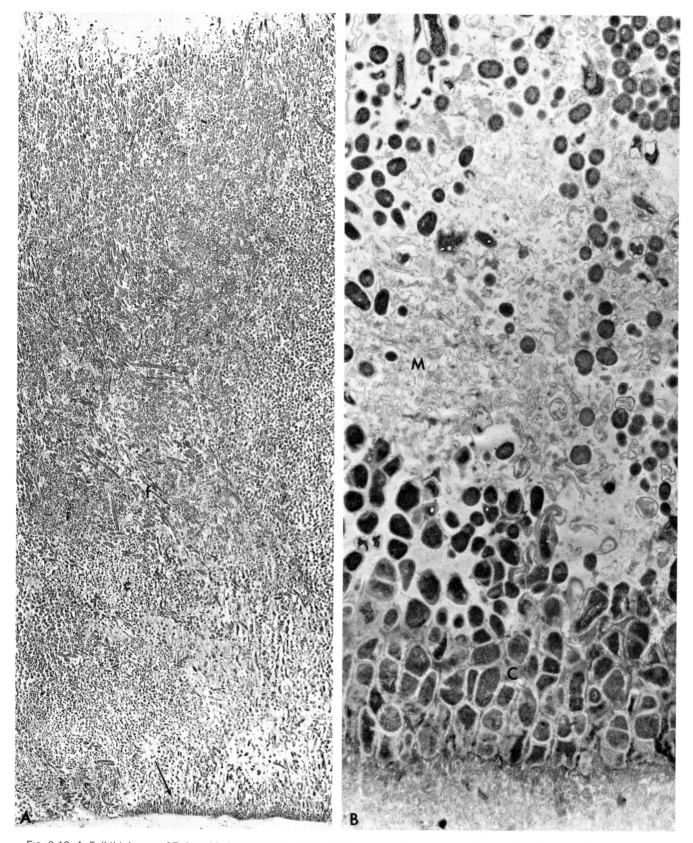

Fig. 6-10. *A. Full thickness of 7-day-old plaque grown on the mesial aspect of a human maxillary incisor. Note the densely packed, heterogeneous microbial nature of the structure, the condensed microbial layer at the tooth-plaque interface (arrow), and the <u>colonies of cocci</u> (c) <u>and filamentous microorganisms</u> (f) (magnification 725 ×). (Schroeder, H. E., and De Boever, J.: The structure of microbial dental plaque. In Dental Plaque. W. D. McHugh, editor. Edinburgh, E. & S. Livingstone Ltd., 1970.) B. Seven-day human plaque illustrating the condensed microbial layer (C) and regions with dense accumulations of membranes (M) and dead cell debris (magnification 8,250 ×). (Courtesy Dr. H. E. Schroeder.)*

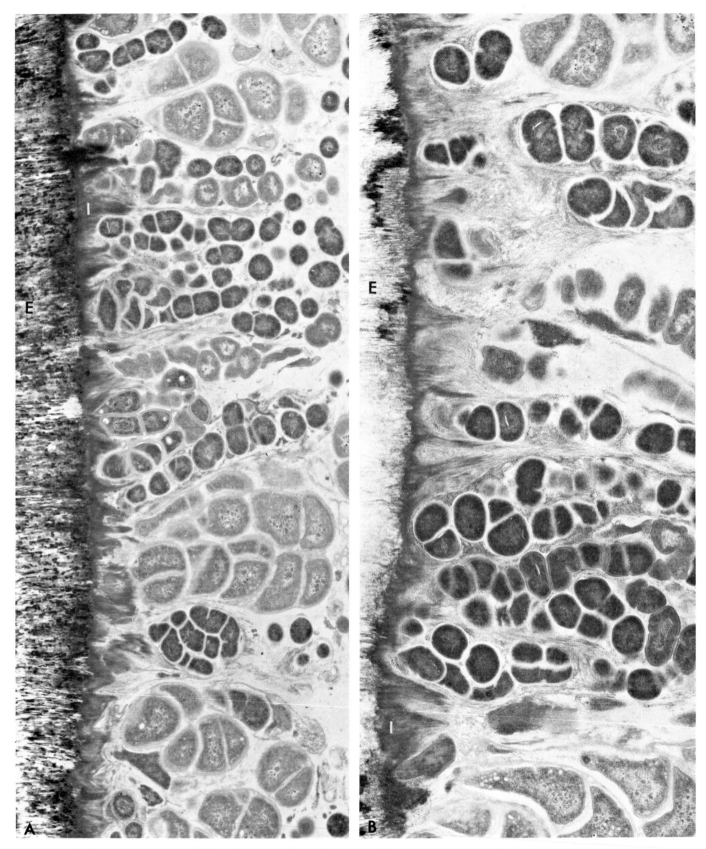

FIG. 6-11. *The interface region of 7-day-old human plaque. The enamel (E) has not been decalcified completely, in order to preserve the interface relationships. The interface material (I) is electron-dense and faintly fibrillar and exhibits a deeply scalloped surface with partially embedded microorganisms. The interface material forms a continuous layer between the microorganisms and the tooth surface. In some areas, the interface material appears to extend into the microbial layer and is continuous with the extracellular matrix. Colonization by at least two different forms of microorganisms is apparent (A, magnification 9,000 ×; B, magnification 18,750 ×). (Courtesy Dr. H. E. Schroeder.)*

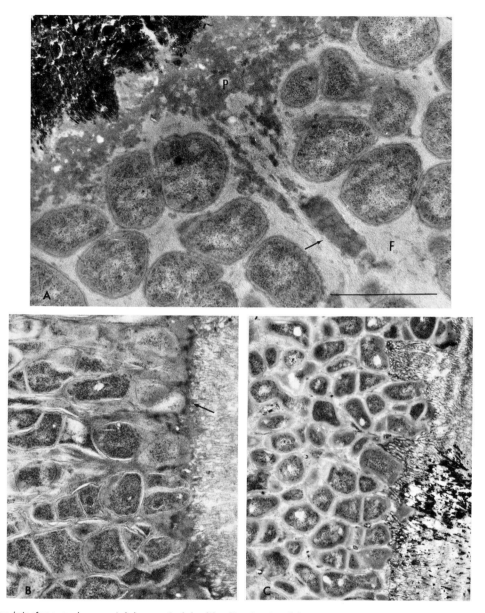

FIG. 6-12. *A. The interface region containing material with ultrastructural features similar to pellicle (P). Note the moth-eaten appearance indicative of partial digestion and the presence of similar material within the fibrillar plaque matrix (F) (magnification 22,400 ×). (Frank, R. M., and Houver, G.: An ultrastructural study of human supragingival dental plaque formation. In Dental Plaque. W. D. McHugh, editor. Edinburgh, E. & S. Livingstone Ltd., 1970.) B. Interface in which only isolated patches of electron-dense material remain (magnification 12,250 ×). (Courtesy Dr. H. E. Schroeder.) C. Plaque microorganisms in direct contact with the enamel surface and embedded within it (magnification 12,600 ×). (Courtesy Dr. H. E. Schroeder.)*

interface material observed most frequently is an electron-dense, granular material, the structure of which closely resembles pellicle (Fig. 6-11). The interface may consist of a thick layer of globular material with microorganisms completely embedded and with projections extending far into the microbial layer (Fig. 6-12A). On the other hand, it may be an electron-dense scalloped sheet (Figs. 6-9, 6-11) or a thin dense discontinuous sheet (Fig. 6-13A), or in some instances only vestiges of the material may remain (Fig. 6-12B).

In some plaque, the interface material is absent completely, and the microorganisms rest directly on the naked enamel rods (Fig. 6-12C); in others, a film of dental cuticle, previously exposed to the oral fluids and colonized, may form the interface material (Fig. 6-13B). The relationship of various forms of interface material to plaque growth and maturation and to pathologic alteration of the tooth surface and gingiva is not known, even though it appears reasonable to suspect that the intact interface may provide a diffusion

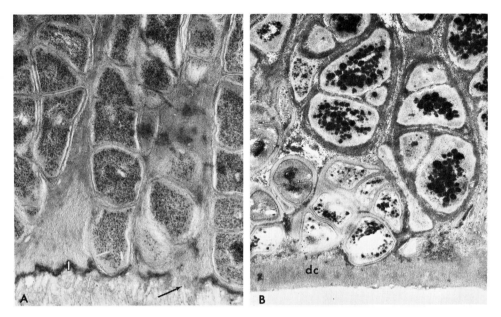

FIG. 6-13. *Seven-day old human plaque. A. The tooth-plaque interface material (I) is discontinuous, and matrix material is in direct contact with the enamel surface (arrow). The density of the matrix material varies markedly (magnification 21,875 ×). B. Homogeneous felt-like material probably dental cuticle (dc) forming the interface between microorganisms and the surface. The preparation has been stained for saccharides, and densely positive granules are seen within the cells (magnification 17,850 ×). (Courtesy Dr. H. E. Schroeder.)*

barrier that provides a measure of protection to the underlying enamel surface. Alternatively, the acquired pellicle may facilitate bacterial adhesion, survival, and colony growth. Much more work will be required to determine which is the case.

Microbial or Cellular Layer

Adjacent to the tooth-plaque interface may be a region of closely packed coccoid organisms with little extracellular matrix material which has been called the "condensed microbial layer" (Fig. 6-10A).[184] The thickness of the layer varies considerably from one region to another, and it may be entirely absent. Its presence is probably a consequence of plaque initiation by discrete colonies of microorganisms that are subsequently buried by further colonization and growth.

A predominant feature of the microbial layer of mature plaque is its extensive variation. The microbial layer may be composed of coccoid and short rodlike microorganisms or of mixtures of several different forms (Figs. 6-8, 6-10A, 6-14). The surface region is of special interest, since it is the area in contact with the oral fluids and in many instances with the gingival tissues. The surface region (Figs. 6-7, 6-15) contains an equally dense microbial population as does the deeper layer, and there is less insoluble extracellular material.[184] The free surface is the region where future growth by apposition occurs (Fig. 6-7D). Dead leuko-

cytes, food debris, and sloughed epithelial cells may be seen covering the free plaque surface.

Extracellular Matrix

Plaque microorganisms are embedded in a complex extracellular matrix containing material elaborated by the bacteria and substances from the saliva. Materials comprising plaque matrix are derived from several sources (Fig. 6-16). This material is of special interest for several reasons:

1. It serves as a framework to bind the microorganisms into a coherent mass and virtually makes possible the existence of plaque.
2. It serves as an extracellular storage site for fermentable carbohydrates.
3. It alters the diffusion of substances into and out of the structure.
4. It may contain numerous inflammation-inducing and other toxic substances such as proteolytic enzymes, antigenic substances, endotoxin, mucopeptide, and low-molecular-weight metabolites.

Plaque matrix has been studied extensively by light and electron microscopy, and many of the components have been resolved. However, it is important to remember that preparation of the material for microscopy requires steps that leach out many of the soluble

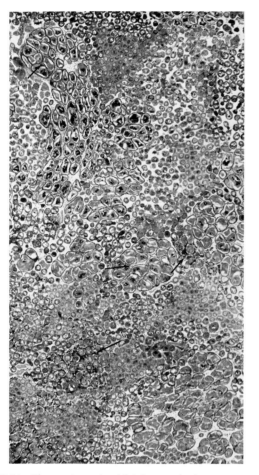

FIG. 6-14. *The major microbial layer of plaque composed almost completely of cocci. Note the persistence of discrete colonies (arrows), each embedded in its own unique extracellular matrix (magnification 2,995 ×). (Courtesy Dr. H. E. Schroeder.)*

substances and only the insoluble matrix components remain. This has favorable and unfavorable consequences. Although the preparative techniques contribute to the identification of matrix components by distinguishing between the insoluble and soluble substances, they also bring about the loss of many components and the artifactual production of apparently empty extracellular spaces.

The presence in plaque matrix of glycoproteins, sugars, proteins and lipids has been shown histochemically,[135,142,143,207] and several morphologically distinct components of plaque matrix have been observed with the electron microscope. The composition of plaque matrix appears to depend, to a great extent, upon the species and strain of microorganism present (Figs. 6-17, 6-18). For example, in regions where gram-negative microorganisms predominate, large accumulations of membrane-bound vesicles, which appear to arise by budding from the cell membranes, may be seen (Fig. 6-18A,C). Since the vesicles arise from gram-negative microorganisms, they may contain endotoxin. In many other regions, plaque matrix is dominated by the presence of cell membranes, dead cell ghosts, and debris (Fig. 6-18B). These regions may be rich in mucopeptide and other cell-wall-derived substances.

A large portion of plaque matrix, as seen with the electron microscope, is made up of a fibrillar material of variable size and density (Fig. 6-18D). This material, which is seen in high concentration around colonies of streptococci, especially in the condensed microbial layer, appears to be continuous with the glycoprotein of the tooth-plaque interface (Fig. 6-11). Some of the material is insoluble in water, but it can be solubilized

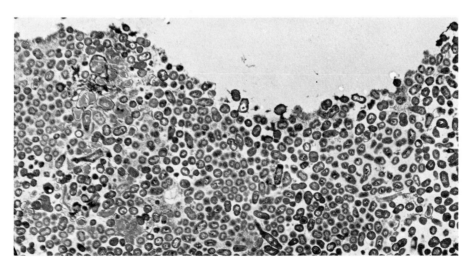

FIG. 6-15. *The oral surface region of a 7-day plaque containing cocci and short rods, and free of nonbacterial surface materials. Compare with that illustrated in Figure 6-9 (magnification 4,200 ×). (Courtesy Dr. H. E. Schroeder.)*

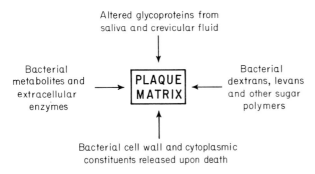

FIG. 6-16. *Substances making up plaque matrix.*

by treatment with alkali.[70] It does not react with thiosemicarbazide-osmium, a staining procedure considered to be positive for dextrans with alpha-1-6 linkages. Cultures of *Streptococcus mutans* grown in sucrose-containing broth,[70] as well as plaque from animals infected with this microorganism produce a material with identical morphologic and chemical features (Fig. 6-19). Thus, the evidence indicates that the fibrillar material is the alpha-1-3-linked glucan.[85] This material provides a part of the structural framework for plaque and has been referred to as *skeletal* glucan in contrast to the alpha-1-6-linked *storage* glucan.

Chemical studies of plaque matrix are based on the fact that the bulk of the low-molecular-weight substances, the soluble proteins, and some of the glucans can be removed by extraction with water, whereas the insoluble matrix components can be extracted with

alkali together with some cell-wall material and intracellular components. The matrix components, especially water-insoluble glucans, can be further separated from the alkali extracts by ethanol precipitation.[20,22,49,85,107,141,191,215,216] Interpretation of the results of the chemical studies has been made difficult by the complexity and heterogeneity of the starting material, by partial degradation of the components during fractionation, by failure to effectively separate extracellular, cell wall, and intracellular components, and by difficulties encountered in identification. In spite of these difficulties, several important components of plaque matrix have been isolated and partially characterized.

An exhaustive analysis of plaque collected from 3,500 school children was reported recently (Fig. 6-20).[85] Plaque contains about 80 percent water. Of the dry material, about 29.6 percent is soluble in water and 25 percent is low-molecular-weight dialyzable substances. The water-soluble fraction contains carbohydrates, nitrogenous substances, and proteins. High-molecular-weight glucans, present in the soluble fractions account for about 1 percent of the total dry weight of the plaque; 5.6 percent of the dry weight consists of water-soluble low-molecular-weight carbohydrates, principally glucose and oligosaccharides, presumably derived from enzymatic breakdown of alpha-1-6-linked dextrans. The glucose present in this fraction accounts for more than 40 percent of the total glucose present in pooled plaque. Thus, plaque con-

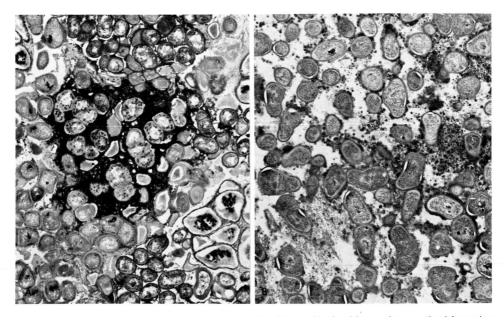

FIG. 6-17. *Features of plaque matrix. A. Human plaque stained by the thiosemicarbazide-osmium method for polysaccharide. Note the discrete colony of microorganisms containing dense, positively staining granules that may be glycogen embedded in a matrix of extracellular polysaccharide (magnification 7,980 ×). B. Sparse granules and globules of polysaccharide in plaque matrix (magnification 10,500 ×). (Courtesy Dr. H. E. Schroeder.)*

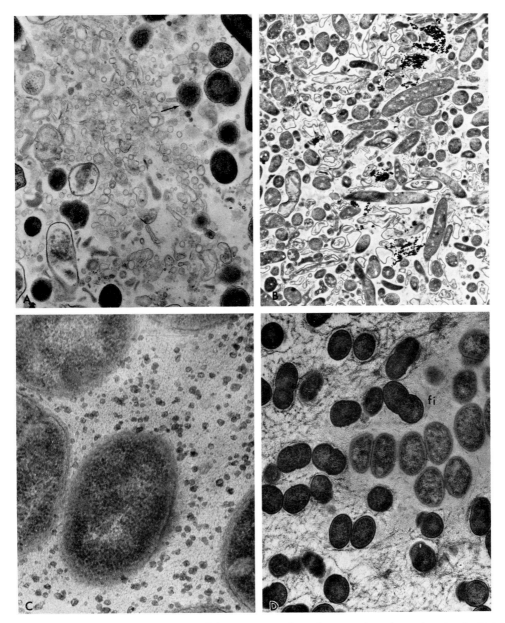

FIG. 6-18. *Features of plaque matrix. A. A region containing gram-negative microorganisms (arrow) and a dense accumulation of membranes which are presumably derived from bacteria and may therefore contain endotoxin or other cell-wall components (magnification 16,500 ×). B. Matrix with numerous dead cell ghosts and membranes and dense deposits presumably calcium salt deposit (magnification 4,875 ×). (A and B courtesy Dr. H. E. Schroeder.) C. Matrix near the oral surface of 3-day old plaque showing numerous dense vesicles of unknown composition in a finely fibrillar matrix. D. Section from 3-day-old human plaque with finely fibrillar material (fi) and coarse material surrounding cocci (magnification 9,000 ×). (C and D from Frank, R. M., and Houver, G.: An ultrastructural study of human supragingival dental plaque formation.* In *Dental Plaque. W. D. McHugh, editor. Edinburgh, E. & S. Livingstone Ltd., 1970.)*

tains a surprisingly high component of fermentable sugar, indicating that microbial activity is not limited by the supply of fermentable substrate.

Altered salivary glycoproteins and bacterial substances are also present in the water-soluble fraction of plaque.[111] Extracts contain both rhamnose and muramic acid sugars not found in saliva, but present in bacterial cells. Salivary glycoproteins contain sialic

acid, fucose, and hexosamine. However, some investigators have failed to find fucose and sialic acid in plaque matrix.[26] Furthermore, the major hexose of salivary glycoprotein is galactose, while glucose and fucose predominate in plaque matrix. Thus, it is likely that plaque bacteria use salivary glycoprotein as substrate and that the carbohydrate side chains are cleaved from molecules by bacterial enzymes. Indeed,

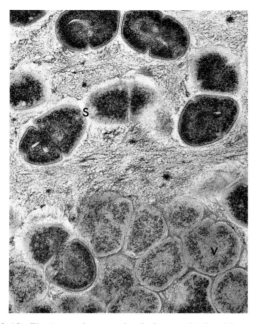

FIG. 6-19. *Electron micrograph of plaque obtained from gno-tobiotic rats infected with* Streptococcus mutans (S) *and* Veillonella (V). *Note the presence of fibrillar matrix material, presumably the alpha-1-3-linked glycan surrounding the streptococci. The features of the material resemble closely the fibrillar material often observed in human plaque. (Guggenheim, B., and Schroeder, H. E.: Biochemical and morphological aspects of extracellular polysaccharides produced by cariogenic streptococci. Helv. Odontol. Acta, 11:131, 1967.)*

some oral microorganisms elaborate sialidase and glucosidase.[163]

The water-insoluble component, which can be fractionated by alkali extraction, makes up 67.1 percent of the total dry material.[85] About one half of this material is insoluble in 1 M KOH and contains, principally, bacteria and cell-wall materials. The material solubilized by alkali treatment contains about two thirds of the water-insoluble carbohydrate material. A large proportion of this material, shown to make up about 1.35 percent of the total dry weight, is precipitable with ethanol and contains alpha-1-3-linked glucans. This substance, sometimes referred to as mutan, is thought to be a major part of the insoluble fibrillar matrix of plaque. Plaque bacteria do not have enzymes capable of hydrolyzing mutan.

In addition to the altered salivary glycoproteins, hexose polymers, lipid membranes, and dead cell debris, matrix also contains enzymes derived from microorganisms. These include proteases,[196] collagenase,[51] hyaluronidase,[186] and beta-glucuronidase.[187]

MICROBIOLOGY OF PLAQUE

There have been but few comprehensive bacteriologic surveys of the complex flora of dental plaque,

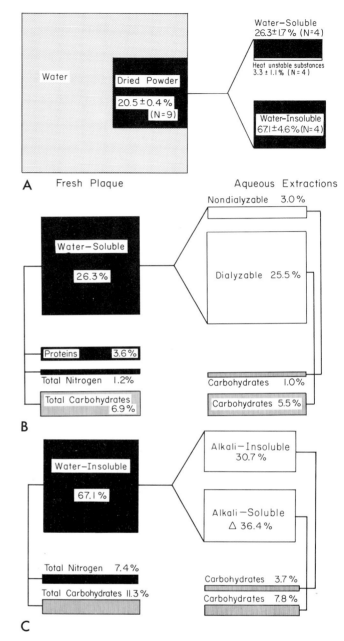

FIG. 6-20. *The composition of pooled human plaque. A. Proportions of water, dried powder, water-soluble and water-insoluble components expressed as percentage of fresh plaque weight. B. Composition of the water-soluble plaque fraction; the values are calculated as the percentage of plaque dry weight. C. Composition of the water-insoluble plaque fraction; the values are calculated as the percentage of plaque dry weight. (Hotz, P., Guggenheim, B., and Schmidt, R.: Carbohydrates on pooled dental plaque. Caries Res., 6:103, 1972. By permission of S. Karger AG, Basel.)*

despite its obvious importance in the induction of both dental caries and periodontal disease. In those few studies technical and conceptual difficulties regarding sampling, cultivation, enumeration, and identification have been encountered. Furthermore, the data available derive almost completely from supragingival plaques.

One major problem has been the use of pooled instead of discrete plaque samples. In early studies directed toward identification of odontopathic and periodontopathic microorganisms, no differences were detected in the plaque flora of affected and normal individuals.[55,56] However, pooled plaque samples from numerous teeth of several individuals were used. More recently, it has become apparent that, at least in some cases, microorganisms with pathogenic potential localize on specific tooth surfaces to an unexpected extent.[33,93] For example, while one surface of a given tooth may be infected with *Streptococcus mutans*, the remaining surfaces of the same tooth may remain free of infection for months. Thus, pooling material from many surfaces would be expected to obscure specific associations between microorganisms and pathologic lesions.

An additional problem in the analysis of plaque flora has been low viability of the microorganisms under various standard culture conditions. Even with enriched culture media and special culture conditions, the yield of viable counts in the early studies represented only about 20 percent of the microorganisms observed in plaque by direct microscopy.[54] Extensive efforts have been directed toward enhancing viability, especially of the anaerobic flora. Special techniques developed for this purpose include dispersal of plaque samples under anaerobic conditions, the use of pre-reduced suspending media, and use of the benzyl viologen roll tube to isolate unusually strict anaerobes. By using these techniques along with specialized culture media, over 70 percent of the organisms observed by direct microscopy can be cultivated.[178]

The population of microorganisms present in plaque changes greatly during growth and maturation of the structure. Most bacteriologic studies in man have been done during the first one to three weeks of plaque growth. Only limited information is available on aged plaque, the type that is most likely to be associated with inflammatory gingival and periodontal disease. During the first 1 to 2 weeks of plaque accumulation, there is a transition from a flora that consists predominantly of gram-positive aerobic cocci and rodlike microorganisms to one characterized by the presence of anaerobic, gram-negative organisms with an increase in filamentous microorganisms and spirochetes (Fig. 6-21).

Early plaque is composed almost entirely of gram-positive cocci, short rods,[127,169,206] *Neisseria*, and *Nocardia*.[169] Spirochetes are not seen for at least the first 3 days of plaque growth.[206] Viable counts vary from 50 to 100 percent, and viability decreases with increasing time.[206] The density of microorganisms in-

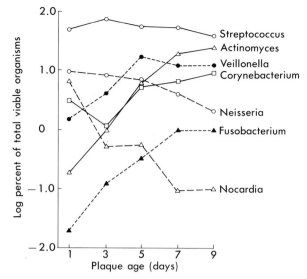

FIG. 6-21. *Relative proportions of selected organisms in developing plaque. Aerobes (– – –), facultative microaerophiles (———), and anaerobes (------). (Adapted from Ritz, H. L.: Microbial population shifts in developing human dental plaque. Arch. Oral Biol., 12:1561, 1967.)*

creases with time; the total number of microorganisms per milligram of plaque increased from 91 to 117×10^6 between days 1 and 3.

When plaque is allowed to grow unhindered on human teeth, three distinct phases of floral transition can be observed.[127] During phase I, the first 24 hours, discrete colonies composed of 80 to 90 percent gram-positive cocci and short rods appear. During phase II, the next 2 to 4 days, rods and filamentous microorganisms appear, and there is a relative reduction in numbers of cocci. These organisms are predominantly *Leptothrix* and *Fusobacteria*. Transition to phase III is gradual and occurs after 6 to 10 days. At this time vibrios and spirochetes appear, and there is a relative increase in the size of the gram-negative anaerobic population. The relative bacterial populations characteristic of plaque at days 1 and 9 are shown in Table 6-5.

Bacterial synergism and antagonism resulting from local environmental conditions may play a major role in the distribution and relative population sizes of microorganisms in plaque.[164] Microorganisms exhibit a strong tendency to localize within specific regions of plaque during maturation. Using specific antiserum, Ritz has shown that while *Streptococci* are present throughout plaque, *Neisseria* locate preferentially near the surface, and *Veillonella* in the central and deeper regions.[168,169] Thus anaerobic organisms may be able to survive only in the deep areas where, after a certain thickness of plaque has been produced, oxygen tension is low. Other organisms such as spirochetes, which have special nutritional and other requirements, may

TABLE 6-5. *Pathogenic Constituents of Dental Plaque*

1. Inflammation-inducing Substances
Various chemotatic substances (polypeptides)
Activators of the complement cascade
Histamine
2. Substances Inducing Direct Tissue Damage

Proteases	Indole
Collagenase	Ammonia
Hyaluronidase	Hydrogen sulfide
Beta-glucuronidase	Toxic amines
Neuraminidase	Organic acids
Chondroitin sulfatase	

3. Substances Inducing Indirect Tissue Damage

Endotoxin	Altered host constituents
Peptidoglycan	Bacterial antigens
Polysaccharide	

be able to grow only after appropriate environmental conditions have been established.

The foregoing discussion pertains specifically to supragingival plaques from smooth surfaces of teeth. It is now abundantly clear that the morphology, composition, and flora of smooth surface plaques, pit and fissure plaques, and plaque material from periodontal pockets differ greatly. In experimentally produced fissures in human teeth, the initial deposit is made up almost completely of fibrous plant material derived from food stuffs. However, by day 3, the fissure is colonized by bacteria and yeast. At the entrance to the fissure, the flora is predominately rapidly multiplying gram-positive cocci. Remnants of the fibrous plant material are still present after 2 to 4 weeks, but by about 60 days the fissures are filled principally with gram-positive cocci. With the further passage of time, microbial viability appears to decrease as evidenced by the presence of increasing amounts of cell wall material and dead cell debris.

The morphology and microbiology of subgingival plaque have not been studied adequately, although several major efforts are underway currently.[159,160,212] The subgingival plaque is in contact with the tooth, but not necessarily adherent to it. The surface in contact with the soft tissues is made up of sloughed epithelial cells, polymorphonuclear leukocytes, and dead cell debris. Immediately subjacent to the surface, the plaque is made up almost entirely of fine unidentified filamentous microorganisms and spirochetes. Interspersed among these are large aggregates of specific microorganisms that have been referred to as bristle

brush structures. These structures, which closely resemble a test-tube brush, are made up of gram-negative filaments and flagellated rods oriented at right angles to a large rod that forms the central core. Bristle brush structures are present in pockets associated with both slowly and rapidly progressing periodontal disease. In some patients, gram-negative rods make up over 60 percent of the total flora present, and they are considered to have etiologic significance. However, the pathogenic potential of these organisms has not yet been studied. The evidence available indicates that the flora observed in periodontal pockets may correlate with the extent and severity of disease; the more gram-negative, anaerobic, and motile the flora, the more severe and rapid the disease state.

PATHOGENIC CONSTITUENTS OF PLAQUE

Complex interactions of the host, microorganisms, and diet lead to pathologic alterations of the teeth and their surrounding supporting tissues, and eventually to tooth loss. In spite of the wealth of data now available, it has not been possible to demonstrate an association between specific plaque substances and the induction and progress of inflammatory lesions of the supporting tissues. Indeed, current data suggest that the active pathogenic substance may have many components, each of which may act upon the host along a different pathway and possibly at a different stage of the disease. Several substances that have pathogenic potential have been detected in plaque (Table 6-5). These include inflammation-inducing substances, bacterial products that may induce direct tissue damage, and substances that may activate destructive mechanisms within the host tissues or paralyze the host's defense mechanisms.

Inflammation-inducing Substances

Substances with the capacity to induce acute exudative phenomena in the vessels of the microcirculation and cause leukocyte chemotaxis are present in dental plaque. Observations of humans and dogs on whose teeth plaque has been allowed to accumulate have revealed a positive correlation between plaque accumulation and leukocyte and fluid exudation from the gingival sulcus.[6,7,204] The presence of chemotactic substances has been demonstrated in culture fluids of plaque microorganism and in whole human saliva, and active chemotactic agents have been extracted from dental plaque.[117,203] These substances have not yet been characterized.

Bacterial Products Inducing Direct Tissue Damage

Microorganisms present in plaque elaborate numerous enzymes with the potential to damage directly the tissues of the host with which they come in contact. These include proteases,[76,196] collagenase,[51] hyaluronidase,[186] beta-glucuronidase,[187] neuraminidase,[109,163] and chondroitin sulfatase.[186] In addition to these substances, low-molecular-weight metabolites such as organic acids, ammonia, indole, toxic amines, and hydrogen sulfide [192] may be present in high concentration.

Substances Inducing Indirect Tissue Damage

The destructive aspects of the inflammatory and immunologic responses of the host have only recently become apparent, and they are still poorly understood. These aspects of inflammatory periodontal disease are discussed in detail in the section on pathogenic mechanisms. Plaque contains numerous substances that activate destructive host mechanisms. These include endotoxins of gram-negative bacteria,[189] peptidoglycan, and polysaccharide of gram-positive microorganisms and foreign antigenic determinants present on the surfaces of microorganisms and in their products as well as the altered host glycoprotein components. While investigators currently attach great significance to the possible role of antigenic substances in plaque in the induction of inflammatory gingival and periodontal disease, essentially no information is available regarding which plaque constituents may be responsible.

CONTROL OF DENTAL PLAQUE

The central role played by bacteria colonizing the teeth in the induction of dental caries and inflammatory gingival and periodontal disease has been firmly established,[192] and it appears likely that the capacity to control bacterial colonization of the teeth may lead to the prevention of these important diseases.[119] As a consequence of this concept, there has been a major effort to find methods and agents that are effective in the long-term control of plaque and calculus in human populations. Colonization of the teeth involves specific, yet poorly understood, interactions of certain oral microorganisms, glycoproteins from saliva, and gingival fluid with the tooth surface. The coherence of plaque, indeed its virtual existence, is dependent upon the integrity of the extracellular plaque matrix. Thus, possible techniques for plaque control have generally been directed toward (1) alteration of interaction at the tooth surface, (2) disaggregation of plaque matrix,

(3) suppression of the oral flora, or (4) disruption of plaque matrix by chemical, enzymatic, or mechanical means.[183]

Alteration of Interactions at the Tooth Surface

Adherence of microorganisms to the tooth surface appears to be an important and possibly an essential step in plaque formation. Thus, one likely means of plaque control would be to alter the adherence properties of the tooth surface. Since absorption and adherence are functions of the surface energy and charge, chemical agents that alter the surface characteristics have been tested. Treatment with sodium fluoride alters the capacity of hydroxyapatite powder to absorb both proteins and microorganisms.[37,63] However, plaque accumulation is not suppressed in human populations using fluoridated drinking water.[100] Equally unsuccessful has been the use of films of silicone and ion exchange resin.[115,179] Generally, the effects of these agents are rapidly masked on the tooth surface by deposition of salivary substances. While effective agents have not yet been found, the possibilities have by no means been exhausted. For example, the possible use of solid-state proteolytic enzymes does not appear to have been considered.

Disaggregation of the Plaque Matrix

Plaque matrix consists of high-molecular-weight carbohydrate polymers, altered salivary and serum glycoproteins, membranes and other dead cell debris, and numerous other uncharacterized substances. The matrix contributes organizational support to the plaque structure much in the same way the connective tissue substances serve in the tissues of higher multicellular organisms. Thus, a disaggregation or dissolution of the matrix could be expected to cause a reduction in plaque accumulation. Urea, a nonspecific denaturing agent, and various enzymes such as trypsin, chymotrypsin, lipase, amylase, and elastase have been used for disaggregation of the plaque matrix without notable success.

The glucans, a family of related carbohydrate polymers, are an important constituent of plaque matrix. These high-molecular-weight branched polymers make an ideal extracellular binding material, and they appear to be responsible to a great extent for the adherence and tensile properties of plaque. While polymers of fructose and glucose containing alpha-1-6-linkages can be hydrolyzed and used as an energy source by plaque bacteria, enzyme systems essential for utilization of the glucans containing alpha-1-3-linkages are not present, and these substances accumulate. Measures directed toward inhibition of the production of insoluble glucans or hydrolysis of those already present in plaque have been used as possible plaque-control techniques. While the administration of crude dextranase and mutanase preparations in drinking water tend to retard plaque formation and the development of caries and periodontal lesions in rodents,[41,42,67,69,102] these substances used in various vehicles have not been effective in man.[14,88,96,121,161]

Suppression of Plaque Flora

Mature dental plaque consists almost completely of microorganisms, and gram-positive streptococci appear to play an important role in the initial colonization of the tooth surface. Thus numerous antibiotic and other chemical antibacterial agents have been tested for their effectiveness in plaque control. Wide-spectrum antibiotics, penicillin, and other chemical agents effective against gram-positive microorganisms are effective in the control of plaque in rodents.[40,96,97,108,140,156] However, in human populations these agents have produced remarkably inconsistent results. Perhaps some of these inconsistencies may be a consequence of the variation in the populations studied, the criteria of measurement, the routes of administration, or the large number of drugs tested. Harvey showed that systemic administration of spiramycin resulted in improved periodontal health,[74] and several investigators have shown that penicillin or tyrothricin dentrifrices suppressed caries activity in school children.[81,180,217] Furthermore, Mitchell and his colleagues, and Collins suppressed plaque formation by topical application of vancomycin.[13,21,152,153,211] Similar results have been obtained with other antibiotics.[80,199]

On the other hand, Littleton and White observed no suppression of plaque in children given systemic penicillin,[120] and Dossenbach and Mühlemann were unable to achieve suppression of calculus formation with penicillin lozenges.[32] McFall and Jensen and their colleagues were unable to suppress plaque accumulation in humans using vancomycin.[89,144] Löe and his co-workers effectively suppressed plaque formation with daily rinses of the broad-spectrum antibiotic, tetracycline, but after 3 days an overgrowth of yeast colonies was observed.[128]

The data available currently indicate that the use of antibiotics for the control of dental plaque by suppression of the oral flora is not a sound prophylactic procedure. Suppression of one segment of the flora, such as the gram-positive organisms, appears to result in their replacement with other organisms equally capable of plaque formation. This fact, along with the acknowledged risk of the development of resistant bacterial strains and of hypersensitivity of the host appear to preclude the use of these drugs for long-term plaque control in human populations.

A new and exciting conceptual basis for the use of antibiotics and other antibacterial substances in plaque control has been presented recently.[130,131] In rodents and to some extent in humans the presence of *Streptococcus mutans* appears to be associated with plaques that have the capacity to induce smooth-surface caries.[64,95] The caries-inducing potential of this microorganism is considered to be associated with its ability to produce an alpha-1-3-linked dextran, to generate acid, and to form plaque.[50,52,64,85,95] *Streptococcus mutans* exhibits a relatively low propensity for adherence to tooth surfaces and when in competition with other microorganisms it becomes implanted only with difficulty.[93,94,106,139] Once implantation has been achieved there is little tendency for spread from one surface to another.[33] Thus, complete eradication of the *Streptococcus mutans* from the oral cavity by antibiotics or other chemotherapeutic agents could conceivably lead to long-term protection against the formation of caries-inducing plaque. While this concept serves as the basis for current extensive experimental studies, its validity has not yet been proved.

The possibility of suppression of the plaque flora by drugs other than antibiotics has been of interest since it was first proposed by Miller.[151] The concept was espoused by Hartzell,[73] and the effectiveness of organic mercurials was demonstrated by Hanke.[72] More recently, several chemical antimicrobial agents, including chloramine-T, cetylpyridinium chloride, benzalkonium chloride and chlorhexidine salts have been used.[31,62,124,125,165,183,201,211]

Chlorhexidine has been of special interest. This agent, when used twice daily as a mouth rinse, at a concentration of 0.2 percent, prevents bacterial colonization of the teeth in human subjects refraining from all other oral hygienic measures.[125] The substance effectively dissolves plaque, and its use results in the transient resolution of well-established gingivitis in dogs and humans,[118] and in caries prevention in laboratory animals.[103,129,165] Chlorhexidine is particularly effective in suppressing microorganisms on the tooth surface. Immediately after use, there is a general suppression of the oral flora,[181] but bacterial populations of the saliva and gingiva return rapidly to normal levels while suppression at the tooth surface continues. This selectivity appears to result from adsorption of the agent to the tooth surfaces, where it continues to be active. Various aspects of chlorhexidine research have recently been summarized.[202]

Although chlorhexidine appears to be the most effective means of chemical plaque control currently available,[61,90,182] its effectiveness in long-term control of plaque seems to be doubtful. Recent observations in dogs[71] and humans indicate that plaque formation eventually returns to original levels, even though routine use of the agent is continued.

Mechanical Disruption of Plaque

The effectiveness of daily mechanical cleansing of the teeth by tooth brushing and other ancillary means has long been recognized.[101] In spite of intensive efforts to devise other means of plaque control, mechanical cleansing remains the only effective method available at the present time (see Chapter 15).

References

1. Armstrong, W. G.: Origin and nature of the acquired pellicle. Proc. Roy. Soc. Med., 61:923, 1968.
2. Armstrong, W. G.: The composition of organic films formed on human teeth. Caries Res., 1:89, 1967.
3. Armstrong, W. G.: Amino acid composition of the acquired pellicle on tooth enamel. Nature (London), 210:197, 1966.
4. Armstrong, W. G., and Hayward, A. F.: Acquired organic integuments of human enamel: a comparison of analytical studies with optical, phase-contrast and electron microscope examinations. Caries Res., 2:294, 1968.
5. Arnim, S. S.: The use of disclosing agents for measuring tooth cleanliness. J. Periodontol., 34:227, 1963.
6. Attström, R., and Egelberg, J.: Presence of leukocytes within the gingival crevices during developing gingivitis in dogs. J. Periodont. Res., 6:110, 1971.
7. Attström, R., and Egelberg, J.: Emigration of blood neutrophils and monocytes into the gingival crevices. J. Periodont. Res., 5:48, 1970.
8. Baumhammers, A., and Stallard, R. E.: Salivary mucoprotein contribution to dental plaque and calculus. Periodontics, 4:229, 1966.
9. Bekker, I.: Aristotelis opera, ex recensione Immanuelis Bekker, accedunt indices sylburgiani, Typographio Academico, Oxonii. (Translated into English from Tome). "Problemata" problem 22, Section 14, p. 186, 1837.
10. Björn, H., and Carlsson, J.: Observations on a dental plaque morphogenesis. Odontol. Revy, 15:23, 1964.
11. Black, G. V.: Dr. Black's conclusions reviewed again. Dental Cosmos, 40:440, 1898.
12. Bladen, H., et al.: Plaque formation in vitro on wires by gram-negative oral microorganisms (viellonella). Arch. Oral Biol., 15:127, 1970.
13. Bowen, W. H.: The prevention or control of dental plaque. In Dental Plaque. W. D. McHugh, Ed. Edinburgh, E & S Livingstone Ltd., 1970, pp. 283–286.
14. Caldwell, R. C., et al.: The effect of a dextranase mouthwash on dental plaque in young adults and children. J. Am. Dent. Assoc., 82:124, 1971.
15. Carlsson, J.: A numerical taxonimic study of human streptococci. Odontol. Revy, 19:137, 1968.
16. Carlsson, J.: Presence of various types of nonhemolytic streptococci in dental plaque in other sites in the oral cavity in man. Odontol. Revy, 18:55, 1967.
17. Carlsson, J., and Egelberg, J.: Effect of diet on early plaque formation in man. Odontol. Revy, 16:112, 1965.
18. Carlsson, J., and Egelberg, J.: Local effect of diet on plaque formation and development of gingivitis in dogs, II. Effect of high carbohydrate versus high protein-fat diets. Odontol. Revy, 16:42, 1965.
19. Carlsson, J., et al.: Establishment of Streptococcus salivarius in the mouths of infants. J. Dent. Res., 49:415, 1970.
20. Carlsson, J., and Sundström, B.: Variation in composition of early dental plaque following ingestion of sucrose and glucose. Odontol. Revy, 19:161, 1968.
21. Collins, J. F.: Effect of vancomycin on plaque after periodontal surgery. J. Dent. Res., 49:1478, 1970.
22. Critchley, P., et al.: The polymerisation of dietary sugars by dental plaque. Caries Res., 1:112, 1967.
23. DaCosta, T., and Gibbons, R. J.: Hydrolysis of leven by human plaque streptococci. Arch. Oral Biol., 13:609, 1968.
24. Davies, R. M., et al.: Chlorhexadine in the prevention of gingivitis. In Prevention of Periodontal Disease. J. G. Estoe, et al., Eds. London, Henry Kimpton, 1971, pp. 224–229.
25. Dawes, C.: Is acid-precipitation of salivary proteins a factor in plaque formation? Arch. Oral Biol., 9:375, 1964.
26. Dawes, C., and Jenkins, G. N.: Studies related to the formation of dental plaque. Abs. 362, 41st General Meeting, IADR, 1963.
27. Dawes, C., Jenkins, G. N., and Tonge, C. H.: The nomenclature of the integuments of the enamel surface of teeth. Br. Dent. J., 115:65, 1963.
28. Dental Plaque, Vol. 1. W. D. Mchugh, Ed., Edinburgh, E & S Livingstone Ltd., 1970.
29. Dick, D. S., and Shaw, J. H.: The infectious and transmissible nature of the periodontal syndrome of the rice rat. Arch. Oral Biol., 11:1095, 1966.
30. Dobell, C. Antony van Leeuwenhock and His "Little Animals." New York, Harcourt, Brace and Co., 1932.
31. Draus, F. J., Leung, S. W., and Miklos, F.: Toward a chemical inhibitor of calculus. Dent. Prog. 3:79, 1963.
32. Dossenbach, W. F., and Mühlemann, H. R.: Effect of penicillin and ricinoleate on early calculus formation. Helv. Odontol. Acta, 5:25, 1961.
33. Edmann, D. C., et al.: Dental floss for interproximal implantation and sampling Streptococcus mutans. 50th General Meeting IADR, Abs. 73, 1972.
34. Egelberg, J.: Local effect of diet on plaque formation and development of gingivitis in dogs, III. Effect of frequency of meals and tube feeding. Odontol. Revy, 16:50, 1965.

35. Ellen, R. P., and Gibbons, R. J.: M-protein associated adherence of *Streptococcus pyogenes* to epithelial surfaces: prerequisite for virulence. Infect. Immun., 5:826, 1972.

36. Ericson, T.: Adsorption to hydroxyapatite of proteins and conjugated proteins from human saliva. Caries Res., 1:52, 1967.

37. Ericson, T., and Ericsson, Y.: Effect of partial fluorine substitution on the phosphate exchange and protein absorption of hydroxyapatite. Helv. Odontol. Acta, 11:10, 1967.

38. Estoe, J. E., Picton, D. C. A., and Alexander, A. G., Eds.: The Prevention of Periodontal Disease. Henry Kimpton, London, 244 pp., 1971.

39. Fitzgerald, R. J.: Plaque microbiology and caries. Ala. J. Med. Sci., 5:239, 1968.

40. Fitzgerald, R. J.: Influence of antibiotics on experimental rat caries. *In* Advances in Experimental Caries Research. R. F. Sognnaes, Ed. Washington, D.C., American Association for the Advancement of Science, 1955, pp. 187–196.

41. Fitzgerald, R. J., et al.: The effects of a dextranase preparation of plaque and caries in hamsters, a preliminary report. J. Am. Dent. Assoc., 76:301, 1968.

42. Fitzgerald, R. J., Spinell, D. M., and Stoudt, T. H.: Enzymatic removal of artificial plaques. Arch. Oral Biol., 13:125, 1968.

43. Fitzgerald, R. T.: Dental caries research in gnotobiotic animals. Caries Res., 2:139, 1968.

44. Foley, G., and Rosebury, T.: Comparative infectivity for guinea pigs of fusospirochetal exudates from different diseases. J. Dent. Res., 21:375, 1942.

45. Frank, R. M., and Brendel, A.: Ultrastructure of the approximal dental plaque and the underlying normal and carious enamel. Arch. Oral Biol., 11:883, 1966.

46. Frank, R. M., and Houver, G.: An ultrastructural study of human supragingival dental plaque formation. *In* Dental Plaque. W. D. McHugh, Ed. Edinburgh, E & S Livingstone Ltd., 1970, pp. 85–108.

47. Fukui, K., Fukui, Y., and Moriyama, T.: Neuramidinase activity in some bacteria from the human mouth. Arch. Oral Biol., 16:1361, 1965.

48. Genco, R. J., Evans, R. T., and Ellison, S. A.: Dental research in microbiology with emphasis on periodontal disease. J. Am. Dent. Assoc., 78:1016, 1969.

49. Gibbons, R. J., and Banghart, S. B.: Synthesis of extracellular dextran by cariogenic bacteria and its presence in human dental plaque. Arch. Oral Biol., 12:11, 1967.

50. Gibbons, R. J., and Fitzgerald, R. J.: Dextran-induced agglutination of *Streptococcus mutans*, and its potential role in the formation of microbial dental plaque. J. Bacteriol., 98:341, 1969.

51. Gibbons, R. J., and Macdonald, J. B.: Degradation of collagenous substrates by *Bacteroides melaninogenicus*. J. Bacteriol., 81:614, 1961.

52. Gibbons, R. J., and Nygaard, M.: Interbacterial aggregation of plaque bacteria. Arch. Oral Biol., 15:1397, 1970.

53. Gibbons, R. J., and Nygaard, M.: Synthesis of insoluble dextran and its significance in the formation of gelatinous deposits by plaque-forming streptococci. Arch. Oral Biol., 13:1249, 1968.

54. Gibbons, R. J., Socransky, S. S., and Kapsimalis, B.: Establishment of human indigenous bacteria in germ free rats. J. Bacteriol., 88:1316, 1964.

55. Gibbons, R. J., et al.: Studies of the predominant cultivatable microbiota of dental plaque. Arch. Oral Biol., 9:365, 1964.

56. Gibbons, R. J., et al.: The microbiota of the gingival crevice area of man, II. The predominant cultivatable organisms. Arch. Oral Biol., 8:281, 1963.

57. Gibbons, R. J., and Spinell, D. M.: Salivary-induced aggregation of plaque bacteria. *In* Dental Plaque. W. D. McHugh, Ed. Edinburgh, E & S Livingstone Ltd., 1970, pp. 207–215.

58. Gibbons, R. J., and van Houte, J.: Selective bacterial adherence to oral epithelial surfaces and its role as an ecological determinant. Infect. Immun., 3:567, 1971.

59. Gibbons, R. J., van Houte, J., and Liljemark, W. F.: Some parameters effecting the adherence of S. salivarius to oral epithelial surfaces. J. Dent. Res., 51:424, 1972.

60. Gibbons, R. J., and van Houte, J.: On the formation of dental plaques. J. Periodontol., 44:347, 1973.

61. Gjermo, P., Baastad, K. L., and Rölla, G.: The plaque-inhibiting capacity of 11 antibacterial compounds. J. Periodont. Res., 5:102, 1970.

62. Gjermo, P., and Rölla, G.: Experiments with chlorhexidine containing dentifrices. IADR 49th General Session, Abstract No. 148, p. 89, 1971.

63. Glantz, P. O.: On wettability and adhesiveness. Odont. Revy, 20 (Supplement 17):1, 1969.

64. Gold, W.: Dental caries and periodontal disease considered as infectious diseases. Adv. Appl. Microbiol., 11:135, 1970.

65. Greene, J. C., and Vermillion, J. R.: The simplified oral hygiene index. J. Am. Dent. Assoc., 68:7, 1964.

66. Guggenheim, B.: Extracellular polysaccharides and microbial plaque. Int. Dent. J., 20:657, 1970.

67. Guggenheim, B., Regolati, B., Mühlemann, H. R.: Caries and plaque inhibition by mutanase in rats. Caries Res., 6:253, 1972.

68. Guggenheim, B.: Streptococci in dental plaque. Caries Res., 2:147, 1968.

69. Guggenheim, B., et al.: Effect of dextranase on caries in rats harbouring an indigenous cariogenic bacterial flora. Arch. Oral Biol., 14:555, 1969.

70. Guggenheim, B., and Schroeder, H. E.: Biochemical and morphological aspects of extracellular polysaccharides produced by cariogenic streptococci. Helv. Odontol. Acta, 11:131, 1967.

71. Hamp, S.-E, Lindhe, J., and Löe, H.: Long term effect of chlorhexidine on developing gingivitis in the Beagle Dog. J. Periodont. Res., 8:63, 1973.

72. Hanke, M. T.: Studies on the local factors in dental caries. I. Destruction of plaques and retardation of

bacterial growth in the oral cavity. J. Am. Dent. Assoc., 27:1379, 1940.

73. Hartzell, T. B.: Prophylaxis and pyorrhea. J. Am. Dent. Assoc., 19:260, 1932.

74. Harvy, R. F.: Clinical impressions of a new antibiotic in periodontics. Spiramycine. J. Can. Dent. Assoc., 27:576, 1961.

75. Hassell, T. M.: Construction of micro antimony electrodes for use in radio telemetry of plaque pH. Helv. Odontol. Acta, 15:50, 1971.

76. Hausmann, E., and Kaufman, E.: Collogenase activity in a particular fraction from Bacteroides melanogenicus. Biochem. Biophys. Acta, 194:612, 1969.

77. Hay, D. I.: The adsorption of salivary proteins by hydroxyapatite and enamel. Arch. Oral Biol., 12:937, 1967.

78. Hay, D. I., Gibbons, R. J., and Spinell, D. M.: Characteristics of some high molecular weight constituents with bacterial aggregating activity from whole saliva and dental plaque. Caries Res., 5:111, 1971.

79. Hay, D. I., Gibbons, R. J., and Spinell, D. M.: Observations on bacterial aggregating component in human saliva. 49th General Meeting IADR, Abs. 355, 1971.

80. Hazen, S. P., Rokita, J., and Volpe, A. R.: Histologic study of a potential plaque inhibiting agent. IADR 49th General Meeting. Chicago. March 18–21, Abs. 285, p. 124, 1971.

81. Hill, T. J., and Kniesner, A. H.: Penicillin dentifrice and dental caries experience in children. J. Dent. Res., 28:263, 1949.

82. Hillman, J. D., van Houte, J., and Gibbons, R. J.: Adsorption of bacteria to human enamel powder. Arch. Oral Biol., 15:899, 1970.

83. Horton, J. E., Lieken, S., and Oppenheim, J. J.: Human lymphoproliferative reaction to saliva and dental plaque deposits: an in vitro correlation with periodontal disease. J. Periodontol., 43:522, 1972.

84. Horton, J. E., et al.: Bone resorbing activity in supernatant fluid from cultured human peripheral blood leukocytes. Science, 177:793, 1972.

85. Hotz, P., Guggenheim, B., and Schmid, R.: Carbohydrates on pooled dental plaque. Caries Res., 6:103, 1972.

86. Ivanyi, L., and Lehner, T.: Stimulation of lymphocyte transformation by bacterial antigens in patients with periodontal disease. Arch. Oral Biol., 15:1089, 1970.

87. Ivanyi, L., Wilton, J.M.A., and Lehner, T.: Cell-mediated immunity in periodontal disease; cytotoxicity, migration inhibition and lymphocyte transformation studies. Immunology, 22:141, 1972.

88. Jensen, S. B., and Löe, H.: The effect of dextranase on plaque and gingivitis in man. In The Prevention of Periodontal Disease. J. E. Eastoe, D. C. A. Picton, and A. G. Alexander, Eds. London, Henry Kimpton, 1971.

89. Jensen, S. B., et al.: Experimental gingivitis in man. IV. Vancomycin induced changes in bacterial plaque composition as related to development of gingival inflammation. J. Periodont. Res., 3:284, 1968.

90. Johnson, N. W., and Kenney, E. B.: Effects of topical application of chlorhexidine on plaque and gingivitis in monkeys. J. Periodont. Res., 7:180, 1972.

91. Jones, S. J.: A special relationship between spherical and filamentous microorganisms in mature human dental plaque. Arch. Oral Biol., 17:613, 1972.

92. Jones, S. J.: Natural plaque on tooth surfaces: A scanning electron microscope study. Apex, J. Univ. Coll. Hosp. Dent. Soc., 5:93, 1971.

93. Jordan, J. V., et al.: Observations in the implantation and transmission of Streptococcus mutans in human beings. J. Dent. Res., 51:515, 1972.

94. Jordan, H. V., Keyes, P. H., and Howell, A.: An in vitro method for assessing the plaque formation and carious lesions. Arch. Oral Biol., 11:793, 1966.

95. Keyes, P. H.: Research in dental caries. J. Am. Dent. Assoc., 76:1357, 1968.

96. Keyes, P. H.: Evaluation of two topical application methods used to assess the antidental caries potential of drugs in hamsters. J. Oral Ther. Pharmacol., 2:285, 1966.

97. Keyes, P. H., et al.: Bio-assays of medicaments for the control of dentobacterial plaque, dental caries and periodontal lesions in Syrian hamsters. J. Oral Ther. Pharmacol., 3:157, 1966.

98. Kirk, E. C.: A consideration of the question of susceptibility and immunity to dental caries. Dental Cosmos, 52:729, 1910.

99. Kleinberg, I.: Biochemistry of the dental plaque. Adv. Oral Biol., 4:43, 1969.

100. Koch, G., and Lindhe, J.: The state of the gingivae and caries-increment in school-children during and after withdrawal of various prophylactic measures. In Dental Plaque. W. P. McHugh, Ed. Edinburgh, E & S Livingstone, Ltd., 1970, pp. 271–281.

101. Koch, G., and Lindhe, J. I.: The effect of supervised oral hygiene on the gingiva of children. The effect of sodium fluoride. J. Periodont. Res., 2:64, 1967.

102. König, K. G., and Guggenheim, B.: In-vivo effects of dextranase on plaque and caries. Helv. Odontol. Acta, 12:48, 1968.

103. Kornman, K. S., Clark, W. B., and Kreitzman, S. N.: Caries control by hibitane. IADR 49th General Meeting. Abs. 784, p. 248, 1971.

104. Krasse, B.: A review of the bacteriology of dental plaque. In Dental Plaque. W. P. McHugh, Ed. Edinburgh, E & S Livingstone, 1970, pp. 199–206.

105. Krasse, B.: The proportional distribution of Streptococcus salivarius and other streptococci in various parts of the mouth. Odontol. Revy, 5:203, 1954.

106. Krasse, B., Edwardsson, S., and Svensson, I.: Implantation of caries-inducing streptococci in the human oral cavity. Arch. Oral Biol., 12:231, 1967.

107. Krembel, J., Frank, R. M., and Deluzarche, A.: Fractionation of human dental plaques. Arch. Oral Biol., 14:563, 1969.

108. Larson, R. H., Zipkin, I., and Fitzgerald, R. J.: Effect of dehydroacetic acid and tetracycline on caries activity and its transmission in the rat. J. Dent. Res., 42:95, 1963.

109. Leach, S. A.: Plaque chemistry and caries. Ala. J. Med. Sci., 5:247, 1968.

110. Leach, S. A.: Release and breakdown of sialic acid from human salivary mucin and its role in the formation of dental plaque. Nature, 199:486, 1963.

111. Leach, S. A., et al.: Salivary glycoproteins as components of the enamel integuments. Caries Res., 1:104, 1967.

112. Leach, S. A., and Saxton, C. A.: An electron microscopic study of the acquired pellicle and plaque formed on the enamel of human incisors. Arch. Oral Biol., 11:1081, 1966.

113. Lenz, H., and Mühlemann, H. R.: In-vivo and in-vitro effects of saliva on etched or mechanically marked enamel after certain periods of time. Helv. Odontol. Acta, 7:30, 1963.

114. Lenz, H., and Mühlemann, H. R.: Repair of etched enamel exposed to the oral environment. Helv. Odontol. Acta, 7:47, 1963.

115. Leung, S. W.: Calculus—its formation and possible prevention. Pa. Dent. J., 27:3, 1960.

116. Liljemark, W. F., and Gibbons, R. J.: Ability of veillonella and neisseria species to attach to oral surfaces and their proportions present indigenously. Infect. Immun. 4:264, 1971.

117. Lindhe, J., and Heldén, L.: Neutrophilic chemotactic activity elaborated by dental plaque. J. Periodont. Res., 7:297, 1972.

118. Lindhe, J., et al.: Influence of topical application of chlorhexidine on chronic gingivitis and gingival wound healing in the dog. Scand. J. Dent. Res., 78:471, 1970.

119. Lindhe, J., Lundgren, D., and Nyman, S.: Considerations of prevention of periodontal disease. Periodont. Abstracts, No. 2. 18:50, 1970.

120. Littleton, N. W. and White, C. L.: Dental findings from a preliminary study of children receiving extended antibiotic therapy. J. Am. Dent. Assoc., 68:520, 1964.

121. Lobene, R. R.: A clinical study of the effect of dextranase on human dental plaque. J. Am. Dent. Assoc., 82:132, 1971.

122. Löe, H.: A review of the prevention and control of plaque. In Dental Plaque. W. D. McHugh, Edinburgh, Ed. E & S Livingstone, Ltd., 1970, pp. 259–270.

123. Löe, H.: Present day status and direction for future research on the etiology and prevention of periodontal disease. J. Periodont., 40:678, 1969.

124. Löe, H., and Schiött, C. R.: The effect of mouth rinses and topical application of chlorhexidine on the development of dental plaque and gingivitis in man. J. Periodont. Res., 5:79, 1970.

125. Löe, H., and Schiött, C. R.: In International Conference on Periodontal Research. J. Periodont. Res., Supplement No. 4, pp. 38–39, 1969.

126. Löe, H., and Silness, J.: Periodontal disease in pregnancy. I. Prevalence and severity. Acta Odontol. Scand., 21:533, 1963.

127. Löe, H., Theilade, E. and Jensen, S. B.: Experimental gingivitis in man. J. Periodontol. 36:177, 1965.

128. Löe, H., et al.: Experimental gingivitis in man. J. Periodont. Res., 2:282, 1967.

129. Löe, H., van der Fehr, F. R., and Schiött, C. R.: Inhibition of experimental caries by plaque prevention. The effect of chlorhexidine mouth rinses. J. Dent. Res., 80:1, 1970.

130. Loesche, W. J., et al.: Effect of topical Kanamycin sulfate on plaque accumulation. J. Am. Dent. Assoc., 83:1063, 1971.

131. Loesche, W. J., Hockett, S. N., and Syed, S. A.: The predominant cultivable flora of tooth surface plaque removed from institutionalized subject. Arch. Oral Biol., 17:1311, 1972.

132. Macdonald, J. B., Socransky, S. S., and Gibbons, R. J.: Aspects of the pathogenesis of mixed anaerobic infections of mucous membranes. J. Dent. Res., 42:529, 1963.

133. Mandel, I. D.: Plaque and calculus. Ala. J. Med. Sci., 5:313, 1968.

134. Mandel, I. D.: Dental plaque: nature, formation, and effects. J. Periodontol., 37:357, 1966.

135. Mandel, I. D., Levy, B. M., and Wasserman, B. H.: Histochemistry of plaque formation. J. Periodontol. 28:132, 1957.

136. Manganiello, A. D., et al.: Attempts to increase the viable recovery of organisms in human dental plaque. 49th General Meeting of the IADR, Abs. 501, 1971.

137. Manly, R. S.: A structureless recurrent deposit on teeth. J. Dent. Res., 22:479, 1943.

138. Mayhall, C. W.: Concerning the composition and source of the acquired enamel pellicle of human teeth. Arch. Oral Biol., 15:1327, 1970.

139. McCabe, R. M., Keyes, P. H., and Howell, A.: An in vitro method for assessing the plaque forming ability of oral bacteria. Arch. Oral Biol., 12:1653, 1967.

140. McClure, F. J., and Hewitt, W. L.: The relation of penicillin to induced rat dental caries and oral L. acidophilus. J. Dent. Res., 25:441, 1946.

141. McDougall, W. A.: Studies on the dental plaque. IV. Levans and the dental plaque. Aust. Dent. J., 9:1, 1964.

142. McDougall, W. A.: Studies on the dental plaque. I. The histology of the dental plaque and its attachment. Aust. Dent. J., 8:261, 1963.

143. McDougall, W. A.: Studies on the dental plaque. II. The histology of the developing interproximal plaque. Aust. Dent. J., 8:398, 1963.

144. McFall, W. T., Shoulars, H. W., and Carnevale, R. A.: Effect of vancomycin in the inhibition of bacterial plaque formation. IADR General Meeting p. 195. Abs. No. 632, 1968.

145. Meckel, A. H.: The formation and properties of organic films on teeth. Arch. Oral Biol., 10:585, 1965.

146. Mergenhagen, S. E.: Endotoxic properties of oral bacteria as revealed by the local Schwartzman reaction. J. Dent. Res., 39:267, 1960.

147. Middleton, J. D.: Human salivary proteins and artificial calculus formation in vitro. Arch. Oral Biol., 10:227, 1965.

148. Middleton, J. D.: Methyl pentoses in human saliva and dental plaque. Nature, *202*:392, 1964.

149. Mikx, F. H. M., et al.: Establishment of defined microbial ecosystems in germ-free rats. I. Caries Res., *6*:211, 1972.

150. Miller, W. D.: The presence of bacterial plaques on the surface of the teeth, and their significance. Dental Cosmos, *44*:425, 1902.

151. Miller, W. D.: Further contributions on the subject of dental caries. I. Caries of enamel. II. Caries of cement. III. Caries of dentine at neck of tooth. IV. Caries of dentine. V. Parasites in non-carious teeth. Independent Pract., *4*:301, 1883.

152. Mitchell, D. F., and Baker, B. R.: Topical antibiotic control of necrotizing gingivitis. J. Periodontol., *39*:81, 1968.

153. Mitchell, D. F., and Holmes, L. A.: Topical antibiotic control of dentogingival plaque. J. Periodontol., *36*:202, 1965.

154. Mühlemann, H. R.: *In vivo* measurements of dental calculus. Ann. N.Y. Acad. Sci., *153*:164, 1968.

155. Mühlemann, H. R., and De Boever, J.: Radiotelemetry of the pH of interdental areas exposed to various carbohydrates. *In* Dental Plaque. W. D. McHugh, Ed. Edinburgh, E & S Livingstone Ltd., 1970, pp. 179–186.

156. Mühlemann, H. R., et al.: The cariostatic effect of some antibacterial compounds in animal experimentation. Helv. Odontol. Acta, *5*:18, 1961.

157. Mühlemann, H. R., and Schroeder, H. E.: Dynamics of supragingival calculus formation. Adv. Oral Biol., *1*:175, 1964.

158. Newman, H. N.: Structure of approximal human dental plaque as observed by scanning electron microscopy. Arch. Oral Biol., *17*:1445, 1972.

159. Newman, M. G., Socransky, S. S., and Listgarten, M. A.: Relationship of microorganisms to the etiology of periodontosis. IADR Program Abstracts No. 2, 324, 1974.

160. Newman, M. G., et al.: Characterization of bacteria isolated from periodontosis. IADR Program Abstracts, No. 325, 1974.

161. Nyman, S., Lindhe, S., and Jansson, J. C.: The effect of a bacterial dextranase on human dental plaque formation and gingivitis development. Odontol. Revy, *23*:243, 1972.

162. Page, R. C., Davies, P., and Allison, A. C.: The role of macrophages in periodontal disease. *In* Host Resistance to Commensual Bacteria. T. MacPhee, Ed. Edinburgh, Churchill Livingstone, pp. 195–201, 1972.

163. Perlitsh, M. J., and Glickman, I.: Salivary Neuramidinase: I. The presence of neuramidinase in human saliva. J. Periodontol., *37*:368, 1966.

164. Regolati, B., Guggenheim, B., and Mühlemann, H. R.: Synergisms and anatagonisms of two bacterial strains superinfected in conventional Osborne-Mendel rats. Caries Res., *6*:211, 1972.

165. Regolati, B., König, K. G., and Mühlemann, H. R.: Effects of topically applied disinfectants on caries in fissures and smooth surfaces of rat molars. Helv. Odontol. Acta, *13*:28, 1969.

166. Renggli, H.: Zahnbeläge und Gingivale Entzündung unter dem Einfluss eines Antibakteriellen Mundspülmittels. Thesis. Zürich, K. Schippert & Co., 1966.

167. Ritz, H. L.: The role of aerobic Neisseriae in the initial formation of dental plaque. *In* Dental Plaque. W. D. McHugh, Ed. Edinburgh, E & S Livingstone, Ltd., 1970, pp. 17–26.

168. Ritz, H. L.: Fluorescent antibody staining of *Neisseria, Streptococcus* and *Veillonella* in frozen sections of human dental plaque. Arch. Oral Biol., *14*:1073, 1969.

169. Ritz, H. L.: Microbial population shifts in developing human dental plaque. Arch. Oral Biol., *12*:1561, 1967.

170. Rizzo, A. A.: Absorption of bacterial endotoxin into rabbit gingival pocket tissue. Periodontics, *6*:65, 1968.

171. Rizzo, A. A., Hampp, E. G., and Mergenhagen, S. E.: Spirochaetal abscesses in hamster cheek pouch. Arch. Oral Biol., *5*:63, 1961.

172. Rizzo, A. A., and Mergenhagen, S. E.: Histopathologic effects of endotoxin injected into rabbit oral mucosa. Arch. Oral Biol., *9*:659, 1964.

173. Rölla, G.: Adsorption of dextran to saliva-treated hydroxyapatite. Arch. Oral Biol., *16*:527, 1971.

174. Salton, M. R. J.: The Bacterial Cell Wall. New York, Elsevier, 1964.

175. Saxton, C. A.: An electron microscope investigation of bacterial polysaccharide synthesis in human dental plaque. Arch. Oral Biol., *14*:1275, 1969.

176. Saxton, C. A.: Scanning electron microscopic study of formation of dental plaque. Caries Res., *7*:102, 1973.

177. Saxton, C. A., and Critchley, P.: An electron microscope investigation of the effect of diminished protein synthesis on the morphology of organisms in dental plaque *in vitro*. *In* Dental Plaque. W. D. McHugh, Ed. Edinburgh, E & S Livingstone, pp. 109–129, 1970.

178. Sayed, S. A., and Loesche, W. J.: Survival of human dental plaque flora in various transport media. Appl. Microbiol., *24*:638, 1972.

179. Schaffer, E. M., Schindler, C. W., and McHugh, R. B.: The effects of two ion exchange resins on the inhibition of calculus-like deposits *in vitro*. J. Periodontol., *35*:296, 1964.

180. Schiere, F. R.: The effectiveness of a tyrothricin dentifrice in the control of dental caries. J. Dent. Res., *36*:237, 1957.

181. Schiött, R. C., et al.: The effect of chlorhexidine mouth rinses on the human oral flora. J. Periodont. Res., *5*:84, 1970.

182. Schiött, C. R. and Löe, H.: The sensitivity of oral streptococci to chlorhexidine. J. Periodont. Res., *7*:192, 1972.

183. Schroeder, H. E.: Formation and Inhibition of Dental Calculus. Berne, Hans Huber Publishers, 1969, p. 145.

184. Schroeder, H. E., and De Boever, J.: The structure of microbial dental plaque. *In* Dental Plaque. W. D. McHugh, Ed. Edinburgh, E & S Livingstone, Ltd., 1970, pp. 49–74.

185. Schroeder, H. E., and Hirzel, H. C.: A method of studying dental soft plaque morphology. Helv. Odontol. Acta, 13:22, 1969.

186. Schultz-Haudt, S. D., Bibby, B. G., and Bruce, M. A.: Tissue-destructive products of gingival bacteria from nonspecific gingivitis. J. Dent. Res., 33:624, 1954.

187. Schultz-Haudt, S. D., and Scherp, H. W.: Production of hyaluronidase and beta-glucuronidase by *Viridans* streptococci isolated from gingival crevices. J. Dent. Res., 34:924, 1955.

188. Schuster, G. S., Hagashi, J. A., and Bahn, A. N.: Toxic properties of the cell wall of gram-positive bacteria. J. Bacteriol., 93:47, 1967.

189. Schwartz, J., Stinson, F. L., and Parker, R. B.: The passage of tritiated bacterial endotoxin across intact gingival crevicular epithelium. J. Periodontol. 43:270, 1972.

190. Schwartz, R. S., and Massler, M.: Tooth accumulated materials: A review and classification. J. Periodontol. 40:413, 1969.

191. Silvermann, G., and Kleinberg, I.: Fractionation of human dental plaque and characterization of its cellular and acellular components. Arch. Oral Biol., 12:1387, 1967.

192. Socransky, S. S.: Relationship of bacteria to the etiology of periodontal disease. J. Dent. Res., 49(Suppl. No. 2):203, 1970.

193. Socransky, S. S., et al.: The microbiota of the gingival crevice area of man. I. Total microscopic and viable counts of specific organisms. Arch. Oral Biol., 8:275, 1963.

194. Socransky, S. S., and Manganiello, S. D.: The oral microbiota of man from birth to senility. J. Periodontol., 42:485, 1971.

195. Socransky, S. S., et al.: Development of early dental plaque. 49th General meeting, IADR, Abs. 502, 1971.

196. Söder, P. O.: Proteolytic activity of dental plaque material, Part IV. Lysis of hemoglobin, amino acid esters and synthetic poly-α-amino acid. Odont. Tidskr., 75:237, 1967.

197. Sönju, T., and Rölla, G.: Chemical analysis of pellicle formed in two hours on cleaned human teeth *in vivo*. Rate of formation and amino acid analysis. Caries Res., 7:30, 1972.

198. Sönju, T., and Rölla, G.: Chemical analysis of acquired pellicle formed in two hours on cleaned human teeth *in vitro*. Caries Res., 7:30, 1973.

199. Stallard, R. E., et al.: The effect of an antimicrobial mouth rinse on dental plaque, calculus and gingivitis. J. Periodontol., 40:683, 1969.

200. Stephan, R. M.: The dental plaque in relation to the etiology of caries. Int. Dent. J., 4:180, 1953.

201. Stralfors, A.: Disinfection of dental plaques in man. In Caries Symposium, Zurich. Proceedings International Symposium. H. R. Mühlemann and K. König; Eds. Berne, Hans Huber, pp. 154–161, 1961.

202. Symposium on chlorhexidine in the prophylaxis of dental diseases. H. Löe, Ed. J. Periodont. Res. Suppl., 12:1, 1973.

203. Tempel, T. R., et al.: Factors from saliva and oral bacteria, chemotactic for polymorphonuclear leukocytes: their possible role in gingival inflammation. J. Periodontol., 41:71, 1970.

204. Theilade, J., Egelberg, J., and Attström, R.: Vascular permeability to colloidal carbon in chronically inflammed gingiva. J. Periodont. Res., 6:100, 1971.

205. Theilade, J., and Mikkelsen, L.: Electron microscopic study of formation of dental deposits on mylar films during the initial 3-hour period. 18th ORCA Congress, 1971.

206. Theilade, E., and Theilade, J.: Bacteriological and ultrastructural studies of developing dental plaque. *In* Dental Plaque. W. D. McHugh, Ed. Edinburgh, E & S Livingstone, Ltd., 1970, pp. 27–40.

207. Turesky, S., Renstrup, G., and Glickman, I.: Histologic and histochemical observations regarding early calculus formation in children and adults. J. Periodontol., 32:7, 1961.

208. Van Houte, J., Gibbons, R. J., and Banghart, S.: Adherence as a determinant of the presence of *Streptococcus salivarius* and *Streptococcus sanguis* on the tooth surface. Arch. Oral Biol., 15:1025, 1970.

209. Van Houte, J., Gibbons, R. J., and Pulkkinen, A. V.: Adherence as an ecological determinant for streptococci in the human mouth. Arch. Oral Biol., 16:1131, 1971.

210. Van Houte, J., and Jansen, H. M.: Levan degradation by streptococci isolated from human dental plaque. Arch. Oral Biol., 13:827, 1968.

211. Volpe, A. R., et al.: The long term effect of an antimicrobial formulation on dental calculus formation. J. Periodontol., 41:463, 1970.

212. Williams, B. L., Pantalone, R. M., and Sherris, J. C.: Subgingival microflora and periodontitis. J. Periodont. Res., 11:1, 1976.

213. Williams, J. L.: A contribution to the study of pathology of enamel. Dental Cosmos, 39:169, 1897.

214. Williams, R. W., and Gibbons, R. J.: Inhibition of bacterial adherence by secretory immunoglobulin A: a mechanism of antigen disposal. Science, 177:697, 1972.

215. Wood, J. M.: The state of hexose sugar in human dental plaque and its metabolism by the plaque bacteria. Arch. Oral Biol., 14:161, 1969.

216. Wood, J. M.: The amount, distribution and metabolism of soluble polysaccharides in human dental plaque. Arch. Oral Biol., 12:849, 1967.

217. Zander, H. A.: Effect of a penicillin dentifrice on caries incidence in school children. J. Am. Dent. Assoc., 40:569, 1950.

7

Structure and Pathogenesis

7
Structure and Pathogenesis

ROY C. PAGE
AND HUBERT E. SCHROEDER

Pathogenesis can be defined as the unfolding of a disease process, or the sequence of events in the development of a disease from its earliest beginnings. Concepts of pathogenesis are based to a large extent upon the natural history of the disease and upon its histopathologic and ultrastructural features.

Until recently there was insufficient information upon which to develop a unified concept of the pathogenesis of inflammatory gingival and periodontal disease. Indeed, views have been uniquely divergent, with emphasis being placed upon the multifactorial nature of the disease. This need be the case no longer. The structural manifestations of the advanced stage of the disease were described accurately over half a century ago;[33,79,89] the natural history of the disease, at least as it occurs in the beagle dog, has been clarified;[37,60] and recently the events occurring during the initial and early stages of the disease were described.[6,39,40,56,62,64,65,69,70,87] Thus, while the observations are far from complete and many of the details remain unclear, the overall features of the pathogenesis are beginning to emerge. It is our intent to organize and present selected portions of the available data in order to make these principal features apparent. This approach has admitted shortcomings and constraints, especially in that coverage is incomplete; however, these are outweighed by the clarity introduced.

The periodontium is the primary seat of several inflammatory lesions that may differ from one another etiologically and in their natural histories, but which may exhibit similar clinical and histopathologic manifestations. Among the better defined of these are acute necrotizing ulcerative gingivitis; hormonal, nutritional, and drug-related gingivitis; periodontosis or juvenile periodontitis; and inflammatory gingivitis and periodontitis associated with the accumulation of microbial plaque. In addition, the supporting structures are affected by several atrophic and degenerative diseases such as occlusal traumatism, alveolar atrophy, and desquamative gingivitis. However, the plaque-associated inflammatory lesion makes up the bulk, by far, of the lesions encountered by the dentist, and it is the only lesion for which sufficient information is available to develop even an elementary understanding of its pathogenesis. Thus, the discussion that follows relates to the plaque-associated inflammatory lesion only.

HISTORIC PERSPECTIVE

Efforts directed toward gaining an understanding of the pathogenesis of inflammatory gingival and periodontal disease span more than a century. These studies can be divided roughly into three categories: clinical observation, structural analysis, and experimental manipulation and quantitative measurement.

Clinical Observation

During the initial period, which extended throughout most of the nineteenth century, the predominant technique used was clinical observation, and efforts were directed almost completely toward documentation of the clinical signs and symptoms of the disease, classification, delineation of associated etiologic factors, and development of techniques for treatment.[10,13,25,31,34,55,57,58,78] The observations of these early investigators established several important points: (1) the disease is not homogeneous, but rather it is a combination of several different diseases with a common manifestation; (2) both local and systemic factors are involved in the etiology; (3) the lesion is basically a form of suppurative inflammation with associated resorption of the alveolar bone; (4) pus formation and exudation are the common features of advanced disease; and (5) debridement, stabilization of the teeth, and oral cleanliness are important aspects of successful treatment.

Structural Analysis

It was not until the turn of the nineteenth century, that investigators began to examine the microscopic structure of the naturally occurring lesion. During the ensuing 50 years, numerous papers appeared, describing structural features of advanced spontaneous periodontal disease.[3,4,8,11,15,27,33,44,79,84,89] These studies established the cardinal histopathologic features of the advanced stages of the disease, as well as its route of progress. Little attention was directed toward study of the initial lesion.[7,43,47,86]

During the past decade, the increased resolving power of the electron microscope has been brought to bear on the problem, and this has provided an insight into many of the cellular and ultrastructural alterations seen in man and other animals.[16,17,18,42,46,52,61,70,71,81,82,88]

Experimental Manipulation and Quantitative Measurement

A more recent development has been the application of an experimental approach and quantitative analytic techniques to problems of pathogenesis. The histopathologic and ultrastructural features of experimental gingivitis have been examined in both cross-sectional and longitudinal studies,[40,56,87] and morphometric techniques have been adapted to problems of quantitative analysis of the components of the affected tissues.[62,63,67,68] Further studies employing these techniques have led to a redefinition of the nature of the early inflammatory lesion and have permitted, for the first time, a better understanding of the temporal progression of events in the pathogenesis.[6,56,65,69,70]

EARLY CONCEPTS OF PATHOGENESIS

One of the earliest concepts of the pathogenesis held that proliferation and apical migration of the cells of the epithelial attachment (junctional epithelium) with pocket formation are the initial and most significant pathologic changes associated with inflammatory gingival and periodontal disease.[22,23,33,79,89] Attention appears to have been focused upon this aspect of the disease by the intense interest of oral histologists in determining the nature of the normal epithelial attachment apparatus.[21,49,83,85] Much of the early work was directed toward discovering the basic cause of the proliferation and migration, and this objective became synonymous with that of understanding the pathogenesis of the disease.

Numerous hypotheses were devised to account for the proliferation and apical migration. Gottlieb considered a limited amount of alveolar atrophy and recession of the marginal bone to be a normal consequence of aging and continuous eruption of the teeth.[21] He felt that pocket formation and "pyorrhea" were a consequence of irregularity or accentuation of this normal process. This idea was strongly opposed by James and Counsell.[33] In 1946, Gottlieb presented his concept of "cementopathia."[23] According to this hypothesis, interference with continuous cemental deposition results in a lack of attachment of the collagen fibers of the gingival and periodontal ligaments to the root surface and permits migration of the epithelial cells apically with pocket formation. On the other hand, Goldman noted that migration of the epithelial cells along the root surface could not occur so long as the dense connective-tissue fibers underlying the attachment apparatus were intact, and he postulated an initial degenerative change in these fibers followed by epithelial-cell proliferation and migration.[20] Still another view was expressed by Aisenberg and Aisenberg, who showed that tongues of epithelial cells migrate apically between presumably normal connective-tissue bundles, and they proposed that the epithelial cells might exert a lytic effect upon the underlying connective tissues.[1]

The importance of the epithelial proliferation and migration as the initial and cardinal event was questioned by Fish.[11] He maintained that long before this event occurred, an accumulation of inflammatory cells could be observed just deep to the junctional epithelium where proliferation subsequently occurs. Fish and James and Counsell referred to this area as the primary zone of injury.[11,33] Their work served to divert attention from the proliferative phenomena and direct it toward alterations within the underlying connective tissues.

In spite of its conceptual limitations and a large body of evidence to the contrary, the idea that epithelial proliferation and apical migration with pocket formation are a cardinal event in pathogenesis of periodontal disease continues to pervade current thought. For example, attention is still focused upon the prime importance of pocket depth in evaluation of periodontal status, and most therapeutic measures are directed toward reduction in the pocket depth. In light of our present understanding of the destructive aspects of inflammation and immunologic reactions and of recent advances in definition of the morphologic features of gingivitis and periodontitis, this view should be reexamined. Generally, the data support the idea that epithelial proliferation and migration and pocket formation may only be secondary features of one stage of a multifaceted disease process. Indeed, the enhanced exudation, the infiltration and transformation of lymphoid cells, and the early loss of connective tissue substance, which occur prior to pocket formation, may be more important pathogenic aspects of the disease than pocket formation, especially from the point of view of arresting its progress.

STAGES IN THE PATHOGENESIS

The natural history of inflammatory gingival and periodontal disease is not well understood, and important aspects of its pathogenesis remain unknown. It has been assumed, especially by epidemiologists and clinicians, that gingivitis progresses with time to destructive periodontal disease. Although this assumption remains unproved and it appears that, at least in some cases, this progression does not occur,[2,61] recent data indicate that the early stages of periodontitis are manifested as gingivitis. For example, when plaque is allowed to accumulate on the teeth of the dog, gingivitis develops within a matter of days, and with the passage of years progresses to periodontitis.[37,60] In addition, the prevalence of spontaneous periodontitis beginning as gingivitis in the dog increases with increasing age.[30]

While current data are incomplete and many of the details of the progression from incipient gingivitis to advanced periodontitis are unclear, the overall features

of the pathogenesis are beginning to emerge. On the basis of the clinical manifestations and measurement of gingival exudate, the chronic plaque-associated lesion has been subdivided into three stages. These are subclinical gingivitis, clinical gingivitis, and periodontal breakdown.[24] However, the distinguishing features of these stages have not been defined clearly. Analysis of the histopathologic and ultrastructural features of the disease permits a more clear-cut subdivision into *initial*, *early*, *established*, and *advanced* stages.[53] While this subdivision too is somewhat arbitrary, it is generally supported by the morphologic data, and it permits focusing attention upon important pathologic aspects of the disease and upon associated pathogenic mechanisms.

The Initial Lesion

One of the major problems in understanding the pathogenesis of periodontal disease has been the inability to distinguish clearly between normal and pathologically altered tissues. In other words, it has not been possible to determine exactly when the disease begins. This problem was first acknowledged almost a half century ago,[33] and it has still not been resolved completely. In the absence of definitive evidence, it has been held, generally, that features characterizing the initial lesion merely reflect enhanced levels of activity of mechanisms of host defense normally operative within the gingival tissues.

In experimental situations in which the tissues of humans and dogs have been kept relatively free of plaque, small numbers of leukocytes may be observed migrating towards the gingival sulcus and residing within the junctional epithelium. In addition, a few isolated lymphocytes and plasma cells may be associated with blood vessels of the subepithelial plexus and

TABLE 7-1. *Features of the Initial Lesion*

1. Classic vasculitis of vessels subjacent to the junctional epithelium

2. Exudation of fluid from the gingival sulcus

3. Increased migration of leukocytes into the junctional epithelium and gingival sulcus

4. Presence of serum proteins, especially fibrin extravascularly

5. Alteration of the most coronal portion of the junctional epithelium

6. Loss of perivascular collagen

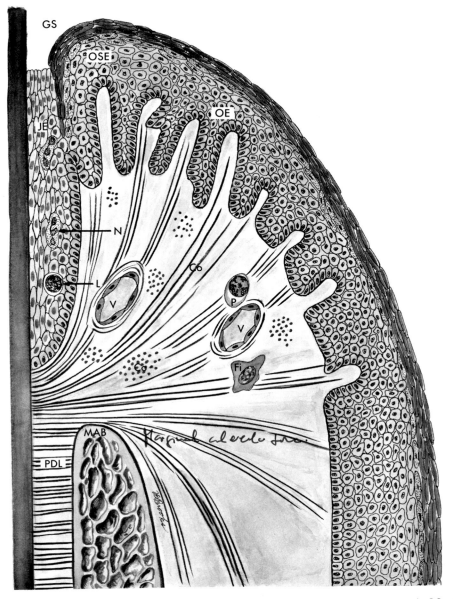

FIG. 7-1. *Schematic illustration of the normal marginal gingiva as it appears on the buccal aspect of a tooth. GS, gingival sulcus; OE, oral epithelium; OSE, oral sulcular epithelium; JE, junctional epithelium; N, neutrophilic granulocyte; L, lymphocyte; V, vessel of the gingival plexus; Co, collagen fibers in long and cross section; Fi, fibroblast; P, plasma cell; MAB, marginal alveolar bone; PDL, periodontal ligament.*

deep within the connective tissue.[6,56] These are not accompanied by manifestations of tissue damage perceptible in the light microscope or ultrastructurally, they do not form an infiltrate, and therefore their presence is not considered to indicate pathologic change. The junctional epithelium uniformly joins the connective tissue without rete ridges, and it is supported by dense, highly oriented connective tissue fiber bundles (Fig. 7-1).[5,6,51,56] In these tissues, the earliest developments following the beginning of plaque accu-

mulation are characteristic of a classic acute exudative inflammatory response.[5,37,48,56,65] The characteristics of this initial lesion are listed in Table 7-1 and are illustrated schematically in Figure 7-2.

The initial lesion is localized to the region of the gingival sulcus. The tissues affected include a portion of the junctional epithelium, the oral sulcular epithelium, and the most coronal portion of the connective tissue. Rarely is a fraction of gingival connective tissue exceeding 5 to 10 percent involved, although as pocket

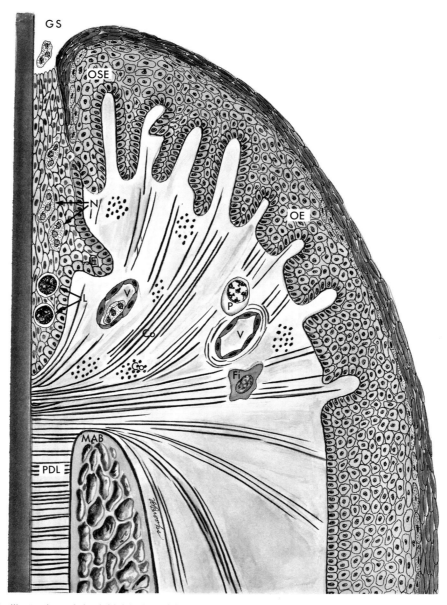

FIG. 7-2. *Schematic illustration of the initial lesion. GS, gingival sulcus; OE, oral epithelium; OSE, oral sulcular epithelium; JE, junctional epithelium; N, neutrophilic granulocytes; L, lymphocyte; V, vessel of the gingival plexus; Co, collagen fiber bundles in long and cross section; Fi, fibroblast; P, plasma cell; MAB, marginal alveolar bone; PDL, periodontal ligament.*

formation occurs during the subsequent stages of the disease, the oral sulcular and junctional epithelia are converted to pocket epithelium and the reaction site extends both apically and laterally. During the initial stage, the vessels of the gingival plexus become engorged and dilated, and large numbers of polymorphonuclear leukocytes migrate into the junctional epithelium and gingival sulcus (Fig. 7-2). A few macrophages and blast-transforming lymphocytes may appear within the junctional epithelium and in the connective tissue. A portion of the perivascular collagen may

disappear, and the resultant space becomes occupied by fluid, serum proteins, and inflammatory cells. Fibrin is especially apparent.[53] While immunoglobulins, especially IgG and complement, are probably present in the extravascular gingival tissues,[9,19] there is insufficient evidence to determine the role, if any, that these substances may play at this stage in the pathogenesis. As shown in Figure 7-3, significant increases in the levels of leukocyte migration and fluid exudation occur by day 2 in experimental gingivitis in the dog. In humans and other species, there are dilation of the

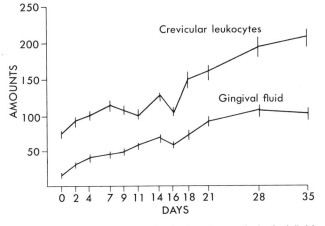

FIG. 7-3. *Amounts of crevicular leukocytes and gingival fluid during developing gingivitis in dogs. Vertical lines indicate the standard error of the mean. (From Attström, R., and Egelberg, J.: Presence of leukocytes within the gingival crevices during developing gingivitis in dogs. J. Periodont. Res., 6:110, 1971.)*

vessels of the gingival plexus, adherence of leukocytes to the vessel walls (Figs. 7-4C,D), and migration of leukocytes through the wall into the connective tissues (Fig. 7-5). The gingival sulcus contains migrating leukocytes, sloughed epithelial cells, and microorganisms (Figs. 7-4A,B, 7-6, 7-7A). In the superficial regions of the junctional epithelium, intact and degenerating neutrophils may be seen (Figs. 7-7B, 7-8A). The extracellular space is occupied by granular material of unknown composition and dead-cell debris (Fig. 7-7B). Within the deeper regions of the junctional epithelium, numerous intact neutrophils and other leukocytes may be present (Fig. 7-8B).

The initial lesion may be a response to the generation of chemotactic and antigenic substances in the region of the gingival sulcus.[38,80] In fact, the acute inflammatory phenomenon can be provoked simply by applying plaque-derived chemotactic substances to the gingival margin.[26]

The initial lesion emerges within a matter of 2 to 4 days when previously normal, infiltrate-free gingival tissue is resubjected to the accumulation of microbial plaque.[6,56] Under less strict experimental conditions, the initial lesion as described earlier may not be observed at all. Instead, a preestablished chronic lymphoid infiltrate resembling the early lesion may be present in an otherwise healthy gingival tissue.[39,40,69] This tissue, when reacting to the onset of plaque accumulation, mimics the initial lesion in that it responds with an exacerbation of acute exudative inflammation that is superimposed upon the lymphoid infiltrate. These tissues manifest clinical signs and symptoms of gingivitis earlier than previously normal, infiltrate-free tissue.[65]

The Early Lesion

The early lesion overlaps with and evolves from the initial lesion with no clear-cut dividing line.[56,65] Features of the early lesion were first described by James and Counsell (1927) as follows:

In the early stage lymphocytes are the characteristic cells. They are diffusely arranged immediately under the epithelium at the zone of injury (subjacent to the junctional epithelium) occupying the papillae formed by the proliferated epithelium and also the adjacent corium. The lymphocytic infiltration remains localized and does not extend deeply into the tissues. This stage may be seen in young subjects and even with temporary teeth. Later stages show the presence of plasma cells.[33]

More recently, the early lesion has been studied morphologically, and its characteristic manifestations have been measured stereologically.[62,69,70] The hallmarks of the early lesion are listed in Table 7-2 and illustrated schematically in Figure 7-9.

The early lesion in humans appears at the site of the initial lesion within 4 to 7 days following the beginning of plaque accumulation (Table 7-3).[56] In essence, it is the result of the formation and maintenance of a dense lymphoid cell infiltrate within the gingival connective tissues.

Acute exudative inflammatory phenomena persist in the early lesion. The exudation of serum components as measured by gingival fluid flow and the number of crevicular leukocytes reach their maximum and level off between 6 and 12 days after the onset of clinical gingivitis.[37] The quantity of sulcular fluid appears to be indicative of the size of the reaction site within the connective tissue.[39,59,65] Although the oral sulcular epithelium and the oral epithelium generally do not become infiltrated, the junctional epithelium contains

TABLE 7-2. *Features of the Early Lesion*

1. Accentuation of the features described for the initial lesion

2. Accumulation of lymphoid cells immediately subjacent to the junctional epithelium at the site of acute inflammation

3. Cytopathic alterations in resident fibroblasts, possibly associated with interactions with lymphoid cells

4. Further loss of the collagen fiber network supporting the marginal gingiva

5. Beginning proliferation of the basal cells of the junctional epithelium

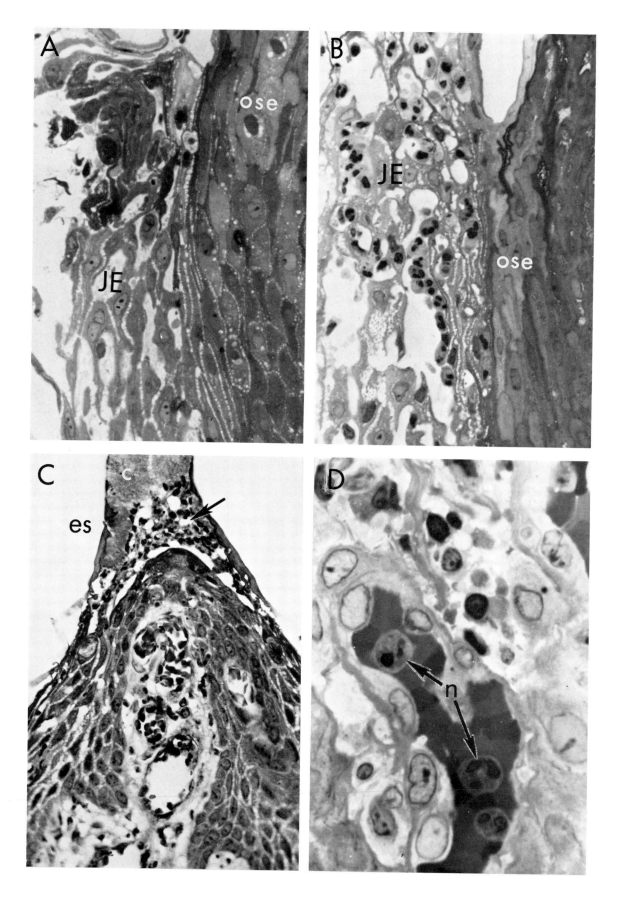

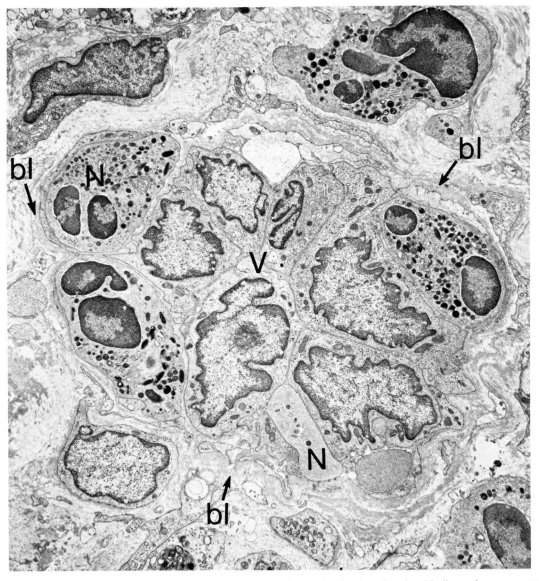

FIG. 7-5. *A collapsed blood vessel in the connective tissues subjacent to the junctional epithelium of a marmoset. Several neutrophils (N) have migrated from the vessel (V) and are located between the endothelial cells and the basal lamina (bl) (magnification 6300 ×). (Schectman, L. R., et al.: Host tissues response in chronic periodontal disease. J. Periodont. Res., 7:195, 1972.)*

FIG. 7-4. *The initial lesion in inflammatory gingival and periodontal disease. A. Biopsy from the free marginal gingiva adjacent to the gingival sulcus of a human free of plaque and of manifestations of disease. Note the sloughing surface of the junctional epithelium (JE) and the oral sulcular epithelium (ose) (magnification 500 ×). B. Biopsy from the free marginal gingiva adjacent to the gingival sulcus of a human in whom plaque was allowed to accumulate for 2 days. Large numbers of leukocytes are present in the junctional epithelium (JE) but the oral sulcular epithelium (ose) is free of infiltrating cells (magnification 500 ×). C. Biopsy from the inter-proximal region of an adult marmoset exhibiting clinical manifestations of early gingival inflammation. Note the presence of calculus (c) adjacent to the enamel space (es) with a dense band of leukocytes (arrow) interposed between the deposit and the epithelial tissue. Many of the vessels in the connective tissue contain adhering leukocytes (magnification 640 ×). D. Section through a vessel located subjacent to the junctional epithelium in a biopsy taken from a human 2 days after the cessation of plaque control. Note the presence of neutrophils (n) within the vessel and possibly adherent to the wall (magnification 1250 ×). (A, B, and D—Payne, W. A., et al.: Histopathologic features of the initial and early stages of experimental gingivitis in man. J. Periodont. Res., 10:51, 1975. C—Schectman, L. R., et al.: Host tissues response in chronic periodontal disease. J. Periodont. Res., 7:195, 1972.)*

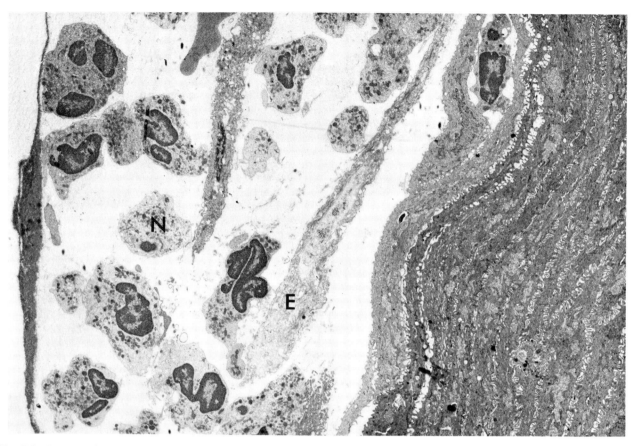

FIG. 7-6. *Electron microscopic view of the contents of the gingival sulcus of a human exhibiting early inflammatory gingival disease. Note the large number of neutrophils (N) and sloughing epithelial cells (E) within the sulcus (magnification 5700 ×). (Lange, D., and Schroeder, H. E.: Cytochemistry and ultrastructure of gingival sulcus cells. Helv. Odontol. Acta, 15(Suppl. 6):65, 1971.)*

a variably increased number of transmigrating neutrophilic granulocytes and infiltrating mononuclear cells including lymphocytes, macrophages, plasma cells, and mast cells.[64] The leukocytes insinuate between the epithelial cells and may be present in numbers sufficiently large as to disrupt the continuity of the epithelial barrier (Figs. 7-10, 7-11A–H).

The area of affected connective tissue can be distinguished clearly from the surrounding normal tissue by the presence of inflammatory cells and the decreased collagen content (Figs. 7-10, 7-11, 7-12, 7-13). The percent cell composition of the infiltrated connective-tissue zone, exclusive of vascular structures, is fibroblasts 14.8, neutrophilic granulocytes 2.6, monocytes and macrophages 2.1, plasma cells 2.0, small lymphocytes 39.3, medium lymphocytes 34.9, immunoblasts 1.9, and mast cells 2.4 (Figs. 7-14, 7-15). While neutrophilic granulocytes densely infiltrate the junctional epithelium and gingival sulcus and a few may be observed within the blood vessels, they are seen only infrequently within the substance of the connective tissues.[33] The largest portion of the infiltrating cells

(about 74 percent) are lymphocytes, and many of these are intermediate in size, an indication that blast transformation and differentiation into sensitized T- and B-lymphocytes and plasma cells may be occurring (Fig. 7-15). A significant number can be identified as immunoblasts.

The collagen fiber content of the affected tissue is reduced (Figs. 7-13, 7-14, Table 7-4). There is a reduction in collagen content of about 70 percent relative to the noninflamed connective-tissue zone.[12,50,69] This alteration, which occurs at an early stage of the disease, affects especially the dentogingival and circular fiber groups that normally support the junctional epithelium. The loss of collagen may therefore be a major factor in the continuing loss of tissue integrity and normal gingival function as the disease progresses.

Specific cytopathic alterations occur in the fibroblasts of the infiltrated connective-tissue zone (Figs. 7-10, 7-11, 7-15, 7-16).[52,69,70,72,73] While the fibroblasts are equally numerous in the infiltrated and noninfiltrated regions of the gingival connective tissues, the fibroblasts in the pathologically altered tissues exhibit a

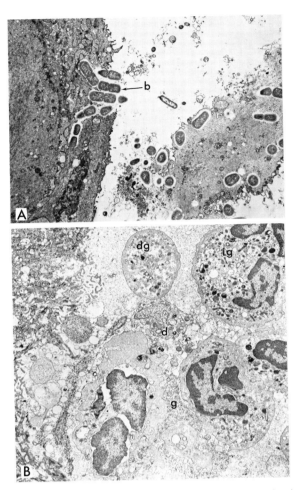

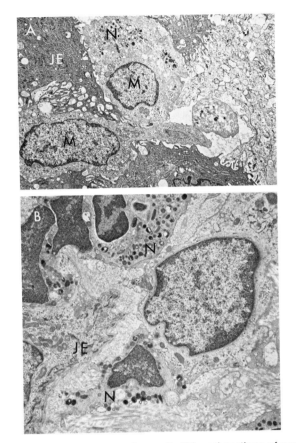

FIG. 7-7. *Electron micrographs of gingival sulcus of adult marmoset. A. Bacteria (b) associated with sloughed junctional epithelial cells (magnification 2,600 ×). B. Intact (ig) and degenerating (dg) granulocytes within the junctional epithelium near the base. Note the granular intercellular material (g) and dead cell debris (d) (magnification 2,900 ×). (Page, R. C., et al.: Host tissue response in chronic periodontal disease. J. Periodont. Res., 7:283, 1972.)*

FIG. 7-8. *A. Two mononuclear cells (M) and portions of neutrophils (N) just beneath the surface of the junctional epithelium (JE) of the mandibular left first molar of a marmoset. The epithelial cell at the upper right is a sloughing surface cell (magnification 3,150 ×). (Page, R. C., et al.: Host tissue response in chronic periodontal disease. J. Periodont. Res., 7:283, 1972.) B. The junctional epithelium (JE), noted on the left side of the picture, is separated from the connective tissues by a basement lamina, and contains a portion of a neutrophil. An apparently intact neutrophil (N) is present in the connective tissues uppermost in the picture, and a portion of a neutrophil (N) with extracellular lysosomal granules is noted in the lower portion (magnification 2,850 ×). (Schectman, L. R., et al.: Host tissues response in chronic periodontal disease. J. Periodont. Res., 7:195, 1972.)*

TABLE 7-3. *Cellular and Tissue Changes Accompanying Microbial Plaque Accumulation in Humans*

TIME	GRANULAR LEUKOCYTES PER UNIT AREA JUNCTIONAL EPITHELIUM	SMALL MONONUCLEAR CELLS PER UNIT AREA OF CONNECTIVE TISSUE	AREA OF COLLAGEN ALTERATION	AREA OF LEUKOCYTE INFILTRATION
Day 0	0.32 (0.38)[a]	11.50 (3.76)[a]	2.35 (1.13)[a]	6.10 (2.79)
Day 1	1.64 (1.35)	12.25 (5.71)	5.04 (2.00)	5.94 (3.63)
Day 4	1.63 (1.10)	23.87 (5.68)	4.36 (1.44)	10.11 (11.73)
Day 8	2.87 (1.26)	30.73 (17.42)	9.74 (4.87)	14.18 (5.95)

From Payne, W. A., et al.: Histopathologic features of the initial and early stages of experimental gingivitis in man. J. Periodont. Res., *10*:51, 1975.
[a] Reported as the Mean (SD)

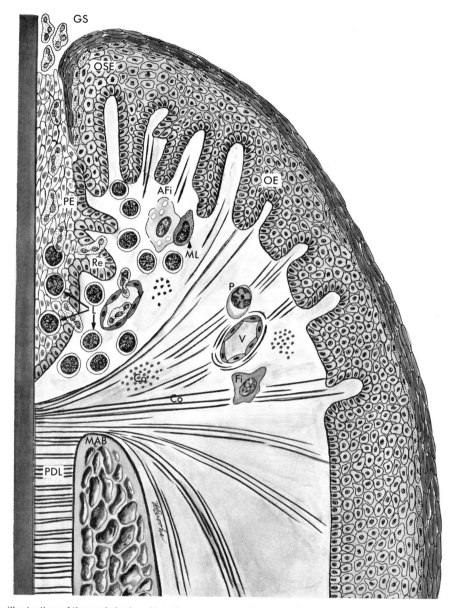

FIG. 7-9. *Schematic illustration of the early lesion. Note the presence of increased numbers of leukocytes in the junctional epithelium and gingival sulcus and the accumulation of lymphocytes in the connective tissues immediately subjacent to the junctional epithelium. Fibroblasts within the zone of infiltration appear to be cytopathically altered and a large portion of the collagen has been lost. GS, gingival sulcus; OSE, oral sulcular epithelium; OE, oral epithelium; PE, pocket epithelium; AFi, altered fibroblast; Re, developing rete ridges of the pocket epithelium; L, lymphocytes; ML, medium-sized lymphocytes possibly representing blast-transforming cells; P, plasma cells; V, vessels; Co, collagen bundles; MAB, marginal alveolar bone; PDL, periodontal ligament.*

FIG. 7-10. *Histopathologic features of the early gingival lesion in man. Note the enamel space (es), surface deposit (d), junctional epithelium (JE), oral sulcular epithelium (OSE), residual collagen fibers (Co), vessels of the gingival vascular plexus (V). Large numbers of leukocytes, predominantly neutrophils, are present between the cells of the junctional epithelium and in the gingival sulcus. The numbers of these cells are so great as to disrupt the continuity of the junctional epithelium in some areas (see arrow lower left-hand corner, B). In the subjacent connective tissues vasculitis is evidenced by the prominence of the vascular plexus, and the collagen bundles have been replaced by a dense infiltrate of inflammatory cells. Most of these cells are lymphocytes. The line of demarcation between infiltrated and noninfiltrated connective tissue is reasonably distinct in A. (Compare with Fig. 1-3, illustrating a relatively normal gingival sulcus) (Epon-embedded 1 micron sections; magnification (A) 100 ×, (B) 150 ×).*

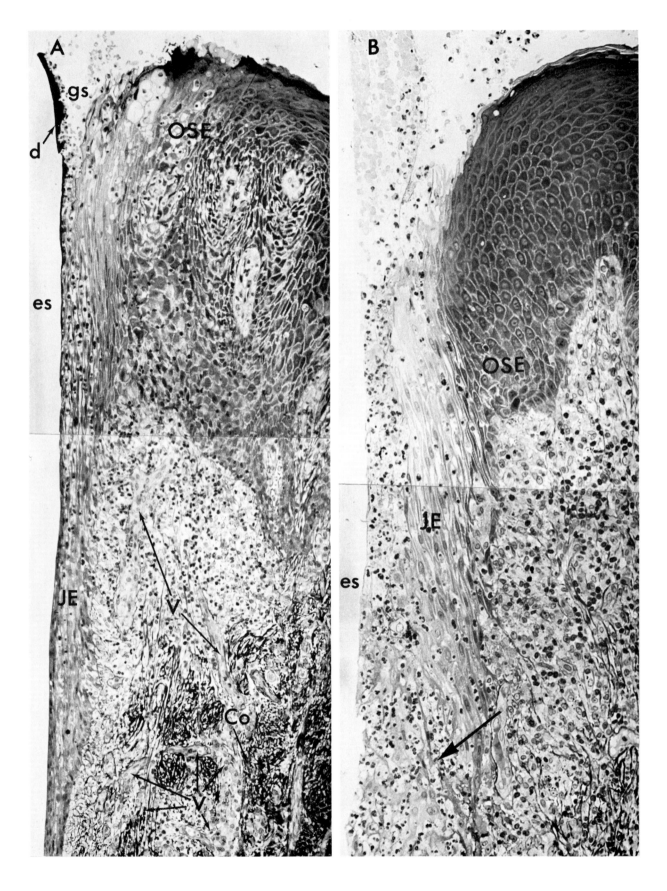

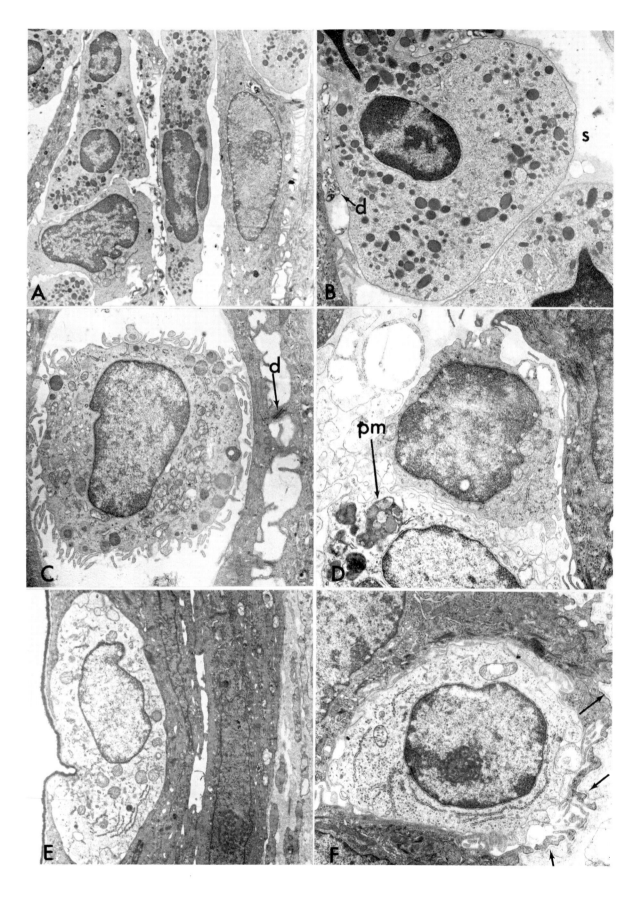

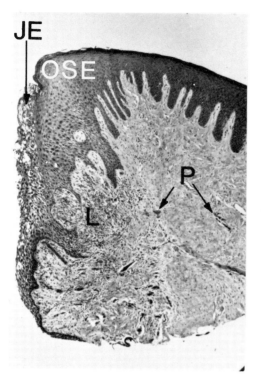

FIG. 7-12. *Characteristic features of a* <u>biopsy specimen</u> *taken after* <u>4 days of plaque accumulation</u>. *Note the oral sulcular epithelium (OSE), the residual junctional epithelium (JE) and the rather distinct line of demarcation between them. The plaque-associated leukocyte infiltrate (L) is present subjacent to the junctional epithelium, and the location of vessels deep within the gingival connective tissue with associated inflammatory cells is indicated by (P). Paraffin section stained with Gomori trichrome (magnification 50 ×). (Payne, W. A., et al.: Histopathologic features of the initial and early stages of experimental gingivitis in man. J. Periodont. Res., 10:51, 1975.)*

mitochondria frequently with loss of cristae, and rupture of the plasma membrane. These alterations are characteristically exhibited by sick or dying cells. The changes do not appear to be a consequence of defective tissue fixation and processing, since they are not seen in fibroblasts or other cells of the normal tissues, nor in the nonfibroblastic cells in the lesion. These cytopathic alterations appear to be associated with the activity of lymphoid cells. There is a positive correlation between the increasing numbers of medium-sized lymphocytes and immunoblasts and increasing fibroblast size.[69] Furthermore, lymphocytes were observed frequently in intimate contact with the altered fibroblasts.

Recently it was shown that peripheral blood lymphocytes obtained from patients with inflammatory gingival disease are sensitized to antigenic substances in human dental plaque.[28,29,32] These cells undergo blast transformation when cultured *in vitro* in the presence of plaque antigens, and fluids from these cultures exert a cytotoxic effect on gingival fibroblasts.[29] The morphologic and morphometric data now available support the idea that a phenomenon similar to that observed *in vitro* may be occurring in the gingival tissues in humans during the early stage of inflammatory gingival and periodontal disease.[70] If this is the case, a form of cellular hypersensitivity to plaque-derived antigens may be an important component in the development of the early lesion.

The Established Lesion

The distinguishing feature of the established lesion is a predominance of plasma cells within the affected connective tissues at a stage prior to extensive bone loss. Lesions of this type appear to be extremely widespread in human and animal populations and have been described by many investigators.[11,33,43,52,79] The lesion has been described by James and Counsell as follows:

threefold increase in size relative to those in the normal tissue (Fig. 7-14). Furthermore, distinctive cytologic alterations are present. These include electron lucency of the nucleus suggestive of a reduced chromatin content, frequent absence of nucleoli, widely dilated cisternae of the endoplasmic reticulum, swollen

FIG. 7-11. *Cells encountered in the junctional epithelium in biopsy specimens from humans during the early stage of gingival and periodontal inflammatory disease. A. Neutrophils located near the gingival sulcus in the junctional epithelium (magnification 4500 ×). (Lange, D., and Schroeder, H. E.: Cytochemistry and ultrastructure of gingival sulcus cells. Helv. Odontol. Acta, 15(Suppl. 6):65, 1971. B. Two neutrophils within the junctional epithelium and surrounded by intercellular space (s) and debris (d) (magnification 9900 ×). C. A mast cell located within the junctional epithelium. Note the presence of dense granules and the microvilli of the plasma membrane. These are distinguishing characteristics of mast cells. A desmosome (d) is seen connecting two epithelial cells (magnification 6900 ×). D. Two mononuclear cells within the junctional epithelium. One of these contains masses of phagocytized material (pm) and is therefore likely to be a macrophage. The other cell probably belongs to the lymphoid series (magnification 9000 ×). E. A "clear cell," not further identified, in the junctional epithelium in contact with the tooth surface (magnification 5900 ×). F. A mononuclear cell located in the basal layer of the junctional epithelium. Note the basal lamina (arrows). The cell exhibits rosettes of ribosomes, scattered mitochondria, a few lamallae of rough endoplasmic reticulum, a pale nucleus with a large nucleolus, and an irregular cell surface. These features are consistent with identification of the cell as an immunoblast (magnification 6900 ×).*

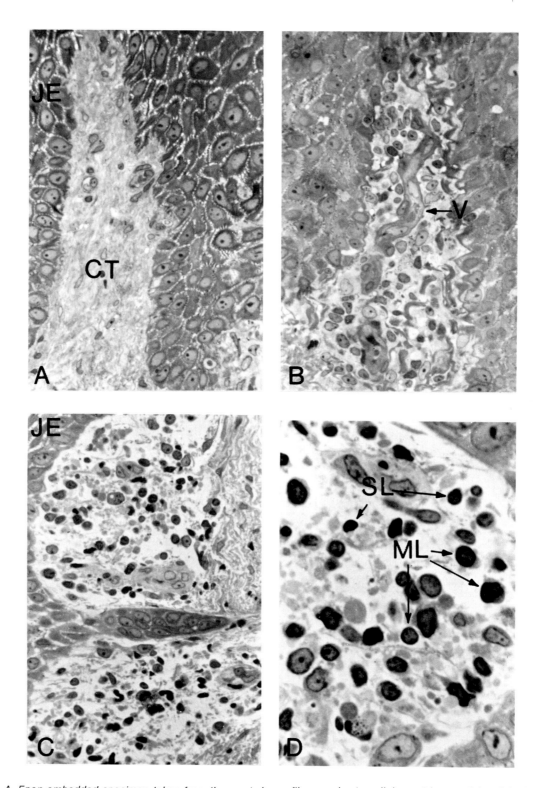

FIG. 7-13. *A. Epon-embedded specimen taken from the most coronal portion of the connective tissue lateral to the gingival sulcus prior to the beginning of plaque accumulation and illustrating the normally dense collagenous tissue along with a very few cells which occupy the connective tissues (CT) subjacent to the junctional epithelium (JE) (magnification 250 ×). B. Epon-embedded specimen taken from a region comparable to (A) after 8 days of plaque accumulation. Note the increased cellularity and the decreased collagen fiber content of the connective tissues. An enlarged blood vessel (V) courses the central portion of the connective tissue core (magnification 250 ×). C. Epon-embedded specimen taken from the region lateral to the base of the gingival sulcus after 8 days of plaque accumulation. Note the disruption of the col-lagen fibers and extracellular matrix material and the infiltrate of mononuclear cells of various sizes in the connective tissue (magnification 250 ×). D. Epon-embedded specimen taken from the region of the base of the gingival sulcus after 8 days plaque accumulation illustrating the features of the infiltrate. The cells are clearly mononuclear and do not exhibit features characteristic of plasma cells. Some of the cells exhibit features typical of small lymphocytes (SL), including a small, round, densely basophilic nucleus with scanty cytoplasm, and others exhibit features consistent with their being medium-sized lymphoid cells (ML) (magnification 625 ×). (Payne, W. A., et al.: Histopathologic features of the initial and early stages of experimental gingivitis in man. J. Periodont. Res., 10:51, 1975.)*

TABLE 7-4. *Total Collagen Content of Human Gingiva*

	DENSITY COLLAGEN FIBERS/mm³[a]	μg HYDROXYPROLINE[b] PER μg DRY CONNECTIVE TISSUE
Noninfilterated Connective Tissue	565.71 ± 72.29	0.091 ± 0.012
Infilterated Connective Tissue	160.75 ± 74.06	0.037 ± 0.009

[a]Schroeder, H. E., Münzel-Pedrazzoli, S., and Page, R. C.: Correlated morphometric and biochemical analysis of gingival tissue in early chronic gingivitis in man. Arch. Oral Biol., *18*:899, 1973.

[b]Flieder, D. E., Sun, C. H., and Schneider, B. C.: Chemistry of normal and inflamed human gingival tissues. Periodontics, *4*:302, 1966.

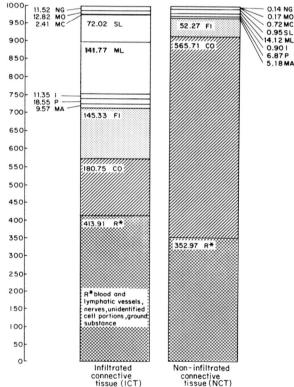

FIG. 7-14. *Average volumetric density (mm³) of tissue components residing in 1 cm³ of infiltrated (ICT) and noninfiltrated (NCT) gingival connective tissue. NG, Neutrophilic granulocyte; MO, monocytes; MC, macrophages; I, immunoblasts; P, plasma cells; MA, mast cells; SL, small lymphocytes; ML, medium lymphocytes; FI, fibroblasts; CO, Collagen; R, lymphatic and blood vessels, nerves, unidentified cell portions, and ground substance. (Schroeder, H. E., Münzel-Pedrazzoli, S., and Page, R. C.: Correlated morphometric and biochemical analysis of gingival tissue in early chronic gingivitis in man. Arch. Oral Biol., 18:899, 1973.)*

Later stages show the presence of plasma cells. These are seen first around the vessels of the subgingival (junctional) epithelium. They eventually almost entirely supercede the lymphocytes of the early stage, and their deep infiltration is confined to the vessels of the corium. Later they are seen to spread in diffuse masses from the zone of injury along the perivascular channels to the bone of the alveolar crest.[33]

The characteristic features of the established lesion are listed in Table 7-5 and illustrated schematically in Figure 7-17. As in the earlier stages, the lesion is still centered around the bottom of the sulcus and is confined to a relatively small portion of the gingival connective tissue. However, plasma cells are not confined to the reaction site; they also appear in clusters along the blood vessels and between collagen fiber bundles deep within the connective tissues. Although most of the plasma cells produce IgG (Fig. 7-18), a small number contain IgA; cells containing IgM are seen rarely.[9,19]

TABLE 7-5. *Features of the Established Lesion*

1. Persistence of the manifestations of acute inflammation

2. Predominance of plasma cells but without appreciable bone loss

3. Presence of immunoglobulins extravascularly in the connective tissues and in junctional epithelium

4. Continuing loss of connective tissue substance noted in the early lesion

5. Proliferation, apical migration, and lateral extension of the junctional epithelium; early pocket formation may or may not be present

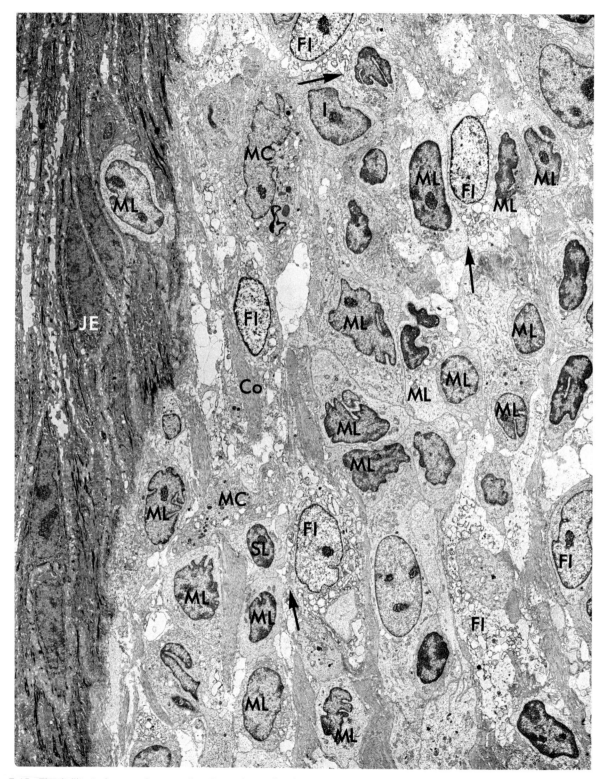

FIG. 7-15. *The infiltrated area of connective tissue immediately subjacent to the junctional epithelium (JE) in a human biopsy specimen illustrating characteristic features of the early stage of the lesion. Medium lymphocyte (ML), fibroblast (FI), small lymphocyte (SL), macrophage (MC), immunoblast (I), and collagen fibers (Co). Note the predominance of lymphoid cells, nuclear alterations and vacuolization of the fibroblasts, and the paucity of collagen fibers. In many areas (arrows) lymphoid cells intimately contact pathologically altered fibroblasts (original magnification 9,000 ×). (Schroeder, H. E., Münzel-Pedrazzoli, and Page, R. C.: Correlated morphometric and biochemical analysis of gingival tissue in early chronic gingivitis in man. Arch. Oral Biol., 18:899, 1973.)*

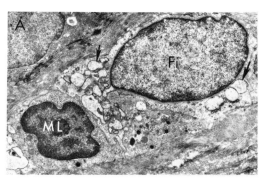

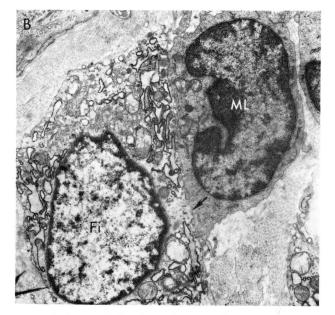

FIG. 7-16. *A. Electron micrograph of a fibroblast (Fi) located adjacent to the pocket epithelium in a young chimpanzee. A medium-sized lymphocyte (ML) is in intimate contact with the fibroblast and appears to have invaginated its surface. Alterations of the fibroblast consist of dilation of the granular endoplasmic reticulum (arrows) and enlargement of the mitochondria which lack cristae and appear empty (original magnification 3,900 ×). (Page, R. C., Ammons, W. F., and Simpson, D. M.: Host tissue response in chronic inflammatory periodontal disease. IV. The periodontal and dental status of a group of aged apes. J. Periodontol., 46:144, 1975.) B. Fibroblast-lymphoid cell interaction in the gingival connective tissues of a human during the early stage of inflammatory gingival and periodontal disease. Fibroblast (Fi) with closely neighboring lymphocyte (ML) residing in the infiltrated connective tissue. Note the electron lucency, dilated cisternae of rough endoplasmic reticulum and mitochondrial alterations in the fibroblast, and the well-preserved lymphocyte structures. In one area (arrow) the two cells may communicate, although this cannot be clearly established morphologically (magnification 6,900 ×). (Schroeder, H. E., and Page, R. C.: Lymphocyte-fibroblast interaction in the pathogenesis of inflammatory gingival disease. Experentia, 28:1228, 1972.)*

In addition to plasma cells, features described for the earlier stages of the lesion are still present, frequently in an accentuated form (Fig. 7-19). The junctional and oral sulcular epithelium may proliferate and migrate into the infiltrated connective tissue and along the root surface with conversion to pocket epithelium (Fig. 7-19). In some cases, the pocket epithelium may be thick and exhibit a tendency toward keratinization (Figs. 7-20A, 7-21), but more frequently it becomes thin and ulcerated (Fig. 7-19A,B). Vascular proliferation is a prominent feature in some animal species.[36,65]

If pocket epithelium is present, blood vessels loop high within the epithelium and may be separated from the external environment by only one or two epithelial cells (Fig. 7-19B). Large amounts of immunoglobulin are present throughout the connective and epithelial tissues,[9,19] and there is evidence for the presence of complement and antigen-antibody complexes, especially around the blood vessels.[19] A subpopulation of degenerating plasma cells may be encountered (Fig. 7-22).[14,51,73] Continuing loss of collagen is apparent in the zone of infiltration (Figs. 19C, 20B); in other more

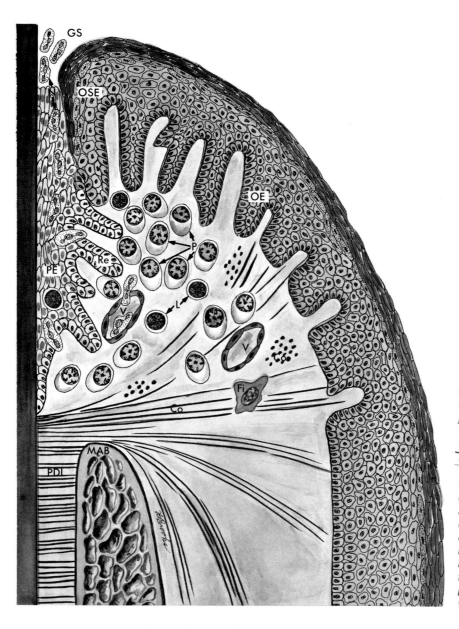

FIG. 7-17. *Schematic illustration of features of the established lesion. The junctional epithelium is being converted into a pocket epithelium and there is beginning pocket formation. Plasma cells predominate the lesion. There is a continuing collagen loss although the alveolar bone and periodontal ligament are not yet affected to any significant extent. GS, gingival sulcus; OSE, oral sulcular epithelium; OE, oral epithelium; PE, pocket epithelium; Re, rete ridges of pocket epithelium; V, blood vessels; Co, collagen bundles; Fi, fibroblasts; L, lymphocytes; N, neutrophilic granulocytes; MAB, marginal alveolar bone; PDL, periodontal ligament.*

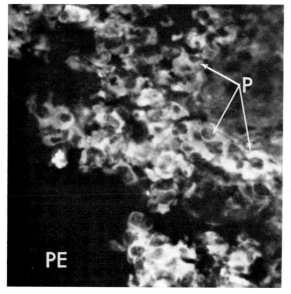

FIG. 7-18. *A section of human gingiva treated with fluorescent anti-IgG antisera to demonstrate the population of IgG-producing plasma cells (P) in the connective tissues immediately deep to the pocket epithelium (PE) (magnification 400 ×). (Courtesy Dr. J. Clagett.)*

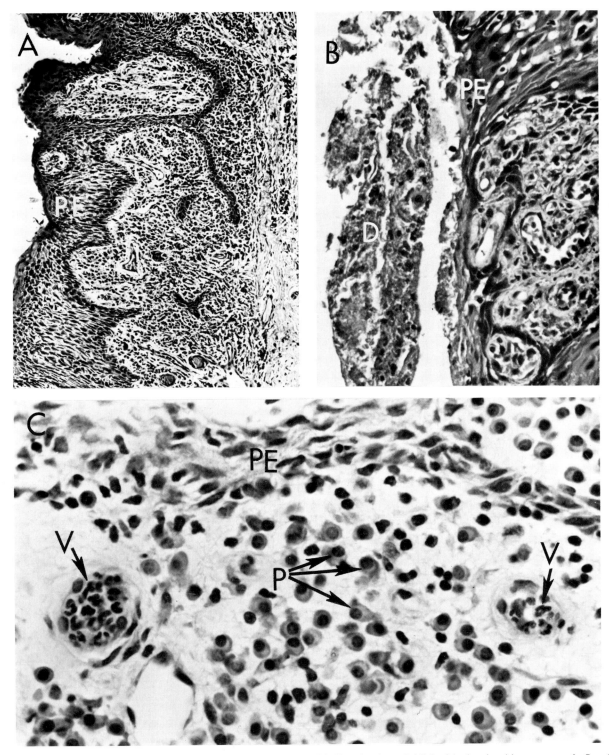

FIG. 7-19. _Characteristic alterations in the zone of the pocket epithelium in the established lesion in chimpanzees._ A. Paraffin-embedded section showing the pocket epithelium (PE) and the adjacent connective tissue densely infiltrated with plasma cells. Note the long extension of epithelium into the connective tissue (hemotoxylin-eosin stain; magnification 50 ×). B. Paraffin-embedded section from a periodontal pocket. Note the deposit (D) made up of degenerating cells and microorganisms. In some areas the pocket epithelium (PE) is only one or two cells thick and blood vessels closely approach the surface deposit. Some of the vessels are engorged with leukocytes (hemotoxylin-eosin stain; magnification 125 ×). C. Features of the connective-tissue zone subjacent to the pocket epithelium. Note the strands of pocket epithelium (PE) and two blood vessels (V) engorged with neutrophilic granulocytes. There is a dense plasma cell (P) infiltrate with a few scattered lymphocytes (hemotoxylin-eosin stain; magnification 800 ×). (Page, R. C., Ammons, W. F., and Simpson, D. M.: Host tissue response in chronic inflammatory periodontal disease. IV. The periodontal and dental status of a group of aged great apes. J. Periodontol., 46:144, 1975.)

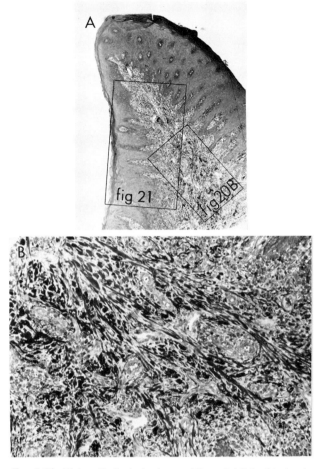

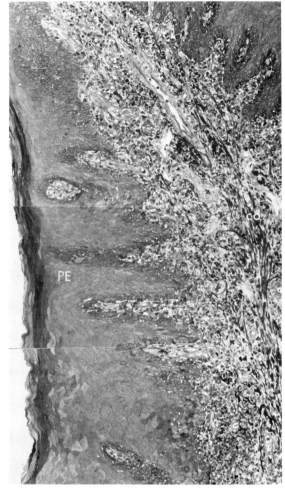

FIG. 7-20. Histopathologic features of the established lesion in a 39-year-old chimpanzee exhibiting gingivitis but without radiographic evidence of bone loss. A. Epon-embedded section from a biopsy. Note that most of the connective tissue has been replaced by a cellular infiltrate and vascular proliferation (magnification 50 ×). (See higher magnification in Fig. 7-21). B. Higher power view from A. Note the strands of residual collagen bundles separated by nests of inflammatory cells which are usually associated with blood vessels (magnification 150 ×). (Page, R. C., Ammons, W. F., and Simpson, D. M.: Host tissue response in chronic inflammatory periodontal disease. IV. The periodontal and dental status of a group of aged great apes. J. Periodontal., 46:144, 1975.)

FIG. 7-21. Higher power view of a portion of the biopsy shown in Figure 7-20A. Most of the collagen fibers (co) have been replaced by plasma cells; the connective tissue papillae loop high within the epithelium. In contrast to the thin, sometimes ulcerated pocket epithelium illustrated in Figures 7-19A,B, the pocket epithelium (PE) here is generally thick, and in some areas keratinization has occurred (magnification 150 ×). (Page, R. C., Ammons, W. F., and Simpson, D. M.: Host tissue response in chronic inflammatory periodontal disease. IV. The periodontal and dental status of a group of aged great apes. J. Periodontol., 46:144, 1975.)

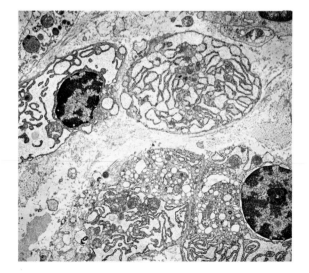

FIG. 7-22. A group of plasma cells demonstrating various stages of degeneration. The primary changes are early nuclear pyknosis, severe dilation and fragmentation of granular endoplasmic reticulum, and formation of numerous cytoplasmic vesicles, presumably arising from the Golgi complex. Portions of endoplasmic reticulum with ribosomes still attached can be seen within the extracellular space (magnification 2,850 ×). (Page, R. C., Ammons, W. F., and Simpson, D. M.: Host tissue response in chronic inflammatory periodontal disease. IV. The periodontal and dental status of a group of aged great apes. J. Periodontal., 46:144, 1975.)

distant regions, fibrosis and scarring may begin to occur. Whether the established lesion is reversible and whether, or under what conditions, it progresses to an advanced lesion remain unknown, although the problem is being studied.[66] Indeed, it appears that most established lesions do not progress.[41,52,74,75,76,77]

The Advanced Lesion

Features of the advanced inflammatory periodontal lesion have been described classically in clinical terms.[13,31,58,79] These may include periodontal pocket formation, surface ulceration and suppuration, fibrosis of the gingiva, destruction of the alveolar bone and periodontal ligament, tooth mobility and drifting, and eventual tooth exfoliation. In other words, the advanced lesion represents frank and overt periodontitis. The histopathologic and some of the ultrastructural features of the advanced lesion have been described.[8,11,14,15,18,27,33,44,45,52,54,71,84,89]

Characteristics of the advanced lesion are listed in Table 7-6 and are illustrated schematically in Figure

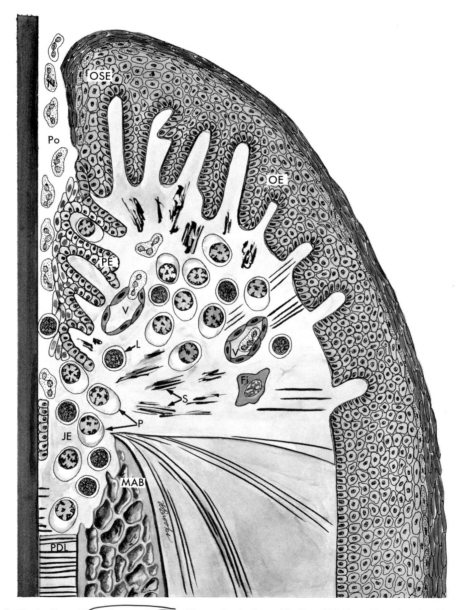

FIG. 7-23. *Schematic illustration of the advanced lesion. The oral sulcular epithelium (OSE) and junctional epithelium (JE) have been converted into pocket epithelium (PE), and a deep periodontal pocket (Po) filled with inflammatory cells and debris has formed. Portions of the marginal alveolar bone (MAB) and periodontal ligament (PDL) have been destroyed. Plasma cells (P) with scattered lymphocytes (L) dominate the lesion, and the blood vessels (V) may exhibit adhering leukocytes. A large part of the collagen within the affected connective tissues has been lost and in some areas fibrotic, scarlike collagenous material (S) may be observed. A small strand of relatively normal junctional epithelium (JE) frequently persists near the base of the pocket.*

7-23. Plasma cells predominate in the lesion, although lymphocytes and macrophages are also present. Signs of acute vasculitis persist in the presence of chronic fibrotic inflammation (Figs. 7-24, 7-25, 7-26). Clusters of plasma cells reside deeply within the connective tissues between remnants of collagen fiber bundles and around blood vessels (Fig. 7-26). The lesion is no longer localized; it may extend apically as well as laterally to form a variably broad band around the necks and roots of the teeth. The size of the band depends upon the extent of the disease, the amount of periodontal tissue

recession, and the pocket depth. While the highly organized fiber bundles of the marginal gingiva lose their characteristic orientation and architecture completely (Fig. 7-25),[51] the transseptal fiber bundles appear to be continuously regenerated as the lesion progresses apically.[53] This band of fibers appears to separate the coronally located infiltrate from the remaining alveolar bone, even when the interdental bone septum has been resorbed to the apical third of the root. Within the hypercellular infiltrated tissue portion, collagen fibers are practically absent (Figs. 7-24C,

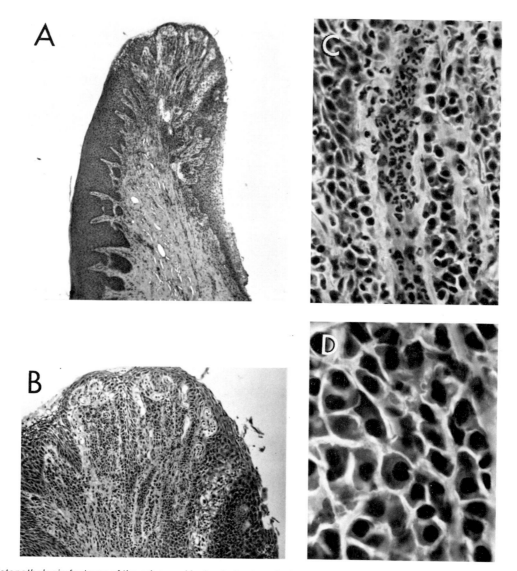

FIG. 7-24. *Histopathologic features of the advanced lesion in the beagle dog. (Paraffin-embedded and stained with hemotoxylin and eosin). A. Low power view of the lateral pocket wall. Note the extensive proliferation and extension of the pocket epithelium and the dense infiltrate extending from the pocket epithelium into the oral epithelium (original magnification 12.5 ×). B. Higher power view from A. Pocket epithelium extends onto the oral epithelial surface, and long fingers of epithelium extend into the connective tissues (magnification 25 ×). C. Higher power view from B. Note the blood vessel completely engorged with granulocytes in the central part of the section and surrounded by plasma cells (magnification 125 ×). D. A higher power view from C demonstrating the dense accumulation of plasma cells (magnification 500 ×).*

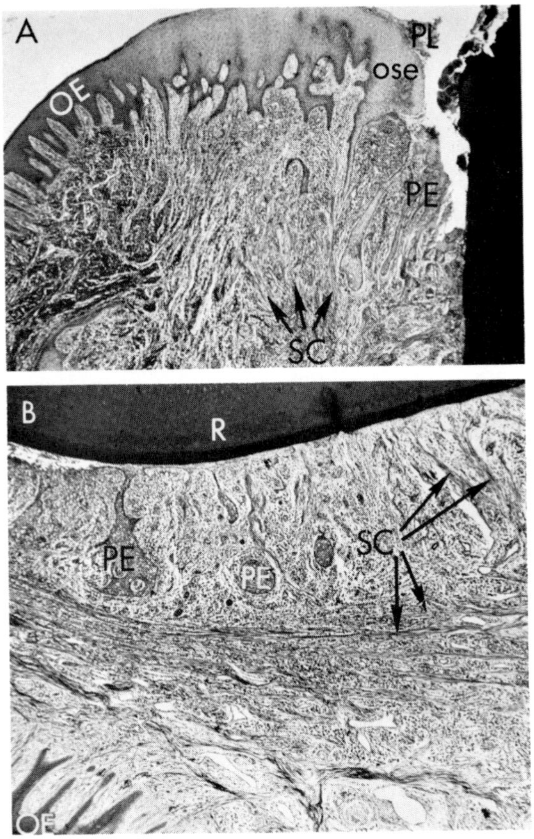

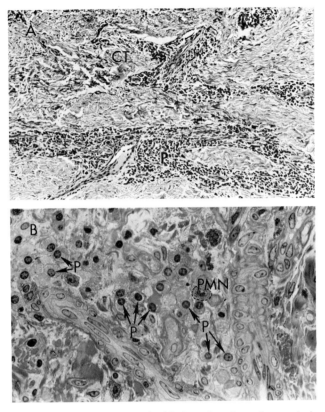

FIG. 7-25. *Paraffin-embedded section through the marginal periodontium and tooth of a specimen taken from a human autopsy illustrating the features of advanced periodontal disease (van Gieson's stain; magnification 25 ×). A. The oral epithelium (OE) and the oral sulcular epithelium (ose) are intact. The pocket epithelium (PE) exhibits areas of ulceration, and long projections extend into the deep connective tissues. The periodontal pocket contains calculus adherent to the root surface, and residual plaque (PL) is apparent on the surface of the soft tissue. The connective tissue has been almost totally replaced by a dense infiltrate of inflammatory cells and an accumulation of dense, disoriented scarlike collagen (SC). B. Horizontal section through a specimen similar to that shown in A taken from a region about one half of the way to the most apical extent of the pocket. The edge of the tooth root (R) and a small portion of the oral epithelium (OE) can be seen. The most prominent feature is the presence of strands of scarlike collagen (SC) running circumferentially around the tooth and at right angles to it and separated by zones of inflammatory cells. Projections of pocket epithelium (PE) are also apparent.*

FIG. 7-26. *A. A paraffin-embedded section from the central portion of an interdental papilla region of a chimpanzee. Note the perivascular islands of plasma cells (P) associated with blood vessels interspersed with dense scarlike collagenous (CT) material (magnification 75 ×). (Page, R. C., et al. Host tissue response in chronic periodontal disease. J. Periodont. Res., 7:283, 1972.) B. A section similar to A except embedded in Epon and illustrating two blood vessels with the surrounding plasma cells (P) and scattered polymorphonuclear granulocytes (PMN) (magnification 400 ×). (Page, R. C., Ammons, W. F., and Simpson, D. M.: Host tissue response in chronic inflammatory periodontal disease. IV The periodontal and dental status of a group of aged great apes. J. Periodontol., 46:144, 1975.)*

TABLE 7-6. *Features of the Advanced Lesion*

1. Persistence of features described for the established lesion

2. Extension of the lesion into alveolar bone and periodontal ligament with significant bone loss

3. Continued loss of collagen subjacent to the pocket epithelium with fibrosis at more distant sites

4. Presence of cytopathically altered plasma cells in the absence of altered fibroblasts

5. Formation of periodontal pockets

6. Periods of quiescence and exacerbation

7. Conversion of the bone marrow distant from the lesion into fibrous connective tissue

8. Widespread manifestations of inflammatory and immunopathologic tissue reactions

7-25A), while dense fibrosis may be apparent in the surrounding area. Strands of the proliferating pocket epithelium extend apically along the root surfaces and fingerlike projections extend into the deep connective tissues. Bone destruction (Figs. 7-27 and 7-29), presumably by osteoclastic resorption (Fig. 7-28), begins along the crest of the alveolar bone usually in the interdental septum around the communicating blood vessels.[33,44,84] As the marrow spaces are opened, both red

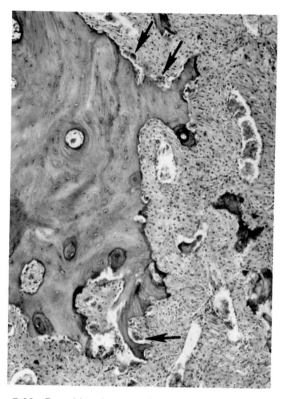

FIG. 7-28. *Resorbing bone surface. Note the presence of osteoclasts (arrows) located in Howship's lacunae, the moth-eaten surface, and the replacement of the bone by fibrous connective tissue (magnification 50 ×). (Courtesy Dr. B. Moffett.)*

and white marrow become hypercellular, undergo fibrosis, and become transformed into scarlike connective tissue.

Periods of acute exacerbation and quiescence occur and they determine, to some extent, the histopathologic picture seen. Frank tissue necrosis is generally not observed. Many of the features resemble closely those of other long-term chronic inflammatory diseases of connective tissue of unknown etiology, such as rheumatoid arthritis.

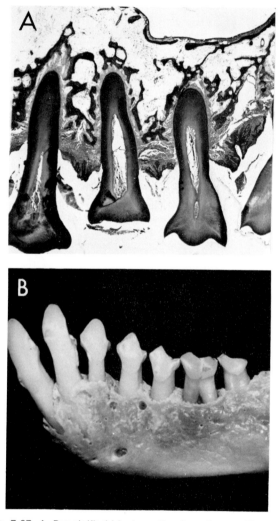

FIG. 7-27. *A. Decalcified block section from the maxillary left quadrant of an adult marmoset, exhibiting advanced inflammatory periodontal disease. There has been extensive resorption of the alveolar bone and the lamina dura along with loss of the periodontal ligament (hematoxylin-eosin stain; original magnification 10 ×). B. Defleshed lower left mandible of an adult marmoset with advanced periodontal disease. Note the abnormal porosity of the buccal and interproximal cortical bone resulting from enlargement of the nutrient foramina, marginal resorption, and formation of dehiscences on the buccal aspect of the canine and lateral incisor. (Page, R. C., et al.: Host tissue response in chronic periodontal disease. J. Periodont. Res., 7:283, 1972.)*

References

1. Aisenberg, M. A., and Aisenberg, A. D.: A new concept of pocket formation. Oral Surg., *1*:1047, 1948.
2. Ammons, W. F., Schectman, L. R., and Page, R. C.: Host tissue response in chronic periodontal disease. I. The normal periodontium and clinical and anatomic manifestations of periodontal disease in the marmoset. J. Periodont. Res., *7*:131, 1972.
3. April E. C., de: A proposito de las celulas reticulohistocitarias que conforman el sistema reticuloendotelial. Rev. Odontol., *42*:115, 1954.
4. Arnim, S. S., and Holt, R. T.: The defense mechanisms of the gingiva. J. Periodontol., *26*:79, 1955.

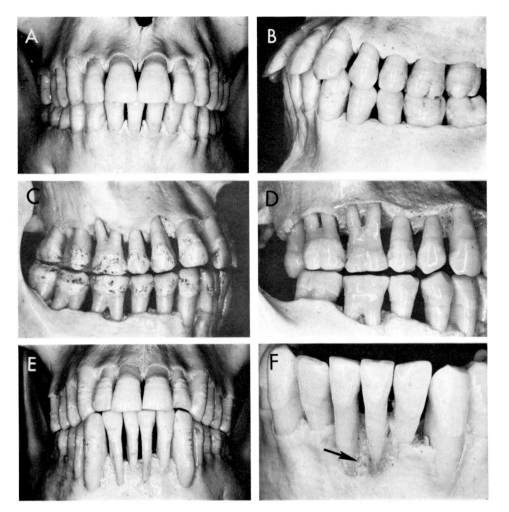

FIG. 7-29. *Gross morphology of the alveolar bone in the advanced stages of inflammatory periodontal disease. A. and B. Normal bone architecture of an adult human. Note the gentle scalloping of the alveolar margin. The margin mimics the contours of the cementoenamel junction and is removed from it apically only 2 to 3 mm. C. and D. There is marked apical recession affecting one half to two thirds of the total root length with grossly abnormal surface contours and furcation involvement. Deposits are present on most of the root surfaces. E. and F. Recession of the bone margin affecting the mandibular anterior teeth. Note the moth-eaten surface (arrow). (Courtesy Dr. W. Avery.)*

5. Attström, R.: Studies on neutrophil polymorphonuclear leukocytes at the dento-gingival junction in gingival health and disease. J. Periodont. Res., 6:(Suppl 8), 1971.

6. Attström, R., Graf-de Beer, M., and Schroeder, H. E.: Clinical and stereologic characteristics of normal gingiva. J. Periodont. Res., 10:115, 1975.

7. Bernier, J. L.: The histological changes of gingival tissues in health and periodontal disease. Oral Surg., 2:1194, 1950.

8. Box, H. K.: Studies in Periodontal Pathology. University of Toronto Press, Toronto, 1924.

9. Brandtzaeg, P.: Local formation and transport of immunoglobulins related to the oral cavity, *In* Host Resistance to Commensal Bacteria. T. MacPhee, Ed. Edinburgh, Churchill Livingstone, 1972, p. 116.

10. Davies, C. G.: Gum and alveolar diseases. Dental Cosmos, 21:192, 1879.

11. Fish, E. W.: Parodontal disease: The pathology and treatment of chronic gingivitis. Br. Dent. J., 58:531, 1935.

12. Flieder, D. E., Sun, C. N., and Schneider, B. C.: Chemistry of normal and inflamed human gingival tissues. Periodontics, 4:302, 1966.

13. Fox, J.: The Natural History and Diseases of the Teeth. Part II. London, Cox, 1833, p. 93.

14. Freedman, H. L., Listgarten, M. A., and Taichman, N. S.: Electron microscopic features of chronically inflamed human gingiva. J. Periodont. Res., 3:313, 1968.

15. Fullmer, H. M.: A histochemical study of periodontal disease in the maxillary alveolar processes of 135 autopsies. J. Periodontol., 32:206, 1961.

16. Gad, T.: Periodontal disease in dogs. I. Clinical investigation. J. Periodont. Res., 3:272, 1968.

17. Garant, P. R., and Mulvihill, J. E.: The fine structure of

gingivitis in the beagle. III. Plasma cell infiltration of the subepithelial connective tissue. J. Periodont. Res., 7:161, 1971.

18. Gavin, J. R.: Ultrastructural features of chronic marginal gingivitis. J. Periodont. Res., 5:19, 1970.

19. Genco, R. J., et al.: Antibody-mediated effects on the periodontium. J. Periodontol., 45:330, 1974.

20. Goldman, H.: The topography and role of the gingival fibers. J. Dent. Res., 50:331, 1951.

21. Gottleib, B.: Der Epithelansatz am Zahne, Dtsch. Mschr. Zahnheilk., 39:142, 1921.

22. Gottlieb, B., and Orban, B.: Biology and Pathology of the Tooth and Its Supporting Mechanism. Trans. by M. Diamond. New York, Macmillan, 1938.

23. Gottlieb, B.: A new concept of periodontoclasia. J. Periodontol., 17:723, 1946.

24. Hamp, S. E., Lindhe, J., and Löe, H.: Long term effect of chlorhexidine on developing gingivitis in the Beagle dog. J. Periodont. Res., 8:63, 1973.

25. Harlan, A. W.: Treatment of pyorrhea alveolaris. Dental Cosmos, 25:517, 1883.

26. Helldén, L., and Lindhe, J.: Enhanced emigration of crevicular leukocytes mediated by factors in human dental plaque. Scand. J. Dent. Res., 81:123, 1973.

27. Hopewell-Smith, A.: Pyorrhea alveolaris—its pathohistology. I. Preliminary note. II. Concluding remarks. Dental Cosmos, 53:397, 981, 1911.

28. Horton, J. E., Leikin, S., and Oppenheim, J. J.: Human lymphoproliferative reaction to saliva and dental deposits: an in vitro correlation with periodontal disease. J. Periodontol., 43:522, 1972.

29. Horton, J. E., Oppenheimm, J. J., and Mergenhagen, S. E.: A role for cell mediated immunity in the pathogenesis of periodontal disease. J. Periodontol., 45:351, 1974.

30. Hull, P. S., Soames, J. V., and Davies, R. M.: Periodontal disease in a beagle dog colony. J. Comp. Pathol., 84:143, 1974.

31. Hunter, J.: The natural history of the human teeth. In Surgical Works, Vol. II, Part I. J. F. Palmer, Ed. London, Longman, Rees, Orme, Brown, Green, and Longman, 1835, pp. 79–81.

32. Ivanyi, L., and Lehner, T.: Stimulation of lymphocyte transformation by bacterial antigens in patients with periodontal disease. Arch. Oral Biol., 15:1089, 1970.

33. James, W. W., and Counsell, A.: A histologic investigation into "so-called pyorrhea alveolaris." Br. Dent. J., 48:1237, 1927.

34. Koecker, L.: An essay on the devastation of the gums and the alveolar processes. Phila. J. Med. Phys. Sci., 2:282, 1821.

35. Lange, D., and Schroeder, H. E.: Cytochemistry and ultrastructure of gingival sulcus cells. Helv. Odontol. Acta, 15(Suppl. 6):65, 1971.

36. Lavine, W. S., Page, R. C., and Padgett, G. A.: Host response in chronic periodontal disease. V. The dental and periodontal status of mink and mice affected by Chediak-Higashi syndrome. J. Periodontol., in press.

37. Lindhe, J., Hamp, S. E., and Löe, H.: Experimental periodontitis in the beagle dog. J. Periodont. Res., 8:1, 1973.

38. Lindhe, J., and Helldén, L.: Neutrophilic chemotatic activity elaborated by dental plaque. J. Periodont. Res., 7:297, 1972.

39. Lindhe, J., et al.: Clinical and stereologic analysis of the course of early gingivitis in dogs. J. Periodont. Res., 9:314, 1974.

40. Listgarten, M. A., and Ellegaard, B.: Experimental gingivitis in rhesus monkeys. J. Periodont. Res., 8:199, 1973.

41. Lovdal, A., Arno, A., and Waerhaug, J.: Incidence of manifestations of periodontal disease in light of oral hygiene and calculus formation. Acta Odontol. Scand., 56:21, 1958.

42. Mazzella, W. J., and Vernick, S. H.: The ultrastructure of normal and pathologic human gingival epithelium. J. Periodontol., 39:5, 1968.

43. McHugh, W. D.: Some aspects of the development of gingival epithelium. Periodontics, 1:239, 1963.

44. Melcher, A. H.: The pathogenesis of chronic gingivitis. I. The spread of the inflammatory process. Dent. Pract., 12:2, 1962.

45. Melcher, A. H.: Some histological and histochemical observations on the connective tissue of chronically inflamed human gingiva. J. Periodont. Res., 2:127, 1967.

46. Mulvihill, J. E., et al.: Histologic studies of the periodontal syndrome in rice rats and the effects of penicillin. Arch. Oral Biol., 12:733, 1967.

47. Mutschelknaus, R.: Das marginale Parodontium. Klinische, Histologische und histochemische Untersuchungen. München, C. Hanser Verlag, 1968.

48. Oliver, R. C., Holm-Pedersen, P., and Löe, H.: The correlation between clinical scoring, exudate measurements and microscopic evaluation of inflammation of the gingiva. J. Periodontol., 40:201, 1969.

49. Orban, B.: Zhanfleischtasche und Epithelansatz. Z. Stomatol., 29:858, 1931.

50. Page, R. C.: Macromolecular interactions in the connective tissues of the periodontium. In Developmental Aspects of Oral Biology. H. Slavkin and L. Bavetta, Eds. New York, Academic Press, 1972, pp. 291–308.

51. Page, R. C., et al.: Collagen fiber bundles of the normal marginal gingiva. Arch. Oral Biol., 19:1039, 1974.

52. Page, R. C., Ammons, W. F., and Simpson, D. M.: Host tissue response in chronic inflammatory periodontal disease. IV. The periodontal and dental status of a group of aged great apes. J. Periodontol., 46:144, 1975.

53. Page, R. C., and Schroeder, H. E.: Pathogenesis of inflammatory periodontal disease. A summary of current work. Lab. Invest., 33:235, 1976.

54. Page, R. C., et al.: Host tissue response in chronic periodontal disease. III. Clinical, histopathologic and ultrastructural features of advanced disease in a colony-maintained marmoset. J. Periodont. Res., 7:283, 1972.

55. Patterson, J. D.: The catarrhal nature of pyorrhea alveolaris. Dental Cosmos, 27:669, 1885.

56. Payne, W. A., et al.: Histopathologic features of the

initial and early stages of experimental gingivitis in man. J. Periodont. Res., *10:*51, 1975.

57. Rawls, A. O.: Pyorrhea alveolaris. Dental Cosmos, 27:265, 1885.

58. Riggs, J.: Suppurative inflammation of the gums and absorption of the gums and alveolar process. Pa. J. Dent. Sci., 3:99, 1876.

59. Rüdin, H. J., Overdiek, H. F., and Rateitschak, K. H.: Correlation between sulcus fluid rate and clinical and histological inflammation of the marginal gingiva. Helv. Odontol. Acta, *14:*2126, 1970.

60. Saxe, S. R., et al.: Oral debris, calculus, and periodontal disease in the beagle dog. Periodontics, 5:217, 1967.

61. Schectman, L. R., et al.: Host tissues response in chronic periodontal disease. II. Histologic features of the normal periodontium, and histopathologic and ultrastructural manifestations of disease in the marmoset. J. Periodont. Res., 7:195, 1972.

62. Schroeder, H. E.: Quantitative parameters of early human gingival inflammation. Arch. Oral Biol., *15:*383, 1970.

63. Schroeder, H. E.: Morphometric study of early gingivitis in man. *In* The Prevention of Periodontal Disease. J. E. Eastoe, D. C. A. Picton, and A. G. Alexander, Eds. London, H. Kimpton, 1971, p. 196.

64. Schroeder, H. E.: Ultrastructure des lésions gingivales précoces. Rev. Fr. Odontostomatol., *20:*103, 1973.

65. Schroeder, H. E., Graf-de Beer, M., and Attström, R.: Initial gingivitis in dogs. J. Periodont. Res., *10:*128, 1975.

66. Schroeder, H. E., and Lindhe, J.: Conversion of a stable established gingivitis into periodontitis. Arch. Oral Biol., in press.

67. Schroeder, H. E., and Münzel-Pedrazzoli, S.: Application of stereologic methods to stratified gingival epithelia. J. Microsc., *92:*179, 1970.

68. Schroeder, H. E., and Münzel-Pedrazzoli, S.: Correlated morphometric and biochemical data on gingival tissue. I. Morphometric model, tissue sampling and application and test of stereologic procedures. J. Microsc., *99:*301, 1973.

69. Schroeder, H. E., Münzel-Pedrazzoli, S., and Page, R. C.: Correlated morphometric and biochemical analysis of gingival tissue in early chronic gingivitis in man. Arch. Oral Biol., *18:*899, 1973.

70. Schroeder, H. E., and Page, R. C.: Lymphocyte-fibroblast interaction in the pathogenesis of inflammatory gingival disease. Experientia, *28:*1228, 1972.

71. Selvig, K. A.: Ultrastructural changes in cementum and adjacent connective tissue in periodontal disease. Acta Odontol. Scand., *24:*459, 1966.

72. Simpson, D. M., and Avery, B. E.: Pathologically-altered fibroblasts within lymphoid infiltrates in early gingivitis. J. Dent. Res., *52:*1156, 1973.

73. Simpson, D. M., and Avery, B. E.: Histopathologic and ultrastructural features of inflamed gingiva in the baboon. J. Periodontol., *45:*500, 1974.

74. Soumi, J. D., et al.: The effect of controlled oral hygiene procedures on the progression of periodontal disease in adults: results after two years. J. Periodontol., *40:*416, 1969.

75. Soumi, J. D., et al.: The effect of controlled oral hygiene procedures on the progression of periodontal disease in adults: results after third and final year. J. Periodontol., *42:*152, 1971.

76. Soumi, J. D., Leatherwood, E. C., and Chang, J. J.: A follow-up study of former participants in a controlled oral hygiene study. J. Periodontol., *44:*662, 1973.

77. Soumi, J. D., et al.: The effect of controlled oral hygiene procedures on the progression of periodontal disease in adults: radiographic findings. J. Periodontol., *42:*562, 1971.

78. Talbot, E. S.: Pyorrhea alveolaris. Dental Cosmos, 28:689, 1886.

79. Talbot, E. S.: Interstitial Gingivitis or So-called Pyorrhea Alveolaris. Philadelphia, S. S. White Dental Mfg. Co., 1899.

80. Tempel, T. R., et al.: Factors from saliva and oral bacteria, chemotatic for polymorphonuclear leukocytes: their possible role in gingival inflammation. J. Periodontol., *41:*71, 1970.

81. Theilander, H.: Permeability of gingival pocket epithelium. Int. Dent. J., *14:*416, 1964.

82. Theilander, H.: Epithelial changes in gingivitis. J. Periodont. Res., 3:303, 1968.

83. Waerhaug, J.: The gingival pocket. Odont. Tidskr., Suppl. 1, 1952.

84. Weinmann, J. P.: Progress of gingival inflammation into the supporting structures of the teeth. J. Periodontol., *12:*71, 1941.

85. Weski, O.: Rontgenographische-Anatomische Studien aus dem Gebiete der Kieferpathologie II. Die chronischen marginalen Entzundungen des Alveolarfortsatzes mit besonderer Berucksichtigung der Alveolarpyprrhoe. Vjschr. Zahnheilk., *37:*1, 1921.

86. Zachinsky, L.: Range of histologic variation in clinically normal gingiva. J. Dent. Res., *33:*580, 1954.

87. Zachrisson, B. W.: A histological study of experimental gingivitis in man. J. Periodont. Res., 3:11, 1969.

88. Zachrisson, B. W., and Schultz-Haudt, D. S.: A comparative histological study of clinically normal and chronically inflamed gingiva from the same individuals. Odont. Tidskr., *76:*179, 1968.

89. Znamensky, N. H.: Alveolar-pyorrhea—its pathological anatomy and its radical treatment. Br. Dent. J., 23:385, 1902.

8

Pathogenic Mechanisms

Components of the Host Defense System

The Microcirculation

Mast Cells

The Phagocytic Cells

Neutrophils

Macrophages

The Lymphoid System

B- and T-Lymphocytes

Lymphokines

Antibodies and Immune Complexes

Complement and Clotting

Fibroblasts

Pathogenic Immune Reactions

Type I Reactions

Type II Reactions

Type III Reactions

Type IV Reactions

Immunopathology of Chronic Inflammatory
Gingival and Periodontal Disease

Humoral Factors

Cell-mediated Hypersensitivity

Mast Cells

Prostaglandins

Microcirculation and the Immune System

8

Pathogenic Mechanisms

There is general agreement that chronic inflammatory gingival and periodontal disease is caused ultimately by microbial plaque or by specific microorganisms in the gingival sulcus and periodontal pocket (see Ch. 4). Remarkable progress has been made in controlling some, but not all, microbial diseases. The forms that have been the most readily controlled are the acute infections such as smallpox, diphtheria, scarlet fever, and measles in which the pathogenesis and host response are reasonably straightforward. In the acute infections, the pathologic manifestations of the disease, even death itself, may be caused directly by the microorganisms through invasion of the tissues and elaboration of toxins and other noxious substances leading to cell death and tissue necrosis. In most cases the host response provoked is protective, and amplification of the pathogenicity via the host defense mechanisms does not occur. Therefore, only an elementary understanding of the etiology and host response mechanisms is required to achieve control. An early milestone in control of infectious disease was the observation in 1798 by Jenner that the human body could be induced to protect itself against smallpox by exposure to crusts from cowpox lesions. It seems likely that Jenner understood neither the infectious etiology of smallpox nor the immune response he was able to provoke to protect against it; it is virtually certain that he had no hint that the immune response to antigenic challenge could contribute to disease or cause disease as well as protect against it.

Compared with progress in control of the acute infections, diseases with major chronic inflammatory and immunopathologic components remain poorly understood. Among these diseases are tuberculosis, the pneumoconioses, poststreptococcal kidney and heart diseases, rheumatoid arthritis, and some forms of malignant tumors. In diseases of this type, the pathogenesis is much more complex; the inciting agent, whether or not it is of microbial origin, appears to be predominantly pathogenic because of its capacity to activate host response mechanisms in such a manner that they may become more destructive than protective. Except for better methods of detection and diagnosis and, in some cases, improved techniques of surgical treatment, almost no progress has been made in management of diseases of this type. It now seems reasonably clear that control and prevention of these diseases require a sophisticated and detailed understanding of host defense mechanisms and the means whereby they may go awry. Evolution of the idea that these mechanisms can be deleterious as well as beneficial has been a recent development, and our current understanding remains vague. This lack of understanding has severely hampered progress. Chronic gingival and periodontal disease is a member of the family of chronic diseases with major inflammatory and immunopathologic components, and our past lack of progress in coming to understand the disease is a reflection of our deficiency in understanding of host response mechanisms.

During the past two decades, rapid progress has been made in basic biomedical research, and a wealth of new information has become available. Of particular importance to the field of periodontal disease research have been advances in immunology and immunopathology and in our understanding of the inflammatory process. The modern approach to research into the pathogenesis of periodontal disease dates back approximately a decade, and it has involved the application of these advances in basic biology and pathology specifically to the periodontal problem, as well as investigation into mechanisms that may be of unique importance in the periodontium. While few advances affecting the periodontal status of the population as a whole or individual patient care have been made so far, a large body of basic new information has been acquired.

This rapid pace has had both beneficial and unfavorable consequences. The new data provide the foundation for new insights into pathogenesis and etiology of the lesions as well as into the basic underlying mechanisms. There seems little doubt that these will lead to major advances in the care of patients and in prevention and control of the disease. However, progress has come so rapidly and from such a broad spectrum of disciplines in the basic sciences that assimilation of the information by the profession and integration of it into the concepts upon which we base diagnosis and treatment have not been possible. Indeed, the vocabulary alone is staggering, and it is difficult for individuals not actively doing research in the field to maintain awareness and understanding of the information available. Furthermore, the speed with which change comes about makes interpretation of the information available at the moment and compilation into textbook form an extremely risky task. In spite of these problems, it is our intent to summarize current information and to do so in terms that can be easily understood by the student or by the practicing dentist.

COMPONENTS OF THE HOST DEFENSE SYSTEM

Inflammatory gingival and periodontal disease begins in the marginal gingiva lateral to the sulcus and, as the disease progresses, extends into the deep connective tissues and bone. The principal pathologic tissue alterations include proliferation and migration of the junctional epithelium and its conversion to pocket epithelium, inflammation, immunopathologic changes, connective-tissue alterations, and bone resorption (see Ch. 7). Certainly additional changes such as alterations in the ground substance occur, but these have not been adequately described and defined for discussion here. The normal periodontal connective tissues contain blood and lymphatic vessels, fibroblasts, mast cells and macrophages, and there is a continuous, although low-level, transmigration of leukocytes. All these cells and structures participate in the normal host defense reaction mounted at the beginning of plaque accumulation, and they have the potential to participate in the ensuing damage to the tissues.

The Microcirculation

The microcirculation, which is made up of the arterioles, capillaries, postcapillary venules, and veins, is the site of the initial response to injury (Fig. 8-1). The events have been described in detail.[135] In general, the structure of the microcirculation of the periodontal tissues is similar to that of the dermis, although the organization is not the same.[49-53,102,122,123,170] The vessels are lined by intact endothelial cells joined to one another by tight junctions and without structurally demonstrable pores. These rest on a basement lamina, made up predominantly of collagen and glycoprotein synthesized by the endothelial cells. Around some of the capillaries and venules another cell, the pericyte, may be observed embedded within the basement lamina material. While the exact function of the pericyte

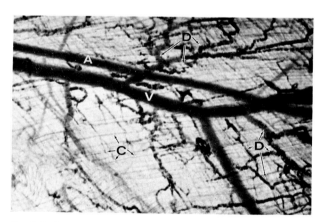

FIG. 8-1. *Specimen of the cremaster muscle of a rat previously injected intravenously with carbon particles and subsequently exposed locally to histamine. The specimen demonstrates that the enhancement of vascular permeability induced by histamine occurs almost exclusively at the postcapillary venule. (A) artery; (V) vein; (C) capillary bed; (D) postcapillary venules. Note that the carbon particles have escaped the vessel lumen at the postcapillary venule and are trapped in the vessel wall. (Prepared by Dr. D. Lagunoff.)*

is not known, it seems likely to play a role in regulating luminal size and blood flow, since it contains contractile elements. The arterioles differ in structure from capillaries, venules, and veins in that they are invested with one or more elastic laminae and a coat of smooth-muscle cells. The veins have a structure similar to the arterioles except that there is no elastic lamina.

In normal vessels, cells rarely cross the intact vascular wall, and fluid transport occurs predominantly in the region of the capillary and venule. Transport across the vascular wall has been studied extensively in muscle. Substances the size of albumin, about 75 nm in diameter, readily pass the vascular wall, but there is a cutoff at 90 nm and a second cutoff at about 700 nm. Fluid transport appears to occur predominantly through a system of pinocytotic vesicles. Substances within the vascular lumen fill invaginations of the luminal surface of the endothelial cell membrane to form vessicles; these bud off, pass through the cytoplasm to the adventitial surface of the cell where they fuse with the cell membrane, open, and discharge their contents onto the basement lamina.

Injury results in an immediate response by the microcirculation (Fig. 8-1). Initially, there is a fleeting constriction of the vessels followed immediately by vasodilation and slowing of the blood flow, with remarkable changes in the properties of the vessel wall. The luminal surface of the endothelial cells becomes sticky, the vascular permeability, especially of the postcapillary venule, is greatly enhanced, and the constituents of the plasma, regardless of their size, pass from the vessels into the extravascular spaces (Fig. 8-1). The polymorphonuclear leukocytes adhere to the sticky endothelial cell walls, send pseudopodia between the cells, and begin to open up the intercellular junctions (Fig. 7-5). The neutrophils emigrate from the vessels, and their movement to the site of injury is directed by chemotactic agents. These events are accompanied by aggregation of platelets and activation of the clotting cascade and the plasmin system. Both intravascular and extravascular clotting may occur. As a consequence of these events, an inflammatory exudate composed of all of the constituents of the blood serum, fibrin, red cells, and granulocytes forms. At this stage, the response is referred to as an acute inflammation. A response of this type is observed in the gingiva of humans within 2 to 4 days following the beginning of plaque accumulation.[187] Depending upon the nature and magnitude of the injury and the character of the host response, the lesion can be resolved rapidly and the tissue will be restored to normal, or it may evolve into a chronic inflammatory lesion. In the latter case, the site becomes populated by macrophages and lymphoid cells within a few days.

The changes in the microcirculation and the formation of an acute inflammatory exudate are induced by chemical substances released at the site of injury or challenge. These substances are generally referred to as the mediators of the inflammatory response, and their activity is evaluated experimentally by measuring their capacity to induce chemotaxis and to enhance vascular permeability. Histamine is a potent mediator of acute inflammatory responses. Enhanced vascular permeability induced by histamine is manifested by the postcapillary venule (Fig. 8-1). Histamine is produced by mast cells (Fig. 1-22C) by the decarboxylation of histidine, and it is stored in the granules of these cells. Large numbers of mast cells located near the blood vessels release their granular contents upon injury. Histamine is also released from aggregating blood platelets and from injured endothelial cells. The substance is an important mediator of allergic inflammation and may also participate in most other forms of acute injury.

The kinins, a family of small peptides generated as indicated in Figure 8-2, are another group of vasoactive substances released during injury and participating in the acute phase of inflammation.[38] Injury activates Hageman factor, which in turn activates the clotting cascade and the generation of plasmin.[200] Both activated Hageman factor and plasmin have the capacity to convert the proenzyme kallikreinogen into an active enzyme kallikrein, and the latter cleaves the active peptide from kininogen, an alpha-2 macroglobulin of the serum. This proenzyme is also present in neutrophils and can be released from them in active form. The active peptide has a short half-life and is inactivated by a kinase also found in serum and neutrophils. The kinins are extremely potent vasoactive and chemotactic substances.

Complement activation, which is likely to occur in inflamed gingival tissue and at the site of most injuries, results in the generation of potent vasoactive peptides. One of these, C5a, is both a chemotactic agent and an enhancer of vascular permeability, and another, C3a, causes mast cell degranulation. The prostaglandins comprise another group of potent vasoactive sub-

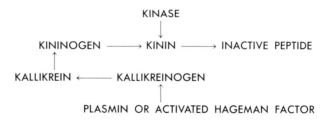
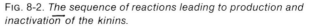

FIG. 8-2. *The sequence of reactions leading to production and inactivation of the kinins.*

stances present in inflamed gingiva in relatively high concentrations. All these substances may participate in the acute inflammatory response occurring within a few days following the beginning of plaque accumulation.

Mast Cells

Mast cells are widely distributed in the dermis and other connective tissues. They are found particularly in the vicinity of the blood vessels. The cells are normal residents of the junctional epithelium and gingival connective tissues, where they appear to be randomly dispersed.[8,9,215,216] The normal function of mast cells remains undefined. The cells are characterized by the presence of large electron-dense granules, which bind basic dyes and exhibit metachromasia (Fig. 1-22C). The granules are made up of heparin, histamine or serotonin, and proteases. The proteases exist in an active rather than a precursor form, and they have substrate specificities resembling chymotrypsin and trypsin.[12,131,249] Granule contents can be released from mast cells into the extracellular compartment without loss of cell viability. Indeed, the cells appear to be able to re-synthesize granule constituents. Stimuli leading to the release of the granule substances include factors released from serum by endotoxin,[105] injury, and exposure to certain toxins and other bacterial substances. Immunologic reactions also may lead to degranulation. Mast cells carry on their surfaces receptors for cytophlic IgE antibody;[128] antibody-carrying cells encountering the antigen for which the antibody is specific undergo degranulation with the release of histamine. This reaction is the basis of anaphylaxis, and it may also participate in other forms of allergic inflammation. The release of histamine can be inhibited by the presence of prostaglandins, and the production and release of the prostaglandins by eosinophils in inflammatory lesions may be one way in which mast-cell activity is controlled.[108] Mast cells in the junctional epithelium and gingival connective tissues may participate in the acute inflammatory response by serving as a source of histamine.

The Phagocytic Cells

NEUTROPHILS

Neutrophils account for about 60 percent of the total circulating leukocytes. They require approximately 3 days to mature in the bone marrow, and they circulate for only about 12 hours. In normal adult humans, about 75 grams of these cells are used and replaced each day. Neutrophils are the first line of defense against all forms of injury and challenge, and they are present in essentially all inflammatory lesions.

The primary protective function of neutrophils is to accumulate at sites of injury or challenge and to engulf, kill, and digest microorganisms and to destroy other noxious substances. Normal neutrophilic function is essential to life, as evidenced by the occurrence of massive and frequently fatal infections in individuals without normal neutrophil protection, such as in patients with agranulocytosis, neutropenia, or the Chékiak-Higashi syndrome.

By virtue of their use of the glycolytic and hexose monophosphate shunt pathways for energy production, neutrophils can operate in environments of low oxygen tension and acid pH usually found in injured tissues. Hydrogen peroxide and lactic acid, the end products of these metabolic pathways, participate in the functional activities of the cells. Mature neutrophils have little capacity to synthesize proteins; instead they carry in granular form all the substances required for phagocytosis and for killing microorganisms (Figs. 7-6, 7-7, 7-8). The *specific granules* contain lysozyme, alkaline phosphatase, and lactoferrin, and the *azurophil granules* contain the acid hydrolases, cationic proteins, and myeloperoxidase, all of which participate in the phagocytosis, killing, and digestion of microorganisms and other noxious substances. For example, myeloperoxidase in the presence of hydrogen peroxide can kill microorganisms by halogenation of the cell wall.

Neutrophils are ameboid and have the capacity to respond to a number of chemotactic agents. Initially, they are trapped at sites of inflammation by injury-induced changes in the microcirculation. Subsequently, chemotactic agents direct movement of the cells to the sites of damage. Most bacteria, including those of dental plaque, have the capacity to produce peptides to which neutrophils respond chemotactically.[244] In addition, C5a, activated-C5,6,7 generated by complement activation, and the kinins induce chemotaxis by neutrophils. Thus, substances generated by injured tissues, as well as substances produced by microorganisms, attract neutrophils.

In spite of their role in host defense, neutrophils also participate in tissue destruction. The necrosis and destruction of small blood vessels and of the perivascular connective tissues that occur in Arthus (type III) reactions require the presence of neutrophils.[35] The connective tissue lysis and bone destruction accompanying acute pus-forming infections are probably caused in large part by neutrophil-derived substances. For example, the injection of microorganisms into normal rabbits results in the formation of an abscess and massive tissue destruction, while in leukopenic rabbits the infection disseminates and may cause death, but there is little or no tissue destruction at the site of injection.[64,242] In addition to the various bactericidal substances, neutrophils carry potent acid hydrolases and a collagenase having the capacity to destroy collagen and other connective-tissue substances and to induce bone resorption.[47,132,247] Neutrophils participating in an acute inflammatory response may die and release these enzymes into the connective-tissue substance. In addition, viable cells ingesting immune complex or some bacterial substances, release hydrolytic enzymes.[35,97,99,243,259,260] Some activities of neutrophils tend to cause a persistence of the inflammatory reaction. For example, enzymes released by neutrophils can cleave the complement component C5 to produce C5a and activated-C5,6,7 and can also activate the kinin-producing system.[54,254] These reactions would in turn attract additional inflammatory cells, magnifying the inflammatory effects of the initial stimulus and perpetuating inflammation. Reactions of this type may underlie the chronicity of gingival inflammation.

MACROPHAGES

The mononuclear phagocytes originate in the bone marrow and are transported throughout the body as peripheral blood monocytes. Upon arrival in the tissues, monocytes differentiate into macrophages (Fig. 1-23B). These cells, which can continue to divide at sites of inflammation,[238] have a long half-life and possess all organelles necessary for the synthesis of protein.

Since the time of Metchnikoff, macrophages have been considered an important part of the host defense system, predominantly because of their capacity to ingest, kill, and digest microorganisms and other foreign substances. This capacity is dependent to a great extent upon their interrelationship with the other leukocytes, the immune system, and complement. Mononuclear phagocytes are probably attracted to sites of inflammation by products of other cells. For example, lymphocytes responding to antigen or mitogen produce and release potent agents inducing macrophage chemotaxis,[234,255] as well as substances retaining them at these sites and leading to their activation.[43,144,157,162,224] On the other hand, macrophages release a proteinase with the capacity to split C5 to produce substances that attract neutrophils.[233] Prior interaction of foreign substances with specific antibody and with complement enhances phagocytic activity by macrophages.

Recently it has become apparent that macrophages participate in a much broader range of activities than had been previously suspected. Macrophages are an integral and essential component of the normal immune response. Both B- and T-lymphocytes respond to antigen and mitogen after processing and presentation by macrophages. Stimulated macrophages produce substances that regulate the immune response.[57] Some of these appear to potentiate the lymphocyte's response;[28,74] others suppress the response.[28,29,163,172] The prostaglandins and cyclic adenosine monophosphate (cAMP) may be involved in these reactions. Gemsa and his associates have shown that cultures of macrophages exposed to prostaglandins produce and release large amounts of cAMP,[71] a compound that plays a major role in regulation of lymphocyte responses.[21,98,229,230,241] Furthermore, there is evidence that macrophages have the capacity to produce prostaglandins,[158] and this family of substances may also regulate lymphoid-cell activity. Macrophages may also play a regulatory role in fibroblast function. As shown in Table 8-1, media from cultures of macrophages maintained *in vitro* contain substances that have the capacity to reduce the synthesis of both collagen and noncollagenous proteins by fibroblasts in culture by 50 percent. Macrophage-derived substances may also affect cell proliferation.[29]

The capacity of macrophages to participate in the tissue destruction of chronic inflammatory lesions has only recently been realized. The cells can undergo activation either by direct interaction with bacterial substances or immune complex,[30,45,178,179] or indirectly in the presence of lymphokines (Fig. 8-3).[43,143,144,157,162,182,183] The activated cells enlarge and exhibit decreased mobility,[43,144] a greater tendency to adhere to culture vessel surfaces,[157] increased levels of oxidative activity and protein synthesis,[161,162]

TABLE 8.1. *Effect of Macrophage-derived Substances upon the Ability of Fibroblasts to Synthesize Collagen*

CULTURE MEDIUM	HYDROXYPROLINE SYNTHESIZED, DPM/PLATE
Incubated control medium	6,763 (1,419)
Macrophage culture medium	3,760 (1,031)

Fibroblasts from mouse gingiva were plated into 60-mm plastic Petri dishes in Waymouth medium containing 10 percent fetal calf serum and allowed to become confluent. Macrophage cultures from mouse peritoneal cavity were established as described by Davies, Page and Allison[45] in Waymouth medium with 10 percent calf serum and incubated for 48 hours, after which the medium was transferred to the fibroblast cultures. (^{14}C)proline (2 μCi/ml) was added, and incubation continued for 24 hours; the entire culture was hydrolyzed and the radioactivity in hydroxyproline was determined using an amino acid analyzer equipped with a stream-splitting device and a radioactivity counter. (Unpublished data of Page et al.)

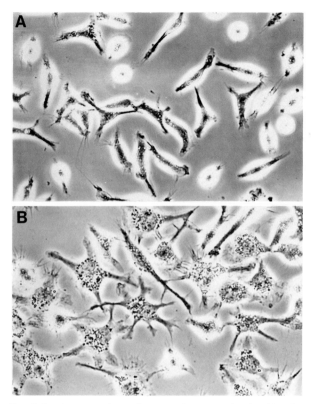

FIG. 8-3. *Mouse peritoneal macrophages maintained* in vitro *in medium 199 with 10 percent newborn calf serum for 48 hours. A. Control cells. B. Cells activated by lymphokine (Pantalone, R. M., and Page, R. C.: Lymphokine induced production and release of lysosomal enzymes by macrophages. Proc. Natl. Acad. Sci. USA, 72:2091, 1975.)*

and enhanced phagocytic capacity and ability to kill microorganisms.[63,130,143,144,148]

While these activities may be predominantly protective, activated cells appear to play a central role in the tissue destruction accompanying delayed-hypersensitivity (type IV) reactions and other forms of chronic inflammation. Macrophages activated with bacterial substances, immune complexes, or lymphokines synthesize and secrete lysosomal hydrolases and neutral proteases such as lysozyme (Table 8-2).[1,30,45,80,178,179,182,183] In addition, macrophages activated either with endotoxin or by lymphokines produce and secrete collagenase (Table 8-3).[183,251,252] Cells exhibiting these properties are otherwise viable and healthy. The enzymes released have the capacity to induce the tissue damage of the type seen in chronic inflammatory and immunopathologic reactions, including periodontal disease.

The Lymphoid System

Only a brief outline of the normal structure and function of the immune system will be presented here for the purposes of refreshing the memory of the reader. Detailed information can be found in the references listed.[11,54,103] The immune system is made up of cells derived from the bone marrow and located in the circulating blood and lymph; in the various lymphoid tissues including the lymph nodes, tonsils, spleen, and Peyer's patches in the gut; and in lymphoid cells scattered more or less randomly throughout the connective tissues or at sites of chronic inflammation. The overall structure of the lymphoid system is illustrated in Figure 8-4.

TABLE 8-2. *Enzyme Levels and Distribution in Mononuclear Phagocyte Cultures Exposed to Lymphokines*

ENZYME	CONTROL LYMPHOCYTE CULTURE MEDIUM		STIMULATED LYMPHOCYTE CULTURE MEDIUM	
	TOTAL ACTIVITY	PERCENT IN MEDIUM	TOTAL ACTIVITY	PERCENT IN MEDIUM
β-glucuronidase	2.5 (0.2)[a]	12.8	4.8 (0.3)	77.1
β-galactosidase	2.0 (0.1)	4.9	2.9 (0.2)	74.2
Acid phosphatase	20.9 (1.8)	10.5	58.4 (1.5)	58.6
N-acetyl-β-D-glucosaminidase	23.8 (2.1)	13.9	56.1 (2.3)	81.5
Cathepsin D	36.4 (5.9)	11.7	189.5 (11.5)	79.2

Pantalone, R. M., and Page, R. C.: Lymphokine induced production and release of lysosomal enzymes by macrophages. Proc. Natl. Acad. Sci., USA, 72:2091, 1975.
[a]Total enzyme activity reported as mean ± (S.D.) nMoles product/μg protein/h.

TABLE 8-3. *Effect of Lymphokines on Collagenase Production and Secretion from Mononuclear Phagocytes*

	COLLAGENASE ACTIVITY, CPM RELEASED				
CULTURE CONDITIONS	DAYS IN SERUM-FREE MEDIUM				
	1	2	3	4	5
199 + 10% NBCS[a]	30 (1.7)[b]	41 (2.3)	32 (4.1)	48 (2.3)	59 (2.7)
1.5 mg/ml CLS	34 (1.1)	44 (3.0)	42 (2.4)	63 (1.0)	57 (7.4)
1.5 mg/ml SLS	87 (1.3)	322 (8.6)	869 (27.0)	895 (12.9)	146 (2.9)
1.5 ml/ml SLS + Cycloheximide	33 (2.6)	31 (1.0)	41 (7.4)	33 (07)	48 (3.9)

Pantalone, R. M., and Page, R. C.: The production and secretion of collagenase and lysosomal hydrolases by macrophages activated with lymphokines (unpublished).

[a]NBCS—New born calf serum; CLS—Control lymphocyte supernatant; SLS—Stimulated lymphocyte supernatant.

[b]Mean values ± (S.D.) for two separate experiments. Cultures were maintained as described in the experimental procedures section.

Control gels incubated in the presence of 0.01% trypsin released 131 (±11) CPM.

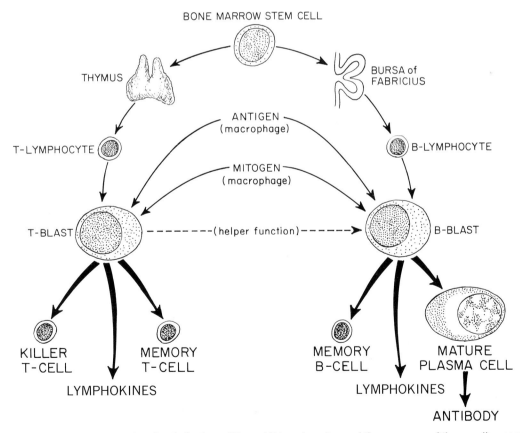

FIG. 8-4. *A schematic diagram illustrating the derivation of B- and T-lymphocytes and the response of these cells upon exposure to antigen or mitogen in the presence of macrophages.*

B- AND T-LYMPHOCYTES

There are two distinct but interrelated parts of the lymphoid system: (1) Humoral immunity is a function of lymphoid cells, which in birds differentiate under the influence of the bursa of Fabricius which in humans is presumed to be represented by the gut-associated lymphoid tissue. These cells, referred to as B-lymphocytes, upon exposure to antigen, give rise to mature plasma cells, which produce the bulk of the circulating immunoglobulin. (2) Cell-mediated immune reactions are carried out by the T-lymphocytes, which differentiate under the influence of the thymus. Both B- and T-lymphocytes acquire the ability to respond to antigen during their differentiation, and both circulate as lymphocytes through the blood and lymph.[81] The lymphoid cells and substances produced by them, including antibodies and lymphokines, interact intimately with other systems, including the microcirculation, the clotting system, and the complement cascade, and with other cells, including macrophages, polymorphonuclear leukocytes, mast cells, fibroblasts, and bone cells. The sum total of these interactions is recognized as the host defense and wound repair reactions to challenge and injury. The manifestations of these reactions are dependent to a large extent upon the nature and magnitude of the insult and the extent of participation of the various parts.

Upon gaining entrance to the body, antigen is transported through the lymph or blood to the lymph nodes or spleen where it becomes associated with macrophages. The antigenic substance is taken up by these cells, which process it in a manner that is not currently understood and present it to the reactive lymphocytes in a form to which they can respond. Within 1 to 2 days following exposure, the cells begin to undergo blastogenesis, a process by which they enlarge greatly, sometimes produce and secrete lymphokines, and undergo mitosis. This response, which may last for up to 2 weeks, gives rise to a large population of antigen-sensitive cells. Some of these cells, having the morphology of small lymphocytes, are the memory cells responsible for the anamnestic response observed upon a second encounter with the same antigens. A portion of the stimulated cells leaves the lymph nodes and spleen via the blood stream, where they comprise the short-lived lymphocyte population. They may localize at the site of injury or antigen deposition as well as in the lungs and in the wall of the gut where they differentiate into mature plasma cells. Some of the sensitized B-cells remain within the spleen and lymph nodes to form clones of mature antibody-producing plasma cells. Stimulated T-lymphocytes give rise to a population of cells that do not produce and release antibody but instead carry on their surfaces specific antigen-recog-

nition sites. These cells recirculate and participate in a variety of reactions, including immune surveillance, the discrimination between self and nonself antigens, and a helper function in antibody production by B-cells. Some of the sensitized T-lymphocytes, referred to as effector or killer T-cells, have the capacity to kill target cells carrying the antigenic determinates to which they are sensitive through cell-cell interactions. These, or additional subpopulations of sensitized lymphocytes, produce and secrete lymphokines. Both B- and T-lymphocytes have the capacity to respond nonspecifically to mitogens in much the same manner as they respond to antigens.

The humoral arm of the immune system is most effective in defense against various bacterial infections. Antibody effects include the following: (1) Toxins and other noxious antigenic substances are inactivated and neutralized by combining with specific antibody to form immune complexes. These complexes are much more readily ingested by phagocytes and eliminated than is antigen alone. (2) Specific antibody combines with surface determinants on invading bacteria to form an immune complex that activates complement and leads to bacteriolysis. (3) Antibodies coat or opsonize bacteria and other foreign substances, either specifically or nonspecifically, greatly enhancing the likelihood of phagocytosis by neutrophils and macrophages. The cellular immune system functions in a considerably different manner. This system is effective against viral, fungal, and some bacterial infections, especially by the intracellular parasites such as mycobacterium and in allograft rejection and tumor resistance. The system functions through direct cell-cell interactions resulting in cytolysis and through the release of lymphokines that recruit other lymphoid cells, activate other effector systems such as the macrophages, affect the microcirculation, or cause destruction directly (see Table 8-4).

LYMPHOKINES

Transforming B- and T-lymphoid cells produce and secrete numerous substances other than immunoglobulin responsible for a variety of biologic activities.[13,19,82,83,189,190] These substances are generally referred to as the "soluble mediators" or lymphokines. When the lymphokines were first described, they were considered to derive only from stimulated sensitized T-lymphocytes and to be the effector molecules carrying out delayed hypersensitivity reactions. More recent information shows that, in some cases, lymphokine production may occur independently from DNA synthesis and mitosis, an indication that only certain subpopulations of cells may be involved or that activated

TABLE 8-4. *Products of Activated Lymphoid Cells*

LYMPHOKINE	ACTIVITY
Migration inhibitory factor	Inhibits migration of normal macrophages
Macrophage aggregation factor	Causes macrophages to aggregate
Macrophage activating factor	Induces unactivated macrophages to become activated
Macrophage fusion factor	Causes macrophages to fuse and form giant cells
Macrophage chemotactic factor	Exerts chemotactic effect on macrophages
Macrophage disappearance factor	*In vivo* causes macrophages to adhere to peritoneal wall
Lymphotoxin	Kills a variety of cultured cells nonspecifically
Proliferation inhibition factor	Inhibits proliferation of cultured cells
Cloning inhibition factor	Inhibits proliferation of clones of cultured cells
Mitogenic factor	Induces blastogenesis in normal lymphocytes
Potentiating factor	Potentiates blastogenesis in antigen-stimulated cultures
Cell cooperation or helper factor	Increases the number or rate of formation of antibody-producing cells in culture
Inhibition factor	Inhibits migration of human granulocytes of peripheral blood buffy coat
Interferon	Prevents replication of viruses
Antifungal factor	Inhibits growth of yeast *in vitro*

cells may have the capacity to produce lymphokines only during a restricted period following stimulation. In addition, it is now clear that B- as well as T-lymphocytes have the capacity to produce lymphokines.[145,146] Some of the lymphokines considered to be of special importance in inflammatory gingival and periodontal disease include cytotoxic factor, chemotactic factor, and osteoclast activating factor. Cell culture and other methods used to study the production and biologic activity of lymphokines have been described in detail.[39,107,112,183,248]

LYMPHOKINES AFFECTING MACROPHAGES. Dramatic effects are induced in the morphology and functional properties of monocytes and macrophages by substances released from sensitized lymphocytes responding to antigen or mitogen (Fig. 8-3; Tables 8-2, 8-3). These include macrophage activation factor (MAF),[143,157,162] macrophage migration inhibition factor (MIF),[13,44,149,206,224,256] macrophage chemotactic factor (CF),[234,255] macrophage secretion factor (MSF),[182,183] and other less well-defined activities such as substances causing aggregation or fusion of macrophages to form giant cells.

The lymphocyte-derived substances affecting macrophages are responsible to a great extent for the features characteristic of the delayed hypersensitivity (type IV) reactions. They have the net effect of chemotactically attracting and retaining monocytes at the site of the lesion and activating the cells upon their arrival. The activated macrophages produce and secrete numerous substances, including lysosomal enzymes and neutral proteases such as collagenase and lysozyme, plasminogen activator, and prostaglandins; these substances likely play a major role in the perpetuation of the chronic inflammatory lesions and in tissue destruction.

CYTOTOXIC FACTOR (LYMPHOTOXIN). Sensitized lymphocytes activated by antigen or nonsensitized lymphocytes responding to mitogen, synthesize and secrete a substance which is nonspecifically cytotoxic to other neighboring cells. This material is generally referred to as lymphotoxin (LT).[83,104,127,262] Lymphotoxin can be differentiated chromatographically from MIF and MAF and appears to be a distinct molecule.[40,209] The mechanism by which it mediates cytolysis remains unclear, although the data indicate that it may cause membrane damage in target cells, with consequent osmotic changes. Lymphotoxin may be important in some of the alterations occurring in inflammatory gingival and periodontal disease. Cultured human peripheral blood lymphocytes from individuals with chronic periodontal disease exposed to dental plaque produce and secrete a lymphotoxin with the capacity to cytopathically alter and kill fibroblasts maintained *in vitro*.[106,107]

Chemotactic Factor (CF). Transforming lymphoid cells also release a factor, which has been purified and to which mononuclear cells are chemotactic.[255]

Osteoclast Activating Factor (OAF). A factor elaborated by human peripheral blood leukocytes, (probably B-cells), maintained in culture and exposed to dental plaque, and termed osteoclast activating factor (OAF) has recently been described.[107] This factor when placed in cultures of fetal bones induces the release of calcium, the appearance of large numbers of osteoclasts, and morphologic features characteristic of bone resorption. Of all the mediators currently identified, this one is likely to be the most important with regard to bone loss in chronic periodontitis.

Other Factors. As noted in Table 8-4, several additional biologically active factors are produced by activated lymphoid cells. These include substances stimulating and/or inhibiting proliferation of lymphoid cells[74] and a factor serving a helper function in antibody production by B-cells.[57,74,109]

ANTIBODIES AND IMMUNE COMPLEXES

A major portion of the circulating immunoglobulin is produced by mature plasma cells, although some may be made by lymphocytes. Any given plasma cell makes an immunoglobulin with but a single specificity, although stimulated cells may produce IgM at an early stage of differentiation prior to the production of either IgG or IgA by the fully differentiated cell. Antibody to some antigens can be produced by plasma cells in the absence of T-lymphocytes, but production of antibody to others such as haptens bound to protein carrier molecules requires the T-cell helper function (Fig. 8-4). The nature of the relationship between T-cells and antibody-producing B-cells is not currently understood, although a soluble substance that can serve the helper function has been described.[57,109]

Five separate immunoglobulin molecules have been identified and partially characterized. A thorough discussion of the structure of the immunoglobulin molecules can be found in Eisen's textbook.[54] The general structural plan, which is similar for the various molecules, is illustrated in Figure 8-5, which presents the structure of immunoglobulin G (IgG), the most abundant immunoglobulin in man. This antibody type constitutes over 85 percent of the total immunoglobulin of normal and hyperimmune sera and is responsible for protection against most infecting agents that are disseminated by the blood, including bacteria, viruses, parasites, and fungi. It is produced by plasma cells located in all of the lymphoid tissues except the thymus, and has a relatively long half-life of approximately 23 days. The molecules can readily cross the vascular endothelial wall to yield a high concentration in the extravascular fluids. Large quantities of IgG are present in normal and inflamed gingiva. IgG antibodies bind efficiently to soluble and insoluble antigens, and the resultant immune complexes have the capacity to activate complement (Fig. 8-6).

IgG molecules have an overall shape of a Y, and each molecule has a molecular weight of approximately 150,000 daltons (Fig. 8-5). Each is made up of two identical heavy and two identical light polypeptide chains of 50,000 and 25,000 daltons each, respectively, and joined to each other by disulfide bonds. A flexible or hinge region is located near the midpoint of the heavy chains, permitting the conformational changes associated with antigen binding to occur. Each

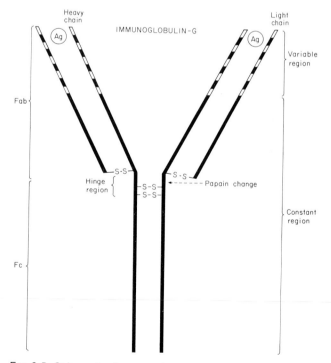

Fig. 8-5. *Schematic diagram of the immunoglobulin molecule IgG illustrating the heavy and light chains, variable and constant regions, antigen binding sites, the Fc and Fab fragments, and location of the interchain disulfide bonds.*

molecule has two antigen-binding sites which confer on the molecules the ability to cross-link and aggregate antigen. Subclasses of IgG have been identified on the basis of minor differences in the amino acid composition of the heavy chains. These are referred to as IgG1, 2, 3, and 4, and they make up 70, 19, 8, and 3 percent, respectively, of the IgG of sera. These subclasses differ functionally in some respects, but the differences are not yet clearly understood.

Immunoglobulin M (IgM), the largest of the immunoglobulin molecules with a molecular weight of 900,000 daltons, consists of five tetrameric subunits. Because of their size, IgM molecules are confined largely to the intravascular space. IgM is likely to be of greatest importance during the primary immune response induced by the initial exposure to a foreign antigen. During this period both IgM and IgG are produced, but within a few days the levels of IgM reach maximum and begin to decrease while the levels of IgG continue to rise. IgM antibodies are probably of considerable importance in normal host defense as well as in immunopathologic reactions (Fig. 8-6). IgM molecules agglutinate particulate antigens such as bacteria effectively and have the capacity to bind and activate complement. IgM-producing plasma cells are present in inflamed human gingiva in small numbers.

Immunoglobulin D (IgD) was discovered as a rare myeloma protein that failed to react with specific antisera against the other immunoglobulins, and it was subsequently found to be a minor component (approximately $\frac{1}{50}$th the level of IgG) of normal sera. The major portion of IgD is bound to the surface of cells, where it may serve as a receptor site for antigen. Little is known about the function of the molecule, and there is currently no information regarding its participation in the defense of the periodontium or in periodontal disease.

Cells producing immunoglobulin A (IgA), the antibody present in most secretions, are found in the salivary glands, gut mucosa, kidney, respiratory mucosa, and, in very small numbers, in normal and inflamed gingiva. Secretory IgA differs structurally from the other immunoglobulins and from serum IgA in that it has an additional polypeptide chain, or secretory piece, which presumably permits the antibody to traverse the secretory epithelium of various glands and become a part of normal secretions. IgA is the predominant antibody in human saliva, and it may play a role in determining the constituents of the oral flora. IgA specific for oral microorganisms can bind to antigenic determinants on the surface of bacterial cells and lead to alteration of adherence properties, to aggrega-

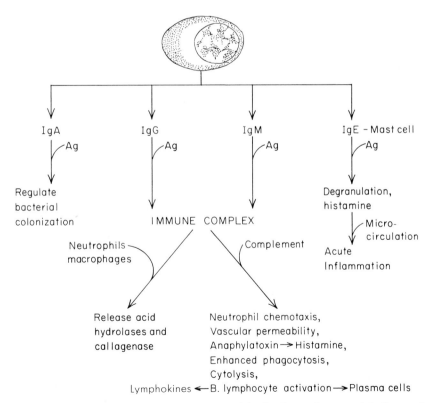

FIG. 8-6. Schematic diagram illustrating the biologic activities of four of the five known immunoglobulins produced by mature plasma cells.

tion, and to cell death. However, IgA-containing immune complexes cannot fix complement.

Immunoglobulin E (IgE), or reaginic antibody, is also present in sera only in trace amounts. It is produced predominantly by cells in the lining of the respiratory and intestinal tracts. Because antibody of this type has a high affinity for receptors on the surface of mast cells, it is known as cytophilic (cell-loving) antibody. This antibody is an important participant in acute allergic inflammation and may be a significant component of acute inflammatory periodontal disease.

The interaction of antigen and specific antibody results in the formation of immune complex (Fig. 8-6). This reaction may be beneficial. Since complex formation may inactivate and neutralize toxins and other noxious antigenic substances, it may convert soluble antigens that are difficult to inactivate into insoluble aggregates or precipitates that are easily destroyed by phagocytic cells, and it may tag invading microorganisms and other foreign particles, greatly enhancing phagocytosis and cytolysis. In addition, immune complexes have the capacity to activate other host effector systems such as the complement cascade and the phagocytes, thereby greatly enhancing the general defense mechanisms.

Although neither the antigen nor the antibody molecules alone may be detrimental, the immune complex resulting from their combination may be pathogenic.[48] Whether the net result of immune-complex formation is beneficial or detrimental is dependent upon several factors, including the location, antibody type, ratio of antigen to antibody, solubility, amount, and the frequency of production. The pathogenicity of immune complexes and their biologic activities reside in the antibody molecule rather than in the antigenic component, although the amount of antigen present is important. Complexes formed in moderate antigen excess are the most active. However, aggregated immunoglobulin not containing antigen exhibits many of the pathogenic properties of complexes.

There are several avenues through which immune complex can participate in the induction and enhancement of pathologic alteration of tissue:[36,48] (1) Possibly the most thoroughly studied pathway is activation of the complement sequence, with generation of numerous biologically active substances that may perpetuate the inflammatory response. (2) Immune complex can lead to the conversion of plasminogen to plasmin with consequent lysis of fibrin clots and to the direct release of kinin from kininogen, stimulating additional inflammation (Fig. 8-2).[36,48] (3) Ingestion of immune complex may stimulate the phagocytic cells to produce and release kallikrein and a variety of hydrolytic enzymes.

(4) Complexes of antigen and IgE on the surfaces of mast cells cause degranulation, thereby releasing histamine, which is a potent vasoactive substance enhancing inflammation, heparin, which may enhance bone resorption, and proteases, which may participate in the degradation of the extracellular matrix. (5) Immune complexes may enhance or block lymphoid-cell response to antigenic stimulation.[126,173]

Complement and Clotting

Following the discovery of complement by Buchner in 1893, Pfeiffer and Bordet elucidated the relationship between complement activity and antibody in bacterial cell lysis.[11] They noted that sera from guinea pigs previously immunized to cholera vibrios had the capacity to lyse the organisms *in vitro*. Comparable activity was not present in sera of nonimmunized animals, an indication that specific antibody is required. However, heating sera from immunized animals to 56°, a condition not altering antibody reactivity, destroyed its ability to lyse microorganisms. This property could be restored by adding to the mixture sera from either immune or nonimmune animals. Thus a nonantibody heat-labile substance was required. This substance was called alexin and subsequently was referred to as complement.

The complement system consists of eleven proteins accounting for about 10 percent of the total human serum globulin. Upon activation these proteins interact in a cascade fashion, generating a variety of biologically active substances and terminating in lysis of the antibody-tagged cells (Fig. 8-7). It appears likely that each step in the complement sequence is influenced by inhibitors that are also present in the serum.

The complement cascade can be activated by a variety of substances, the most important of which is immune complex or aggregated immunoglobulin.[75,154,232] There are two independent pathways of activation (Fig. 8-7). In the *direct pathway*, substances such as immune complexes containing IgG or IgM, certain aggregated immunoglobulins, plasmin, kallikrein, and trypsin react with the first component of complement (C1) to activate the entire series of reactions. The *alternate pathway* is activated by the cleavage of C3 by exposure to bacterial lipopolysaccharide (endotoxin), zymosan (yeast cell wall), certain aggregated immunoglobulins, plasmin or trypsin, without the participation of the previous steps in activation. Other alternate pathways include the cleavage of C3 by properdin and the cleavage of C5 by trypsin or lysosomal enzymes. The properdin pathway is not well worked out, but it appears to consist of at least three

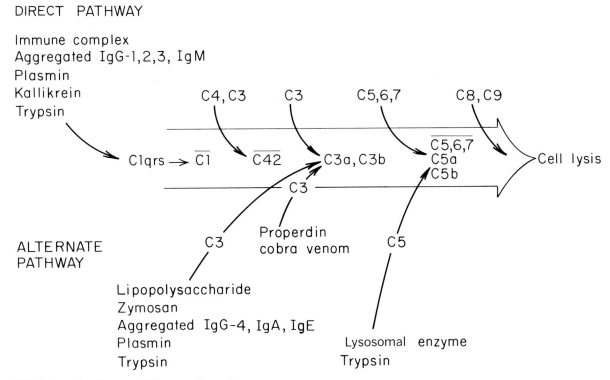

FIG. 8-7. Schematic diagram of the complement sequence.

proteins. Cobra venom, a substance sometimes used experimentally to make animals complement-deficient, probably operates via the properdin pathway. Although immune complexes containing IgA, IgE, and IgG4 cannot activate complement by the direct pathway, aggregates of these immunoglobulins can activate complement by the direct pathway.

The complement system, which can be viewed as an amplifier and effector of the immune system, is likely to participate in the host response to injuries and challenges of all types. The third component of complement (C3) plays a key role in the amplification process. Once a single enzymatically active complex of C4 and C2 has been formed, large numbers of C3 molecules can be cleaved. In addition, both C3 and C5 can be cleaved by the indirect as well as by the direct pathway. Thus, literally hundreds of potent effector molecules inducing a variety of biologic events, such as chemotaxis of leukocytes and greatly enhanced phagocytosis, can derive from a single antibody molecule present in an immune complex and be capable of activating complement. In addition, complement activation results in lysis of antibody-tagged cells, an event that does not occur with antibody alone.

The principal reactions that have been attributed to complement activation include anaphylaxis, immune adherence, and opsonization causing enhanced phago-

cytosis and bacterial lysis. These events are initiated by biologically active molecules produced during the complement reaction sequence. Some of these products, along with their activities, are listed in Table 8-5.

Complement activation is tied intimately to all of the other participants in the host response to injury (Fig. 8-8). Hageman factor, which is activated by injury, initiates both the clotting cascade and the conversion of plasminogen to plasmin. Plasmin not only provides a means for fibrinolysis and clot dissolution, but it also has the capacity to cleave C3 and activate the alternate pathway of complement, as well as to cleave C1 and activate the direct pathway. Kallikrein, which is also generated during blood clotting, has the capacity to activate complement along the direct pathway. On the other hand, substances generated from the complement proteins activate and regulate a host of other reactions. C3a enhances vascular permeability and phagocytosis, C3b activates lymphoid cells, and C5a induces histamine release from mast cells and chemotaxis by neutrophils.[232] Thus, complement activation plays a central role in all forms of inflammation.

In addition to the above reactions, which may be predominantly protective and beneficial, severe tissue damage can be induced from the inflammatory response provoked by complement activation. In some situations such as the Arthus (type III) reaction, other-

TABLE 8-5. *Principal Activities of Activated Complement (C) Proteins and Their Fragments*

ACTIVITY	C PROTEIN OR FRAGMENT
Anaphylatoxin: Histamine release from mast cells and increased permeability of capillaries	3a; 5a
Activation of B-lymphocytes	3b
Chemotaxis: Attract polymorphonuclear leukocytes	5a; 5b,6,7
Immune adherence and opsonization: Adherence of Ab-Ag-C complexes to leukocytes, platelets, etc., increasing their susceptibility to phagocytosis by leukocytes and macrophages	3b; 5b
Membrane damage: Lysis of red cells; leakiness in plasma membrane of nucleated cells; lysis of gram-negative bacteria	8; 9

Adapted from Eisen, H. N.: Immunology. An Introduction to Molecular and Cellular Principles of the Immune Responses. New York, Harper & Row, 1974.

wise innocuous immune complexes activate complement and lead to the accumulation of large numbers of leukocytes, enhanced vascular permeability, and the release of quantities of lysosomal enzymes and other substances that destroy normal tissue.

Fibroblasts

The remaining participant in the normal host response mechanisms is the fibroblast. This cell is the principal resident of the normal connective tissue and has the responsibility of synthesizing and maintaining the various collagens, proteoglycans, and other substances comprising the connective tissues (see Ch. 1). Fibroblasts are particularly important in the restoration of structure and function following injury or challenge. In an uncomplicated experimental skin wound, fibroblasts migrate into the site within about 4 to 5 days following wounding, and the production of collagen and other connective tissue substance begins within 5 to 7 days. Usually, by the elapse of 2 to 3 weeks, the collagenous connective tissues have been replaced, and except for a transient increased vascularity which gradually resolves, the part may be restored to normal.[207] Although little or no information is currently available, it is likely that interactions be-

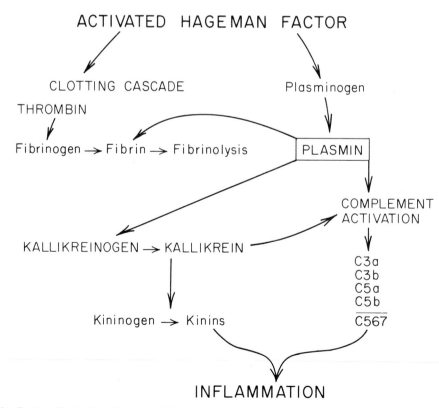

FIG. 8-8. *Schematic diagram illustrating the interrelationships of various host response systems and demonstrating how injury of almost any type, through activation of Hageman factor, can initiate inflammatory and lymphoid-cell responses.*

tween fibroblasts and the leukocytes and lymphoid cells, similar to those that are known to exist between the macrophage and lymphoid cells, occur. As with the other facets of host defense, fibroblast function can go awry. For example, in chronic inflammatory lesions, including chronic periodontal disease, fibrosis with disruption of the normal tissue architecture may be a major component.

PATHOGENIC IMMUNE REACTIONS

While there is no doubt that immune reactions are of major benefit in host defense, the same reactions in some circumstances can be turned against the immunologically competent host with deleterious effects. These are usually referred to as hypersensitivities or allergies. Reactions of this type appear to play a major role in the pathogenesis of chronic inflammatory lesions, possibly including periodontal disease. Reactions in which serum antibodies play a major role usually become apparent within a few hours following antigenic challenge, and they are classified as the *immediate hypersensitivities;* allergic reactions associated with cell-mediated immunity generally require 48 to 72 hours or more to evolve, and they are described as *delayed hypersensitivities.* Hypersensitivity reactions have been classified by Gell and Coombs as types I, II, III, and IV.[70] Important characteristics of each of these types are listed in Table 8-6.

Type I Reactions

Type I reactions are manifest within a few minutes following the injection into the circulation of antigen against which the host has a high tissue load of cytophilic IgE antibody. Mast cells and basophils carrying these antibodies and encountering antigen undergo rapid degranulation, with the release of large quantities of histamine. The released histamine acts on the microcirculation and the smooth muscle of the bronchioles, resulting in anaphylaxis. Systemic anaphylaxis in humans has three components: vascular collapse with increased permeability and widespread peripheral vasodilation, bronchiolar constriction, and laryngeal edema. Local type I reactions resulting from the same mechanism are manifest as urticaria and hay fever. It has been suggested that type I reactions can occur in the periodontal tissues. Gingiva contains large numbers of mast cells, some of which appear to undergo degranulation during inflammation. Small numbers of IgE-producing plasma cells have been detected, and it is likely that plaque-derived antigens can gain

TABLE 8-6. Hypersensitivity

	DESCRIPTOR	DEFINITION	EXAMPLES
Type I	Anaphylactic	Antigen reacts with cells sensitized by γE antibody and releases mediators	Urticaria; hay fever; asthma; anaphylaxis; some food allergies
Type II	Cytotoxic	Antibody reacts with cell-associated antigen, killing cell usually, but not always, with help of C or phagocytic cells	Transfusion reaction; autoimmune hemolytic anemia; autoimmune thrombocytopenia
Type III	Arthus reaction, serum sickness	Antibody reacts with antigen in tissue space or blood stream to cause vasculitis and/or other inflammation; Requires C	Serum sickness; rare iatrogenic Arthus reaction in humans
Type IV	Delayed	Immune lymphocytes react with antigen; Reaction mediated by lymphocytes, macrophages, or their products	Tuberculin reaction; contact dermatitis; autoimmune disease; allograft rejection

Classification of Gell, P. G. H., and Coombs, R. A., Eds.: Clinical Aspects of Immunology. Philadelphia, F. A. Davis, 1968.

entrance to the connective tissue. If reactions of this sort occur in response to plaque accumulation, acute inflammatory response would be expected to result.

Type II Reactions

In type II reactions, antibody reacts with a cell-surface antigen, and, in collaboration with complement and phagocytic cells, the target cell is killed. Blood transfusion reactions are examples of type II hypersensitivity. Some autoimmune diseases in which the immunologic system fails to distinguish between self and nonself antigens and produces antibodies against normal tissue constituents are also examples of type II reactions. Cell destruction is usually mediated by humoral antibody, which in some cases leads to complement activation and cell lysis and in others to opsonization of the cells and their phagocytosis by macrophages. The autoimmune hemolytic anemias and thrombocytopenia are the most completely studied autoimmune states. In these diseases, circulating specific antibody against the red cells or platelets is the cause of the disease. Whether type II reactions occur in the periodontal tissues in periodontal disease is not known. It has been suggested that a mechanism of this type may account for the cytopathic alterations in fibroblasts and plasma cells seen at certain stages of the disease.

Type III Reactions

Type III hypersensitivity is commonly known as the Arthus reaction and was the first example of immune complex hypersensitivity to be described. The lesion results when antigen is introduced into the tissues of a host with a high circulating level of precipitating antibody. In antibody excess, immune complexes form in the walls of the vessels of the microcirculation, leading to activation of the complement cascade. Thus, the onset of the reactions is slower than in types I and II, requiring 4 to 6 hours to reach maximum intensity. Biologically active substances released by activation of the complement sequence provoke an inflammatory reaction of such magnitude that thrombosis and vessel necrosis occur. Most of the observed tissue damage can be accounted for by the activity of hydrolytic enzymes released from neutrophils. Serum sickness, as exemplified by penicillin allergy, is another form of type III reaction; immune complexes form in the circulation in the presence of antigen excess. Circulating immune complexes may be responsible for some of the tissue destruction observed in autoimmune disease, post-streptococcal glomerulonephritis, and rheumatoid arthritis. The role of immune complexes in human periodontal disease has not been resolved at the present time.

Type IV Reactions

Type IV reactions are dependent upon the presence of sensitized cells rather than circulating antibody. In typical experimental reactions, an animal is injected, usually subcutaneously, with small doses of antigen in Freund's adjuvant. The use of larger doses of antigen given via the circulation and without adjuvant encourages the development of humoral rather than cellular hypersensitivity. After the lapse of 5 to 21 days, a second injection is given at a second site; within about 6 hours, swelling, redness and induration appear and increase in intensity, reaching a maximum after 24 to 48 hours and lasting for several days. Frank necrosis may ensue. The lesion is characterized histologically by the intense infiltration of lymphoid cells, many of which appear to be undergoing blast transformation, and macrophages. The cells localize around blood vessels. Lymphokines may be released by the activated lymphoid cells. These substances recruit and activate other lymphoid cells and macrophages and probably account in major part for the tissue damage characteristic of delayed-hypersensitivity reactions. At some stages, inflammatory gingival and periodontal disease exhibits features characteristic of type IV reactions.[181,220] The massive tissue destruction that usually accompanies type IV reactions can be accounted for in major part by the production and secretion of large quantities of acid hydrolases and collagenase by lymphokine-activated macrophages.

IMMUNOPATHOLOGY OF CHRONIC INFLAMMATORY GINGIVAL AND PERIODONTAL DISEASE

The likely participation of various immunopathologic reactions in the pathogenesis of inflammatory gingival and periodontal disease has become apparent within the past decade and a large part of current research effort is aimed in this direction. Several reviews of the field have appeared recently.[4,7,17,37,73,106,133,156,164,192]

Humoral Factors

Plaque-associated inflammatory gingival and periodontal disease begins as an acute inflammation that evolves into a lymphocyte-dominated lesion within about one week (see Ch. 7).[187] A lesion characterized by a predominance of mature plasma cells forms within about 2 weeks and persists through the course of the disease.[181] The gingival tissues in both the normal and the inflamed states are bathed in immunoglobulin produced by the local plasma cells and derived from the blood serum.[23,25] These observations provide strong morphologic support for the idea that humoral factors may play a central role in the pathogenesis of inflammatory periodontal disease.

The identity of the plasma cells populating inflamed human gingiva has been established and the nature of the immunoglobulin partially elucidated. IgG-producing plasma cells make up, by far, the majority of the cell population, with but few cells producing IgM and IgA.[23,25,72,73] In some sections of inflamed human gingiva, an occasional IgE-producing cell may be found.[73] Unusually large quantities of immunoglobulin are present extravascularly; indeed, the quantity is so large that extensive washing is necessary before cell identity can be established. A portion of this immunoglobulin appears to be bound to the collagen fibers, and it is not removed by the usual washing procedures.[73] Most of the immunoglobulin is IgG with almost negligible quantities of IgM and IgA.

The specificity of the immunoglobulin present in the inflamed gingiva and that produced by gingival plasma cells locally remains unclear,[23,25,73,192,214] although a portion of this is specific for plaque-derived microorganisms. Schneider and his associates showed that sections of inflamed gingiva have the capacity to specifically bind oral microorganisms, thus demonstrating the presence of antibody with specificity for the antigens of these organisms.[214] In addition, Berglund showed that immunoglobulin obtained from inflamed gingiva can form immune complex with antigens of plaque microorganisms.[15] There is also evidence for significant quantities of circulating antibody to oral microorganisms.[59,155,167,168,239,240]

In spite of these observations, little is known about the specificity of the immunoglobulin synthesized by the plasma cells present in gingival tissue in periodontal disease. Although a portion of the immunoglobulin produced is specific for oral microorganisms, the bulk of the material has a specificity which, so far, has not been determined. Injection of a purified antigen, egg-white lysozyme, into the gingival tissue of the rabbit leads to the differentiation and accumulation of mature plasma cells. However, fewer than half of these produce lysozyme-specific antibody.[24] The nature of the nonreactive antibody remains unknown. The amount of specific antibody made is a function of the number of antigens applied.[250] For example, it has been suggested that if there were eight immunogenic constituents in plaque, an average of only 5 percent of the plasma cells accumulating would make antibody specific for these antigens.[24] The likelihood that a large number of specific immunogens are present in plaque is high. Thus, it may be expected that the bulk of the immunoglobulin in inflamed gingiva will be nonreactive or of a non-plaque antigen specificity. Alternatively this antibody may be made in response to irrelevant antigens, it may be nonsense antibody, or it may

be antibody made against normal or altered gingival tissue constituents.

Whether humoral factors can participate in the pathogenesis of periodontal disease has been examined experimentally by several investigators. Rizzo and Mergenhagen were able to induce the Shwartzman reaction in oral mucosa of rabbits with endotoxin from an oral microorganism.[202] The same investigators induced delayed hypersensitivity (type IV) reactions on the palatal gingiva of the rabbit by sensitizing with horse serum or with tubercle bacilli and subsequently challenging locally with the same antigens.[201] Repeated administration of the antigens led to the accumulation of large numbers of plasma cells. Similarly, Terner induced the Arthus (type III) reaction in the attached gingiva of rabbits, guinea pigs, and rats, using standard procedures and horse serum as antigen.[245] The effects of topical application of the antigenic substance has also been tested. The repeated application of egg albumin as antigen into the gingival sulcus of the normal mandibular incisor of the rabbit led to the local differentiation of plasma cells and to detectable titers of specific antibody.[203]

The likely participation of the humoral arm of the immune system in the evolution of the periodontal lesion was demonstrated by Ranny and Zander.[199] These investigators sensitized squirrel monkeys by subcutaneous injection of ovalbumin emulsified in Freund's complete adjuvant. Subsequently, the animals were challenged by placement of antigen-soaked threads in the gingival sulcus. The repeated challenge three times each week for 3 months led to the evolution of a lesion similar to that in human inflammatory gingival and periodontal disease.

The work done in humans also appears to support the idea that humoral factors are important. Nisengard and his colleagues have shown that individuals exhibiting periodontitis give a positive immediate hypersensitivity reaction when skin tested with an antigenic preparation from the plaque microorganism *Actinomyces viscosus*.[164-169] In addition, Steinberg found, using tanned red-cell hemagglutination and whole spirochetal cells as antigen, that individuals with periodontal disease exhibit more serum antibody for this antigen than do normal control persons and that individuals with severe disease do not have antibody.[239]

The mechanisms through which humoral factors, specifically immunoglobulin, can participate in the pathogenesis of inflammatory gingival and periodontal disease have not been clarified. It seems likely that the presence of large numbers of plasma cells in inflamed gingiva and the production of specific antibody may be predominantly protective. Antibody would be expected to opsonize microorganisms and enhance their phagocytosis and destruction; additionally, antigens penetrating the gingival tissue would likely be inactivated through immune-complex formation. If antibodies participate in the pathologic tissue alterations accompanying chronic inflammation, they most likely do so through immune-complex formation and type I or type III immunopathologic reactions.

While there are several pathways through which immune complexes can be pathogenic, serious questions remain as to whether they actually play an important role in human inflammatory gingival and periodontal disease. Berglund has shown that immunoglobulin produced by plasma cells in gingiva slices incubated *in vitro* forms immune complex when treated with plaque antigens and that these complexes activate complement.[15] However, the possibility that inadvertently aggregated immunoglobulin rather than immune complex is responsible cannot be ruled out. There is some evidence that complexes may be present in detectable amounts in diseased gingival tissue. Using immunofluorescence techniques, Genco and Krygier found deposits of C3 and IgG at the epithelial-connective tissue interface and between the cells of pocket epithelium.[72] Subsequently, cigar-shaped deposits associated with blood vessels that stained positively for IgM, C3, and C4 and that were not removed by washing the tissue were described.[73] Using similar techniques, Clagett (unpublished) has done extensive studies on both human and dog tissues. As shown in Figure 8-9, lumpy deposits associated with blood vessels and positive for immunoglobulin and complement were found. However, sections exhibiting these deposits were rare. Definitive proof that complexes are present requires detection and identification of the associated antigen; so far, this has not been possible. Therefore,

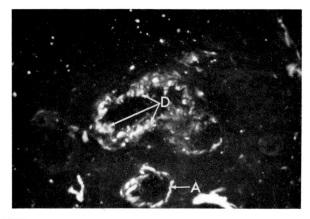

FIG. 8-9. *Photomicrograph of a section of periodontally diseased dog gingiva treated with fluorescent anti-C3 immunoglobulin and demonstrating the location of lumpy deposits within the wall of a small blood vessel (D). In an adjacent arteriole, the autofluorescense (A) of elastin is noted (Original magnification 420 ×). (Courtesy Dr. J. Clagett.)*

the possible significance of immune complexes in periodontal disease currently remains unanswered.

The predominance of plasma cells in the inflammatory periodontal lesion, combined with the failure so far to demonstrate a major role for immune complexes in its pathogenesis, have led to a reevaluation of mechanisms through which B-lymphocytes and plasma cells may participate in tissue damage. There is recent evidence that stimulated B-cells do produce and release lymphokines,[145,146] and these may participate in a major way in the pathogenesis. Whether mature plasma cells have the capacity to produce substances other than immunoglobulins remains unknown.

Cell-mediated Hypersensitivity

Until the work of Ivanyi and Lehner in 1970 and 1971, there was little direct evidence indicating a role for cell-mediated hypersensitivity (type IV reactions) in the pathogenesis of plaque-associated periodontal disease.[112,113,115] However, these investigators were able to show that peripheral blood leukocytes from patients with periodontal disease, maintained *in vitro* in the presence of various plaque antigens, undergo blast transformation. The cells synthesize DNA, release lymphokines, and exhibit cytotoxic reactions (Figs. 8-10, 8-11). Comparable cultures from normal persons free of gingival and periodontal disease do not respond in this manner to plaque antigens. The extent of the response is related to the periodontal status, as measured by the Russell Index; individuals with moderately severe periodontitis respond to a greater extent than do individuals with gingivitis. Furthermore, cells from individuals with advanced periodontitis (Russell Index Score greater than 4) fail to respond and behave as control cultures when the cells are maintained in autologous serum. This failure to respond, however, does not result from an absence of sensitized cells; leukocytes from these individuals, when maintained in culture with serum from normal individuals or individuals with gingivitis or moderately severe periodontitis, do respond. Furthermore, when the serum from the nonresponding periodontally diseased individuals was added to cultures of otherwise responding cells, the response was inhibited. Thus, it was shown that the serum from individuals with advanced periodontitis contains factors that block the lymphoid-cell response. The nature of these factors has not been determined, although immune complexes can cause these effects.[126] Serum antibody may also play a role. Ivanyi, Challacombe, and Lehner demonstrated a positive correlation between lymphocyte stimulation and IgM hemagglutinating antibody titers in patients with mild periodontitis, but not in individuals with severe perio-

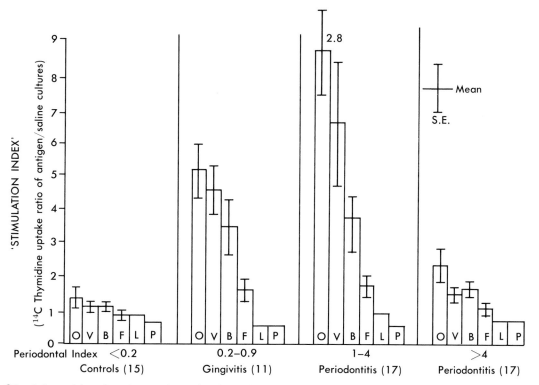

FIG. 8-10. *Stimulation of lymphocyte transformation in patients with gingivitis and periodontitis and in control individuals by ultrasonicates of* Actinomyces viscosus (O), Veillonella alcalescens (V), Bacteroides melaninogenicus (B), Bacteroides fusiformis (F), Lactobacillus acidophilus (L), *and* Proteus mirabilis (P). *Note that the stimulation index of individuals with gingivitis and mild-to-moderate periodontitis to all of the microorganisms from plaque, except lactobacillus, but not from the nonoral microorganism proteus, is significantly greater than the stimulation index from control individuals. (Ivanyi, L., and Lehner, T.: Stimulation of lymphocyte transformation by bacterial antigens in patients with periodontal disease. Arch. Oral Biol., 15:1089, 1970.)*

dontitis.[111] The data were taken to indicate that an IgM class of antibody may play a regulatory role in lymphocyte responses.

The work of Ivanyi and Lehner marks a major advance in our understanding of the inflammatory periodontal lesion. They were the first to document a distinct difference between normal and periodontally diseased individuals with regard to the activities of the immune system or other host defense systems. Subsequent to these observations, Horton and his colleagues confirmed and extended the initial observations.[107] They were able to show not only that peripheral blood leukocytes from periodontally diseased individuals stimulated with plaque or plaque extracts undergo blast transformation as manifested by the uptake of radioactively labeled DNA precursors but also that the cells synthesize and release lymphotoxin.[106,107] This lymphokine has the capacity to kill fibroblasts and other cells maintained in culture.

More recently the possible role of cell-mediated hypersensitivity in the periodontal lesion has been extended by examining reactivity of individuals in whom experimental gingivitis has been induced. Indi-

viduals, otherwise normal, allowing plaque to accumulate for 28 days, exhibited a biphasic response in lymphocyte transformation with two maxima at day 14 and between days 28 and 35 to various gram-negative endotoxin-containing microorganisms, to *Actinomyces viscosus* and to *Lactobacillus acidophilus*. This response returned to normal baseline values by day 56. However, the interpretation of the observations was made complex by the fact that the individuals responded in a similar manner to nonoral microorganisms and substances such as purified protein derivative to which they were not exposed during the period of experimental gingivitis induction. Therefore, it was proposed that accumulating plaque may act as an adjuvant enhancing both related and unrelated cell-mediated immune responses.[134]

At the time of the original Ivanyi and Lehner experiments the response of lymphocytes maintained *in vitro* to antigen by mitogenesis and lymphokine production was considered to be an *in vitro* correlate of cell-mediated or Type IV hypersensitivity.[112] The experiments with periodontal patients were widely taken to mean that cell-mediated hypersensitivity plays an important

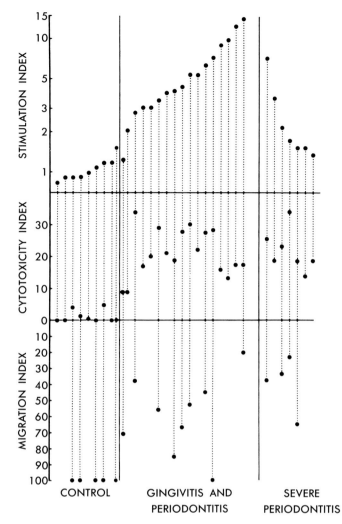

FIG. 8-11. *Comparison of lymphocyte transformation, cytotoxocity, and migration inhibition in patients with periodontal disease and in controls. (Lehner, T.: Cell-mediated immune responses in oral disease. J. Oral Pathol., 1:39, 1972.)*

part in the pathogenesis of inflammatory gingival and periodontal disease. However, at that time this concept was inconsistent with observations from other sources. For example, except for the brief period of about 1 to 2 weeks following the beginning of plaque accumulation, inflammatory gingival and periodontal disease in humans does not resemble a delayed-hypersensitivity response; indeed, throughout the remaining course of the lesion, even if this is several decades, it is predominated by plasma cells, not by other mononuclear cells typical of delayed hypersensitivity reactions.[181,220] Several recent observations have helped to clear up this apparent enigma.

It is now clear that both the B- and T-lymphocytes have the capacity to respond mitogenically and antigenically, and both cell types produce lymphokines and carry out cytotoxicity reactions.[145,146] Indeed, the

data now available indicate that the production of some lymphokines of considerable potential importance in the periodontal lesion, such as osteoclast activating factor, may be the exclusive product of B-lymphocytes. Secondly, microorganisms making up microbial plaque induce mitogenic and antigenic activity in both B- and T-lymphocytes. Some microorganisms such as *Veillonella alcalescens* activate T-cells through a protein component and B-cells through the lipid A fraction of endotoxin;[114] others such as *Actinomyces viscosus* are potent B-lymphocyte mitogens (Table 8-7).[55] Additional substances produced by plaque bacteria stimulate lymphocytes nonspecifically. Levan, a sugar polymer synthesized by plaque bacteria, is a stimulator of B-cells,[114] and individuals with periodontal disease exhibit greater response to this polysaccharide than do normal control individuals. These observations may account for the predominance of plasma cells in the established and advanced stages of inflammatory gingival and periodontal disease.

Mast Cells

Whether mast cells play an important role in host defense reactions in the vicinity of the dento-gingival junction or in inflammatory gingival and periodontal disease remains unknown. Numerous attempts have been made to evaluate the relative numerical density of mast cells in inflamed vs. normal gingiva in order to determine whether degranulation on a significant scale accompanies gingival inflammation.[46,204,225,226,246,267] Although some investigators have claimed an inverse relationship between the population of mast cells and the extent of gingival inflammation, there is as yet no clear-cut answer to the question. The capacity for antigenic degranulation appears to exist in the periodontal tissues, since antigenic substances appear to gain entrance to the gingival tissues (see Ch. 4) and IgE-producing plasma cells appear to be present.[169] Using the electron microscope and human tissues, Barnett has studied the role of these cells in inflammatory disease.[8-10] Large numbers of mast cells were found in pocket epithelium completely separated from the connective tissues. These cells exhibited unusual shapes and morphologic features of high levels of synthetic activity; evidence of degranulation was seen frequently. On the other hand, in the connective tissues, evidence of granule release was rarely seen. The cells were often associated with regions of collagen breakdown, and microvillous contacts between mast cells and collagen fibers were noted.

There appear to be at least three routes through which substances derived from mast cells can participate in the tissue alterations characteristically seen in

TABLE 8-7. *Mitogenic Effect of Homogenates of Actinomyces Viscosus on Mouse Lymphocytes*

SPLEEN CELLS	STIMULATION INDEX (EXPERIMENTAL/CONTROL)		
	B-CELL MITOGEN (LPS)	T-CELL MITOGEN (PHA-P)	A. VISCOSUS
Congenitally[a] T-Cell deficient (B-Cells only)	19.6	1.6	24.9
Normal BALB/cJ (B- and T- Cells)	19.4	53.7	24.5
Experimentally[b] T-Cell Deficient (B-Cells only)	18.2	3.3	23.5

Engel, L. D., et al.: Unpublished data

[a] Nu/Nu BALB/cJ (nude) mice.

[b] Spleen cells treated *in vitro* with anti-T-cell antiserum with complement. 5×10^6 spleen cells/ml were cultured in the presence of 100 μg/ml lipopolysaccharide (LPS) or *Actinomyces viscosus* homogenate (*A. viscosus*) or of 20 μg/ml phytohemagglutinin (PHA-P) for 48 hours. DNA synthesis was assayed during the last 12 hours of incubation.

inflammatory gingival and periodontal disease. However, whether any of these do in fact operate is not known: Tissue bits exposed to heparin *in vitro* produce more collagenase than do tissues free of heparin, and the enzyme has an enhanced level of activity.[211] Thus, at least conceptually, the release of heparin during gingival inflammation may enhance tissue breakdown through elevating levels of collagenase activity. In addition, the neutral proteases derived from mast-cell granules would be expected to digest noncollagenous proteins of the extracellular matrix as well as act on collagen after the initial cleavage by collagenase. Heparin has the capacity to enhance the effectiveness of numerous substances that induce bone resorption *in vitro*.[76] Whether sufficient concentrations of heparin can be reached in the gingival tissue to exert these effects is not known. The vasoactive properties of histamine are well established, and it is clear that this substance is an important component in many inflammatory reactions.

PROSTAGLANDINS

The prostaglandins (PG) are a family of chemically similar fatty acids of molecular weight 300 to 400 daltons and were first described by von Euler.[58] The prostaglandins are produced from prostanoic acid by prostaglandin synthetase (Fig. 8-12).[38,100,257] These substances have a remarkably broad range of biologic activities, and current evidence indicates that they may be of considerable importance in the mechanisms

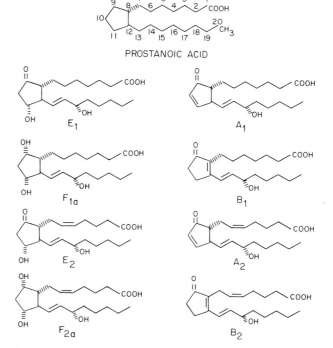

FIG. 8-12. *Chemical structure of the various prostaglandins and their precursor prostanoic acid.*

underlying the inflammatory periodontal lesion as well as in many other forms of chronic inflammation. The prostaglandins are generally classified as local or cellular hormones. Since they are produced and liberated locally at many sites within the body, they have a short range of activity and, with the exception of prostaglandin-A (PGA), they can be inactivated rapidly.[191,198,212] The prostaglandins appear to be important channels of intercelluar communication.

The capacity to produce prostaglandins is reported to be almost ubiquitous throughout the animal kingdom with regard to species and cell type,[100] although the data available on this point are not definitive. Prostaglandin production has been demonstrated by cultures of spleen cells,[61] macrophages,[158] fibrosarcoma cells,[136] fibroblasts,[89] and eosinophils.[108] Prostaglandin production by spleen cells is enhanced 2- to 10-fold by mitogen stimulation. Prostaglandins are found in high concentration in inflamed human gingiva,[78] and in various inflammatory exudates.[2,78,84,263]

The prostaglandins have been implicated as both mediators and modulators of numerous biologic processes, including acute and chronic inflammation,[2,22,42,78,84,117-120,151,237,263] normal and pathologic immune reactions,[21,33,98,101,129,229,230,241] connective-tissue alterations and fibrosis,[20,121,124,147,150,188,194,197,261] and pathologic bone resorption.[91,125,197]

The basic mechanism through which the prostaglandins exert their action is not fully understood, although it appears likely that they activate the adenyl cyclase enzyme system leading to the conversion of adenosine triphosphate (ATP) to cyclic adenosine monophosphate (cAMP), which, in turn, mediates the specific cellular events. Several different lines of evidence support this idea.[71,89,121,147,230] The better defined effects of the prostaglandins and elevated levels of cAMP induced by them will be described.

Microcirculation and the Immune System

Exposure of the skin of humans or experimental animals to prostaglandins causes a prolonged erythema with vasodilation, elevated vascular permeability, and

enhanced neutrophil chemotaxis.[42,117-120,236,258,264] In addition, eosinophils respond to many stimuli by liberating prostaglandins which, in turn, inhibit the release of histamine from mast cells,[108] presumably by elevating the mast cell levels of cAMP.[152] Thus, the prostaglandins may mediate some facets of acute inflammation and modulate allergic inflammatory responses.

The prostaglandins may play an important, although as yet poorly defined, role in immune reactions. Exposure to prostaglandin reduces the nonspecific mitogenic response and the specific antigenic response of lymphoid cells.[21] In some cases, the magnitude of the suppression is greater than 90 percent (Table 8-8). Both B- and T-lymphocytes are affected, although the effects on T-cells appear to be of a greater magnitude than those on B-cells. The suppressor effects are probably mediated through cAMP.[33,98,101,229,230,241] The ability of activated macrophages to inhibit lymphoid cell responses may reside in their capacity to produce prostaglandins.[29,172]

Connective-Tissue Cells

In addition to the suppression of mitogen- and antigen-induced lymphoid cell proliferation, prostaglandins also have the capacity to reduce proliferation of other cells. As shown in Table 8-9, PGE_2 at 10^{-5} M suppresses mitosis of cultures of human gingival fibroblasts about 50 percent. Similar effects have been noted in bone cultures,[194] and they can be induced in fibroblasts by elevation in the levels of cAMP.[150]

The synthetic activity of fibroblasts and bone cells in culture is modulated by the presence of prostaglandins or by elevation in the levels of cAMP. The magnitude and direction of the effects of these substances upon synthetic activity remain controversial. Blumenkrantz and Sondergaard reported that both PGE and PGF

TABLE 8-8. *Effect of Prostaglandin on Mitogenically Stimulated Human Peripheral Blood Leukocytes*

STIMULANT	ETHANOL CONTROL	PGE2 AT 10^{-5} M	PERCENT INHIBITION
PHA-P (25 µg/ml)	145.8 (5.7)[a]	12.1 (0.3)	91.7
Endotoxin (10 µg/ml)	2.6 (0.2)	1.5 (0.05)	42.3
A. viscosus (50 µg/ml)	3.5 (0.3)	1.0 (0.05)	71.2
A. viscosus (100 µg/ml)	3.3 (0.3)	1.0 (0.1)	69.6
Unstimulated control	0.8 (0.004)	0.6 (0.003)	25.0

Page, R. C., et al.: Unpublished data.
[a] Reported as cpm $\times$ 10^3.
PHA-P: Phytohemagglutinin-P, a mitogen for human T-lymphocytes.
A. viscosus: Actinomyces viscosus homogenate.

TABLE 8-9. *Effect of Prostaglandin on the Mitosis of Human Gingival Fibroblasts Maintained in Culture*

	CPM ^{3}H/plate after 48 hours (S.D.)
Control cultures	444,411 (49,925)
PGE$_2$ (10^{-5} M)	217,587 (7,472)

Ko, D., Page, R. C., and Narayanan, A. S. Unpublished data.
Human gingival fibroblasts were plated in Dulbecco-Vogt medium containing 10 percent calf serum on to 60-mm plastic Petri dishes at 0.5 × 10^6 cells per plate, and allowed to adhere. Fresh medium containing 10^{-5} M PGE$_2$ was added along with 5 µCi/ml tritiated thymidine. After 48 hours' incubation, the cells were harvested, and the radioactivity incorporated was measured.

TABLE 8-10. *Effect of Prostaglandin on the Synthetic Activity of Human Gingival Fibroblasts Maintained in Culture*

	CPM ^{14}C/plate (S.D.) × 10^{-3}	
SYNTHETIC ACTIVITY	CONTROL	PGE$_2$ 10^{-6} M
Total synthetitic activity	3,388 (67)	1,700 (53)
Proline incorporated	146 (12)	76 (2)
Hydroxyproline	14 (1)	7 (0.2)

Unpublished data of Ko, D., Page, R. C., and Narayanan, A. S.
Human gingival fibroblasts were plated in Dulbecco-Vogt medium containing 10 percent calf serum onto 60-mm plastic Petri dishes at 0.5 × 10^{-6} cells per plate and allowed to become confluent. (^{14}C)proline and (^{14}C)lysine, 2 µCi/ml each, were added to the cultures, and incubation was continued for 24 hours. The cells and the culture medium were harvested, dialyzed vs. 0.5 M acetic acid, hydrolyzed, and the total radioactivity incorporated measured by liquid scintillation counting. Proline and hydroxyproline were isolated on an amino acid analyzer, and the radioactivity was measured.

effectively stimulated collagen synthesis by cultures of embryonic 10-day-old chick tibia.[20] On the other hand, Raisz and Koolemans-Beynan, using cultures of 21-day-old fetal rat calvaria found that PGE$_2$ inhibited collagen production but did not affect synthesis of noncollagen proteins.[194] Using cultures of cells from human fetal bone (presumed to be fibroblasts) Manner and Kuleba demonstrated that the presence of 1 mM cAMP reduced total protein synthesis by 30 to 50 percent, while collagen synthesis was enhanced by 20 to 35 percent.[150] A similar enhancement by cAMP of collagen production by sarcoma cells in culture was reported by Peterkofsky and Prather.[188]

The results of exposing fibroblasts in culture to prostaglandins are more clear-cut than the results obtained from bone cultures. Prostaglandins reduce fibroblast synthetic activity, presumably by elevating levels of cAMP. The addition of PGE$_1$ at a concentration of 0.2 µg/ml to cultures of fibroblasts results in a rise in cAMP levels.[147] A similar enhancement in levels of cAMP was shown by Kelly and Butcher in cultures of lung fibroblasts, and in this case, release of cAMP to the medium by the cells was observed.[121] Prostaglandins affect synthetic activity by human gingival fibroblasts maintained in culture. PGE$_1$, PGE$_2$ and to a lesser extent PGFα inhibit total synthetic activity, protein synthesis, and collagen synthesis by about 50 percent (Table 8-10). Specific effects on collagen synthesis such as those described above for bone cultures were not seen. The inhibitory effects became maximal within 12 hours where they plateaued and were maintained for at least 36 hours.

Bone Resorption

Of all the biologic effects of the prostaglandins, their role in the induction of bone resorption is likely to be of greatest importance to our understanding of the inflammatory periodontal lesion. The potential of the prostaglandins and other substances as mediators of bone resorption has been investigated using cultures of fetal bones labeled *in vivo* with radioactive calcium.[77,94,125,195] This system appears to yield biologically useful information, since the cultures contain chemically defined medium, the morphology of induced resorption is similar to that seen *in vivo*, and the response of the cultures to parathyroid hormone, vitamin A, metabolites of vitamin D, thyrocalcitonin, and diphosphonate is comparable to that seen in bone.[65,91,193,196] Concentrations of prostaglandin PGE$_1$ or PGE$_2$ in the range of 10^{-6} to 10^{-8} M induce remarkable resorption in these cultures.[125] These effects are inhibited by thyrocalcitonin and cortisol and they appear to be mediated by cAMP.[32]

Participation in Periodontal Disease

A large body of evidence supports the idea that the prostaglandins, especially PGE$_1$ and PGE$_2$, may be involved in chronic inflammatory periodontal disease. Prostaglandins have the capacity *in vitro* to mediate the acute inflammatory response, modulate the immune response, suppress mitotic activity, alter the synthetic activity of various cells, and stimulate bone resorption. Prostaglandins are present in inflamed human gingiva and in periodontal exudates at concentrations sufficiently high to induce most of the biologic activities demonstrated *in vitro*.[78] The subdermal injection of prostaglandin solutions adjacent to bone in the rat over a period of 7 days induces resorption of the bone;[79] thus, prostaglandins appear to exercise properties demonstrated *in vitro* when administered locally *in vivo.*

Some aspects of the periodontal lesion in which prostaglandins may participate include the following: (1) mediation of the acute inflammatory response, which is the earliest manifestation of tissue alteration following the beginning of plaque accumulation, (2) inhibition of both the mitogenic and the antigenic responses of lymphocytes and suppression of the immune response, (3) inhibition of fibroblast mitosis, with consequent failure to replace cytopathologically altered cells in the marginal gingiva, (4) suppression of the synthesis and turnover of collagen and noncollagenous proteins of the connective tissues, and (5) induction of resorption of the alveolar bone.

MECHANISMS OF TISSUE ALTERATION

The chronic inflammatory periodontal lesion is extremely complex at any stage and its pathologic features change with the passage of time (see Ch. 7). It seems unlikely that a single mechanism underlies all aspects of the disease, as no single mechanism can account for all the features observed. Furthermore, it is likely that the etiologic agent activating one mechanism is not the same as that responsible for another. For example, the etiologies and the mechanisms accounting for bone resorption may differ from those related to fibrosis or epithelial proliferation. Thus, we propose to discuss mechanisms that may relate to (1) development of the acute inflammatory response and conversion of the junctional epithelium into pocket epithelium, (2) alterations in the periodontal connective tissues, and (3) bone resorption.

Conversion of the Junctional Epithelium into Pocket Epithelium

During the first few days following the beginning of microbial plaque accumulation, an acute inflammatory response develops,[3,88,137,171,187,217,218] and the normal relationship between the gingival tissue and the calcified tooth surface becomes altered (see Ch. 7). The microcirculation just deep to the junctional epithelium and lateral to the base of the gingival sulcus exhibits a classic exudative acute inflammation.[181] There is an outpouring of serum proteins; the tissues become laden with fibrin and immunoglobulin, large numbers of polymorphonuclear leukocytes transmigrate across the vessels and junctional epithelium, and a large proportion of the perivascular collagen is lost. Abnormally large numbers of nonepithelial cells, including neutrophils, mononuclear cells, mast cells, and plasma cells, appear in the junctional epithelium. The basal epithe-

lial cells begin to proliferate and to extend into the connective tissues and along the root surface with rete ridge formation. Abnormal maturational patterns may appear in the junctional epithelial cells, with keratinization in some cases and cell death in others. Vascular loops extend high into the epithelial tissues and microulcerations appear. These events lead to the conversion of the junctional epithelium to pocket epithelium. This conversion begins in the coronal portion of the junctional epithelium and extends in an apical direction; as the sulcus deepens and a pocket forms, a short strand of reasonably normal junctional epithelium generally persists near the most apical termination.[217]

Mechanisms underlying induction of acute inflammation and conversion of the junctional epithelium into pocket epithelium have not been explained, although several likely possibilities are apparent. Initially the idea that substances elaborated by plaque microorganisms induce the changes directly was considered,[222,223] and the possibility that this does indeed occur has not been ruled out. Plaque microorganisms do elaborate substances, especially enzymes, that have the capacity to break down the extracellular epithelial substances and induce direct cytotoxic effects. However, the realization that the tissues themselves can serve as a source of potentially toxic substances has lead to modification of the idea. Plaque elaborates and releases highly diffusable small peptides which are potent chemotactic agents for polymorphonuclear leukocytes.[138,244] These substances have the capacity to induce an acute inflammation of the type observed, and application of these compounds to the gingival tissues does induce such a reaction. Therefore, these agents may account for the transmigration of neutrophils, enhanced vascular permeability, and the extravasation of serum proteins.

The large population of nonepithelial cells that come to reside in the junctional epithelium during the early stage of the disease may also contribute to the toxic reactions. Large amounts of fluid derived from the serum and containing immunoglobulins (the crevicular fluid) pass through the connective and epithelial tissues, possibly leading to immune-complex formation and the entrance of bacterial antigens. Neutrophils encountering these substances may release their lysosomal enzymes and other proteases, and macrophages may undergo activation with the long-term production of a variety of hydrolases. Approximately half of the leukocytes appearing in the junctional epithelium or pocket epithelium are mononuclear cells,[215,216] and many of these cells appear to be undergoing transformation. If this is the case, lymphotoxin may be released. In addition, there is some evidence that the lymphoid cells may be involved in cytotoxic reactions with the epithelial cells.[159,205]

TABLE 8-11. *Collagen Content of Normal and Periodontally Diseased Beagle Dog Gingiva*[a]

	SALT-SOLUBLE	ACID-SOLUBLE	INSOLUBLE	TOTAL
Normal gingiva	0.05 (0.01)	0.12 (0.04)	8.61 (0.44)	8.79 (0.45)
Diseased gingiva	0.10 (0.05)	0.15 (0.08)	6.10 (1.21)	6.35 (1.21)

Unpublished data of Page, R. C., Lindhe, J., Narayanan, A. S.
[a]Reported as μg hydroxyproline/mg wet tissue (S.D).

Mast cells make up a portion of the nonepithelial cell population in the pocket epithelium, and Barnett has suggested that they too may play a destructive role.[8] Mast-cell granules contain potent trypsinlike neutral proteases. Enzymes of this type are known to dissociate epithelial cells one from another. They are presumed to digest the extracellular substance and to lyse the intercellular junctions. An event of this sort in the junctional or pocket epithelium would be expected to lead to an influx of serum proteins and leukocytes, which could be beneficial in defense against bacterial substances in the gingival sulcus or pocket. However, it seems likely that the reverse passage of bacterial substances into the connective tissues from the pocket would also occur, leading to perpetuation of the lesion.

Mechanisms and substances to account for the initiation of proliferation of the junctional epithelial cells and extension of the vascular loops are not currently known.

The Connective-Tissue Alterations

In normal gingiva, intricately organized groups of collagen fiber bundles, along with the proteoglycans of the ground substance, make up the bulk of the marginal gingiva (see Ch. 1).[176] These fiber bundles provide support to the junction between the gingiva and the tooth surface, they are responsible for the tissue tone, and they enmesh the capillary plexus and microcirculation immediately subjacent to the junctional epithelium. These fibers are essential for the normal function of the marginal gingiva which separates the external environment from the connective tissues. During an early stage of inflammatory gingival and periodontal disease (see Ch. 7), the resident fibroblasts become cytopathically altered,[220] and there are changes in the quality and quantity of the connective-tissue substance.[5,27,66,153] There is a significant net decrease in the total collagen content (Table 8-11).[174, 180,210,221] The magnitude of this decrease within the infiltrated tissue is in the range of 60 to 70 percent (Table 8-12). In both the gingiva and the periodontal ligament, the solubility properties and the pattern of cross-linking of collagen are altered (Table 8-11).[185] In the later stages of chronic periodontitis, fibrosis and scarring become increasingly important aspects of the disease and account for some of the functional aberations and clinical manifestations. These changes in the connective-tissue substance play an important role in the continuing loss of tissue integrity as the disease progresses.

Microorganisms are ultimately responsible for provoking the connective-tissue and other alterations characteristic of gingivitis and periodontitis in hu-

TABLE 8-12. *Total Collagen Content of Human Gingiva*

	DENSITY COLLAGEN FIBERS/mm^{3a} OF CONNECTIVE TISSUE	μg HYDROXYPROLINE[b] PER μg DRY CONNECTIVE TISSUE
Noninfilterated connective tissue	565.71 $\pm$ 72.29	0.091 $\pm$ 0.012
Infilterated connective tissue	160.75 $\pm$ 74.06	0.037 $\pm$ 0.009

[a]Schroeder, H. E., Münzel-Pedrazzoli, S., and Page, R. C.: Correlated morphometric and biochemical analysis of gingival tissue in early chronic gingivitis in man. Arch. Oral. Biol., *18*:899, 1973.
[b]Flieder, D. E., Sun, C. N., and Schneider, B. C.: Chemistry of normal and inflamed human gingival tissues. Periodontics, *4*:302, 1966.

mans.[85,141,208] and in animals.[88,140,213] Since the work of Schultz-Haudt and his colleagues,[223] investigators have considered the idea that hydrolytic enzymes elaborated by plaque microorganisms may enter the gingival tissues and degrade the connective-tissue substance. This idea was given a considerable boost when Macdonald and his co-workers demonstrated that *Bacteroides melaninogenicus*, a resident of human dental plaque, has the capacity to produce collagenase, and several investigators found acid hydrolases capable of digestion of the constituents of the connective tissue present in plaque extracts.[142] However, the possibility that direct toxicity mechanisms of this sort are of major importance became less attractive when it was shown that collagenase can be produced by the periodontal tissues as well as by neutrophils and macrophages populating periodontal lesions. While innumerable potentially toxic substances are present in plaque,[235] it appears unlikely that these substances act only by direct means to induce the connective-tissue alterations. In contrast to acute necrotizing ulcerative gingivitis,[139] microorganisms do not appear to invade the gingival tissues in commonly encountered inflammatory gingival and periodontal disease. Most of the evidence indicates that the presence of plaque initiates immunopathologic and other destructive inflammatory mechanisms in the host and that these, in turn, lead to the observed tissue alterations.[180,181]

Since the total amount of collagen present in a tissue is determined, at least in part, by the relative rates of production and degradation, an alteration in amount may result from an imbalance in these relative rates. Thus, the mechanisms participating in the decrease in the size of the total collagenous component of inflamed gingiva may relate to an overall decrease in the production of collagen or to an accentuated level of collagen degradation. Mechanisms of the latter type, frequently referred to as collagen destruction, are considered to involve accentuated levels of activity of enzymes such as collagenase and acid hydrolase. Only recently have mechanisms relating to depressed rates of collagen production been considered.

MECHANISMS ENHANCING COLLAGEN DESTRUCTION OR DEGRADATION

Most of the data now available indicate that alterations of the connective tissue substance can be accounted for most readily by the activities of cells responding to interaction with plaque-derived substances. This approach to understanding these alterations is illustrated schematically in Figure 8-13. The interaction of these substances with the phagocytic cells appears to be particularly important (Pathways 1 and 5).

Small numbers of neutrophils consistently transmigrate through the normal marginal gingival tissue. However, with the beginning of plaque accumulation, the numbers increase remarkably, and, along with the other manifestations of acute inflammation which characterize the initial stage of inflammatory gingival and periodontal disease, lysosomal granules may appear within the extravascular connective tissues (Fig. 7-8B).[181] Concurrently, there is loss of the perivascular collagen fibers. Whether these events are related remains unclear, although the neutrophils have the capacity to induce the damage observed.[110] In addition to the various bactericidal substances, neutrophils carry potent acid hydrolases and a collagenase having the capacity to destroy collagen and other connective tissue substances.[87] When neutrophils ingest certain bacterial substances including dental plaque (Pathway 5) or immune complexes (Pathway 4b), their hydrolytic enzymes are released.[35,97,99,243,259,260]

Macrophages are present in normal gingival tissues, and the population increases significantly at an early stage of inflammatory gingival and periodontal disease.[219] These cells have the capacity to undergo activation and are considered to be a prime participant in the tissue destruction accompanying chronic inflammation and delayed-hypersensitivity reactions. Although there is virtually no information regarding their activity within the inflamed gingiva, the response of these cells *in vitro* has been studied. When exposed to dental plaque, endotoxin, and streptococcal cell walls (Pathway 1) or to lymphokines (Pathway 2b), the cells undergo activation (Fig. 8-4) and produce and secrete hydrolytic enzymes, including the lysosomal hydrolases, neutral protease, and collagenase (Tables 8-2, 8-3).[45,80,177-179,182,183,251] These enzymes have the capacity to degrade the collagen fibers and proteoglycans of the connective-tissue matrix. In addition, it has been suggested that macrophages, and possibly fibroblasts, have the capacity to resorb collagen fibers by phagocytosis.[184]

The role of collagenase in the observed destruction of collagen in inflammatory gingival and periodontal disease and in chronic inflammatory lesions generally may be especially important. With the possible exception of cathepsin, collagenase is the only enzyme able to cleave the native intact collagen molecule. The enzyme was first detected in the tail of the tadpole,[86] and it has been found subsequently in numerous human and animal tissues. In addition to its presence in neutrophilic leukocytes,[132] and its production and secretion by activated macrophages,[183,251] the enzyme can be produced by cells in bone,[253,265,266] and by normal gingiva.[14,18,67-69,186] The amount of activity that can be detected in bits of inflamed tissue in culture

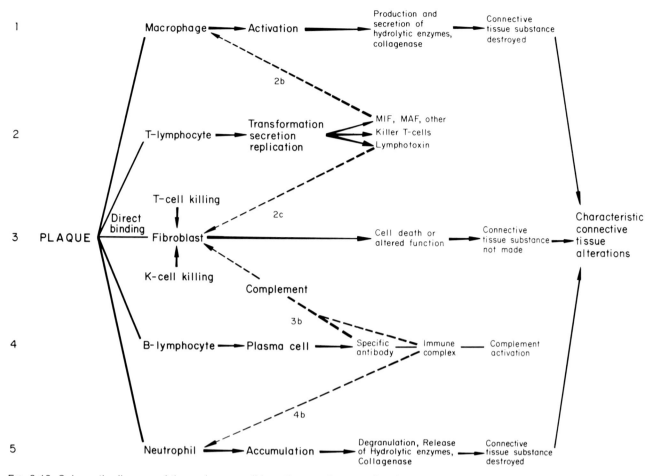

FIG. 8-13. *Schematic diagram of the various possible pathways of connective tissue substance alteration in inflammatory gingival and periodontal disease.*

is greater than in normal clinically noninflamed tissue.[16,60,90,132] These observations have led to the idea that collagenase, along with other neutral proteases and possibly the acid hydrolases, is chiefly responsible for the tissue alterations characteristic of many forms of inflammatory disease.

SUPPRESSION OF COLLAGEN PRODUCTION

Recent observations provide evidence to support the hypothesis, first elaborated over a decade ago,[221] that the loss of connective-tissue substance in inflamed gingiva may be a consequence of depressed collagen production rather than of enhanced collagen destruction. Even in adults gingival collagen turns over at an inordinately high rate (see Ch. 1);[31,34,41,175,228] thus, even a minor decrease in the rate of production could result, with the passage of time, in a decrease in collagen content.

Experimental evidence indicates that a decreased production does occur in human gingiva immediately following the beginning of plaque accumulation.[116]

Premolar interdental papillae taken from 10 young adults after 3 weeks of intensive plaque control and again after 10 days of plaque accumulation were diced into small cubes and placed in culture in the presence of radioactively labeled amino acids under conditions leading to maximum synthetic activity. Although the total synthetic activity of the plaque-exposed gingival tissue was greater than that of the control normal tissue, the amount of collagen produced by the plaque-exposed tissue was reduced relative to the control by about 30 percent. A similar result of about the same magnitude was found in labeling experiments done *in vivo* in marmosets with early periodontitis (Page, Levy, and Narayanan, unpublished).

There appear to be at least three pathways through which the level of collagen production can be decreased, and all of these operate through the gingival fibroblast. As noted previously, cytopathic alterations have been observed in these cells at an early stage of inflammatory disease (Figs. 7-14, 7-15).[220,227] Direct binding of plaque substances by fibroblasts (Pathway 3) may induce cytopathic alterations and inhibit collagen

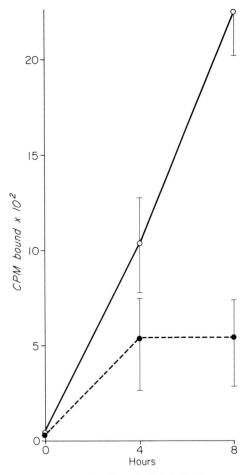

FIG. 8-14. *The binding of radioactively labeled homogenates of* Actinomyces viscosus *by mouse gingival fibroblasts maintained in culture. The medium contained 25 μg/ml homogenate. In cultures containing 0.1 percent sodium azide (_ _ _ _ _), a compound which inhibits ingestion by the cells but does not prevent binding to the cell membrane, the uptake of radioactivity reached a plateau at 4 hours. In cultures not containing azide (_____), binding continued linearly for 8 hours. Thus, the cells appear to bind and to injest the labeled bacterial substance. (Engle, L. D.: Unpublished observations.)*

synthesis. As shown in Fig. 8-14 and Tables 8-13 and 8-14 gingival fibroblasts maintained *in vitro* do avidly bind microbial substances, including homogenates of *Actinomyces viscosus*, although the treated cells synthesize protein and collagen at a normal rate. Therefore, direct binding does occur, but the pathway does not appear to account for collagen loss.[56] Microorganisms from dental plaque can interact *in vitro* with T-lymphocytes antigenically to induce blastogenesis (Pathway 3)[107,112] with the production of lymphokines[106] and the generation of cytotoxic cells. Fibroblast cytotoxicity may result from the direct nonspecific action of lymphotoxin, or from the direct cell-cell interaction of T-lymphocytes sensitized to bacterial antigens displayed on the surface of the gingival fibro-

TABLE 8-13. *Cytotoxicity Assays on Human Gingival Fibroblasts Previously Exposed to Homogenates of* Actinomyces Viscosus *or Dental Plaque*

ASSAY	CONTROL	AVIS	PLAQUE
LDH[a]	283 (25)	341 (9)	396 (3)
Microcytoxicity[b]	59 (4)	55 (4)	N.D.

Engel, L. D., et al.: Unpublished.
Human gingival fibroblasts were cultured for 72 hours in the presence of 25 μg/ml *Actinomyces viscosus* (AVIS) or plaque homogenates.
[a] Lactic dehydrogenase, a cytoplasmic enzyme that leaks from damaged cells, was not decreased in the treated cells.
[b] The mean number of fibroblasts remaining in microtest wells was not significantly altered by exposure to AVIS homogenate.

blasts (Pathway 2c). Specific antibody may bind to bacterial antigens on the fibroblast surface, with activation of the complement sequence and cell lysis (Pathway 3b) or killing by immune complex-dependent lymphoid cells (K-cells).[23] Whether these pathways are operative *in vivo*, or indeed whether some of them can be made to operate *in vitro*, remains unknown.

In addition to the pathways illustrated, the possible role of the prostaglandins in inhibition of collagen synthesis at sites of inflammation must be considered. The exact source of the prostglandin in inflamed gingiva is not known, although biologically significant concentrations are present.[78] Prostaglandins E_1, E_2, and F-α all affect fibroblast function.

ALTERATION OF THE COLLAGEN TYPE

As periodontal disease progresses, fibrosis and scarring become of increasing importance. These features account for the thickening of the gingiva and the

TABLE 8-14. *Effects of Binding of Homogenates of* Actinomyces Viscosus *to Human Gingival Fibroblasts upon Their Ability to Synthesize Collagen and Noncollagenous Protein*

	HYPRO	PROLINE	HYP/PRO-HYP
Control	6.8 (1.6)[a]	156 (32)[a]	4.2
A. viscosus-treated	9.7 (2.5)	176 (12)	5.2

Monolayers of human gingival fibroblasts were cultured in the presence of 50 μg/ml *Actinomyces viscousus* homogenate for 48 hours in medium containing 2 μCi/ml (^{14}C)-proline. Incorporation of label and hydroxylation of proline, indications of collagen synthesis, were slightly increased in the exposed cultures.
[a] Reported as CPM/plate $\times 10^{-3}$.

aberrant architecture necessitating surgical treatment. The nature of the accumulating fibrotic material is not known, although it appears to be collagenous. Thus, one mechanism of importance underlying the collagenous alterations may be the production of abnormal collagens or the production of normal molecules in abnormal amounts. Collagens making up normal gingival and periodontal tissue have not yet been characterized, although the data available indicate that type I is the principal constituent, with type III as a minor component.[6,26,160] Fibroblasts derived from normal interdental papillae of young adults and maintained *in vitro* synthesize both types I and III collagens with the proportion of type III molecules ranging from 5 to 20 percent. Cells obtained from periodontally diseased gingiva, on the other hand, may not synthesize type III molecules at all, and about 20 to 30 percent of the material made appears to be an abnormal, previously undescribed molecule.[160] Whether this material exists in inflamed periodontal tissues and just what its significance may be remain unclear.

Bone Resorption

Loss of alveolar bone is the most critical aspect of inflammatory periodontal disease with regard to tooth loss. Bone formation and turnover during growth and in the normal adult are not well understood, and there is virtually no information about the behavior of bone in inflammatory pathological situations. In periodontitis, bone loss may be of a generalized horizontal type in which all the teeth are affected more or less equally, or isolated bone craters affecting single teeth may be seen. While substances derived from microbial plaque or specific microorganisms residing in periodontal pockets are ultimately responsible for triggering bone loss, the means by which this occurs remains an enigma. It has been presumed that the resorption is a consequence of osteoclastic action, although this point has not been documented. Microbial substances may affect bone directly, causing differentiation of osteoclasts and resorption, or these substances may inhibit bone formation. Furthermore, the effects of microbial substances may be achieved through activation of other cells such as lymphocytes and macrophages to produce substances that affect bone. The latter possibility currently seems the most attractive.

Although there has been great interest and a flurry of research in attempting to achieve bone regeneration with grafts and transplants, until recently almost no research effort had concentrated on the basic mechanisms underlying alveolar bone resorption. The development by Raisz and his colleagues of a tissue-culture system in which bone resorption can be studied has

been an important catalyst.[77,91,125,193,195] Basically, this system involves the maintenance of embryonic long bones previously labeled with radioactive calcium in culture along with the addition of various putative bone resorption agents.

Substances of three types have been identified as inducers of bone resorption *in vitro*. These include microbial material from dental plaque, substances extracted from gingiva, and factors generated by activation of the immune system and complement cascade. The first type includes endotoxin derived from gram-negative bacteria, lipoteichoic acid from the cell wall of gram-positive microorganisms, and a soluble extract of whole plaque (Table 8-15).[91-94] The activity of endotoxin and lipoteichoic acid resides in the glycolipid portion of the molecule. Heparin, a component of mast cells that is released during injury, does not have the capacity to induce bone resorption directly, although it is a potent enhancer of resorption by endotoxin and other microbial substances.[76] Other substances classically associated with the acute inflammatory response, including bradykinin, histamine, and lysosomal enzymes, are unable to stimulate resorption.[91]

Goldhaber has shown that extracts of normal and periodontally diseased human gingiva exert bone resorption activity in the *in vitro* system, although the nature of the active substance has not been determined.[77] The prostaglandins, which are present in inflamed gingiva and in the exudate of periodontal pockets in high concentrations, are potent inducers of bone resorption.[78,79]

Complement-sufficient serum, but not complement-deficient serum, has the capacity to induce resorption, presumably through its activation by immune complex.[95,197] Complement activation leads to an in-

TABLE 8-15. *Induction of Bone Resorption in Culture by Various Substances*

SUBSTANCE	^{45}Ca RELEASE, EXPERIMENTAL/CONTROL
Endotoxin	3.30 (0.15)
Lipoteichoic acid	1.96 (0.22)
Plaque extract	3.69 (0.18)
Parathyroid hormone	3.24 (0.22)

Hausmann, E.: Potential pathways for bone resorption in human periodontal disease. J. Periodontal., 45:388, 1974.

Embryonic rat limb bones prelabeled with ^{45}Ca were precultured for 24 hours and incubated for 2 days. The ratio of ^{45}Ca released by experimental as compared with control bones is based on that released during days 2 and 3 after a 24-hour preculture period. The ratio determined for each agent represents ^{45}Ca release from 8 experimental and 8 control bones.

crease in prostaglandin levels in the cultures that parallels increased resorption; both prostaglandin production and bone resorption can be prevented by the addition of indomethacin, an inhibitor of prostaglandin synthetase, to the culture medium.[197] Whether bacterial substances such as endotoxin that induce bone resorption act via the alternate pathway of complement activation and prostaglandin production remains unknown.

Activation of the immune system also appears to have the potential for causing bone resorption. Horton and his colleagues have shown that peripheral blood leukocytes from normal or periodontally diseased individuals stimulated with the mitogen phytohemagglutinin, and leukocytes from individuals with periodontal disease stimulated with plaque antigens undergo blast transformation and produce a lymphokine which is a potent stimulator of bone resorption (Table 8-16).[107] This substance, which has not been further characterized, has been called osteoclast activating factor (OAF).

SUMMARY

Although it is generally agreed that bacterial substances in dental plaque comprise the primary etiologic agent responsible for gingival and periodontal

TABLE 8-16. *Induction of Bone Resorption* in vitro *by a Factor Released from Activated Lymphoid Cells*

ADDITIONS TO LYMPHOID CELL CULTURES	^{45}Ca RELEASE FROM BONE IN CULTURE BY LYMPHOID CELL SUPERNATANT
Control culture medium	
None	0.93 (0.04)
PHA	0.88 (0.03)
Antigen	0.99 (0.04)
Lymphoid cell culture medium	
None	1.30 (0.02)
PHA	1.48 (0.03)[a]
Antigen	2.97 (0.17)[a]

Horton, J. E., et al.: Bone resorbing activity in supernatant fluid from cultured human peripheral blood leukocytes. Science, *177*:793, 1972.
Leukocyte cultures were from an individual with chronic periodontitis and were maintained for 6 days in the presence of phytohemagglutinin (PHA) or plaque-derived antigen in autologous plasma. The supernatants were then transferred to bone cultures.
[a]$P < 0.01$.

disease, many significant features of the disease cannot be accounted for by these substances alone. For example, neither the broad spectrum of host susceptibility observed among individuals and various animal species, nor the variation in prevalence and extent of the disease from tooth to tooth can be accounted for by bacterial factors alone. Furthermore, the well-documented fact that prevalence and extent of the disease increase linearly with increasing age is more likely to be a consequence of intrinsic host-related factors than of extrinsic bacterial substances. Thus, the response of the defense mechanisms of the host appears to play an overriding role in the pathogenesis of the disease. Indeed, the data currently available indicate that substances derived from microorganisms are pathogenic because they have the capacity to activate certain host defense mechanisms that serve as amplifiers and induce the tissue damage observed.

Numerous pathways that may lead to pathologic tissue alterations in chronic inflammatory lesions have been identified. Most of these observations have been made in *in vitro* systems, and whether they function in the gingival tissues in inflammatory periodontal disease remains undetermined, although the likelihood appears to be high. Substances derived from microorganisms present at the dentogingival junction and in the periodontal pocket appear to have the capacity to traverse the junctional epithelium and enter the gingival tissues in both normal and pathologically altered tissues. These substances can interact with several different types of cells. They can exert an antigenic effect on previously sensitized cells or a mitogenic effect upon previously nonsensitized cells. While these effects may be in part protective, they may also wreak havoc on the tissues in which the reactions are occurring, especially if they go uncontrolled. Some of the possible deleterious pathways are illustrated in Figures 8-15 and 8-16.

Antigenic activation of previously sensitized B- and T-lymphocytes results in blastogenesis, with the production of lymphokines, the differentiation of mature antibody-producing plasma cells and cells with the capacity to kill target cells carrying the sensitizing antigen, and the generation of memory cells (Fig. 8-4). Many of these same responses can be induced by mitogens in nonsensitized lymphoid cells. Individuals with periodontal disease have circulating cells that can undergo these responses, including lymphokine production, and microbial plaque can induce them. Lymphoid cells, especially B-lymphocytes and plasma cells, predominate throughout the course of the inflammatory periodontal lesion. Plaque contains numerous antigens as well as potent B-cell mitogens. Thus, there is a large body of circumstantial evidence

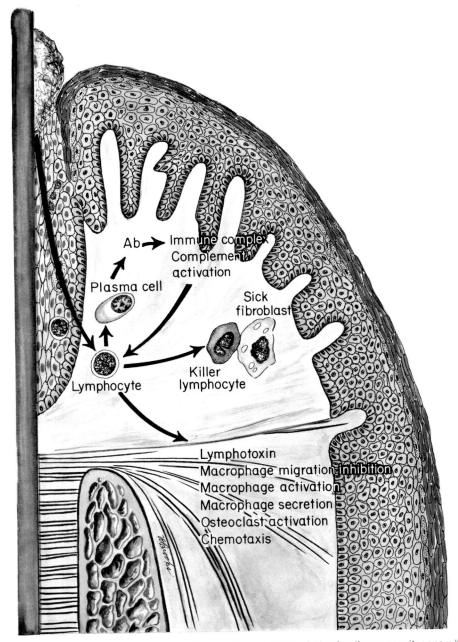

FIG. 8-15. *Schematic diagram of the possible pathways of interaction of plaque-derived antigens or mitogens with lymphoid cells in the periodontal tissues, along with some of the possible consequences.*

that reactions of the type illustrated in Figures 8-13 and 8-14 do occur.

The relative magnitude of the beneficial vs. detrimental effects of the events described above in tissues is not known, although numerous potentially destructive pathways are possible (Figs. 8-15 and 8-16). For example, released lymphotoxin may be responsible for the cytopathic alterations of fibroblasts in the gingival tissues or, alternatively, the altered fibroblasts may carry on their surfaces bacterial antigens to which

killer lymphoid cells are sensitized and direct cell-cell interactions may lead to the observed alterations. Transformed lymphoid cells may release osteoclast-activating factor causing extensive bone resorption and also chemotactic factors that attract both neutrophils and monocytes to the reactive site. The monocytes may become activated and produce and secrete lysosomal enzymes and collagenase. These substances have the capacity to induce destructive changes within the connective-tissue substance that are characteristic of

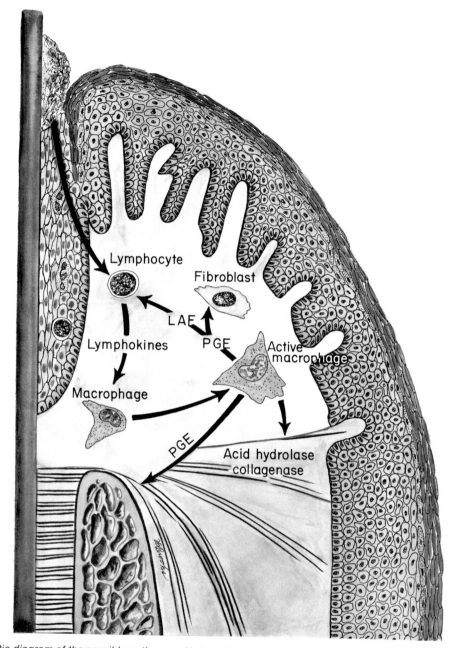

FIG. 8-16. *Schematic diagram of the possible pathways of interaction of plaque-derived antigens or mitogens with lymphoid cells in the periodontal tissues, along with some of the possible consequences.*

the disease. In addition, activated macrophages appear to have the capacity to produce prostaglandins, and these substances can lead to bone resorption, decreased levels of bone formation, and inhibition of fibroblast activity. At sites where bone and connective-tissue turnover are unusually high, as is apparently the case in the periodontium, these events could prove highly deleterious.

Antigenic stimulation can also lead to differentiation of mature plasma cells and the local production of specific antibody. In the presence of plaque antigens, immune-complex formation and the activation of the complement sequence, degranulation of mast cells and enhancement and perpetuation of the inflammatory response may be expected to occur.

Several potential control pathways are apparent. Some of these may lead to amplification and intensification of the response, but others would tend to suppress activity. For example, in addition to enhancing the inflammatory response, immune-complex formation and activation of the complement sequence would generate C3b, a substance with the capacity to activate additional B-cells. Thus, immune-complex formation could tend to perpetuate the reaction by enlarging the plasma-cell population. Another such pathway may operate through the macrophage (Fig. 8-16). Stimulated lymphocytes lead to accumulation and activation of macrophages and the production of lymphocyte-activating factor (LAF) enhancing the reactivity of the lymphoid cells. On the other hand, some of the same pathways appear to have the potential to dampen or control the various interactions. For example, although the prostaglandins may cause bone resorption and decreased bone and collagen production, they are also potent inhibitors of blastogenesis of both B- and T-lymphocytes. Thus, their release may tend to bring the reactions under control.

Major advances have been made in recent years in the available information regarding normal host defense mechanisms, inflammatory and immunopathologic aspects of tissue destruction, and mechanisms underlying chronic inflammation. Most of this new information has been obtained from cell and tissue-culture systems, and most of it is currently only at the stage of phenomenology. Indeed, in only rare instances have the biologically active factors or substances been isolated, identified, and characterized biochemically. Furthermore, the activities of these various substances and cells *in vivo* in actual chronic inflammatory lesions have not been studied to any great extent, and whether they participate in inflammatory periodontal lesions has not been established. Indeed, scientists investigating the host aspects of chronic periodontitis today are afflicted with a phlethora of possible mechanisms and pathways that could be important in its pathogenesis and that can, at least conceptually, account for the tissue damage and alterations seen. The major tests now faced are the determination of which of these possibilities are real and the development of means by which the pathways can be modified to produce the most desirable results.

References

1. Ackerman, N. R., and Beebe, J. R.: Release of lysosomal enzymes by alveolar mononuclear cells. Nature, *247*:475, 1974.
2. Anggard, E., and Jonsson, C. E.: Efflux of prostaglandins in lymph from scalded tissue. Acta Physiol. Scand., *81*:440, 1971.
3. Attström, R.: Studies on neutrophil polymorphonuclear leukocytes at the dento-gingival junction in gingival health and disease. J. Periodont. Res., *8*(Suppl):1, 1971.
4. Bahn, A. N.: Microbial potential in the etiology of periodontal disease. J. Periodontol., *41*:603, 1970.
5. Balazs, E. A., and Rogers, H. J.: The amino sugar-containing compounds in bones and teeth. The Amino Sugars IIA, 263, 1965.
6. Ballard, P. B., and Butler, W. T.: Proteins of the periodontium. Biochemical studies on the collagen and noncollagen proteins of human gingiva. J. Oral Path., *3*:176, 1974.
7. Baram, P., and Arnold, L.: Immunologic aspects of periodontal disease. J. Periodontol. *41*:617, 1970.
8. Barnett, M. L.: The fine structure of human epithelial mast cells in periodontal disease. J. Periodont. Res., *8*:371, 1973.
9. Barnett, M. L.: Mast cells in the epithelial layer of human gingiva. J. Ultrastruct. Res., *43*:247, 1973.
10. Barnett, M. L.: The fine structure of human connective tissue mast cells in periodontal disease. J. Periodont. Res., *9*:84, 1974.
11. Bellanti, J. A.: Immunology. Philadelphia, W. B. Saunders Co., 1971.
12. Benditt, E. P., and Lagunoff, D.: The mast cell: its structure and function. Prog. Allergy, *8*:195, 1964.
13. Bennett, B., and Bloom, B. R.: Reactions in vivo and in vitro produced by a soluble substance associated with delayed-type hypersensitivity. Proc. Nat. Acad. Sci., USA, *59*:756, 1968.
14. Bennick, A., and Hunt, A. M.: Collagenolytic activity in oral tissues. Arch. Oral Biol., *12*:1, 1967.
15. Berglund, S. E.: Immunoglobulins in human gingiva with specificity for oral bacteria. J. Periodontol., *42*:546, 1971.
16. Beutner, E. H., Triftshauser, C., and Hazen, S. P.: Collagenase activity of gingival tissue from patients with periodontal disease. Proc. Soc. Exp. Biol. Med., *121*:1082, 1966.
17. Bickley, H. C.: A concept of allergy with reference to oral disease. J. Periodontol., *41*:302, 1970.
18. Birkedal-Hansen, H., et al.: Bovine gingival collagenase: demonstration and initial characterization. J. Oral Pathol., *3*:232, 1974.
19. Bloom, B. R., and Bennett, B.: Mechanisms of a reaction in vitro associated with delayed-type hypersensitivity. Science, *153*:80, 1966.
20. Blumenkrantz, H., and Sondergaard, J.: Effect of prostaglandins E_1 and F_{1a} on biosynthesis of collagen. Nature [New Biol.], *239*:246, 1972.
21. Bourne, H. R., Epstein, L. B., and Melmon, K. L.: Lymphocyte cyclic adenosine monophosphate (AMP) synthesis and inhibition of phytohemagglutinin-induced transformation. J. Clin. Invest., *50*:10a, 1971.
22. Bourne, H. R., Lichtenstein, L. M., and Melmon, K. L.: Pharmacologic control of allergic histamine release in vitro: evidence for an inhibitory role of 3′,5′-adenosine monophosphate in human leukocytes. J. Immunol., *108*:695, 1972.
23. Brandtzaeg, P.: Local factors of resistance in the gingival area. J. Periodont. Res., *1*:19, 1966.

24. Brandtzaeg, P.: Local formation and transport of immunoglobulins related to the oral cavity. *In* Host Resistance to Communsal Bacteria. T. MacPhee, Ed. Edinburgh, Churchill Livingstone, 1972, pages 116–150.

25. Brandtzaeg, P., and Kraus, F. W.: Autoimmunity and periodontal disease. Odont. Tidskr., 73:281, 1965.

26. Butler, W. T., et al.: Proteins of the periodontium. Identification of collagens with the $\alpha 1(I)_2\alpha_2$ and $\alpha 1(III)_3$ structures in bovine periodontal ligament. J. Biol. Chem., 250:8907, 1975.

27. Cabrini, R. L., and Carranza, F. A.: Histochemistry of periodontal tissues. A review of the literature. Int. Dent. J., 16:466, 1966.

28. Calderon, J., and Unanue, E. R.: Two biological activities regulating cell proliferation found in cultures of peritoneal exudate cells. Nature, 253:359, 1975.

29. Calderon, J., Williams, R. T., and Unanue, E. R.: An inhibitor of cell proliferation released by cultures of macrophages. Proc. Nat. Acad. Sci., 71:4273, 1974.

30. Cardella, C. J., Davies, P., and Allison, A. C.: Immune complexes induce selective release of lysosomal hydrolases from macrophages. Nature, 247:46, 1974.

31. Carneiro, J. Synthesis and turnover of collagen in periodontal tissues. Symp. Int. Soc. Cell Biol., 4:247, 1965.

32. Chase, L. R., and Aurbach, G. D.: The effect of parathyroid hormone on the concentration of adenosine 3′,5′-monophosphate in skeletal tissue *in vitro*. J. Biol. Chem., 245:1520, 1970.

33. Chisari, F. V., and Edington, T. S.: Human T lymphocyte "E" rosette function. I. A process modulated by intracellular cyclic AMP. J. Exp. Med., 140:1122, 1974.

34. Claycomb, C. K., Summers, G. W., and Dvorak, E. M.: Oral collagen biosynthesis in the guinea pig. J. Periodont. Res., 2:115, 1967.

35. Cochrane, C. G.: The arthus phenomenon: a mechanism of tissue damage. Arthritis Rheum., 10:392, 1967.

36. Cochrane, C. G.: Mechanisms involved in the deposition of immune complexes in tissues. J. Exp. Med., 134:75, 1971.

37. Cohen, S., and Winkler, S.: Cellular immunity and the inflammatory response. J. Periodontol., 45:348, 1974.

38. Collier, H. O. S.: Introduction to the actions of kinins and prostaglandins. Proc. R. Soc. Med., 64:1, 1971.

39. Cooperband, S. R., and Green, J. A.: Production and assay of a lymphocyte derived "proliferation inhibition factor" (PIF). *In In Vitro* Methods in Cell-Mediated Immunity. B. R. Bloom and P. R. Glade, Eds. Academic Press, New York, 1971, p. 381.

40. Coyne, J., et al.: Guinea pig lymphotoxin (LT). II. J. Immunol., 110:1630, 1973.

41. Crumbley, J. P.: Collagen formation in normal and stressed periodontium. Periodontics, 2:53, 1964.

42. Crunkhorn, P., and Willis, A. L.: Interaction between prostaglandins E and F given intradermally in the rat. Br. J. Pharmacol., 41:507, 1971.

43. David, J. R.: Delayed hypersensitivity in vitro: its mediation by cell-free substances formed by lymphoid cell-antigen interaction. Proc. Nat. Acad. Sci., USA, 56:72, 1966.

44. David, J. R., and David, R.: Assay for inhibition of macrophage migration. *In In Vitro* Methods in Cell-Mediated Immunity. B. R. Bloom and P. R. Glade, Eds. Academic Press, New York, 1971, p. 249.

45. Davies, P., Page, R. C., and Allison, A. C.: Changes in cellular enzyme levels and extracellular release of lysosomal acid hydrolases in macrophages exposed to group A streptococcal cell wall substances. J. Exp. Med., 139:1262, 1974.

46. Dienstein, B., Ratcliff, P. A., and Williams, R. K.: Mast cell density and distribution in gingiva biopsies: a quantitative study. J. Periodontol., 38:198, 1967.

47. Dingle, J. T.: The extracellular secretion of lysosomal enzymes. *In* Lysosomes in Biology and Pathology. J. T. Dingle and H. B. Fell, Eds. Amsterdam, North Holland Publishing Co., 2:421, 1969.

48. Dixon, F. J.: Antigen-antibody complexes and autoimmunity. Ann. N.Y. Acad. Sci., 124:162, 1965.

49. Egelberg, J.: Blood vessels at the dento-gingival junction. J. Periodont. Res., 1:163, 1966.

50. Egelberg, J.: Permeability of the dento-gingival blood vessels. I. Application of the vascular labelling method and gingival fluid measurements. J. Periodont. Res., 1:180, 1966.

51. Egelberg, J.: Permeability of the dento-gingival blood vessels. II. Clinically healthy gingivae. J. Periodont. Res., 1:276, 1966.

52. Egelberg, J.: Permeability of the dento-gingival blood vessles. III. Chronically inflamed gingivae. J. Periodont. Res., 1:287, 1966.

53. Egelberg, J.: Permeability of the dento-gingival blood vessels. IV. Effect of histamine on vessels in clinically healthy and chronically inflamed gingivae. J. Periodont. Res., 1:297, 1966.

54. Eisen, H. N.: Immunology. An Introduction to Molecular and Cellular Principles of the Immune Responses. New York, Harper & Row, 1974.

55. Engel, L. D., Clagett, J., and Page, R. C.: Response of mouse spleen cells to Actinomyces viscosus antigens. Fed. Am. Soc. Exp. Biol. Abstracts, 1975.

56. Engel, L. D., and Page, R. C.: Interaction and effects of bacterial components on gingival fibroblasts. Programs and Abstracts 52nd Gen. Mtg. IADR, Abs. #492, 1974.

57. Erb, P., and Feldman, M.: Role of macrophages in vitro induction of T-helper cells. Nature, 254:352, 1975.

58. Euler, W. S. von: Uber die spezifische blutdracksenkende Substanz des menschlichen Prostata-und Samenblasensekretes. Klin. Wochenschr., 14:1182, 1935.

59. Evans, R. T., Spaeth, S., and Mergenhagen, S. E.: Bacteriocidal antibody in mammalian serum to obligatory anaerobic gram-negative bacteria. J. Immunol. 97:112, 1966.

60. Evanson, J. M., Jeffery, J. J., and Krane, S. M.: Human collagenase: Identification and purification of an en-

zyme from rheumatoid synovium in culture. Science, *158*:499, 1970.

61. Ferraris, V. A., and DeRubertis, F. R.: Release of prostaglandin by mitogen- and antigen-stimulated leukocytes in culture. J. Clin. Invest., *54*:378, 1974.

62. Fleider, D. R., Sun, C. N., and Schneider, B. C.: Chemistry of normal and inflamed human gingival tissues. Periodontics, *4*:302, 1966.

63. Fowles, R. E., et al.: The enhancement of macrophage bacteriostasis by products of activated lymphocytes. J. Exp. Med., *138*:952, 1973.

64. Freedman, H. L., Taichman, N. S., and Keystone, J.: Inflammation and tissue injury. II. Local release of lysosomal enzymes during mixed bacterial infection in the skin of rabbits. Proc. Soc. Exp. Biol. Med., *125*:1209, 1967.

65. Friedman, J., Au, W. Y. W., and Raisz, L. G.: Responses of fetal rat bone to thyrocalcitonin in tissue culture. Endocrinology, *82*:149, 1968.

66. Fullmer, H. M.: A histochemical study of periodontal disease in the maxillary alveolar process of 135 autopsies. J. Periodontol. *32*:206, 1961.

67. Fullmer, H. M., and Gibson, W.: Collagenolytic activity in the gingivae of man. Nature, *209*:728, 1966.

68. Fullmer, H. M., et al.: The origin of collagenase in periodontal tissues of man. J. Dent. Res., *48*:646, 1969.

69. Fullmer, H. M., Taylor, R. W., and Guthrie, R. W.: Human gingival collagenase: Purification, molecular weight and inhibitor studies. J. Dent. Res., *51*:349, 1972.

70. Gell, P. G. H., and Coombs, R. R. A., Eds.: Clinical Aspects of Immunology. Philadelphia, F. A. Davis Co., 1968.

71. Gemsa, D., et al.: Release of cyclic AMP from macrophages by stimulation with prostaglandins. J. Immunol., *144*:1422, 1975.

72. Genco, R. J., and Krygier, G.: Localization of immunoglobulins, immune cells and complement in human gingiva. J. Periodont. Res. 10 (Suppl):30, 1972.

73. Genco, R. J., et al.: Antibody-mediated effects on the periodontium. J. Periodontol., *45*:330, 1974.

74. Gery, I., and Waksman, B. H.: Potentiation of the T-lymphocytes response to mitogens. J. Exp. Med., *136*:143, 1972.

75. Gewurz, H.: The immunologic role of complement. Hosp. Practice, *2*:45, 1967.

76. Goldhaber, P.: Heparin enhancement of factors stimulating bone resorption in tissue culture. Science, *147*:407, 1965.

77. Goldhaber, P.: Tissue culture studies of bone as a model system for periodontal research. J. Dent. Res., 50 (Suppl. 2):278, 1971.

78. Goodson, J. M., Dewhirst, F. E., and Brunetti, A.: Prostaglandin E$_2$ levels and human periodontal disease. Prostaglandins, *6*:81, 1974.

79. Goodson, J. M., McClatchy, K., and Revell, C.: Prostaglandin-induces resorption of the adult rat calvarium. J. Dent. Res., *53*:670, 1974.

80. Gordon, S., Todd, J., and Cohn, Z. A.: In vitro synthesis and secretion of lysozymes by mononuclear phagocytes. J. Exp. Med., *139*:1228, 1774.

81. Gowans, J. L.: Immunobiology of the small lymphocyte. Hosp. Practice, *3*:34, 1968.

82. Granger, G. A.: Lymphokines—the mediators of cellular immunity. Ser. Haematol., *4*:8, 1972.

83. Granger, G. A., and Kolb, W. P.: Lymphocyte in vitro cytotoxicity: Mechanisms of immune and non-immune small lymphocyte mediated target L cell destruction. J. Immunol., *101*:111, 1968.

84. Greaves, M. W., Sondergaard, J., and MacDonald-Gibson, W.: Recovery of prostaglandins in human cutaneous inflammation. Br. Med. J., *2*:258, 1971.

85. Greene, J. C.: Oral hygiene and periodontal disease. Am. J. Public Health, *53*:913, 1963.

86. Gross, J., and Lapiere, C. M.: Collagenolytic activity in amphibian tissues: A tissue culture assay. Proc. Nat. Acad. Sci., USA, *48*:1014, 1962.

87. Hamp, S. E., and Folke, L. E. A.: The lysosomes and their possible role in periodontal disease. Odont. Tidskr., *76*:353, 1968.

88. Hamp, S. E., Lindhe, J., and Löe, H.: Long term effect of chlorhexidine on developing gingivitis in the beagle dog. J. Periodont. Res., *8*:63, 1973.

89. Hamprecht, B., Jaffe, B. M., and Philpott, G. W.: Prostaglandin production by neuroblastoma, glioma and fibroblast cell lines: stimulation by N^6, O^2-dibutryl adenosine $3'5'$-cyclic monophosphate. FEBS Lett., *36*:193, 1973.

90. Harris, E. D., Dibona, D. R., and Krane, S. M.: Collagenase in human synovial fluid. J. Clin. Invest., *48*:2104, 1969.

91. Hausmann, E.: Potential pathways for bone resorption in human periodontal disease. J. Periodontol., *45*:338, 1974.

92. Hausmann, E., Raisz, L. G., and Miller, W. A.: Endotoxin: stimulation of bone resorption in tissue culture. Science, *168*:862, 1970.

93. Hausmann, E., Weinfeld, N., and Michaels, S.: Lipopolysaccharide diphosphonate interaction on bone in tissue culture. Arch. Oral Biol., *17*:1381, 1972.

94. Hausmann, E., Weinfeld, N., and Miller, W. A.: Effects of lipopolysaccharides on bone resorption in tissue culture. Calcif. Tissue Res., *9*:272, 1972.

95. Hausmann, E., et al.: Effects of sera on bone resorption in tissue culture. Calcif. Tissue Res., *13*:311, 1973.

96. Hausmann, E., and Weinfeld, N.: Human dental plaque: stimulation of bone resorption in tissue culture. Arch. Oral Biol., in press.

97. Hawkins, D.: Neutrophilic leukocytes in immunologic reactions: evidence for the selective release of lysosomal constituents. J. Immunol., *108*:310, 1972.

98. Henney, C. C., Bourne, H. R., and Lichtenstein, L. M.: The role of cyclic $3'$-$5'$ adenosine monophosphate in the specific cytolytic activity of lymphocytes. J. Immunol., *108*:1526, 1972.

99. Henson, P. M.: Interaction of cells with immune complexes: adherence, release of constituents, and tissue injury. J. Exp. Med., *134*:114, 1971.

100. Hinman, J. W.: Prostaglandins. Ann. Rev. Biochem., *41*:161, 1972.

101. Hirschhorn, R., Grossman, J., and Weissmann, G.: Effect of cyclic 3'-5' adenosine monophosphate and theophylline on lymphocyte transformation. Proc. Soc. Exp. Biol. Med., *133*:1361, 1970.

102. Hock, J., and Nuki, K.: A vital microscopy study of the morphology of normal and inflamed gingiva. J. Periodont. Res., *6*:81, 1971.

103. Holborow, E. J.: An ABC of Modern Immunology, 2nd ed., Boston, Little, Brown & Co., 1973.

104. Holm, G., Perlmann, P., and Werner, B.: Phytohaemagglutinin-induced cytotoxic action of normal lymphoid cells on cells in tissue culture. Nature, *203*:841, 1964.

105. Hook, W. A., Snyderman, R., and Mergenhagen, S. E.: Further characterization of a factor from endotoxin-treated serum which releases histamine and heparin from mast cells. Infect. Immun., *5*:909, 1972.

106. Horton, J. E., Oppenheim, J. J., and Mergenhagen, S. E.: Elaboration of lymphotoxin by cultured human peripheral blood leukocytes stimulated with dental-plaque deposits. Clin. Exp. Immunol., *13*:383, 1973.

107. Horton, J. E., et al.: Bone resorbing activity in supernatant fluid from cultured human peripheral blood leukocytes. Science, *177*:793, 1972.

108. Hubscher, T.: Role of the eosinophil in the allergic reactions. II. Release of prostaglandins from human eosinophilic leukocytes. J. Immunol., *144*:1389, 1975.

109. Hunter, P., and Kettman, J. R.: Mode of action of a supernatant activity from T-cell cultures that nonspecifically stimulated the humoral immune response. Proc. Nat. Acad. Sci., USA, *71*:512, 1974.

110. Ishikawa, I., Cimasoni, G., and Ahmad-Zadeh, C.: Possible role of lysosomal enzymes in the pathogenesis of periodontitis. A study on cathepsin D in human gingival fluid. Arch. Oral Biol., *17*:111, 1972.

111. Ivanyi, L., Challacombe, S., and Lehner, T.: The specificity of serum factors in lymphocyte transformation in periodontal disease. Clin. Exp. Immunol., *14*:191, 1973.

112. Ivanyi, L., and Lehner, T.: Stimulation of lymphocyte transformation by bacterial antigens in patients with periodontal disease. Arch. Oral Biol., *15*:1089, 1970.

113. Ivanyi, L., and Lehner, T.: Lymphocyte transformation by sonicates of dental plaque in human periodontal disease. Arch. Oral Biol., *16*:1117, 1971.

114. Ivanyi, L., and Lehner, T.: The significance of serum factors in stimulation of lymphocytes from patients with periodontal disease. Int. Arch. Allergy, *41*:620, 1974.

115. Ivanyi, L., Wilton, J. M. A., and Lehner, T.: Cell-mediated immunity in periodontal disease: cytotoxicity, migration inhibition and lymphocyte transformation studies. Immunology, *22*:141, 1972.

116. Jensen, S. H., Page, R. C., and Narayanan, A. S.: Effects of plaque accumulation on gingival collagen and protein production. Programs and Abstracts, 53rd Gen. Mtg. IADR, London, Abs. #L15, 1975.

117. Juhlin, L., and Michaelsson, G.: Cutaneous vascular reactions to prostaglandins in healthy subjects and in patients with urticaria and atopic dermatitis. Acta. Derm. Venereol., *49*:251, 1969.

118. Kaley, G., and Weiner, R.: *In* Prostaglandin Symposium of the Worcester Foundation for Experimental Biology. P. W. Ramwell and J. E. Shaw, Eds. New York InterScience, 1968, pp. 321–328.

119. Kaley, G., and Weiner, R.: Effect of prostaglandin E_1 on leukocyte migration. Nature [New Biol.], *234*:114, 1971.

120. Kaley, G., and Weiner, R.: Prostaglandin E_1: A potential mediator of the inflammatory response. Ann. N. Y. Acad. Sci., *180*:338, 1971.

121. Kelly, L. A., and Butcher, R. W.: The effects of epinephrine and prostaglandin E_1 on cyclic adenosine 3'-5'-monophosphate levels in WI-38 fibroblasts. Clinc. Invest. *53*:3098, 1974.

122. Kindlova, M.: Development of vessels in the marginal periodontium in rats. J. Dent. Res., *47*:507, 1968.

123. Kindlova, M.: The development of the vascular bed of the marginal periodontium. J. Periodont. Res., *5*:135, 1970.

124. Kischer, C. W.: Effects of specific prostaglandins on development of a chick embryo skin and down feather organ in vitro. Dev. Biol., *16*:203, 1967.

125. Klein, D. C., and Raisz, L. G.: Prostaglandins: Stimulation of bone resorption in tissue culture. Endocrinology, *86*:1436, 1970.

126. Klein, W. J.: Lymphocyte mediated cytotoxicity in vitro. Effect of enhancing antisera. J. Exp. Med., *134*:1238, 1971.

127. Kolb, W. P., and Granger, G. A.: Lymphocyte in vitro cytotoxicity: characterization of human lymphotoxin. Proc. Nat. Acad. Sci., USA, *61*:1250, 1968.

128. König, W., and Ishizaka, K.: Association of receptors for mouse IgE with the plasma membrane of rat mast cells. J. Immunol., *113*:1237, 1974.

129. Koopman, W., Gillis, M. H., and David, J. R.: Prevention of MIF activity by agents known to increase cellular cyclic AMP. J. Immunol., *110*:1609, 1973.

130. Krahenbuhl, J. L., Rosenberg, L. T., and Remmington, J. S.: The role of thymus derived lymphocytes in the in vitro activation of macrophages to kill Lysteria monocytogenes. J. Immunol., *111*:992, 1973.

131. Lagunoff, D.: The properties of mast cell proteases. Biochem. Pharmacol., Suppl., 221–227, 1968.

132. Lazarus, G. S., et al.: Human granulocyte collagenase. Science, *159*:1483, 1968.

133. Lehner, T.: Cell-mediated immune responses in oral disease: A review. J. Oral Pathol., *1*:39, 1972.

134. Lehner, T., et al.: Sequential cell-mediated immune response in experimental gingivitis in man. Clin. Exp. Immunol., *16*:481, 1974.

135. Lepow, I. H., and Ward, P. A., Eds.: Inflammation. Mechanisms and Control. New York, Academic Press, 1972.

136. Levine, L., et al.: Prostaglandin production by mouse fibrosarcoma cells in culture. Inhibition by indo-

methacin and aspirin. Biochem. Biophys. Res. Commun. *47*:888, 1972.

137. Lindhe, J., Hamp, S. E., and Löe, H.: Experimental periodontitis in the beagle dog. J. Periodont. Res., *8*:1, 1973.

138. Lindhe, J., and Helldén, L.: Neutrophilic chemotatic activity elaborated by dental plaque. J. Periodont. Res., *7*:297, 1972.

139. Listgarten, M. A.: Electron microscopic observations on the bacterial flora of acute necrotizing ulcerative gingivitis. J. Periodontol., *36*:328, 1965.

140. Listgarten, M. A., and Ellegaard, B.: Experimental gingivitis in rhesus monkeys. J. Periodont. Res., 10 (Suppl):13, 1972.

141. Löe, H., Theilade, E., and Jensen, S. B.: Experimental gingivitis in man. J. Periodontol., *36*:177, 1965.

142. Macdonald, J. B., Socransky, S. S., and Gibbons, R. J.: Aspects of the pathogenesis of mixed anaerobic infections of mucous membranes. J. Dent. Res., *42*:529, 1963.

143. Mackaness, G. B.: The immunological basis of acquired cellular resistance. J. Exp. Med., *120*:105, 1964.

144. Mackaness, G. B.: The relationship of delayed hypersensitivity to acquired cellular resistance. Br. Med. Bull., *23*:52, 1967.

145. Mackler, B. F., et al.: Induction of lymphokine production by EAC and of blastogenesis by soluble mitogens during human B cell activation. Nature, *249*:834, 1974.

146. Mackler, B. F., et al.: Blastogenesis and lymphokine synthesis by T and B lymphocytes from patients with periodontal disease. Infect. Immun., *10*:844, 1974.

147. Maganiello, V., and Vaughan, M.: Prostaglandin E_1 effects on adenosine $3':5'$-cyclic monophosphate concentration and phosphodiesterase activity in fibroblasts. Proc. Nat. Acad. Sci., USA, *69*:269, 1972.

148. Magliulo, E., et al.: Enhanced in vitro phagocytic power of macrophages from PPD-stimulated skin sites in human subjects hypersensitive to PPD. Clin. Exp. Immunol., *14*:371, 1973.

149. Manheimer, S., and Pick, E.: The mechanism of action of soluble lymphocyte mediators. I. A pulse exposure test for the measurement of macrophage migration inhibitory factor. Immunology, *24*:1027, 1973.

150. Manner, G., and Kuleba, M.: Effect of dibutryl-cyclic AMP on collagen and noncollagen protein synthesis in cultured human cells. Conn. Tissue Res., *2*:167, 1974.

151. Marx, J. L. Prostaglandins: Mediators of inflammation. Science, *177*:780, 1971.

152. May, C. D., Levine, B. E., and Weissmann, G.: Effects of compounds which inhibit antigenic release of histamine and phagocytic release of lysosomal enzyme on glucose utilization by leukocytes in humans. Proc. Soc. Exp. Biol. Med., *133*:758, 1970.

153. Melcher, A. H.: Some histological and histochemical observations on connective tissue of chronically inflamed gingiva. J. Periodont. Res., *2*:127, 1967.

154. Mergenhagen, S. E.: Complement as a mediator of the inflammatory response: Interaction of complement with mammalian and bacterial enzymes. J. Dent. Res., *51* (Suppl 2):251, 1972.

155. Mergenhagen, S. E., DeAraujo, W. C., and Varah, E.: Antibody to leptotrichia buccalis in human sera. Arch. Oral Biol., *10*:29, 1965.

156. Mergenhagen, S. E., and Scherp, H. W., Eds.: Comparative Immunology of the Oral Cavity. DHEW pub. No. 73-438, 1973.

157. Mooney, J. J., and Waksman, B. H.: Activation of normal rabbit macrophages by supernatants of antigen-stimulated lymphocytes. J. Immunol., *105*:1138, 1970.

158. Morley, H.: Prostaglandins and lymphokines in arthritis. Prostaglandins, *8*:315, 1974.

159. Movius, D. L., Rogers, R. S., and Reeve, C. M.: Lymphocyte-mediated cellular immunity and the pathogenesis of periodontal disease. Program and Abstracts, 52nd Gen. Mtg. IADR, Abs. #498, 1974.

160. Narayanan, A. S., and Page, R. C.: Biochemical characterization of collagens synthesized by fibroblasts derived from normal and periodontally diseased human gingiva. J. Biol. Chem., 1976.

161. Nath, I., Poulter, L. W., and Turk, J. L.: Effect of lymphocyte mediators on macrophages in vitro. A correlation of morphological and cytochemical changes. Clin. Exp. Immunol., *13*:455, 1973.

162. Nathan, C. F., Karnovsky, M. L., and David, J. R.: Alterations of macrophage functions by mediators from lymphocytes. J. Exp. Med., *133*:1356, 1971.

163. Nelson, D. S.: Production by stimulated macrophages of factors depressing lymphocyte transformation. Nature, *246*:306, 1973.

164. Nisengard, R.: Immediate hypersensitivity and periodontal disease. J. Periodontol., *45*:344, 1974.

165. Nisengard, R. J., and Beutner, E. H.: Immunologic studies of periodontal disease. V. IgG type antibodies and skin test responses to actinomyces and mixed oral flora. J. Periodontol., *41*:149, 1970.

166. Nisengard, R. J., and Beutner, E. H.: Relation of immediate hypersensitivity to periodontitis in animals and man. J. Periodontol., *41*:223, 1970.

167. Nisengard, R. J., Beutner, E., and Hazen, S. P.: Bacterial hypersensitivity and periodontal disease. J. Periodontol., *39*:46, 1968.

168. Nisengard, R. J., Beutner, E. H., and Hazen, S. P.: Immunologic studies of periodontal disease. IV. Bacterial hypersensitivity and periodontal disease. J. Periodontol., *39*:329, 1968.

169. Nisengard, R. J., Beutner, E. H., and Gauto, M.: Immunofluorescence studies of IgE in periodontal disease. Ann. N. Y. Acad. Sci., *177*:39, 1971.

170. Nuki, K., and Hock, J.: The organization of the gingival vasculature. J. Periodont. Res., *9*:305, 1974.

171. Oliver, R. C., Holm-Pedersen, P., and Löe, H.: The correlation between clinical scoring, exudate measurements and microscopic evaluation of inflammation of the gingiva. J. Periodontol., *40*:201, 1969.

172. Opitz, H. G., et al.: Inhibition of H-thymidine incor-

poration of lymphocytes by a soluble factor from macrophages. Cell. Immunol., *16*:379, 1975.

173. Oppenheim, J. J.: Modulation of in vitro lymphocyte transformation by antibodies. Enhancement by antigen-antibody complexes and inhibition by antibody excess. Cell. Immunol., 3:341, 1972.

174. Page, R. C.: Macromolecular interactions in the connective tissues of the periodontium. *In* Developmental Aspects of Oral Biology. H. Slavkin and L. Bavetta, Eds. New York, Academic Press, 1972.

175. Page, R. C., and Ammons, W. F.: Collagen turnover in the gingiva and other mature connective tissues of the normal marmoset Saguinus oedipus. Arch. Oral Biol., *19*:651, 1975.

176. Page, R. C., et al.: Collagen fibre bundles of the normal marginal gingiva in the marmoset. Arch. Oral Biol., *19*:1039, 1974.

177. Page, R. C., Davies, P., and Allison, A. C.: Effects of dental plaque on the production and release of lysosomal hydrolases by macrophages in culture. Arch. Oral Biol., *18*:1481, 1973.

178. Page, R. C., Davies, P., and Allison, A. C.: Pathogenesis of the chronic inflammatory lesion induced by group A streptoccocal cell walls. Lab. Invest., *30*:568, 1974.

179. Page, R. C., Davies, P., and Allison, A. C.: The role of the mononuclear phagocyte in chronic inflammatory disease. J. Reticuloendothel. Soc., *15*:413, 1974.

180. Page, R. C., and Schroeder, H. E.: Biochemical aspects of connective tissue alterations in inflammatory gingival and periodontal disease. Int. Dent. J., *18*:899, 1973.

181. Page, R. C., and Schroeder, H. E.: The pathogenesis of chronic inflammatory periodontal disease. Lab. Invest., *33*:235, 1976.

182. Pantalone, R. M., and Page, R. C.: Lymphokine induced production and release of lysosomal enzymes by macrophages. Proc. Natl. Acad. Sci., USA, *72*:2091, 1975.

183. Pantalone, R. M., and Page, R. C.: The production and secretion of collagenase and lysosomal hydrolases by macrophages activated with lymphokines. Submitted J. Reticuloendothel. Soc., 1976.

184. Parakkal, P. F.: Involvement of macrophages in collagen resorption. J. Cell Biol., *41*:345, 1969.

185. Paunio, K.: Periodontal connective tissue biochemical studies of disease in man. Soumen Hammas Laakariseuran Toimituksia, *65*:251, 1969.

186. Paunio, K., and Mäkinen, K.: Studies on hydrolytic enzyme activity in the connective tissue of the human periodontal ligament. Observations apart from areas of inflammation. Acta. Odontol. Scand., *27*:153, 1969.

187. Payne, W. A., et al.: Histopathologic features of the initial and early stages of experimental gingivitis in man. J. Periodont. Res., *10*:51, 1975.

188. Peterkofsky, B., and Prather, W. B.: Increased collagen synthesis in Kristen sarcoma virus-transformed BALB 3T3 cells grown in the presence of dibutryl cyclic AMP. Cell, 3:291, 1974.

189. Pick, E., et al.: Interaction between "sensitized lymphocytes" and antigen in vitro. I. The release of a skin reactive factor. Immunology, *17*:741, 1969.

190. Pick, E., and Turk, J. L.: The biological activities of soluble lymphocyte products. Clin. Exp. Immunol. *10*:1, 1972.

191. Piper, P. J., and Vane, J. R.: Release of additional factors in anaphylaxis and its antagonism by anti-inflammatory drugs. Nature, *223*:29, 1971.

192. Platt, D., Crosby, R. G., and Dalbow, N. H.: Evidence for the presence of immunoglobulins and antibodies in inflamed periodontal tissues. J. Periodontol., *41*:215, 1970.

193. Raisz, L. C.: Bone resorption in tissue culture. Factors influencing the response to parathyroid hormone. J. Clin. Invest., *44*:103, 1965.

194. Raisz, L. G., and Koolemans-Beynen, A. R.: Inhibition of bone collagen synthesis by prostaglandin E_2 in organ culture. Prostaglandins, *10*:377, 1974.

195. Raisz, L. G., and Niemann, I.: Effect of phosphate, calcium and magnesium on bone resorption and hormonal responses in tissue culture. Endocrinology, *85*:446, 1969.

196. Raisz, L. G., et al.: 1.25-dihydroxycholecalciferol: a potent stimulator of bone resorption in tissue culture. Science, *175*:768, 1972.

197. Raisz, L. G., et al.: Complement-dependent stimulation of prostaglandin synthesis and bone resorption. Science, *185*:789, 1974.

198. Ramwell, P. W., and Shaw, J. E.: Biological significance of prostaglandins. Rec. Prog. Horm. Res., *26*:139, 1970.

199. Ranny, R. R., and Zander, H. A.: Allergic periodontal disease in sensitized squirrel monkeys. J. Periodontol., *41*:12, 1970.

200. Ratnoff, O. D.: The interrelationship of clotting and immunologic mechanisms. Hosp. Practice, *6*:119, 1971.

201. Rizzo, A. A., and Mergenhagen, S. E.: Studies on the significance of local hypersensitivity in periodontal disease. Periodontics, 3:271, 1965.

202. Rizzo, A. A., and Mergenhagen, S. E.: Local Shwartzman reaction in rabbit oral mucosa with endotoxin from oral bacteria. Proc. Soc. Exp. Biol. Med., *104*:580, 1968.

203. Rizzo, A. A., and Mitchell, C. T.: Chronic allergic inflammation induced by repeated deposition of antigen in rabbit gingival pockets. Periodontics, 4:5, 1966.

204. Robinson, L. P., and DeMarco, T. J.: Alteration of mast cell densities in experimentally inflamed human gingiva. J. Periodontol., *43*:614, 1972.

205. Rogers, R. S., Movius, D. L., and Reeve, C. M.: Lymphocyte-epithelial cell interactions in oral inflammatory disease. Program and Abstracts, 53rd Gen. Mtg. IADR, Abs. #L267, 1975.

206. Rosenberg, S. A., et al.: Guinea pig lymphotoxin (LT). I. In vitro studies of LT produced in response to antigen stimulation of lymphocytes. J. Immunol., *110*:1623, 1973.

207. Ross, R.: Wound healing. Sci. Am., 220:40, 1969.

208. Russell, A. L.: Epidemiology of periodontal disease. Int. Dent. J., 17:282, 1967.

209. Russell, S. W., et al.: Purification of human lymphotoxin. J. Immunol., 109:784, 1972.

210. Rysky de, S., Cattaneo, V., and Montanari, M. C.: Determination Quantitative des Exasamines et de L'ydroxyproline dans les inflammations gingivates chroniques. Bull. Group Int. Rech. Sci. Stomatol., 12:359, 1969.

211. Sakamoto, S., Goldhaber, P., and Glimcher, M. J.: Mouse bone collagenase: The effect of heparin on the amount of enzyme released in tissue culture and on the activity of the enzyme. Calcif. Tissue Res., 12:247, 1973.

212. Samuelsson, B., et al.: Metabolism of prostaglandins. Ann. N.Y. Acad. Sci., 180:138, 1971.

213. Saxe, S. R., et al.: Oral debris, calculus, and periodontal disease in the beagle dog. Periodontics, 5:217, 1967.

214. Schneider, T. F., et al.: Specific bacterial antibodies in the inflamed human gingiva. Periodontics, 4:53, 1966.

215. Schroeder, H. E.: Ultrastructure des lesions gingivales precoces. Rev. Fr. Odontostomatol., 20:103, 1973.

216. Schroeder, H. E.: Transmigration and infiltration of leucocytes in human junctional epithelium. Helv. Odontol. Acta, 17:6, 1973.

217. Schroeder, H. E., Graf-de Beer, M., and Attström, R.: Initial gingivitis in dogs. J. Periodont. Res., 10:128, 1975.

218. Schroeder, H. E., et al.: Structural constituents of clinically normal and slightly inflamed dog gingiva. A morphometric study. Helv. Odontol. Acta, 17:70, 1973.

219. Schroeder, H. E., Münzel-Pedrazzoli, S., and Page, R. C.: Correlated morphometric and biochemical analysis of gingival tissue in early chronic gingivitis in man. Arch. Oral Biol., 18:899, 1973.

220. Schroeder, H. E., and Page, R. C.: Lymphocyte-fibroblast interactions in the pathogenesis of inflammatory gingival disease. Experientia, 28:1228, 1972.

221. Schultz-Haudt, S. D., and Aas, E.: Observations on the status of collagen in human gingiva. Arch. Oral Biol., 2:131, 1960.

222. Schultz-Haudt, S., Bibby, B. G., and Bruce, M. A.: Tissue-destructive products of gingival bacteria from nonspecific gingivitis. J. Dent. Res., 33:624, 1954.

223. Schultz-Haudt, S., Dewar, M., and Bibby, B. G.: Effects of hyaluronidase on human gingival epithelium. Science, 117:653, 1953.

224. Seravalli, E., and Taranta, A.: Release of macrophage migration inhibitory factor(s) from lymphocytes stimulated by streptococcal preparations. Cell. Immunol. 8:40, 1973.

225. Shapiro, S., Ulmansky, M., and Scheuer, M.: Mast cell population in gingiva affected by chronic destructive periodontal disease. J. Periodontol., 40:276, 1969.

226. Shelton, L. E., and Hall, W. B.: Human gingival mast cells. Effects of chronic inflammation. J. Periodont. Res., 3:214, 1968.

227. Simpson, D. M., and Avery, B. E.: Histopathologic and ultrastructural features of inflamed gingiva in the baboon. J. Periodontol., 45:500, 1974.

228. Skougaard, M. R., Levy, B. M., and Simpson, J.: Collagen metabolism in skin and periodontal membrane of the marmoset. J. Periodont. Res., (Suppl 4):28, 1969.

229. Smith, J. W., et al.: Cyclic adenosine 3′-5′-monophosphate in human lymphocytes. Alterations after phytohemagglutinin stimulation. J. Clin. Invest., 50:432, 1971.

230. Smith, J. W., Steiner, A. L., and Parker, C. W.: Human lymphocyte metabolism. Effects of cyclic and noncyclic nucleotides on stimulatin of phytohemagglutinin. J. Clin. Invest., 50:442, 1971.

231. Snyderman, R.: Role for endotoxin and complement in periodontal tissue destruction. J. Dent. Res., 51 (Suppl 2):356, 1972.

232. Snyderman, R., Phillips, J. K., and Mergenhagen, S. E.: Biological activity of complement in vivo: Role of C5 in the accumulation of polymorphonuclear leukocytes in inflammatory exudates. J. Exp. Med., 134:1131, 1971.

233. Snyderman, R., Shin, H. S., and Dannenberg, A. M.: Macrophage proteinase and inflammation. Production of chemotatic activity from the fifth component of complement by macrophage proteinase. J. Immunol., 109:896, 1972.

234. Snyderman, R. H., Shin, H. W., and Hausmann, M. H.: A chemotatic factor from mononuclear phagocytes. Proc. Soc. Exp. Biol. Med., 138:378, 1971.

235. Socransky, S. S.: Relationship of bacteria to the etiology of periodontal disease. J. Dent. Res., 49 (Suppl 2):203, 1970.

236. Solomon, L. M., Juhlin, L., Kirschenbaum, M. B.: Prostaglandin on cutaneous vasculature. J. Invest. Dermatol., 51:280, 1968.

237. Sondergaard, J., and Greaves, M. W.: Recovery of a pharmacologically active fatty acid during the inflammatory reaction involved by patch testing in allergic conta dermatitis. Int. Arch. Allergy Appl. Immunol., 39:56, 1970.

238. Spector, W. G.: The macrophage in inflammation. Ser. Haematol., 3:132, 1970.

239. Steinberg, A. I.: Evidence for the presence of circulating antibodies to an oral spirochete in the sera of clinic patients. J. Periodontol., 41:213, 1970.

240. Steinberg, A. I., and Gershoff, S.: Quantitative differences in spirochetal antibody observed in periodontal disease. J. Periodontol., 39:286, 1968.

241. Strom, T. B., et al.: Alteration of the cytotoxic action of sensitized lymphocytes by cholinergic agents and activators of adenylate cyclase. Proc. Nat. Acad. Sci., USA, 69:2995, 1972.

242. Taichman, N. S., Freedman, H. L., and Uriuhara, T.: Inflammation and tissue injury. I. The response to intradermal injections of human dentogingival plaque

in normal and leukopenic rabbits. Arch. Oral Biol., *11:*1385, 1966.

243. Taichman, N. S., Pruzanski, W., and Ranadive, N. S.: Release of intracellular constituents from rabbit polymorphonuclear leukocytes exposed to soluble and insoluble immune complexes. Int. Arch. Allergy Appl. Immunol., *43:*182, 1972.

244. Tempel, T. R., et al.: Factors from saliva and oral bacteria, chemotatic for polymorphonuclear leukocytes: Their possible role in gingival inflammation. J. Periodontol., *41:*71, 1970.

245. Terner, C.: Arthus reaction in the oral cavity of laboratory animals. Periodontics, *3:*18, 1965.

246. Terner, C.: Histological categories of the clinically healthy gingiva. J. Periodontol., *38:*211, 1967.

247. Vaes, G.: Hyaluronidase activity in lysosomes of bone tissue. Biochem. J., *103:*802, 1967.

248. Valentine, F.: Lymphocyte transformation: the proliferation of human blood lymphocytes stimulated by antigen in vitro. *In In Vitro* Methods in Cell-Mediated Immunity. B. R. Bloom and P. R. Blade, Eds. New York, Academic Press, 1971.

249. Vensel, W. H., Komender, J., and Barnard, E. A.: Non-pancreatic proteases of the chymotrypsin family. II. Two proteases from a mouse mast cell tumor. Biochem. Biophys. Acta, *250:*395, 1971.

250. Vos-Cloetens, C., De Minsart-Baleriaux, V., and Urgain-Vansanten, G.: Possible relationships between antibodies and non-specific immunoglobulins simultaneously induced after antigenic stimulation. Immunology, *20:*955, 1971.

251. Wahl, L. M., et al.: Collagenase production by endotoxin-activated macrophages. Proc. Nat. Acad. Sci., USA, *71:*3598, 1974.

252. Wahl, L. M., et al.: Collagenase production by lymphokine-activated macrophages. Science, *187:*261, 1975.

253. Walker, D. G., Lapiere, C. M., and Gross, J.: A collagenolytic factor in rat bone promoted by parathyroid extract. Biochem. Biophys. Res. Commun., *15:*397, 1964.

254. Ward, P. A., and Hill, J. H.: C5 chemotatic fragments produced by an enzyme in lysosomal granules of neutrophils. J. Immunol., *104:*535, 1970.

255. Ward, P. W., Remold, H. G., and David, J. R.: Leukocatic factor produced by sensitized lymphocytes. Science, *163:*1079, 1967.

256. Ward, P. A., Remold, H. G., and David, J. R.: The production of antigen-stimulated lymphocytes of a leukotatic factor distinct from migration inhibitory factor. Cell. Immunol., *1:*162, 1970.

257. Weeks, J. R.: Prostaglandins. Ann. Rev. Pharmacol., *12:*317, 1972.

258. Weiner, R., and Kaley, G.: Influence of prostaglandin on the terminal vascular bed. Am. J. Physiol., *217:*563, 1969.

259. Weissmann, G., Dukor, P., and Zurier, R. B.: Effect of cyclic AMP on release of lysosomal enzymes from phagocytes. Nature [New Biol.], *231:*131, 1971.

260. Weissmann, G., et al.: Mechanism of lysosomal enzyme release from leukocytes exposed to immune complexes and other particles. J. Mep. Med., *134:*149S, 1971.

261. Whitehouse, M. W., and Bostrom, H.: Biochemical properties of anti-inflammatory drugs. VI. Biochem. Pharmacol., *14:*1173, 1965.

262. Williams, T. W., and Granger, G. A.: Lymphocyte *in vitro* cytotoxicity: lymphotoxins of several mammalian species. Nature, *219:*1076, 1968.

263. Willis, A. L., et al.: Release and actions of prostaglandins in inflammation and fever: Inhibition by anti-inflammatory and antipyretic drugs. *In* Prostaglandins in Cellular Biology. P. W. Ramwell and B. B. Pharris, Eds. 1972.

264. Willoughby, D. A.: Effects of prostaglandins PGF_{2a} and PGE_1 on vascular permeability. J. Pathol., *96:*381, 1968.

265. Woods, J. F., and Nichols, G.: Collagenolytic activity in mammalian bone. Science, *142:*386, 1963.

266. Woods, J. F., and Nichols, G.: Distribution of collagenase in rat tissues. Nature, *208:*1325, 1965.

267. Zachrisson, B. U.: Mast cells of the human gingiva. II. J. Periodont. Res., *2:*87, 1967.

9

Acute Inflammatory Periodontal Disease

9

Acute Inflammatory Periodontal Disease

Periodontal diseases are generally considered to be chronic. Every feature seems to point to essential chronicity, from the usual insidious course of the disease on a gross clinical level to the cellular infiltrate within the affected tissues. There are, nevertheless, acute inflammatory periodontal diseases.

These acute inflammatory diseases are not so numerous or so common as to create more than a small area of concern or to require more than simple treatment and are not comparable to the chronic lesion in importance. They are, however, not to be glossed over. There are two specifically acute periodontal diseases: (1) acute periodontal abscess, and (2) necrotizing ulcerative gingivitis. These are in no way related to each other in either pathology or etiology.

THE ACUTE PERIODONTAL ABSCESS

The accepted view of an acute periodontal abscess is that it occurs when a common suppurating pocket is occluded, shutting off drainage. This may be true in some lesions, but it is a rather simplistic view of the problem. The explanation does not take into account the tendency of lesions in furcations to exacerbate, in pockets in patients with diabetes mellitus, or in pockets adjacent to teeth under the extremely heavy occlusal stress of particularly pernicious bruxism. These pockets are not always occluded, yet they have a tendency to acute exacerbation.

Signs and Symptoms of the Acute Periodontal Abscess

All the classic signs of acute inflammation are sometimes present with the acute periodontal abscess, but swelling, redness, and pain are not always found. On occasion, the signs are masked and subtle. In the standard abscess, adenopathy, extrusion of the tooth involved, loosening, and tenderness to even slight percussion are most common. A slight elevation of temperature is an occasional finding.

Diagnosis presents some problems, and localization of the lesion is not always easy. Treatment constitutes an emergency, since pain is acute and the patient has great difficulty in eating and even in bringing the teeth together in casual closure. The therapist is confronted with a patient who is in great pain, is visibly apprehensive of any manipulation, and is obviously stressed to a great degree. He may be toxic and somewhat febrile. Sometimes the periodontal lesion is combined with pulpitis, and in that contingency the signs are equivocal. Percussion and palpation are the most reliable diagnostic aids.

Etiology of the Periodontal Abscess

The periodontal abscess exhibits all the clinical signs of an acute infection, but whatever infection is present is endogenous to the oral cavity (Fig. 9-1). The development of the acute exacerbation occurs from an alteration in the tissues immediately adjacent to the affected tooth. Occlusion of the orifice of a periodontal pocket, diabetes, and bruxism or clenching are factors that can enter into such an alteration.

OCCLUSION OF THE ORIFICE OF A DEEP PERIODONTAL POCKET. This is the classic cause of the periodontal abscess. While it is true that, in treatment, most periodontal abscesses respond dramatically to penetration into the pocket by one means or another with the concomitant evacuation of pus and the release of pressure, the blockage of the lumen of the pocket is only one of the causes of the swelling and pain and the bacterial flora found in these lesions. Precisely what influence in the local environment induces a sharply localized purulent exudate is only one of the mysteries confronting us. With the injudicious use of the various irrigating devices, periodontal abscesses are common. It seems that the force of the irrigating stream of water forcing the ordinary bacterial contents deeper into the

tissues can and does generate periodontal abscesses. The presence of bacteria from a quiescent chronic lesion deep into the connective tissues undoubtedly alters the nature of response. An acute lesion may result.

DIABETES. Microabscesses in gingiva in patients suffering from advanced diabetes mellitus have been observed widely. These are not, however, the same thing as the clinical entity known as the periodontal abscess. The tendency to purulent infections by diabetics makes them prone to acute periodontal abscesses (Fig. 9-2). The appearance of several of these acute lesions should raise the possibility of covert diabetes in the patient who should be referred to a competent internist for an accurate evaluation of his carbohydrate metabolism. A surprising number of diabetics are revealed who were never aware of their illness.

PERNICIOUS BRUXISM OR CLENCHING. The arrangement of tissues in the furca of the multirooted tooth makes them especially vulnerable to heavy occlusal forces. The periodontal ligament within the furca lies confined between the furca and the bony septum so that abnormal forces, either intrusive or torquing, place it between the hammer and the anvil, so to speak, of two hard tissues.

The usual response of soft tissue to such trauma is to swell. Again, because of the arrangement of tissue, any enlargement causes an extrusion of the tooth which aggravates the trauma. If there is a lesion of the attachment apparatus, the response can be acute exacerbation of the pocket and a resultant periodontal abscess.

The long-range result of such trauma is resorption of the tip of septal bone within the furca. It is for this reason that most authorities believe that there is a

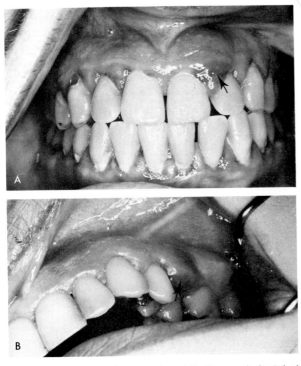

FIG. 9-1. *Periodontal abscess. A and B. Two periodontal abscesses (arrows) revealing swelling and acute inflammation.*

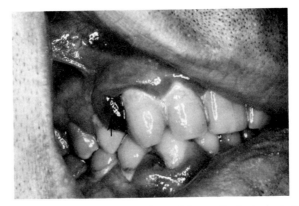

FIG. 9-2. *Periodontal abscess (arrow) in a patient who proved to be an uncontrolled diabetic.*

causal connection between furcation invasions and occlusal traumatism. While this is likely true to some extent, the short-term response is the major concern. Occasionally, a patient will report with multiple periodontal abscesses in a number of widely separated teeth in more or less simultaneous exacerbation. In every patient with multiple abscesses massive trauma was present, usually because of heavy clenching of teeth or bruxism or both.

Treatment of the Periodontal Abscess

The first objective in treating the acute lesion is to establish drainage. As with many acute pyogenic infections, the release of pressure through the evacuation of pus has a salutary effect on the lesion. Pain is relieved, swelling is resolved, the extruded tooth returns to its normal position, mobility is reduced, the pericementitis no longer gives acute pain on occlusion, and in general the patient begins to feel better.

Drainage may be established in one of two ways: (1) by finding the orifice of the occluded pocket and by gently distending the aperture so that instrumentation may make the evacuation of pus possible, or (2) by traditional incision and drainage.

Finding the opening into the pocket is not always easy. Because of the distension of the tissues, any entry is difficult. The most effective method requires the careful circumferential probing of the base of the sulcus in the gingiva surrounding the tooth, using a fine probe with *gentle* but insistent pressure. Frequently the probe will drop into a cavernous cavity and pus will exude.

Having once entered the opening, it is easily widened to admit a flat, narrow periodontal file, which not only serves to open the aperture more extensively but also begins the debridement of the root. The file is easily followed by a slender curet, which usually finishes the job of distending the orifice of the pocket and makes possible the evacuation of copious amounts of pus. Pocket distension is made easier from the outset by the reduction of internal pressure in the pocket by pus evacuation. Pursued to a logical conclusion by easy stages, the acute phase can be subverted, and the pocket can be reduced to a standard chronic lesion within a few days.

The second approach to management of an acute periodontal abscess is by incision and drainage, with no attempt to enter the aperture of the pocket. This method is faster and is at times more painful. The incision has a tendency to heal and close, once again creating an occluded periodontal pocket. To avoid such a contingency, the operator should extend and distend the incision as much as possible. Most periodontists insert a drain of rubber dam material to keep the incision open for subsequent drainage. If the patient is febrile, it is often useful to initiate a course of antibiotic therapy, using all the standard precautions as to dosage and duration.

In both approaches, the complete evacuation of the contents of the pocket is highly desirable to end the acute phase. The rate of bone loss due to the acute inflammatory infiltrate is rapid and extensive. While this loss is sometimes reversed after the successful treatment of the pocket, all possible precautions should be taken to avoid reexacerbation of the lesion. Therefore, when the acute phase is treated, it should be done completely and effectively.

After the acute phase has subsided, a chronic inflammatory lesion is left and must be treated. Many fine clinicians believe that the sooner the lesion is treated definitively, the better the chances for a reversal of the loss of bone and attachment. Prichard reported that there is strong clinical evidence, admittedly subjective, but convincing, nevertheless, that there is a certain advantage in treating the pocket promptly after the acute exacerbation has subsided.[18]

The topography of these pockets is often intrabony, since such a form is more prone to occlusion of the aperture and to subsequent acute flare-up than is one with a wide aperture and little or no confining bony walls. This feature provides an occasional favorable morphologic arrangement for a reversal of bone and attachment loss, which responds to early pocket therapy with a reconstitution of lost bone and attachment. While not proven, there is a strongly held opinion that the response is partly due to some factor created or enhanced by the recent acute episode.

The treatment of the pocket includes the usual standard methods of flap reflection, debridement to remove exuberant granulation tissue and all other accretions, plus the adequate preparation of the root surface and the bony walls within the pocket. No bone should be reduced or removed at this stage, even if it appears to be necessary for pocket elimination. The reason for this is our inability to predict precisely how much bone we can expect to gain within the defect. If bone is to be removed, it should be done as a second-stage procedure after basic pocket therapy has been completed and evaluated.

The administration of antibiotics is a standard rational approach to supportive treatment of the periodontal abscess. The use of tetracycline is common and effective. Care must be taken that an effective level in the blood stream is achieved (1 gram per day) and that it is taken long enough (at least 4 to 5 days) to insure against the dangers of inadequate administration of an antibiotic.

NECROTIZING ULCERATIVE GINGIVITIS

Necrotizing ulcerative gingivitis has had an interesting and checkered history since it was described by Vincent in 1896 and Plaut in 1894.[17,22] Although the number of cases appearing in a practice is exceedingly small, the nature of the disease excites interest far beyond its importance in the general periodontal spectrum.

It has been only several decades since necrotizing ulcerative gingivitis, then known as Vincent's infection, was considered a highly contagious quasivenereal disease, requiring isolation or at least segregation of patients suffering from it. Very likely the spirochete found in great numbers on the oral lesions of necrotizing ulcerative gingivitis alarmed a profession and public with little knowledge of the disease.

In the first World War, necrotizing ulcerative gingivitis achieved a certain notoriety because of an extensive incidence and was referred to as trench mouth. It was then that it achieved its reputation for contagious properties and virulence. Subsequent experience with the disease proved its reputation in these directions unfounded.

Incidence

All writers on the subject of necrotizing ulcerative gingivitis refer to the sudden onset of the disease as being one of its salient features, and this is probably true. All acute diseases have a sudden onset. What is of greater interest is the age span of susceptible individuals. There is a remarkably consistent age group in early adulthood, with the incidence being higher in the 18- to 30-year age group. There have been confirmed reports of patients as young as 14 years and as old as the 30's.

The reader will unquestionably learn of cases of necrotizing ulcerative gingivitis in children—some as young as 5 or 6 years. None of these cases has ever been established as necrotizing ulcerative gingivitis. These children are most likely suffering from either primary herpetic gingivostomatitis or aphthae or even the infinitely more serious Stevens-Johnson syndrome. All these diseases have prominent features of pain, adenopathy, necrosis, fever, and, in extreme cases, prostration. In only rare cases of necrotizing gingivitis is the patient this ill. By far the majority has little or no malaise and rarely any fever.

Symptomatology
NECROSIS

Necrotizing ulcerative gingivitis is, as its name connotes, a gingival disease characterized by necrosis and ulceration (Fig. 9-3). Surface necrosis is easily recognized by the grayish-white membrane that is so characteristic that the disease was once known as ulceromembranous gingivitis, but this sign is not always limited to or even visible on the surface. More common is necrosis within the gingival sulcus, now greatly distended by edema and gingival enlargement. It is not always as apparent as one would like to believe, but it is not too difficult to discover on careful examination of the papillary area of the gingiva.

The gingival papilla is the most common area of involvement. Most marginal gingival necrosis and inflammation result from direct extension from two adjacent interproximal papillae. When this occurs, the marginal tissue sometimes gives the moth-eaten appearance so commonly described as one of the features

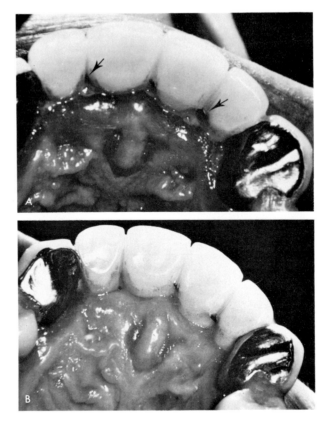

FIG. 9-3. *Acute necrotizing ulcerative gingivitis. A. Precurettage. Note the interproximal papillary destruction even between pontics (arrows). Necrosis can be clearly seen interproximally. B. Postsubgingival curettage in the same area.*

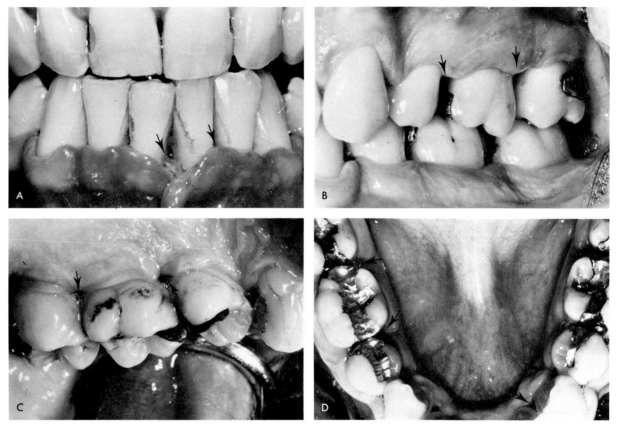

FIG. 9-4. *Acute necrotizing gingivitis. Note the predilection of the disease for the interproximal papillae, giving the gingiva a "punched out" appearance. The interproximal involvement is pathognomonic to acute necrotizing ulcerative gingivitis. A. A gingival crater adjacent to a completely destroyed interproximal papilla (arrows). B, C, and D. Different views and locations (arrows) of gingival craters typical in acute necrotizing ulcerative gingivitis.*

of necrotizing gingivitis. The papilla itself appears to be punched out and partially or completely destroyed by necrosis, creating the gingival craters commonly seen (Fig. 9-4).

Gingival interproximal craters are almost pathognomonic of necrotizing gingivitis. In many patients, there is some soft tissue at the base of the crater, but commonly there is none. Probing will give the response of palpating bone with a labial and lingual curtain of gingiva and of the adjacent roots bordering the lesion (Fig. 9-5). These craters are common and frequently persist for many years. In gingival examination, they remain as mute testimony to the gingival history of the patient. This adds an interesting peripheral feature in the psychologic makeup of the patient.

Extension of necrosis or ulceration to the alveolar or buccal mucosa or palate has been occasionally described, but not by a knowledgeable observer. What is probably being described is a herpetiform lesion, which is often confused with necrotizing ulcerative gingivitis because of the painful response and because

of the necrosis and ulceration present. They should easily be differentiated (Fig. 9-6).

PAIN

Gingival pain is a common feature and is generally pathognomonic of necrotizing gingivitis. Again, as in necrosis, the pain is limited to the interproximal papilla. This may not have been emphasized in the history, but it becomes quite noticeable when the gingivae are examined. Even with gentle probing the pain response is exaggerated.

An interesting sidelight is that we have never seen a dentition that is totally involved. It is possible, therefore, to compare the patient's pain response in an involved papilla with that in an uninvolved papilla, and the difference is great and inescapable. There is also a pain response to instrumentation, no matter how circumspect the operator is. There is, however, a quality and character to pain. The pain incident to instrumentation is dull and definitely endurable. A skillful

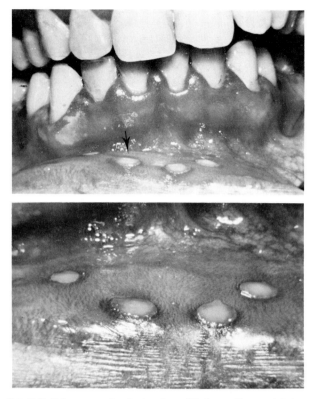

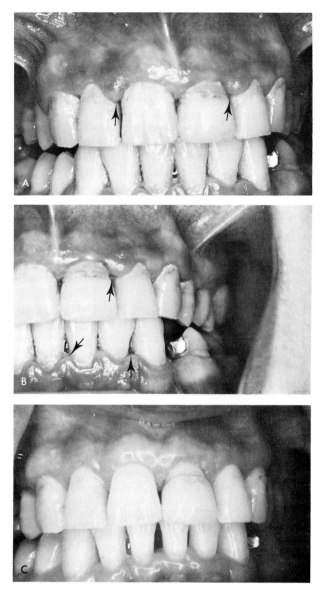

FIG. 9-6. *Primary acute gingivostomatitis (sometimes mistaken for acute necrotizing gingivitis). Note the evenly distributed gingivitis with necrotic areas in fundus of vestibular trough and on the inner surface of the lower lip. There is no interproximal involvement with necrosis. (Courtesy Dr. H. Selipsky.)*

FIG. 9-5. *Acute necrotizing ulcerative gingivitis. A. General gingival cratering. Note especially the upper lateral incisor-central incisor interproximals on both right and left (arrows). B. Gingival craters in lower anterior as well as in the upper left central incisor-lateral incisor interproximal (arrows). C. After complete therapy, which included subgingival curettage and a gingivoplasty one month after the curettage was completed.*

operator using slender curets can keep pain to a bearable minimum without the help of an anesthetic.

FETOR ORIS AND OTHER OCCASIONAL SYMPTOMS

There is a characteristic odor to some cases of fulminating necrotizing gingivitis. It is of little importance diagnostically, since it is more often absent than not. In these days of the ubiquitous use of mouthwashes and deodorants, it is less likely that odor will be present.

Other symptoms mentioned in the older literature were salivation and a peculiar sensation of teeth "feeling like wooden pegs." For some reason these are no longer reported. Probably they were exaggerated responses of imaginative patients.

ELEVATED TEMPERATURE

The older literature, again, contains reports of elevated temperature—with Wilson reporting temperatures as high as 103°F.[23] After examining several hundred sufferers from acute necrotizing ulcerative gingivitis since then, this has not been found to be true. In a number of studies, some involving as many as 1,000 subjects, temperature rise has been limited to 1°F and, in some cases, actually dropped a degree. In other words, elevation of temperature is inconclusive and inconsequential even when it occurs.

In contrast, many patients suffering from acute herpetic gingivostomatitis have elevated temperatures.

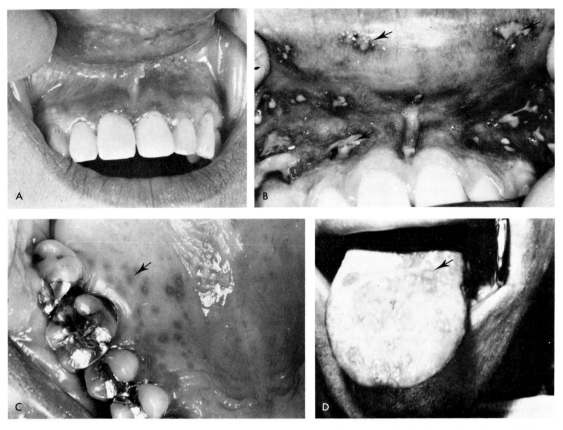

FIG. 9-7. *Acute herpetic gingivostomatitis with multiple vesicles and aphthae generally distributed. A. Acute primary gingivostomatitis: the gingivae are beefy red with no discernible differentiation between gingiva and mucosa. B. Another patient suffering from herpetiform vesicles on the lip and alveolar mucosa (arrows). Note that there is no gingival involvement. C. Aphthae on the flat surface of the palate (arrow). D. Vesicles on the tongue (arrow).*

Multiple vesicles and aphthae generally distributed will be found in these patients (Fig. 9-7). All of these lesions are painful. No affinity for interproximal tissue can be found, and none of the lesions is found with acute necrotizing ulcerative gingivitis.

MICROBIOLOGY

The early reports on acute necrotic gingivitis stressed the microbiologic aspect of the disease. Upon this factor rested the entire concept of the contagious nature of so-called Vincent's infection.

The fusiform bacillis and the spirochete implicated from the initial description of the disease have had a number of other organisms added such as a nonspecific gram-negative anaerobe, a facultative diphtheroid, and two bacteriodes plus the versatile *Bacteroides melaninogenicus*. More recent studies, however, suggest that the spirochete plays an important part after all.

The disease is not transmissible in animals as a gingival disease. Microbiologists traditionally inject cultures of the fusospirochete subcutaneously into the groin of a rabbit or guinea pig, eliciting the standard abscess formation from which the fusospirochetal strain could be cultured.

Listgarten, as well as Hamp and Mergenhagen, found that the spirochete and the fusiform bacilli were indispensable ingredients of the bacterial flora causing the necrotic lesions.[9,11] Listgarten, however, revealed still more uncertainty with his observations based upon electron microscopic examination of the spirochete involved in acute necrotizing ulcerative gingivitis. It exhibits differences from standard laboratory strains of the *Treponema microdentium* and the fusiform bacillis.

Goldhaber points out that all injuries, wounds, or lesions, including neoplastic lesions in the oral cavity, are invaded by a fusospirochetal infection.[6] Thus it is that the diagnosis of acute necrotizing ulcerative gingivitis by microscopic examination of a bacterial smear is made at some risk to the patient. A positive smear is certainly not diagnostic of the disease under discussion. It may, in fact, delay the early diagnosis and treatment of more serious diseases.

There is no question, on the other hand, but that the

pain and necrosis are due to the bacterial component. This is easily and quickly proved by the dramatic relief from pain and the temporary halting of the progress of necrosis after administering an antibiotic.

The hypothesis, widely held by investigators into this area, is that essentially the tissues are somehow altered by the disease and that bacterial invasion is secondary and incidental. This has been found to be true in other diseases as well.

THE PSYCHOGENIC FACTOR

While mentioned in many reports, emotional stress has been examined only in its most obvious forms. This is not surprising, since only a single psychoanalyst in collaboration with two periodontists brought the necessary insight and skills to the problem in its several aspects. The study by Moulton and her associates was done on a group of patients with periodontal disease.[15] While only six suffered from acute necrotizing ulcerative gingivitis, they formed a subgroup who were seriously neurotic in specific ways. All six had serious problems in emotional adaptability to their respective life situations.

It is interesting to note that the psychogenic aspect often reveals itself in the routine treatment of patients suffering with necrotizing gingivitis. One is struck with the hostile and dour personality of many of them. Here we must utter a word of caution. In the examination of patients suffering from acute necrotizing ulcerative gingivitis, the history may encourage the examiner to investigate the psychogenic factor with too great a specificity. It should be kept in mind that all the therapist may do with profit is to establish that such a factor exists. It adds nothing to his understanding of the case to press for details which, if revealed, would disturb the patient and serve to alienate him from the therapist. The periodontist is not a psychiatrist. A number of painful episodes have occurred when the rules of caution and reserve have been violated.

A number of other etiologic factors have obvious psychologic components. Pindborg, among others, considers smoking a contributing factor.[16] He cites the overwhelming majority (57 to 1) of smokers over nonsmokers in his sample of patients in his study. Goldhaber confirms these data and supports Pindborg's contention.[5] Neither worker, however, seems to have considered that smokers, especially heavy smokers, are more emotionally inadequate than their nonsmoking opposite numbers to begin with.

The entire subject of personality analysis is a large one, not too easily classified. It should be clear, however, that simplistic approaches can be misleading. For example, during World War II, according to one report, the number of patients suffering from acute necrotizing ulcerative gingivitis repeatedly increased just prior to field exercises in training.[21] Another report found no correlation between an increased number of army patients, field exercises, and bivouac, but did find a significant number of outbreaks of the disease in new recruits entering the army and in those who went on furlough.[6] This again points to emotional stress on confronting a radical change in life style and in meeting demands made upon the individual.

The emotional factor is unquestionably a strong one in the etiology of necrotizing ulcerative gingivitis, but it must not be taken to be the only one. There are a number of patients from whom no such history can be gleaned. It is possible to make too much of the psychiatric aspect of periodontal disease by bending facts to fit the case.

SMOKING

Pindborg, in a study conducted in the Norwegian Army Forces, has established a relationship between smoking and necrotizing gingivitis.[16] This is an interesting observation. The relationship between cigarette smoking and emotional needs has been mentioned.

The use of tobacco has been implicated as an etiologic factor for many years. The basis upon which it acted, ostensibly, was that it lowered the resistance of the gingival tissues so that the normal flora became more virulent. The mechanism by which this occurred was somewhat vague at best and even moralistic at worst. Although the connection is undoubtedly valid and is well supported by statistical evidence, the method by which it works is not understood. Whether smoking is a contributing factor or whether it has a direct role in acute necrotizing ulcerative gingivitis, we do not know.

Treatment of Acute Necrotizing Ulcerative Gingivitis

The microbial aspects of acute necrotizing ulcerative gingivitis dominated therapy for many years and, to a limited extent, still do today. Early on, when the spirochete excited all sorts of visions of venereal overtones, arsenicals were widely used. Salvarsan and neosalvarsan were pressed into service and were applied to the ulcers and areas of necrosis in the affected gingiva. The results were far from spectacular. It must be remembered that an acute lesion such as necrotizing gingivitis cannot have too long a life, so that even the mild debridement of careful swabbing had some effect, however minimal.

The next important agents used were the oxidizing

agents, since the anaerobic character of the bacteria involved seemed to be an acceptable rationale for using them. Chromic acid was a great favorite. While it performed no great miracles in cure, it did etch the roots adjacent to the craters and yielded an abundant harvest of carious and decalcified roots. In spite of its ravages, however, chromic acid enjoyed a vogue which spanned two decades.

Beust, on the other hand, reported that the acute lesion can best be treated with debridement.[1] This was an extremely radical position at that time and for many years later. The standard belief held by authorities was that any manipulation of the infected gingiva incident to instrumentation not only spread the lesions to heretofore uninvolved areas, but was actually a dangerous course to take, since it subjected the patient to possible Vincent's angina. This fear proved to be completely groundless. In fact, many operators performed repeated excursions with curets into involved areas that were adjacent to uninvolved gingivae and found the procedure to be entirely safe. In not a single patient did acute necrotizing gingivitis spread to as little as a single previously uninvolved papilla. On the contrary, the outcome was quick rehabilitation of the affected gingiva. What emerged as a result was that immediate

subgingival root curettage to the most complete level possible became the basic treatment for acute necrotizing ulcerative gingivitis. That is not to say that all or almost all therapists immediately have accepted root curettage as the treatment of choice. Inevitably, however, more and more dentists turn to root curettage, no longer frightened by the unsupported accounts of increased spread of infection and virulence (Fig. 9-8).

The question of pain in the tissues was raised earlier in this chapter. Many therapists thought that the involved tissues were so tender that the manipulation and tissue displacement, to say nothing of the sulcular curetting by the offset blade of the curet, would be more than most patients could bear. Local anesthesia was out of the question, of course. In practice, it was found that pain caused by careful curettage was much exaggerated. While the gingivae are unquestionably tender, careful use of curets with as little displacement of tissue as possible makes the procedure only slightly painful and easily endured. Even the little pain inflicted is not a sharp sensation. It is much like a moderate soreness and does not seem to be particularly unpleasant. Continued curettage seems to cause less, not more, pain in the gingiva.

Curettage causes the gingivae to bleed easily. This

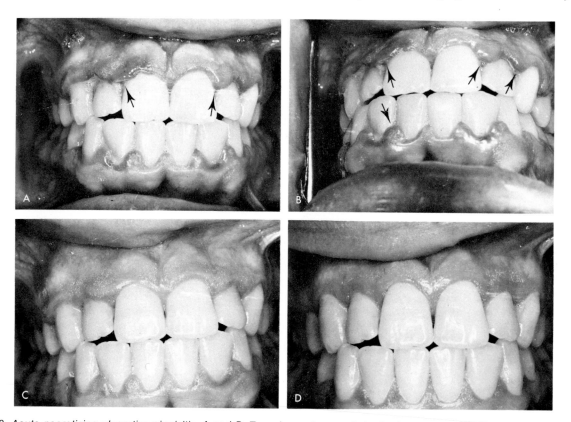

FIG. 9-8. *Acute necrotizing ulcerative gingivitis. A and B. Two views of necrosis in the interproximal areas of the upper anterior segment (arrows). C. The same patient one week later after subgingival curettage. D. Three months later after the post-curettage gingivoplasty has healed.*

lavage and the removal of the enormous masses of bacteria lying upon the surface seem to have a spectacular effect upon the tissues. Reinforced by frequent flushing, rinsing the tissues every hour of the first day with one tablespoon of 3 percent hydrogen peroxide mixed with one tablespoon of warm water usually yields complete relief from pain and halts necrosis of the gingivae.

Vigorous follow-up of both curettage and lavage is most important. It is highly desirable for the therapist to see the patient daily for 2 or 3 days until the roots of the teeth have become smooth and clean from repeated application of curets by the dentist and of the toothbrush and related instruments by the patient.

Correction of Gingival Aberrations

In certain mild manifestations of acute necrotizing ulcerative gingivitis, it is possible with vigorous treatment and with good patient cooperation to achieve a complete remission from the disease. In such a situation, even the gingival craters heal and become once again properly shaped papillae, performing their normal function.

Unfortunately, remission does not always occur. In fact, in some patients, some corrective surgery is necessary to eliminate the gingival craters that are often the result of necrotizing gingivitis. While it is true that the disease is no longer present, the gingival abnormalities constitute a nidus for the retention of debris and for the initiation of a train of events ending in progressive periodontal breakdown.

In common with other acute diseases, the active course of acute necrotizing gingivitis is relatively short. Two weeks is the upper limit of the duration of the infection. Treatment of the gingivae with repeated curetting can and does extend beyond this period, but the infection and ulceration are no longer present, nor is pain any longer a factor to reckon with. A month, therefore, is an ample time lapse after the acute infection to apply corrective surgery to the gingivae, if it is required.

The actual procedures incident to the correction of these abnormalities are simple. They consist primarily in the reshaping of the gingiva through gingivoplasty.

Steel blades, shears, rotary abrasives, and any other convenient modality are used to reshape the gingiva surgically. As in all gingivoplasties, the difficulties encountered are engendered by the tiny quantities of tissue to be excised. This is why scalpels alone are rarely sufficient to finish the task. To manage small tabs of gingiva, iris and tenotomy shears are useful. Properly used, they may be effective, even interproximally, to a considerable degree. Even the steel blade, such as

the kidney-shaped gingivectomy knife, is most useful as a scraper. It is used at right angles to the surface of the gingiva to achieve an undulating contour after the gingival margin has been thinned properly with the same instrument and interproximal gingival reshaping has been done.

Care must be taken to observe the basic principles of gingivoplasty. Reverse gingival architecture must be eliminated, obviously at the expense of labial and lingual marginal gingiva, so that the papillae can be reconstituted.

Postoperative care of the wound is standard. Most operators use a surgical dressing to cover the wound. This is almost always required in the long-beveled external gingival incisions used in corrective surgery. Patients will experience pain during eating and brushing if the tissues are left unprotected. The dressing may be removed after 5 to 7 days.

Unfortunately, most patients suffering from acute necrotizing ulcerative gingivitis do not follow through to complete corrective treatment. The reasons are (1) the lack of assurance that the disease, once treated, will not recur, and (2) the general lack of interest and motivation in most patients because of their ages and temperaments. In this connection, it is useful to establish clearly that much of the responsibility for cure rests with the patient. Recurrent acute episodes are far from rare. In fact, the old and discredited chronic necrotizing gingivitis was no more than a series of recurrent acute exacerbations (Fig. 9-9). There is no chronic acute necrotizing ulcerative gingivitis.

The possibility of recurrence must be impressed upon the patient. Having discharged his responsibility thoroughly in the initial bout, the therapist need feel no guilt for the reexacerbation.

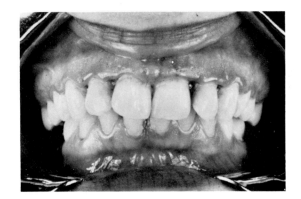

FIG. 9-9. *Acute necrotizing ulcerative gingivitis. This illustrates the typical appearance of a recurrent acute necrotizing gingivitis.*

References

1. Beust, T. B.: Oral manifestations and treatment of Vincent's infection. J. Dent. Res., *10:*97, 1930.

2. Emslie, B. D.: Cancrum oris. Dental Pract. Dent. Res., *13:*481, 1963.

3. Giddon, D. B., Zackin, S. J., and Goldhaber, P.: Acute necrotizing gingivitis in college students. J. Am. Dent. Assoc., *68:*381, 1964.

4. Goldberg, H., et al.: Emotional status of patients with acute gingivitis. N.Y. Dent. J., *22:*308, 1956.

5. Goldhaber, P.: Study of acute necrotizing ulcerative gingivitis. Abstract #35, I.A.D.R. Abstracts, 1957.

6. Goldhaber, P.: Periodontal Therapy, 4th ed. Goldman and Cohen, 1968, pp. 198, 199.

7. Goldhaber, P., and Giddon, D. B.: Present concepts concerning the etiology and treatment of acute necrotizing ulcerative gingivitis. Int. Dent. J., *14:*468, 1964.

8. Grupe, H. E., and Wilder, L. S.: Observations of necrotizing gingivitis in 870 military trainees. J. Periodontol., *27:*255, 1956.

9. Hamp, E. G., and Mergenhagen, S. E.: Experimental infections with oral spirochetes. J. Infect. Dis., *109:*43, 1961.

10. Hiatt, W. H.: Regeneration of the periodontium after endodontic therapy and flap operation. Oral Surg., *12:*1471, 1959.

11. Listgarten, M. A.: Electron microscopic observations of the bacterial flora of acute necrotizing ulcerative gingivitis. J. Periodontol., *36:*328, 1965.

12. Listgarten, M. A., and Socransky, S. S.: Ultrastructural characteristics of a spirochete in the lesion of acute necrotizing ulcerative gingivostomatitis (Vincent's infection). Arch. Oral Biol., *9:*95, 1964.

13. MacDonald, J. B., Gibbons, R. J., and Socransky, S. S.: Bacterial mechanisms in periodontal disease. Ann. N.Y. Acad. Sci., *85:*467, 1960.

14. MacDonald, J. B., et al.: Pathogenic components of an experimental fusospirochetal infection. J. Infect. Dis., *98:*15, 1956.

15. Moulton, R., Ewen, S., and Thieman, W.: Emotional factors in periodontal disease. Oral Surg., *5:*833, 1952.

16. Pindborg, J. J.: Gingivitis in military personnel with special reference to ulceromembranous gingivitis. Odont. Tidskr., *59:*407, 1951.

17. Plaut, H. C.: Studien zur bakteriellen diagnostik der diphtherie und der anginen. Dtsch. Med. Wochenschr, *20:*920, 1894.

18. Prichard, J. F.: Management of the periodontal abscess. Oral Surg., *6:*474, 1953.

19. Prichard, J. F.: Regeneration of bone following periodontal therapy. Oral Surg., *10:*247, 1957.

20. Schluger, S.: The etiology and treatment of Vincent's infection. J. Am. Dent. Assoc., *30:*524, 1943.

21. Schluger, S.: Necrotic ulcerative gingivitis in the Army; incidence, communicability and treatment, J. Am. Dent. Assoc., *44:*671, 1949.

22. Vincent, H.: Sur l'etiologie et sur les lesions anatomo-pathologiques de la pourriture d'hopital. Ann. Inst. Pasteur, *10:*448, 1896.

23. Wilson, J. R.: Etiology and diagnosis of bacterial gingivitis including Vincent's disease. J. Am. Dent. Assoc., *44:*671, 1952.

10

Diabetes Mellitus

Diabetes mellitus is a syndrome of abnormal elevations of blood glucose due to a relative or absolute lack of insulin, at times associated with changes in electrolytes and water. Alterations in lipid and protein metabolism are part of this syndrome. Vascular changes characterized by accelerated nonspecific atherosclerosis and more specific microangiopathy, particularly involving the eye and kidney, are frequent manifestations. It is now evident that the mere labeling of a patient "diabetic" does not in itself define the etiology or the biochemical, hormonal, or histologic abnormalities that may be present.

EPIDEMIOLOGY

It is estimated that there are some four million individuals in the United States with diabetes. This approximates some 2 percent of the total population. Of these individuals, roughly half are undiagnosed.[34] The difficulty in acquiring exact figures is due to lack of agreement as to what constitutes the minimal requirement for the diagnosis. Since absolute diagnostic criteria are still lacking, many questions remain unanswered, one of which is the meaning of the increasing frequency of abnormal glucose tolerance in old age.

Age

The prevalence increases rapidly with increasing age so that in the age range 45 to 70, the prevalence of diabetes is about 5 percent.[39] In the diabetic population, some 4 out of every 5 diabetics are over 45 years old,[1,74] with peak prevalence being reached at age 65 to 74.[38,39]

Family History

Diabetes is more common among the relatives of diabetics than among similar relatives of nondiabetics. A positive family history may be elicited in up to 50 percent of all newly diagnosed patients.[54] Although the evidence derived from studies of family aggregates and twins affirms the importance of genetic factors in the etiology of diabetes, the exact mode of inheritance of the diabetic trait or traits is still to be clarified.[54,55]

Obesity

The prevalence is seven times greater among those who are 50 percent overweight than among those of normal weight.[26] Obesity and carbohydrate intolerance tend to coexist in man, and prolonged obesity may unmask genetic diabetes.[3,75]

10
Diabetes Mellitus

ELAINE D. HENLEY

Large Babies

Mothers who deliver babies weighing over 9 to 10 pounds are at increased risk for the future development of diabetes.[37,44,48]

CLASSIFICATION

In an attempt to define the disease, diabetes mellitus, it has proved useful to classify the natural history of this syndrome into four stages.[19] These arbitrary and artificial divisions are based solely on the presence or absence of hyperglycemia and on the degree of measurable abnormalities of glucose metabolism. This classification does not include the existence, degree, or severity of the other abnormalities found in this disease, nor does it imply that all diabetics progress unrelentingly from stage 1 through stage 4 (Table 10-1). Fluctuations between these various stages in a given patient are not uncommon, and varying degrees of regression as well as progression of carbohydrate intolerance often occur.

Prediabetes

The earliest stage, prediabetes, is also called potential diabetes (World Health Organization).[13] It identifies the individual who will eventually develop diabetes and defines the interval of time from conception until the demonstration of impaired glucose tolerance.[8] Normal glucose tolerance is present under all conditions. This theoretical stage can only be identified with certainty, in retrospect, and only after the individual manifests evidence of decreased glucose tolerance.[74] Prediabetes may be suspected to be present in the nondiabetic identical twin of a diabetic,[52] or in the offspring of two diabetic parents.[14]

Latent Diabetes

The next stage, suspected diabetes, has been variously called latent (World Health Organization), or subclinical.[19] Under usual circumstances, fasting and postprandial blood sugars are normal as is the glucose tolerance test. Diabetes, however, may be suspected in a woman who now has normal glucose tolerance but who has had a history of gestational diabetes which is characterized by elevated blood sugars during pregnancy,[4,43] or in an individual with a history of abnormal blood sugars associated with the stress of an acute illness, injury, or surgery. Suspected diabetics respond abnormally to oral cortisone-glucose tolerance tests.[19]

Chemical Diabetes

Chemical or latent diabetes, also termed asymptomatic or subclinical diabetes, defines the stage during which the patient is without signs or symptoms of the disease. Fasting blood sugars are usually normal, although minimally elevated fasting and postcibal blood sugars can occur at times. This stage differs from suspected diabetes in that the oral glucose tolerance is always abnormal. A cortisone-glucose test is unnecessary for diagnosis.

Overt Diabetes

Clinical or overt or frank diabetes is the most advanced of these defined stages. There is always fasting and postprandial hyperglycemia. The classic symptoms

TABLE 10-1. *Stages in the Natural History of Diabetes Mellitus*

| | FASTING BLOOD SUGAR | GLUCOSE TOLERANCE TEST | CORTISONE GLUCOSE TOLERANCE TEST | TERMS EMPLOYED | |
				AMERICAN DIABETES ASSOC.	WORLD HEALTH ORGANIZATION
Prediabetes	Normal	Normal	Normal	Prediabetes	Potential diabetes
Subclinical	Normal	Normal or abnormal during pregnancy; stress	Abnormal	Suspected diabetes	Latent diabetes
Latent	Normal or Mildly abnormal	Abnormal	Abnormal	Chemical or Latent	Asymptomatic or Subclinical
Overt	Abnormal	Abnormal	Abnormal	Overt	Clinical

of polydipsia, polyphagia, and weight loss are due to marked glucosuria and polyuria with the associated loss of calories and water. Since fasting as well as random blood and urine sugars are always elevated, a glucose tolerance test is never needed for diagnosis. Many obese adult patients, however, do not develop this acute symptomatic state. These individuals, with maturity-onset diabetes, who comprise 60 percent of the total diabetic population,[22] are for the most part only minimally symptomatic. In this group, when fasting blood sugars are mildly or equivocally elevated, an abnormal two-hour postprandial blood sugar will usually confirm the diagnosis.

Clinically, it has been helpful to divide overt diabetes into the ketotic and nonketotic forms of the disease. Generally, the ketotic form occurs in children or young adults and has been variously called growth onset or juvenile type or ketosis-prone or insulin-dependent diabetes. This insulin-requiring form can also occur in mature adults, the majority of whom are normal weight or lean. The nonketotic form tends to occur in obese middle-aged adults and has been referred to as maturity onset or adult type or nonketosis-prone diabetes mellitus.

The young lean ketosis-prone individuals, who comprise only some 5 to 10 percent of the entire diabetic population, have little or no effective endogenous insulin and therefore require insulin therapy for survival. Overweight, middle-aged diabetics, on the other hand, have relatively elevated endogenous insulin levels compared with lean normals (Fig. 10-1).[29,50] Obesity, per se, has been shown to be associated with elevated levels of endogenous insulin, probably as a consequence of tissue resistance to its effect.[5,30] Thus, the adult-onset obese patient with comparatively mild carbohydrate intolerance usually does not require exogenous insulin for survival. Weight reduction in these individuals will invariably improve glucose tolerance.

There are, however, many exceptions to these customary divisions. Very mild diabetes may abruptly become severe, necessitating insulin therapy, and regression from insulin dependency to latent or even prediabetic stages has been reported.[19,45,47]

PATHOPHYSIOLOGIC ABNORMALITIES

The prevalence of periodontal disease is increased in patients with diabetes mellitus.[23,24,35,77] The development of a reproducible and reliable method of scoring periodontal disease,[56] and information regarding the early biochemical and histologic aberrations occurring in the asymptomatic diabetic helped clarify this relationship. The findings of periodontal disease in Chinese hamsters (Cricetulus) who develop spontaneous hered-

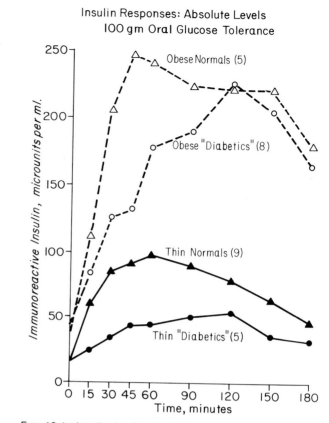

FIG. 10-1. *Insulin levels of obese and thin persons. (From Badade, J. D., Bierman, E. L., and Porte, D., Jr.: The significance of basal insulin levels in the evaluation of the insulin response to glucose in diabetic and nondiabetic subjects. J. Clin. Invest., 46:1553, 1967.)*

itary diabetes led to studies that confirmed this association in human patients.[10] A positive association has been found between the severity of periodontal disease and the age of the patient, the duration of known diabetes, the degree and frequency of variations or fluctuations in blood sugar, and the severity of complications and late manifestations of this disease.[21]

Susceptibility and Response to Infection

Despite frequent remarks to the contrary, it is clinically apparent that the incidence of both systemic and localized bacterial infections is not increased in controlled diabetic patients without vascular disease. No defect in host defense has been found in diabetics without significant hyperglycemia or ketoacidosis.[6,15,27] Although common asymptomatic skin or urinary tract infections have not been found to be increased in diabetics compared with normals,[40,49] symptomatic pyogenic infections when they occur tend to be more severe and persistent. There is clinical evidence, however, that diabetics are more susceptible to superficial

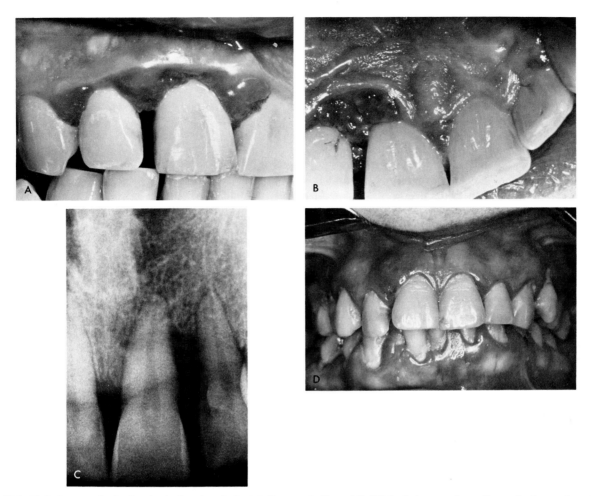

FIG. 10-2. *Diabetes as a factor in gingival and periodontal disease. A, B, and C. Clinical views and a radiograph of a portion of the upper incisor area of an uncontrolled diabetic. D. The same area after control was established but with no gingival or periodontal therapy administered, not even a simple prophylaxis. Improvement in the gingiva was rapid, but the inflammation did not disappear and required the same treatment as that for a nondiabetic patient.*

monilial infections than are nondiabetics.[25] The inability of the decompensated or untreated diabetic patient to cope with established infection has been shown to be related to altered host defenses.[9] Phagocytosis is impaired in both hyperglycemia and ketoacidosis,[16] and chemotaxis of polymorphonuclear leukocytes is impaired in the absence of insulin.[41]

Surgical healing in the controlled diabetic without vasculopathy is no different from nondiabetic operative wound healing (Fig. 10-2).[10]

Vascular Disease

Diabetics have a higher prevalence of vascular disease, including coronary artery involvement, than nondiabetics of similar age and sex.[42] Vascular abnormalities develop not only at an earlier age but in a more diffuse and extensive pattern than in nondiabetics. Statistically, evidence of vascular involvement becomes apparent with increasing frequency in juvenile diabetics 15 years after diagnosis, regardless of the patient's age or insulin requirement. Ninety-two percent of a group of diabetic children studied for 20 years at the Joslin Clinic were found to have some degree of vascular disease.[77]

Vascular lesions occur in large-sized and medium-sized vessels (arteriosclerosis), small arteries (arteriolosclerosis), and capillaries (microangiopathy). The arteriosclerotic process in the diabetic does not differ morphologically from that in nondiabetics, except that it is more diffuse, involves segmental occlusions, and early obliterates lower extremity vessels.[65] These differences are responsible for the increased incidence of gangrene found in diabetics.[2]

The capillary microangiopathy is generally considered specific to diabetes. It is associated with an increase in endothelial basal lamina thickness.[60] Basal lamina changes can occur in all tissues, although involvement of the eye, kidney, and peripheral nerves has been emphasized as constituting the so-called diabetic triopathy. The exact etiology and significance of basal lamina thickening is still not settled. It has been reported to be present in some individuals with potential diabetes or prediabetes.[59] However, some investigators have been unable to confirm this finding and postulate the relation of the thickening to accelerated cell turnover that probably occurs in diabetics.[72] Still others find convincing evidence that the basal lamina thickening is a consequence of abnormal metabolism.[62,63,64] Basal lamina thickness is found to be increased in diabetics in direct relationship to the duration of the disease.[46] Similar changes in basal lamina thickness have been found to occur normally with aging.[78]

In adult onset disease, symptomatic angiopathy may at times antedate the diagnosis of diabetes. Patients, thus, may initially manifest coronary artery disease or distal lower extremity gangrene. Diabetic retinopathy has been found on opthalmoscopic examination in approximately 10 percent of newly diagnosed patients over the age of 50.[61] Not only is diabetic retinopathy one of the leading causes of blindness today, but the presence of several retinal changes is also of prognostic significance in diabetics of all ages. Approximately 65 percent of patients with proliferative retinopathy and less than 50 percent of newly diagnosed blind diabetics survive more than 5 years.[7] Since microangiopathic lesions tend to develop in parallel in various organs, patients with severe retinopathy have a high probability of also having advanced kidney lesions.[66] Uremia as a result of nephropathy is a common cause of death in diabetics. It can occur in patients with mild carbohydrate intolerance who have never received insulin as well as in growth-onset diabetes. It is found with increasing frequency as the duration of diabetes increases.

Neurologic Disease

Disorders of the nervous system, which includes the brain, spinal cord, and autonomic and peripheral nerves, occur in diabetes mellitus. Controversy exists regarding the exact etiology of the neurologic abnormalities. Metabolic derangements have been strongly implicated, especially in the polyneuropathies,[72] but there is also some evidence that implicates microangiopathic changes.[17] Involvement of the sensory, motor, or autonomic systems, singly or in combination, gives varied findings and symptoms.

The clinical syndromes include polyneuropathy, mononeuropathy, amyotrophy, and autonomic neuropathy.

Polyneuropathy, which is usually symmetrical with sensory loss, involves predominantly the distal extremities. Symptoms of numbness and tingling, associated with diminished sensation in the hands and especially the feet, occur. When there is a marked loss of sensation, trophic ulcers of the feet and Charcot-type changes (neuropathic arthropathy) occur in the joints of the lower extremities. There is often evidence of a preexisting sensory neuropathy when diabetes is first diagnosed in elderly persons. Although the rate of progression varies, return of function rarely occurs.

Mononeuropathy affects one or sometimes more peripheral nerves. Motor, sensory, as well as autonomic involvement leads to paralysis which is often painful. Extraocular muscle palsies, especially involving cranial nerves III and VI, as well as foot drop involving the lateral popliteal nerve occur most commonly. The onset is sudden and recovery is usual.

Diabetic amyotrophy or asymmetric motor neuropathy usually involves muscles of the pelvic girdle and thighs. There are associated weakness and muscle wasting. In this uncommon neuropathy, slow improvement may occur following control or treatment of the diabetes.

Autonomic neuropathy is usually associated with polyneuropathy. Gastrointestinal disturbances with diarrhea and atony of the esophagus and stomach may be present. Bladder dysfunction, retrograde ejaculation, and impotence, as well as orthostatic hypotension, anhidrosis, and vasomotor instability, are some of the autonomic abnormalities that give rise to symptoms.

DIAGNOSIS

The *asymptomatic patient* suspected of having diabetes will have a fasting blood sugar that is only mildly abnormal or borderline elevated. A postprandial blood sugar can often be helpful in confirming the diagnosis. A blood sugar drawn 2 hours after a large meal, in nondiabetics should be in the same range as normal fasting values. In mild asymptomatic diabetics, it is frequently elevated. The use of a 75 or 100 gram glucose load should not be used unless the patient is adequately prepared for several days with a 250 to 300 gram carbohydrate diet prior to testing, similar to the preparation for an oral glucose tolerance test. A high carbohydrate diet will increase insulin secretion in normal subjects, and carbohydrate restriction for any reason such as from prolonged bed rest,[32] illness with anorexia, dieting, or inability to chew will give a false positive result to the test.

The symptomatic patient is diagnosed without difficulty when there is a history of polyuria, polydipsia, polyphagia, and weight loss. Some patients, however, have significant but less dramatic symptoms. Fatiguability, nocturia, vaginitis, or skin infections may be the only complaint. Unless the patient has been on a prolonged fast, all blood and all or most urine sugars will be abnormal at this time. Since a random blood sugar level, with or without a corresponding urine sugar level, will be elevated, a diagnostic glucose tolerance test is never indicated.

APPROACHES TO TREATMENT

It is clear to those clinicians who have diabetic patients, that despite optimal medical care and meticulous daily management, some diabetics will develop all the late irreversible lethal sequelae of this syndrome. Even when a diabetic is apparently well controlled, there are intervals throughout each day or week when hyperglycemia of varying degrees occurs. Fluctuations in plasma lipoproteins and episodes of protein breakdown associated with accelerated gluconeogenesis no doubt occur concomitantly.

Controversy exists as to whether the more tragic late manifestations occurring in diabetes mellitus, such as the various forms of renal disease, the neurologic deficits, and loss of vision, might be prevented or at least delayed by control or improved management of these metabolic changes. As knowledge about diabetes continues to accrue, perhaps some of these late manifestations can be forestalled. Recommendations by the Committee on Food and Nutrition of the American Diabetes Association concerning changes in dietary composition may prove helpful in attaining this goal.[12] Likewise, since infection causes further fluctuations and elevations of blood sugar as well as increased morbidity in diabetes, patients should be vigorously encouraged to take special precautions, not only to prevent infections, but to seek prompt treatment when they occur, since infections of any type or severity can lead to hyperglycemia and ketosis. During treatment for such infections, which include severe periodontal disease, individuals ordinarily treated with diet alone or diet and oral agents may require insulin therapy until the infection is brought under control.

Diet

Diet continues to be one of the most important factors in the control of the hyperglycemia of diabetes. There is no agreement among physicians as to what constitutes the ideal diabetic diet. Rigid carbohydrate restriction is no longer encouraged.[12] Current medical opinion, in an attempt to reduce the premature vasculopathy, including the risk of coronary artery disease, advises the dietary restriction of lipids, especially saturated fats and cholesterol-containing foods. Optimally, the diet should be nutritious, maintain or restore normal body weight, and minimize rapid and marked fluctuations in blood sugar. Obese patients should be rigorously encouraged to lose weight, and children must be given adequate calories for normal growth and development. In insulin-dependent diabetes, it is essential that the total caloric intake, the distribution of food throughout the day, and the timing of meals and snacks remain reasonably constant from day to day.

Insulin

Insulin is mandatory in the treatment of ketoacidosis and acute-onset symptomatic disease. It is necessary in the majority of juvenile-onset patients and in women with gestational diabetes. It is indicated for patients who cannot be controlled by diet alone and for patients with neuropathy.

Most commercial insulins (U40, U80) contain about 95 percent pure insulin. Recently, "single peak" insulin (U100) which is 99 percent pure has been marketed. In the near future a "single component" insulin of 100 percent purity will also be available.

Three types of insulin are marketed: short-acting, intermediate, and long-acting insulin (Table 10-2). Although most patients will be adequately controlled on a single morning dose of intermediate-acting insulin alone or mixed with short-acting insulin, many patients, especially adolescents and young adults, may require a mixture of short- and intermediate-acting insulin twice daily, in the morning before breakfast and again before supper. The prescribed doses are tailored to each individual's needs. Usually the dose must be increased during illness, infection, emotional stress, or surgical procedures. When the patient is unable to eat normally as a result of oral surgery, an increased dose of insulin may still be necessary. In contrast, the usual insulin dose is decreased with the initiation of regular exercise or generally increased physical activity. Although the acknowledged goal of therapy is normalization of blood sugar, this is rarely, if ever, feasible because of the problems inherent in the use of exogenous insulin administered once or twice daily. If rigid blood sugar control (euglycemia) is attempted, insulin-induced hypoglycemia with its attendant hazards is an inevitable result. Hypoglycemia, depending on the depth and duration, can cause coma with irreversible brain damage and even death, sometimes without the usual early symptomatic warnings of hunger, sweating, tremulousness, and mental confusion.

Oral Hypoglycemic Agents

Five oral hypoglycemic antidiabetic preparations are available by prescription in this country (Table 10-3). Four are sulfonylureas, and all are similar in chemical structure to sulfanilamide. They are pre-

TABLE 10-2. *Insulin Preparations*

TYPE OF INSULIN	ACTION	PEAK HOURS*	DURATION HOURS*
Regular; crystalline zinc	Rapid	4–6	6–12
Semilente	Rapid	4–6	12–16
NPH insulin (Isophane)	Intermediate	8–12	18–24+
Lente (30% semilente + 70% Ultralente)	Intermediate	8–12	24+
Globin	Intermediate	8–12	18–24+
Ultralente	Long	16–18	30–36+
Protamine zinc PZI	Long	14–20	24–36+

*Depends on size of dose and individual treated.

sumed to act by stimulating the beta cells of the pancreatic islets to increase insulin secretion and by potentiating the effectiveness of endogenous insulin.[33] The fifth agent, a biguanide, differs in structure and mechanism of action, but the exact mode of action has not been clearly elucidated.[31] These agents have been used widely for nearly 20 years in the treatment of recently diagnosed mild maturity diabetes.

The results of a recent large prospective study involving multiple participating diabetic centers, the University Group Diabetes Program, has led some physicians to question the significance or validity of the published results, and others to question the clinical use of these agents.[20,28,51,57,58,67-70] The report of the Committee for the Assessment of Biometric Aspects of Controlled Trials of Hypoglycemic Agents confirmed the validity of the protocol and findings of the University Group Diabetes Program.[53] The study revealed that there was no evidence of beneficial effects from the use of tolbutamide or phenformin in the patients studied. It also showed that there was an increased number of cardiovascular deaths in the diabetics taking these drugs, compared with those on diet alone or on diet plus insulin injections.[52,67-70] Since the efficacy and safety of these preparations continues to be controversial, increased and stringent attention should instead be given to diet and weight reduction.

References

1. Bauer, M. L., et al.: Characteristics of persons with diabetes. National Center for Health Statistics. U.S. Public Health Service Publication, 1000 Series 10, Number 40. Washington, D.C., Government Printing Office, 1969.
2. Bell, E. P.: Arteriosclerotic gangrene of the extremities in diabetic and nondiabetic persons. Am. J. Clin. Pathol., 28:27, 1957.

TABLE 10-3. *Oral Hypoglycemic Agents*

TYPE	GENERIC NAME	TRADE NAME	USUAL DURATION OF ACTION (HOURS)
Sulfonylurea	Tolbutamide	Orinase	Short 6–12
Sulfonylurea	Tolazamide	Tolinase	Medium 6–18
Sulfonylurea	Acetohexamide	Dymelor	Medium 12–24
Sulfonylurea	Chlorpropamide	Diabinese	Long 24–60
Phenethylbiguanide	Phenformin	DBI	Short 4–6
	Phenformin Time-Dispersal	DBI-TD	Medium 8–12

3. Bierman, E. L., Bagdade, J. D., and Porte, D., Jr.: Obesity and diabetes: the odd couple. Am. J. Clin. Nutr., 21(12):1434, 1968.

4. Brudenell, M., and Beard, R.: Diabetes in pregnancy. Clin. Endocrinol. Metabolism. 1:3, 674, 1972.

5. Butterfield, W. J. H., and Whickelow, M. J.: Effect of diet, sulfonylureas and pheniformin on peripheral glucose uptakes on diabetics and obesity. Lancet, 2:785, 1968.

6. Bybee, J. D., and Rogers, D. E.: The phagocytic activity of PMN leukocytes obtained from patients with diabetes mellitus. J. Lab. Clin. Med., 64:1, 1964.

7. Caird, F. I., Pirie, A., and Ramsell, T. F.: In Diabetes and the Eye. Edinburgh, Blackwell Scientific Publications, 1968, pp. 94–98.

8. Camerini-Davalos, R. A.: Prevention of diabetes mellitus. Med. Clin. North Am., 49:865, 1965.

9. Chernew, I., and Braude, A. I.: Depression of phagocytosis by solutes in concentrations found in the kidney and urine. J. Clin. Invest., 41:1945, 1962.

10. Cohen, L. S., Fekety, F. R., and Cluff, L. E.: Studies on the epidemiology of staphylococcal infections. VI. Infections in the surgical patient. Ann. Surg., 159:321, 1964.

11. Cohen, M. M., Shklar, G., and Yerganian, G.: Periodontal disease in the Chinese hamster (Cricetulus griseus) with hereditary diabetes mellitus. Diabetes, 15:531, 1966.

12. Committee on Food and Nutrition, American Diabetes Association: Special report: Principles of nutrition and dietary recommendations for patients with diabetes mellitus. Diabetes, 20:633, 1971.

13. Conn, J. W., and Fajans, S. S.: The prediabetic state. A concept of dynamic resistance to a genetic diabetogenic influence. Am. J. Med., 31:839, 1961.

14. Cooke, A. M., et al.: Conjugal diabetes. Diabetologia, 2:145, 1966.

15. Crosby, B., and Allison, F., Jr.: Phagocytic and bacterial capacity of polymorphonuclear leukocytes recovered from venous blood of human beings. Proc. Soc. Exp. Biol. Med., 123:660, 1966.

16. Drachman, R., Root, R., and Wood, W. B.: Studies on the effect of experimental diabetes mellitus on antimicrobial defense. I. Demonstration of defect in phagocytosis. J. Exp. Med., 124:227, 1966.

17. Fagerberg, S. E.: Studies on the pathogenesis of diabetic neuropathy. Acta Med. Scand., 157:401, 1957.

18. Fajans, S. S., and Conn, J. W.: An approach to the prediction of diabetes mellitus by modification of the glucose tolerance test with cortisone. Diabetes, 3:296, 1954.

19. Fajans, S. S., and Conn, J. W.: Prediabetes, subclinical diabetes and latent chemical diabetes. Interpretations, diagnosis and treatment. In On the Nature and Treatment of Diabetes. B. S. Leibel and G. S. Wrenshall, Eds. International Congress Series No. 84, 1965, pp. 641–656.

20. Feldman, R., et al.: Oral hypoglycemic drug prophylaxis in asymptomatic diabetes. In Diabetes. W. J. Malaisse and J. Pirart, Eds. Excerpta Medica. New York, American Elsevier Pub. Co. 1974, pp. 574–587.

21. Finestone, A. J., and Boorujy, S. R.: Diabetes and periodontal disease. Diabetes, 16:336, 1967.

22. Fisher, G. F., and Vavra, H. M.: Diabetes Source Book. U.S. Public Health Service Publications, May, 1964, p. 1168.

23. Gottsegen, R.: Dental and oral considerations in diabetes mellitus. N.Y. State J. Med., 62:289, 1962.

24. Gottsegen, R.: Dental and oral aspects of diabetes mellitus. In Diabetes Mellitus: Theory and Practice. M. Ellenberg and H. Rifkin, Eds. New York, McGraw-Hill, 1970, pp. 770–779.

25. Johnson, J. E., III: Infection and diabetes. In Diabetes Mellitus: Theory and Practice. M. Ellenberg and H. Rifkin, Eds. New York, McGraw-Hill, 1970, p. 739.

26. Joslin, E. P.: The treatment of diabetes mellitus. In Diabetes Mellitus. E. P. Joslin, et al. Philadelphia, Lea & Febiger, 1959, p. 211.

27. Kass, E.: Hormones and host resistance to infection. Bacteriol. Rev., 24:177, 1960.

28. Keen, H., Jarrett, R. J., and Fuller, J. H.: Tolbutamide and arterial disease in borderline diabetics. In Diabetes. W. J. Malaisse and J. Pirart, Eds. Excerpta Medica. New York, American Elsevier Pub. Co., 1974, pp. 588–601.

29. Kipnis, D. M.: Insulin secretion in diabetes mellitus. Ann. Intern. Med., 69:891, 1968.

30. Kipnis, D. W.: Does diabetes begin with insulin resistance? In Early Diabetes. R. A. Camerini-Davalos and H. W. Cole, Eds. New York, Academic Press, 1970, 171.

31. Lebovitz, H. E., and Feldman, J. M.: Oral hypoglycemic agents. Mechanisms of action. Diabetes Mellitus, Dx and Rx, Vol. III, American Diabetic Association, 1971.

32. Lipman, R. L., et al.: Impairment of peripheral glucose utilization in normal subjects by prolonged bedrest. J. Lab Clin. Med., 76:221, 1970.

33. Loubatieres, A. L.: Complementary arguments in favor of the betacytotrophic action of the hypoglycemic sulfamides. In Early Diabetes by R. A. Camerini-Davlos and H. S. Cole. New York, Academic Press, 1970, pp. 411–420.

34. McDonald, G. W., and Fisher, G. F.: Diabetes prevalence in the United States. Public Health Reports, 82:334, 1968.

35. MacKenzie, R. S., and Millard, A. D.: Interrelated effects of diabetes, arterioscleroses and calculus on alveolar bone loss. J. Am. Dent. Assoc., 66:19, 1963.

36. Malaisse, W. J., and Pirart, J., Eds: Diabetes. Excerpta Medica. New York, American Elsevier Pub. Co., 1974, pp. 612–623.

37. Malins, J. M., and Fitzgerald, M. G.: Childbearing prior to the recognition of diabetes. Diabetes, 14:175, 1965.

38. Malins, J. M.: Diabetes in the population. Clin. Endocrinol. Metabolism, 1:3, 645, 1972.

39. Malins, J. M.: Diabetes; screening for disease. Lancet, 2:1367, 1974.

40. Minchew, B. H., et al.: Studies on the epidemiology of staph infections. VII. Bull. Johns Hopkins Hosp., 114:414, 1964.

41. Mowat, A. G., and Baum, J.: Chemotaxis of PMN leukocyte from patients with diabetes mellitus. N. Engl. J. Med., *284:*621, 1971.

42. Ostrander, L. D., Jr., et al.: The relationship of cardiovascular disease to hyperglycemia. Ann. Int. Med., *62:*1189, 1965.

43. O'Sullivan, J. B.: Gestational diabetes and its significance. *In* Early Diabetes. R. A. Camerini-Davalos and H. S. Cole, Eds. New York, Academic Press, 1970, p. 339.

44. O'Sullivan, J. B., Gillis, S. S., and Tenny, B. O.: Gestational blood glucose levels in normal and potentially diabetic women related to the birth weight of their infants. Diabetes, *15:*466, 1966.

45. O'Sullivan, J. B., and Hurwitz, D.: Spontaneous remission in early diabetes mellitus. Arch. Int. Med., *117:*769, 1966.

46. Pardo, V., et al.: Incidence and significance of muscle capillary basement lamina thickness in juvenile diabetes. Am. J. Pathol., *68:*67, 1972.

47. Peck, F. B., Sr., Kurtley, W. R., and Peck, F. B., Jr.: Complete remission of severe diabetes. Diabetes, *7:*93, 1958.

48. Pedersen, J.: The Pregnant Diabetic and her Newborn. Problems and Management. Copenhagen, Munksgaard, 1967.

49. Pometta, D., et al.: Asymptomatic bacteriuria in diabetes mellitus. N. Engl. J. Med., *276:*1118, 1967.

50. Porte, D., Jr., Bagdade, J. D., Bierman, E. C.: The critical role of obesity in the interpretation of serum insulin levels. Early Diabetes. R. A. Camerini-Davalos and H. W. Cole, Eds. New York, Academic Press, 1970, 191.

51. Prout, T. E.: The UGPD controversy clinical trials versus clinical impression. Diabetes, *21:*1035, 1972.

52. Prout, T. E.: Adverse effects of the oral hypoglycemic drugs. *In* Diabetes. W. J. Malaisse and J. Pirart, Eds. Excerpta Medica. New York, American Elsevier, 1974, pp. 612–623.

53. Report of the Committee for the Assessment of Biometric Aspects of Controlled Trials of Hypoglycemic Agents. J.A.M.A., *231:*583, 1975.

54. Rimoin, D. L.: Inheritance in diabetes mellitus. Med. Clin. North Am., *55:*807, 1971.

55. Rimoin, D. L.: *In* Diabetes. W. J. Malaisse and J. Perart, Eds. Excerpta Medica. New York, American Elsevier Pub. Co., 1974, pp. 346–350.

56. Russell, A. L.: A system of classification and scoring for prevalence surveys of periodontal disease. J. Dent. Res., *35:*350, 1956.

57. Schwartz, T. B.: The tolbutamide controversy, a personal perspective. Ann. Intern. Med., *75:*303, 1971.

58. Selzer, H. S.: A summary of criticisms of the findings and conclusions of the UGPD study. Diabetes, *21:*976, 1972.

59. Siperstein, M. D., Unger, R. H., and Madison, L. C.: Studies of muscle capillary basement membrane in normal subject, diabetic and prediabetic patients. J. Clin. Invest., *47:*1973, 1968.

60. Siperstein, M. D., Unger, R. H., and Madison, L. C.: Further electron microscopic studies of diabetic microangiopathy. *In* Early Diabetes. R. A. Camerini-Davalos, and H. S. Cole, Eds. New York, Academic Press, 1970, 261.

61. Soler, N. G., et al.: Retinopathy at diagnosis of diabetes, with special reference to patients under 40 years of age. Br. Med. J., *3:*567, 1969.

62. Spiro, R. G.: Glycoproteins, their biochemistry, biology and role in human disease. N. Engl. J. Med., *281:*991, 1969.

63. Spiro, R. G.: Chemistry and metabolism of basement membrane. *In* Diabetes Mellitus: Theory and Practice. M. Ellenberg and H. Rifkin, Eds. McGraw-Hill, 1970, pp. 210–220.

64. Spiro, R. G.: Glycoproteins and diabetic microangiopathy. *In* Joslin's Diabetes Mellitus. A. Marble *et al.*, Eds. Philadelphia, Lea & Febiger, 1971.

65. Strandness, D. E., Jr., and Priest, R. E.: Combined clinical and pathological study of diabetic and nondiabetic peripheral arterial disease. Diabetes, *12:*366, 1964.

66. Thomsen, A.: The Kidney in Diabetes Mellitus. Copenhagen, Munksgaard, 1965.

67. University Group Diabetes Program: A study of the effects of hypoglycemic agents on vascular complications in patients with adult onset diabetes. I. Design, methods and baseline results. Diabetes, *19*(Suppl. 2):747, 1970.

68. University Group Diabetes Program: A study of the effects of hypoglycemic agents on vascular complications in patients with adult onset diabetes. II. Mortality results. Diabetes, *19*(Suppl. 2):789, 1970.

69. University Group Diabetes Program: A study of the effects of hypoglycemic agents on vascular complications in patients with adult onset diabetes. III. Clinical implication of UGDP results. J.A.M.A., *218:*1400, 1971.

70. University Group Diabetes Program: A study of the effects of hypoglycemia agents on vascular complications in patients with adult onset diabetes. IV. A preliminary report on phenformin results. J.A.M.A., *217:*777, 1971.

71. Vracko, R., and Benditt, E. P.: Basal lamina, The scaffold for orderly cell replacement. J. Cell Biol., *55:*406, 1972.

72. Ward, J. D.: Diabetic neuropathy. Clin. Endocrinol. Metabolism, *1:*3, 809, 1972.

73. West, K.: Response to cortisone in prediabetes. Diabetes. *9:*379, 1960.

74. West, K. M.: Epidemiology of diabetes. *In* Diabetes Mellitus: Diagnosis and Treatment. American Diabetes Association, Vol. III, 1971, pp. 121–126.

75. West, K. M.: Epidemiologic evidence linking nutritional factors to the prevalence and manifestations of diabetes. Acta Diabetol. Lat. *9*(Suppl. 1):405, 1972.

76. White, P.: Childhood diabetes. Diabetes, *9:*345, 1960.

77. Williams, R. C., Jr., and Mahan, C. J.: Periodontal disease and diabetes in young adults. J.A.M.A., *172:*776, 1960.

78. Williamson, J. R., et al: Microvascular disease in diabetes. Med. Clin. North Am., *55*(4):847, 1971.

Section II
Clinical Management

11

Examination Procedures and Recording of Data

11

Examination

Procedures

and

Recording

of

Data

Examination of the patient and the logical and orderly recording of pertinent data are critical procedures in periodontics. It must be kept in mind that we are recording deviations from the normal. This will be developed to a somewhat greater degree later in the chapter, but mention of this fact is always in order.

One cannot record what one does not see; faulty and incomplete treatment planning and execution flow inexorably from incomplete, careless, and slipshod methods in examination and observation.

On the other hand a concise, well-coordinated and designed examination makes for logical treatment planning. Rational therapy can only be the product of complete information and of the proper organization of effort. In addition, certain habits in procedure are formed during initial contact with the case. Careful attention to detail should be applied throughout the entire period of management. In a very real sense, examination and observation never end. An opinion once formed is sometimes changed at a later date on the basis of closer observation. The examination is important, since all therapy hinges upon the results of the effort and its efficient organization. It must not be hurried or superficial if it is to yield good results. The patient has sought and surely deserves careful attention to his illness. A hurried screening is not a proper examination.

A useful sequence to be followed during the examination procedures is illustrated in Figure 11-1. The outline is taken from the examination and treatment planning syllabus of the Department of Periodontics of the University of Washington. Although it is subject to variation in approach, it is essentially basic and straightforward.

THE HISTORY

Ordinarily the first order of business in an examination is the patient's history. This portion of the examination is usually organized into three general parts— (1) the chief complaint, (2) the specific dental or oral history, and (3) the general systemic history.

The Chief Complaint

Periodontal disease is so insidious that it may be lacking in symptoms in the early and moderately advanced case. Gingival bleeding is not a consistent attendant, nor is mobility to be expected in any but the most seriously involved teeth. It is, nevertheless, important to ask each patient whether he suffers from any of the common symptoms of periodontal disease. Inflammation, bleeding, exudation, mobility, and migration are all dramatic occurrences, which the patient

HISTORY AND EXAMINATION

Sequence of Procedure

II. CHIEF COMPLAINT

Summary statement

III. PRESENT ORAL ILLNESS AND HISTORY OF ILLNESS

A. History of Present Illnesses

Signs and symptoms present, e.g., pain, bleeding, odor, taste, food impaction or retention

B. Past Dental History

1. Name(s) of dentist(s)
2. Frequency of dental visits
   a. date of last prophylaxis
   b. frequency of prophylaxis
3. History of previous periodontic, restorative, endodontic, prosthodontic, orthodontic, or oral surgical treatment
4. Episodes of N.U.G., "canker sores" and periodontal abcesses
5. Family dental history
   a. history of familial caries and/or periodontal disease
   b. any unusual finding concerning loss of teeth in parents or siblings
   Destructive habits
   a. clenching teeth
   b. bruxism (grinding of teeth)
   c. chronic biting of lip, cheek, or tongue
   d. tongue thrusting
   e. mouth breathing
   f. foreign object doodling
   g. cigarette or pipe smoking

C. Oral Hygiene

1. Toothbrushing
   a. type and age of brush (have patients bring old brush in for inspection
   b. method
   c. frequency (number of times a day)
   d. by whom and when was instruction given
   e. patient's estimate of time spent brushing teeth (patient's actual brushing time should be noted later just before first oral hygiene instruction)
2. Auxiliary aids
   a. disclosing tablet, ever used? used now?
   b. mouth mirror
   c. floss
   d. toothpicks

   e. other accessories in current use (e.g., electric toothbrush, water pik) and how used, how often, etc.

D. Oral Image

1. Overall importance of natural teeth to patient
2. Relative importance of function and esthetics to patient

IV. MEDICAL HISTORY AND EXAMINATION

See Health Questionnaire and Health Questionnaire Comment Sheet. Add here in red any factors which should be considered in treatment or prognosis of the periodontal condition, e.g., rheumatic fever, diabetes

V. ROENTGENOGRAPHIC EXAMINATION

Suggested technique for X-ray exam. Make a series of circuits, concentrating on one aspect at a time. Move on each circuit from UR to UL, to LL to LR

A. Evaluation of quality of X-rays being examined by observing the reproduction of

1. Occlusal surfaces
2. Contacts

B. Peripheral areas: body of maxilla and mandible

1. Character of trabeculation
2. Atypical radiolucent or radiopaque areas
3. Maxillary sinus
   a. close proximity of sinus floor to teeth or edentulous ridge
   b. clarity

C. Apical third of root regions, changes in periapical region, lamina dura and periodontal ligament space

D. Middle third of root region

1. Changes in the lamina dura and p.d. ligament
2. Presence of retained root fragments

E. Coronal third of root region

1. Character of the alveolar crest
   a. crestal density
   b. horizontal resorption
   c. vertical resorption
   d. mesio-distal slope of alveolar crest
   e. cratering

FIG. 11-1. *A useful sequence for the student to follow in taking the history and examination.*

f.   suspected intrabony defects
g.   hemisepta
h.   furcation involvements

2.   Retained root fragments

F.   Teeth Proper

1.   Anatomical factors
a.   root form
b.   root size
c.   crown-root ratio
d.   root proximity (parallelism)
e.   convergence of roots of separate teeth
f.   impactions
g.   contact relationships

2.   Pathological changes
a.   crown caries, new or recurrent
b.   root caries, new or recurrent
c.   root resorption, external or internal
d.   crown or root fracture hypercementosis

3.   Endodontic treatment

VI.   INTRAORAL EXAMINATION

A.   Extraoral head, face and neck examination

Intraoral examination

1.   Soft tissues
a.   lips; cheek mucosa; vestibules; e.g., scarring of cheek at level of occlusal plane
b.   palate and pharynx-mucosa
c.   tongue - inspection and palpation - pull out, using gauze
d.   floor of mouth - inspection and bimanual palpation
e.   saliva - amount and consistency
f.   breath odor
g.   mouth breathing
h.   oral hygiene - summary statement on effectiveness

2.   Gingiva
a.   color
b.   form marginal, papillary
c.   consistency
d.   texture
e.   bleeding or exudation
f.   adequacy of attached gingiva

3.   Teeth
a.   sensitivity
b.   clinical crown size
c.   hypoplasia of enamel

d.   caries, immediate danger
e.   quality of restorations present
f.   contacts, form
g.   embrasures, form
h.   signs of habits involving teeth
extreme tooth wear (bruxism)
intruded teeth (pipe smoking)
evidence of fingernail biting

4.   Occlusion and temporomandibular joint. Note findings of potential importance in diagnosis or prognosis of treatment. E.g., extreme occlusal wear, soreness of teeth, jaws tired, especially on waking, T.M.J. popping, crackling, or clicking

VII.   CHARTING

A.   Follow systematic sequence. Employ a number of circuits, examining and charting for one function at a time. If facial and lingual charting are needed proceed from facial UR to UL, palatal UL to UR, lingual LR to LL, facial LL to LR. Otherwise proceed facial UR to UL, then facial LL to LR.

B.   Suggested circuits
1.   Missing, impacted or unerupted teeth
2.   Tooth position; buccoversion, lingoversion, rotation, extrusion
3.   Tooth restorations; full or partial dentures, FPD
4.   Tooth contacts and marginal ridge discrepancies
5.   Carious lesions
6.   Amount of subgingival deposit
7.   Overhanging restorations
8.   Sensitive teeth; brush or instrument contact, percussion
9.   Tooth mobility
10. Food retention; food impaction plunger cusps (check models)
11. Pocket (or sulcus) depth
12. Furca involvements
13. Position of mucogingival junction
14. Position of freni of significance
15. Position of vestibular fornix

VIII.   DIAGNOSTIC OPINION

A.   Periodontal disease(s) where present, be specific as to name

B. List all other diseases and/or conditions present which will influence prognosis or treatment of the periodontal disease(s) listed under A. E.g., caries, diabetes, tongue thrust, mouth breathing, gross facial asymmetry.

IX. PROGNOSIS

A. General prognosis for the dentition (excellent, good, fair, poor) with listing of reasons for prognosis given.

B. Specific prognosis of individual teeth or groups of teeth when this varies from A, with reasons for the individual tooth prognosis.

X. ETIOLOGY

A. General
The major factors contributing to the disease(s) present

B. Specific
The factor(s) contributing to lesion(s) present at specific sites.

will notice if they are present in an area that he can easily see or are of a magnitude that will intrude on his consciousness.

Frequently the patient will respond in an equivocal fashion—sometimes even embarrassed to report such apparently trivial complaints as a "bad taste" in the mouth, vague feelings of discomfort, or the "teeth feel sore" in the morning. On occasion, however, more definite complaints will be offered in response to the query on a chief complaint. Migration of teeth, frequently noticed by the patient when contact relationship is lost in anterior teeth or when a previously regular alignment becomes irregular and crowded or flared, is by no means uncommon as the chief complaint.

When the patient complains of acute symptoms, the orderly progress of history taking and recording is dropped momentarily in order to deal with the acute lesion. It must be emphasized, however, that the interruption is just that, and that the therapy directed to relieving the patient of pain or to reducing the emergency is simply an interregnum in the examination.

The intrusion of a periodontal emergency is, however, by no means the rule. The chief complaint for most patients consists of low-grade physical symptoms with, perhaps, evidence of a long-standing periodontal disease. A surprising number complain of gingival recession or bad breath or tooth migration. An even greater number have no chief complaint at all. This places a heavy responsibility upon the dentist to seek out disease when there is no subjective evidence of it and to reveal to the patient any pathologic condition discovered.

Often the chief complaint will reveal much to the examiner about his patient. It must be kept in mind that the patient may sometimes express his discomfort in imprecise terms and may even ramble, but it is always rewarding to hear him out.

Although many therapists begin history taking with the general history—and no great principle is in-

volved—the oral history frequently serves as a good beginning. It seems to be logical to the patient and sometimes makes him more communicative.

The Oral History

After the chief complaint has been recorded, the oral and dental histories are taken. This is usually not too difficult insofar as stimulating a response from the patient is concerned, but sifting of pertinent data from a mass of trivia requires skill.

The extensive and searching history commonly irks the student, who may regard the time expended as wasteful and generally unrewarding. Many patients ramble on at great length, but the experienced historian learns to control the length of responses by skillful questioning. Histories need not be as interminable as they seem to beginners to be. There is no better way to develop skill as a questioner, however, than by taking a complete history.

The objectives in recording the history of the patient with obvious or incipient periodontal disease may be somewhat different from those sought by the general diagnostician. In the latter case, the primary task is to establish the cause of the chief complaint and to uncover any possible underlying disease. In the periodontal patient, the disease is fairly obvious and is easily discovered, and the chief complaint is vague or nonexistent. The objectives in taking the history of a periodontal patient are:

1. To provide a proper and complete background to the state of chronic destructive periodontal disease at that given moment. Is the disease still fairly active? Is it relatively quiescent? Has the patient suffered from juvenile periodontitis? Has he been treated before? How extensively? Why did he fail? Surely no one would question the necessity for this information.

2. To reveal any possible oral or systemic disease

directly related to periodontal disease, the treatment of which may modify therapy. Diabetes mellitus is an example.

3. To facilitate following the course of the patient's periodontal disease after active therapy has been completed.

4. To provide a strong position for the examiner in any possible malpractice litigation and to establish a general impression of competence with medical and dental colleagues.

In taking the history it is best, at least for the inexperienced examiner, to question the patient in a systematic manner, inquiring first about the purely dental part of the history, using a written or memorized list of inquiries. An excellent beginning is to inquire about missing permanent teeth and the reason for their loss. A considerable difference exists in the treatment planning for patients who have lost teeth because of caries, accident, ulceration, or loosening and pyorrhea. It would be misleading to classify patients as irredeemably of one type or another, since almost no patient is. Nevertheless, it is most helpful to know whether your patient is caries prone, even though caries is not, at the moment, of paramount interest to you. A patient who is particularly prone to caries, even into middle age, may not be a prime candidate for periodontal surgery that might result in some root exposure.

On the other hand, a patient who has lost teeth through loosening and "pyorrhea" and who has not sought help earlier may not be a good periodontal patient either. Much has been made in recent years of something called the "oral image" of the patient. What is meant by asking a patient about his oral image is simply to ask him how important teeth—or at least natural teeth—are to him. Such a question, properly posed, can reveal a great deal about the patient. For example, one would ordinarily think that the prospect of the loss of all the natural teeth would be most shocking to a young person, particularly a young woman in the twenties. Strangely enough, the patient to whom the loss of teeth is most distressing—often to the point that the possibility cannot be tolerated at all—is frequently the menopausal woman. There are several perfectly good reasons for this, and they warrant definite consideration.

Without going into inordinate detail on this subject, it should be recognized that the mouth is psychologically one of the most highly charged organs in the body. It is the earliest organ of perception of the newborn and remains an important psychosexual factor throughout the life of the individual. As dentists we invade the oral cavity, traumatize its components by grinding, incision, and abrasion and yet maintain a rather superficial interest in personality traits of our patients and their responses to our treatment. Many patients who have neglected their teeth throughout their lives suddenly become desperate to retain them when faced with the possibility of their loss.

This rather common clinical situation is offered in this context merely to point up the importance of intangibles. One cannot treat a patient merely by enumerating and recording clinical signs and symptoms. Emotional reactions of patients constitute an area much neglected and glossed over.

In questioning a patient, it is not rare to invade certain emotional and psychologic areas that touch sensitive feelings. There is a temptation to pursue this course of questioning, prompted by some curiosity in addition to purely professional interest; but it might not be amiss here to offer a word of caution. While it is perfectly proper for the examiner to establish a possible emotional basis for necrotizing ulcerative gingivitis, for example, or for bruxism or for a sudden loss of interest in maintenance, it might not be wise to delve too deeply. The dentist is not a psychiatrist, and without the skill, training, or ability to manage such a patient competently, emotional storms generated by searching questions can be disturbing.

It is, of course, well within our area of competence to establish the existence of an emotional factor, but there is no need to go further. Reference to competent professional help in a skillful and understanding manner is all that is required in such a situation.

Information elicited from the patient in regard to his total dental experience is also revealing. For the specialist it reveals the attitude of the patient in relation to the profession, and specifically, to the referring dentist. To the general practitioner it may provide the underlying reason for the patient's seeking him out for professional help in preference to a dentist he has seen already. The stated reasons may or may not be the actual ones. Specific incidents of note should be listed and recorded when deemed useful.

During the taking of the oral history, a standard system of questioning should be established. Questions on prior therapy—periodontal, orthodontic, or general—are rewarding. Past response to local and general anesthesia is important and useful. Information on bleeding, odor, bad taste, pain, food impaction, and the incidence and frequency of canker sores is all grist to the diagnostic mill.

In our experience, the use of complex history charts, with all the items to be dealt with listed within the small space provided for a possible positive reply, leaves much to be desired. This type of chart is conducive to checking off certain items that seem to apply. This can be productive as a patient-response type of questionnaire and is useful in setting the stage for a definitive general history, which will be discussed later in this chapter. For the recording of useful data, we recommend a simple chart that provides enough room for ample, uncramped recording. An illustration of a chart of this nature is included in the illustrations in this chapter.

HABITS

Included in an oral history should be a good searching record of the oral habits practiced by the patient. Clenching and grinding—while not habits, strictly speaking—can very well be included in this category. The results of bruxism will depend upon the occlusal relationship of the incisors. If they are in an edge-to-edge relationship, the incisor crowns will be worn down to a fraction of their former length (Fig. 11-2). If the patient has a deep overbite, the palatal surfaces of the crowns of the upper incisors will be worn thinner, but not shorter, until they become chipped and fractured at their incisal edges.

Lip biting, inserting foreign objects between the teeth, cheek biting, and occupational abuse of the teeth by musicians, seamstresses, and others are all items that must be recorded (Figs. 11-3, 11-4, 11-5). Mouth breathing is extremely common in children (Fig. 11-6). Many items in a history of oral habits are occlusal in nature. Activities that involve a tooth-to-tooth contact or tooth contact with a hard substance naturally fall into an occlusal category because they are frequently involved in occlusal traumatism. Habit, by definition, is repetitive, and dental or periodontal damage is a fairly common result. The information gleaned from the oral history must be correlated with

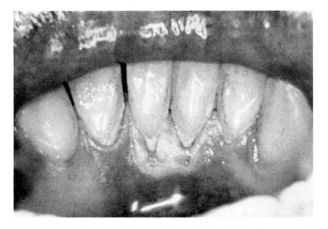

FIG. 11-3. *Nail scratching on the gingiva. Note the area of hyperkeratosis on the lingual surface of the lower gingiva. The patient cultivated this habit in an attempt to remove lingual calculus on the incisor teeth.*

the occlusal analysis in the intraoral physical examination. That is its principal purpose.

All of the above information should be collected before the systematic intraoral examination is begun. After the oral history, a good orderly progression is to the general systemic history.

General Systemic History

There is no doubt that every case of periodontal disease has a systemic factor in its essential etiology. This factor, however, is inextricably bound to such areas as resistance to disease, to general immune reactions, and to enzyme chemistry with which we are only superficially familiar. It is not in a vain hope that some

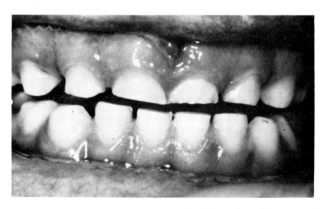

FIG. 11-2. *A rather extreme example of bruxism. Because of the occlusal relationship of the incisors, the teeth are wearing into an edge-to-edge relationship, and the incisor crowns are worn down to a fraction of their former length.*

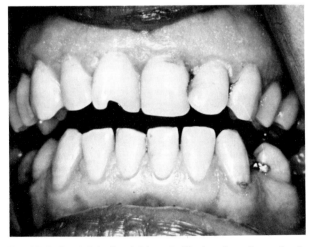

FIG. 11-4. *A notch in the right central incisor from the patient's habit of opening bobby pins over an 18-year period.*

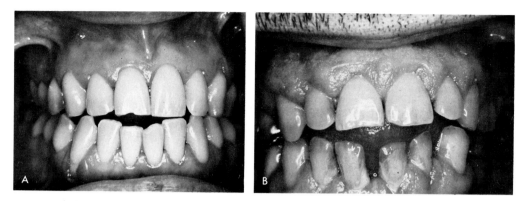

FIG. 11-5. *Open bite because of tongue thrust. A. Open bite. Note wear patterns on teeth no longer in occlusion. B. Upper and lower teeth are splayed and separated by the abnormal swallowing pattern in thrusting the tongue between the teeth.*

mysterious etiologic factor will be revealed that the general history is so integral a part of a *routine* history. This portion of the history is most important in disclosing known systemic factors of interest in the patient's physical condition and is important to the therapist in his management of whatever disease is present.

ALLERGIES

Allergies, to mention a most common finding in a large number of patients, can be of considerable importance to the examiner. In a number of procedures, drugs of various kinds are used either to prevent infec-

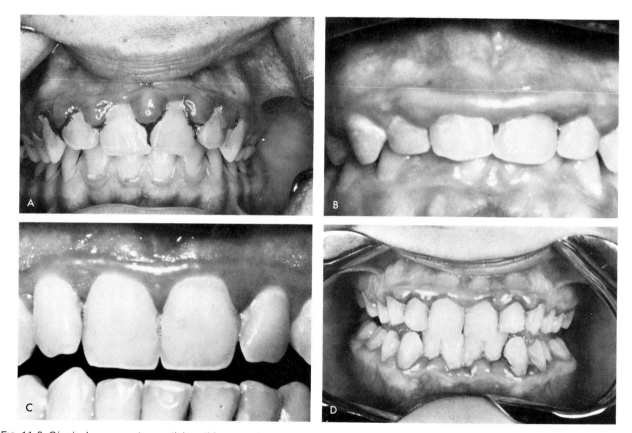

FIG. 11-6. *Gingival response to mouth breathing at various stages of maturity. A linear marginal fibrosis is frequently seen because of the constant low-grade irritation by the surface drying of the tissue and the generally productive nature of the tissue of young and growing patients. A. Gingival response in a 14-year-old girl. Menarche at 12 years. Note the difference between the upper and lower gingiva. B. Mouth-breathing hyperplasia in an 18-year-old young woman. C. Mouth-breathing hyperplasia in a 20-year-old man. D. Mouth-breathing hyperplasia in a 22-year-old woman.*

tion or to induce anesthesia or to control pain. A number of patients are sensitive to many of the drugs used for these purposes. The need for prior knowledge of the specific allergen is obvious.

CARDIOVASCULAR DISEASE

Many patients seeking periodontal therapy are suffering or have suffered from some cardiovascular disease. It is important to establish the possible existence of essential hypertension or the date of the last coronary episode, anginal attack, or cerebrovascular accident. It is well to consult the patient's physician of record, but in order to come to some useful conclusion it is important for the dentist to have some general idea of the systemic disease with which he is confronted and at the same time to be able to convey to the physician some idea of the procedure he intends to perform. For a consultation to be useful, the physician should be given information in terms that he can understand. He should not be expected to know what our surgical procedures consist of and how stressful they are. The decision to halt anticoagulant administration temporarily must be made by the physician, and the responsibility is obviously his. The dentist should be as helpful as possible.

A history of coronary disease is certainly no contraindication for periodontal therapy. The patient, however, must be treated with some consideration for the condition from which he suffers. Most patients having a history of a coronary episode are on anticoagulent therapy, and this becomes an important factor to reckon with in treatment. Periodontal surgery obviously must be discussed with the patient's internist. On occasion, even subgingival root curettage causes extensive bleeding in cardiac patients receiving bishydroxycoumarin (Dicumerol).

ANGINA PECTORIS. The patient suffering from occasional episodes of angina pectoris will require some mild preoperative sedation. Periodontal therapy is, however, by no means contraindicated. Precautions must be taken to make certain that the office drug supply contains the proper chemotherapeutic aids for the acute attack.

RHEUMATIC FEVER. The patient who has a history of rheumatic fever in childhood may be suffering from cardiac valvular damage. It is possible to treat such patients with no compromise in achievement levels by altering the treatment plan. An antibiotic is plainly necessary whenever the tissues are subjected to instrumentation. The reason for this precautionary measure is the well-known phenomenon of a transient bacter-

emia, primarily *Streptococcus viridans*, which has a peculiar affinity for damaged heart valves or artificial heart valves on which it forms colonies. These can be quite dangerous. For this reason, the number of individual treatments should be as few as possible, and the duration of each visit should be extended as much as is practical. In this fashion, the number of courses of antibiotics will be minimal. It must be kept in mind that probing is relatively traumatic and may be instrumental in causing temporary septicemia so dangerous to patients who are suffering from cardiac valvular damage. Probing, therefore, is definitively included in the procedures to be performed under the protective cover of an antibiotic.

DIABETES

All procedures used in periodontic therapy may be used on the diabetic patient, but with certain precautions, and these are critically important. First, a history of diabetes mellitus is established during the patient interview. On occasion, should the patient not mention a history of diabetes, a well-taken history may reveal evidence to the examiner of the existence of some unsuspected imbalance in the patient's carbohydrate metabolism. As with the cardiac patient, reference to a medical consultant is recommended if the referring dentist lacks some basic knowledge of the problem. An understanding of the various tests to be applied and their relative sensitivity and reliability will aid the dentist in his communication with his medical colleague. This is particularly true in so common a disease as diabetes mellitus, with which every dentist is bound to come into contact.

HEMORRHAGIC DISEASE

The interest of the periodontist in hemorrhagic disease is primarily in the clotting mechanism which, when deficient, has a profound effect on therapy and treatment planning. The history in this instance becomes critical. Most patients have had some surgical experience, and they are quite accurate in their responses to questions on these experiences. It is remarkable that many operators are as fortunate as they seem to be in avoiding serious consequences of dental extractions and other surgical procedures that are routinely performed, when no prior history has been taken. The consequences of trusting to luck may be disastrous, and only one bad guess in an entire career is too many, particularly since the evidence is so easy to obtain.

While bleeding episodes are uppermost in the mind of the therapist, they are by no means the only concern. A major emergency can occur with the careless prescription of the pyramidines for analgesia and of the sulfonamides for control of infections (both classes of drugs, by the way, are commonly used) without giving serious thought to possible responses of the white blood cells. Intermittent leukopenia is by no means rare as a result of the ingestion of certain drugs.

INFECTIOUS OR SERUM HEPATITIS

Infectious and serum hepatitis are serious liver diseases thought to be frequently transmitted by nonsterile hypodermic needles. The lumens of hypodermic needles are extremely difficult to sterilize by ordinary methods. With the advent of disposable needles, this vector has been essentially eliminated. A history of a past episode of infectious hepatitis, however, should occupy a prominent place in the patient's chart. It must be remembered that there are other modes of transmission of infection than by hypodermic needle, and a patient remains a carrier for many years after clinical cure.

PSYCHOGENIC FACTORS

Enough has been alluded to psychogenic factors to indicate that the oral cavity is a highly charged organ. Because of the length of time for treatment and because of the necessary manipulation of the tissues in the mouth, the periodontist becomes an important figure to the psychologically dependent patient. Serious errors in patient management and blunders in therapy naturally follow from an uninformed or overconfident approach in treatment.

Treatment of the Patient with Systemic Disease

In nearly all cases of even serious systemic disease there are no essential contraindications to periodontal surgery. Modifications must, of course, be made in the treatment of some patients and in a few cases, such as patients with hemorrhagic diseases or Dilantin hyperplasia, periodontal objectives are altered and become secondary to other treatment directed toward the more critical health problem (Fig. 11-7). None of these modifications will be made, however, in the absence of definite information on the general systemic disease of the patient.

Some periodontists use a "yes" and "no" choice questionnaire in which a reasonably complete "system" history of a superficial nature can be compiled using the prototype Cornell Medical Index or one of its several variants (Fig. 11-8). This consists of a number of

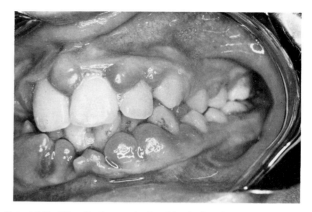

FIG. 11-7. *Dilantin hyperplasia. Gingival enlargement of this nature occurs in 13 to 15 percent of patients taking Dilantin (sodium diphenylhydantoin).*

questions ingeniously arranged in groups of related symptoms, so that the circling of a "yes" or "no" becomes a simple procedure, requiring little explanation. Such a questionnaire can be given to the patient before the formal history is taken so that the responses may be scanned by the examiner and his questioning may be adapted and oriented by the data in the questionnaire. A series of "no"-circled responses will reveal little about the patient except that he is a comparatively healthy person.

"Yes" responses should be regarded differently. They should alert the examiner and direct specific and searching attention to the organ or system implicated. For example, should a patient circle "yes" to the question, "Do you suffer from shortness of breath?" some thought should be given to further questioning, to eliminate or establish the possibility of cardiovascular disease or emphysema, or even neurasthenia. A whole series of interesting possibilities comes to mind, none involved with etiology, but all having a most important bearing upon the case management. To choose another example, a "yes" reply to the question, "Do you have to urinate during the night?" should make the examiner aware that the related questions are designed to probe into the question of diabetes, with the precautions required for the rendering of complete periodontal therapy and with the etiologic qualifying factors which diabetes furnishes.

THE ORAL EXAMINATION

Clinical observation is most rewarding. The time to begin to learn how to examine a patient is at the beginning—by learning how to evaluate gingival tissues and how to determine their relative health and their *visible* response to irritation and disease.

Chart No._____

SCHOOL OF DENTISTRY
UNIVERSITY OF WASHINGTON

HEALTH QUESTIONNAIRE

Answers to the following questions are for our records only. Naturally they will be considered confidential and will become part of your permanent dental record.

Date_____

Name_____ Date of birth_____

Height_____ Weight_____ Occupation_____

Circle the Highest Year You Completed in School /1 2 3 4 5 6 7 8/ /1 2 3 4/ /1 2 3 4/ /1 2 3 4 5 6/
Elementary School *High* *College* *Post-College*

Circle if you are . . . Single, Married, Widowed, Separated, Divorced

Physician's Name_____

Physician's Address_____ Physician's Phone_____

What is *your* estimation of your general health? (circle one) Good, Fair, Poor

Why are you now seeking dental treatment?_____

DIRECTIONS

If your answer is YES to the question asked, put a circle around (YES) NO

If your answer is NO to the question asked, put a circle around YES (NO)

Please answer all questions.

1. Do you think that your teeth are affecting your general health in any way?	YES	NO
2. Are you dissatisfied with the appearance of your teeth?	YES	NO
3. Are you worried about receiving dental treatment?	YES	NO
4. Do you have difficulty in chewing your food?	YES	NO
5. Do you have sensitive teeth?	YES	NO
6. Do you have bleeding gums?	YES	NO
7. Have you ever had sores in the mouth or on the lips that are slow to heal?	YES	NO
8. Do you have difficulty in opening your mouth wide?	YES	NO
9. Do you now have or have you ever had sinus trouble?	YES	NO
10. Have you ever had any injury to your face or jaws?	YES	NO
11. Have you been examined by your physician within the last year?	YES	NO
12. Are you being treated for any condition by a physician now?	YES	NO
13. Have you been taking any medicines within the past year?	YES	NO
14. Has there been any change in your general health in the past year?	YES	NO

OPEN TO NEXT PAGE

FIG. 11-8. *Health history form found useful in the University of Washington clinical departments. "Yes" answers to these questions require specific questioning and possible consultations.*

15. Have you lost or gained weight in recent months?   YES   NO

16. Have you ever been seriously ill?   YES   NO

17. Have you ever been hospitalized?   YES   NO

18. Have you ever had surgery (an operation)?   YES   NO

19. Have you ever had a blood transfusion?   YES   NO

20. Have you ever had x-ray or surgery treatment for a tumor, growth, or other conditions about your head, mouth, or on your lips?   YES   NO

21. Have you ever been treated for a growth or tumor in any other part of your body?   YES   NO

22. Are you frequently ill?   YES   NO

23. Do you often feel exhausted or fatigued?   YES   NO

24. Have you ever had any of the following diseases or conditions:

A. Jaundice (yellow skin & eyes)	YES	NO	I. Diabetes (sugar disease)	YES	NO
B. Hepatitis	YES	NO			
C. Tuberculosis	YES	NO	J. Measles	YES	NO
D. Venereal disease	YES	NO	K. Chicken pox	YES	NO
E. Heart attack	YES	NO	L. Mumps	YES	NO
F. Stroke	YES	NO	M. Polio	YES	NO
G. Ulcers	YES	NO	N. Rheumatic fever	YES	NO
H. Epilepsy	YES	NO	O. Scarlet fever	YES	NO

25. As a child, did you have growing pains or twitching of the limbs?   YES   NO

26. Have you ever had painful or swollen joints?   YES   NO

27. Have you ever been told by a physician that you have a heart murmur?   YES   NO

28. Do you now have or have you ever had any heart trouble?   YES   NO

29. Do you have high blood pressure?   YES   NO

30. Do you bleed for a long time when you cut yourself?   YES   NO

31. Do you bruise easily?   YES   NO

32. Do you have any blood disorder such as anemia (thin blood)?   YES   NO

33. Do you have any chest pain on exertion?   YES   NO

34. Are you ever short of breath on mild exertion?   YES   NO

35. Do your ankles ever swell?   YES   NO

36. Do you have a persistent cough?   YES   NO

37. Do you ever have asthma?   YES   NO

38. Do you ever have hay fever?   YES   NO

39. Do you have any allergies (to food, cat's fur, dust, etc.)   YES   NO

GO TO NEXT PAGE

40. Do you ever have hives or skin rash? YES NO

41. Have you ever experienced an unusual reaction to any of the following drugs:

A. Penicillin	YES	NO	D. Iodine	YES	NO
B. Barbiturates (sleeping pills)	YES	NO	E. Sulfa drugs	YES	NO
C. Aspirin	YES	NO	F. Other medicines	YES	NO

42. Have you ever experienced an unusual reaction to a dental anesthetic ("Novocaine Injection")? YES NO

43. Do you often have to get up at night to urinate? YES NO

44. During the day, do you usually have to urinate frequently? YES NO

45. Are you thirsty much of the time? YES NO

46. Has a doctor ever said you had kidney or bladder disease or infection? YES NO

47. Has a doctor ever said you had liver disease? YES NO

48. Do you have any numbness or tingling in any part of your body? YES NO

49. Has any part of your body ever been paralyzed? YES NO

50. Do you ever have fits or convulsions? YES NO

51. Do you have a tendency to faint? YES NO

52. Do you have frequent severe headaches? YES NO

53. Do you consider yourself to be a nervous person? YES NO

54. Do you suffer from severe nervous exhaustion? YES NO

55. Do you often feel unhappy and depressed? YES NO

56. Do you often cry? YES NO

57. Are you easily upset or irritated? YES NO

58. *Women*—Are you pregnant at the present time? YES NO

59. *Women*—Are you in or have you passed through the menopause (change of life)? YES NO

60. *Women*—Have you had a hysterectomy or ovariectomy? YES NO

The method by which this critical skill will be mastered is twofold:

1. Repeated experience in examining tissue within the various shades of the normal range.
2. Constant recording of even the slightest deviation from this normal range, in the most punctilious manner.

This approach lacks the attractive character of revelation, but there appears to be no adequate shortcut to success.

Familiarity with Normal

Nothing will make the examiner more aware of disease than a thorough familiarity with the normal (Figs. 11-9, 11-10). Subtle changes in the surface characteristics of gingiva can be noticed only by someone with a clear concept of normal and aware of any slight deviation from it. This awareness is not easy to come by. The most encouraging feature of the problem is that all seriously motivated dentists who apply themselves to the problem seem to master it. That is not to say that all periodontists are uniformly good observers.

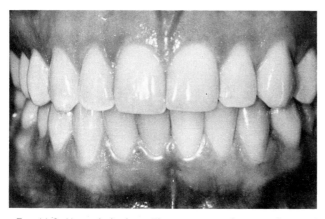

FIG. 11-9. *Normal gingivae. There are enough areas of normal gingiva in the mouth of this young woman to fall within the range of normal.*

To become a good observer requires considerably more than ability to delineate subtle differences in tissue quality and texture. All periodontists can, however, "see" in the true periodontal sense. One inevitable conclusion to be drawn is that constant and repeated examination of gingival tissues enables us to see. Another conclusion is that appreciation of the normal range is most important, since it furnishes the baseline from which the variations diverge (Fig. 11-11).

The description of the normal healthy oral mucosa can be used to set up baseline criteria for establishing a standard by which (pathologic) variations can be measured.

THE VESTIBULAR FORNIX

The vestibular trough or fornix is formed by the alveolar mucosa on one side and the buccal and labial mucosa on the other, forming a simple continuum of tissue. This trough—often erroneously referred to as the mucobuccal fold—is of great interest to the periodontal surgeon. There are clinical situations in which

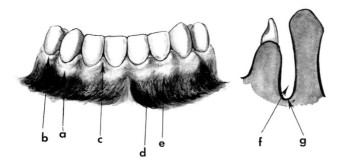

FIG. 11-10. *Normal gingivae (drawing). Anatomic features: the attached gingiva (a), the free gingival margin (b), the interproximal papilla (filling the interproximal embrasure) (c), the alveolar mucosa (d), the mucogingival junction (e), the vestibular trough or fornix (f), the fundus of the vestibular trough (g).*

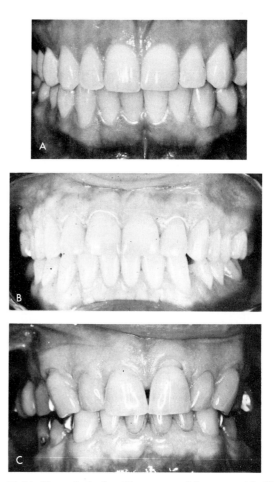

FIG. 11-11. *Normal gingiva. The range of the normal is illustrated to a degree. A. Normal gingiva in a 19-year-old woman. B. The gingiva of a 30-year-old woman. C. The gingiva of a 70-year-old man.*

the vestibular fornix is too shallow to permit adequate surgical correction of gingival deficiencies without making special provision for its extension and alteration. While the surface characteristics of the vestibular trough are similar to those of the adjacent mucosa on both sides, the fundus of the trough properly delimits the labial and buccal extent of the oral cavity. It should be kept in mind that the extension of the trough is at the expense of displaced connective tissue, which normally occupies the space created.

GINGIVA

In examining the rather simple tissue complex comprising the gingiva, several salient features are present in health.

1. The gingiva is firmly attached to underlying structures except for the marginal edge, which is free.

2. The surface of the gingiva is characterized by stippling, except for the marginal edge, which is

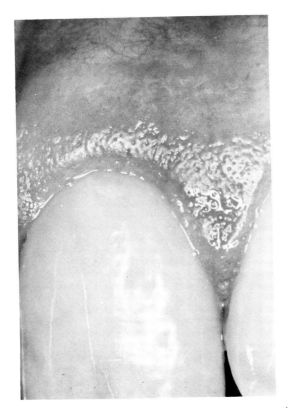

FIG. 11-12. *A normal interproximal papilla. Note the moderately coarse stippling in the body of the gingiva, but the tip of the free margin is not keratinized. The interproximal embrasure is filled by the papilla up to the contact point.*

smooth (Figs. 11-12, 11-13). The surface characteristic is more clearly seen by drying the tissue.

3. The tissues of the interproximal papilla are similar, both in its body and in its tip, to those of the labial gingiva. The major variant is the form of the papilla which is, in health, pyramidal or conical, so that the embrasure between adjacent teeth is effectively filled and occluded against retention of debris.

4. The color range of the gingiva, both marginal and

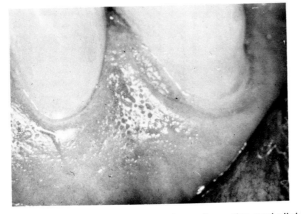

FIG. 11-13. *Normal papilla. Note plaque formation and slight tooth brush abrasion.*

papillary, is from pale pink to a light red. It is misleading to attempt to describe a single color value as normal. The exact color of the gingiva in health depends upon the complexion of the individual and the amount of keratin on the surface.

Brunettes have darker gingiva, frequently characterized by patches of dark-brown-to-yellow pigment, caused by the presence of melanin in the stroma. Blondes and individuals with fair skin have gingiva which is lighter in color and generally finer in texture.

The reader will remember that there is a steady migration of the cells comprising the stratified squamous epithelial cover to the gingiva toward the surface where, through metaplasia, keratin is formed. The rate of keratin formation and the thickness of the layer of keratin will qualify the color of the gingiva. Since keratin is gray and opalescent, a thick layer upon a red mucosa will appear light pink to visual examination. The converse is, of course, also true; the thinner the layer of keratin, the deeper the color of the gingival tissue. In adult women the keratin is thinner than in adult men. Young people are, as one would expect, endowed with thinner gingival keratin than are older people.

5. The apical border of the gingiva blends with the adjacent oral mucosa, which is usually referred to as alveolar mucosa. This consists of loose areolar tissue containing many elastic fibers. Its surface characteristics are in sharp contrast to those described for the neighboring gingival or masticatory mucosa. Here the surface is smooth and glistening, with no stippling and no keratin or other factor modifying its basic red color. Blood vessels are easily noted lying close to the surface. It is easily moved about when the lips or cheeks are distended or retracted. These are important characteristics and should be carefully noted by the reader. They have a profound effect upon case management.

6. The line of union between the gingiva and the alveolar mucosa is called the mucogingival junction or line. It is a blending of two disparate tissues and otherwise is totally unremarkable. The mucogingival line is referred to frequently, particularly in discussion of surgical procedures of various types.

7. Following the alveolar mucosa apically on the buccal and lingual aspects, it soon forms the vestibular trough or fornix throughout both upper and lower arches. The mucosa then imperceptibly blends with the buccal and labial mucosa. It must be understood that there is no difference in surface texture between the buccal and labial mucosa on the one side and vestibular or alveolar mucosa immediately adjacent.

8. On the lingual aspect, the gingival zone and alveolar mucosa and the mucosa of the floor of the mouth are similar to their counterparts on the labial

and buccal sides, with the important exception of the numerous ducts and large vessels that are immediately subjacent to the surface and impart to this surface its irregular appearance and bluish color.

The palate, on the other hand, presents an altogether different appearance. The entire palatal mucosa appears to be a continuum of the gingiva. It possesses the same firm attachment to the underlying bone, similar surface characteristics with the exception of the rugae and, in general, appears to be a very similar tissue to gingiva, although there are some differences that need not concern us here.

On the vestibular aspects of the arches and on the lingual side of the lower arch as well the normal gingiva consists of a marginal band of keratinized tissue of variable width. This averages 5 to 6 mm, but it frequently all but disappears in certain areas. This zone of masticatory mucosa is of critical importance to the health of the gingiva and is just as critical in the treatment of disease. Yet mere quantity or dimensions are no indication of the relative health of the tissue. It is not only possible but common to find, in the lower premolar region on the vestibular surface, a zone of keratinized gingiva of 1 to 2 mm, and yet gingival breakdown in this area is uncommon. Other areas seem to require much more marginal protection from the demands of function, so that the band of gingiva is much wider.

Common Abnormalities of the Gingiva

The gingiva and the tissues immediately adjacent comprise much of the total area with which the periodontist is concerned in treatment. The variations from normal are the things that the periodontist treats. Without going into great detail about the gross changes in the gingiva beyond that required for case documentation, it is quite enough for our present purpose to state that these disease processes are generally three in number: (1) inflammatory (Fig. 11-14), (2) necrotizing, and (3) dystrophic. Only a brief and superficial description will be attempted.

INFLAMMATORY PROCESSES

Enlargement of the marginal gingiva, with accompanying color changes and the alteration of basic architectural features, constitutes the classic picture of gingival inflammation (Fig. 11-15). No longer is the gingiva knife-edged marginally, with sharp pointed papillae filling the dental embrasures. Gone are the delicate festoonings so typical of healthy gingiva. Stippling of the surface departs; color deepens to a deep red and even to a deep violet in many cases.

On a light microscopic level, the cells associated with chronic inflammation are infiltrated. Plasma cells and lymphocytes especially are so densely distributed as to mask the stroma. Fluid engorgement occurs, contributing to the enlargement and architectural alteration mentioned above. Enzymes that are released destroy part of the fiber-attachment apparatus which is so critical in fixing and holding the gingival margin and papilla firmly and securely about the necks of the teeth. The destruction of gingival fibers also contributes to the blunting and rounding of all marginal edges (Fig. 11-16).

When these alterations in form, color, texture and tonus take place, the gingiva cannot meet the demands

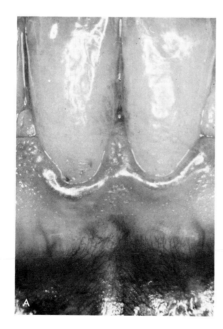

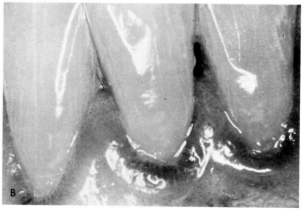

Fig. 11-14. *Gingival inflammation. A. Beginning marginal gingivitis. Note the early cervical caries as well. B. Advanced gingivitis with edema, enlargement, and hyperemia. Note the prominent vessels in the free margin of the gingiva.*

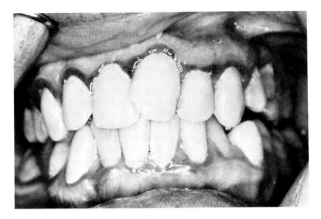

FIG. 11-15. *Marginal gingivitis with a rather dramatic response to cervical plaque retention.*

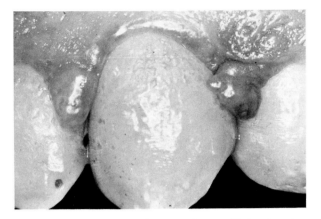

FIG. 11-17. *Variations from the norm. One papilla is edematous and enlarged and extrudes from the embrasure, thus acting as an entrapping mechanism instead of as a part of the deflecting contour of normal gingiva. The polypoid mass extruding on the distal of the canine is a fibrotic response of gingiva to long-standing low grade irritation. It is a pseudopapilla emanating from the gingival sulcus.*

of function. Instead of deflecting the invasive debris, it becomes entrapped, initiating and exacerbating an inflammatory lesion.

Early variations from the norm are naturally more subtle than is the process described, and all intermediate stages become proportionately easier to discern and record. The inflammatory lesion must, however, become obvious indeed, if it intrudes upon the vision of one who does not look for it. The habit of recording on the chart *all* deviations from normal form, color, and texture is a good one to cultivate. Not only is the record more complete, but it serves to direct attention to the most important single problem in preventative periodontics—the early lesion (Fig. 11-17). The loss of stippling and a smooth, glistening surface that should have a velvety texture, a red or bluish blush on a papilla that should be pink, a flaccid and flabby margin that should be firm, and a noticeable purulent exudate are important notations to be made. The fact that they are common is no reason to accept them as the norm (Fig. 11-18).

A later variation in the inflammatory response of gingiva to irritational factors is the thickening and marginal blunting of the tissues involved. Stippling and color on the other visible surfaces may or may not be normal in appearance. Such gingiva are referred to as fibrotic (Fig. 11-19).

PRECOCIOUS INFLAMMATORY GINGIVAL AND PERIODONTAL DISEASE

Although so-called periodontosis is discussed in another context, some mention of it should be made under examination procedures. For many years periodontal disease in children and in young adults was considered to be degenerative in nature and not inflammatory until late in the course of the syndrome. In

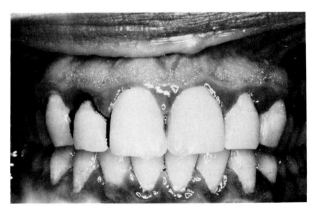

FIG. 11-16. *Papillary gingivitis. Some marginal gingivitis is present, but the papillae are somewhat more heavily involved.*

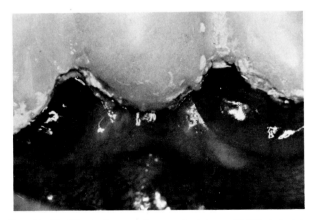

FIG. 11-18. *Gingival cyanosis marginal to an ill-fitting poorly fabricated temporary bridge.*

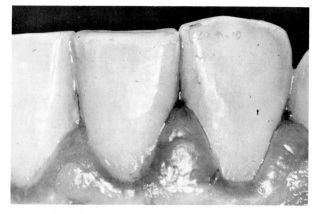

FIG. 11-19. *Fibrotic gingivae. Gingival thickening and enlargement are due to chronic inflammation.*

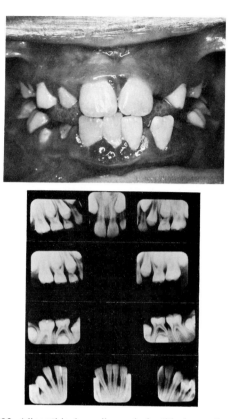

FIG. 11-20. *Idiopathic juvenile periodontitis in an 8-year-old girl. Note the mixed dentition. The patient was a perfectly normal child in all other respects. There is no lack of inflammatory signs. In the radiographs, note the resorption adjacent to newly erupted teeth. Note also the beginning furcal invasion in a newly erupted molar.*

spite of an enormous amount of effort expended by many skilled investigators, no degenerative factor could be incontrovertibly identified. There have been many hypotheses, but all have been found deficient in one aspect or another.

Juvenile periodontitis certainly does not ordinarily resemble the usual case of this disease found in a middle-aged patient. It is sometimes deficient in visual signs of gingival inflammation. What seems to be innocuously normal-looking gingiva actually proves on probing to be involved to a considerable degree in chronic destructive periodontal disease. This is not always the case. Some patients reveal gingival inflammation to a dramatic degree. A typical and peculiar tissue response common in a number of other diseases usually associated with middle age when found in children—diabetes, neoplasia, and some herpetiform diseases—come to mind readily.

Therapy might or might not be altered, but that does not change the essential pathologic conditions (Figs. 11-20, 11-21, 11-22, 11-23, 11-24).

NECROTIZING CHANGES IN THE GINGIVA

Several oral diseases are characterized by areas of necrosis. Most common among these (see Chapter 9) are (1) acute necrotizing ulcerative gingivitis (Fig. 11-25) and (2) aphthae and other herpetiform lesions of the oral mucosa (Fig. 11-26). The necrotic area of an aphthous ulcer has a deep red border. There are other more serious diseases of the mouth that are herpetiform in nature. Reference is made to Stevens-Johnson syndrome and other dermatologic diseases with oral symptoms. These are not within the purview of the periodontist, however, and do not affect the gingivae in a specific manner.

It is important to differentiate between acute nec-

rotizing ulcerative gingivitis and aphthae and herpetiform ulcers of the oral mucosa. Once differentiated, the data should be clearly recorded (Fig. 11-27).

DYSTROPHIC LESIONS OF THE PERIODONTIUM

Lesions in which the inflammatory response occupies a relatively minor role, if it plays any part at all, are few in number. Two syndromes are commonly classified in this category: gingival recession and occlusal traumatism. In a very real sense, both of these may be essentially traumatic in nature.

GINGIVAL RECESSION. In gingival recession, the marginal gingiva is distinctly apical to its normal position at the cementoenamel junction (Fig. 11-28). This recession sometimes takes the form of an arched curve, with its most apical position over the root prominence. One of the causes, more common in past years than presently seen, is traumatic toothbrushing, usually, but not always, with a horizontal stroke. This type of gingival recession is usually localized where the stroke

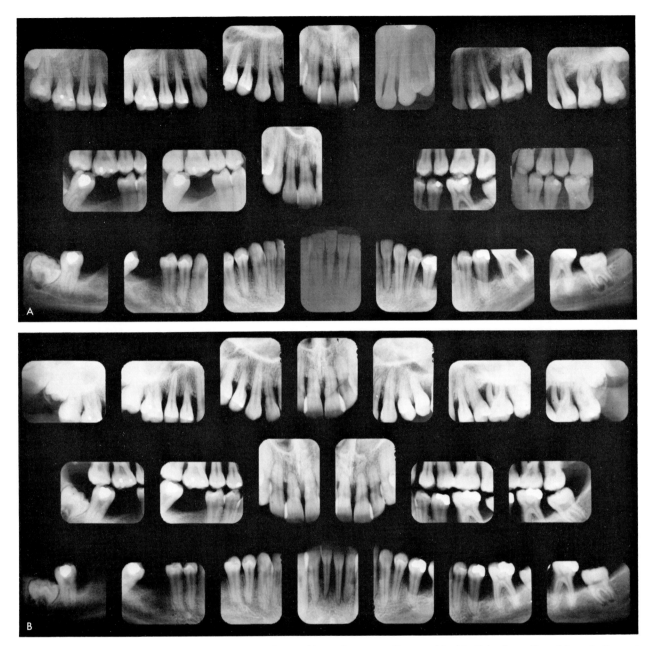

FIG. 11-21. *Juvenile periodontitis. A. Full-mouth radiographic series on a 13-year-old girl. Note the rather thin spindly roots, especially in the upper premolars. B. Full-mouth series of radiographs in the same patient one year later (at age 14).*

is most vigorous, on the labial aspects of the canine and premolar areas on the side opposite the hand used for brushing (the left side in right-handed individuals and the right side in left-handed individuals). While not limited to these areas by any means, they are affected most. More common are gingival clefts, some of which are the results of too vigorous scrubbing.

The upper or lower first molars are frequently rotated slightly so that the mesiobuccal line angles of the mesiobuccal root of the upper molar, or of the mesial root of the lower molar are exposed buccally through the cortical plate of the alveolar process. When this exposure extends to and through the marginal border of the bone, it is called a dehiscence. When a marginal isthmus of bone is still in place, the midroot exposure is called a root fenestration. It is uncommon to find a skull without a single area of fenestration or dehiscence anywhere. These areas of bone inadequately covering the root prominences are commonly involved in gingival recession (Fig. 11-28B). Gingiva alone, it appears, is inadequate covering for an exposed root in a relatively prominent position. Another area of gingival recession

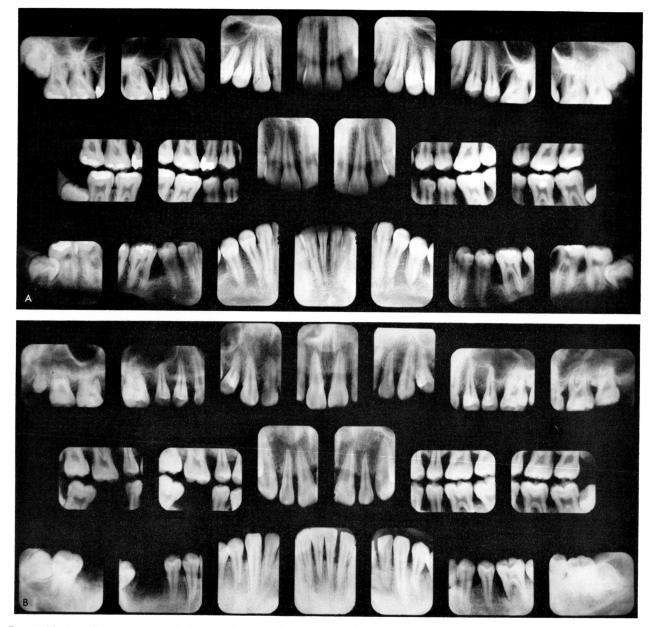

FIG. 11-22. *Juvenile periodontitis. A. Full-mouth series of radiographs of a 16-year-old young male patient. B. Full-mouth series of radiographs of the same patient 8 months later.*

commonly believed to be idiopathic is the gingiva over the palatal root of some upper molars, usually the first molar. Observation will reveal that in most cases the lower opposing molar has been lost and the upper tooth has extruded somewhat and has been tilted buccally. When the palatal root is widely flaring, it moves into prominence through the palate. When a root is not covered by bone and is shielded only by gingiva, even normal forces may result in a gingival recession.

Generalized gingival recession appears in mouths in which the roots of the teeth are large and well-formed, but which are invested in alveolar processes that are slender and poorly endowed with sufficient bone to cover the roots adequately. Many of these are involved in lingual recessions in relatively sheltered areas.

Gingival recession is not a simple dimensional phenomenon to be recorded by a numerical designation. The variants are many, and it is important to record them. Pockets are charted with six measurements in the circumferential probing of each root. With gingival recession, however, a swift rendering of the general

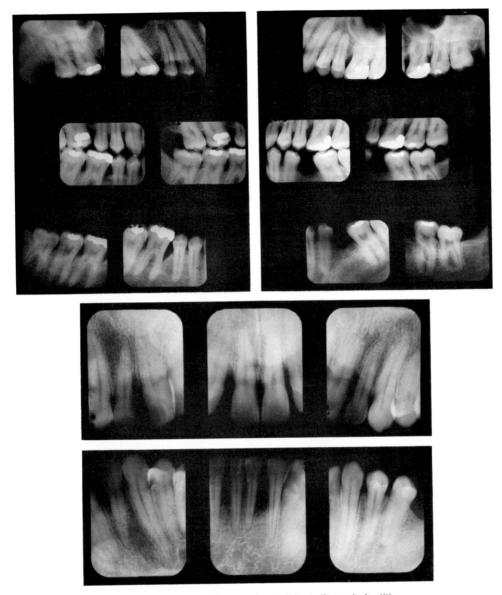

FIG. 11-23. *Radiographic survey of mouth a 20-year-old man who had juvenile periodontitis.*

shape of the recession, with the single numerical recording of maximal extent on the facial and lingual surfaces, is sufficient.

It can be readily seen that arched recession, in which the mesial and distal level of the gingival margin may be relatively undisturbed, is a different matter from a flat recession of the same dimension, but which indicates a fairly horizontal attachment loss circumferentially, and is more serious in many ways. There are, as may be imagined, many variations in these two general configurations. A swift delineation of the form and position of the gingival margin in the diagram of the teeth goes far to clarify the situation. One may be puzzled, for example, by a shallow pocket depth record on a given surface of a molar, coupled with a

furcation invasion that would normally require much greater depth for exposure. If the form of the gingival recession is recorded on the diagram, the situation would be clarified.

OCCLUSAL TRAUMATISM. Occlusal traumatism is a common affliction of the human dentition. The subject has been treated more completely in Chapter 5.

RECORDING DATA

In taking the history and in the recording of the findings of the clinical examination an orderly and systematic sequence of questioning of the patient and setting down of findings is the key to efficient manage-

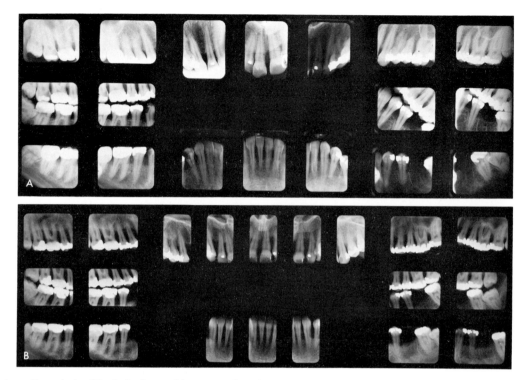

FIG. 11-24. *Juvenile periodontitis. A. Radiographic survey of surviving dentition of a 22-year-old man. B. Radiographic survey of the same patient 3 years later, at age 25.*

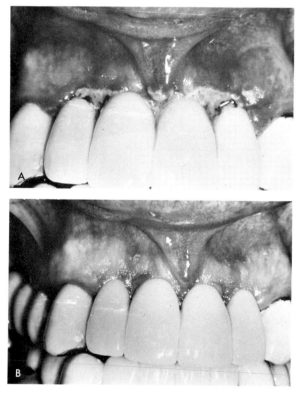

FIG. 11-25. *Acute necrotizing ulcerative gingivitis. A. Note the typical interproximal necrosis, even in a pontic area. B. After a single debridement.*

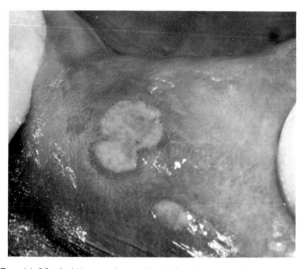

FIG. 11-26. *Aphthous ulcers. Note the sharply delimited zone of necrosis with a deep border. Note also that these ulcers occur on relatively flat surfaces.*

ment. The evaluation of irritational and other etiologic factors such as ill-fitting prostheses, calculus, and overlapping teeth should be indicated on the diagram as completely as possible. All must be carefully described in the narrative portion of the clinical examination record (Figs. 11-29 through 11-37).

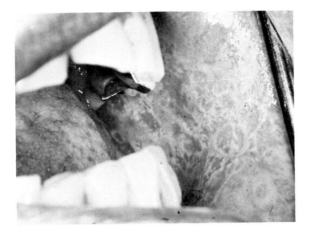

FIG. 11-27. *Lichen planus on the buccal mucosa and tongue. Areas of hyperkeratosis are frequently alarming to the patient. They should be carefully recorded and annotated.*

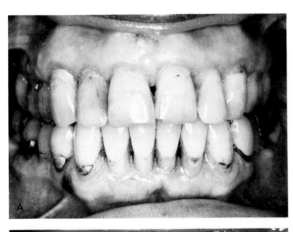

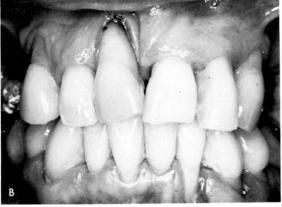

FIG. 11-28. *Gingival recession. A. Generalized gingival recession. The upper left lateral incisor gingival contour is an example of a flat or horizontal recession while enough papillary gingiva remains to be considered fairly "arched." B. The upper right central incisor and the lower left lateral incisor are clearly recessions over dehiscences.*

The Periodontal Chart

The periodontal chart, which is an integral part of every examination form, consists of a schematic rendering of the teeth and roots in buccal, lingual, and occlusal views. Some diagrams have a series of parallel horizontal lines, usually 2 mm apart, beginning at the cementoenamel junction, to permit the examiner to plot out pocket depth and shape with reasonable accuracy against the dimensional lines.

Easier to record and to read is the method using a simple numerical expression of pocket depth apical to the area measured (Fig. 11-38). For example, most examiners use six measurements (in millimeters) about the circumference of each tooth, although continuous circumferential measurement is the rule. Distal, mid-root, and mesial depths are recorded with a millimeter probe from a buccal and lingual approach. Some periodontists use a line on the root in a rough approximation of the number expressed. Whether or not a line is used, however, the greatest advantage of this numerical system over the graphic recording is that it can be dictated to the assistant in a systematic fashion, in a series of six numbers for each tooth in a given order. In this manner, the mouth may be charted for pocket depth quickly but with enough accuracy for good treatment planning. Special and peculiar pockets may, of course, be recorded as a special measurement on the chart as the occasion requires.

USES OF THE PERIODONTAL CHART

The setting down of a considerable mass of information and the graphic representation of clinical features of a periodontally involved mouth serves to answer several needs, all of them important.

1. A basis is provided for a therapeutic approach, in that the current illness of the organ is recorded in a systematic fashion. It makes possible a rational treatment plan.
2. A ready reference is provided for the operator throughout and following the entire course of therapy. (It would be optimistic to suppose that the treatment plan adduced from the chart and history is so precise and accurate that no further reference is necessary to the record, but merely to the plan.)
3. It establishes a moment in the history of the patient when the signs and symptoms were as they were recorded, and provides a baseline, as it were, from which all variations can be plotted. "Improvement" and "regression" are relative terms, and a point of reference is critically im-

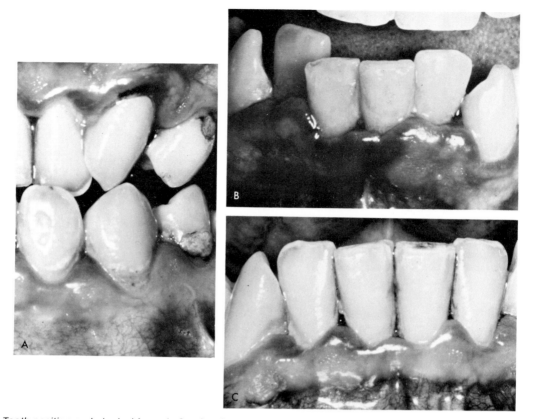

FIG. 11-29. Tooth position and gingival form. A. Overlapping teeth create difficult situations for the interproximal papilla because of invasion of the interproximal embrasure. B and C. Parallel root proximity as suggested in these incisors is far more serious than overlapping when they become involved with periodontal disease.

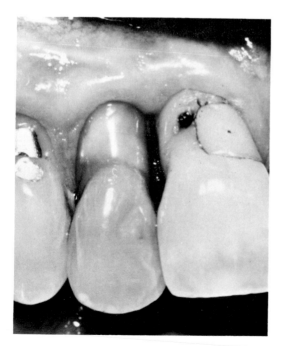

FIG. 11-30. Parallel root proximity. Note how different the interproximal tissue is from the distal and mesial aspect of the lateral incisor.

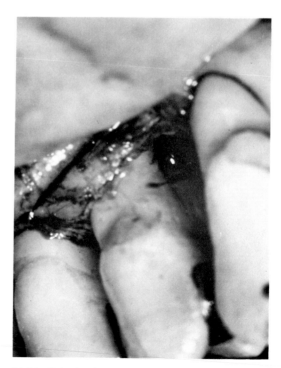

FIG. 11-31. Calculus in the fluting of a premolar.

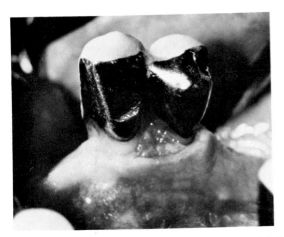

FIG. 11-32. *Clasp impingement from an ill-fitting partial denture.*

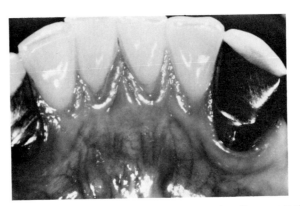

FIG. 11-34. *Partial denture clasp impingement on the marginal gingiva.*

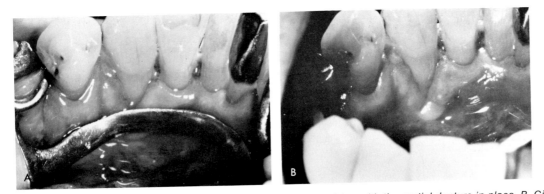

FIG. 11-33. *Lingual bar impingement on the gingiva. A. Position of the lingual bar with the partial denture in place. B. Gingiva and mucosa under the bar.*

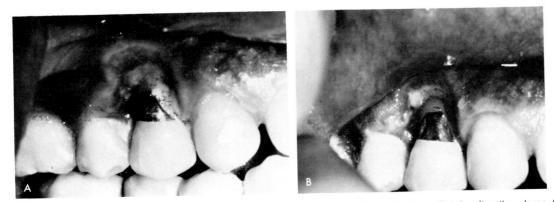

FIG. 11-35. *Gingiva crushed and lacerated by impingement of a rubber dam clamp. A. Immediately after the clamp had been removed. B. Three days later. Permanent injury is sometimes inflicted on the gingiva by the improper use of rubber dam clamps and tooth separators.*

portant in making value judgments meaningful. Total cure and total failure rarely occur in the short run and, more than the neophyte realizes, the periodontist deals in trends and tendencies. The need for a basic record against which to plot these tendencies is self-evident.

The chart is carried forward, after the actual symbolic representation, with an evaluation of the general systemic findings against the picture of periodontal disease and of the various other factors entering the case. Many of these considerations will be discussed more fully under treatment planning, in Chapter 13.

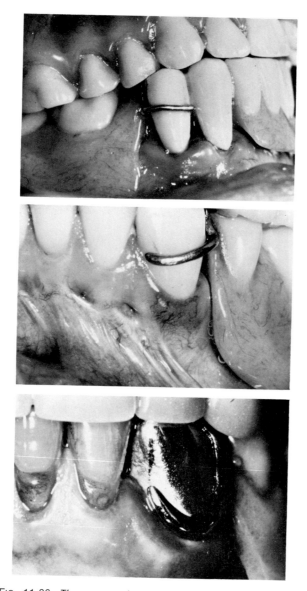

FIG. 11-36. *Three examples of poorly designed removable partial dentures with clasps and saddles that inflict gingival and periodontal damage.*

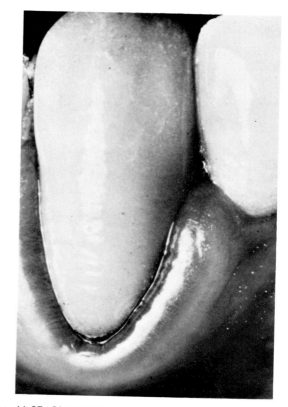

FIG. 11-37. *Gingival response to a Ceramco crown with poor gingival fit.*

The treatment plan itself is entered in the chart. The treatment plan must, in order to be effective, correlate all the useful data collected in the examination. Not only is the extent of periodontal destruction important, but the systemic findings as well as the dental history must all be taken into consideration by the therapist.

Radiographs

Well-angulated, properly exposed dental radiographs in sufficient number (18 to 20) including bitewing films are important in any searching periodontal examination. A number of anatomic structures and relationships are critical to the periodontal surgeon, especially in any procedure that is not limited to the marginal tissues.

The large maxillary sinuses dipping close to the crest can present an unwelcome surprise if they are inadvertently invaded when the periodontist is reducing what he believes to be a marginal mass of bone. Many of these areas appear to be large buccal bone masses, which later prove to be quite thin.

Mandibular canals are another potential hazard in certain procedures. Impacted teeth in the surgical field are commonly exposed when the operator had no intention of removing them.

The radiograph is not too satisfactory a diagnostic instrument in periodontal lesions. It is not a question of its being misleading. Whenever the radiographic film reveals a shadow suggesting radiolucency, it almost always reflects an area of bone resorption. As corroborative evidence it is excellent (Fig. 11-39). The difficulty lies with radiographs that show no shadows but instead suggest undamaged alveolar and supporting bone. There is no assurance that resorptive lesions do not exist—sometimes of spectacular size and extent—which make a tooth with a hopeless prognosis appear sound (Figs. 11-40, 11-41).

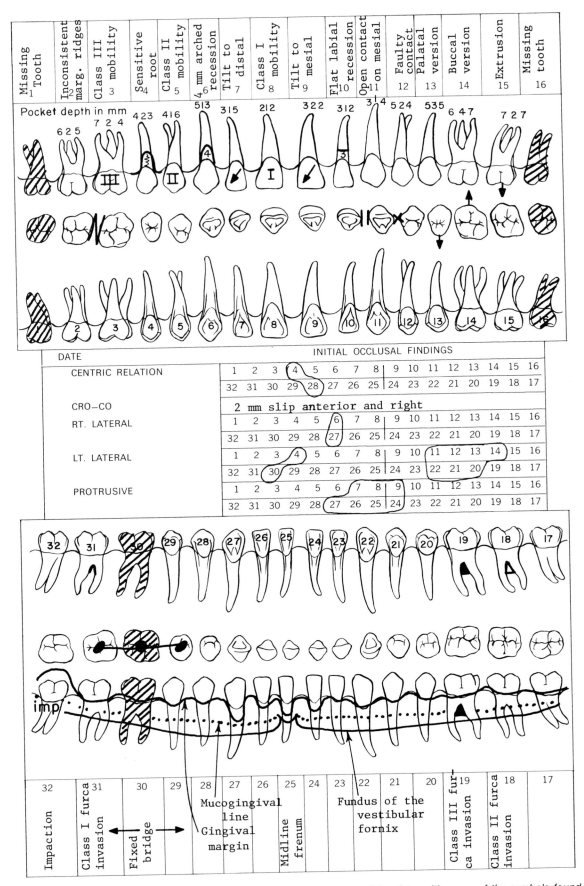

FIG. 11-38. *A standard chart in use at the University of Washington School of Dentistry with some of the symbols found useful.*

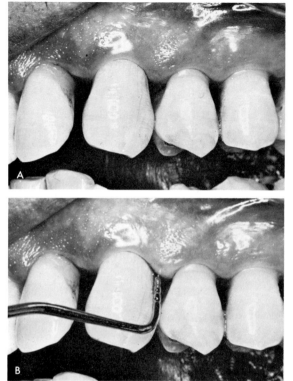

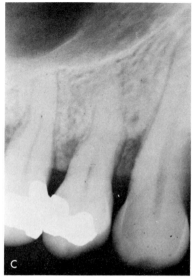

Fig. 11-39. *Probing of periodontal pockets. A. The canine and premolar area (mirror view). B. The radiograph of the area. C. Insertion of the probe to midplane on the distal of the canine.*

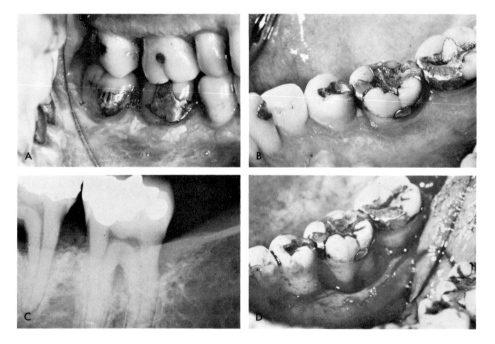

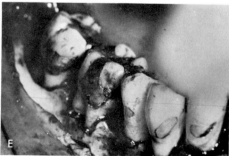

Fig. 11-40. *The unreliability of radiographic evidence. A. Buccal view of the molar region (the epithelial dysplasia need not concern us here). B. Lingual view of the same area. C. Radiographic view of the second molar. D. Lingual view with flaps reflected. E. Buccal view of the second molar with flaps reflected. Note the cavernous resorptive lesion on the second molar.*

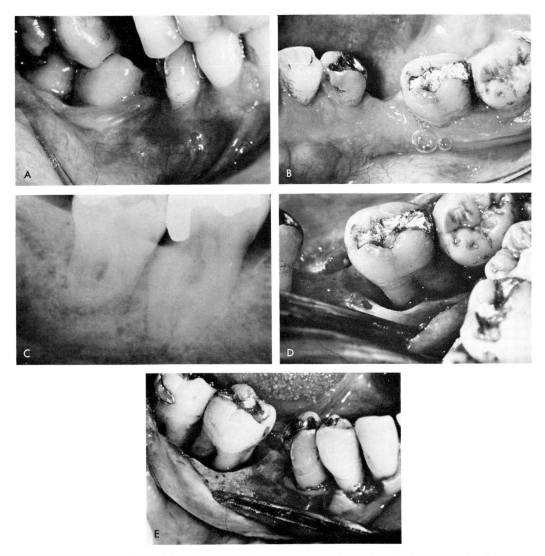

FIG. 11-41. *The unreliability of radiographic evidence and surface observations alone in the diagnosis of periodontal disease.*
A. Buccal view of a lower molar region. B. Lingual view of a lower molar region. C. Radiographic view of the region. D. Lingual view
with flaps reflected. E. Buccal view of the same area with flaps reflected.

Periodontal Probe

The unreliability of radiographs and purely visual criteria is the reason that nothing can supplant the periodontal probe as a diagnostic instrument (Fig. 11-42). Properly used, it has no peer in the periodontal examination. More sound data can result from its skillful use than from any other source.

PERIODONTAL POCKETS

It is surprising how a simple and direct procedure such as probing can become complicated by misconceptions. The probing for pockets and the recording of lesion measurements are basic requirements for any

kind of treatment planning and projection. In too many instances, the probe is merely inserted in several sample areas, and the number of millimeters is set down (Fig. 11-43). In practice, it has been found that the gentle circumferential traverse of the probe, lightly but searchingly in contact with the base of the pocket throughout its entire extent, reveals much that might be overlooked in a series of disparate insertions and measurements. Sudden dips in attachment, deepened zones over root prominences, where they are uncommon, or line-angle detachments are most useful records to have.

The actual record may, and probably must, be the usual six spot measurements, but the method of arriving at these dimensions is not necessarily limited by the

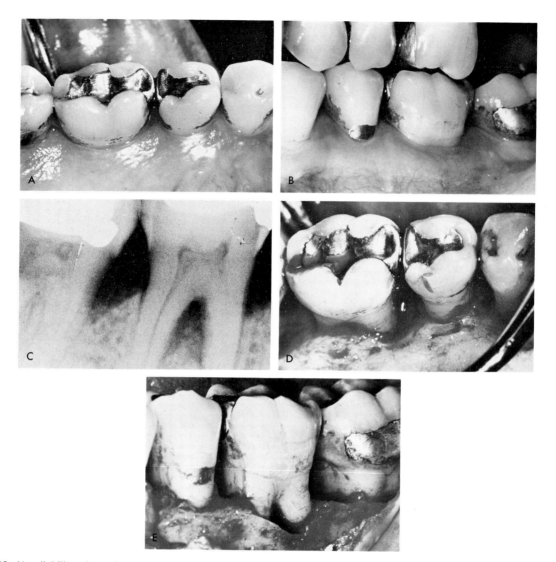

FIG. 11-42. *Unreliability of purely visual criteria. A and B. Normal-appearing gingiva on both buccal and lingual aspects with restorations of high quality. C. Radiographic view of the same area. D and E. With flaps reflected to expose both the buccal and lingual areas, the extensive periodontal destruction can be seen. Only periodontal probing can reveal these lesions to their full extent.*

number recorded. The continuous circumferential probe is favored by most clinicians. The only areas in which such a probing cannot be easily performed is on the proximal surfaces. The probe's shank soon ends the circumferential probe at the contact point. The instrument must be inserted at an angle, and it is in this insertion that the neophyte encounters difficulty.

The principal difficulty lies in the mistaken concept that all probing must be perpendicular. The frequently invoked dictum of parallelism to the long axis of the tooth occurs in so many rules in dentistry that it is carried over into periodontal probing. Insistence on this principle limits interproximal probing to vertical insertions on either side of the proximal contacts. Be-

cause of the ubiquity of the bony crater and the proximal col-shaped pockets, the deepest penetration of the lesion is usually midway between the buccal and lingual plates interproximally. This is the area that cannot be probed with a vertical insertion (Figs. 11-44, 11-45, 11-46, 11-47).

The only solution to this dilemma is to angle the probe insertion so that the deepest penetration is achieved. This is usually in the midplane. The actual linear discrepancy between a vertical probing and one angled to the extent made necessary by the contact area is actually less than 0.25 mm. In addition, there is nothing sacrosanct about a numerical expression of pocket depth. It is basically a useful guide to therapy

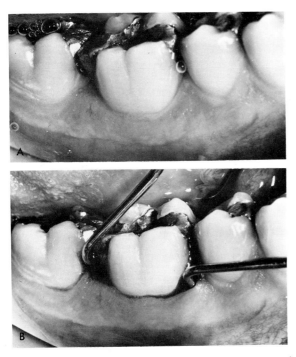

FIG. 11-43. *A. Innocuous-appearing gingiva in a lower molar region. B. Probes in place revealing pockets to the apex of the root.*

and a measure of the success of therapy. If the insertion is always made at the same angle, the guide remains useful.

RECORDING PERIODONTAL POCKETS. In recording data about periodontal pockets, so necessary to treatment, some measurement must be made of sulcular depth that is due to gingival enlargement and not to resorption of a portion of the attachment apparatus. In the diagrammatic charting of the mouth, symbols should be used to indicate such gingival enlargement and even overgrowth when it occurs, so that the actual pocket depth, expressed in millimeters, can be viewed in proper context.

FURCAL INVASIONS

Periodontal pockets commonly involve and include resorptive lesions in the alveolar bone. These resorptive processes, as they extend apically, invade the root functions that normally exist in molars and in some premolar teeth. These special features in a periodontal pocket are called furcal invasions or furca involvements. These lesions are important in both case management and treatment planning, as well as in special maintenance procedures. It is for this reason that they should be described fully, with all variations in form and extent. The most efficient and, at the same time,

most graphic rendering of the extent and form of furcal invasions can be the symbolic rendering and recording on the chart. There is, for example, considerable difference between a beginning invasion, where the probe will reveal a mere dip into the notchlike depression for a millimeter or two, and a patent resorptive defect that extends well into the interfurca so that there are a floor, sides, and a roof to the lesion. Then there is the even more extensive resorption amounting to a through-and-through invasion, such that the defect extends from a buccal to a lingual aspect on a lower molar, or from buccal to distal and/or mesial direction on an upper molar (Fig. 11-48).

RECORDING FURCAL INVASIONS. In most charts, furcal invasions are drawn in by outlining the particular furca involved. In a further effort to clarify the extent of the invasion, Easly and Drennen suggested that the furca be merely outlined with heavy lines in beginning invasions. These are commonly referred to as Class I furcation invasions. In somewhat deeper and more patent penetrations, a base may be drawn to the chevron-shaped outline so that a triangular space is suggested. These are Class II invasions. In invasions that traverse the interfurcal zone so that it is involved in a through-and-through resorptive lesion (for instance, from buccal through to the lingual aspect on a lower molar or from the buccal through to the mesial or distal aspect, or both, on an upper molar) the symbol is a shaded triangle. This last is called a Class III invasion. It becomes obvious that the graphic rendering on the schema or diagram is at once clearer and more useful, since few if any therapists read through a long and necessarily detailed verbal description before each visit of the patient. All, however, examine the diagram in the chart quite carefully and attempt to visualize the area under immediate consideration.

It is for this reason that the examiner should relegate as much information as possible to the diagram. Symbols become most important for this purpose, and a series of graphic symbols is recommended.

Proximal Contact

The proximal contact provides the principal defense against food impaction and invasion, with the subsequent damage to the tissues apical to it. There are several important aberrations in this contact relationship that should appear on the chart.

THE OPEN CONTACT. Open contact relationships can vary from a barely perceptible one to a diastema. The symbol most commonly used is the placing of two parallel lines between the adjacent teeth in question.

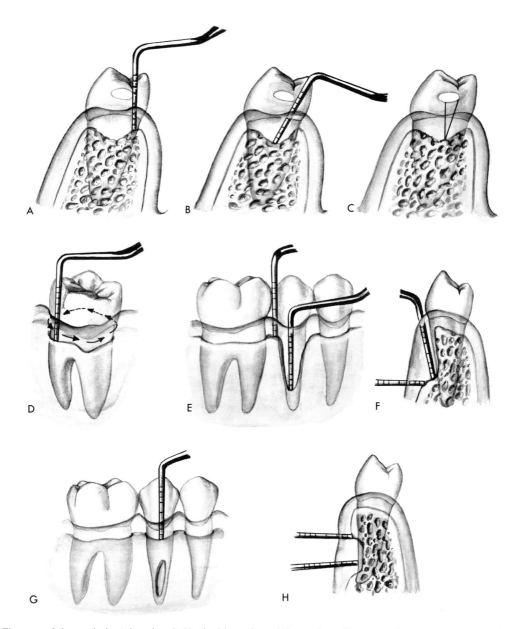

FIG. 11-44. *The use of the periodontal probe. A. Vertical insertion of the probe adjacent to the contact area results in inaccurate pocket depth measurement, since the tip of the instrument reaches only the crest of a bony crater. B. Proper insertion of the probe (searching out the deepest recesses of destruction) and yet trying to negotiate the probing as vertically as the contact area will allow. C. Using average dimensions in an 8 mm-pocket the difference between a plumb-line measurement and one angled to the extent required by the contact area is less than 0.1 mm. D. Probing sulcular depth should be circumferential, thus skipping no area at the bottom of the sulcus. E. Probing sharply deviant pocket depths. F. Probing and sounding (under anesthesia) a dehiscence to determine its extent and the thickness of the marginal bone. G. The false security of probing a root with the overlying bone fenestrated. H. Sounding through mucosa (anesthetized) for the form and extent of the fenestration.*

THE POOR OR FAULTY CONTACT. Where the relation of two adjacent teeth is bad, there are a number of possibilities in their proximal arrangement, all potentially troublesome.

A faulty contact relationship may be fairly firm and by no means open, but may be a poor defense for the papilla apical to it. Teeth with a labial or buccal or lingual inclination, which places them at a considerable variance to the prevailing alignment adjacent, invariably have poor proximal contact relationship with their neighbors. Observation will reveal that it requires more than firmness to provide adequate contact protection. The anatomic arrangement of adjacent marginal ridges to deflect the thrust of the bolus and to direct food onto the occlusal table and into the fossae of the teeth is a most important property of correct

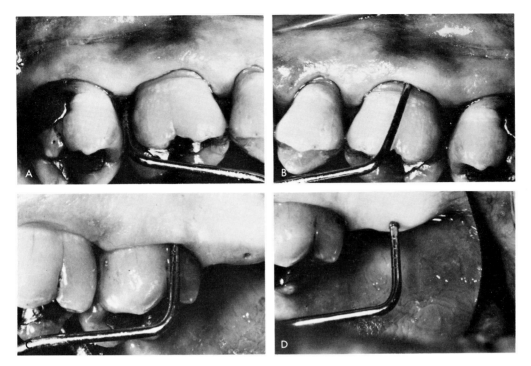

FIG. 11-45. *Probing periodontal pockets. A. Interproximal probing. Note the angle of insertion, which is as vertical as possible. B. Midbuccal probe insertion. The probe is sometimes followed by a curet or a curved explorer to define furcation invasions. C. Palatal probe insertion. D. Sounding the tuberosity pad to determine the thickness of the tuberosity and the location of the underlying bone.*

functional anatomy. The actual degree of firmness of the contact is just one factor of several in the protective arrangement. The graphic symbol for poor contact is frequently an *X* placed at the point of contact on the chart.

INCONSISTENT MARGINAL RIDGES. This term, though not precisely descriptive, is usually reserved for adjacent marginal ridges at differing occlusal levels. Such a poor contact relationship occurs where one tooth is extruded or intruded in relation to its neighbor. Here again, the actual degree of firmness in the contact is not effective alone to protect the underlying structures from trauma, from food impaction, or from food retention.

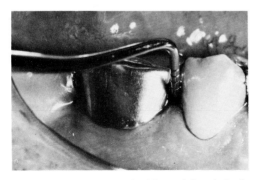

FIG. 11-46. *Probing innocuous-looking sulci and gingiva adjacent to a poorly fitting gold crown.*

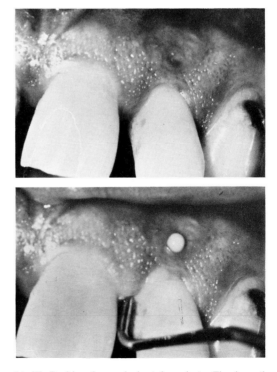

FIG. 11-47. *Probing for periodontal pockets. The insertion of the probe into the periodontal pocket causing pus to flow from the opening of the fistulous tract.*

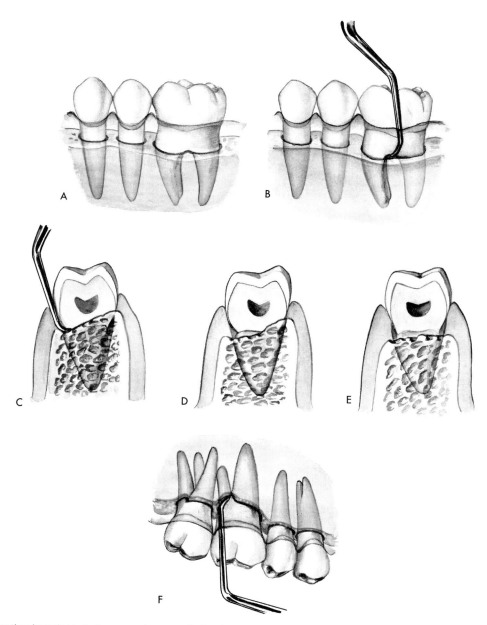

FIG. 11-48. *Furcation invasions. A. Lower molar area. B. Beginning furcal invasion with a curet used as a probing device. C. Cross hemisection of a lower molar showing an incipient or Class I furcal invasion with the toe of a curet inserted. D. A cross hemisection of a lower molar illustrating a patent or Class II furcal invasion. E. A cross hemisection of a lower molar illustrating a communicating or Class III furcal invasion. F. A distal furcal invasion in an upper molar with a curet used as a probing device.*

The symbol *N* placed between the two affected teeth on the chart is sometimes used and is fairly descriptive. Any clearly defined symbol would do as well.

MALPOSED AND TILTED TEETH. Unfortunately, related to faulty contacts and usually incident to them is the malposed tooth. This is certainly a common feature in dentistry. It assumes special importance in periodontics, however, because of the many critical etiologic and therapeutic connotations of malposition. For example, if the tooth is in buccal version, the question of

adequate buccal bony plate is a strong qualifying factor in flap reflection and in the location of a vertical relaxing incision. Another example is the slightly rotated lower canine. Because of the long oval cross section of this tooth and the common drifting of the lateral incisor against it, root proximity is a common finding. This is a seriously unfavorable arrangement in the presence of periodontal disease. A third and common example is the deep mesial pocket on the mesial aspect of a mesially tilted second molar into the space of an unreplaced missing first molar. Examples of the importance of charting this aberration in position are easy to find in large numbers.

The symbol that we use on the chart to mark the tooth in question is an arrow slanting in the direction of the tilt.

EXTRUSIONS AND INTRUSIONS. These malpositions have been mentioned in the context of the faulty contact. They are usually annotated on the chart by arrows pointing in the direction of the variation. Any symbols will do, just so they are clear and as graphically suggestive as possible.

FOOD IMPACTIONS AND RETENTIONS. These are also graphically designated on the chart by properly placed arrows directed into the invaded gingiva. Ordinarily, a simple arrow pointing into the offending contact or gingiva can represent food retention. A tailed arrow, on the other hand, may represent food impaction. Some periodontists mark the outline of the cusp of the tooth in the opposing jaw with a simple chevron to mark the impacting plunger cusp.

HOPELESSLY INVOLVED TEETH, IMPACTIONS, AND DOUBTFUL TEETH. These symbols are variously drawn on the sample charts used in illustration.

Occlusal Examination

Occlusal factors are of great importance in the general examination of the patient. Premature contact in centric occlusion and in lateral excursions, working and nonworking side encumbrances, excursive aberrations are all noted by the careful and skilled observer. The examination of the occlusion and the recording of the data are performed at the same time as is that of the other tissues and their functional relationships. Practical considerations dictate their separation into ordered areas of interest. The orderly recording of occlusal findings is discussed in Chapter 12.

References

1. Allen, D. L., McFall, W. J., Jr., and Hunter, G. C.: Periodontics for the Dental Hygienist, 2nd ed. Philadelphia, Lea & Febiger, 1974.
2. Asgis, A. J.: Clinical and oral case recording. Am. J. Med. 41:47, 1935.
3. Ash, M. M.: Third molars as periodontal problems. Dent. Clin. North Am., March, 1964, p. 51.
4. Beagrie, G. S., and James, G. A.: The association of posterior tooth irregularity and periodontal disease. Br. Dent. J., 113:239, 1962.
5. Bernier, J.: The Registry of Dental and Oral Pathology as an aid in oral diagnosis. Am. J. Orthod., 28:385, 1942.
6. Black, A. D.: Examination and diagnosis by the dentist. J. Am. Dent. Assoc., 18:62, 1931.
7. Burnette, E. W.: Limitations of roentgenograms in periodontal diagnosis. J. Periodontol., 42:293, 1971.
8. Easly, J. R., and Drennen, G. A.: J. Can. Dent. Assoc., 35:104, 1969.
9. Everett, F. G., and Fixott, H. C.: The use of an incorporated grid in the interpretation of dental roentgenograms. Oral Surg., 16:1016, 1963.
10. Goldman, H. M., and Cohen, D. W.: Periodontal Therapy. St. Louis, The C. V. Mosby Co., 1968.
11. Hirschfeld, I.: Diagrammatic recording of periodontal disease. J. Am. Dent. Assoc., 18:1927, 1931.
12. Hirschfeld, I.: The importance of casts in periodontia practice. J. Am. Dent. Assoc., 20:1223, 1933.
13. Hirschfeld, L.: A calibrated silver point for periodontal diagnosis and recording. J. Periodontol., 24:94, 1953.
14. Kerr, D. A., Ash, M. M., and Millard, H. D.: Oral Diagnosis, 3rd ed. St. Louis, The C. V. Mosby Co., 1970.
15. Lovett, D. W.: Radiodontic aspects of oral diagnosis. J. Am. Dent. Assoc., 27:421, 1940.
16. Maynard, J. G.: The periodontal probe. Va. Dent. J., 46:20, 1969.
17. Morris, M. L.: The diagnosis, prognosis and treatment of the loose tooth. Oral Surg., 6:1037, 1953.
18. Morris, M. L.: Artificial crown contours and gingival health. J. Prosthet. Dent., 12:1146, 1962.
19. Muhlemann, H. R.: Ten years of tooth mobility measurements. J. Periodontol., 31:110, 1960.
20. O'Leary, T. J., Shannon, I. L., and Prigmore, J. R.: Clinical and systemic findings in periodontal disease. J. Periodontol., 33:243, 1962.
21. Prichard, J. F.: The role of the roentgenogram in the diagnosis and prognosis of periodontal disease. Oral Surg., 14:182, 1961.
22. Sicher, H., and DuBrul, E. L.: Oral Anatomy, 6th ed. St. Louis, The C. V. Mosby Co., 1975.
23. Silha, R. E.: Paralleling long cone technique. Dent. Radiogr. Photogr., 41:3, 1968.
24. Smith, J. H.: The interdental gingival topography and its role in periodontal disease. Texas Dent. J., 82:20, 1964.
25. Tennenbaum, B., and Karshan, M.: Blood studies in periodontoclasia. J. Dent. Res., 23:190, 1944.
26. Tibbetts, L. S.: Use of diagnostic probes for detection of periodontal disease. J. Am. Dent. Assoc., 78:549, 1969.
27. Updegrave, W. J.: Higher fidelity in intraoral roentgenography. J. Am. Dent. Assoc., 62:1, 1961.
28. Wahl, N.: Oral Signs and Symptoms. A Diagnostic Handbook. Springfield, Ill., Charles C Thomas, 1969.
29. Wright, W. H.: Local factors in periodontal disease. Periodontics, 1:163, 1963.
30. Wuehrmann, A. H.: The Long Cone Technic. Practical Dental Monographs. Chicago, The Year Book Medical Publishers, July, 1957.
31. Zegarelli, E. V., and Kutcher, A. H.: Keratosis of the mouth: hyperkeratosis and leukoplakia. Southern Calif. Dent. Assoc. J., 27:345, 1959.

12

Diagnosis of Occlusally
Related Disturbances

12
Diagnosis
of
Occlusally
Related
Disturbances

The dental profession is becoming increasingly aware that functional occlusal disturbances may lead to disorders such as periodontal disease, temporomandibular joint dysfunction, occlusal attrition, or a combination of these manifestations. Since most dentists are general practitioners and most dental therapy is provided by them, the knowledge of functional occlusion and treatment of occlusal disturbances should be a basic requirement, not only for the specialists in periodontics and restorative dentistry but especially for the general practitioner.

We accept that many adult occlusal and periodontal problems are initiated during childhood and adolescence, and it is the general practitioner and rarely the periodontist who treats the majority of these young patients. Consequently, training in recognizing the signs and symptoms of periodontal disease and the conditions from which it arises, together with training in procedures for therapy, should be made available to the profession as a whole. Only in this manner can the treatment of the overwhelming proportion of the population be undertaken.

Many dentists resist treating functional occlusal disturbances, even though they recognize their presence and prevalence, because they are faced with a problem involving the function of the entire mouth rather than with a single tooth or segment. Dentists must accept the fact that the single-tooth concept is outdated and that greater emphasis must be placed on the total-mouth concept, and schools of dentistry must provide training in this concept at the undergraduate and postgraduate levels.

Occlusal function is the final expression of the stomatognathic system, and as part of this system it should be treated by methods that are biologically and technologically sound. The functional relationships of single teeth to their antagonists must be examined in addition to their pathologic condition. Once the dentist has accepted this requirement, he will better comprehend the relationship of good dental function to the total health and comfort of the masticatory apparatus.

Controversies abound in the study and treatment of functional occlusion. Most of the ideas in this chapter are not new or original but represent a compilation and at times a modification of accepted concepts of several recognized authorities on this subject. The material is organized in a sequence both practical and applicable not only for specialists but especially for general practitioners who encounter patients with occlusal problems in the course of their routine examinations.

CHARACTERISTICS OF NORMAL FUNCTIONAL OCCLUSION

There is some disagreement over how teeth should function. In our opinion, a wide range of functional and static occlusal relationships can function in health. Many patients have morphologic malocclusions that vary from the classic relationships and yet manifest no subjective symptoms or recognizable pathologic signs. For them, the occlusion is physiologically acceptable, at least for the present, and no alterations need to be made.

Criteria are more difficult to set for functional than for morphologic normality, and consequently it may be difficult to decide whether a given occlusion is pathologic. It is possible for dental arches to be esthetically aligned but for the teeth to clash grossly in functional excursions, while a gross morphologic occlusal deformity may function well and remain healthy.

An occlusion cannot be examined or discussed without first understanding the important basic positions that the mandible may assume relative to the maxilla and distinguishing between mandibular border movements and physiologic functional movements.[19] The literature related to this aspect of occlusion is voluminous. However, it is not within the scope of this chapter to treat the physiology of occlusion in all its detail. Excellent textbooks cover this material accurately.[20,21] Consequently, it will suffice to describe that portion of the occlusal physiology pertaining especially to functional analysis and to adjustment of occlusion of the natural dentition by selective grinding.

Basic Mandibular Positions

The three most important basic mandibular positions are postural or rest position, centric occlusion position, and centric relation position.

POSTURAL OR REST POSITION

The postural or rest position is the position from which normal functions start. The opposing teeth should not make contact in this position. It is defined as the habitual postural position of the mandible when the patient is resting comfortably in the upright position and the condyles are in a neutral, unstrained position in the glenoid fossae.[1] Sicher and DuBruhl state that the rest position is determined by resting muscle tonus which is constantly maintained by a reflex contraction of a proportionate number of fibers in the muscle.[23] This position is, however, variable and can be affected mainly by the body and head positions and occasionally by a number of pathologic conditions,

overwork, or nervous tension. It is not possible, therefore, to record for any one patient an accurate measurement of the "normal" interocclusal distance or free-way space, which is the distance between mandibular and maxillary teeth in this physiologic resting position, because this varies with the position itself. The free-way space is not a single entity but a range and may vary from 1 mm to 9 mm in a single individual.[6,19,25] Even patients with an interocclusal distance as great as 8 to 10 mm have been observed to be free of any functional disturbance.[21]

The significance of postural position and the interocclusal distance becomes apparent mainly during prosthetic restoration. The consequences of excessively opening or excessively closing the bite by restorative means are well understood. A certain amount of interocclusal space is a basic requirement. Opening the bite excessively prevents the muscles of mastication from ever relaxing; excessive closure causes overrelaxation. In either case the neuromuscular tonus is disturbed. However, selective grinding of the natural dentition during occlusal adjustment procedures probably does not change this significantly. Occasionally, a dentition will have been extensively restored, and the natural interocclusal space has been obliterated by excessively opening the bite. It is doubtful whether this condition can be treated successfully by selective grinding and in most cases the restorations, either fixed or removable, have to be remade to a vertical dimension that is physiologic to the patient.

CENTRIC OCCLUSAL POSITION AND CENTRIC RELATION POSITION

Differing interpretations of the terms *centric occlusal position* and *centric relation position* have been a source of confusion to the dental profession for many years. In fact, the word *centric* may be the most controversial term in dentistry. This can partly be blamed on semantics, but it is mainly attributable to differences in concept. Because it is often used differently by different authors, it is doubtful that the serious differences in concept will ever be resolved. The generally accepted definitions are applied here.

Centric occlusal position, also referred to as "habitual centric," "intercuspal position," and "acquired centric," is a tooth-to-tooth (mandibular-to-maxillary) relationship and is the position assumed by the mandible when there is maximum intercuspation. Consequently, centric occlusion refers to the manner of tooth contact at the centric occlusal position and will hereafter be abbreviated to CO (Fig. 12-13B).

Centric relation position, also referred to as "hinge position," "terminal hinge position," "retruded position," and "terminal hinge interocclusal position," is the position assumed by the mandible relative to the maxilla when the condyles are in their rearmost, midmost position in the glenoid fossae. Centric relation is a bone-to-bone relationship (condyle-to-glenoid fossa), and the manner in which the teeth make contact when the mandible assumes the most closed position in centric relation is referred to as centric relation occlusion, hereafter abbreviated to CRO (Fig. 12-13A).

Probably the most important and most basic requirement in examining, analyzing, adjusting, or restoring occlusions is the ability to locate precisely and to register CRO.

Basic Mandibular Movement

During normal function the mandible moves by a combination of rotation and translation of the condyles in the glenoid fossae. When the mandible moves or is manually guided on paths determined by the extreme limits of ligaments and structures of the temporomandibular joints, a characteristic pattern develops that can be measured and registered. The positions that the mandible assumes anywhere on these boundary paths are called ligamentous or border positions.[21] Posselt has shown that these positions are constant and reproducible for each individual and can be traced in both sagittal and horizontal planes (Figs. 12-1, 12-2).[19] They constitute the envelope of motion. Parts of the superior boundaries of this envelope, in both sagittal

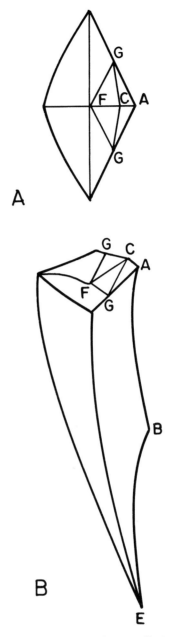

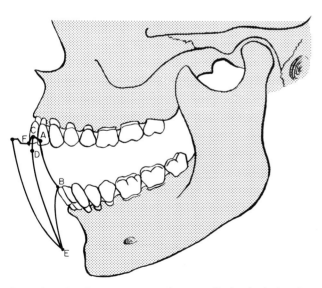

FIG. 12-1. *Border movement of a mandibular incisal point, traced in sagittal plane. CRO position (A); path of terminal hinge movement (A–B); CO position (C); path of mandibular shift from point of initial contact to maximum intercuspation (A–C); path of incisal guidance (C–F); rest position (D); maximum opening (E).*

FIG. 12-2. *A. Border movement of a mandibular incisal point and enclosed area recorded in horizontal plane. CRO position (A); CO position (C); lateral movement from CRO position (A–G); lateral movement from CO position (C–G) edge-to-edge incisal position (F). B. Lateral view of a three-dimensional tracing of the border movement of a mandibular incisal point. Path of terminal hinge position devoid of any muscular activity (A–B); path of mandibular movement when muscular activity causes a forward translation (B–E).*

and horizontal planes, are determined by the contact relationship of the teeth and as such represent occlusal rather than ligamentous positions (Fig. 12-2). All other mandibular movements constituting normal functions are within this envelope and are relatively unimportant in occlusal adjustment.

Only a part of the border movements is clinically significant in routine examination, analysis, and adjustment of occlusion. It is extremely important to execute accurately and precisely the posterior border movement constituting the path followed by the mandible while in centric relation and the occlusally determined portion of the envelope of motion if occlusal analysis and adjustment procedures are to be correctly performed.

POSTERIOR BORDER MOVEMENT

The mandible moves by a combination of rotation and translation. In executing the posterior border movement, the first portion (A–B, Fig. 12-1) is pure rotation (hinge movement). When the mandible reaches approximately 2 to 2.5 cm of opening, the lateral pterygoid muscles react and cause a forward translation (B–E, Fig. 12-1) of the mandible. It is the pure hinge movement (A–B), devoid of any muscular activity, that is important in accurately locating and registering occlusal contacts at the CRO position. This border movement is not natural, and most patients need precise guidance by the dentist in order to perform it accurately. The most common error in occlusal analysis, adjustment, and rehabilitation leading to iatrogenic occlusal disharmony stems from the dentist's inability to recognize the precise CRO position, to guide the patient's jaw to, and register the position accurately in wax in order to transfer the mandibular casts of the patient's jaws to an articulator.

OCCLUSALLY DETERMINED GLIDING MANDIBULAR MOVEMENTS

Several components are clinically significant. In the sagittal plane, one component represents the mandibular shift from CRO to CO (A–C, Fig. 12-1). During the examination procedure the magnitude of this shift is readily seen once the CRO position has been located and the patient is asked to bite hard. With this the mandible usually skids from the point of initial contact in CRO to the maximum intercuspation (Fig. 12-13). The significance of the shift is explained later. The remainder of the occlusally determined sagittal border path of the mandible during protrusive movement is the line (C–F, Fig. 12-1). The character of this segment is determined initially by the pattern of incisal contacts made by the mandibular anterior teeth as they pass from CO over the lingual surfaces of the maxillary anterior teeth and finally by posterior occlusal contacts, if any, during extreme protrusive movement. In order to register contact relationships and to determine

occlusal interferences during protrusive excursion, it is imperative that the patient perform this movement accurately.

In the horizontal plane, the boundaries determined by tooth contact as the mandible moves laterally from CRO position (A–G, Fig. 12-2) are significant in properly locating and registering the manner of tooth contact during lateral mandibular excursions. The side to which the mandible moves is called the working side, and the opposite side is the balancing side (often referred to as the nonworking side). This movement constitutes a combination of condylar rotation and translation. The working condyle not only rotates in a horizontal plane but in most cases has a slight lateral shift (Bennett shift). This shift may be straight out laterally, laterally and protrusively, or laterally and retrusively. Any of these movements may also have a superior or inferior component. The balancing condyle translates forward, downward, and inward the manner being determined by the shape of the glenoid fossa.

During examination and registration of working and balancing contacts, the dentist must guide the patient's jaw to prevent any anterior translation of the working condyle that is due to contraction of the lateral pterygoid muscle on the working side. This guidance is equally important while registering lateral relationships of the mandible to the maxilla for the purpose of articulator analysis.

The superior boundaries determined by the gliding relationships of such teeth are also significant, as it is usually on these paths that parafunction such as grinding occurs. Careful examination of the dentition often reveals the pattern of grinding. It is easy to distinguish, with the aid of accurate study casts, the retrusive, working, or nonworking facets from normal wear patterns (Fig. 12-3).

Differing Concepts of Mandibular Positions

Some of the conflicting concepts concerning centric relation occlusion and centric occlusion and lateral and protrusive excursions are the following:

CENTRIC RELATION OCCLUSION AND CENTRIC OCCLUSION

1. Mandibular positions at CRO and CO should coincide.[12,24]
2. Mandibular positions at CRO and CO need not coincide.
3. CRO position should be a stable position with a range of cuspal noninterference from CRO to CO.[21]

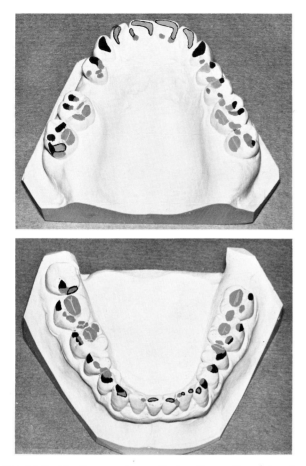

FIG. 12-3. *Maxillary and mandibular diagnostic casts of a dentition suffering from long history of bruxism, showing many centric facets (grey), working facets (black), and protrusive facets (grey with black outline). Many of the broad centric facets act also as cross-tooth and cross-arch nonworking facets during lateral excursive movement.*

4. A mandibular shift from CRO to CO can be ignored if it is 1 mm or less, without a lateral component, and unassociated with any recognized signs and symptoms of occlusally related disturbances.[19]

LATERAL EXCURSION

1. A maximum number of cusps should make contact on both the working and nonworking sides with both cross-tooth and cross-arch balancing contacts.[9,22]
2. Maximum cuspal contact (group function) should only be on the working side, with disclusion or no contact on the nonworking side.[4]
3. Cuspid rise on the working side should cause a disclusion of all other teeth on both working and nonworking sides.[12]

4. Noninterfering group function should exist on both working and nonworking sides during the initial phase of lateral excursion (1 to 2 mm) with subsequent cuspid rise or group function on the working side which will effect a disclusion on the nonworking side.

PROTRUSIVE EXCURSION

1. Maximum cuspal contact of both anterior and posterior teeth with their antagonists is desirable.[22]
2. Contact of as many anterior teeth as possible with disclusion of the posterior teeth is desirable.[12]

Currently Accepted Beliefs

Ideal functional occlusions are characterized by a harmonious interaction between the teeth, periodontium, and the temporomandibular joints and their associated musculature. The entire masticatory system has a stable neuromuscular pattern; were it not so, functional disorders could be triggered by even slight occlusal interferences. Chewing should be equally easy on both sides and unassociated with pain.

Preferably, CRO and CO should coincide. However, most people, regardless of age, exhibit an anterior shift from CRO to CO.[11,19] If this shift is slight (1 mm or less) and has no lateral component, the discrepancy neither necessarily contributes to nor precedes occlusally related disturbances. If it is greater than 1 mm or has a lateral component, or both, it is potentially pathologic because cuspal interferences require muscle and temporomandibular-joint adaptation and therefore the occlusion may require adjustment.[20]

During normal function there should be no deflecting interference upon closure, and the teeth should make contact in stable cusp-to-fossa or cusp-to-flat-plane relationships in either the CO position or the CRO position, if these positions coincide. Any cuspal contacts or unbalanced inclined planes are potentially damaging to the masticatory apparatus, especially under parafunctional circumstances. Bilaterally distributed stress in the intercuspal position should be experienced by most of the teeth, and this stress should be directed axially in the posterior teeth.

There should be a free-way space at the resting position of about 2 to 3 mm, but it may be much wider. This is necessary to prevent muscle fatigue and cuspal contact during speech.

Optimally, a cuspid rise should cause a slight disclusion of all teeth on both the working and the nonworking sides during lateral mandibular excursions

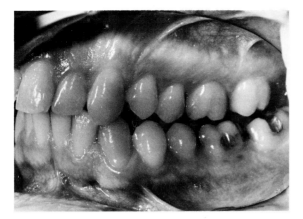

FIG. 12-4. *Dentition in which the posterior teeth are discluded by the cuspid during lateral excursion. Also referred to as cuspid rise.*

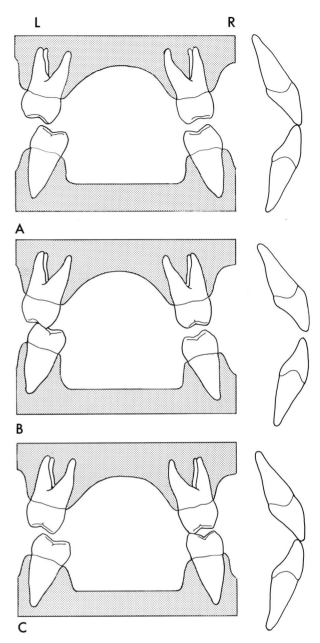

FIG. 12-6. *Types of contact relationship during lateral excursion. A. Cuspid rise ideally effecting slight disclusion of posterior teeth on both working (R) and nonworking (L) sides. B. Cross-arch deflective nonworking contact (L) preventing normal cuspid function. C. Cross-tooth nonworking contact (R) which is also undesirable.*

(Figs. 12-4, 12-6A). With slight cuspid wear, a simultaneous gliding contact (group function) of the posterior teeth on the working side may result (Fig. 12-5). This is acceptable if no cross-tooth or cross-arch contacts are present (Fig. 12-6B,C). No working-side contact of the incisors should prevent cuspid function.

During protrusive function there should be no contacting posterior teeth deflective or otherwise (Fig. 12-7). Ideally a maximum number of anterior teeth and the mandibular first premolars should be made to contact with their antagonists and effect a complete disclusion of the remaining posterior teeth.

These concepts apply to younger patients as well. Although most children and young adults seem to have tissue vitality sufficient to resist manifestations of disease related to occlusion, disharmonies allowed to remain into adulthood can result in pathogenesis.[5,11,21]

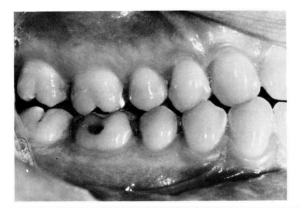

FIG. 12-5. *Dentition in which cuspid wear has effected group functional contact of posterior teeth on the working side during lateral excursion.*

Deviations from Normal Occlusal Patterns

The dentist will often encounter patients with morphologic or functional occlusal patterns that seem to contradict these rules. For example, deflective interference may be present but unassociated with obvious signs of functional disturbances. Whether prophylactic

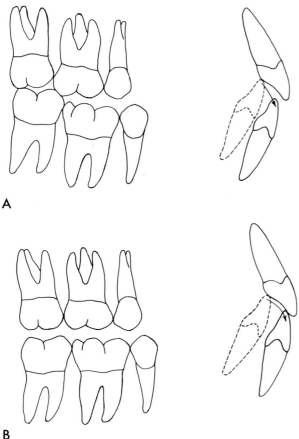

A

B

Fig. 12-7. *A. Deflective posterior interference preventing contact of anterior teeth during protrusive excursion (undesirable). B. Normal disclusion of posterior teeth during protrusive excursion.*

correction of functional malocclusion is wise for such patients is a matter of opinion and often greatly depends on the dentist's ability to recognize subtle but significant signs and symptoms related to occlusal disturbance. Consequently a complete history and examination are essential to the accuracy of any diagnosis of occlusal disturbances.

EXAMINATION OF THE OCCLUSION

For the routine patient the format should be simple and precise and need not be time-consuming. An effective chart for recording the data, developed by Yuodelis, is shown in Figure 12-8. Prerequisites for the occlusal examination are a complete intraoral radiographic survey and accurate casts for studying the morphology and position of the teeth (wear facets, interproximal contact relationships), interarch relationships, and arch form. With these, the importance of subjective symptoms can better be judged.

In most cases the clinical examination, complete radiographic survey, and study casts are usually sufficient to make the correct diagnosis and to develop an appropriate treatment plan. The more complex case, however, may require special aids, such as articulated casts, to evaluate a functional disturbance.

Occlusal History

A concise and accurate history should be taken prior to the clinical examination, the extent and detail depending mainly on the absence or presence of occlusally related symptoms. This is to establish the patient's reason for seeking treatment and to record chronologically the events that may have caused or contributed to these complaints.

Significance of Parafunctional Habits

The close relationship of parafunctional habits and occlusal traumatism and other manifestations of distress has been emphasized. The dentist should determine whether the patient is aware of occlusally related symptoms and should not necessarily accept his lack of awareness as a sign that disturbances do not exist, since many patients are unaware of signs such as mobility or unusual wear and therefore require further examination. Questioning should include the past or present history of symptoms such as pain in the teeth, periodontium, or temporomandibular joint and associated musculature, important symptoms that may be related to parafunctions such as nocturnal or diurnal bruxism, and lip or cheek biting. Oral habits are common at any age and are a major concern in the diagnosis, treatment planning, and correction of occlusally related disorders. They can be brought to light by such questions as: "Are your teeth together upon awakening? Do your jaws feel tired in the morning or evening? Do you have squeaky fillings?" Any positive answers may indicate bruxism. Patients are often unaware of parafunctional habits, and it may be necessary to ask whether people sleeping in the same room complain of grinding. Since parafunctional habits are commonly associated with psychologic disorders,[13] it is most important to learn whether the spouse, employer, parents, or friends may be causing psychologic stress associated with the occlusal disorder. The patient may require psychotherapy in addition to dental therapy. Serious tension problems or psychic disturbances must be recognized as early as possible, since they must be controlled if treatment of the occlusal disturbance is to be successful.

EXAMINATION OF OCCLUSION

Name Mrs. R. S. T.   Chart No. 1341   Date 2/21/72

Occlusal History (occlusal complaints, habits, pertinent physical and psychological findings from health questionnaire)
Patient admits to nocturnal and diurnal bruxism--mostly of a clenching nature.

Extra-oral Examination (facial asymmetries, mandibular deviations, TMJ dysfunction, pain)
Clicking of right TMJ concomitant with slight left lateral mandibular deviation on wide opening. No associated pain.

Intra-oral Examination: Angle's classification 1 Interoccl. clearance 2-4 mm

Ant. overbite 4 mm   Ant. overjet 2 mm Migrations slightly procumbent anteriors

Wear (degree, distribution, etiology) slight wear of posterior teeth

Sensitivity (thermal, percussion) generalized thermal sensitivity
Intra-arch form and alignment (occlusal plane, extrusions, crossbites, arch collapse, etc.)
Tooth #17 extruded; stepped occlusal plane between mandibular anterior segment and right posterior segment resulting in an exaggerated curve of Spee.

Radiographic Examination (bone support, alteration of periodontal ligament, root resorption, pulpal death, etc.)
Generalized widening of PDL spaces; hemiseptal bone loss in 2, 3, 15 regions.

INITIAL OCCLUSAL FINDINGS

CENTRIC RELATION OCCLUSION																
1	2	3	4	5	6	7	8	9	10	11	(12)	13	14	15	16
32	31	30	29	28	27	26	25	24	23	22	(21)	20	19	18	17

CRO - CO HORIZONTAL 2mm ant., 1mm left   VERTICAL Ant. 4 mm

RIGHT LATERAL																
1	(2)	(3)	(4)	(5)	(6)	7	(8)	9	10	11	12	13	14	15	16
32	(31)	(30)	(29)	(28)	(27)	26	(25)	24	23	22	21	20	19	18	17

LEFT LATERAL																
1	(2)	(3)	4	5	6	7	8	9	10	(11)	12	(13)	14	15	16
32	(31)	(30)	29	28	27	26	25	24	23	(22)	21	(20)	19	18	17

PROTRUSIVE																
1	2	3	4	5	(6)	(7)	8	(9)	10	11	12	13	14	(15	16
32	31	30	29	28	(27)	(26)	25	(24)	23	22	21	20	19	18	17)

MOBILITY																
-	I	-	I	I	-	I	I	II	I	-	I	II	I	-	-
1	2	3	4	5	6	7	8	9	10	11	12	13	14	15	16
32	31	30	29	28	27	26	25	24	23	22	21	20	19	18	17
-	-	I	I		II	I		I	II	-	-	I	-	-	-

Occlusal Treatment Plan (1) CRO: Eliminate shift from CRO to CO; (2) Rt Lateral: maintain group function; eliminate 8/25 contact; (3) Left Lateral: establish cuspid rise; eliminate cross-arch balancing contacts; (4) Protrusive: improve group function; eliminate posterior balancing contact 15/17.

Extraoral Examination

Seat the patient in a semireclining position with his head properly supported and slightly tipped back (Fig. 12-9). Note any facial asymmetries or gross abnormalities and relate them to their cause. Ask the patient to open and close his mouth. Observe signs of temporomandibular joint dysfunction, such as lateral deviations of the jaw (Fig. 12-10), limited opening, and clicking or popping of the temporomandibular joint. These symptoms may be associated with pain. Palpate the muscles of mastication for soreness.

Intraoral Examination

Unless the dentist is adept at recognizing the signs and symptoms of occlusal disorders, their clinical manifestations will frequently elude him. No single sign in itself can be considered diagnostic but should be related carefully to other diagnostic measures, such as functional analysis and radiographic and historical findings.

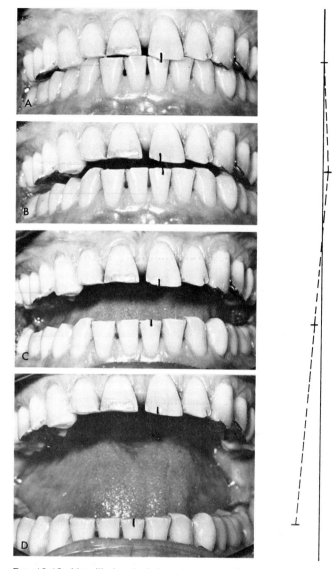

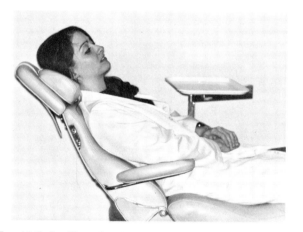

FIG. 12-9. *Position of patient for functional occlusal analysis. Note that the head is slightly tipped back. This same position is also fundamental for all occlusal adjustment procedures.*

FIG. 12-10. *Mandibular deviation during opening and closing related to temporomandibular joint dysfunction. Note progressive lateral deviation of the mandible at different stages of opening. A. Teeth in centric occlusion. B. Teeth in centric relation occlusion. C. Moderate opening. D. Full opening. (Courtesy Dr. W. Kaldahl)*

FIG. 12-8. *Completed chart used in examination of occlusion. Interpretation of occlusal findings:*
Centric Relation Occlusion: *Initial contact in CRO position is between maxillary and mandibular left first premolars ($^{12}/_{21}$).*
CRO-CO, Horizontal and Vertical: *The mandible appears to shift 2 mm anteriorly and 1 mm left laterally from CRO to CO in a horizontal plane, and the difference in vertical dimension between CRO and CO in the incisor region is 4 mm.*
Right Lateral: *Maxillary and mandibular central incisors, cuspids, premolars and first and second molars contact in right lateral excursion, starting from the CO position. There are no cross-arch nonworking contacts.*
Left Lateral: *Maxillary and mandibular cuspids and second premolars contact in left lateral excursion. There are also cross-arch nonworking contacts between the first and second molars.*
Protrusive: *Mostly group function as well as posterior nonworking contact between the maxillary left second molar and the mandibular third molar.*
Mobility: *Generalized mobility ranging from $^1/_2$ (−) to II, indicated above or below the respective tooth numbers.*

PROCEDURE

Prior to examining the functional occlusion, determine the static relation of the teeth in CO and record the interocclusal clearance, overlap (overjet), and overbite. With the help of accurate study models, examine the teeth for excessive variations in occlusal planes, extrusions, crossbites, arch collapse, and open bites and record the effects of these abnormalities.

Note the degree and distribution of wear facets and relate them to the age of the patient. Although occlusal wear is not always associated with traumatized periodontal support or hypermobility, it is nonetheless pathognomonic of bruxism (Fig. 5-16) and is only rarely the result of abrasive foods. Patterns of increased occlusal wear are often concomitant with increased tooth mobility and sometimes migration. Wear facets are readily recognized by examination of the occlusal surfaces of accurate stone casts (Fig. 12-3). Facets can often be matched to their opposites and consequently related to a particular pattern of mandibular movement, which in turn provides information concerning the mode of bruxism or other habits that caused the wear. Wear facets associated with tooth migration are usually related to patterns of bruxism beyond the normal functioning range or to habits such as pencil chewing and nail or lip biting. Migration of unworn teeth may be associated with tongue habits, cheek biting, lip sucking, or atypical swallowing habits (Fig. 5-21). Wear should also be related to the radiographic picture of the bone support. Such signs as bone loss (Fig. 5-20D), pulpal death (Fig. 5-17),[10] changes in width of the periodontal ligament space (Figs. 5-1, 5-9), root resorption (Fig. 5-14), and even root fracture (Fig. 5-19) may be associated with occlusally related disturbances.

SENSITIVITY

Examine the teeth for sensitivity to thermal changes or percussion, a condition often concomitant with increased mobility. A mobile tooth has a duller percussion sound than does a normal tooth because the periodontal space has widened.

PERIODONTAL CHANGES

Examine the periodontal tissues for signs of pathogenesis. There is no scientific evidence that gingival changes such as clefts or festoons are manifestations of occlusal traumatism. It is, however, at present widely accepted that occlusal traumatism in the presence of local factors such as microbial dental plaque, poor restorations, and food impaction can cause increased pocket formation and bone resorption, although alone it does not cause gingival inflammation.[8,21] The histopathology and significant relationship of occlusal traumatism and periodontal disease are discussed in Chapter 5.

Tooth Mobility

Excessive tooth mobility is recognized as an alarming sign of a disturbed attachment apparatus and is most often due to loss of alveolar bone, alteration of the width of the periodontal ligament space, or a combination of these factors. During examination procedures it is important to distinguish between normal physiologic mobility and pathologic tooth mobility.

NORMAL PHYSIOLOGIC MOBILITY

Even teeth free from periodontal disturbance demonstrate slight mobility, which is normal and physiologic and varies with the type of tooth. With few exceptions, such as teeth with incomplete root formation or congenitally shortened or excessively tapered roots, physiologic tooth mobility is not readily discernible to the eye by the commonly used method of measurement.

Studies have shown that physiologic tooth mobility is affected most commonly by variable factors such as number, size, shape, and distribution of roots, time of day, and normal function.

Having less total surface area of root attachment, incisors are, in most cases more mobile than molars, cuspids, and premolars. It has also been shown that tooth mobility is greatest immediately upon arising and decreases progressively during waking hours.[16] This has been explained as being due to slight extension of the tooth from the socket resulting from a lack of functional contact during sleep. A significant decrease in tooth mobility results from chewing.[17]

PATHOLOGIC TOOTH MOBILITY

Pathologic tooth mobility readily discernible to the eye when force is applied to the tooth in a lateral direction is a significant sign of periodontal disturbance.[15] It is, in fact, the most common sign. Several variables contribute to pathologic mobility. The most common are widening of the periodontal ligament space (Fig. 5-1), loss of alveolar bone support (Fig. 5-26), or a combination of these (Fig. 5-9). Factors usually responsible for excessive widening of the periodontal ligament space are:

1. Parafunctional habits and occlusal interferences, alone or in combination, both of which may result in occlusal traumatism.
2. Gingival conditions resulting in severe inflammation caused by irritants such as microbial dental plaque.
3. Transient factors affecting the gingiva or periodontal attachment apparatus or both, such as traumatic injury or surgical, restorative, or endodontic procedures.

With elimination of the cause, excessive mobility patterns are reversible when healing of the attachment apparatus and surrounding gingival tissue is complete.

Factors responsible for insufficient alveolar bone support are:

1. Periodontitis resulting in excessive horizontal or vertical bone loss (Fig. 5-2).
2. Injudicious osseous resection during periodontal surgery (Fig. 5-22) or tooth extraction.
3. Excessive apical root resorption concomitant with orthodontic and endodontic therapy or of an idiopathic nature (Fig. 5-14).
4. Congenitally short, slender, or tapered roots (Fig. 5-4).

It is evident that any of these factors may cause a permanent increase in tooth mobility. If the amount of alveolar support is excessively embarrassed, severe occlusal traumatism will result and necessitate therapeutic splinting.

MEASUREMENT OF TOOTH MOBILITY

The most commonly accepted clinical method is to hold the crown of the tooth between the forefinger and an instrument and apply force (Fig. 12-11). The degree of tooth movement is estimated and can be scored from I to III with increments of one half marked as [–]. Interpretation of the values is as follows:

  0 = Clinical mobility within normal range
[–] = Clinical mobility considered slightly more than physiologic but less than 1 mm buccolingually
  I = Clinical mobility approximately 1 mm buccolingually
 II = Clinical mobility approximately 2 mm buccolingually but with no mobility in an apical direction
III = Clinical mobility greater than 2 mm buccolingually in addition to mobility in an apical direction

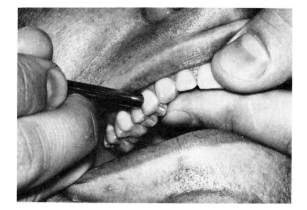

FIG. 12-11. *Position of instrument handle and operator's forefinger when estimating degree of tooth mobility.*

Pathologic mobility should always be related to radiographic evidence of pathogenesis and to pocket-depth measurements to see if it is caused by parafunctional stress alone or by a combination of occlusal traumatism and loss of supporting bone.

RECORDING OF FUNCTIONAL OCCLUSION

The purpose of the functional examination is to determine whether occlusal interferences exist during centric relation closure and mandibular border movements. A superficial examination or a static analysis of the teeth in CO is insufficient because many diagnostic signs of occlusal disharmonies may not be uncovered. The chart "Examination of Occlusion" (Fig. 12-8) provides a standardized format for recording occlusal contacts in CRO and during right and left lateral and protrusive border movements of the mandible. The magnitude and direction of mandibular slide from CRO to CO and degree of mobility can also be recorded on this chart. The use of such a chart will ensure a uniform and adequate occlusal examination of each patient.

Armamentarium

1. Chart, "Examination of Occlusion"
2. Red and green dental tape (Madam Butterfly ³/₄", #40 inking; Wm. Dierickx, Seattle)
3. Cotton rolls or 2" × 2" gauze
4. Dental mirror
5. Hand mirror
6. Occlusal-tape forceps (Miller articulating paper forceps, Misdom-Frank, New York)

Examination of Centric Relation Occlusion and Centric Occlusion

One of the most important prerequisites in the study of occlusion is the ability to locate the CRO position precisely. For the inexperienced, this is often difficult and incorrectly executed. The procedure is also difficult if the patient has temporomandibular-joint problems or tense jaw muscles.

There are several methods for obtaining an accurate record of CRO. It matters little which method is used, as long as the procedure is accurate. (Accuracy is verified by locating precisely the same initial point[s] of contact between the mandibular and maxillary teeth over and over again.) If there is a large discrepancy between CRO and CO, there is usually a single mandibular tooth making the initial contact with the maxillary arch. If there is no discrepancy between CRO and CO or if the difference is slight, several teeth may make the initial contact.

The method we prefer for determining CRO position and marking the point of initial contact varies only slightly from that described by Ramfjord and Ash.[21]

PROCEDURE FOR DETERMINING CRO POSITION

Seat the patient in a slightly reclined, comfortable position. Adjust the headrest so that the head is properly supported and tipped back slightly (Fig. 12-9). Ask the patient to relax his body as much as possible and to look straight forward. Place your right thumb over the labial aspect of the patient's mandibular incisors and your forefinger under his chin. The thumb must be positioned high enough so that upon closure it will prevent the teeth from contacting (Fig. 12-12A). Inform the patient that you will guide his jaw in an up-and-down hingelike motion. Ask him not to assist actively but to allow his jaws and muscles to respond passively. If he attempts actively to open and close his jaws, the mandible will likely seek the CO position and a false recording will result.

From an opened position and with slight retrusive pressure, guide the patient's jaw to a rearmost, midmost, ligamentous position. Move the jaw up and down to be sure that the arc has pure hingelike qualities. Bring the teeth gradually closer together until the contact of the maxillary anterior teeth (CRO) is felt or heard (Fig. 12-12B). Repeat the hingelike movement until you are certain that the same initial point of contact is always precisely the same.

If the patient experiences difficulty in performing a pure hingelike movement, it is helpful to demonstrate this movement on your own jaw. Occasionally it is necessary to have the patient practice for a few min-

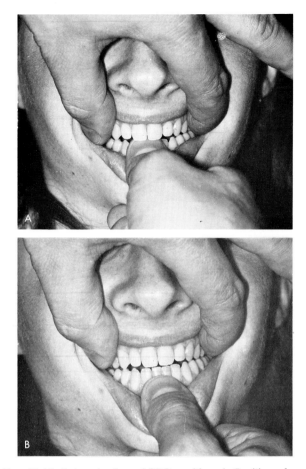

FIG. 12-12. *Determination of CRO position. A. Position of operator's right thumb and forefingers when executing the hinge movement of the mandible. Thumb prevents tooth contact during closure. Note also position of left thumb and forefinger for exposure of the maxillary teeth. B. Lowered position of right thumb to allow initial tooth contact in CRO position. The thumb is lowered only when the patient can execute a pure hingelike movement of the mandible.*

utes each day in front of a mirror. On a subsequent appointment much of the difficulty is usually overcome.

REGISTRATION OF POINTS OF INITIAL CONTACT

When you are certain that the point of initial contact (CRO) can be precisely located, dry the teeth carefully with gauze or air. (Teeth must always be dried immediately before using dental tape in order to get good results.) Place a two-inch strip of red dental tape between the teeth, on the side making the initial contact, with the aid of occlusal-tape forceps. Guide the mandible in a hingelike rearmost and midmost position, as described. Tap the patient's teeth together so that the points of initial contact are marked by the ribbon. Note these contacts on the chart by circling the appropriate pair(s) of teeth (Fig. 12-8). Since in most

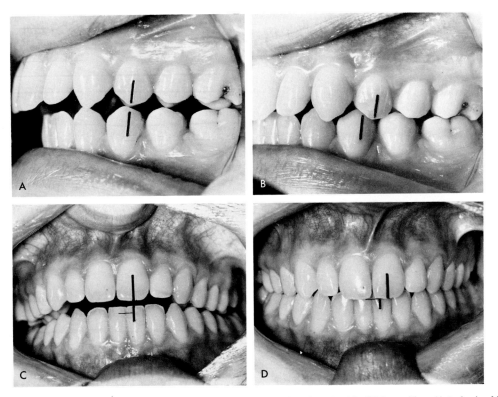

FIG. 12-13. *Examination of CRO and CO positions. A. Lateral view of occlusal contact in CRO position. Note lack of interdigitation. B. Lateral view of occlusal contact in CO position. Note degree of horizontal shift between the two positions. C. Anterior view of initial tooth contact in CRO position. Note amount of opening in the incisor region. D. Anterior view of occlusal contact in CO position. Note degree of lateral shift between CRO and CO position.*

cases only one pair of teeth will be making this contact, it is wise to suspect that the mandible is slightly anterior to the CRO position if there is more than one pair marked.

Enter the magnitude (mm) and direction (anterior, right, left) of any shift from CRO to CO in the appropriate place on the chart. Observe the direction of the slide carefully, recalling that a straight forward slide in the absence of any signs of occlusal traumatism is less significant than one with a lateral component (Fig. 12-13). Examine the teeth making the initial contact for such signs of trauma as hypersensitivity, hypermobility, or wear facets. Also, examine teeth receiving the impact at the end of the slide, since they are often more traumatized than the teeth that provide the path of the slide.[21] Note the amount of opening in the incisor region between CRO and CO (Fig. 12-13C,D).

Registrations of Lateral and Protrusive Border Excursions

Excursive movements during mastication rarely start or end at the CRO position but remain on a path from CO. Therefore, during the examination of these excursions it is necessary to guide the patient's jaw from the

CO position, even though there is a detectable difference between CRO and CO. During deglutition and bruxism the jaw may reach the CRO position, as evidenced by the pattern of retrusive-position wear facets on some dentitions.

PROCEDURE

Place green dental tape between the teeth on the right side and guide the patient's jaw to the right. Circle on the chart the numbers of the green-marked contacting teeth (Fig. 12-8). Next, place green tape between the teeth on the left and guide the jaw toward the right side while exerting pressure on the left side of the jaw in an occlusal direction (Fig. 12-14). This provides positive contact and greater accuracy. In order not to confuse broad centric occlusion contacts with nonworking contacts, place red tape between the teeth on the nonworking side and have the patient tap lightly in the acquired CO position so that CO contacts are superimposed in red on the green.

Repeat the same steps to detect contacts during left lateral excursion with concomitant nonworking side contacts, circling the respective sets of teeth on the chart. It is important to detect accurately and to record any cuspal contacts and deflective interferences on

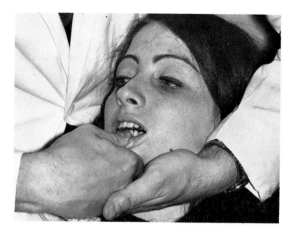

FIG. 12-14. *Registering border excursions. Position of operator's hands to exert pressure upward on the mandible, to facilitate accurate marking of teeth that make contact on the nonworking side.*

the nonworking side, since these are generally considered by authorities on occlusion to be potentially traumatic.[12,21,26]

Occasionally, the patient may experience difficulty in performing smooth lateral gliding movements. In these instances, it is most helpful to allow him to observe his efforts in a hand mirror. If the difficulty persists, it is usually attributable to a splinting action of certain muscles, most often the lateral pterygoids. This may be a protective reflex to avoid occlusal interferences such as overerupted teeth (usually third molars), severe marginal ridge discrepancies, steep cuspal inclines, or teeth in complete lingual or buccal version.

Examine protrusive border excursions of the mandible by marking the protrusive gliding contacts with green tape. Initiate the protrusive excursion from CO position and guide the jaw forward without any lateral deviation. A hand mirror often facilitates this procedure. Mobile teeth can be splinted with the index finger so that accurate markings can be obtained. Place red tape between the maxillary and mandibular anterior segments and have the patient tap his teeth lightly in CO position. The CO points of contact will be superimposed on the green protrusive contacts. Circle the appropriate sets of teeth on the chart. Check with green tape any posterior teeth that contact during the protrusive movement and record by circling the respective sets of teeth on the chart.

ARTICULATOR ANALYSIS

The information gathered thus far is usually sufficient to determine whether any occlusal factors should be considered as immediate or potential problems, but for accurate analysis, diagnosis, and treatment plan-

ning for a disturbance that may be related to occlusion it may be necessary to mount and to analyze the casts on an appropriate semiadjustable articulator. Whether this is required often depends on the previous experience and training of the dentist. A novice should use such an articulator for all patients with functional occlusal problems until he is experienced enough to decide which cases he can accurately diagnose and plan treatment for without it. There are several advantages. Articulated casts are invaluable for patient- as well as self-education, offering the opportunity to observe static and functional relations of the cusps from both lingual and buccal viewpoints. The dentist does not have to contend with the annoying problems of the tongue, cheeks, saliva, or with any patient psychoses, and when extensive restorative dentistry in addition to major occlusal adjustment or orthodontic therapy is contemplated, the use of articulated casts is indispensable to the inexperienced and a great aid to the experienced dentist.

Of the several types of semiadjustable articulators available, the Whip-Mix articulator with the Quick-Mount face-bow has been used for occlusion instruction for the past several years (Fig. 12-16). It is accurate for this purpose, yet simple to master. There are several techniques for mounting casts as an aid to accurate occlusal analysis. The following is presently taught by the authors.

Alginate Impressions

Obtaining accurate impressions and stone casts is critical, so one must adhere to the principles of a good impression technique.

ARMAMENTARIUM

1. Alginate
2. Rim-lock trays (unperforated)
3. Rubber bowl and spatula

PROCEDURE

The patient's mouth must be clean and free from calculus and debris. If not, scale the teeth and polish them. Position the patient in the dental chair so that the mandible is parallel to the floor for taking the lower impression, and the maxilla parallel to the floor for taking the upper impression. Select rim-lock trays that fit the patient's upper and lower arches. Try them in place to make sure the selection is correct. Select an alginate that will not stick to the teeth and result in fuzzy cusps on the cast. Use the manufacturer's directions as a guide in determining the water/powder ratio and temperature of the water. Add the powder to the water in a plaster bowl and spatulate until the mix is smooth and creamy. This should occur within the time limit suggested by the manufacturer. Prior to inserting the loaded tray, wipe some alginate over the occlusal surfaces, forcing the alginate into the grooves and sulci in order to prevent bubbles in the finished impression. Hold the tray steady in the mouth until the alginate sets. Remove the tray by placing an index finger at the periphery and snapping the impression free from the teeth. Rinse it. The impression is acceptable if there has been no tooth contact with the tray and no tears or large bubbles appear in critical areas. If the impression has to be stored for a short time before pouring, wrap it in a wet towel or place it in a humidifier.

Stone Casts

ARMAMENTARIUM

1. White artificial stone (Vel-Mix; Kerr Mfg., Romulus, Michigan)
2. Rubber bowl and spatula
3. Colored stone (pink Vel-Mix)
4. Large camel's-hair brush
5. Vibrator
6. Model trimmer

PROCEDURE

Trim any excess alginate at the periphery of the tray and reduce excessively deep palatal vaults with a sharp blade. Sprinkle colored stone into the impression and wash it out with tap water and a soft brush to remove any mucus from the impression and to give a better surface to the stone cast (Fig. 12-15A). Wet, fold, and shape a paper towel to block out the lingual area of the lower impression. Mix white artificial stone according to the manufacturer's directions. The addition of slurry to the water used will hasten the setting time and make the technique easier. Shake and blow the excess water out of the impression and carefully vibrate the stone into the impression. Do *not* invert the impressions; if this is done, moisture tends to rise to the upper surface and to create porous cusp tips. Add excess stone to the base of the cast in the form of three retentive knobs which will aid in the mounting procedure (Fig. 12-15B). After the initial set, trim any excess stone that would lock the cast to the tray, and either wrap the poured impression in a wet towel or place it in a humidifier. After the stone has set, separate the casts from the impressions under water to facilitate removal of the casts from the impressions and make possible the pouring of accurate duplicate casts. Trim the casts,

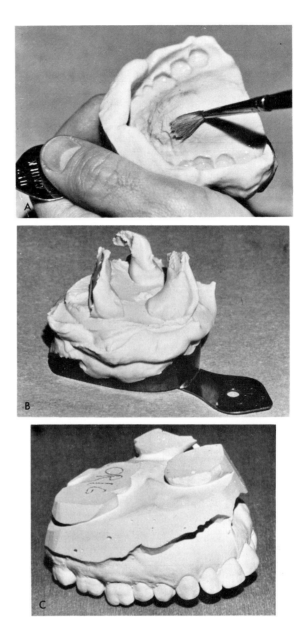

FIG. 12-15. *Making casts for occlusal analysis. A. Removal of mucus by sprinkling colored stone into impression and washing it out with water and a soft brush. B. Impression poured with stone and retentive knobs added. C. Cast trimmed for articulator mounting. (Courtesy Dr. G. Schultz.)*

flattening the base, but leaving the knobs for retention in mounting (Fig. 12-15C). Trim the periphery close to the teeth (not with the angles and corners of orthodontic casts).

Face-Bow Transfer of Maxillary Cast

The Quick-Mount face-bow adapted for use with the Whip-Mix articulator allows the operator to record estimated axis-orbital relations for the upper cast both

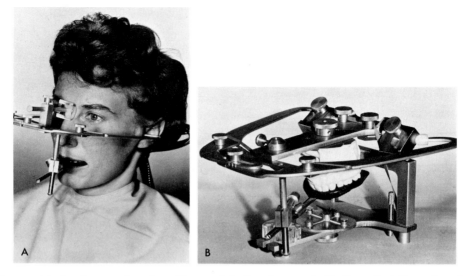

FIG. 12-16. *Face-bow registration for mounting of maxillary cast. A. Face-bow applied to the patient. The external auditory meatuses and the nasion are the three points of reference. B. Face-bow applied to the articulator to relate the maxillary cast which is secured to the upper member of the articulator. (Courtesy Dr. G. Schultz.)*

simply and with acceptable accuracy (Fig. 12-16). For greater precision the hinge axis may be located, but it is doubtful that this is necessary for diagnosis of occlusal problems in the majority of cases. Precision is dependent primarily upon the accuracy of the CRO wax record and the mounting of the mandibular casts, rather than on the hinge-axis location and transfer.

ARMAMENTARIUM

1. Whip-Mix articulator
2. Quick-Mount face-bow (Whip-Mix Corp., Louisville, Kentucky)
3. Articulator rings (Whip-Mix)
4. Trimmed models
5. Hard baseplate wax (Moyco; J. Bird Moyer, Philadelphia)
6. Rubber bowl and spatula
7. Impression plaster

PROCEDURE

The instructions as outlined by the manufacturer for the use of the Whip-Mix articulator and Quick-Mount face-bow should be followed closely.

Recording Centric Relation Occlusion

ARMAMENTARIUM

1. Trimmed models
2. Aluwax cloth form wafers (Aluwax Denture Products Co., Grand Rapids, Michigan)

3. Ash's #7 relief metal (Claudius Ash & Sons, Inc., Niagara Falls, New York)
4. Surgident Copr Wax rims (Surgident, Ltd., Los Angeles)
5. Trimming scissors
6. Scalpel with #21 Bard Parker blade

PROCEDURE

Carefully examine the casts to be sure all nodules have been removed. Wet the upper cast, warm a double thickness of Aluwax wafer (waxed cloth form) over a flame and press it into place on the upper cast, making imprints of the cusp tips (Fig. 12-17A). With a pair of scissors, trim the wafer 1 mm outside the outline of the cusp imprints (Fig. 12-17B). Cut a strip of Ash's #7 soft metal to reinforce the wafer in its center. Trim and position the metal so that it is 4 mm inside the imprints of the upper lingual cusps (Fig. 12-17C). Cut the lower side to the approximate shape of the lower arch, double the metal over the posterior end of the wafer so that the wax is sandwiched between, and with sticky wax seal the edges of the metal to the wax wafer.

Adjust the dental chair so that the patient is in the same semireclining position as described for locating CRO (Fig. 12-9). Warm the wax wafer in hot water and place it in the mouth by fitting the maxillary imprints in the wax over the upper teeth. Support the wafer against the upper arch with the left thumb and second finger in the premolar region. Support the mandible by placing the right thumb over the labial aspects of the mandibular incisors and the forefinger under the patient's chin (Fig. 12-17D). Tell the patient

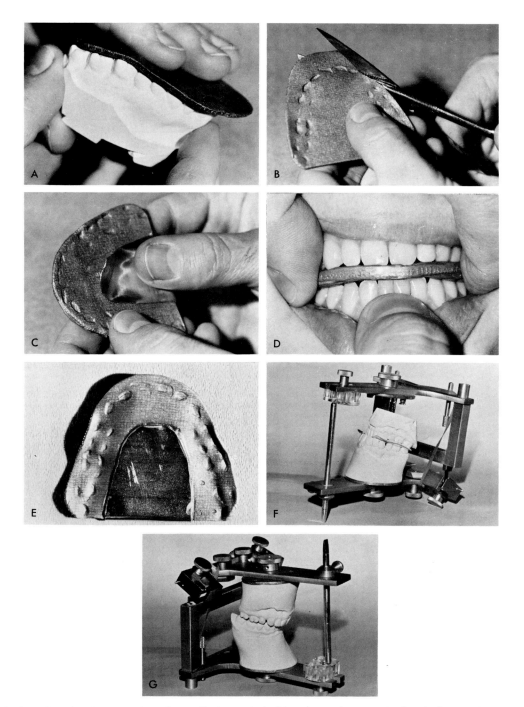

FIG. 12-17. *CRO registration for mounting of mandibular cast. A. Placement of wax wafer for shallow occlusal imprints of the maxillary teeth from the cast to facilitate accurate positioning of the wafer in the mouth. B. Trimming the wafer 1 mm outside the cusp imprints. C. Soft metal trimmed and positioned so that it lies approximately 4 mm in from the maxillary imprints and doubled over the posterior end of the wafer. D. The wafer held against the maxillary teeth with the left thumb and forefinger. The right thumb and forefinger are positioned to guide the mandible to CRO position. E. Proper depth of occlusal imprints. A clear imprint should be obtained without perforation of the wax wafer. F. Placement of centric relation wafer and mandibular cast on previously secured maxillary cast. G. Secured mandibular cast in CRO position relative to maxillary cast.*

to relax his tongue completely so that it will not warp the bite. Gently guide his jaw in a centric relation hingelike movement in the same manner as described for examination of CRO. Tell him to close lightly into the wax while in centric relation position and to maintain this contact while you chill the record with cold air. If the patient has a fairly deep overbite, add a strip of Aluwax where necessary to gain contact with the posterior teeth so that the wafer is not warped badly anteriorly. If the overbite is severe, cut off the anterior portion of the wafer so that the anterior teeth do not touch it. To remove the wafer without distortion, support it first against the upper and then against the lower teeth as the patient opens slightly and then closes lightly. Remove the wafer and chill it slightly in cold water. Replace it in the mouth and again guide the jaw to tap gently in CRO. Remove and examine the wax record carefully to see that it fits both casts accurately. If the wafer contacts soft tissue, either trim the cast in this region or trim the wafer with a sharp blade. If the cusp imprints are too deep, trim the wax carefully and again take the record to the mouth to be sure it has not been distorted (Fig. 12-17E). If the wafers must be stored for a short period, place them on a wet sponge in a humidifier to prevent distortion. Aluwax is relatively soft, and records made from it are easily warped by rough handling or changes in temperature.

Mounting the Mandibular Casts

The CRO wax record is used to relate the mandibular to the maxillary cast on the articulator. This is the most critical step of the mounting procedure. To make sure that the wax record has not warped, check that each cast fits into the wax imprints precisely. Open the incisal pin approximately 5 mm to compensate for the thickness of the wax bite. Invert the articulator and place the wax bite on the previously mounted maxillary cast. Carefully set the mandibular casts in the imprints and close the articulator to see if there is sufficient vertical space to accept the cast (Fig. 12-17F). If not, further trim the base. Hold the mandibular cast firmly in place while an assistant secures it to the lower member of the articulator with a soft mix of impression plaster (Fig. 12-17G).

Verify the accuracy of the mounting by comparing the point(s) of initial contact in CRO; they should be precisely in the same place on the articulated casts as in the mouth. The magnitude and direction of slide from CRO to CO should also be the same. If not, then

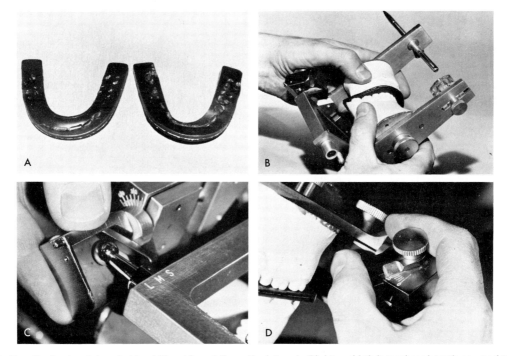

FIG. 12-18. *Setting the horizontal and side-shift guides of the articulator. A. Right and left lateral registrations used to set both the horizontal condylar guide and the side-shift guide (Bennett movement) of the articulator. B. The lateral interocclusal record is placed between the mounted casts after the holding screws on the advancing condylar side have been loosened. C. The horizontal condylar guide is rotated downward until it contacts the condylar element and is set by tightening the holding screw. D. The side-shift guide is set by bringing it into contact with the condylar element and tightening the holding screw. (Courtesy Dr. G. Schultz.)*

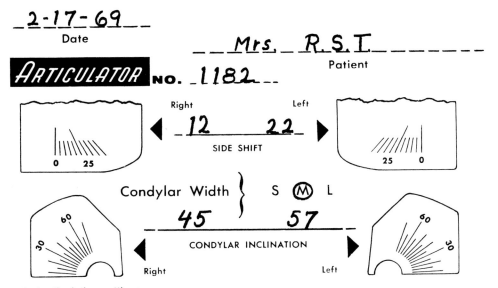

FIG. 12-19. *Record of articulation settings.*

the CRO records and mandibular cast mounting should be repeated.

Setting the Articulator

Take right and left lateral interocclusal records with Surgident Copr Wax rims especially prepared for this (Fig. 12-18A). Set the condylar inclinations and side shift according to the instructions of the articulator manufacturer (Fig. 12-18B–D). The resultant condylar guidance settings are only a close approximation but sufficiently accurate for the objectives of articulator analysis. Make a notation of these settings and file it with the patient's chart for future reference (Fig. 12-19).

CASE ANALYSIS

Cuspal contact relationships during CRO, CO, and all excursions can now be viewed not only from the buccal but also from the lingual aspect, a decided advantage made possible by the articulated casts. Record contacts with red and green tape in the same manner as described for the intraoral examination of occlusion and compare with the initial charting of the occlusion. Locate interferences causing mandibular deflections, determine their magnitude and direction, evaluate, and record. Check for faceting teeth making initial contact as well as those making contact during and at the end of the mandibular slide and relate the faceting to the mobility and radiographic findings. Note the presence of plunger cusps.

It is not surprising to find that contact relationships of the articulated casts differ from those of the teeth during excursions. Closer and keener observation usually discloses cuspal contacts and deviations that may previously have passed unnoticed during examination of the natural dentition.

From this analysis the diagnosis can be verified. Determine whether the patient is in need of treatment for occlusal disorders, and to what degree, and whether the treatment requires correlated restorative or orthodontic therapy. Recall, however, that the teeth and periodontium of younger patients are subject to changes during growth and development. Often in younger patients teeth not in occlusion or slightly malposed have no need of occlusal restoration, tooth movement, or occlusal correction. Further growth, development, and function will correct many of the occlusal conditions that would require treatment in adults.

References

1. Academy of Denture Prosthetics: Glossary of Prosthodontic Terms, 3rd ed. J. Prosthet. Dent., *20:*447, 1968.
2. Ahlgren, J., and Posselt, U.: Need of functional analysis and selective grinding in orthodontics: A clinical and electromyographic study. Acta Odontol. Scand., *21:*187, 1963.
3. Avant, W. E.: Using the term, 'centric.' J. Prosthet. Dent., 25:12, 1971.
4. Beyron, H. L.: Optimal occlusion. Dent. Clin. North Am., 13:537, 1969.
5. Fabrick, R. W.: Occlusal therapy in adolescents. Dent. Clin. North Am., *13:*451, 1969.
6. Garnick, J. J., and Ramfjord, S. P.: Rest position: An

electromyographic and clinical investigation. J. Prosthet. Dent., *12:*895, 1962.

7. Glickman, I.: Inflammation and trauma from occlusion, co-destructive factors in chronic periodontal disease. J. Periodontol., *34:*5, 1963.

8. Glickman, I.: The significance of trauma from occlusion in periodontal disease—a new concept. Curr. Dent. Comment, Feb., 1969.

9. Granger, E. R.: Practical Procedures in Oral Rehabilitation. Philadelphia, J. B. Lippincott Co., 1962.

10. Ingle, J. I.: Alveolar osteoporosis and pulpal death associated with compulsive bruxism. Oral Surg., *13:*1371, 1960.

11. Ingervall, B.: Studies of mandibular positions in children. Odontol. Rev., *19:*413, 1968.

12. Lauritzen, A. G.: Atlas of Occlusal Analysis. Colorado Springs, HAH Publications, 1974.

13. Lipke, D., and Posselt, U.: Parafunctions of the masticatory system (bruxism). J. West. Soc. Periodont., *8:*133, 1960.

14. Mann, A. W., and Pankey, L. D.: Oral rehabilitation, Part I. J. Prosthet. Dent., *10:*135, 1960.

15. O'Leary, T. J.: Tooth mobility. Dent. Clin. North Am., *13:*567, 1969.

16. O'Leary, T. J., Rudd, K. D., and Nabers, C. L.: Factors affecting horizontal tooth mobility. Periodontics, *4:*308, 1966.

17. O'Leary, T. J., et al.: The effect of mastication and deglutition on tooth mobility. Periodontics, *5:*26, 1967.

18. Pankey, L. D., and Mann, A. W.: Oral rehabilitation, Part II. J. Prosthet. Dent., *10:*151, 1960.

19. Posselt, U.: Studies in the mobility of the human mandible. Acta Odontol. Scand., *10:*suppl. 10, 1952.

20. Posselt, U.: Physiology of Occlusion and Rehabilitation, 2nd ed. Philadelphia, J. B. Lippincott Co., 1968.

21. Ramfjord, S. P., and Ash, M. M.: Occlusion, 2nd ed. Philadelphia, W. B. Saunders Co., 1971.

22. Shore, N. A.: Occlusal Equilibration and Temporomandibular Joint Dysfunction. Philadelphia, J. B. Lippincott, Co., 1959.

23. Sicher, H., and Dubruhl, E. L.: Oral Anatomy, 5th ed. St. Louis, C. V. Mosby, 1970.

24. Silverman, M. M.: Occlusion in Prosthodontics and in the Natural Dentition. Washington: Mutual, 1962.

25. Tallgren, A.: Changes in adult face height due to aging, wear and loss of teeth and prosthetic treatment. Acta Odontol. Scand., *15:*suppl. 24, 1957.

26. Yuodelis, R. A., and Mann, W. V., Jr.: The prevalence and possible role of non-working contacts in periodontal disease. Periodontics, *3:*219, 1965.

13

Periodontal Treatment Planning

Initial Therapy
    Coronal Scaling and Polishing
    Microbial Dental Plaque Control
    Root Curettage
    Gingival Curettage
    Reduction of Iatrogenic Irritants
    Minor Tooth Movement
    The Temporal Factor in Treatment Planning
    Reevaluation
The Surgical Phase
    The Surgical Treatment Plan
    Definitive Occlusal Adjustment
The Maintenance Phase
Special Cases in Planning Therapy

13
Periodontal Treatment Planning

One of the most important uses of the history, the chart, and the data worthy of record is the formulation of a workable treatment plan. Obviously, the orderly and logical progression of treatment and application of methods is an indispensable component of the total case workup.

A precise blueprint of proposed treatment can be attempted after the clinical condition of the dentition has been projected by the chart, but it must be understood that the treatment plan that emerges must be regarded as an aid to rational treatment and not as a straitjacket. The operator must be ready at all times to depart from the plan, if necessary, should the clinical situation warrant such a change.

At an earlier time the task for the treatment planner was simpler. The available methods were fewer, and their arrangement in the plan was a more direct affair. At the present writing, however, the number of techniques are many and overlapping. Some have been discarded because of limited usefulness; others have been incorporated in a differing approach so that the construction of a treatment plan requires not only a knowledge of available methods and skills but also a keen temporal sense. Timing becomes important so that treatment time is not extended by waiting for tissue responses that are long in coming from procedures that might have been performed early in therapy.

INITIAL THERAPY

In almost every case a number of steps may be taken prior to more definitive approaches. These are designed to reduce or eliminate etiologic factors on a clinical level. Since irritational factors play such a large role in the etiology of periodontal disease, their reduction or elimination may turn out to be a rather large order, since these irritational factors may prove to be iatrogenic factors, malposed teeth, or habit, as well as plaque and calculus, which are usually considered the standard etiologic factors.

Coronal Scaling and Polishing

Assuming that no dental emergency intrudes into the orderly treatment plan, the first task in case management is general debridement and the thorough indoctrination of the patient in control of microbial dental plaque. These are obvious expedients since, in the light of our present knowledge, plaque constitutes the primary irritational factor in the etiology of periodontal breakdown.

The removal of gross supragingival calculus and the polishing of the teeth are always the procedures used to begin therapy. Not only do these elicit some initial response from the gingiva, but they are preliminary to indoctrination in plaque control.

Microbial Dental Plaque Control

The elimination and control of plaque are probably the most critical procedures in therapy. An enormous amount of effort will be expended in pocket elimination in the treatment to follow. The primary benefit gained is that the elimination of pockets, often by resective methods, makes possible more adequate maintenance on the part of the patient. The introduction of plaque control early in treatment is, therefore, as logical as it is effective.

Root Curettage

Root curettage is, as has been mentioned, the basic therapy in periodontics. It can be combined ideally with plaque control in a team effort by the therapist, his staff, and the patient.

Certain changes occurring in the tissues may be observed at this time and may qualify the rest of the treatment plan. To elicit the maximum response of the tissues to the elimination or reduction of irritational factors, iatrogenic mechanisms should be eliminated as one of them.

Gingival Curettage

Gingival curettage, meaning the curettement of the sulcular wall of the gingiva, was once far more widely used than it is today. Originally intended to remove ulcerated lining epithelium, it was always suspect as a formal technical method to be included in a treatment plan. The reason for this was that, although no one objected to the "scarring down" of an individual papilla or two which was somewhat refractory in response to root curettage by reversing the curet for several strokes for gingival curettage, a full mouth procedure under anesthesia could be far more effectively done (if deemed necessary) by a clean incisional procedure of internally beveling the gingiva with a scalpel in place of scraping and scratching the sulcular gingiva with a curet.

Reduction of Iatrogenic Irritants

The elimination of overhanging restorations is no longer the task it was in the past, since high speed rotary instruments serve well in the correction of many of these deficiencies. Much more difficult, however, is the correction of open contacts and faulty contacts

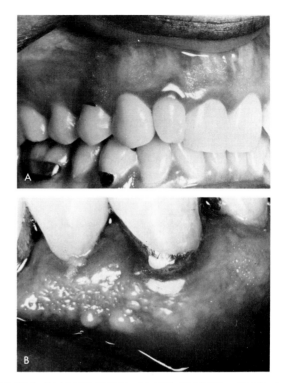

FIG. 13-1. *Iatrogenic factors. A and B. Gold foil restorations of high quality and good marginal fit are associated with marginal gingival inflammation and damaged periodontal support because of trauma inflicted on the gingiva by the rubber dam clamp. The damage is irreversible in these two examples, and the mere removal of the etiologic factor will not suffice to ensure healing. Initial therapy should include treatment for these lesions.*

when they are due to (1) substandard restorative dentistry, and (2) malposed teeth.

To correct the first, a variable number of restorations must be replaced, either on a temporary or a permanent basis depending upon the restorative treatment plan to follow periodontal therapy (Fig. 13-1). Malposed or malaligned teeth require some form of orthodontic correction. Within the context of periodontal therapy this has come to be called minor tooth movement. Chapter 21 deals with the subject in greater detail.

Minor Tooth Movement

In recent years minor tooth movement has gone from an adjunctive role in periodontal therapy to one that appears to be assuming major proportions. As might be expected, such a development has created a certain amount of controversy in periodontal circles. The concern here is the justification for inserting a time-consuming procedure into a periodontal treatment plan. A brief examination of the positions taken by the various protagonists is in order.

A number of patients are referred by periodontists to orthodontists to enlist their services in prescribed tooth movement. In other patients the periodontist may have attempted the task himself. In either expedient it sometimes happens that extensive banding in fairly complex applications is required to achieve the desired result. The time involved in this portion of treatment is frequently protracted, and this too has added fuel to the controversy on the propriety or advisability of including minor tooth movement in routine periodontal therapy.

Benefits have been claimed for moving teeth bodily into healthy bone not involved with periodontal lesions and by so doing eliminating or reducing bony resorptive lesions, making pocket elimination by other means unnecessary. Thus far the evidence has not been conclusive in spite of some apparent success in individual cases.

The Temporal Factor in Treatment Planning

In the construction of a treatment plan, the temporal factor must, of course, be taken into account. A course of therapy that is ongoing in its active management phase for one or two years seems to require a special set of circumstances. However that may be, should a major alteration in the position of teeth be considered, it is in the initial phase that orthodontics should be used. It would, of course, be more convenient after pocket elimination and mucosal repair have been achieved, but that course is not advisable. Obviously bone reshaping, if indicated, should be postponed until after tooth movement has been completed. The bone reduced for osseous resection might be needed for root investment in a new position.

Care must be taken to ensure a high order of maintenance of the tissues during tooth movement. Bands and appliances create difficulties for the patient in maintaining plaque control at an optimum level, but perform he must.

Careful observation on the part of the periodontist must be maintained throughout movement for variations in embrasure form as well as for a transitory occlusal traumatism which may occur.

Reevaluation

The constant reexamination of the marginal tissues is indispensable in periodontal therapy. The establishment of reevaluation of effort and response at this moment in a standard treatment plan connotes a formal and recorded reevaluation. Pocket depth should be re-recorded on a fresh basis, and the mucogingival picture should be reassayed in relation to the procedures to follow as well as to the demands to be made upon the tooth or teeth in the given area.

Further therapy should be projected on the basis of the charting at reevaluation. The periodontist has a firmer grasp of the case at this point. He knows the responsive potential of the gingiva as well as the performance level of his patient. Both factors are critical to success. The decision to proceed into a surgical phase on the one hand or into definitive curettage on the other may be made at this point in a surprisingly large number of patients. Many periodontists set up provisional treatment plans at the initial examination to be made definitive at the time of reevaluation. Whether this is done on a routine basis is beside the point. At the moment of the formal reevaluation, the periodontist is in a position of commitment to therapy that will have an important bearing on the outcome of treatment.

The periodontist has certain advantages at this time. The decisions to be made are on the whole simpler than those made at the initial examination. The gingiva is sound, and pocket depth has been reduced by debridement techniques so that a plan can be drawn for procedure at this point, taking tissue responses and patient performance on responses into consideration (Fig. 13-2).

THE SURGICAL PHASE

The entry into the surgical phase of total therapy is made in the expectation of pocket elimination and mucosal repair. Once the necessity for one or both of these objectives has been established in the revised treatment plan made at the formal reevaluation, the periodontist is now confronted by a bewildering array of choices to attain his therapeutic aims. He is not only charged with the performance of certain procedures, but their sequence is of considerable importance.

The Surgical Treatment Plan

The multiplicity of choices from available surgical procedures to accomplish therapeutic objectives on a variety of lesions in the attachment apparatus can appear to be a complicated task. In practice the bringing together of the lesion and the method designed to treat it are made complex by the number of variables encountered. These variables fall, however, into categories that may be best projected by using the case method, that is, by describing actual clinical situations and by constructing a surgical treatment plan to solve the problems described. Four varied cases are described.

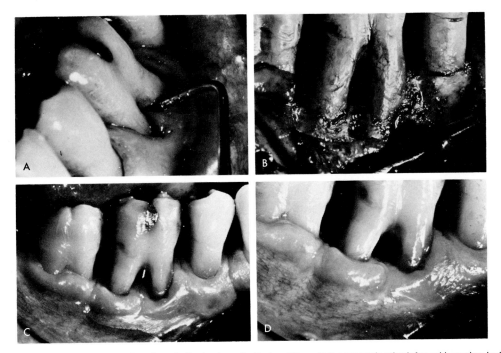

FIG. 13-2. *Furcal invasions in treatment planning. A. Probe inserted into a Class III (communicating) furcal invasion before treatment. B. Surgical exposure of the area. Note the scarring of the roots by many bouts of prior instrumentation. Note the deep scratch in the furca. C. Odontoplastic rounding of the furcal crotch and polishing of the roots to make maintenance easier. D. Close-up view of C. Note the midbuccal grooving in the tooth to facilitate cleaning and polishing by the patient. This treatment plan should include odontoplasty.*

Case 1: The first case under consideration presented no unusual problems in pocket elimination. The operator had reason to believe that standard methods would be successful in achieving a good postoperative result. There were, however, problems with the gingiva. On examination and recording mucosal features of interest it was noted that there was a serious lack of gingiva both in the upper right and left canine and in the premolar regions.

In drawing up a treatment plan the gingival consideration was prominent in the mind of the therapist because both first molars were missing and there was a restorative program waiting to be initiated after the completion of periodontal therapy. The premolars were involved with Class V caries, and the periodontist assumed, correctly, that these teeth would be restored with full crowns.

The need for an adequate band of marginal gingiva in these areas was apparent. The important question was choosing the method. A new and more adequate band of gingiva can be induced to form by using one of several procedures:

1. Apically repositioned full-thickness flaps leaving some marginal bone exposed
2. Apically positioned split-thickness flaps with the periosteal side carefully plucked so that it is thin and firm
3. Rotated pedicle flaps (partial or full-thickness)
4. Free autogenous gingival grafts

The choice among these four methods depends upon the local factors present:

1. The presence or absence of bone over the root prominences and, if present, its thickness and dimension
2. The width of gingiva desired
3. The availability of gingiva

It should be kept in mind that in either of the apically positioned flaps (full- or split-thickness) the mucogingival repair can be incorporated into the basic periodontal pocket eliminating procedure as a single operation. If, however, the decision is made to solve the problem with a free autogenous gingival graft, sometimes a two-staged operation is needed. This obviously must be taken into consideration in planning a progression of treatment. As a general rule when two-stage operations or time-consuming procedures are in the plan, they are done early in the surgical phase.

The rotated single pedicle graft is also feasible in

full- or split-thickness grafts. However, it depends upon an adjacent source, such as a saddle area, for gingiva. Also, only one or two teeth can be provided with gingiva by this method.

Let us assume that in our theoretical patient careful preoperative sounding revealed that on the left side the buccal plate of bone was extremely thin over the root prominences. This finding would automatically preclude the raising of full-thickness flaps over the area, since the cost in labial plate resorption could be high.

Since the area deficient in gingiva involves several teeth, the rotated pedicle is eliminated even if a source is available. Two choices remain: (1) an apically positioned split-thickness flap leaving the marginal bone covered with the split remnant of the original gingiva (which was deemed deficient) or (2) a free autogenous gingival graft.

The first of our remaining choices may or may not be available. If the original zone of gingiva was so miniscule that doubling its dimension by splitting it and adding one split layer apically to another is not sufficient, then the free gingival graft must be considered as a useful alternative and the best solution to the problem. This is especially true for full crown preparations requiring several millimeters of additional gingiva to ensure against minor accidents in instrumentation. The more permanent subgingival irritant of the crown margin is an even more important factor to be considered.

Since the free gingival graft is a two-stage procedure, the therapist should consider doing the upper premolar grafts coupled with major lower quadrant correction to conserve healing time. Such a coupling of method helps in the overall expeditious management of the case. It means that restoration may proceed much sooner.

Case 2: In this hypothetical case the soft and hard tissue lesions are of a commonly found variety. Bony craters are present in the posterior segments. There is, however, a deep cryptlike lesion with three bony walls on the distal aspect of the upper right cuspid. This lesion definitely endangers the cuspid if it cannot be induced to heal by reconstitution of its lost attachment. Since the posterior segments require resective surgery which may reduce somewhat the total amount of bony support, the retention of the cuspid assumes overriding importance. The loss of a cuspid is a serious matter in any dentition, but in this patient it is particularly damaging to the overall prognosis.

The topography of the bony lesion is such that the width of its mouth at the crest of bone is a bit on the wide side, and some doubt exists in the mind of the therapist of his ability to induce an adequate bone fill

and attachment repair by the standard treatment using only an open curettage approach.

The therapeutic decision to be made here is to use one of three materials available:

1. Ground bone to be obtained from adjacent bone reduced incident to crater leveling and from interradicular grooving in osseous resection
2. Swaging of the distal bony wall of the lesion against the root
3. A bone-marrow graft from either the tuberosity or the hip

The most promising method with the least tissue loss in the event of failure is desired. This relegates the second method, swaging, to a subordinate position, since success is not ensured and failure would incur the loss of the proximal septum on the distal aspect of the cuspid. In short, success is doubtful and failure is expensive.

The first approach, autogenous ground bone powder, is promising in some cases. Its success rate is, however, on the low side, although it carries no great penalty for failure and can be redone if the mere exposure does not cost a thin buccal or lingual wall via resorption in healing. Therefore, if the buccal and lingual walls of bone are adequately thick so that reentry is not impossible, this approach can be relegated to second place only because its success rate is low.

This more or less commits the periodontist to attempt repair by using an autogenous bone and marrow graft from the tuberosity or iliac crest. The advantage of the tuberosity as a source is obvious. It is accessible and adjacent to the surgical field. The question then arises as to the size and adequacy of the tuberosity and its contents to the task at hand. If the tuberosity can provide enough grafting material, it should be considered the source of the graft. This latter takes a bit more doing, and adequate preparation must be made for the procedure of obtaining the graft material and having it ready at the time of operation. The decision must be made whether to use a fresh or frozen graft.

After these decisions have been made and procedureal schedules have been established, care must be taken not to endanger actual performance by unrecognized contingencies. For example, in reviewing the topography of the upper right quadrant the periodontist may discover that from the premolars distally there is a generally narrow zone of gingiva of 3 mm throughout. The original treatment plan called for a full-thickness flap approach, here necessitated by crater leveling, with an apically positioned flap to extend the zone of attached gingiva.

The apically positioned flap is inconsistent with tight

and snug closure distal to the cuspid. This means that a vertical releasing incision must be made on the buccal side of the interproximal gingiva between the premolars so that the flap distal to the release can be apically positioned while the cuspid-premolar interproximal gingiva can be snugly closed. If a classic intrabony debriding approach is feasible, then exposed bone margins should impose no great barrier to healing, since many of these, when properly managed, prove successful. The use of an autogenous bone and marrow graft, however, imposes snug closure and thus the two-level approach when a graft is used in conjunction with a buccal repositioned flap. A footnote should be made in the treatment plan that a mucosal repair may be required for the area where the attempt for a repair in the intrabony lesion was made at a later date. These areas treated in such a manner sometimes heal with an irregular gingival margin.

The lessons to be learned from Case 2 are several. First, establish procedures specifically before operation. Do not fall into a trap of a standard approach. Always remember that the initial incision most often commits the operator to a given flap design which then cannot be altered. Second, the time spent in exploring contingencies is well spent. Contingencies have a way of becoming unavoidable courses of procedure. Third, attempts should always be made to provide for failure of techniques. That is not to say that these methods should be avoided. It does mean, however, that the fate of a critical tooth cannot be taken for granted if high risk methods must be used. A tooth committed to such a procedure will have to be discounted in the prognosis.

Case 3. Another projected case has the following clinical features: In spite of deep pockets with resorptive lesions in bone generally distributed throughout the dentition, the patient was treated with definitive curettage and plaque control for 3 years because he could not afford complete therapy and a subsequent periodontal prosthesis.

The financial factor was eliminated when the patient received a legacy, and definitive therapy, including an extensive periodontal prosthesis, became acceptable. The patient is most anxious to retain his teeth and will do what is required to accomplish that end. In spite of the fact that this patient has been under frequent reevaluation, a new examination is in order to construct a new and different treatment plan to conform to the new conditions.

The patient is 50 years old and has proved to be a fine performer in maintenance procedures. He has completely intact arches. In spite of deep pockets, tooth mobility is minimal to absent. In the original treatment plan, the contiguity of the arch was considered a great advantage in spite of extremely deep lesions in every area of the mouth.

The construction of an extensive fixed prosthesis will allow for (1) the removal of teeth deemed hopeless even though they have been successfully maintained, and (2) the fabrication of an occlusion for more efficient function within the ability of the tissues to support.

In reexamination, different criteria of achievement must be considered. A new factor has been added, namely, responsibility for the survival of a costly restoration in addition to the hoped-for improvement in the patient's periodontal condition. The architect of the new treatment plan will no longer enjoy the simplicity of a simple treatment plan.

Doubtful teeth are now regarded with more doubts and less hope. Great care is taken to select the surviving teeth so that the retained abutments are secure. There is some danger, when determining sound teeth for survival, in overlooking one of the basic principles in periodontal prognosis—the performance level in plaque control by the patient and the availability of all areas for maintenance. It is sometimes incomprehensible to see a fine performer in tissue maintenance and plaque control become less successful when a complex restoration is inserted. Also, while not the subject of periodontal prognosis strictly interpreted, embrasure and pontic design are critical to this subject and these are altered in a large restorative treatment plan.

Other factors come into play. The question arises, "When in therapy should the complex prosthesis be introduced?" The general answer to this question is that the most propitious time is after the surgical phase has been completed and the tissues have healed. As in all general principles there are logical exceptions in its application. Temporary stabilization, with the missing teeth restored, is a useful expedient when the periodontist believes that mobility or the presence of hopelessly involved teeth seriously compromises the fate of the remaining teeth. Temporary stabilization, when introduced into treatment, is usually done early in therapy in order to reap maximum advantage from time elapsing prior to the presurgical reevaluation.

Temporary stabilization was dispensed with in Case 3 since mobility was not a factor and the arch was intact.

In going over the surgical phase of the treatment plan, pocket elimination is, as ever, a most important consideration, but other aspects of the case merit special consideration. Reference is made here to potentially troublesome furcation invasions and to root proximities.

One of the many details to be considered is the added handicap to good maintenance posed by the presence of a solder joint, even though the union may be at the contact point area with good embrasure form. No longer can the patient slip the strand of unwaxed dental floss directly through a contact point. It must be strung through with the aid of a device made for this purpose. Not only is an added task involved but that task is multiplied by a large number of soldered contact points in a large restoration involving the entire arch. Some patients no longer do as well with maintenance after a large complex restoration as they did before without it.

Root proximities become particularly troublesome when the teeth in question must be crowned, as connecting members of a reconstruction and the constricted interproximal embrasure must endure two adjacent crown margins. This sometimes makes necessary the extraction of one of the teeth involved.

Root amputations, of upper molars especially, sometimes do poorly when incorporated into a reconstruction. This seems to be particularly true when the crown is preserved with an altered root support. Individual roots do better when used as abutments. This is likely the explanation for the better record of hemisected lower molars. They do quite well as "premolars" (Fig. 13-3).

In planning the amputation of a root of a multirooted tooth it is highly desirable to have the endodontic treatment done in advance. While roots of vital teeth may be resected with impunity most of the time, there are occasional troublesome responses. It is, therefore, useful to resect roots of endodontically treated teeth. Resection must be planned and arranged for during the presurgical period of treatment.

When teeth clearly need root resection, even these are sometimes resected and removed in the periodontal presurgical period. This is done to avoid some of the complications of resection and stump preparation while flaps are reflected and debris incident to the operation may fall into the wound. Incorporation of some of the dust from old restorations commonly causes an ugly tattoo in the healing gingiva (Fig. 15-3).

More important than any of these considerations, however, is the amount and condition of bone in the central area of the alveolar process between the roots. The buccal aspect of the palatal root, particularly, can be troublesome if it is not well invested in bone. The exploration of this detail is an integral part of treatment planning.

In the final analysis of Case 3, there remains the problem of the patient who has mastered maintenance in a given set of conditions who is now called upon, after years of good performance, to alter his methods and application to a new anatomic situation with altered embrasures, portions of teeth that prove more

difficult to maintain, and root surfaces that are enclosed in crowns.

The technical requirements are extremely high, and the demands made upon craftsmanship of the restorative dentist are considerable. In such a clinical situation the actual treatment plan is dictated by the financial circumstances of the patient and operates over an unusually long period with a hiatus of several years between definitive curettage and the surgical and restorative phases.

Case 4. Let us assume that the patient is 30 years of age, male, with a significant history of rheumatic fever in childhood with some evidence of cardiac valvular damage, with mitral stenosis. Periodontal examination is complete and searching and was performed under antibiotic protection, since the history revealing the cardiac valvular damage preceded the probing.

Examination revealed that the patient was suffering from advanced periodontal disease, probably a survivor of a case of juvenile, precocious periodontitis or so-called periodontosis. Pockets were generalized and were of variable depth, but vertical resorptive lesions were common, especially in the premolar and molar regions in all four posterior segments.

Calculus was not a significant feature, but plaque was extremely heavy throughout. Personal care consisted of the usual two brushings per day with a medium-texture natural-bristle toothbrush of commercial design using a vertical stroke with a slight horizontal motion on the lingual surfaces of the upper and lower posteriors.

The dental arches were almost intact with only the four third molars missing.

The occlusion was in Class I relationship and did not present unusual features in adjustment.

It was obvious that standard pocket elimination by resection would be too destructive in this case. Inductive methods using marrow or ground bone chips were not deemed feasible because of the enormous mass of material required and the physical condition of the patient.

The decision was reached to reflect flaps throughout and institute open curettage, removing exuberant granulation tissue and establishing a high level of maintenance.

In referring to the physical condition of the patient it became apparent that all procedures had to be accomplished under adequate antibiotic protection. The first effect on treatment planning is the reduction of the number of separate visits for manipulative therapy. This means that consolidation is in order. Such an expedient can be carried too far, however, in lengthy sessions that may exhaust the patient—particularly when his general condition is taken into account. Not

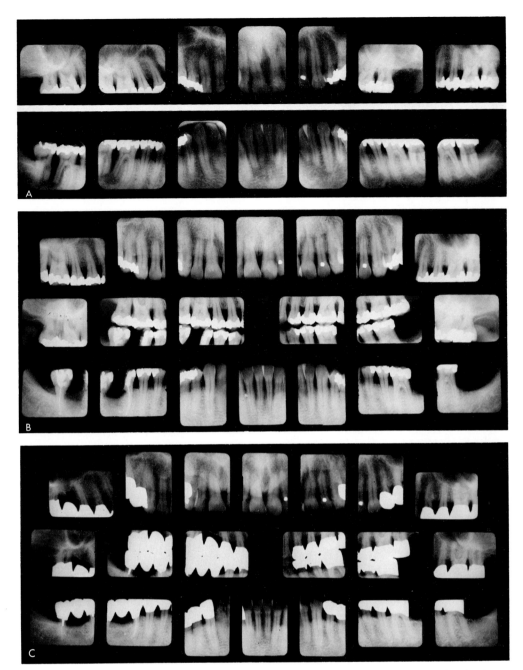

Fig. 13-3. *Three full-mouth series of radiographs spanning 7 years revealing fairly standard treatment planning in a complex case of chronic destructive periodontal disease. A. Preoperative radiographs of a 35-year-old male patient. (The premolar and molar exposures on the patient's upper left arch were reversed.) The upper right first molar was deemed hopeless because of extremely deep lesions on both mesial and distal aspects with communicating furcal invasions (Class III) on the mesial, distal, and buccal aspects. In addition, the distobuccal root of the upper right first molar was in dangerous proximity to the mesiobuccal root of the upper right second molar. A root amputation of the distobuccal root of the upper right first molar was considered and rejected because, while two furcal invasions would be eliminated by the amputation, there was little support remaining interradicularly on the first molar to make retention a feasible course. In addition, retention of the first molar compromised the maintenance of the second molar. The first molar was sacrificed subsequently. The distal root of the lower right first molar and the mesial root of the lower right second molar were extensively involved and already undergoing root resorption. On the lower left side the second molar was extracted as a hopeless tooth with ineradicable pockets on both mesial and distal aspects in addition to internal resorption. All the other teeth were retained. The patient then moved because of an employment transfer. B. A full mouth series of radiographs of the same patient taken 7 months after the initial series (A). This series revealed a mini-crotch remaining in the lower right first molar and incomplete treatment of the upper arch because of the move by the patient. C. Five years after periodontal therapy and restorative treatment. The periodontal condition has stabilized and the patient is doing well. The point to remember is that it is good judgment, in the opinion of the authors, to treat for maximum pocket elimination those patients who require periodontal protheses. Treatment planning includes full and partial extraction of teeth as well as retention of teeth with damaged support. (Restored by Dr. G. Schultz.)*

only are some procedures consolidated, but others are eliminated. For example, presurgical preparation is entirely eliminated except for plaque control. It must be remembered that even probing must be done under a protective antibiotic regimen.

Occlusal adjustment is not a serious factor in this case. It is managed in routine fashion. Surgery, however, is quite another matter. These operations can be performed in single quadrants, and the mouth can be treated in four surgical visits after initial examination and the institution of plaque control.

It will be found that gingivoplasty is indicated for many of these patients after the basic corrective surgery is finished and the tissues have healed. The therapist should, however, keep certain important facts in mind:

1. It may be necessary to compromise optimum results because of the handicaps encountered, since pocket elimination under such circumstances may not be possible and deep sulci may have to be accepted postoperatively.
2. Because of the compromises in treatment, the maintenance phase is critical. Plaque control must be meticulous, and subsequent visits to the periodontist for curettage must be frequent.
3. Long protracted surgical management is stress-producing and should not be resorted to. Single-quadrant operative sites are more safely borne by the patient with mitral stenosis.

Four cases have been briefly presented with some attention given to the salient aspects that placed the treatment plan somewhat out of the routine projection and arrangement of therapeutic method. It will be noted again that only the surgical phase was considered in this sequence. The nonsurgical aspects of treatment lend themselves to a more orderly and routine approach.

Routine measures are more easily enumerated and set down in the sequence in which they are to be applied. In planning treatment it is good practice to choose as simple and as straightforward an order of techniques as possible, using logic and common sense liberally.

Definitive Occlusal Adjustment

In planning for postsurgical therapy it is best to review any occlusal adjustment previously done at this time. Teeth frequently shift slightly in their positions after surgical intervention with the usual postoperative mobilities encountered at that time. There is, of course, a wide range of choice in the sequence in the plan to perform occlusal adjustment. Almost any position in the progression of method in the average case has its devotees. Some master clinicians even adjust an occlusion during visits used for surgery when the anesthetic (the diversion of the attention of the patient from the problem of occlusion for the more stressful surgery in progress) effectively decreases the likelihood of a positive occlusal sense.

Although a good case can be made for presurgical occlusal adjustment, the correction of occlusal discrepancies after surgical procedures is favored by a narrow margin. However, early or late, adjustment must be carefully planned for and performed.

THE MAINTENANCE PHASE

The maintenance of the tissues by the patient is an ongoing struggle from the outset. Many sources stress that constant effort by the patient is necessary for the survival of the dentition. While this may be the new norm of general dental activity, it has been standard procedure in periodontic practice and must be as carefully planned as is any other aspect of treatment. Frequency, character, and extent of the recall are important.

Just as there is no such thing as a standard patient, just so there should be no routine recall regimen. Some patients require four appointments a year with both hygienist and periodontist; others are adequately maintained with visits for coronal scaling and polishing alternating with curettage and spaced three months or even more apart. Each patient requires a precise prescription within the treatment plan.

Usually patients are divided into three general classes or types.

Type I
1. Examination procedures and the recording of data
   a. X-ray evaluation
   b. Mucosal and gingival topography
   c. Periodontal lesions record
   d. Plaque and calculus assay
2. Initial therapy
   a. Coronal scaling and polishing
   b. Start of plaque control regimen
   c. Patient performance evaluation
3. Root curettage—number of operative periods
4. Occlusal adjustment
   a. Initial
   b. Definitive
5. Reevaluation and reexamination of patient performance

6. Establishment of recall regimen and frequency

Type I is the simplest approach to the periodontal problem. It is designed as definitive therapy for patients with gingival inflammation or beginning periodontal disease.

Type II
1. Examination and the recording of data
2. Initial therapy
   a. Coronal scaling and polishing
   b. Establishment of plaque control regimen
3. Root curettage (presurgical)
4. Initial occlusal adjustment
5. Reevaluation
6. Surgical therapy
   a. Pocket elimination
   b. Mucosal repair including gingivoplasties where required because of coarse healing patterns
7. Definitive occlusal adjustment
8. Reevaluation
9. Establishment of the maintenance program

Type III
1. Examination, case workup, recording of pertinent data
2. Initial therapy
   a. Coronal scaling and polishing
   b. Plaque control
3. Root curettage (presurgical or definitive)
4. Minor tooth movement
5. Maintenance
6. Reevaluation
7. Surgical regimen
   a. Pocket elimination
   b. Mucosal repairs and gingivoplasties, if required
8. Definitive occlusal adjustment
9. Postsurgical reevaluation and reoperation when necessary
10. Establishment of the maintenance regimen

SPECIAL CASES IN PLANNING THERAPY

Periodontic therapy is not so predictable and routine as to permit setting down an order of procedure that will be more than a guide in the most general sense. There are cases in which two-stage surgical procedures require that mucosal correction precede any other surgical procedures so that enough gingiva is present for special purposes.

In bone induction, for example, it is important to have as good a gingival seal of the interproximal areas as possible. To accomplish this, the initial incision of the gingiva must be festooned from the buccal and lingual margins sharply into the interproximal areas to provide rather long papillae. These interproximal tissue extensions then meet when the flaps are co-opted and may be securely sutured together with an interrupted suture to provide a snug closure and, it is hoped, an effective seal.

In order to festoon the gingiva in the initial cut, there must be a wide zone of gingiva to begin with so that the mucogingival line is not crossed or even approached too closely. Hence the mucosal repair (free autogenous gingival graft or pedicle graft) must be done before the definitive surgical procedures are attempted.

Another special case in treatment planning is the patient with serious systemic disease. Patients who are on anticoagulant treatment for some cardiovascular disease must be carefully managed both in the magnitude of the surgical procedure and in timing. The patient's cardiologist should be consulted on the joint management of the surgical phase. He will be highly cooperative in most cases if reasonable requirements are set. The level of performance may have to be scaled downward in serious cases if the stress of the planned technique cannot be comfortably borne by the patient.

There is a tendency on the part of the operator to minimize the stress inflicted on the patient by periodontal surgery, since many procedures are done on an outpatient basis. The loss of blood alone in a protracted, single-quadrant procedure equals that lost in a major general surgical operation. General surgeons routinely tie off severed blood vessels, or bleeders, early in the operation; the periodontal surgeon does not. Since the latter does not deal with large vessels, he ties off "bleeders" only postoperatively and, in many cases, many hours postoperatively after considerable bleeding on the part of the patient.

A third class of special case in treatment planning involves interruptions in the continuity of treatment. These are quite common and present no great problem in management, except that it is easy to forget to schedule extra sessions devoted to plaque control and evaluation. Patients commonly backslide during these periods. On occasion the hiatus lasts for a long time— many months. This occurs commonly with some patients in retirement who divide their time between two homes in different climates. Treatment plans must be worked out to fit into the migratory schedule of the patient.

Because of the many-faceted nature of periodontal therapy, its orderly progress is endangered by aimless and indecisive use of various techniques. A definite plan is a basic necessity; the time spent in such planning is a small fraction of that wasted in poorly directed efforts.

References

1. Amsterdam, M.: Periodontal prosthesis. Alpha Omegan, Dec. 1974.

2. Crumley, P. J.: Clinical periodontics, the effect of recent research. Academy Review, *12:*11, 1964.

3. Morris, M. L.: Periodontal aspects of restorative dentistry. Dent. North Am., Clin. Nov. 1963.

4. Prichard, J. F.: Philosophy of practice. Periodontics, *3:*32, 1965.

5. Prichard, J. F.: Management of soft tissue in periodontal surgery. Bull. Acad. Gen. Dent., Dec. 1967.

6. Prichard, J. F.: The etiology, diagnosis and treatment of the intrabony defect. J. Periodontol., *38:*455, 1967.

14

Periodontal Prognosis

How Long Has the Tooth (or Entire Dentition) Been So Seriously Involved?

How Old Is the Patient?

How Many Teeth Are Present?

How Much Bony Support Remains to the Tooth?

How Critical Is the Survival of the Tooth to the Treatment Plan?

Can a Strategic Retreat Be Made if One Key Tooth Fails?

Can the Arch Be Restored with a Fixed Prosthesis?

How Much Can the Climate of the Mouth Be Changed?

How Extensively Do Parafunctional Demands Affect the Dentition?

How Well Can the Patient Control Plaque Formation?

Are the Skills Available for an Optimum Treatment Plan?

14
Periodontal
Prognosis

In every dentition seriously involved with periodontal disease several difficult decisions must usually be made regarding the survival or possible sacrifice of a variable number of teeth. The fate of the dentition sometimes rests upon the decision of the therapist. Patients almost always ask for reassurance on the chances of retaining natural teeth and usually express their questions in the form of an expressed doubt on the advisability of proceeding with therapy.

It is no great task to predict the fate of palpably hopeless teeth or of teeth with slight involvement. These obviously are either hopeless or in no danger. The difficult evaluations are those which must be made on teeth that are seriously involved with periodontal disease and that may be lost or saved depending upon a number of factors.

It is difficult to teach therapeutic judgment without many years of success and failure in treating a large number of patients. Great progress can be made, however, in establishing certain criteria against which to measure questionable teeth.

Periodontics is one of the areas of dentistry that is especially directed to the total mouth concept. What is meant by this is that success or failure is not measured on a tooth-by-tooth basis such as is the case in operative dentistry. The prime objective of therapy is to maintain the mouth in health throughout the life of the individual.

The implications of this total mouth concept are that it is not necessary to "save" every tooth for therapy to be a success. The loss of one or of several teeth does not detract from the relative success of the treatment, so long as the dentition can be restored to good function with good chances of long-term survival. Unquestionably this explains the close relationship between restorative dentistry and periodontics. This relationship has given rise to the establishment of periodontal prosthetics as a separate and rapidly developing field in dentistry.

Although periodontists address themselves to the entire dentition, often survival depends upon the retention in health of certain key teeth that make restoration feasible. In a surprising number of patients these key teeth are indeed critical, and it is to those that we will address our attention for much of this chapter. There are, of course, other considerations, but these will be dealt with in turn.

The most effective method in dealing with key teeth desperately involved, is to subject them to sharp scrutiny. This is best realized by the posing of a series of searching questions and attempting to answer them satisfactorily.

It should always be kept in mind that all problems do not have solutions in the present state of the art. The posing of the question and the facing up to the problem is the only avenue toward a solution. That is why it has often been said that questions are more important than answers. A facile and incomplete answer can often shut off further search.

Failure, also, is a prime teacher on the possibilities of therapy. It must, however, be fairly faced and carefully documented to be of value. Prognosis is not one of the black arts—it is a system of therapeutic projection based upon successes and failures of the past.

1. HOW LONG HAS THE TOOTH (OR ENTIRE DENTITION) BEEN SO SERIOUSLY INVOLVED?

On the face of it, this question does not seem to be of enough importance to make a difference. If, however, it is assumed that the progress of periodontal destruction has been so slow over the last few years as to be virtually arrested, then it must be admitted that the prospect for the future is brighter than it would be if the downhill phase were short and of recent origin.

It is difficult at times to obtain definite information on resistance to periodontal breakdown. The response of the patient is not a reliable source. Neither, unfortunately, is the case history or data obtained from former dentists. Histories and charts are usually casual affairs. In many instances the best sources of information are old roentgenograms (Fig. 14-1A). Although roentgenographic evidence is far from being conclusive, a good working comparison can be made between old and recent roentgenograms, since the same kinds of evidence are being compared. If, on comparison, the difference between the old and new series is slight, then the inference can be made that the resorptive lesions are progressing relatively slowly and should yield to therapy (Fig. 14-1B). In other words, the prognosis would be favorable.

If, on the other hand, the comparison of roentgenograms reveals that there is a definite and considerable difference in the bone level surrounding the teeth, the periodontist then must assume that periodontal destruction has been steady and relatively rapid. Even more alarming is the distinct possibility that the resorptive process is continuing. The prognosis in such a case is poor.

The hard fact is that little is known of the essential pathogenesis of periodontal disease. The therapist does well with patients in whom the disease has been reduced to a low state of chronicity. There is little evi-

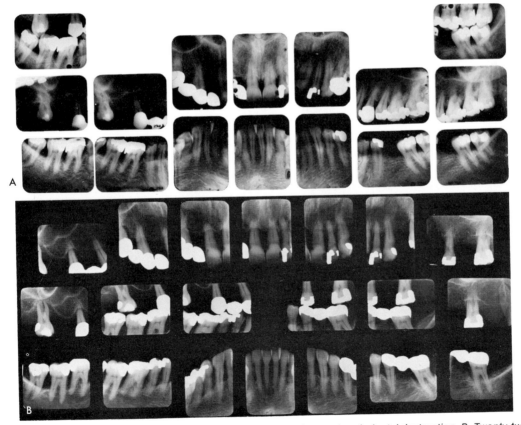

FIG. 14-1. *A. Radiographs of the dentition of a 33-year-old woman with advanced periodontal destruction. B. Twenty-two years later. The patient (now 55 years old), who has had dental cleaning about every 3 years, is seeking periodontal therapy for the first time. Note the missing teeth and progression of periodontal destruction. The dentition has not been totally destroyed, however, and even the upper arch can be partially salvaged with the aid of extensive periodontal prosthesis.*

dence of this obtainable, except by the history of the course of destruction. Roentgenograms provide objective evidence that may be valuable.

2. HOW OLD IS THE PATIENT?

The age of the patient is an important factor in prognosis. The older the patient, the better the prognosis. The reasons for this are not difficult to understand. With advancing age, the inflammatory response is diminished, and the resorptive processes are slowed. Another factor comes into play here. While little is understood about the patient's resistance to periodontal disease, such a thing exists and is a very real quality to reckon with. Obviously resistance to periodontal breakdown must be higher in an older patient than in one considerably younger, given similar amounts of breakdown in both. There is yet another aspect to be considered. The older the patient, the fewer are the years remaining for the dentition to serve. It is for this reason that treatment planning for the younger patient is directed to far more definitive solutions to therapeutic problems in many cases. The result must serve for a long time, and the natural history up to this time has been bad. In the older patient, the reverse is true, and a certain amount of conservatism in therapy is in order.

3. HOW MANY TEETH ARE PRESENT?

The greater the number of teeth present, the fewer are the demands made upon individual teeth in the arch. Tooth position in the arch becomes important. While numbers are most helpful, the arrangement of the remaining teeth is often critical, particularly when there are a number of missing teeth or hopelessly involved teeth. The presence of key teeth in strategic locations is of great value to a more favorable prognosis. This is particularly true in patients in which the disease is serious. A full complement of teeth, or at least most members in the arch present, in a continuum of teeth, presents fewer problems. Drifting is minimal in such an arch and the occlusion is more stable than it would be if interdental gaps are present. Extrusion and arch collapse are minimized.

4. HOW MUCH BONY SUPPORT REMAINS TO THE TOOTH?

The old query about bony support is usually answered with a formula such as two thirds of one half of the investing bone as the minimal amount. All of these formulas are relatively useless because a number of facets of the question are ignored by the formula approach. For example, what is the root form? It is obvious that a thick, club-shaped root is far more securely anchored per linear unit of measure than is a thin spindle-shaped root. Root length itself enters here. Because many teeth with rather extensive resorption of alveolar bone have long roots, the *relative* resorption does not express the actual alveolar support. Even expressing the crown-root ratio is not too rewarding.

Tooth position can be a serious complication in many patients, regardless of the proportional bone loss. Root proximity may be another complication. One of the worst examples of the difficulties presented by root proximity occurs in the upper canine-first premolar interproximal zone where, with even a slight rotation, the palatal aspects of both roots converge. Not only is the converging dangerous, but the palatal constriction in this region, because of arch form, makes pocket elimination difficult to achieve. In addition, the first premolar has deep proximal root surface fluting that often enters into a furcation involvement and makes maintenance impossible. One of these teeth, usually the first premolar, is doomed even though the pocket depth is unremarkable.

The difficulties incidental to tooth position alone have by no means been exhausted. The extruded tooth may carry with it some alveolar support in its extrusion. If a formula is applied, the verdict may be a favorable one—a verdict one may have cause to regret. Questions should be raised and answered as to the effect of the extrusion on the interproximal embrasures. Are they so badly constricted, because of the aberrant contact relationship, that adequate restoration of the arch is impossible? Although vital extirpation of the pulp can make possible extensive occlusal reduction to create a workable occlusal plane, can the resultant stunted crown form be a useful one?

Extrusions are not the only anatomic variables that must be taken into account in the prognosis of the effect of therapy. Teeth may be in normal positions and yet present impossible obstacles to pocket elimination. For example, a lower second molar may have a deep infrabony lesion on its buccal aspect. Because of a horizontally flaring external oblique ridge and a shallow vestibule, it becomes obvious that pocket elimination by resective means is impossible. Should inductive methods fail, the prognosticator is faced with a possible compromise of retaining a tooth with a residual deep pocket that will have to be carefully and faithfully maintained by both patient and operator. A new question arises: Are both equal to the task?

Now to compound the dilemma, suppose that the tooth is to be a terminal abutment of a large fixed prosthesis with a two- or three-tooth edentulous span immediately adjacent. This question must be resolved before committing the patient to a costly restoration or to a removable prosthesis. How much will a unilateral distal extension saddle restoration compromise the longevity of the dentition? To answer this question, the periodontist must look to the condition of the remaining teeth and the design of the prosthesis in addition to all other factors. The futility of seeking a formula becomes apparent.

5. HOW CRITICAL IS THE SURVIVAL OF THE TOOTH TO THE TREATMENT PLAN?

Here again the answer is never simple. The key tooth, commonly regarded as indispensable, may be seriously depleted of support. Sometimes the fate of other teeth depends upon the survival of the key tooth. Whether the key tooth is indeed critical depends, in a large number of patients, upon the size of the edentulous span on either side of it. The greater the size of the span (or spans), the more support is needed. The introduction of tooth and metal implants may make this problem less vexing, but at the present state of the art this is not the case.

In thinking of a key tooth the periodontist is usually considering the periodontal prosthesis. In many cases the arch may be terminated in the second premolar region. Judicious use of the securely supported cantilevered pontic is also to be considered.

6. CAN A STRATEGIC RETREAT BE MADE IF ONE KEY TOOTH FAILS? ARE THERE ALTERNATIVE ABUTMENTS NEARBY? HOW LONG IS THE SPAN?

All these questions are germane to a useful restorative treatment plan. Often the survival of the dentition of an arch depends upon the restorative treatment plan to hold the whole together as a functioning unit. Accomplishing this requires the blending of all the methods available to general dentistry and of special skills applied in the most sophisticated approach to the restorative problem (Fig. 14-2).

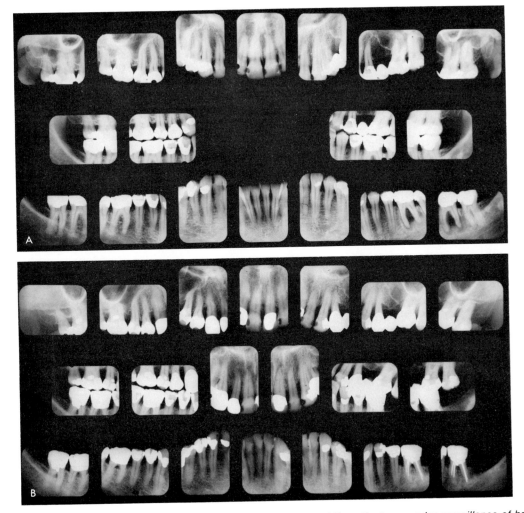

FIG. 14-2. *The decline and very nearly complete destruction of a dentition while patient was under surveillance of her dentist. A. Radiographic examination of the patient on June 1, 1950. B. Radiographic examination of the patient on March 14, 1969. This was the date of reference to a periodontist.*

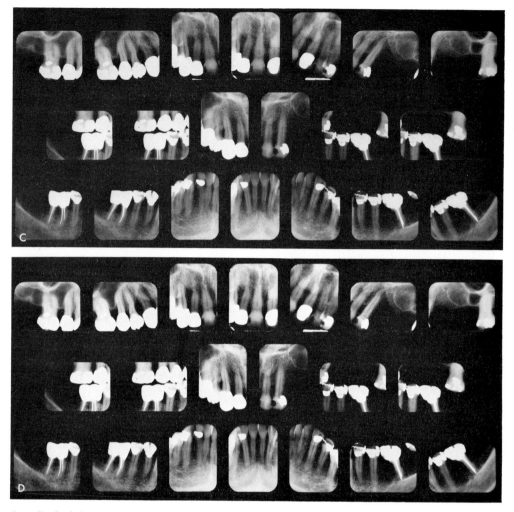

FIG. 14-2 (continued). *C. Subsequent full-mouth series of radiographs of the patient taken on November 13, 1971. D. The last available full-mouth series of radiographs taken on February 7, 1972.*

7. CAN THE ARCH BE RESTORED WITH A FIXED PROSTHESIS?

This question addresses itself to one of the basic problems in restorative dentistry—the demands made upon abutment teeth. Some definition of the removable partial denture is in order. What is usually meant in this context is the distal extension partial denture—either unilateral or, more commonly, bilateral. This connotes no serviceable posterior abutments. It also means that one of the principal abutments is the saddle area. Since this is made up of mucosa and underlying soft tissue, it is compressable because of the displacement of the fluid content of the tissue upon which the appliance is to rest. This is not the place to discuss this property of the behavior of mucosa under a free-end saddle. It is sufficient to state that with one or more of the abutments made up of mucosa, the torquing and displacement of the dental abutments is greater than if all the abutments were firm teeth. Stated differently, a removable prosthesis makes greater demands upon the remaining teeth than do fixed replacements.

The displacing effects of a removable denture are palliated somewhat by splinting the remaining teeth together for greater resistance to displacement. The degree of resistance varies, but splinting does not eliminate displacement as a serious factor.

It is a safe assumption that a retreat to a removable partial denture reduces the life expectancy of the remaining natural teeth in the arch. It is a bad prognostic sign if such a retreat is unavoidable.

Inevitably the complex removable appliance that makes use of splinting segments of abutment teeth and adequate distal abutments will be cited in rebuttal. This sort of partial denture, sometimes resorted to by skilled restorative specialists to provide cross-arch stabilization via a palatal band, is not the restoration referred to here. These appliances are usually entirely

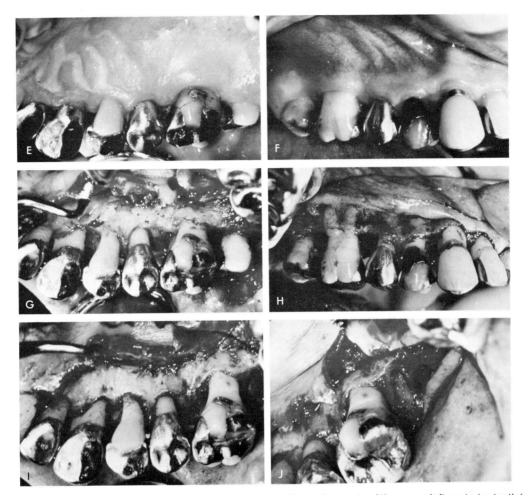

FIG. 14-2 (continued). *E and F. The presurgical view of the palatal and buccal aspects of the upper left posterior teeth (mirror views are shown). G and H. Flaps reflected and the area partially debrided. I and J. Complete debridement and extraction of the malposed second molar.*

tooth-borne and not tissue-borne. They may be regarded in the same light as fixed bridges.

8. HOW MUCH CAN THE CLIMATE OF THE MOUTH BE CHANGED?

The evaluation of the etiologic factors involved in the patient's condition is brought into prominence by the question about changing the climate of the mouth. Since evaluation is limited to determining the effects of local irritational factors on the tissues and since the level of periodontal disease seen is an expression of the response of tissue to injury, as well as a measure of the magnitude of the irritant, some appreciation of the magnitude of the task becomes clear. Essentially tissue change is the primary reason why prognosis is such a difficult task. It must be the product of extensive experience with the subtleties of tissue changes in altered functional environment.

It is obvious that when the patient seeks treatment the dentition is in a downhill phase. In order to reasonably expect a favorable long-term result, a series of changes in the oral milieu must be forthcoming. If not, it would be unsupported optimism to expect a favorable result.

There are several areas in which changes must occur. If local factors include occlusal forces that are amenable to correction, then a serious etiologic factor can be dealt with. If a redistribution of destructive occlusal forces, either by adjustment of the natural dentition or by resurfacing an entire occlusion plus stabilizing weak members, can be effected, then a distinct improvement in the dental climate is not only possible but likely. This is a favorable prognostic sign—sometimes a critical one in borderline cases. If the soft tissue response is one of a definite hyperemia with the classic inflammatory picture complete with irritational factors, then a good response can be expected with debridement, maintenance, and good dentistry. Not nearly so favorable is the prognosis for the

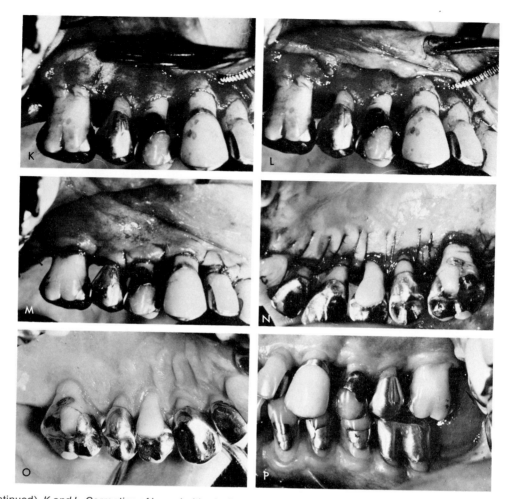

FIG. 14-2 (continued). *K and L. Correction of irregularities in the bone profile. M and N. Flap closure and suturing. O and P. Two-year postoperative views of buccal and palatal aspects of the area. (Treated by Dr. S. Sapkos and J. Townsend.)*

dentition with pale and flaccid gingiva, an adequate occlusal relationship, good contact relationship, good dentistry, and little or no plaque or other irritational factors. A dentition that is failing periodontally leaves little room for optimism. In such cases the factors are not understood and cannot be changed, and the prognosis must be a guarded one.

9. HOW EXTENSIVELY DO PARAFUNCTIONAL DEMANDS AFFECT THE DENTITION?

The deleterious effects of bruxism and clenching are widely known. Also, the percentage of the general population that grinds and clenches its teeth in nonfunctional activity is extremely large. All sources agree that the great majority of people are the victims of occlusal neurosis, as it is called by some. Childhood bruxism is easily corroborated, and the dentitions of older people are commonly worn down in the typical fashion common to nocturnal grinders. Even aboriginal skulls reveal heavy bruxism in the wear patterns of the teeth.

With so ubiquitous a compulsion, two minor qualifying questions arise: (1) if so wide a population sample is a victim of bruxism, can the activity be deemed abnormal, and (2) why is not periodontal destruction even more widely distributed than it apparently is? Both questions have a single answer. Bruxism has a large range of intensity and duration. The constant nocturnal and sometimes diurnal clamping and grinding of the dentition is obviously a greater contributing factor to breakdown than is occasional grinding. In other words, it is a matter of degree as well as the presence of the neurosis in the first place.

Every periodontist has the experience of examining a patient who suffers from many local irritational factors operating upon the tissues and yet shows remarkably little breakdown. Usually such a patient is a member of the minority who do not grind their teeth, or only slightly grind them. The *degree* of bruxism is a critical factor in a prognosis.

10. HOW WELL CAN THE PATIENT CONTROL PLAQUE FORMATION?

Success or failure in almost every case hinges on the control of plaque formation. It is an error to assume cooperation in this complex area which depends heavily upon the psychologic makeup of the patient. Many otherwise meticulous well-groomed people simply cannot maintain their dentitions adequately over a long period. Instruction, threats, and all other motivational approaches fail. Admittedly these are extreme cases.

There are always patients who appear to be hopeless in plaque control, but who become ideal maintainers with adequate instruction. They are not many but are just numerous enough to make generalization dangerous. This problem is dealt with in Chapter 30. It is touched upon here because of its overwhelming importance. If the therapist has a patient who is not a good maintainer, he has no patient at all. The treatment will inevitably go on to failure. The converse is true. Miracles in therapeutic success attend the good patient.

11. ARE THE SKILLS AVAILABLE FOR AN OPTIMUM TREATMENT PLAN?

Central to the solution of any problem is the ability to bring to bear methods and techniques available for use. There is no magic, however, in any method. The effectiveness of technique lies in its performance, as well as in its applicability. Although precise and well-directed treatment planning is important, skillful and efficient performance is just as important. Needless trauma to flaps, dehydration of the tissues, rough or inept execution of the procedures involved, and imprecise wound closure are all heavy contributors to therapeutic failure or to substandard postoperative results. While this is costly enough in even routine procedure where some margin for error exists, in the desperately involved case of periodontal disease it is all too often the difference between success and failure. Like all other skills, periodontal skills are not difficult to develop. Constant practice and careful examination of failure are the only roads to success.

It is easy for the critic to ascribe all failure to lack of skill. It cannot be argued, however, that skills are most important. It must be kept in mind that restorative skills are every bit as important as are basic periodontal skills. Good therapy is ineffective in the face of poor restorative sequels.

References

1. Awwa, I., and Stallard, R. E.: Periodontal prognosis. Educational and psychological implications. J. Periodontol., *41:*183, 1970.
2. Beube, E. E.: Correlation of degree of alveolar bone loss with other factors for determining the removal or retention of teeth. Dent. Clin. North Am., *13*(No. 4): 1969.
3. Corn, H., and Marks, M. A.: Strategic extractions in periodontal therapy. Dent. Clin. North Am., *13*(No. 4): 1969.
4. Derbyshire, J. C.: Patient motivation in periodontics. J. Periodontol., *41:*630, 1970.
5. Dummett, C. O.: Significant considerations in the prognosis of periodontal disease. J. Periodontol., *22:*77, 1951.
6. Everett, F. G., and Stern, I. B.: When is tooth mobility an indication for extraction? Dent. Clin. North Am., *13*(No. 4): 1969.
7. Kay, S., Forscher, B. K., and Sackett, L. M.: Tooth root length-volume relationships. An aid to periodontal prognosis. I. Anterior teeth. Oral Surg., *7:*735, 1954.
8. Morris, M. L.: The diagnosis, prognosis and treatment of the loose tooth. Oral Surg., *6:*1037, 1953.
9. Prichard, J. F.: Management of the periodontal abscess. Oral Surg., *6:*474, 1953.
10. Prichard, J. F.: Regeneration of bone following periodontal therapy. Oral Surg., *10:*247, 1957.
11. Prichard, J. F.: The infrabony technique as a predictable procedure. J. Periodontol., *28:*202, 1957.
12. Prichard, J. F., Simon, P., and Lorimer, J. W.: Periodontal prosthesis in occlusal trauma. J. Periodontol., *29:*131, 1958.
13. Prichard, J. F.: The role of the roentgenogram in the diagnosis and prognosis of periodontal disease. Oral Med., Oral Surg., Oral Path., *14:*182, 1961.
14. Prichard, J. F.: Advanced Periodontal Disease, 2nd ed. Philadelphia, W. B. Saunders Co., 1972.
15. Saxe, S. R., and Carman, D. K.: Removal or retention of molar teeth: the problem of the furcation. Dent. Clin. North Am., *13*(No. 4): 1969.
16. Slatten, R. W.: An evaluation of factors determining prognosis in inflammatory and retrogressive periodontal disease. A Series. J. Periodontol., *25:*30, 1954.
17. Staffelino, H. J.: Surgical management of the furca invasion. Dent. Clin. North Am., *13*(No. 4): 1969.
18. Sternlicht, H. C.: Prognostic considerations in periodontal disease. Tex. Dent. J., *82:*11, 1964.
19. Wade, A. B.: Causes in failure in treatment of localized pocketing. Dent. Health, *4:*9, 1965.

15

Plaque Control

15

Plaque Control

WALTER B. HALL
AND GORDON DOUGLASS

Oral hygiene is the key to prevention and successful treatment of inflammatory periodontal disease. Many failures in periodontal therapy and other forms of dental treatment can be attributed to inadequate oral hygiene. These are failures not only of the patient but also of the dentist who does not understand the relationship of the oral environment to plaque accumulation and fails to provide methods of plaque control specifically adapted to the needs of the individual patient. One primary objective of dental and periodontal therapy is the creation and maintenance of smooth tooth and root surfaces and soft tissue contours so as to reduce plaque accumulation and to permit easy plaque removal. If he is to achieve success, the clinician must have a thorough knowledge of factors related to plaque accumulation and distribution and of techniques of removal and control. Traditionally, efforts at plaque control have been considered a hurdle the patient must surpass before the beginning or at the end of treatment. In our view this is an incorrect approach; we present oral hygiene as an integral part of dental and periodontal therapy. It is our aim to describe the techniques and procedures generally useful in plaque control, to point out changes that must be made in the standard methods in order to maintain health in the periodontal patient, to discuss the close relationship between the oral environment and plaque accumulation, and to describe the effects of therapeutic alteration of the oral environment upon plaque growth and distribution.

FACTORS INFLUENCING PLAQUE FORMATION AND DISTRIBUTION

The events occurring in early plaque formation and growth are described in Chapter 6. On a previously clean tooth surface, plaque formation begins with pellicle deposition and bacterial colonization along the gingival margin and in the pits and fissures on the tooth surface. After colonization occurs, the plaque mass becomes thicker and extends over the surface by selective adherence of microorganisms from the saliva to the plaque surface and by microbial multiplication. For reasons that are not completely clear, the extent of plaque growth varies considerably from one region of the mouth to another. Plaque accumulation is greatest on the interproximal surfaces, less on the lingual and palatal surfaces, and still less on the facial surfaces. Furthermore, the posterior teeth generally accumulate more plaque than the anterior teeth, and the mandibular lingual surfaces have more plaque than the comparable maxillary surfaces (Fig. 15-1).[4] Many of these differences appear to be a consequence of tooth contour and position. The height of contour on the palatal

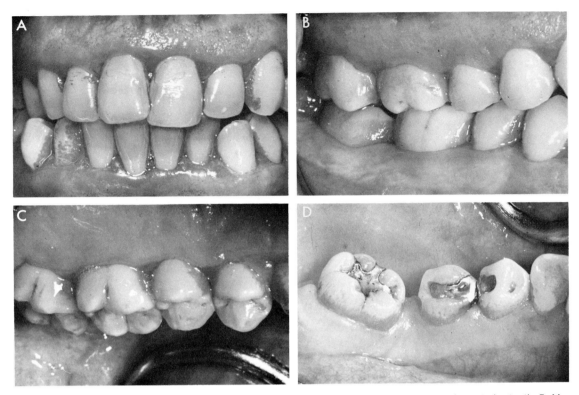

FIG. 15-1. *Variation in the distribution of plaque from one area of the mouth to another. A. Less on the anterior teeth. B. More on the posterior teeth. C. Less on the facial tooth surfaces. D. More on the lingual surfaces of the mandibular teeth.*

surfaces of the maxillary teeth is at the gingival margin, and most of the surface is subjected to friction by food and the tongue, whereas the height of contour of the lingual surfaces of the mandibular teeth is located near the occlusal surface, and the teeth are inclined lingually to produce an undercut area gingivally which tends to accumulate plaque.

The ultimate extension of plaque on the tooth surface is affected by the anatomy, position, and surface characteristics of the teeth, by the architecture of the gingival tissue and its relationship to the teeth, and by friction at the tooth surface from the diet, lips, and tongue. Plaque retention is enhanced by the presence of calculus, defective restorations, carious lesions, and other factors producing a rough surface (Fig. 15-2). The axial contours of the teeth are also important in determining the extent to which plaque accumulation occurs. In dogs, teeth with axially overcontoured crowns accumulate much more plaque and develop more marginal gingival inflammation than the natural teeth or teeth with undercontoured crowns.[11,12] Even subtle changes in tooth position may enhance plaque retention. Abnormal tooth position produces accentuated axial contours, abnormal marginal ridge relationships, and altered embrasure form, all of which lead to plaque growth and increased difficulty in plaque re-

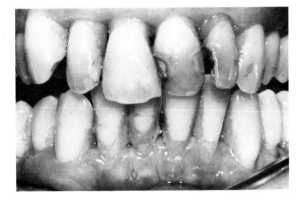

FIG. 15-2. *Irregularities of the tooth surface—defective restorations, calculus, and exposure of the cementoenamel junction—that increase plaque retention.*

moval (Figs. 15-3–15-6). Contrary to widespread belief, fibrous foods such as carrots and apples do not greatly influence the accumulation of plaque at its usual sites (Fig. 15-7). Their effect is limited to the incisal and occlusal surfaces of the teeth. While dietary consistency may determine, at least in part, whether plaque will extend over the chewing surfaces and the more occlusal portions of the buccal and lingual surfaces of the teeth, it appears to have little effect upon events occurring below the height of contour where

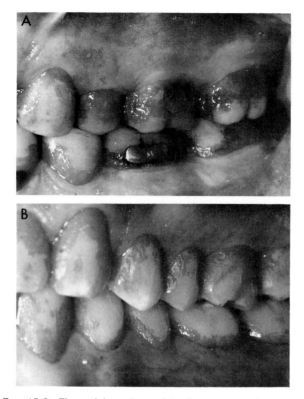

FIG. 15-3. *The axial contour of teeth causes variations in plaque accumulation and distribution. Note increase in plaque below the height of contour.*

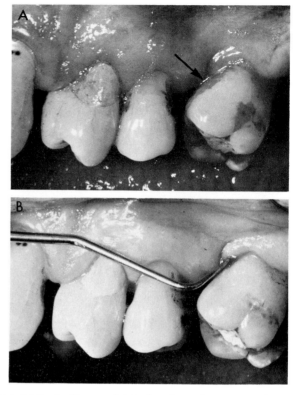

FIG. 15-5. *A. Plaque distribution (arrow) on second molar which is inclined mesially into the space from which the first molar was extracted. B. An adjacent periodontal pocket.*

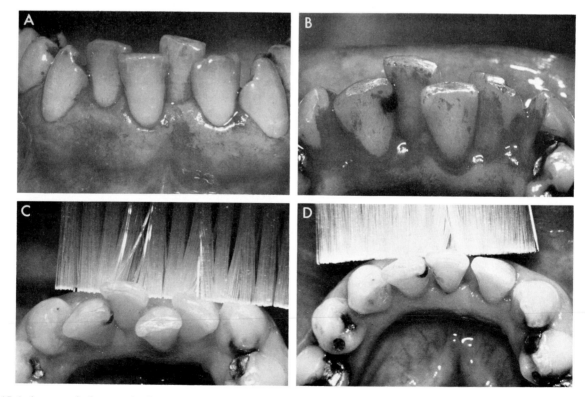

FIG. 15-4. *Increased plaque retention as a result of tooth misalignment and overlap. A. Facial surfaces. B. Lingual surfaces. C. Plaque removal by usual means difficult or impossible. D. Reduction in plaque retention by tooth brushing following extraction of one incisor and realignment of the remaining teeth by minor tooth movement.*

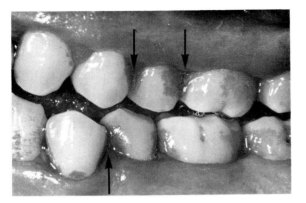

FIG. 15-6. *Increased plaque retention (arrows) on second premolar that is tilted palatally.*

the greatest bulk of plaque accumulates and where plaque is the most deleterious to the marginal gingival tissues.[8,9]

The anatomic relationship of the gingival tissues to the tooth surface is probably the most important of all factors influencing the extent of plaque growth and the

difficulty encountered in plaque control. Thick tissue ledges provide protected niches in which plaque growth is encouraged (Fig. 15-8). Ledges preclude successful plaque removal by preventing the close adaptation of toothbrush bristles to the region of the gingival sulcus. Hyperplastic gingiva, such as that seen in cases of Dilantin (diphenylhydantoin) hyperplasia, gingival fibromatosis, and in some cases of chronic fibrotic periodontal disease, may create pseudopockets that cannot be cleansed by tooth brushing, dental floss, or other currently available means (Fig. 15-9). While the normal gingival sulcus is shallow and reasonably self-cleansing (see section Chapter I), periodontal pockets are routinely filled with sloughed epithelial cells, dead leukocytes, and myriads of microorganisms (Figs. 15-10; 7-6). The use of water-jet devices has been recommended for these areas. However, it is quite clear that the damage created by high-pressure irrigation may more than outweigh the benefits gained. Irrigation devices frequently seed microorganisms more deeply into the tissues, leading to abscess forma-

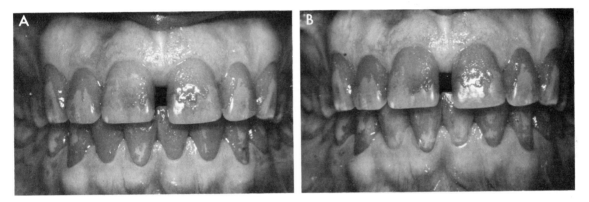

FIG. 15-7. *The effect of fibrous foods on plaque. A. A 10-day plaque accumulation in an otherwise normal individual before consumption of fibrous food. B. After eating fibrous food. Note that some of the plaque on the labial aspect of the lower incisor has been removed.*

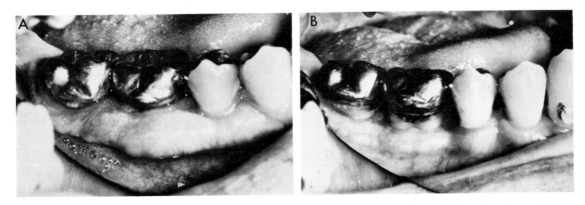

FIG. 15-8. *Abnormal contour of the clinical crown and the adjacent periodontal tissues enhance the tendency toward plaque growth and prevent effective plaque removal. A. Two overcontoured full crowns, associated with a thick bone ledge that make the area of the tooth adjacent to the gingival margin virtually inaccessible to the toothbrush bristles. B. After periodontal surgery to thin the bone ledge and eliminate the pocket depth, making the area accessible to the toothbrush. However, the poorly contoured crowns and the carious lesions at the buccal crown margins continue to encourage plaque accumulation. (Courtesy Dr. J. Schwartz.)*

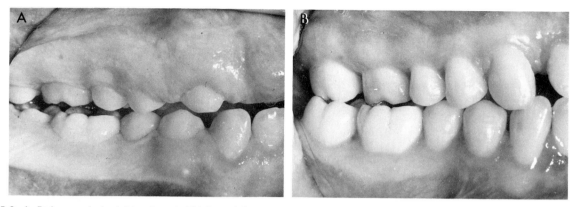

FIG. 15-9. *A. Before periodontal treatment. Thickened, hyperplastic gingiva in an individual with hereditary gingival fibromatosis partially obscures the surfaces of the teeth and makes effective plaque removal extremely difficult. B. Following periodontal surgery. The oral environment has been modified to reduce the tendency toward plaque growth and to achieve effective plaque control.*

tion. Thus, the presence of periodontal pockets greatly accentuates the problem of plaque retention, and there is currently no readily available means by which the patient can routinely maintain periodontal pockets free of plaque.

Periodontal therapy provides numerous opportunities to reduce the magnitude of plaque accumulation

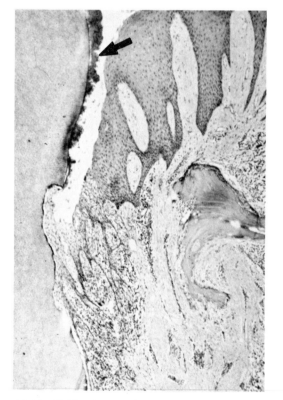

FIG. 15-10. *Light micrograph of section of gingiva. Even though the patient was maintaining what appeared clinically to be a satisfactory level of plaque removal, the periodontal pocket was filled with microorganisms (arrow). (hemotoxylin-eosin stain; original magnification 40 ×.) (Courtesy Dr. M. Dragoo.)*

and resolve problems of plaque removal by improving the oral environment. Root planing results in smooth, easily cleaned root surfaces. Standard surgical therapy permits reduction of thick hard- and soft-tissue ledges, resulting in restoration of a knife-edge gingival margin (Figs. 15-8, 15-9). Furthermore, periodontal pockets can be converted into shallow, self-cleansing gingival sulci, thereby exposing the root surfaces for easy access (Figs. 15-8, 15-9). Open contacts, overlapping teeth (Fig. 15-4), and marginal ridge discrepancies leading to food impaction and abnormal occlusal function can be corrected by minor tooth movement, and axial contours can be improved. Odontoplasty can be used to reduce axial contours and to create sluiceways leading into furcation areas and flutings.

The creation of an improved oral environment extends far beyond the area of periodontal treatment (Chapter 26). The construction of proper contours and the location and adaptation of margins and functional occlusal characteristics of individual restorations, crowns, bridges, splints, and other oral appliances may create an oral environment that is relatively resistant to plaque accumulation and in which plaque control can be achieved by simple routine procedures. Alternatively, when contours are constructed improperly, they may lead to conditions that cannot be maintained even by intensive effort by either the dentist or the patient (Fig. 15-8).

The intimate relationship between dental and periodontal treatment and the ultimate ability of the patient to maintain plaque control must be a primary consideration in any therapeutic endeavor. In essence, any modification in the oral environment will either enhance or decrease the tendency for plaque accumulation and the ultimate ability of the patient and dentist to achieve control. Thus, the influence of treatment of any kind upon the plaque status of the patient and the overall oral environment is a paramount consideration.

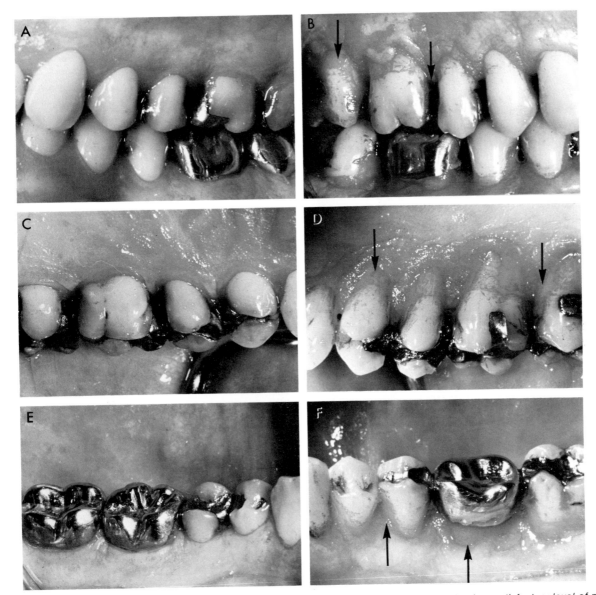

FIG. 15-11. *The effect of alteration of the oral environment upon the ability of the patient to maintain a satisfactory level of plaque control by toothbrushing and the use of dental floss. Periodontal surgery was done on one side of the mouth. A, C, and E. A fairly effective level of plaque control was maintained on the unoperated side. B, D, and F. The presurgical methods and techniques have been completely ineffective on the operated side. The normal anatomic relationship of the gingiva to the tooth has been radically changed. Surfaces such as the palatal aspects of the maxillary molars which usually are relatively self-cleansing are now longer, poorly contoured, and exhibit exposed fluted areas (D) and the size of the area between the height of contour of the tooth surface and the free gingival margin, which is most prone to plaque accumulation, has been greatly enlarged on all of the teeth. In addition, the embrasure areas are open and susceptible to plaque growth. The arrows point to enlarged root surfaces and fluting areas between the free gingival margin and the height of contour when there is an increase in plaque retention.*

While periodontal therapy is a means by which the capacity to achieve plaque control can be greatly enhanced by eliminating periodontal pockets, tissue ledges, and tooth surfaces serving as reservoirs for plaque growth, the potential benefits can be realized only when treatment is accompanied by rigorous instruction in the techniques of oral hygiene (Fig. 15-11). Oral hygiene measures must undergo evolution and change with changing oral conditions.

TECHNIQUES OF PLAQUE REMOVAL

The magnitude of the problem of teaching individuals to accomplish daily plaque control has only recently been recognized. Indeed, it has become patently clear that considerable technical skill is needed and that intensive, individualized training is essential. No single technique or method is universally applicable; plaque control procedures that are eminently successful for one patient may fail completely for another. Techniques and procedures must be adapted to the individual patient; indeed, they frequently must be modified from one site to another in the same patient if optimal results are to be achieved.

The dental and periodontal status of the patient is an important determinant of the techniques and procedures required. For example, the needs of the individual with an incomplete dentition, open interdental contacts, tilted teeth, or fixed or removable prosthetic or orthodontic appliances differ greatly from those of the normal individual or the individual with advanced periodontal disease. Furthermore, needs of an individual patient may vary from one time to another. For example, plaque-control procedures required by the periodontal patient may change radically during the course of periodontal therapy (Fig. 15-11). The instruments and techniques required to adequately debride a tooth surface adjacent to a deep interdental crater or a thick buccal ledge are different from those required to remove plaque from the same tooth surface following successful periodontal surgery.

In addition to the toothbrush, a large variety of instruments to be used by the patient for plaque control have become available in recent years. It is the responsibility of the dentist and the hygienist to learn the advantages and limitations of each of these and to select from among them, sometimes on a trial-and-error basis, instruments that can be effectively used in individual cases, to instruct the patient in their use, and to monitor the result if success is to be permanently achieved.

Toothbrushing

Of all methods of plaque removal, toothbrushing is the most universally used. There appear to be several reasons for this. Brushing is easy, it is socially accepted as the proper means to clean the mouth, and it is a cultural characteristic possibly extending back historically to the subhuman primates. Toothbrushing, using a variety of techniques and brushes, greatly reduces plaque on the buccal and lingual surfaces and, to some extent, on the interproximal surfaces of the teeth (Fig. 15-12). In the periodontal patient as well as in the normal person, the effectiveness of toothbrushing in removing interproximal plaque is related to the shape and size of the embrasure spaces.

Manual and automatic toothbrushes are about equally effective in the removal of dental plaque. In one experiment, subjects were instructed to brush the teeth in the right side of the mouth with either a manual or an electric toothbrush and to use no means of plaque control on the left side (Fig. 15-12). Other subjects used a manual brush on the right side and an electric brush on the left side. Relatively effective plaque control was maintained by both types of brushes (Fig. 15-12A, C, E). In subjects with slightly misaligned teeth, there was some plaque accumulation when brushing was not accompanied by use of dental floss (Fig. 15-12F).

BRUSH DESIGN

Recommended toothbrush design has changed radically during the past few years from large brushes with hard bristles reputed to be effective in stimulating the gums to brushes of various sizes with soft bristles of approximately 0.007 inch diameter (Fig. 15-13). This change has accompanied the emerging appreciation of the importance of plaque as an etiologic agent related to both dental caries and periodontal disease and of the absolute necessity for plaque control in successfully treating these diseases. Soft-bristle brushes offer several advantages: they can be better adapted to the gingival marginal area to permit more effective sulcular and interproximal cleansing;[2,3] soft bristle tips enter the gingival sulcus and tooth surface defects more readily than hard bristles; and vigorous use does not lead to gingival recession and root abrasion as may be the case with the long-term use of hard bristle brushes.[10] Several acceptable brush designs are available, including those with bristles arranged in two or three rows as single tufts and those with multitufts (Fig. 15-14). In most relatively normal persons, the three-row single-tufted brush is probably the most easily positioned and used (Fig. 15-13). However, for those who have undergone full-mouth reconstruction, in whom almost all of the cleansing efforts must be directed toward the zone of the gingival margin, two-row single-tufted brushes seem to be the most effective. When irregularities in tooth position are prominent, single-tufted brushes appear to be more effective than multitufted brushes. In spite of these observations, the means by which the brush is applied and used is probably of far greater importance than are details of brush design.

BRUSHING TECHNIQUES

The toothbrushing techniques recommended for a specific patient are dependent upon the dental and periodontal status of the individual patient. For example, when the gingival margins are located at the cementoenamel junction and the interdental papillae fill the embrasure spaces, the Bass sulcular technique is the method of choice. The brush is angled so that the bristle tips are directed at the gingival sulcus (Fig. 15-15). Light pressure is applied, barely flexing the bristles. The brush is then moved in short, back and

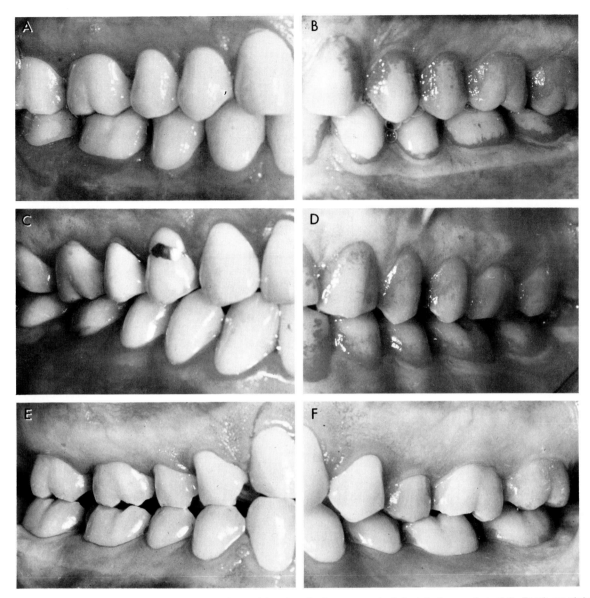

FIG. 15-12. *Effectiveness of manual and automatic toothbrushes in the removal of dental plaque. A and C. Teeth on right side brushed with either a manual or an automatic toothbrush for 10 days. C and D. Teeth on left side after 10 days of no plaque control. E. Teeth on right side after use of a manual brush. F. Teeth on left side after use of an automatic brush. Relatively effective plaque control was maintained by individuals using automatic brushes and those using manual brushes. In cases with slightly misaligned teeth both methods, when not accompanied by the use of floss, resulted in plaque accumulation.*

forth or rotary scrubbing strokes (Fig. 15-16), and guided systematically around the mouth to permit the bristles to scrub the plaque from the exposed tooth surfaces, the sulci, and parts of the proximal surfaces. Lingual to the anterior teeth, the brush may be turned to a vertical position to provide better bristle adaptation, but the motion is kept the same. The sulcular technique cleans the lingual and facial surfaces well, but does not adequately clean the embrasure spaces.

The Bass technique must be altered when disease or therapeutic intervention has led to gingival recession and open interproximal spaces. The extent of

interproximal cleaning can be enhanced by using the Charters' technique in which the brush is placed at the gingival margin at an angle of approximately 45 degrees toward the occlusal surface, a position that forces the bristles into the embrasures, and the brush moved systematically around the mouth in a vibratory motion (Fig. 15-17). The Charters' method is effective in plaque control below the heights of contour of the teeth. When gingival recession has occurred and the embrasures are open, optimal results are obtained by making one complete circuit with the Bass technique and a second complete circuit with the Charters' tech-

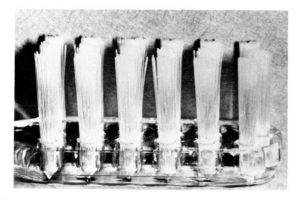

FIG. 15-13. *A toothbrush with soft nylon bristles 0.007 inch in diameter, which have been rounded and polished to prevent tissue damage, is recommended for most toothbrushing techniques.*

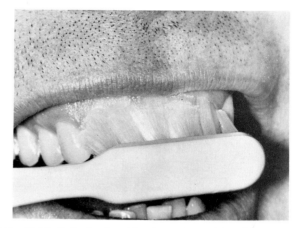

FIG. 15-15. *Sulcular brushing is performed by directing the bristles into the gingival sulcus.*

nique. When this routine is used, the amount of interproximal plaque left to be removed by other means is reduced to a minimum (Figs. 15-18, 15-19).

Unfortunately, some patients do not possess the manual dexterity to perform adequately either the Bass or the Charters' technique. The automatic toothbrush provides a suitable alternative for them. Though often maligned, the electric brush appears to be at least the equivalent of, and in some cases superior to, the manual brush (Fig. 15-12). However, as with the manual brush, considerable care in selection of the correct

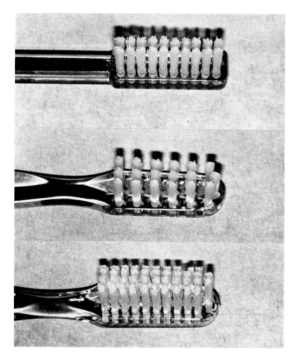

FIG. 15-14. *Soft nylon toothbrushes: (top to bottom) a two-row multitufted, a three-row single-tufted, and a four-row multitufted brush.*

brush and training in its proper use are essential for successful results. Since a vigorous motion with hard-bristle brushes can cause soft-tissue damage and tooth abrasion, patients should be cautioned to select an automatic instrument with relatively mild motion and to use soft-bristle brushes. As in the manual Bass technique, the brush head can be positioned with the bristle tips directed toward the gingival margin, and the brush can be slowly guided around the mouth. Patients who have open embrasures and gingival recession can place the brush in the Charters' position to enhance cleaning potential in the interproximal areas.

Judgment and flexibility must be exercised in selecting an appropriate toothbrush and in choosing the correct method for using it. If a particular patient has effective toothbrushing habits that are not damaging the tissues, his toothbrushing technique should not be changed. For such a person, a change may reduce effectiveness. Patients who have generalized difficulty with toothbrushing are ideal candidates for an automatic brush.

A more common problem is difficulty in adequately brushing specific areas. In these cases, reinstruction with the same methods and instruments may not be fruitful, but application of various techniques in different areas is frequently helpful. For example, at the buccal surfaces of the maxillary second molars, where there is a minimum of vestibular space, a smaller brush may be helpful; on the lingual surfaces of the mandibular molars, an area that is frequently missed in most patients, bending the brush handle may be helpful. In some areas, a back-and-forth motion is much easier than a rotary motion. Generally, the objective should be that of complete daily plaque removal with a minimum of effort, time, and armamentarium, and using the simplest methods possible. Individuals who achieve this goal tend to continue their efforts permanently and

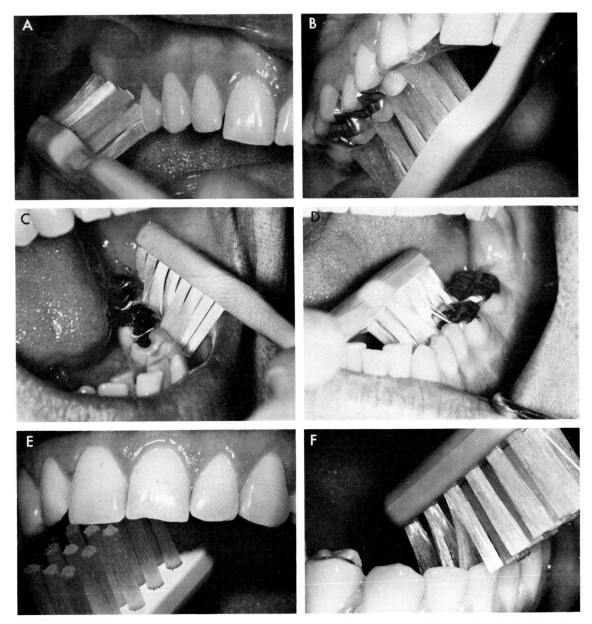

FIG. 15-16. *The correct placement of the brush for sulcular brushing in various segments of the mouth. A–D. The tips of the bristles are placed at the margin of the free gingiva with the brush angled approximately 45° in the posterior segments. E–F. On the lingual or palatal aspect of the incisors the brush is moved to a vertical position to permit better adaptation.*

do not revert to their old habits at the termination of periodontal therapy.

BRUSHING FREQUENCY

Since 24 to 36 hours are required for the accumulation of significant amounts of dental plaque, thorough toothbrushing once each day should be adequate, provided that a high degree of efficiency is achieved. However, the key factor in the effectiveness of plaque control procedures is not the frequency of their application, but rather the thoroughness of their use. Al-

though conceptually plaque removal once a day should be adequate, in actual practice this is usually not the case. Regardless of the instruments and methods used, it is only in rare cases that people are able to remove plaque completely. Therefore, most persons benefit from brushing more frequently than once each day.[7]

Control of Interdental Plaque

Both in normal persons and in patients in whom gingival recession has occurred and the interdental embrasures are open, some form of interdental clean-

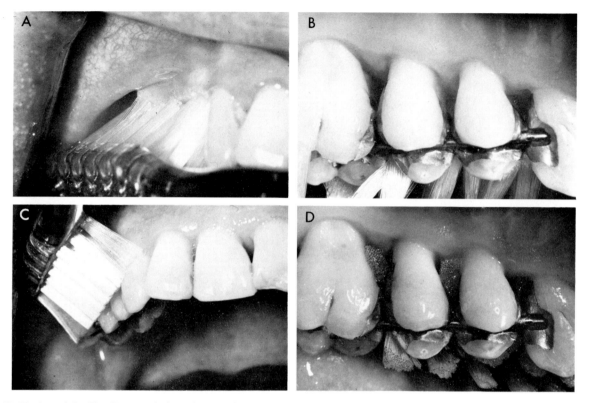

FIG. 15-17. A and B. The Bass technique in a patient with gingival recession. The bristles are adapted to the gingival margin (A) but do not extend very far into the interproximal embrasures (B). C. The toothbrush placed in a Charters' position in the same patient. D. The bristles extend through the open embrasures, giving improved interdental cleansing.

ing is necessary, since even the most effective use of the toothbrush does not remove all of the interdental plaque. Numerous devices for interdental cleaning have been advocated, but these have not received widespread patient acceptance. In general, they are difficult and cumbersome for most patients to use. Thus, the devices chosen in any given case for interdental plaque control must be selected with great care, and the patient must be trained specifically in their use.

FLOSS

Dental floss is the most widely prescribed and probably the most useful interdental cleaning aid. When used regularly and properly for relatively normal dentitions in which the interdental spaces are filled by the interdental papillae, floss is approximately 80 percent effective in removing interdental plaque (Figs. 15-20, 15-21). The presence of the interdental papillae is related to the effectiveness of dental floss. In dentitions in which the positions of interdental papillae have been moved apically by periodontal surgery, the effectiveness of floss is significantly reduced (Fig. 15-22). This loss of effectiveness seems to be related to the lack of papillary guidance which, in the normal denti-

tion, helps to adapt the floss closely to the tooth surface. The potential effectiveness of floss in plaque control procedures has led some clinicians to conclude that floss rather than toothbrushing should be considered as the primary device for plaque removal and that flossing should be taught prior to toothbrushing. In our view, it is better to teach toothbrushing first and then demonstrate to the patient the residual interproximal plaque as a means of reinforcing the need for interproximal cleaning (Fig. 15-23A).

Both waxed and unwaxed types of dental floss are in use. As demonstrated by Arnim and others, unwaxed floss offers several advantages:[1] (1) it is small in diameter and passes more easily through tight interproximal contacts, (2) under tension it flattens out on the tooth surface with each component thread acting separately as a cutting edge to dislodge debris (Fig. 15-23B), and (3) unwaxed floss makes a squeaking noise when used on a clean tooth surface, and this noise can be used to monitor performance. Although unwaxed floss is widely used, the view that it is superior to waxed floss is not universally held.

The correct procedure for using floss is illustrated in Figure 15-24. A 12 to 18-inch length of the material is obtained, wrapped around the middle finger of at least one hand, and positioned over the tips of the index

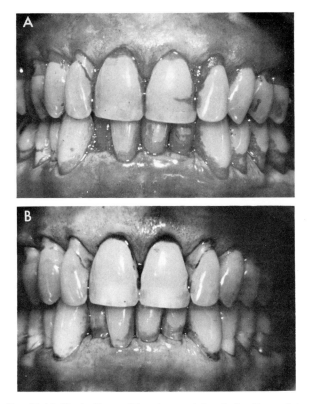

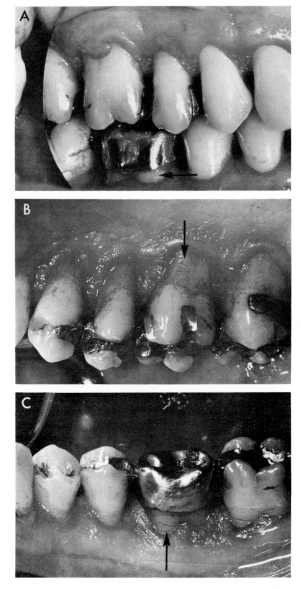

FIG. 15-18. *Illustrations of the plaque status during the maintenance phase following the completion of periodontal treatment. A. The patient was using the sulcular brushing technique, and this was not removing the plaque adequately. B. After adding the Charters' toothbrush position to the sulcular toothbrush position, plaque removal was greatly improved, although complete control has still not been achieved. (Courtesy Dr. T. Wilson, Dallas, Texas.)*

FIG. 15-19. *Plaque status of teeth seen in Figures 15-8 and 15-37 after reinstructing the patient in toothbrushing by both a sulcular and a Charters' position. Plaque removal has improved, particularly below the height of the contour (arrows) on both the buccal and the lingual surfaces (A, B, and C).*

fingers. The two index fingers should be about $3/4$ to 1 inch apart, with the floss grasped firmly between them. The floss is worked between the teeth with a slight buccolingual shoe-shining motion until it passes through the contact area. Then, the floss should be wrapped around one of the teeth and worked apically into the gingival sulcus. The surface is cleaned by moving the floss up and down on the tooth. Once one tooth surface has been cleaned, the floss is adapted around the adjacent tooth surface, and the process is repeated. If shoe-shining movements are used subgingivally, damage to both the hard and soft tissues may occur (Fig. 15-25).

To be effective as a means of interdental plaque control, dental floss should be used daily on all interproximal surfaces, although motivating patients to continue this indefinitely has generally been extremely difficult. A decrease in flossing frequency and effectiveness has been observed in almost all patients examined on a long-term basis. A more expeditious use of floss can be encouraged in several ways: (1) patients

should be trained thoroughly in the correct technique and monitored until they have become successful in interdental plaque control; otherwise they may not be able to remove all of the plaque and they become discouraged; (2) self-monitoring by using the squeaky-clean sound of a plaque-free surface should be encouraged; (3) in individuals who have mastered floss technique before a mirror, a more regular use of floss can be induced by encouraging the use of floss while doing something else such as reading or watching television.

For those who do not have the manual dexterity to

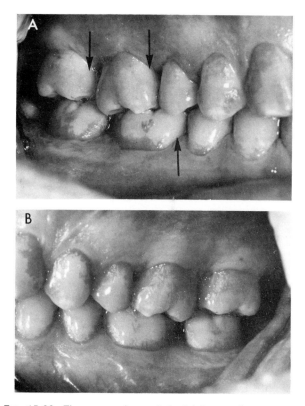

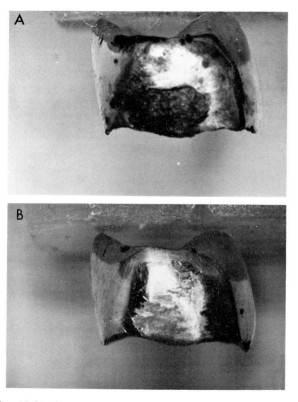

FIG. 15-20. *The comparison of dental floss only to no oral hygiene for a 10-day period. A. Dental floss effectively removes interproximal plaque (arrows). Note that plaque is even reduced on the buccal surfaces of the maxillary molars as a result of wrapping the floss around the teeth. B. No oral hygiene.*

FIG. 15-21. *An experiment in plaque removal. The full crown shown was temporarily cemented on a mandibular first molar. A. The subject was instructed to use only a toothbrush for two weeks. The crown was removed, stained with disclosing solution, and photographed at a fixed focal distance and the plaque area of the proximal surface was measured. B. This process was repeated except that the subject was instructed to use a toothbrush and dental floss. There was an 80 percent reduction in the area of plaque accumulation.*

handle dental floss, the use of a floss holder may be helpful (Figs. 15-26, 15-27). While floss cannot be as closely adapted to the tooth surface with a floss holder as with the fingers, it is easier to use, particularly between the posterior teeth, and the slight reduction in effectiveness is compensated for by the more frequent and continued usage.

Floss-threading devices provide a method for cleaning under fixed bridges, splints, and orthodontic appliances. In using these devices, a piece of floss or yarn is attached and carried under a bridge or splint (Fig. 15-28). Several devices are available, including wire and nylon loops, short plastic strips with eyelets, and plastic strips with hooks. The best floss threaders are those that are easiest to use because the main difficulty with floss threaders has been a lack of continued patient use. The wire and nylon loops are the easiest to use in tight embrasure spaces, and the plastic strips with hooks are the easiest to use in other areas because the floss or yarn is more easily attached. In view of the problem encountered in using floss, it is advisable to create open embrasures under fixed bridges whenever

possible to allow cleaning with devices that are easy to use, such as the Perio-Aid or the interproximal brush.

Although dental floss is effective in interproximal plaque removal in the healthy mouth with a normal relationship between teeth and gingiva, many dentists and hygienists express reservation about flossing effectiveness in surgically treated periodontal patients. Floss is totally ineffective in removing debris from concavities and fluting areas of exposed root surfaces (Fig. 15-29). Therefore, other aids are necessary to clean these critical areas.

TOOTHPICK

The toothpick, mounted in an angled plastic holding device called the Perio-Aid, is the device most widely used to reach furcation areas, root concavities, and fluting areas (Fig. 15-30). The mounted toothpick has been advocated for plaque removal from both interproximal and facial and lingual surfaces. The effective-

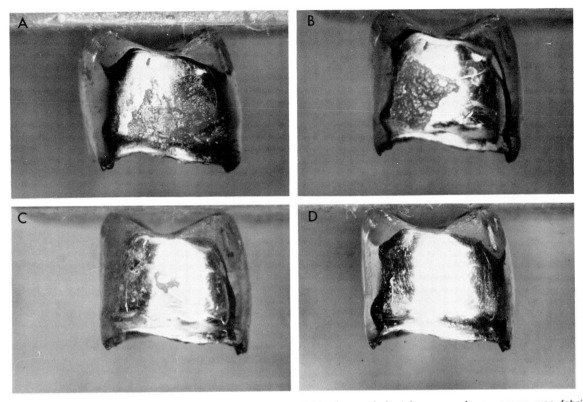

FIG. 15-22. *Repetition of the experiment illustrated in Figure 15-21 after periodontal surgery. A new crown was fabricated, duplicating the original tooth contours, including the fluting. A. Toothbrushing only was done for two weeks. B. The use of both brushing and dental floss for two weeks resulted in a 55 percent reduction in the area of plaque accumulation when compared with that observed in A. C. The use of a toothpick attached to an appropriate handle resulted in an 80 percent reduction in the area of plaque accumulation. D. Use of the interproximal brush reduced the plaque area by 95 percent.*

ness of toothpicks in plaque removal has not been thoroughly evaluated. However, Gjermo and Flötra reported that while toothpicks were not as effective as dental floss in removing interdental plaque from individuals with a healthy periodontium, they were more effective than floss with open embrasures and gingival recession.[6] Our own observations of plaque removal with the Perio-Aid tend to support this idea. The toothpick is especially effective in areas not readily accessible to the brush or floss, although to recommend its general use on all of the teeth may result in decreased effectiveness in the critical fluting and furcation areas where it is most needed (Figs. 15-31, 15-32). If patients are not properly instructed in the use of the Perio-Aid, they may use it in an ineffective manner. To remove plaque effectively, the toothpick must be placed in the specific fluting area and rubbed against the tooth surface (Fig. 15-32).

WATER-JET DEVICES

The use of water-jet devices has been advocated for many years. A wide variety of these, some of which are self-contained while others are designed to attach to the bathroom water faucet, are currently available. Whether water-jet devices are effective is still a controversial matter. Many clinicians believe that they produce beneficial effects in the mouths of patients with extensive bridgework, splints, or orthodontics bands, especially when used as an adjunct to flossing and brushing. There is no doubt that the user may experience a clean feeling following their use. Although the devices may remove food particles and loose debris, they are not effective in removing plaque (Fig. 15-33).[5] That a high pressure jet of water may improve soft-tissue health by washing away damaging bacterial products or by interfering in some as yet undetermined way with plaque ecology has not been ruled out, although there is no evidence in its support. If water-jet devices are to be used at all, it must be as an adjunct to brushes and floss, and great caution must be exercised, especially in individuals with deep periodontal pockets. The high-pressure water jet directed into the pocket may force microorganisms from the pocket into the surrounding tissues and thereby enhance periodontal breakdown.

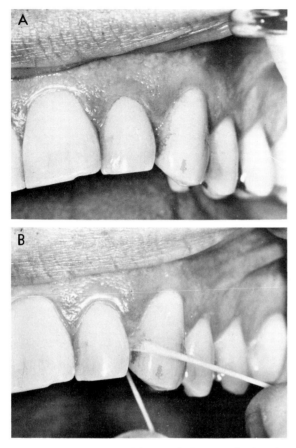

FIG. 15-23. *A. Plaque remaining on the interproximal surfaces of the teeth after toothbrushing. B. Unwaxed dental floss wrapped around the tooth. Note that the multiple fibers splay out.*

INTERPROXIMAL BRUSH

Small brushes resembling miniature test-tube or bottle brushes have recently become available for plaque removal from open embrasures and furcations. These brushes can be obtained with a short wire handle or mounted, by a screw-type or snap-on attachment, to a metal or plastic handle (Fig. 15-34). The latter type is superior since it can be manipulated more easily in the posterior segments of the mouth and in small embrasure spaces. Interproximal brushes appear to be superior to either toothpicks or dental floss for interproximal cleaning in patients with open embrasures.[6] To be effective, they should be used from both the buccal and the lingual sides so that all aspects of the interproximal surfaces are cleaned (Fig. 15-35). The interproximal brush is clearly more effective than either floss or toothpicks in interproximal plaque control in the periodontal patient both immediately postsurgically and during the long-term maintenance period as was shown by a comparison of the three methods (Fig. 15-36).[13] The following results were observed:

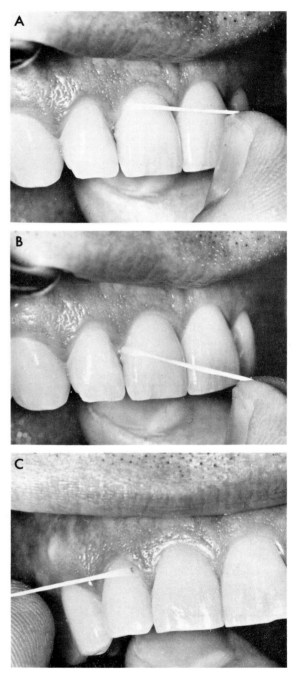

FIG. 15-24. *Procedure for using dental floss. A. Dental floss is wrapped around the tooth and carried into the gingival sulcus. B. Floss is then moved up and down to remove plaque from the sulcus and the proximal tooth surface. C. Next, the floss is wrapped around the adjacent tooth and the up-and-down action is continued.*

1. During the maintenance period, all of the patients were more effective in removing plaque from the buccal and lingual surfaces than from the mesial and distal surfaces of the teeth, regardless of the methods used.

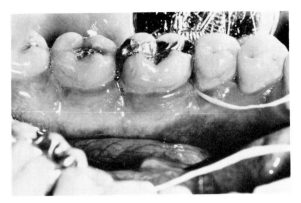

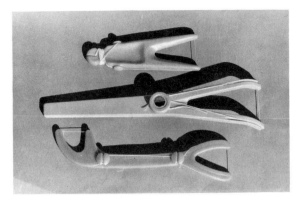

FIG. 15-25. *Floss cuts from "shoe-shining." Buccolingual motion should be avoided while using floss. (Courtesy Dr. W. Ammons.)*

FIG. 15-26. *Floss holders of various designs.*

2. All three programs were equally effective in controlling plaque accumulation on the buccal and lingual surfaces.
3. Both the Perio-Aid and the interproximal brush lead to improved interproximal plaque control, but the interproximal brush was more effective than the Perio-Aid.

Furthermore, we have observed that the results obtained from a variety of therapeutic procedures, including osseous resection, root amputation, and various restorative procedures, are improved by the use of interproximal brushes (Fig. 15-37).

Use of the interproximal brush is not limited to the postsurgical periodontal patient; its use can be initi-

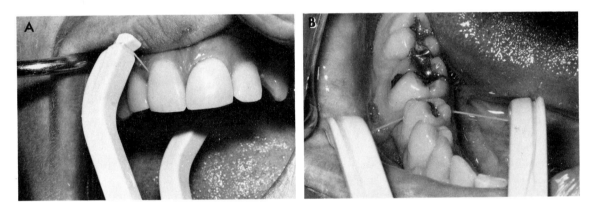

FIG. 15-27. *A. Floss may be carried into the gingival sulcus with a floss holder, but it is not easily wrapped around the tooth. B. Floss holders are particularly useful in reaching the posterior areas.*

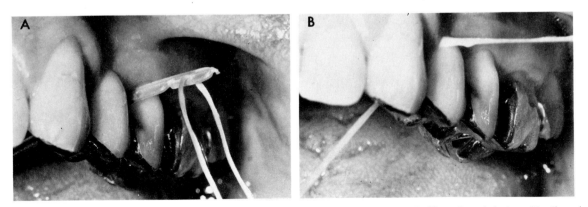

FIG. 15-28. *A. Floss threaders can be used to carry floss beneath fixed bridges and splints. B. Cleansing of abutment teeth and areas beneath pontics with floss.*

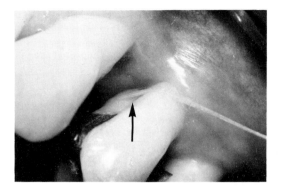

FIG. 15-29. *Fluting and furcation areas (arrow) are missed by dental floss.*

ated at any time there is sufficient embrasure space for brush insertion. For example, if sufficiently open embrasures are created by proper contouring of posterior restorations such as full crowns, pontics, and splints, the interproximal brush can be used easily to control interproximal plaque even in the nonperiodontal patient. Experience has shown rather clearly that patients are much more likely to continue using the interproxi-

mal brush than dental floss or toothpicks on a long-term basis because of the ease of use. In the periodontal patient, improved interproximal cleaning and soft tissue contour can be obtained frequently by instituting use of the interproximal brush in lieu of the interdental stimulator immediately following root planing and curettage.

The Proxabrush or a comparable device should be introduced as soon as possible after periodontal surgery, and in no case later than 2 or 3 weeks after, in order to promote the desired interproximal soft tissue contour as well as maintain interproximal plaque control.

Although the use of interproximal brushes has been extremely beneficial to most individuals whose anatomic relationships permit insertion, there are disadvantages. The brushes are relatively expensive, and they may last for only 1 or 2 weeks. However, as they become more widely used, it is likely that the quality of construction will be improved and the cost will be lowered. Another suggested disadvantage is that interproximal brushes may not enter and clean the interdental gingival sulcus as effectively as dental floss,

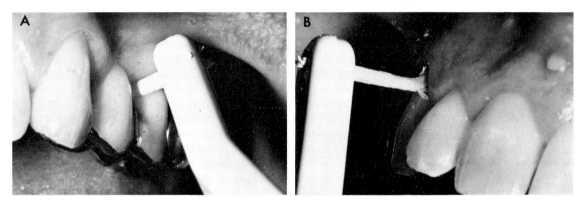

FIG. 15-30. *Using the Perio-Aid. A. Interproximal cleaning. B. Facial-surface cleaning.*

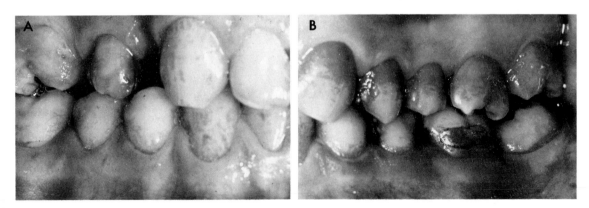

FIG. 15-31. *An experiment in plaque removal. A. The Perio-Aid was used on one side of the mouth for a period of 10 days. B. No oral hygiene measures were taken on the other side. It is apparent that the Perio-Aid alone is ineffective in the control of plaque on the facial surfaces.*

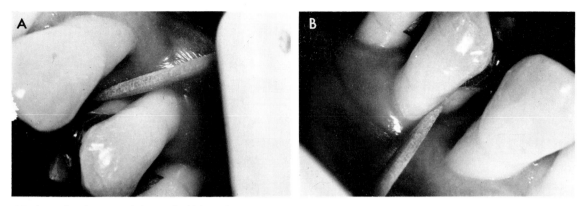

FIG. 15-32. *A. Ineffective use of the Perio-Aid. B. Correct placement of the toothpick in the specific fluting area.*

although this has not been our experience. Where the brush does not clean the sulcus adequately, both the brush and floss can be used.

INTERDENTAL STIMULATORS

Short sticks of wood or nylon and rubber tips of various sizes attached to the toothbrush handle (Fig. 15-38) have been recommended for many years as a means of interdental stimulation and plaque removal.

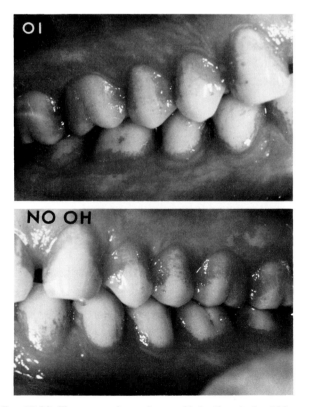

FIG. 15-33. *The comparison of an oral irrigation device (OI) on the right side to no oral hygiene (NO OH) on the left side of the same patient for 10 days. The plaque accumulation is almost identical on both sides.*

Whether there is therapeutic value to soft-tissue stimulation remains unknown. Advocates claim that stimulation increases circulation and keratinization, although there is no evidence to support this claim nor to demonstrate that, if it does occur, the change is beneficial. These aids may be valuable in reshaping the interdental tissue following surgical periodontal therapy. Most interdental stimulators are only minimally effective in removing plaque from the interproximal surfaces, although the wedge-shaped wooden interdental stimulators may be beneficial because of their soft, rough surfaces. These wedges do not effectively clean fluting areas, and they are extremely difficult to insert from the lingual and palatal directions. Thus, these aids are not as effective as floss and the interproximal brush in removal of interproximal plaque.

Adjuncts to Plaque Removal Procedures

Although most patients can clean their mouths adequately with a combination of the toothbrush, dental floss, mounted toothpick, or interproximal brush, additional aids may be used to improve effectiveness and to

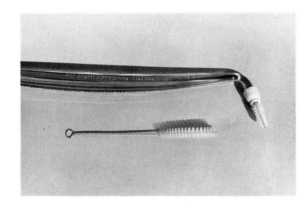

FIG. 15-34. *Two basic types of interproximal brush: tapered brush on the handle (top); brush with short wire handle (bottom).*

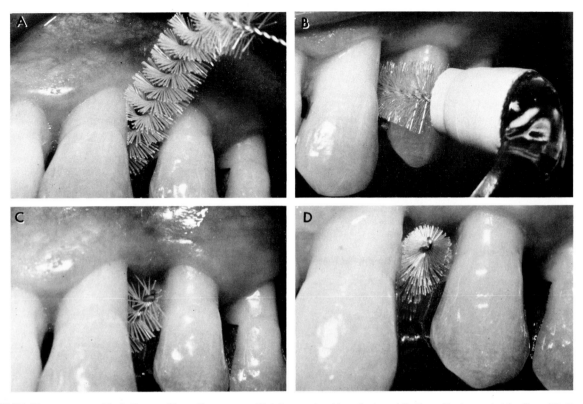

FIG. 15-35. *Plaque removal in fluting and furcation areas with interproximal brush. A and B. From the buccal side. C and D. From the lingual side.*

permit the individual to master the techniques more rapidly.

DISCLOSING AGENTS

Disclosing agents of several types have been employed in dentistry for many years, although they have only recently been given to patients for home use. Arnim incorporated Erythrosin Red (FDC #3) into a tablet which the patient chews and swishes throughout the mouth;[1] the excess dye is removed by a water rinse, leaving plaque strikingly bright red. The primary disadvantage of the tablets is a residual red tongue and lips, which is objectionable to some people. However, the color fades rapidly. More recently, exposure of the teeth to a fluorescein-containing dye and visualization of plaque under an ultra violet light has been used. However, the lighting device is expensive, and small amounts of plaque may be difficult to see. To achieve better visibility and preclude the red color of Erythrosin, FDC Red #3 and FDC Green #3 have been incorporated into a disclosing agent which does not stain the mucosa but leaves mature plaque a dark blue under ordinary light. This dye is a valuable adjunct for patients who have poor eyesight or cannot see suffi-

ciently plaque that has been colored with a standard disclosing agent.

Bacterial plaque is difficult to see, particularly to the untrained eye. Disclosing agents can be used to demonstrate the location of plaque, and they permit patients to evaluate their own performance using various oral hygiene techniques (Fig. 15-39).

Most bathroom lights are inadequate for intraoral illumination. For patients to see plaque adequately at home, a good light source and some type of mirror-light combination are useful in seeing the lingual and posterior tooth surfaces (Fig. 15-40). A special light may be purchased or a flashlight or makeup light may be used. These aids combined with the use of disclosing tablets will enable a patient to evaluate his own progress.

MONITORING PERFORMANCE

Means of evaluation of the amount and distribution of plaque on the teeth of individual patients are essential for teaching plaque control and for evaluating the effectiveness of the measures chosen. Various indices permitting the expression of the plaque status of all the teeth as a single numerical value have been developed.

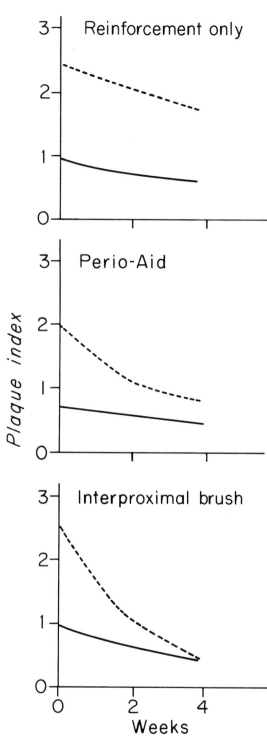

FIG. 15-36. *Comparison of the plaque status, using the Plaque Index, of 12 postperiodontal therapy patients during the maintenance period. Plaque Index scores on the mesial and distal (-----) surfaces and the buccal and lingual (———) surfaces in individuals using standard toothbrushing and dental floss plus educational reinforcement only (uppermost graph), Perio-Aid (middle graph), or the interproximal brush (lower graph).*

Most of these indices were designed initially for use in epidemiologic studies, and they yield valuable information when applied to large populations. However, the numerical score reflects an average distribution of plaque, and it is not informative either to the dentist or to the patient in working toward a solution of problems of plaque control in the individual. In addition, the plaque indices are time-consuming to use, and they do not reflect subtle difference in plaque accumulation.

A pictorial record of plaque distribution, consisting of a diagram upon which the sites of plaque accumulation on all surfaces of the teeth can be rapidly recorded, provides a superior measurement system for the individual patient (Fig. 15-41). The pictorial record allows accurate and rapid visualization of the effectiveness of the oral hygiene regime; patterns of plaque accumulation become readily apparent, and therapeutic decisions can be based on this information. Progress of the patient can be assessed accurately, and necessary modification in his plaque control practices made. For example, if significant amounts of interproximal plaque, but little buccal and lingual plaque are present, more stress can be placed on the use of dental floss or other means of interproximal cleaning.

Evaluation of the tendency of the gingiva to bleed can also be useful to both the dentist and the patient in devising the best means of plaque control. The bleeding index is a count of the number of areas that bleed upon gentle probing. An index of this type is helpful to the dentist in evaluating progress, but it cannot be used as such by the patient. However, the patient can be made aware that healthy gingiva is firm, light pink and does not bleed during or after normal oral hygiene procedures. Furthermore, the patient can be shown that gingival bleeding ceases when plaque control measures are effective.

DEVELOPMENT OF A PLAQUE CONTROL PROGRAM FOR THE PERIODONTAL PATIENT

An elementary understanding by the patient of the nature of inflammatory periodontal disease and the important etiologic relationship of dental plaque to its development and progress is essential if long-term, effective plaque control is to be achieved. Thus, a successful plaque-control plan must include patient education, as well as information regarding the devices available for plaque control and instruction in the techniques of their use. Furthermore, effective plaque control is not a goal which can be attained prior to initiation of periodontal therapy and then neglected by either the dentist or the patient. Periodontal therapy frequently requires a time period of several months

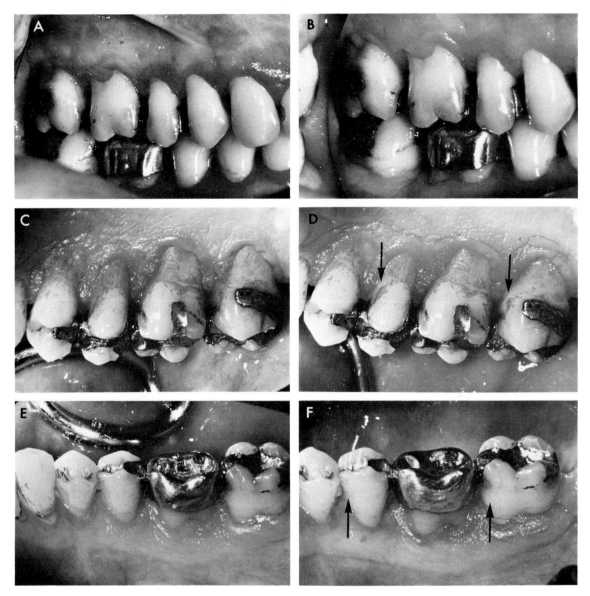

FIG. 15-37. *The effects of the use of the interproximal brush and the Perio-Aid in the postsurgical periodontal patient. The extent of plaque control using toothbrushing and dental floss prior to surgical intervention and following surgical intervention is illustrated in Figs. 15-11 and 15-19. A, C, and E. The results of adding the use of the Perio-Aid. B, D, and F. Adding use of the interproximal brush. Note its effectiveness in the control of interproximal plaque accumulation (arrows).*

during which the oral environment may be drastically altered. Concurrently, the devices and methods used for plaque control must undergo evolution. Plaque-control efforts can be integrated into and coordinated with diagnostic and treatment planning procedures and the initial, surgical, restorative, and maintenance phases of periodontal therapy.

Diagnosis and Treatment Planning

The initial dental and periodontal treatment plan must include a program designed to achieve and to maintain adequate plaque control. This will require (1)

measurement of the initial plaque level and distribution, possibly by a plaque index, pictorial record, or bleeding index to establish baseline values, (2) selection of devices for use in control, (3) education of the patient regarding the relationship of plaque to his dental and periodontal condition, and (4) elementary instruction in the use of plaque control devices.

The goal for the first few plaque control sessions should be education of the patient about the presence and location of bacterial plaque in the mouth and its role in the etiology and progression of periodontal disease. The signs and symptoms of disease such as bleeding and suppuration should be explained. Audio-

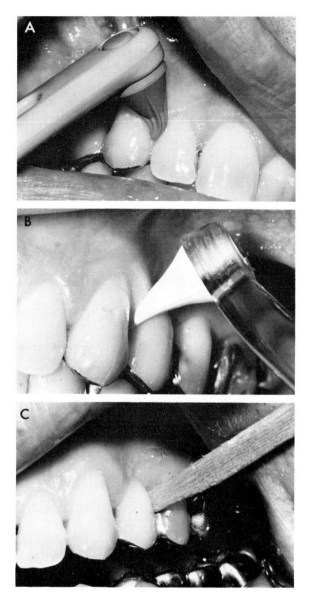

FIG. 15-38. *Types of interdental stimulators. A. Rubber. B. Nylon. C. Wood.*

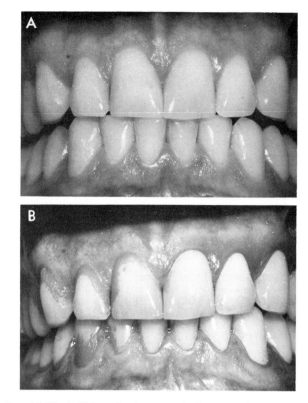

FIG. 15-39. *A. This patient appears to have no plaque on his teeth. B. After using a disclosing tablet, a heavy plaque accumulation is evident on the right side.*

visual aids such as slides and films help to communicate this information. Disclosing agents are particularly useful, since they demonstrate plaque in the patient's own mouth. Establishing an understanding of the reasons for controlling plaque accumulation provides a basis for motivation in learning and practicing an efficient oral hygiene regime.

Initial Therapy

During the initial phases of periodontal therapy, the patient is instructed in detail in the plaque-control techniques selected for him. Basic instructions should be given in toothbrushing and interdental plaque removal. The appointment interval may be daily or weekly, and progress should be reinforced as initial therapy brings a reduction in bleeding and suppuration. If a patient is aware of the changes in his tissues from disease to health, he may become better able to monitor his own oral health status. The patient can use visual aids such as disclosing agents, mirrors, and lights to evaluate his own performance at home. His success should be monitored periodically by the same methods used to establish the initial baseline values.

The goal at this stage is for the patient to be able to perform the basic plaque-control techniques adequately and within a reasonable time. If, after repeated instructions, a patient is still not able to satisfactorily perform a particular plaque control technique, then a different method such as an automatic toothbrush or floss holder should be substituted.

Surgical Therapy

A patient's plaque control procedures must be modified as changes occur in the soft-tissue anatomy following periodontal surgery. When a therapist decides to alter a patient's oral environment surgically, he must be willing also to accept the responsibility for teaching

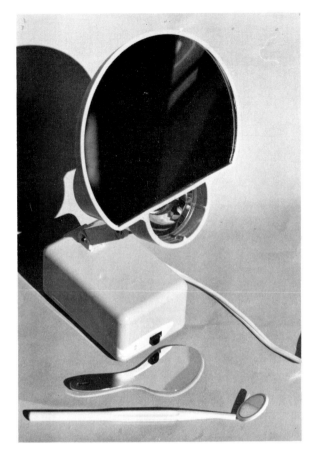

FIG. 15-40. *Intraoral mirrors.*

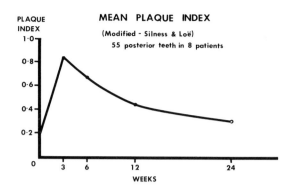

FIG. 15-42. *Mean plaque index for 55 posterior teeth in 8 patients following periodontal surgery. Note that adequate control was not achieved until 12 to 24 weeks. (Courtesy Dr. H. Selipsky, unpublished)*

cleaned with the Perio-Aid. The patient's tooth-brushing techniques can be changed to a combined sulcular and Charters' technique to aid in interproximal plaque removal. These changes should not be taken lightly by the patient or the dentist; they are more important than the original plaque-control techniques in the long-term periodontal health of the patient. Therefore, as much effort should be made by the therapist in the instruction of these additional plaque-removal aids as was made in the original instructions. Even with intensive attention and instruction, there may be a lengthy period following surgery during which the patient may not be able to bring plaque control to presurgical levels (Fig. 15-42).

Restorative Dentistry

An oral environment which can be maintained relatively easily, or one in which intensive efforts by the dentist and the patient at plaque control will meet

the patient to clean the postsurgical environment. To control interproximal plaque, an interproximal brush should be added as a primary interdental cleaning aid during the postsurgical period in patients having open embrasures and flattened papillae. Exposed furcation and fluting areas that require special attention can be

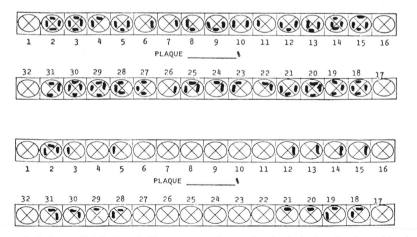

FIG. 15-41. *A pictorial record of plaque distribution. In the uppermost record, prior to instruction in oral hygiene, the overall pattern of plaque accumulation on both the facial and interproximal surfaces is easily seen. In the lower record, it can be seen that after several instructional sessions, the plaque status has improved, but deposits remain on some of the posterior, interproximal, and mandibular lingual surfaces. (Record adapted from O'Leary, T. J., Drake, R. B., and Naylor, J. E.: The plaque control record. J. Periodontol., 43:38, 1972.)*

with failure, can be created by the extensive restorative dentistry that may be needed following periodontal therapy. The restorative phase is an extremely critical period during which the restorative dentist and the periodontist must collaborate closely in the design of restorations that are easy to clean and decrease the tendency for plaque growth (see Chapter 26). Possibly, the restorative stage is the most critical of all periods of periodontal and dental treatment with regard to the need for additional help and instruction in plaque control, since it is at this time that permanent oral hygiene practices will be established. Frequently, patients who have undergone therapy of this type do not receive the help they need to perform adequate oral hygiene.

In places where the embrasures are kept open, the interproximal brush can be used; where closed embrasures are essential, a floss threader or a mounted toothpick may be helpful (Fig. 15-43). The Perio-Aid should be reserved for particular fluting and furcation

areas that are likely to be missed by the other devices. The general use of a mounted toothpick around all margins should not be advocated because of the possibility of tissue damage and recession, particularly where the soft gingival tissues may be unusually thin. In individuals who have difficulty in removing all of the plaque from the sulcus or who have the problem of recurrent caries at the marginal areas, a two-row toothbrush may be useful. The patient should be instructed to brush at the gingival margin with the sulcular technique. The narrowness of the two-row brush improves visibility and emphasizes to the patient the importance of cleaning this critical area.

Maintenance and Recall

Careful monitoring of the effectiveness of the patient's plaque-control efforts is essential during the posttreatment period. Some individuals who initially performed adequately will become lax and revert to their previous habits. During the posttreatment period, the patient should be able to identify and remove plaque from all surfaces of the teeth. He should be able to do this in a reasonably short time without great difficulty or discomfort. He should also be able, at least in part, to evaluate his own gingival health, to be aware of any signs of continuing periodontal breakdown such as swelling or bleeding, and appreciate their significance. When he is unable to achieve these objectives, reeducation, perhaps with different devices and methods of plaque control, is essential if the results of therapy are to be successful.

The relative ability of a patient to achieve a good level of plaque control on his own should be a factor in establishing a recall interval. Patients who have difficulty should be started on a short recall interval of 2 to 3 months, which can be gradually lengthened as they continue to improve. Many patients will achieve good levels of plaque control during therapy and even at their first recall visit, only to lapse into poor plaque control. This type of relapse should not be taken lightly, and at a subsequent visit the significance should be conveyed to the patient. The patient should be reinstructed, and any additions or modifications which might help should be attempted. When a patient does not maintain satisfactory plaque control, recurrence of periodontal disease is likely, regardless of how skillfully the periodontal therapy has been performed.

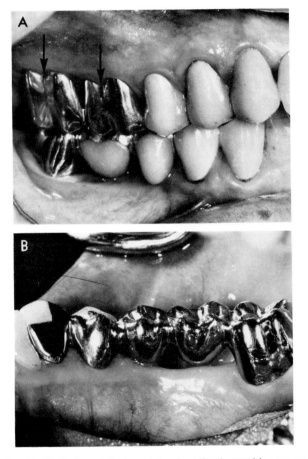

FIG. 15-43. A. A well-designed fixed prothesis provides crown contours that permit sulcular brushing and provide access to furcation areas (arrows). The embrasures are open to provide access for an interproximal brush. B. The pontic contacts the tissue only lightly, providing easy access for cleaning this area.

References

1. Arnim, S. S.: The use of disclosing agents for measuring tooth cleanliness. J. Periodontol., 34:277, 1963.
2. Bass, C. C.: The optimum characteristics of tooth brushes for personal oral hygiene. Dent. Items Int., 70:696, 1948.

3. Bass, C. C.: The necessary personal oral hygiene for prevention of caries and periodontoclasia. J. Louisiana Med. Soc., *101*:52, 1948.

4. Bjorby, A., and Löe, H.: The relative significance of different local factors in the initiation and development of periodontal inflammation. J. Periodont. Res., *2*:76, 1966.

5. Fine, D. H., and Baumhammers, A.: Effect of water pressure irrigation on stainable material on the teeth. J. Periodontol. *41*:568, 1970.

6. Gjermo, P., and Flötra, L.: The plaque removing effect of dental floss and toothpicks: A group comparison study. J. Periodont. Res., *4*:170, 1969.

7. Goldman, H. M.: Effect of single and multiple tooth brushing in the cleansing of the normal and periodontally involved dentition. Oral Surg., *9*:203, 1956.

8. Howitt, B. F., Fleming, W. C., and Simonton, F. V.: Study of effects upon hygiene and microbiology of the mouth of various diets with and without the toothbrush. Dental Cosmos, *70*:575, 1928.

9. Lindhe, J., and Wicen, P. O.: The effects on the gingivae of chewing fibrous foods. J. Periodont. Res., *4*:193, 1969.

10. O'Leary, T. J., et al.: The incidence of recession in young males: relationship to gingival and plaque scores. USAF School of Aerospace Medicine. SAM-TR, 67, 1967.

11. Perel, M. L.: Axial crown contour. J. Prosthet. Dent., *25*:642, 1971.

12. Perel, M. L.: Periodontal considerations of crown contour. J. Prosthet. Dent., *26*:627, 1971.

13. Wilson, T., and Douglass, G.: Unpublished observations, 1972.

Suggested Reading

Alexander, A. G.: The effect of frequency of brushing and the type of bristle used on gingival inflammation, plaque and calculus accumulation. Dent. Pract. Dent. Rec., *20*:347, 1970.

Alexander, A. G.: A study of the distribution of supra and subgingival calculus, bacterial plaque and gingival inflammation in the mouths of 400 individuals. J. Periodontol. *42*:21, 1971.

Arnim, S. S.: How to teach prevention and control of dental disease. Bull. Phila. Co. Dent. Soc., *28*:12, 1963.

Arnim, S. S.: Dental irrigators for oral hygiene, periodontal therapy and prevention of dental disease. J. Tenn. Dent. Assoc., *47*:65, 1967.

Arnim, S. S., and Sandell, P. J.: How to educate high school students in oral hygiene. J. Health Phys. Ed. Recreation. Oct., 1960, page 33.

Arnim, S. S., and Williams, Q. E.: How to educate patients in oral hygiene. Dent. Radiogr. Photogr., *32*:61, 1959.

Barkley, R. F.: A preventive philosophy of restorative dentistry. Dent. Clin. North Am., *15*:569, 1971.

Bass, C. C.: An effective method of personal oral hygiene. J. Louisiana Med. Soc., *106*:100, 1954.

Bass, C. C.: Personal oral hygiene: A serious deficiency in dental education. J. Louisiana Med. Soc., *114*:370, 1962.

Bay, I., Kardel, K. M., and Skougaard, M. A.: Quantitative evaluation of the plaque removing ability of different types of toothbrushes. J. Periodontol., *38*:526, 1967.

Bergenholtz, A., et al.: The toothbrush as an aid in oral hygiene. J. Periodont. Res., Suppl. 1, Abst. No. 18, 1967.

Bernier, J. L., et al.: A Comparison of three oral hygiene measures. J. Periodontol., *37*:267, 1966.

Bhaskar, S. J., Cutright, D. E., and Frisch, J.: Effect of high pressure water jet on oral mucosa of varied density. J. Periodontol., *40*:593, 1969.

Cantor, M. T., and Stahl, S. S.: The effects of various interdental stimulators upon the keratinization of the interdental col. Periodontics, *3*:243, 1965.

Carlson, J., and Egelberg, J.: Effect of diet on the early plaque formation in man. Odontol. Revy, *16*:112, 1965.

Charters, W. J.: Proper home care of the mouth. J. Periodontol. *19*:136, 1948.

Chasens, A. I., and Marcus, R. W.: An evaluation of the comparative efficiency of manual and automatic toothbrushes in maintaining the periodontium. J. Periodontol., *39*:156, 1968.

Clark, J. W., Cheraskin, E. M., and Ringsdorf, W. M.: An ecologic study of oral hygiene. J. Periodontol., *40*:476, 1969.

Crumley, P. J., and Sumner, C. F.: Effectiveness of a water pressure cleansing device. Periodontics, *3*:193, 1965.

Curtis, G. H., McCall, C. M., and Overaa, H. I.: A clinical study of the effectiveness of the roll and Charters methods of brushing teeth. J. Periodontol., *28*:277, 1957.

Derbyshire, J. C.: Methods of effective hygiene of the mouth. Dent. Clin. North Am., March 1964, p. 231.

Derbyshire, J. C.: Patient motivation in periodontics. J. Periodontol., *41*:630, 1967.

Derbyshire, J. C., O'Leary, T. J., and Robinson, E. K.: How patients are taught to practice effective oral hygiene. J. West. Soc. Periodont., *16*:98, 1968.

Di Orio, L., and Madsen, K.: Patient education. Dent. Clin. North Am., *15*:905, 1971.

Egelberg, J.: The local effect of diet on plaque formation and development of gingivitis in dogs. I. Effect of soft and hard diets. II. Effect of frequency of meals and tube feeding. Odontol. Revy, *16*:31, 50, 1965.

Ferris, R. T., and Winslow, E. K.: Reinforcing desired behavior with periodontal patients. Dent. Clin. North Am., *14*:279, 1970.

Fones, A. C.: Home Care of the Mouth. Philadelphia, Lea & Febiger, 1934.

Frandsen, A. M., et al.: The effectiveness of Charters, roll and scrub methods of toothbrushing by professionals in removing plaque. Scand. J. Dent. Res., *78*:459, 1970.

Glickman, I., Petralis, R., and Marke, R.: The effect of powered toothbrushing and interdental stimulation upon microscopic inflammation and surface keratinization of the interdental gingiva. J. Periodontol., *35*:519, 1964.

Hall, W. B.: A basic change in toothbrushing technique is coming. Oregon Dent. J., *34*:2, 1964.

Hazen, S. P.: One and three day calculus formation. Program Abstracts Int. Assoc. Dent. Res., *39*:709, 1960.

Hein, J. W.: A study of the effect of frequency of toothbrushing on oral health. J. Dent. Res., *33*:708, 1954.

Hine, M. K., Wachtl, C., and Fosdick, L. S.: Some observations on the cleansing effect of nylon and bristle toothbrushes. J. Periodontol., 25:183, 1954.

Hirschfield, I.: The Toothbrush—Its Use and Abuse. Brooklyn, New York, Dental Items of Interest Publishing Co., 1939.

Hoover, D. R., and Robinson, H. B. G.: Effect of automatic and hand tooth brushing on gingivitis. J. Am. Dent. Assoc., 65:361, 1962.

Hoover, D. R., and Robinson, H. B.: The comparative effectiveness of the Water Pic in non-instructed population. J. Periodontol., 42:37, 1971.

Horton, J. E., Zimmerman, E. R., and Collings, C. K.: Effect of toothbrushing frequency on periodontal disease measurements. J. Periodontol., 40:14, 1969.

Kinery, M. J., and Stallard, R. E.: The evolutionary development and contemporary utilization of various oral hygiene procedures. J. West. Soc. Periodontol., 16:90, 1968.

Koch, G., and Lindhe, J.: The effect of supervised oral hygiene on the gingiva of children: The effect of tooth brushing. Odontol. Revy, 16:327, 1965.

Krajewski, J.: Current status of water pressure cleansing. J. Col. Dent. Assoc., 42:433, 1966.

Larato, D. C., et al.: The effect of a prescribed method of tooth brushing on the fluctuation of marginal gingivits. J. Periodontol., 40:142, 1969.

Lefkowitz, W., and Robinson, H. B. G.: Effectiveness of automatic and hand brushes in removing dental plaque and debris. J. Am. Dent. Assoc., 62:351, 1962.

Leonard, H. J.: Is massage a valuable treatment in gingivitis and periodontitis? J. Periodontol. 19:63, 1948.

Lightner, L. M., et al.: The periodontal status of incoming Airforce Academy Cadets. USAF School of Aerospace Medicine. SAM-TR-66 August, 1966.

Lilienthal, B., Amerena, V., and Gregory, G.: An epidemiological study of chronic periodontal disease. Arch. Oral Biol., 10:553, 1965.

Lindhe, J., and Koch, G.: The effect of supervised oral hygiene on the gingiva of children; the effect of toothbrushing. J. Periodontol. Res., 1:260, 1966.

Lindhe, J., and Koch, G.: The effect of supervised oral hygiene on the gingiva of children: Lack of a prolonged effect of supervision. J. Periodontol. Res., 2:215, 1967.

Lobene, R. R.: Evaluation of altered gingival health from permissive powered toothbrushing. J. Am. Dent. Soc., 69:585, 1964.

Lobene, R. R.: The effect of a pulsed water pressure cleansing device on oral health. J. Periodontol., 40:667, 1967.

Löe, H.: A review of the prevention and control of plaque. In Dental Plaque. W. D. McHugh, Ed. Edinburgh, E. and S. Livingstone, Ltd., 1970, p. 259.

Löe, H., and Rindom-Schiöt, C.: The effect of suppression of the oral microflora upon the development of dental plaque and gingivitis. In Dental Plaque. W. D. McHugh, Ed. Edinburgh, E. and S. Livingstone, Ltd., 1970, p. 247.

Lövdal, A., Arno, A., and Waerhaug, J.: Clinical manifestations of periodontal disease in light of oral hygiene and calculus formation. J. Am. Dent. Soc., 50:21, 1958.

Lövdal, A., et al.: Combined effect of subgingival scaling

and controlled oral hygiene on the incidence of gingivitis. Acta Odontol. Scand., 19:537, 1961.

Manhold, J.: Hand versus powered brushing. J. Periodontol., 38:23, 1967.

Maslow, A. H.: Motivation and Personality. New York, Harper and Row, 1954.

Massler, M., et al.: Gingivitis in young adult males; lack of effectiveness of a permissive program of tooth brushing. J. Periodontol., 28:111, 1957.

Masters, D. H.: Oral hygiene procedures for the periodontal patient. Dent. Clin. North Am., 13:3, 1969.

Maurice, C. G., and Wallace, D. A.: Toothbrush effectiveness: relative cleansing ability of four toothbrushes of different design. Ill. Dent. J., 26:286, 1967.

McClure, D. B.: A comparison of tooth brushing techniques for the preschool child. J. Dent. Child., 33:205, 1966.

O'Leary, T. J.: Patient motivation in oral hygiene. J. So. Calif. Dent. Assoc., 36:455, 1968.

O'Leary, T. J., and Nabors, C. L.: Instructions to supplement teaching oral hygiene. J. Periodontol., 40:27, 1969.

O'Leary, T. J.: Oral hygiene agents and procedures. J. Periodontol., 41:625, 1970.

O'Leary, T. J., Drake, R. B., and Naylor, J. E.: The plaque control record. J. Periodontol., 43:38, 1972.

Parfitt, G. J.: Cleansing the subgingival space. J. Periodontol., 34:133, 1963.

Rodda, J. C.: A comparison for four methods of toothbrushing. New Zeal. Dent. J., 64:162, 1968.

Selipsky, H. L., Ammons, W. F., and Yuodelis, R. A.: The effect of periodontal therapy upon tooth mobility: III. Osseous surgery and plaque control. Program and Abstract 50th General Meeting IADR Abs. No. 552, 1972.

Silness, J., and Löe, H.: Periodontal disease in pregnancy. II. Correlation between oral hygiene and periodontal condition. Acta Odontol. Scand., 22:112, 1964.

Starkey, P.: A study of four methods of presenting dental health information to patients. J. Dent. Child., 29:11, 1962.

Stillman, P. R.: A philosophy of the treatment of periodontal disease. Dent. Dig., 38:215, 1932.

Sumnicht, R. W.: Research in preventive dentistry. J. Am. Dent. Assoc., 79:193, 1969.

Suomi, J. D., et al.: The effect of controlled oral hygiene procedures on the progression of periodontal disease in adults. J. Periodontol., 42:152, 1971.

Toto, P. D., and Farchione, A.: Clinical evaluation of an electrically powered toothbrush in home periodontal therapy. J. Periodontol., 32:249, 1961.

Toto, P. D., Rapp, G. W., and Goljon, K. R.: The effect of manual and mechanical tooth brushing on oral hygiene caries and conduciveness and pH of the oral cavity. J. Oral Ther. Pharm., 1:612, 1965.

Wilcox, C. E., and Everett, F. G.: Friction on the teeth and the gingiva during mastication. J. Am. Dent. Assoc., 66:515, 1963.

Winslow, E. K., and Ferris, R. T.: Developing desired patient behavior. Dent. Clin. North Amer., 14:269, 1970.

Zaki, H. A., and Bandt, C. L.: Model presentation and reinforcement, an effective method of teaching oral hygiene skills. J. Periodontol., 41:394, 1970.

16

Initial Therapy—
Curettage Techniques

The irritating effect of plaque, calculus, and food debris in various stages of decomposition has been universally observed. Only a few years ago, many workers in the field believed that calculus was the prime etiologic factor in inflammatory periodontal disease and pocket formation. Today we do not quite accept the validity of this concept, but there is no question that calculus and other accretions are associated with periodontitis and that their removal from the crowns and roots of the teeth commonly permits an improvement in the condition of the gingiva. Plaque, of course, has been fairly well established as the basic irritational factor in initiating the lesions of inflammatory periodontal disease. Calculus, with its rough and irritating surface, provides an excellent nidus for plaque formation and retention.

Traditionally, debriding techniques have been divided into two general procedures, (1) coronal scaling and polishing, and (2) subgingival curettage.

DEFINITION OF TERMS

The terms *scaling* and *subgingival curettage* require definition, primarily because of a rather loose usage of the terms. *Scaling* means the splitting or prying of scale from a surface. It connotes a rather forcible though controlled action of a sharp steel instrument designed for the purpose, which is called a scaler. *Curettage* refers to shaving or scraping performed with spoon-shaped instruments called curets. Root curettage in this text means the use of a curet on the root of the tooth. Subgingival curettage means that the curet is used under the gingiva upon the root or upon the sulcular surface of the overlying gingiva. To avoid ambiguity, this text will use the terms *root curettage*, *gingival curettage*, or *subgingival curettage* in the sense of the definitions given above. The line of demarcation between these methods is not clearly drawn, and there is a tendency toward some overlap, but as a large generality the division serves well enough to be useful.

CORONAL SCALING AND POLISHING

The procedure of coronal scaling and polishing is one of the most widely applied techniques in all of dentistry. Practically every routine dental procedure is begun or ended with a cleaning. So common has this technique become that much of the time of the dental hygienist has been devoted to its performance.

Coronal scaling, as its name implies, consists of the removal of accretions from the clinical crowns of the teeth with some extension of effort to the subgingival area immediately apical to the marginal and papillary

16
Initial
Therapy—
Curettage
Techniques

gingiva. Logically enough, the instruments used are scalers of various shapes and some heavy curets which are used as scalers.

Zander has described four modes whereby calculus attaches to the root.[19] They are (1) by a cuticle, (2) by irregularities in the root surface, (3) with some penetration of calculus into the cemental defects and gaps, and (4) into rather sizable resorption bays into the cementum and dentin.

With varying types of attachment comes a variation in the ease or difficulty of removal. For this reason instruments of differing shape, purpose, size, delicacy, and application have been introduced into the armamentarium. Since debridement is the basic method of treatment and is the oldest of all techniques, it is not surprising that an extraordinarily large number of sets of instruments have been introduced. Most of these sets have not adequately met the test of time and of continued use, so that there has been a constant attrition of their number and complexity. One set of scalers (the Carr set) contained nearly 150 instruments (all hoes), which were shaped and designed to be applied to every variant of every root surface in the arch. Needless to say, this set had few devotees. However extreme this set may be, it is interesting to note that present-day instruments have been drastically reduced both in the number of sets available and in the number of instruments offered in each set.

Most therapists mix sets to suit personal preferences and do not use complete sets as their single armamentarium. Some schools assemble sets under their special issue and name for convenience, but there are, nonetheless, basically two general types: (1) scalers which are scaling or splitting instruments, and (2) curets which are basically scrapers or shavers. Each of these general types has a number of modifications, some of which do not seem to resemble the prototype until use and action are examined critically.

Scalers

Scalers are the most varied instruments. They include (1) pick scalers, (2) chisels, (3) hoe scalers, and (4) files (Fig. 16-1).

PICK SCALERS

These instruments take their name from their general appearance. They are sickle-shaped (sickle scalers); hook-shaped with a fairly straight blade, some with right and left application for proximal use (Jacquette scalers); and some that are simple picks with a universal application. They all have certain characteristics in common. They use as a scaling or splitting edge one of the three or four angled edges that they present because of their rectangular or triangular cross sections. Pick scalers are used in either a pull or push motion, using any and all available edges. They are applied at the base of a flake of calculus where it is attached to the root or to the crown of the tooth and are directed to splitting or scaling off a large mass of calculus. The tip of the instrument is slipped under the free gingiva to engage a heavy flake of calculus and, with a vigorous but controlled coronal stroke, the calculus is removed. The Jacquette scalers are particularly applicable to the posterior teeth because of the angles of the necks.

The extent to which such a scaler can be inserted subgingivally is limited by the amount of tissue displacement possible—usually not very much. Because they are coronal in application, root scarring is minimal with these instruments. The same cannot be said, however, for possible gingival laceration. Some care is necessary in the application of the scaler so that the tip or point does not engage the gingiva.

CHISELS

The periodontal chisel occupies a small though important position in the armamentarium. The straight or slightly bent chisel is an old and useful instrument for the rapid and easy dislodgement of calculus sometimes found in heavy masses on the interproximal and lingual surfaces of lower anterior teeth. A carefully controlled push stroke will split and loosen the calculus.

HOE SCALERS

These venerable warriors in periodontal therapy are, as the name suggests, hoe-shaped in that the distal millimeter is bent at right angles to the face of the instrument to form a sharp right-angled cutting edge for the dislodgement of calculus. The hoe scalers are designed with shanks so bent that the instrument may be applied directly to four surfaces of the teeth. This means that most sets of hoes consist of four instruments. There are, however, still some sets of hoes that are designed to fit line angles and to offer some less acutely angled instruments more comfortably applied to anterior teeth.

The hoe is a most useful instrument when properly used and the most dangerous when carelessly applied. Because these instruments have relatively small heads and long shanks, they can be slipped subgingivally in molar pockets to almost the entire extent of the pocket. Molar gingival margins are more flaccid than are those of smaller teeth. Lingual pockets are particularly receptive to the insertion of a hoe, although all

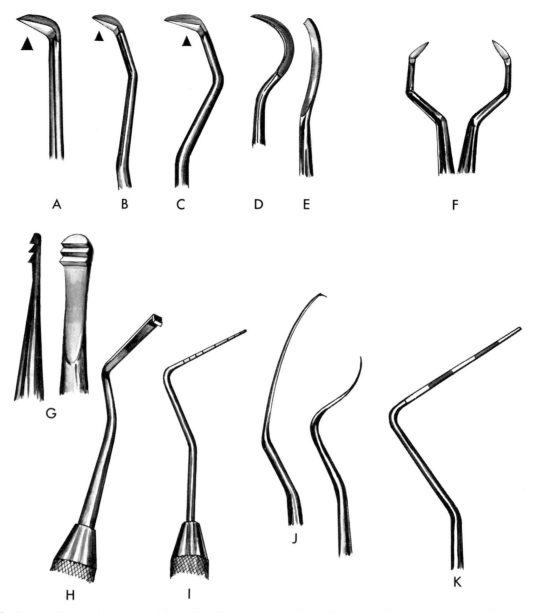

FIG. 16-1. *Scalers, probes, and explorers. A, B, and C. Standard pick scalers with a triangular cross section. D. Sickle scaler with a rectangular cross section. E. The periodontal chisel. F. Jacquette scalers, right and left versions. G. Periodontal files. H. The hoe scaler. I. The Michigan "O" periodontal probe with the Williams scoring. J. Two explorers useful in some aspects of the periodontal examination such as furcal exploring and caries examination. K. The Marquis probe which is designed to facilitate reading pocket depth because of alternating bands of 3 mm in width.*

pockets can be treated by them at times. This property of the hoe makes for a peculiarly useful instrument, in spite of its very real limitations. The hoe has two sharp angles which may groove and cut a root if the blades are slightly tilted. Since the head of the instrument is lost to direct view when it is introduced into a pocket, the operator must be especially careful in using the instrument subgingivally. This is of very real concern. The usefulness and drawbacks of the hoe will be dealt with in greater detail under instrumentation.

FILES

Periodontal files are in a more or less equivocal position in the armamentarium. They are made in all the standard instrument inclinations—facial, lingual, distal, and mesial. Scalers are generally considered to be coarse and powerful instruments designed for heavy duty of a primarily supragingival nature. A file is a series of hoelike blades arranged in an instrument head to present its working face to the root surface. It is designed for only the finest work, in sharp contrast to other scalers, and because of its size, the smallest and flattest of all periodontal instruments other than the probe, it is most easily introduced into pockets having tight marginal gingiva.

Its use is restricted by the difficulty of sharpening it and its lack of transmission of tactile impression of the character of the root. It does not yield any information on smoothness or roughness to the therapist. It has, however, its uses and applications which cannot be quite met by any other instrument and is a valuable adjunct.

Ultrasonic Scaling Device

With the introduction of ultrasound into dentistry in 1953, primarily for cavity preparation, it was inevitable that its use would be extended to debridement. In 1957, Johnson and Wilson, among others, reported on the effective use of a specially designed ultrasonic instrument in scaling teeth. It might be of interest to note that this scaling instrument was the only ultrasonic instrument to survive in dental instrumentation.

The effectiveness of the instrument depends upon the constant flow of water which cools the blunt working tip, in addition to providing part of the force in the dislodgement of calculus. Because of the prime necessity of the water irrigant and the attendant bulk of the apparatus it becomes impossible to use the principle of ultrasonic debridement subgingivally. The enormous heat generated precludes the use of such an instrument without water. The tips of the ultrasonic scaler are also necessarily crude, when compared with a fine, slender curet.

These factors more or less limit the ultrasonic scaler to coronal scaling and to open flap curettage where it is an effective tool. The water coolant acts as a flushing mechanism which clears the field visually. It is a fine, time-saving device for removing gross supragingival calculus, no matter how tenaciously attached, stain, and even subgingival calculus to a limited distance from the margin of the sulcus. Anything deeper into the sulcus must be removed with finer instruments unless flaps are reflected. For this reason, the ultrasonic device should be classified as a scaler and not as a specific instrument used in or capable of total debridement.

Some periodontists use ultrasonic scalers to debride the roots of teeth in the surgical field after gingival flaps have been reflected and the root has been exposed to the level of crestal bone investment. With good aspiration this can be an effective instrument in debridement of roots. The ultrasonic scaler is obviously just as effective in this clinical situation as in any supragingival scaling procedure.

Curets

Curets are the basic periodontal instruments. Over the years they have been refined to an extremely high degree. Basically a curet is a spoon-shaped scraping instrument and its principal use is the same whether it is used on bone, soft tissue, cementum, or ligament (Fig. 16-2). It is used to debride the tissue or tissues upon which it is applied. Through many decades of trial and error, the curet has been firmly established as the ideal general purpose instrument for subgingival debridement. In fact, the entire procedure is called subgingival curettage for this reason. The curet is clearly superior to the hoe and file for subgingival debridement. For example, the hoe cannot reach quite to the deepest point of the pocket because of the dimension of the cutting edge. Fluting in the roots of some teeth presents serious problems to such an instrument on two counts: (1) the fluting may be bridged by the hoe and the deepest portion may be left untouched; and (2) there is danger of root damage in any tilting or angling of the hoe to reach the recess in the root. The curet also is far better adapted to general subgingival use than is the file, which is limited in use and is not a sensitive indicator of the condition of the root.

The question may well be asked, if the curet is so overwhelmingly superior to any other instrument for subgingival debridement, why is any other type of instrument needed? Experience provides the answer to this question. The restricted confines of the periodontal pocket frequently make the use of a small instrument necessary (Fig. 16-3). Curets, which are small and delicate, are ideally suited to shaving and scraping the root surface to render it smooth and clean. It is, however, not uncommon to find calculus accretions subgingivally that are tenaciously attached to the root surface or even locked to the root by invasion of resorption bays and other irregularities in surface characteristics. The inevitable dilemma encountered here of a flake of calculus requiring a powerful instrument for its removal, in confines admitting only delicate curets, is nicely resolved by the use of a hoe to deliver the calculus in a large piece or, in even more restricted space, by the use of the file to crush the large deposit of calculus so that the fragments may be removed by finer instruments.

Curets, however, are basic and are used in various sizes for various purposes. Heavy curets are well suited for supragingival scaling and fine curets for application

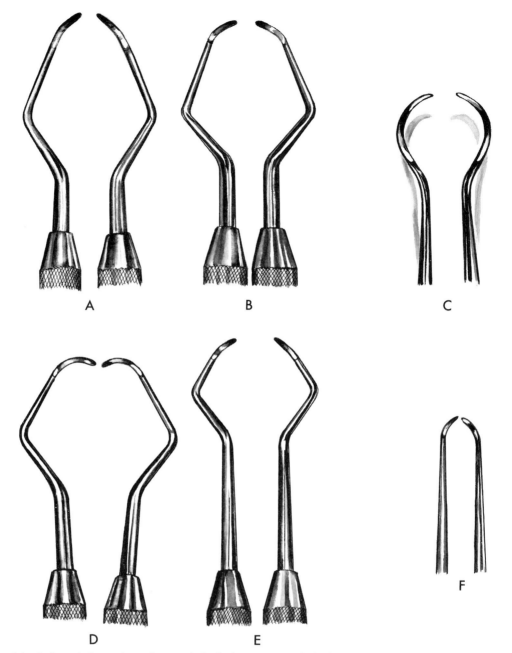

FIG. 16-2. *A useful set of curets for root curettage, subgingival curettage and gingival curettage. A. McCall's 2R and 2L primarily for use on anterior teeth. B. McCall's 4R and 4L for use on premolars and molars. C. McCall's 17 and 18 for circumferential curettage and especially useful on lingual and facial surfaces of posterior teeth. D. Gracey 11 and 12 and E. Gracy 7 and 8 with blades angled so that they are effective with a push and pull motion. F. Hutchinson 1 and 2 especially for labial surfaces in deep narrow pockets of anterior teeth.*

subgingivally. In fact, a useful and well-designed set of curets introduced by the late Dr. Clayton Gracey may be used in both pull and push motions to good effect. Generally, however, curets are used with a pull motion, that is to say, the working blade is carefully inserted to the depth of the pocket and is applied to the root firmly in a coronal stroke.

INSTRUMENTATION

The basic techniques in the application of the various instruments are essentially (1) scaling or splitting of calculus from its attachment to the root and (2) shaving and scraping to render the root smooth. Although scaling is performed with some controlled power, cu-

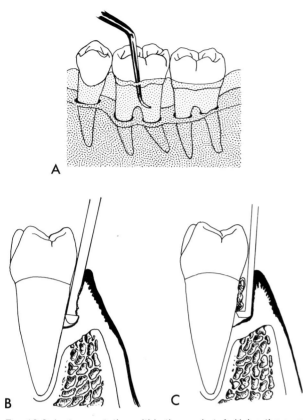

FIG. 16-3. *Instrumentation within the pocket. A. Using the curet in an exploratory stroke to find root roughness and to explore the intrasulcular topography. B. The curet inserted into the deeper recesses of the periodontal pocket. Note that the soft tissue or gingival wall of the pocket is distended by the curet and lies against it in the working stroke. It can be seen that some gingival curettage is attendant on root curettage. C. A hoe scaler inserted subgingivally to engage a mass of calculus. Note that the instrument cannot reach the base of the pocket because of the shape and dimension of its blade.*

rettage is executed with even more control and with a conscious effort to evaluate the condition of the root by tactile means alone. It is for this reason that the two classes of instruments differ somewhat in application and will be considered separately.

Scaling

Scaling consists of the rather forcible removal of visible or easily discovered calculus. It usually, but not always, connotes the removal of considerable masses of calculus, particularly subgingival calculus.

INSTRUMENT GRASP

The scaler is held in a modified pen grasp, which differs from a simple pen grasp mainly by the position of the middle finger on the handle of the instrument. The distal phalanx of the middle finger engages the handle of the instrument on the medial aspect of its tip instead of folding under the pen in the usual writing position (Fig. 16-4). This grasp provides maximum control of the instrument and brings to bear an additional fingertip for increased tactile acuity.

This same finger position is used in both scaling and curettage. It minimizes fatigue from cramped finger positions and conveys maximum tactile sensation from the handle. It must be kept in mind that instrumentation such as this may be performed over extremely long periods—several consecutive hours on a number of patients is common—and such factors as fatigue and finger cramp are of considerable importance. Fatigue is one of the major factors in reducing tactile sensitivity.

FINGER REST

The finger rest is basic to the efficient application of an instrument. In scaling and curettage the rest is somewhat more flexible than it would be in the use of operative instruments, since the usual pull stroke of the instrument is less hazardous than is the usual push stroke used in operative dentistry, but its importance in attaining leverage will be obvious at the outset.

The use of a third finger rest on the teeth is standard (Fig. 16-5). The middle finger rest allows for more power but a more restricted arc of motion and some reduction in tactile sensitivity. There are, however, variations on this anchor. The third finger is used when the curet blade must be somewhat removed from the finger rest. It must be kept in mind that in scaling and curettage the range of effort is an extremely wide one. The operator almost never limits his efforts to a single tooth. For this reason the establishment of a single rest is impossible, and each position of the hand in either of the arches will require a new anchor. Such constant shifting brings into play considerable innovation. A combination of the middle and third finger rest positions is a common expedient (Fig. 16-6).

SCALING MOTION

Much has been made in instrumentation of the rocking motion of the wrist and forearm, with the fingers relegated to a rather passive role of holding the instrument firmly. While the rocking motion is most useful, particularly in the forceful splitting of a tenacious flake of calculus, there is an accompanying contracture of the fingers that is particularly applicable in curettage. Far from causing fatigue, it relaxes the muscles of the

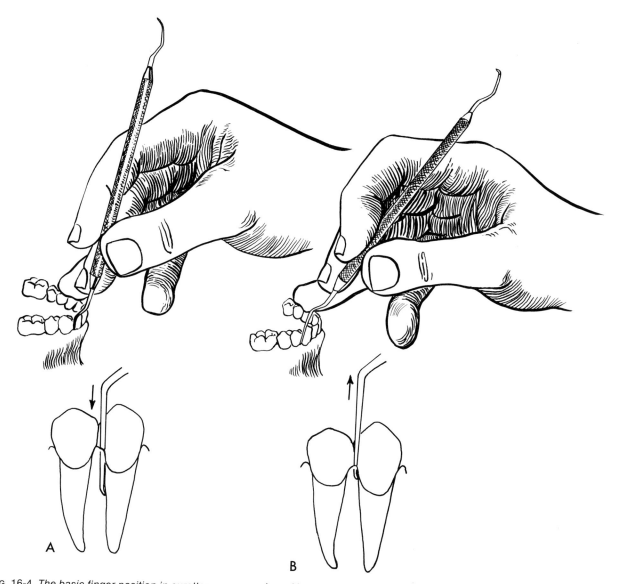

FIG. 16-4. *The basic finger position in curettage, commonly and incorrectly referred to as the pen grasp. The instrument is held with medial side of middle or third fingertip as the stabilizing element in curettage. A. Instrument insertion. This is done in a gentle probing manner to the base of the pocket. B. The basic curetting working or power stroke. Note the contracture of the fingers, which hold the instrument firmly during the rocking motion of the wrist and forearm.*

fingers as only movement can. In addition, considerable tactile acuity is present in a pure finger stroke that is absent to a degree in the rocking motion.

Curettage

Scaling and curettage are frequently similar in approach and application. There are some differences, however, in the use of the curet. The basic curetting procedure begins with the insertion of the curet into the pocket and with a long light stroke—an exploratory stroke to be precise—the character of the root surface is determined, the shape and extent of the pocket is delineated, and the topography of the calcu-

lus, if present, is noted. Palpable masses of calculus are then dislodged and removed with short powerful strokes. The calculus removed, the stroke is now longer and is a distinctly shaving motion, smoothing the root surface so that there are no zones of smooth and rough cementum. It is in this phase of curettage that the texture of the root surface may be sensed via the instrument from the contracture of the grasping fingers.

Much has been made of this tactile sensitivity, since it is the only sensory means by which results from the effort expended can be evaluated. Such sensitivity is definitely not present in the power or working stroke. It is definitely present when the stroke is exploratory and self-consciously an evaluating one. It is a common

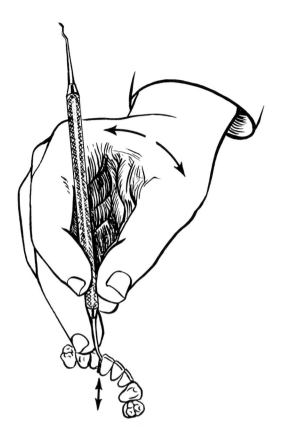

FIG. 16-5. *The middle finger used as a rest.*

error, unfortunately widespread, to limit the curetting stroke to the wrist-rocking working stroke.

Flexibility of approach is most helpful. Rigidity in method has a way of making curettage mechanical and ineffective.

THE CIRCUMFERENTIAL STROKE

Of equal importance is the flexibility that permits the use of the curet in a circumferential direction. This approach is particularly useful in certain instances (Fig. 16-7).

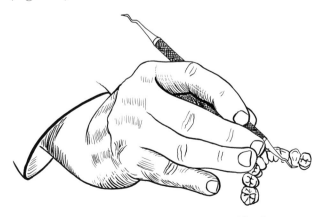

FIG. 16-6. *Middle and third finger rest in combination.*

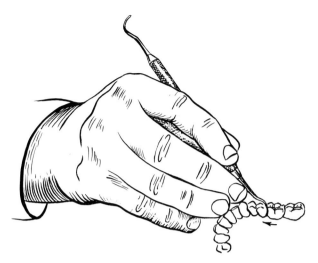

FIG. 16-7. *The circumferential stroke in curettage.*

1. When there is a metal proximal restoration in the tooth, repeated encounters with the blade used with a vertical stroke dull the instrument without accomplishing the objective.
2. Line angles are finished with more control in a circumferential stroke.
3. In deep pockets, the long vertical stroke frequently leaves small islands of calculus cervically, particularly on the interproximal root surfaces. A horizontal circumferential stroke is an excellent adjunct to a vertical stroke in these situations.
4. The horizontal stroke following a series of vertical strokes is an effective expedient in achieving a smooth root surface.

Particularly well-adapted to the circumferential stroke are the McCall's #17 and #18 curets. Other curets may be used.

EVALUATION OF EFFORT

While coronal scaling is relatively easy to judge, since it may be evaluated visually, subgingival curettage, on the other hand, can be checked only by tactile response to exploration. A sharp curet serves this purpose well. Some therapists use a sharp explorer to perform this task. A particularly effective calculus explorer is available in an old curet that has been sharpened to the degree that it is too thin to perform effectively. In this condition, however, it serves better than any other instrument in negotiating a root surface to judge smoothness. It is an error to discard these instruments as useless.

In the final analysis, the response of the gingiva is the essential evaluation of effort, but before this is discussed other important aspects of curettage that affect tissue response should be examined.

GINGIVAL CURETTAGE

Each stroke of subgingival curettage that is *directed* solely at root curettage has as an inevitable consequence curettage of the lining of sulcular tissue by the offset blade of the curet. Some misconception of the relationship of the soft-tissue side of the pocket to the root surface may be prevalent because of the universal practice of regarding the pocket as a *space* between a root and overlying tissue. This convention is reproduced in drawings and illustrative diagrams. There is, however, no actual space. There is merely *detachment*. The overlying soft tissue lies against the root surface, and the introduction of even the finest curet into the pocket distends and displaces it. The curetting stroke directed toward the root also affects the lining of the sulcus because the curet blade has two edges. Gingival curettage is, then, unavoidable as a standard by-product of root curettage. There is little doubt that part of the response of gingiva to curettage is due to the removal of some sulcular epithelial lining incident to the procedure.

Having stated this, we can then proceed to render an opinion on a widespread practice of gingival curettage; that is, the use of the curet specifically on the lining of the sulcular tissue as a separate excursion under local anesthesia. Many skilled therapists perform this extra step which, we believe, might be better accomplished, if deemed advisable, by simple surgical excision, using an internal bevel procedure throughout the mouth. There are several reasons for this opinion:

1. There are neither visual nor tactile criteria for accomplishment. Visual examination of the lining tissue by reflected flap yields no information whatever, and to the eye no difference is discernible between curetted and uncuretted tissue.

2. Tissue stabilization is unreliable in many areas. The finger may be used on buccal and lingual aspects, but proximal tissue is difficult to stabilize. Perforation of gingiva by the toe of the curet is not uncommon.

3. Therapy is needlessly protracted by making this procedure a standard part of treatment planning. The results obtained do not justify, in our opinion, the time expended on this practice.

This position on gingival curettage as a separate and general procedure does not preclude its use in sharply restricted areas, such as in the gingiva of a single tooth. There are sometimes good reasons to avoid surgery in such an area, and there is widespread clinical opinion that a low-grade, indolent inflammatory nidus can exist within the corium. Repeated curettage of the gingiva results in a scarring down of the tissue and in a generally acceptable result in the area. This approach cannot, however, be logically extended to include the total gingiva as a general procedure.

TISSUE RESPONSE TO CORONAL SCALING AND CURETTAGE

The various debridement techniques are so basic to therapy and have been so widely used for so long that it is natural for many differing opinions on the response of the tissues to this therapy to exist. Observation will reveal that skillful and complete debridement yields certain unmistakable benefits (Fig. 16-8):

1. Remission from inflammation, edema, and exudation.
2. Recapture of lost form insofar as it is possible for the tissues to shrink.

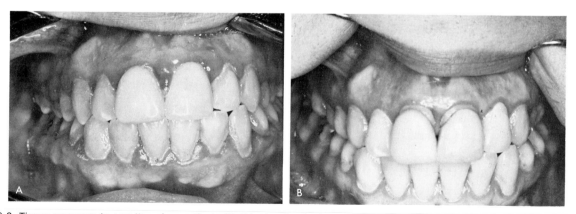

Fig. 16-8. *Tissue response to curettage in a patient with thin, fragile gingiva. A. Preoperative view. Note that the gingiva is enlarged by edema. B. Postoperative view. Debridement resulted in shrinkage. Since there was little or no fibrotic content in the gingiva, shrinkage resulted in a complete remission from inflammation with no residual enlargement. Note that there is a persistent marginal gingivitis in the labial gingiva of the lower anterior teeth and the upper left lateral incisor and canine. Accretions of retained plaque can be clearly seen. Gingivae as thin and as delicate as these are extremely responsive to irritational factors.*

CURETTAGE IN PRESURGICAL PREPARATION OF THE TISSUES

Coronal scaling and subgingival curettage are most extensively used, perhaps, in debriding the crowns and roots of the teeth preparatory to entering a surgical phase of therapy. The reasons lie in the response of gingiva to scaling and curettage, especially when gingival enlargements are mainly the result of edema (Fig. 16-9). Fibrotic changes in older lesions sometimes preclude a total response in the recapture of normal form.

When calculus is present in varying amounts in both supragingival and subgingival locations, the gingiva responds with the classic reaction of chronic inflammation. Inflammation, edema, loss of tonus, exudation, and bleeding on slight manipulation are the common clinical manifestations encountered. Sometimes the inflammation is so generalized that tissue delineation between gingiva and mucosa is difficult.

Assuming that a surgical approach is deemed inevitable because of a variety of factors, presurgical curettage is useful for a number of reasons.

1. The tissue responds favorably to curettage. Shrinkage, resolution of edema and exudation, a return to normal color values, and diminution of bleeding all occur and collectively aid in determining areas that must be corrected by surgery and those that may be resolved by conservative means.
2. Morphologic features in the gingiva and mucosa are more clearly delineated after inflammation has been resolved.
3. Surgery may be performed in a relatively clean field devoid of calculus and plaque.
4. Gingiva is firm to the scalpel and is of good texture to be beveled or split as required.
5. Bleeding from surgery is definitely less than it would be in an inflamed gingiva.
6. Exuberant granulation tissue is rarely present postoperatively.
7. The interval required for its performance provides an insight into the patient's management of brushing and stimulation.

The standards of achievement in presurgical curettage are high, but they are not so demanding as those striven for in *definitive curettage* (Fig. 16-10). The necessary tissue response must be forthcoming so that essentially the roots must be relatively calculus-free. Gingiva that is coarsely grained, stippled, and thick because of fibrotic content will not respond as dramatically to debridement.

If, in reflecting the gingiva and mucosa to perform the periodontal surgery, a remnant of calculus is nestled in a furca, no great failure of effort is implied or felt (Fig. 16-11). Tissue response and field debridement are the principal aims of the operator. For this reason, a zonal approach to a presurgical curettage is practical and preferred. That is, a quadrant-by-quadrant performance is completed, with each area completely curetted and not to be redone (Fig. 16-12).

DEFINITIVE CURETTAGE

A small but significant number of patients are best treated with *subgingival curettage as the total method* insofar as soft tissue management is concerned. In other words, only curettage is to be used and all surgical procedures are to be avoided. These patients fall generally into three types:

1. Patients who are psychologically unable to accept surgery and excisional techniques. These patients have a right to whatever help the periodontist can provide within the limits imposed by the illness of the patient. Periodontists habitually trim therapeutic sails to adapt to the patient's infirmity—from blood dyscrasias to grand mal or cardiovascular disease. Psychic illness is no exception and should be treated in the same fashion. It must be remembered that we are not

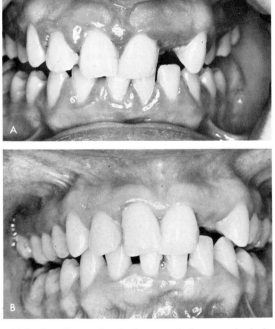

FIG. 16-9. *Curettage of anterior area before surgical phase. A. Precurettage showing enlargement of gingiva from edema. B. Postcurettage view. Shrinkage of gingiva and changes in color, form, and tonus are clearly shown as a result of debridement. Such a response may be expected in gingival enlargements that are mainly the result of edema.*

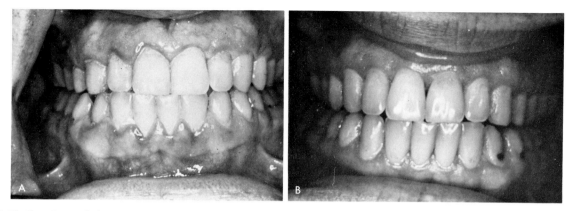

FIG. 16-10. *Curettage of gingivae that are coarsely grained and stippled and thicker because of fibrotic content in its connective tissue. A. Preoperative view. B. Postcurettage view. The response is not dramatic, but there are resolution from edema and shrinkage to the extent of the enlargement originally due to edema.*

engaged in a life-and-death struggle with disease. Our area of effort affords some electives.

2. Patients with an active caries proclivity that persists into middle age. It will be seen in later chapters on periodontal surgery that most pockets are eliminated by achieving a selective recession. This means that the result of excisional surgical therapy is measurable root exposure. In a mouth which is caries-prone it will serve the patient poorly to save the teeth from periodontal disease only to lose them to root caries. For some reason, caries within the sulcus is practically unknown. The obvious rational approach to such a problem is to treat the disease with definitive curettage.

3. In mouths so ravaged by periodontal destruction that every tooth in an arch is involved with extremely deep pockets, the elimination of which would cause excessive root exposure and a sacrifice of supporting tissues which the patient could not afford. In other words, bone may be reshaped to help eliminate pockets if there is sufficient bone to be reshaped and still leave enough to fulfill its supportive role. If not enough bone is present, then hopeless teeth should be extracted and the arch should be restored. If, however, in considering extraction and in the automatic search for an abutment none is suitable, a serious decision must be made—either all the teeth in the arch will be sacrificed or they will be retained. If they are kept, then the only therapeutic method left is definitive curettage. Curettage in many of these cases is surprisingly successful (Fig. 16-13).

In Chapter 21 on surgical method, it will be noted that excision techniques, that is, those procedures that achieve pocket elimination through establishment of a selective recession, are not well suited to very deep lesions. They do most for the patient with moderately extensive pockets. It is natural that as broad an attack be mounted on periodontal disease in its various forms as is possible. Definitive curettage is one of the most important weapons in this attack.

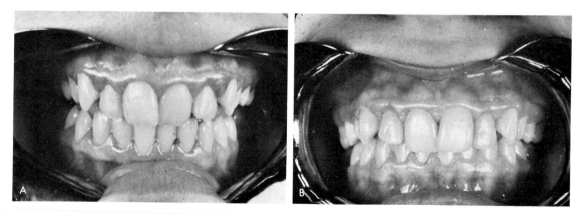

FIG. 16-11. *Curettage revealing an underlying linear marginal fibrosis due to mouth-breathing which was masked by edema preoperatively. A. Preoperative view. B. After subgingival curettage. Note that there has been a resolution of edema and a remission from inflammation, but there is some residual enlargement due to fibrotic changes.*

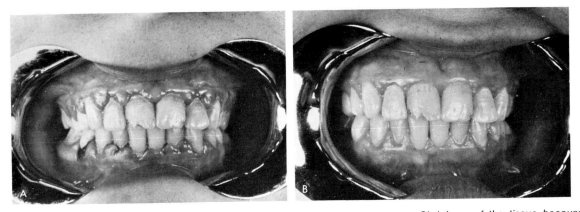

FIG. 16-12. *Curettage. A. Before subgingival curettage. B. After subgingival curettage. Shrinkage of the tissue because of a resolution of edema reveals an underlying fibrotic enlargement.*

TECHNIQUE FOR PERFORMING DEFINITIVE CURETTAGE. Because curettage in this context and application will constitute the central aspect in total therapy a different approach is required than is the case with presurgical curettage. No direct view of the subgingival area is possible for final correction. In a treatment plan calling for definitive curettage, surface texture and smoothness of all roots must be determined by tactile means. It is primarily for this reason that the single circuit approach is usually unsuitable.

Definitive curettage is best done by repeated circuits of the dentition. An attempt should be made to perform a complete circuit in a single visit and plan to repeat in subsequent visits until roots are smooth and not a single area of roughness can be found anywhere in the subgingival areas of the roots exposed by disease. Furcal notches are explored with sharp curets, and every square millimeter of root is carefully searched out in exploratory strokes for curetting.

As the circuits are made, it will be found that exploration is easier and more rewarding. Less and less

curetting is required and more and more exploring is possible. Fatigue—that old enemy of tactile acuity—has been eliminated as a factor.

Patient performance can be much more effectively monitored than in less searching methods. The tissues respond surprisingly well in many patients, and patients become imbued with missionary zeal.

Definitive curettage is not a time-saving expedient. The amount of time expended is roughly the same as that required for a surgical solution. But continuing curettage is sometimes necessary after surgery as well.

It would be a fine thing if periodontal methods were always successful and that no result less than complete cure was the reward for effort. In truth, however, results forthcoming from well-conceived treatment plans and skillful execution are generally successful, but residual pocket depth is not rare and some compromise is a common occurrence.

Both the residual pocket remaining after therapy and the compromise area require maintenance. This means frequent and skillful curettage, and without

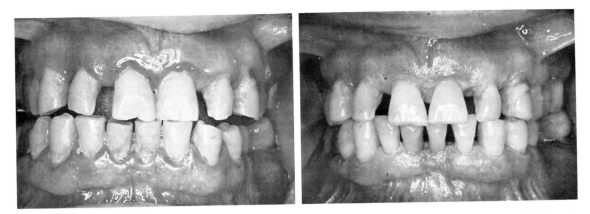

FIG. 16-13. *Curettage in a dentition with thick coarse gingiva. A. Before curettage. B. After curettage. The essential character of the gingiva has not changed, but pocket depth has been reduced.*

development of this basic method to a high degree, such effort is useless and frustrating to both patient and therapist.

PAIN CONTROL IN CURETTAGE

The use of local anesthetic with subgingival curettage is common, particularly with those operators using a quadrant approach. It is more difficult to use a local anesthetic with the repeated-circuit approach so common in definitive curettage. Some periodontists find nitrous oxide, inhalation analgesia, ideal for this purpose as well as for other procedures that are uncomfortable and unpleasant. Dressing changes, needle punctures in the palatal mucosa, removal of temporarily cemented bridges, and similar operations fall into this category. Intravenous analgesia is also used for these procedures, but is best suited to longer operations.

Most periodontists, however, do not require local anesthesia for definitive curettage. Care and delicacy in instrument insertion and use paying particular attention to instrument position so that the end of the curet or scaler does not gouge tissue, are, in the final analysis, the best assurance that pain will not be inflicted. It should be borne in mind that almost all pain in curettage and scaling is soft tissue pain and not root pain. Instrument choice is made on factors of tissue displacement, as well as on effectiveness in calculus removal.

ROOT SENSITIVITY

Root sensitivity is a varying and a common occurrence after curettage. While frequently attributed to root exposure incident to periodontal surgery, it is more often a sequel to curettage, particularly the variety of root sensitivity that is elicited by touch or by certain foods and sweets. The pain in these roots is acute and often excruciating, fortunately subsiding after the stimulus is withdrawn. This pain is always set off by contact of the instrument or chemical at the cementoenamel junction and rarely in more apical areas of an exposed root. Gingival recession is common, and these roots are rarely, if ever, sensitive.

There is another variety of root sensitivity that is sometimes found in newly exposed roots—thermal sensitivity. This type is no particular problem in management, since it gradually diminishes over a period of time; pulpal insulation occurs much like the similar phenomenon occurring with the insertion of metal restoration.

TREATMENT FOR ROOT SENSITIVITY. Unfortunately, no uniformly effective treatment for root sensitivity has yet been found, other than constant and repeated burnishing of the cervical area of the tooth with the toothbrush. This is more easily said than done because contact sets off the pain response. Yet, avoidance allows for the accretion of plaque which increases the sensitivity immeasurably. The patient frequently finds himself in a real dilemma.

There are a number of desensitizing agents available which are variably effective. The various fluorides have long been a favorite, with application on the dried root and burnishing in of the agent on the sensitive area. Prednisolone has been briefly used. Formaldehyde is perhaps the oldest chemical used. Hot glycerine is yet another. Ionization with fluorides has been recommended. Surgical cement dressing applied to the dried root and allowed to remain in contact with the root for a week is another in a long list of panaceas. It is usually true that when there are many remedies none is really specific. This is nowhere so true as in the treatment of root sensitivity.

There is an interesting sidelight on these remedies for root sensitivity. Each agent seems to work well when it is introduced. Shortly afterward the effectiveness falls off sharply, so that it is soon discarded and a newer remedy is tried. This seems to imply a strong placebo effect and this may be the case. The response to pain is such a variable one; with pain thresholds at widely varying levels, it is impossible to test this concept with any exactitude.

According to Hirschfeld the only effective agent that operates over an indefinite period is daily burnishing with the toothbrush. This observation has been amply supported by experience. The primary benefit to be gained by the many agents used is that of temporary desensitivity achieved for a period long enough to permit brushing by the patient. Whatever the reasons, root sensitivity usually does not last long when the patient is faithful in maintenance. The great danger lies with the patient who avoids the sensitive neck until a thick layer of plaque provides a protective film. When the plaque is removed, the tooth is more sensitive than ever.

Although root sensitivity is a serious annoyance, it does not constitute a major factor in the management of the case.

CURETTAGE IN THE TREATMENT PLAN

In discussing therapeutic method, it is most important to establish its position in the orderly treatment of the patient. From much of the first portion of this chapter it may be inferred—and correctly so—that coronal scaling and curettage, plus instruction in procedures to be practiced by the patient, properly constitute initial therapy in practically every case.

It will be found, however, that debridement has no set place in the sequence. It may precede the surgical phase, but it follows it, too. Most patients revert to some slipshod cleansing methods because surgery with its dressing and healing tissue necessitates gentle brushing with minimal standards for a time. The course of active treatment is terminated with coronal scaling and polishing. The maintenance phase of therapy is heavily involved with curettage. With so pervasive and universal an application and with so critical a role in cure it is difficult to avoid placing curettage and general debridement in a position of indispensability. Learning to perform it well is rewarding.

References

1. Bandt, C. L., Korn, N. A., and Schaffer, E. M.: Bacteremias from ultrasonic and hand instruments. J. Periodontol., 35:214, 1964.
2. Beube, F. E.: An experimental study of the use of sodium sulphid solution on treatment of periodontal pockets. J. Periodontol., 10:49, 1939.
3. Bjorn, H., and Lindhe, J.: The influence of periodontal instruments on the tooth surface. Odontol. Revy, 13:355, 1962.
4. Bodecker, C. F.: The difficulty of completely removing subgingival calculus. J. Am. Dent. Assoc., 30:703, 1943.
5. Box, H. K.: Treatment of the Periodontal Pocket. Toronto, University of Toronto Press, 1928.
6. Chaikin, B. S.: Subgingival curettage. J. Periodontol., 25:240, 1954.
7. Clark, S. M.: The effect of ultrasonic instrumentation on root surfaces. J. Periodontol., 39:135, 1968.
8. Green, E., and Ramfjord, S. J.: Tooth roughness after subgingival root planing. J. Periodontol., 37:44, 1966.
9. Hirschfeld, I.: The Toothbrush—Its Use and Abuse. Brooklyn, N. Y., Dental Items of Interest Publishing Co., Inc., 1939.
10. Hirschfeld, L.: Subgingival curettage in periodontal therapy. J. Am. Dent. Assoc., 44:301, 1952.
11. Ingle, J.: Periodontal curettement in the premaxilla. J. Periodontol., 23:143, 1952.
12. James, A. F.: Conservative treatment of periodontal diseases. J. Am. Dent. Assoc., 20:991, 1933.
13. Johnson, W. N., and Wilson, J. R.: The application of the ultrasonic dental units to scaling procedures. J. Periodontol., 28:264, 1957.
14. Kerry, G. J.: Roughness of root surfaces after use of ultrasonic instruments and hand curettes. J. Periodontol., 38:340, 1967.
15. Orban, B., and Manella, V. B.: A macroscopic and microscopic study of instruments designed for root planing. J. Periodontol., 27:120, 1956.
16. Sanderson, A. D.: Gingival curettage by hand and ultrasonic instruments—a histologic comparison. J. Periodontol., 37:279, 1966.
17. Sternlicht, H. C.: Curettage, its place in the treatment of periodontal disease. Tex. Dent. J., 79:4, 1961.
18. Waerhaug, J.: Microscopic demonstration of tissue reaction incident to the removal of subgingival calculus. J. Periodontol., 26:26, 1955.
19. Zander, H. A.: The attachment of calculus to root surfaces. J. Periodontol., 24:16, 1953.

17

Corrective Occlusal Therapy
for the Natural Dentition

17

Corrective Occlusal Therapy for the Natural Dentition

Examination of the functional occlusion as described in Chapter 12 allows the dentist to detect and identify signs and symptoms of occlusally related functional disturbances and disorders. Once such a diagnosis is made, treatment should be directed to the control of any inflammation present and to the correction of faulty functional occlusal relationships. This is especially important if occlusally related disturbances are associated with periodontitis. In such cases, reduction of inflammation by scaling, curettage, and oral physiotherapy should precede definitive occlusal correction, except when occlusal interferences are grossly obvious and require immediate correction. They should then take precedence.

Once inflammation is under control, functional occlusal disturbances may be treated by one or a combination of methods:

1. Occlusal adjustment by selective grinding
2. Control of parafunctional habits
3. Temporary, provisional, or long-term stabilization of mobile teeth to provide support and counteract parafunctional habits
4. Correction of morphologic malocclusion by minor or major tooth movement by orthodontic means, most often considered only if the occlusion cannot be corrected by occlusal grinding or if an improvement of esthetics is desired[13]
5. Occlusal reconstruction by restorative means

The primary object of any of these measures is to redistribute either functional or parafunctional forces upon the teeth, especially forces directed horizontally. The order in which these therapeutic approaches are made is decided by the needs of each individual case. For example, where it is obvious that occlusal adjustment by selective grinding alone cannot improve the functional relationships because of gross morphologic malocclusion, minor or major orthodontic correction should be done first. In some instances, selected extractions and a combination of single restorations, fixed bridges, and occlusal grinding may be required. If mobility is generalized and severe because of occlusal traumatism associated with loss of supporting bone, some form of temporary stabilization may have to be provided prior to adjusting the occlusion by selective grinding.

This chapter will be limited to a discussion of corrective occlusal adjustment of the natural dentition by selective grinding. The remaining forms of occlusal therapy are discussed in Chapters 5, 18, 19 and Section III.

Concepts of Occlusal Adjustment

Although concepts of functional occlusion have changed considerably, the prime objective of occlusal adjustment has not changed much. The objective is to distribute occlusal stresses as evenly as possible over the maximum number of teeth, so that no single tooth, or small number of teeth, is subjected to excessive stress.

The current method of occlusal adjustment of the natural dentition by selective grinding has long been recognized as effective in managing occlusally related disturbances or disorders. It is based on scientific evidence.[2,3,4,8,9,11]

The earlier concept of occlusal adjustment was based erroneously on the full-balance principles of full-denture prosthodontics and met with much disfavor. Proponents advocated reduction of cuspal or anterior inclined planes to provide for simultaneous cuspal contact on both the functioning and nonfunctioning sides during lateral excursions from centric occlusion, and for simultaneous contact of all posterior teeth throughout the protrusive range. Critics of this concept felt that there was no need for natural dentitions to function in the same manner as artificial dentures and that the main reason for full balance in artificial dentures was to maintain stability of the denture base. Grinding the natural dentition to full balance unnecessarily and grossly sacrificed tooth structure, often causing discomfort. They felt that the needless articulative contacts on the nonfunctioning side exerted excessive lateral force on the roots of the teeth making the contacts.

Since most mouths with natural dentition do not display full-balanced contact during all excursive movements, it was only natural that occlusal adjustment procedures should be modified to provide for disclusion of the posterior teeth during excursive gliding movements of the mandible, and a degree of overjet and overbite of the anterior teeth is natural and purposeful in providing this disclusion. It was through these observations of attributes of normal functional occlusion that correct concepts of occlusal adjustment were derived.

Indications for Occlusal Adjustment

It is not always easy to decide when to adjust the occlusion. Often it is more difficult to decide when not to adjust, and this demands the greater discipline and concentration.

The presence of periodontal disease concomitantly with faulty functional occlusal relationships is only one of several indications of the need for occlusal adjustment. Other equally important indications are

1. Evidence of occlusal disharmony in conjunction with parafunctional habits such as nocturnal or diurnal clenching and grinding as manifested by signs of occlusal traumatism, excessive occlusal attrition, temporomandibular-joint dysfunction or any combination of these manifestations.
2. Anticipation of restoration of a significant number of posterior or anterior teeth or both. Occlusal adjustment will allow development of optimal functional relationships prior to the restorative procedures. Failure to correct occlusal disharmony prior to restorative procedures will only result in its perpetuation.
3. Need for improvement of functional occlusal relationships and for stabilization of tooth position during and after orthodontic therapy.
4. Functional occlusal relationships recognized as potentially damaging and in need of correction even when periodontal and temporomandibular-joint disturbances are lacking. This indication for occlusal adjustment is controversial and is considered by some to be prophylactic occlusal adjustment and hence invalid. It is important to emphasize, however, that signs and symptoms of occlusally related disturbances are not always obvious and may remain innocuous for a long time. Diagnosis of such disturbances often depends on the ability of the dentist to recognize these subtle signs. For these reasons, what appears to be prophylactic occlusal adjustment to one may seem corrective to another.

Examples of occlusal relationships considered by most authorities to be inharmonious and potentially damaging are

1. Excessive anterior deflection of the mandible from CRO to CO (more than 1 mm), especially if there is a lateral component (Fig. 12-13) and associated faceting (Fig. 12-3).
2. Deflective balancing interferences on the functioning side (cross-tooth balance) or nonfunctioning side (cross-arch balance), preventing either cuspid rise or simultaneous group function on the functioning side (Fig. 12-6B,C).
3. Posterior deflective balancing interferences, preventing smooth gliding protrusive function (Fig. 12-7).
4. Deflective interferences of posterior functioning

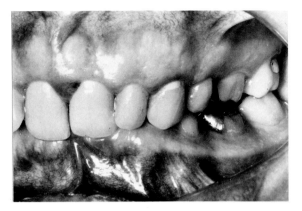

FIG. 17-1. *Deep overbite of anterior teeth which prevents smooth gliding protrusive or lateral excursion.*

cusps or incisors, preventing normal cuspid rise or simultaneous group function on the same side.

5. Deep intercuspation of the posterior teeth (locked bite), preventing smooth gliding movement of the mandible during function (Fig. 5-20).
6. Cross-bite relationships of the cuspids and incisors, resulting in balancing contacts on the nonfunctioning side or a locked bite.
7. Deep overbite with minimal overjet relationship of the anterior teeth, causing locking of the bite (Fig. 17-1).

Several morphologic occlusal irregularities are considered potentially damaging regardless of whether there are associated periodontal disturbances:

1. Marginal ridge discrepancies.
2. Extrusions.
3. Hanging or plunging centric holding cusps.
4. Broad opposing wear facets.
5. Wide occlusal tables resulting from excessive wear.
6. Rotated and crowded teeth.
7. Grossly uneven incisal relationships.

Such conditions may not require definitive occlusal adjustment, but, rather, partial adjustment or localized reshaping and/or restorative or orthodontic correction to improve normal function. More will be said regarding these irregularities later in the chapter.

DIAGNOSTIC ADJUSTMENT OF ARTICULATED CASTS

Once functional malocclusion has been diagnosed and occlusal adjustment is called for, the dentist must determine the extent of adjustment necessary. To gain competence in correct adjustment procedures, he should plan and perform them on the articulated casts,

either prior to or in conjunction with adjustment of the natural teeth. If the final result cannot be visualized with confidence, the adjustment should always be carried through on articulated casts prior to carrying out the same procedure on the patient. Adjustment of the casts may show the occlusal discrepancies to be so great that adjustment of the natural dentition would be unwise and that orthodontic or restorative therapy would be necessary to correct the disorder. Diagnostic adjustment also reveals which occlusal surfaces require only selective reshaping in order to function adequately.

Many occlusal adjustment techniques have been advocated[1,6,8,10,12,15,16] Sound basic principles are far more important than either technique or armamentarium. Whatever method works best in the individual's hands is the method he should use, provided that he adheres to the fundamental rules. The younger the patient, the more conservative the adjustment should be. Developing dentitions have many unpredictable adaptive mechanisms, and faulty anatomic and functional malocclusions are best treated orthodontically in coordination with growth and development. The total occlusal adjustment that is provided for adult occlusions should not be considered unless the eruption of the permanent dentition is complete and the active growth stage is at least nearly complete. Only minor occlusal adjustment of an interceptive nature should be considered during active growth of the developing jaws.

Basic Principles

1. Eliminate deflective occlusal interferences in CRO and excursive mandibular movements, to permit free bilateral and protrusive gliding movements.
2. Maintain or move the force vectors so that they act toward the long axis of the tooth, by eliminating unbalanced cuspal contacts on inclined planes and providing and maintaining stable cusp-to-fossa relationships wherever possible.
3. Improve the occlusal anatomy by creating and maintaining cusp form, eliminating broad facets, narrowing occlusal tables, and creating correct marginal ridge relationships, fossae, spillways, and grooves.
4. Improve or maintain esthetics whenever possible; do not destroy them.

Elimination of Occlusal Interferences

We subscribe to a technique that eliminates occlusal interferences in the field between CRO and CO firstly,

OCCLUSAL ADJUSTMENT CHART

Patient __Mrs. R. S. T.__

Articulator No. ____1182____

Date ____2-25-72____

Condylar Width ____Medium____

	R	L
Condylar Inclination	45	57
Side Shift	12	22

CRO-CO (mm)

Horizontal __2 mm anterior, 1 mm left__

Vertical ____4 mm (incisor region)____

____6 mm (articulator incisal pin)____

Step	Teeth in Contact	Area of Interference	Teeth Adjusted	Step	Teeth in Contact	Area of Interference	Teeth Adjusted
1	12/21	LC, II, MS / BC, II, DS	12/21				
2	14/19	MLC, II, MS / DBC, II, DS	14				
3	4/29	MF / BC	29				

FIG. 17-2. *Example of a grind-in list with sequential steps taken for adjustment of articulated stone casts.*

Step 1. Teeth causing primary interference are the maxillary left first premolar (#12) and the mandibular left first premolar (#21). Area of interference of #12 includes the lingual cusp, inner incline, mesial slope; of #21 it includes the buccal cusp, inner incline, distal slope. Both teeth require grinding.

Step 2. Next teeth to contact are the maxillary left first molar (#14) and the mandibular left first molar (#19). Interfering area of #14 includes the mesiolingual cusp, inner incline, mesial slope; of #19 it includes the distobuccal cusp, inner incline, distal slope. Only #14 requires grinding.

Step 3. Next interference includes the mesial fossa of #4 and the buccal cusp of #29. Tooth #29 requires grinding.

in lateral excursions secondly, and in protrusive excursions lastly. A grind-in list is recommended, especially for the beginner. Listing each sequential step required in adjusting articulated casts makes it much easier to accomplish it on the natural dentition (Fig. 17-2). The terminology for coronal anatomy can be simply abbreviated to provide an effective method of documenting clearly which surfaces have been ground (Fig. 17-3). Red and green dental tape (Madam Butterfly 3/4", #10 inking) is ideally suited for marking the occlusal contacts of the stone casts. The inking is light enough to minimize smudging, yet sufficiently intense to provide clear markings. To reduce the marked areas, any small sharp hand instrument such as a cleoid-discoid instrument or amalgam carver can be used to scrape the casts. An original unmounted set of accurate stone casts should be preserved to judge the extent to which the occlusal surfaces have been reduced. In addition,

the articulated casts should be painted with a pastel-colored poster paint (preferably yellow) prior to adjustment. When the areas of interference are removed by scraping, the yellow paint will outline them clearly and show exactly where on the tooth itself reduction must be made. Comparing the adjusted casts with the original casts is clearer than comparing the adjusted casts with the natural dentition. This allows for a more accurate estimate of the amount of tooth structure to be removed with each adjustment procedure.

Objectives for Adjustment of CRO Position

The dentist should strive toward the following objectives when carrying out the adjustment of the CRO position:

1. The elimination of any anterior or lateral shift of

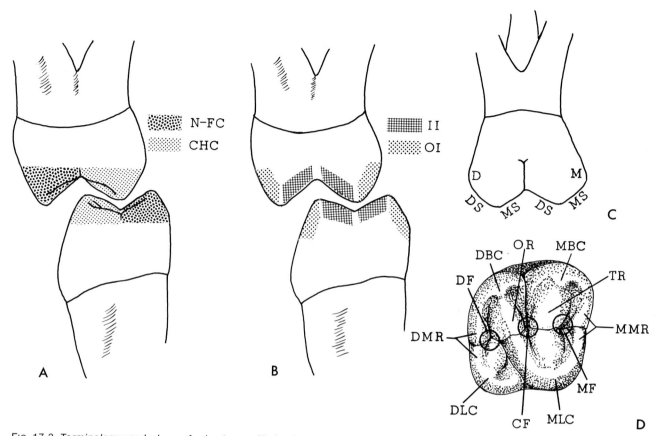

FIG. 17-3. *Terminology used when referring to specific landmarks during occlusal adjustment procedures. A. Centric holding cusps (CHC), the maxillary lingual cusps and the mandibular buccal cusps; nonfunctioning cusps (N-FC), the maxillary buccal cusps and the mandibular lingual cusps. B. Inner inclines (II), cuspal inclines of the teeth directed toward the central groove; outer inclines (OI), cuspal inclines directed away from the central groove. C. MS, mesial slope; DS, distal slope. D. MBC, mesiobuccal cusp; DBC, distobuccal cusp; MF, mesial fossa; DF, distal fossa; CF, central fossa; MMR, mesial marginal ridge; DMR, distal marginal ridge; TR, transverse ridge; OR, oblique ridge; MLC, mesiolingual cusp; DLC, distolingual cusp.*

Sequence for referring to area of interference: the cusp is noted first, the incline second, and the slope last, e.g., BC, II, MS = the buccal cusp, inner incline, mesial slope.

the mandible after initial contact in CRO position (Figs. 17-9, 12-13).

2. A maximum number of centric holding cusps (maxillary-lingual and mandibular-buccal) in contact when in CRO position (Fig. 17-4).

3. A vertical dimension in CRO position that is the same as or slightly more closed than that in CO position (Fig. 17-5).

4. The elimination of deflective interferences between CRO position and CO position, so that the movement is a free gliding movement in a horizontal plane (Fig. 17-9).

5. A cusp-to-fossa relationship, wherever possible, rather than a cusp-to-marginal-ridge relationship (Fig. 17-4).

6. Cusps shaped in such a way that they make contact as closely as possible with the centers of the fossae. In this way the horizontal forces will be directed more toward the long axis of the tooth (Fig. 17-6).

7. Contact between the centric holding cusp tips (rather than broad surfaces) and flat horizontal areas in the centers of the fossae (Figs. 17-6, 17-17). There should be no cusp contact on inclined planes, except on the lingual surfaces of the maxillary anterior teeth, or unless there is a reciprocal contact on a balancing inclined plane. In unworn dentitions, cusp tips often do not reach the bases of the fossae; multiple-point contacts on the balanced reciprocally inclined planes are considered as stable and desirable as centric holding cusps seated on a flat surface perpendicular to the tooth's long axis (Fig. 17-7).

If there is a choice between shortening an interfering cusp and deepening a fossa, the cusp should be

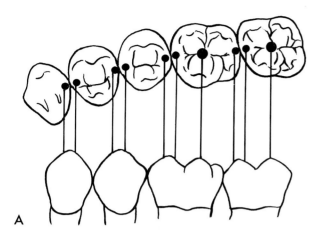

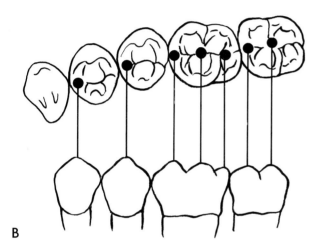

FIG. 17-4. *Centric holding cusps and their respective stops. A. Centric holding stops representing a cusp-to-fossa and/or marginal ridge relationship. B. Centric holding stops, representing a cusp-to-fossa relationship.*

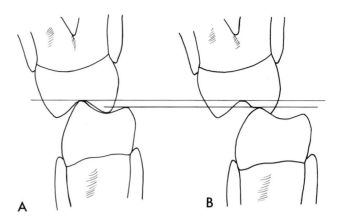

FIG. 17-5. *Correction of prematurities of CRO position. A. Buccolingual view illustrating centric stops at CO position. B. Buccolingual view illustrating incomplete adjustment, resulting in a slightly opened vertical dimension at CRO position. The patient will not function at such a CRO position, but rather will seek the most closed position, in this case, CO position.*

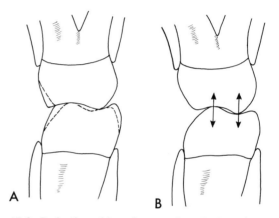

FIG. 17-6. *Reduction of broad areas of contact so that cusp tips contact a flat horizontal area in center of fossa. A. Before adjustment. B. After adjustment.*

shortened; this will provide for easier gliding movements during lateral and protrusive excursions. Cusp tips should not be locked in by deep and narrow fossae (Fig. 17-18). Once CRO has been established, the centric holding cusps should never be ground out of contact.

Objectives for Adjustment of Right and Left Lateral Excursions

The dentist should strive toward

1. A slight cuspid disclusion of the posterior teeth during lateral excursions, except when
   a. The cuspid is worn and there is an existing group function with no evidence of trauma.

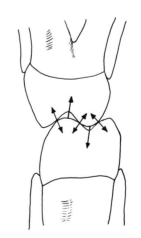

FIG. 17-7. *Illustration of cusp-to-fossa relationship in unworn dentitions. Note that the cusp tip does not reach the base of the fossa and that multiple points make contact on balanced reciprocal inclined planes.*

b. The cuspid is malposed or periodontally weakened. In these cases adjusting to a posterior group function is necessary (Fig. 17-10C).
2. Elimination of cross-arch and cross-tooth balancing contacts or deflective interferences (Fig. 12-6).
3. Elimination of deflective central- or lateral-incisor contacts that prevent cuspid function during lateral excursions. An exception to this is central and lateral incisors that are in group function with the cuspid and show no pathologic signs such as greater-than-normal mobility or excessive wear.

Objectives for Adjustment of Protrusive Excursions

The dentist should strive toward
1. Even distribution of contact during protrusive excursions over as many anterior teeth as possible. There should be no cuspal contact of the posterior teeth, except between the mesial slope of the buccal cusp of the mandibular first premolars and the distal slope of the maxillary cuspid, if these are within practical adjustable range or already in function. Reduction to achieve this should be from the lingual aspect of the maxillary anterior teeth unless there is an anterior prematurity in CRO position, in which case reduction should be from the incisal edge of the mandibular anterior teeth (Fig. 17-12).
2. Reduction of the incisal edges of extruded teeth if they interfere with an even distribution· of contact during protrusive excursion. This will improve the occlusal plane as well as the esthetic qualities of the dentition (Fig. 17-12A, B).
3. Reduction of the crown length of anterior teeth to alleviate a deep overbite. This is often effective in providing for unrestricted protrusive mandibular movement but should be done with caution. Anterior teeth with broad centric relation contacts can be safely shortened without danger of losing centric contact (Fig. 17-8), but if by shortening the mandibular teeth centric contact is lost, the adjusted teeth will often extrude to reestablish their original positions.

Objectives for Improving Occlusal Anatomy

1. The narrowing of occlusal tables (Figs. 17-6, 17-17)
2. Reduction of broad opposing wear facets
3. The correction of marginal-ridge discrepancies,

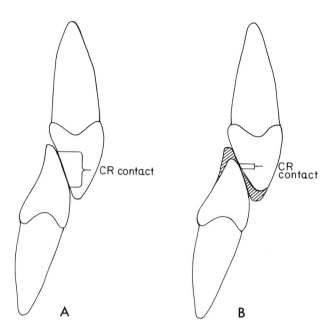

FIG. 17-8. *Adjustment of anterior teeth with deep overbite and minimal overjet. A. Characteristic broad centric contact. B. Area with oblique lines shows amount of reduction that may be necessary to improve anterior function in protrusive range and reduce the area of centric contact.*

and extrusions such as hanging or plunging centric holding cusps (Figs. 17-15, 17-16)
4. The correction of abnormal buccal and lingual contours due to rotation or crowding of teeth
5. The improvement of spillways, supplemental grooves, and marginal ridges
6. Leveling of uneven incisal edges (Fig. 17-12)

Such corrections as listed above are desirable, but should be done at the expense of only nonfunctioning planes and surfaces, so as not to destroy previously attained functional contacts.

OCCLUSAL ADJUSTMENT OF THE NATURAL DENTITION

Except for the armamentarium, the technique and sequence of steps are similar to those for the adjustment of articulated casts. Prior to adjustment, review the objectives for each phase of the procedure as explained earlier.

Armamentarium

1. Red and green dental ribbon (Madam Butterfly $\frac{3}{4}$", #40 inking, Wm. Dierickx, Seattle, Washington)
2. Artus occlusal registration strips (Artus Corp., Englewood, New Jersey)

3. Occlusal ribbon forceps (Miller articulating paper forceps, Misdon-Frank Corp., New York, New York)

4. Diamond stones, friction grip, (e.g., WM 1 & 2 or PDQ 1 & 2, Starlite; Star Dental Mfg. Co., Inc., Philadelphia, Pennsylvania)

5. Polishing stones, friction grip (Green #46 and White #46P, Chayes Dental Instrument Corp., Danbury, Connecticut)

6. Small pumice-impregnated wheels for final polishing

7. Fine powdered-pumice paste

8. Cotton rolls, diameter, $\frac{3}{8}$″, length, $1\frac{1}{2}$″

9. 2″ × 2″ gauze

10. Grind-in list

11. Adjusted articulated casts and marked original casts

Preliminary Preparation of Patient

To control salivation, an antisialalogue such as Banthine (methantheline bromide) can be prescribed (50 mg tablet, one hour prior to the appointment, or two tablets if salivation is profuse). To control remaining salivation, place $\frac{3}{8}$″-diameter cotton rolls or folded 2″ × 2″ gauze in the vestibules of the maxillary and mandibular arches and also beneath the tongue.

Seat the patient in the same comfortable position, with the chair slightly reclined, as during the examination procedure. Adjust the headrest so that the head is slightly tipped back and properly supported (Fig. 12-9).

Prior to each marking procedure, use air, cotton roll, or gauze to make certain the occlusal surfaces on that side are dry. The ribbon must also be dry or it will not mark adequately.

Adjustment of CRO Position

The basic principles and objectives as outlined for adjusting the articulated casts must be followed, although there are no set rules established, because each individual situation is different and requires a different approach.

PROCEDURE

Locate the CRO position. Close the mandible with red occlusal tape between the posterior teeth, first on one side and then on the other, using firm and crisp manipulation to ensure clear marking. Observe the marks left by the tape and decide where to grind. Adjustment is facilitated by following the grind-in list. Determine the amount of tooth structure to be ground

off by referring to the unground stone casts and comparing the same area of the painted, adjusted casts. The main concern is to reduce those cuspal contacts on inclined planes that lack balancing reciprocal contacts to create stable cusp-to-fossa centric holding positions. With a high-speed handpiece and a diamond stone, grind the areas marked on the inclined planes until re-marked contacts indicate a stable holding position in a fossa or until there are reciprocal contacts.

Each time after grinding off marks, wipe off any remaining marks, dry the teeth, and repeat the procedure. There should be a gradual decrease in the shift from CRO to CO position and a noticeably more solid sound when tapping the teeth together as the adjustment progresses. General recontouring of all old restorations can be done at this time to create occlusal embrasures, fossae, marginal ridges, lingual spillways, proper buccal and lingual embrasures, and proximal contact areas. Do not, however, alter the centric stops.

Elimination of most of the mandibular shift from CRO to CO is relatively easy because the major portion of this deflection is caused by only a few gross occlusal interferences. The elimination of the last part of the shift is more difficult because the occlusal tape marks additional contacts with each adjustment. The operator is faced with deciding where and how much of each registered contact to grind and is tempted to terminate the adjustment before all shift has been eliminated. When the CRO-CO shift has been reduced to $\frac{1}{2}$ mm or less, examination and adjustment of the lateral excursions may be undertaken if many of the mandibular centric holding cusps also contact in lateral excursions, as for example in group function on the working side, or if the shift is mainly on a horizontal plane with little vertical compensation. Adjustment of lateral excursions in such circumstances will often aid in elimination of much of the remaining CRO-CO shift, but should not be relied upon to take care of it in every case; and if lateral adjustment is made, centric relation occlusion must afterwards always be checked, and the necessary refinement must be completed.

However, if the remaining portion of the shift is mainly vertical rather than horizontal or if the cuspids and incisors effect a posterior disclusion during mandibular excursions, this last portion of the shift from CRO to CO should be completely eliminated and refined prior to making lateral adjustments.

Refinement of the CRO-CO Range

Never refine the CRO position and the range between CRO-CO with diamond stones. These stones cut too rapidly. Instead, use green and white stones that will afford better control of the degree of cutting and will leave a smoother surface for final polishing procedures.

The refinement procedure is often regarded as the most difficult and time-consuming part of the occlusal adjustment. It need not be, if each step in the following instructions is taken precisely and in proper sequence. Failure to refine contact relationships in the CRO position will inhibit the patient from functioning within the range of CRO-CO, and he will continue to function in the CO position because the jaws are in a more closed position in CO than in CRO position. Patients will always seek the most closed mandibular position, because the more opened CRO position with its many occlusal contacts on inclined planes is functionally uncomfortable.

Whenever possible, refinement of the CRO position should be left for at least a week after gross adjustment of the CRO position has been completed. This will allow for minor changes in tooth position resulting from the elimination of gross interferences and will facilitate the refinement procedure.

PROCEDURE

Make certain that the teeth are dry before placing fresh, dry, green marking ribbon between the teeth on one side. With crisp manipulation, locate the CRO position, and from this position ask the patient to bite hard and purposely slide to the CO position several times. Repeat this on the opposite side. Remove the green ribbon and with fresh, dry, red ribbon precisely mark the CRO contacts on both sides. This will superimpose the red CRO marks over the longer green marks that indicate the CRO-CO range (Fig. 17-9A). Note the amount of closure between the CRO-CO positions (Fig. 17-9B). This will give some indication of how much grinding is necessary. At this stage, limit the adjustment to the centric holding cusps and leave the fossae until later. Note any broad centric holding cusps and reduce the area of all contacts that are more than 1 to 2 mm in diameter, being careful not to reduce the height of the centric holding cusps at this time. (Fig. 17-9C, D).

When the area of contact of the cusp tips is satisfactory, re-mark CRO-CO range and observe the green mark of the path between CRO and CO. Grind each path to the horizontal level of its lower part (which is always at the CO position) (Fig. 17-9E, F). This can be done for the mandibular fossae first and the maxillary fossae next. Re-mark the teeth and repeat refinement, if indicated (Fig. 17-9G). At this stage of refinement, the white polishing stone rather than the green stone may be used in order to prevent overcutting. Without interposing ribbon, guide the jaw to the CRO position

and ask the patient to bite hard. If refinement of the fossae is complete, there should not be any shift to the CO position. Ask the patient to slide to the CO position; visually note if the movement is smooth and on a horizontal plane, with no change in vertical dimension.

Recheck the centric cusp-to-fossa contact relationships with red ribbon and if many cusp tips are not registering, slightly reduce the height of the interfering cusp tips. In most cases it is unnecessary and impractical to expect all possible centric holding cusps to contact, since this would require overadjustment. Smooth all scratched surfaces with the white stone, and further polish all ground surfaces with a pumice-impregnated wheel. Recheck the CRO position and the CRO-CO range. If satisfactory, place a small amount of finely powdered pumice paste (or any commercially prepared prophylactic paste) over the occlusal and incisal regions of the teeth. Ask the patient to close and grind from CRO-CO for a minute or two. This will reduce any roughness caused by surface scratches.

Adjustment of Right and Left Lateral Excursions

If adjustment of right and left lateral excursions is performed at a later appointment and not at the time of adjustment and refinement of the CRO position, mark and check the CRO and CO positions again. Slight tooth movement may necessitate further refinement.

Once satisfactory centric contacts have been created and the anterior and/or lateral slip has been eliminated, consider the type of relationship that should be created in lateral excursions. The objectives for this phase of adjustment should be reviewed. There may be a choice of cuspid rise or posterior group function including the cuspid, or perhaps posterior group function excluding the cuspid. Opposite sides may have different relationships. Which one is developed will depend upon the root form, crown-root ratio, mobility, and location of individual teeth and the possibilities pertaining to each patient's characteristics.

PROCEDURE

With the teeth dry, place green occlusal ribbon between them on the right side. Hold the mandible in CRO position and have the patient close with moderate pressure; then have him slide the mandible toward his right shoulder. Green marks show which teeth are contacting on the functioning side. Switch to red ribbon, leaving the green marks untouched and tap the teeth in CRO position to mark established centric holding contacts. Red marks indicate the centric hold-

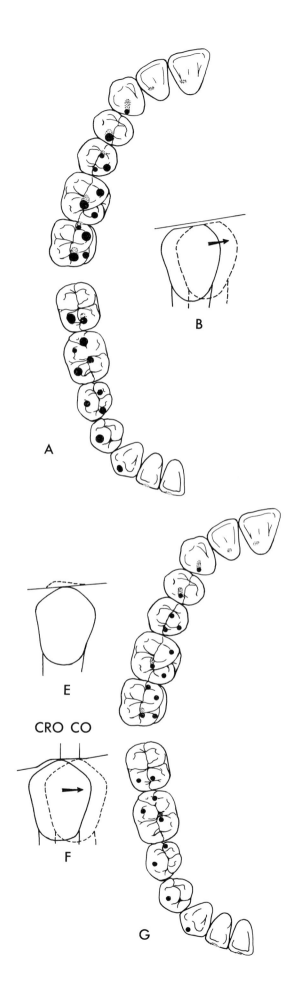

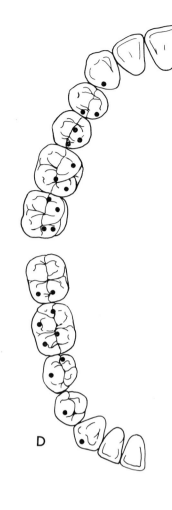

CRO CO

FIG. 17-9. *Steps in refinement of CRO-CO range. A. Occlusal view, showing broad CRO markings (in black) and skid marks to CO position (stippled). B. Broad centric holding cusp skidding on inclined path of CRO-CO range to a more closed position. C. Centric holding cusp narrowed to approximately 2 mm diameter. D. CRO markings (in black) made by narrowed centric holding cusps. E. All inclined planes marked in CRO-CO range are leveled to most closed position. F. Leveled CRO-CO range. G. CRO-CO range re-marked to illustrate simultaneous contact of maximum number of narrowed centric holding cusps in contact with a flattened CRO-CO range, free of all deflection. This allows the patient to function freely within the CRO-CO range.*

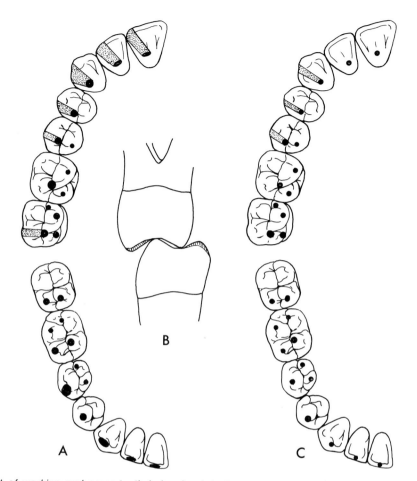

FIG. 17-10. *Adjustment of working and cross-tooth balancing interferences. A. Occlusal view showing CRO markings (black) and marks made during working excursion (stippled). B. Undesirable contacts reduced on inner inclines of the maxillary buccal cusps, with CRO contacts carefully preserved. C. Occlusal view, showing how all excessively broad markings are reduced in width by narrowing the diameter of centric holding cusp and how undesirable excursive contacts are eliminated.*

ing cusps (Fig. 17-10A). To remove interferences, grind only the undesirable green marks that have registered on the inner inclines of the maxillary buccal cusps or lingual surfaces of the upper anterior teeth and all green marks that indicate cross-arch and cross-tooth balancing contacts. This will remove the interferences but leave the centric holding contacts undisturbed (Fig. 17-10B).

Proceed to create on the right side the preferred type of function. For example, if it has been decided to create a cuspid rise in lateral excursion because both cuspids are solid and have good bone support and because the posterior teeth have less support, grind the green marks on the inner inclines of the maxillary posterior buccal cusps. However, if posterior group function is desired, grind the heavier of the green marks until even function is established on as many posterior teeth as is deemed necessary (Fig. 17-10C). Sometimes it is necessary to grind nonworking contacts, if they interfere, prior to correcting the working

side. Never grind the centric holding cusps out of contact. Repeat this procedure with left lateral excursions.

While establishing lateral function, make sure that no anterior teeth are causing interference. If they are, then they should be adjusted.

It is imperative that all cross-arch and cross-tooth balancing contacts be removed, because this category of interference is considered by most authorities to be the most damaging. These contacts should be checked early in the procedure of adjusting right and left lateral excursions and again periodically throughout this grinding procedure. Deflective balancing interferences will prevent acquisition of the desired type of working-contact relationships (Fig. 12-6).

To mark the balancing contacts on the left side, place green ribbon between the left posterior teeth; have the patient close tightly and move the mandible to the right while you exert added pressure on the left side in an occlusal direction (Fig. 12-14). Then have

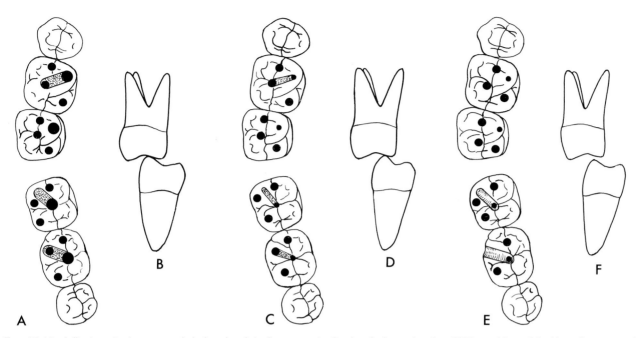

FIG. 17-11. *Adjustment of cross-arch balancing interferences. A. Occlusal view, showing CRO markings (black) and cross-arch balancing contacts (stippled). B. Mesial view in molar region to show broad balancing contact. C. Occlusal view after all broad centric holding cusps have been narrowed to approximately 1 to 2 mm diameter and balancing contacts have been re-marked. D. Mesial view in molar region to show position of narrowed balancing contacts. E. Occlusal view of supplemental grooves created to allow centric holding cusp to pass through without contact. F. Mesial view in molar region to show elimination of cross-arch balancing interference.*

him open; place red occlusal ribbon between the left posterior teeth and mark the CRO position. Grind where necessary to eliminate nonworking interfering cusps and still leave as many centric holds as possible. It may be necessary to create a supplemental groove to allow the interfering centric holding cusp to pass freely without contacting the nonworking side (Fig. 17-11). Occasionally a centric holding cusp must be reduced to eliminate a cross-arch balancing interference if it lies in the pathway of the groove to be created. Repeat these steps, to remove the balancing interferences on the right side. Check the working excursions again to see that removal of balancing contacts has not disturbed the working side. Polish, with white stones and a pumice-impregnated rubber wheel, all surfaces that have been ground.

Adjustment of Protrusive Excursions

Prior to adjustment of protrusive excursions, the desired objectives should be reviewed.

PROCEDURE

To check for optimum protrusive function, place green ribbon between the anterior teeth and have the patient move the mandible into protrusive position to mark protrusive contacts. Place red ribbon between the anterior teeth and mark the CRO position. Adjust interferences by grinding the green marks on the lingual surfaces of the upper teeth, except when the mandibular incisors interfere in CRO position; if they do, shorten the interfering mandibular incisor (Fig. 17-12). If any posterior teeth are in contact during protrusive excursions, these interferences should be removed by grinding the marks on the distal slopes of the upper posterior teeth and the mesial slopes of the lower posterior teeth (Fig. 12-7).

Wipe off all marks, dry the teeth thoroughly, and mark again in CRO position on both sides, to relocate centric stops. General reshaping, faciolingual narrowing, and improvement of incisal planes may now be done, if required. Do not alter either centric stops or previously created lateral function. Smooth all tooth surfaces that have been ground. Have the patient perform excursive movements with nothing between the teeth, to make certain that there are no rough contact areas. After all teeth have been smoothed, wipe off all marks, dry the teeth, and again mark the centric holds. Adjust further if necessary.

The entire occlusal adjustment procedure should be accomplished in several appointments to minimize wear on the patient and muscle fatigue. Patient reaction to the changes can be observed. Removal of pre-

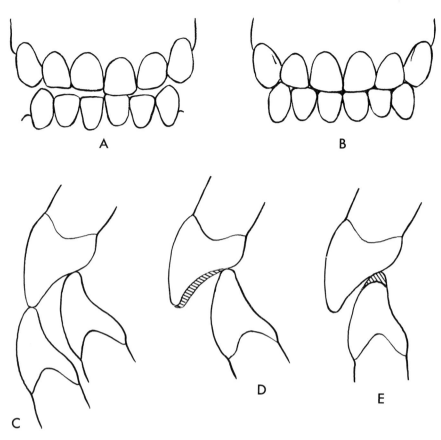

FIG. 17-12. *Adjustment of anterior prematurities in the protrusive range. A. Schematic drawing of mandibular central incisor in protrusive position interfering with maxillary central incisor. B. After adjustment to distribute contact evenly over as many anterior teeth as possible in protrusive position. C. Protrusive gliding contact smooth and free from deflections. D. Area of the lingual surface of the maxillary tooth to be reduced from the point of CRO contact if interfering mandibular tooth is not premature in CRO. This will preserve CRO contact. E. Area of incisal edge to be shortened if the interfering mandibular tooth is also premature in CRO.*

mature contacts will allow teeth to move slightly, and follow-up appointments will be required.

Correction of Occlusal Discrepancies Prior to Restorative Procedures

Prior to any restorative procedure, the dentist should carefully assess the present status of the patient's functional occlusion. He should determine whether the existing occlusion merits perpetuation or calls for modification. Dentitions requiring multiple occlusal restorations either immediately or in the predictable future should have existing occlusal discrepancies corrected prior to the restorative phase of therapy. If the occlusal discrepancies are interferences in CRO position or during various excursive movements, or both, complete occlusal adjustment is mandatory whether or not symptoms related to functional disorders are present. If a healthy occlusal pattern does not exist before restorative treatment, it will undoubtedly be absent following treatment.

Occlusions resisting trauma during childhood and young adulthood may lose their resistance later. It is far simpler to improve and control occlusal harmony during restorative therapy than to adjust occlusions when symptoms appear after the occlusal surfaces are covered with gold or amalgam. If the treatment plan calls for fixed bridgework or multiple inlays, working casts, accurately articulated in the CRO position, will ensure control of the occlusion. Using the articulator is meaningless, however, if inharmonious occlusal relationships are allowed to determine the articulation of the working casts and to effect undesirable occlusal relationships in the new restorations. Thus, the occlusion should be adjusted prior to articulation of the working casts. This is especially important if the restorations are to be constructed by a technician. The practice of depending on the technician to modify inharmonious occlusal conditions on the working stone casts in order to improve the functional aspects of the restorations is dangerous, because it is difficult for the dentist to simulate accurately on the patient's dentition the same degree of reduction that the technician provides on the working casts. Usually overadjustment and loss of functional occlusal contact will result.

Many patients not requiring definitive occlusal adjustment prior to restorative procedures may still require minor correction or alteration of occlusal irregularities, not only in the teeth to be restored, but also in approximating or opposing teeth. Several of the common irregularities that require modification are marginal-ridge discrepancies, extruded teeth, hanging or plunging centric holding cusps, broad opposing wear facets, nonanatomic opposing restorations, wide occlusal tables, and rotated teeth.

MARGINAL-RIDGE DISCREPANCIES

Marginal ridges of posterior teeth that do not direct food into the fossae promote food impaction in the interproximal region (Figs. 17-13, 26-11). Prior to restoring such teeth, the opposing marginal ridges should be leveled, either by grinding if the discrepancy is slight or by restorations if the discrepancy is gross.

EXTRUDED TEETH

A tooth may extrude because of massive coronal breakdown of the opposing tooth or, more frequently, into an edentulous area. These irregularities should be corrected in conjunction with restoration of the edentulous or cariously involved area by grinding and reshaping if the extrusion is slight or by installing an inlay or crown, depending on the severity of the

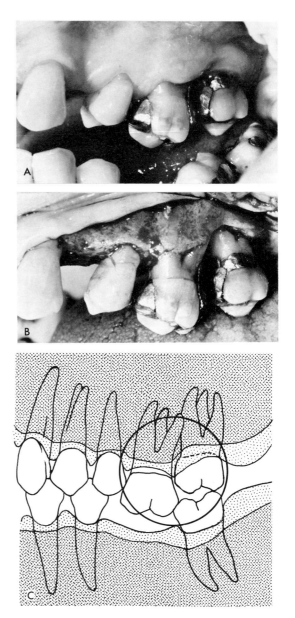

FIG. 17-14. *Severely extruded tooth in need of more than occlusal reduction because of extreme changes in the soft and hard tissues surrounding it and adjacent teeth. A. Presurgical view showing soft tissue and marginal ridge discrepancies. B. View of alveolar bone showing root proximities between first and second molar and associated osseous discrepancies. C. Schematic drawing to show how severe extrusion affects a loss of space and results in root proximities and irregularities in alveolar support.*

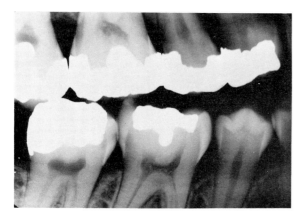

FIG. 17-13. *Mesial tilting of posterior teeth, which caused marginal ridge discrepancies between approximating teeth. Note concomitant angulation of the crestal bone, which should not be interpreted as angular bone loss; it is due to the vertical difference between the cementoenamel junctions. Prior to restoring any of these teeth, the opposing marginal ridges should be leveled, either by grinding if the discrepancy is slight or by restorations if the discrepancy is gross.*

extrusion. Allowing extrusions to remain may result in functional disorders caused by occlusal interferences in the course of excursive jaw movements. Their reduction will also provide for better adaptation to the edentulous ridge of a more functional and esthetic pontic. If the extrusions, such as seen in Fig. 17-14, are so severe that interproximal space is concomitantly lost, orthodontic treatment may be necessary. If orthodontic treatment is not feasible because of excessive loss of interproximal space, extraction of the extruded tooth and replacement with a fixed bridge may be the only choice. If severe reduction of extruded teeth is required, endodontic intervention and surgical exposure of additional root structure may be necessary to improve retention and to allow for a normal interproximal environment for the surrounding hard and soft tissues.

HANGING OR PLUNGING CENTRIC HOLDING CUSPS

Hanging or plunging centric holding cusps are often the result of tipping and extrusion into a grossly carious opposing occlusal surface. Reduction and reshaping are imperative prior to restoring the opposing tooth, if such cusps are to function properly with the restored teeth. Simply reducing the height of the plunging cusp would be insufficient, for this would result in an excessively flattened cusp. Rather, the centric holding area should be predetermined and projected to the height at which it would function best with the new opposing restoration. By correctly reducing the cusp, the dentist may be able to warp the centric contact in any direction (Fig. 17-15). Allowing hanging cusps to remain greatly increases the likelihood of both cross-arch and cross-tooth balancing interferences (Fig. 17-16).

The same modification may apply to grasping cusps that have long and steep inclines. They may also be reduced slightly and reshaped so that they are easily freed from contact during mandibular excursive movements.

BROAD OPPOSING WEAR FACETS

Broad opposing wear facets should be eliminated by reshaping to permit establishment of minimal centric contact areas (Fig. 17-17). It is important to preserve stable centric stops.

NONANATOMIC OPPOSING RESTORATIONS

Existing restorations that have either flat or excessively deep fossae opposing teeth in need of restorative work may be readily modified to improve fossae, cusps, marginal ridges, and grooves, to increase masticatory efficiency, and to improve centric contact relationships. Opposing restorations with excessively deep fossae are best redone, and no attempt should be made to fit a newly restored cusp tip to such a fossa; this will create unfavorable occlusal relationships (Fig. 17-18).

WIDE OCCLUSAL TABLES

Wide occlusal tables are usually a symptom of excessive wear and should be narrowed to maintain good centric holding areas, by reshaping the cusp tips according to the objectives outlined for hanging cusps (Fig. 17-17).

ROTATED TEETH

Moderate reshaping of rotated teeth may improve the occlusion, but not much can be accomplished by grinding. It may also be necessary to construct an onlay or crown for a rotated tooth.

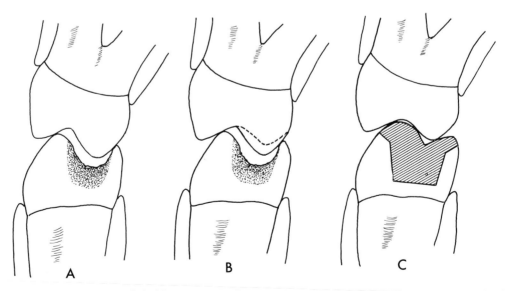

FIG. 17-15. *Adjustment of extruded centric holding cusps. A. Tilted maxillary tooth occluding with a cariously involved surface of an opposing tooth. B. Occlusal surface of maxillary tooth reshaped to shorten lingual cusp so that it will not interfere during excursive movements. C. Restored mandibular tooth, illustrating improved centric contact relationship with reshaped maxillary tooth.*

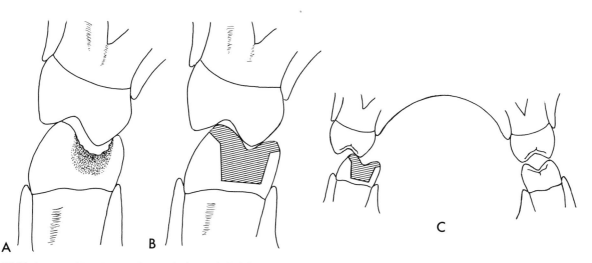

FIG. 17-16. *Incorrect treatment of extruded centric holding cusp. A. Illustration of condition prior to restoration of mandibular tooth. B. Restoration incorrectly constructed to accommodate the extruded maxillary centric holding cusp. C. Cross-arch balancing interference created in lateral excursion because maxillary centric holding cusp was not shortened.*

RESTORATION OF MISSING AND CARIOUS TEETH

Once the dentist is satisfied that the needs of the existing occlusion have been met, he may then begin the restoration of missing or carious teeth. Improper restoration of the occlusal surface, whether with amalgam or gold, can cause functional disorders. It is imperative to follow the principles of good occlusion previously outlined. Overcarving the occlusal anatomy so that centric holding areas are removed is a serious mistake and is especially common if all the carving is completed while the rubber dam is still in place (Fig. 17-19). Centric stops, if removed during cavity preparation, must be restored and preserved; otherwise the teeth may erupt into a new occlusal relationship that may be traumatic to the supporting tissues during

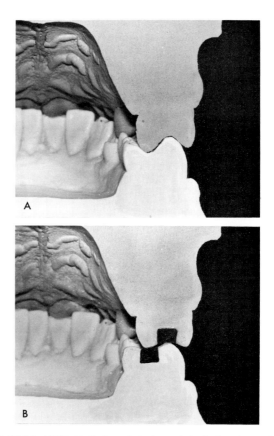

FIG. 17-18. *Midbuccal view of study casts in first molar region, showing reshaping of undesirable grasping centric holding cusps which interfere during lateral mandibular excursions (Same patient as in Fig. 5-20). A. Contact in centric occlusion prior to reshaping of cusps. B. Contact in centric occlusion after reshaping and shallowing of excessively deep fossae by placement of occlusal restorations.*

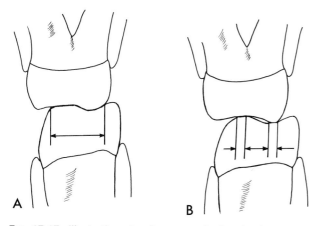

FIG. 17-17. *Illustration showing amount of reshaping necessary to improve functional relationship of severely worn occlusal surfaces. A. Before reshaping. B. After reshaping.*

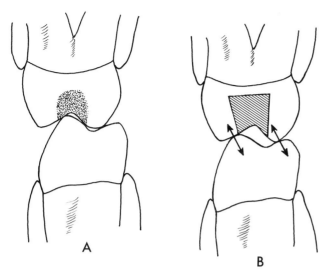

FIG. 17-19. *Improperly carved restoration. A. Prior to restoration. B. Overcarved occlusal surface resulting in an unstable occlusal relationship, since biting forces are not axially directed.*

excursive movements. The centric stops must be restored so that the forces are axially directed.

In young dentitions with little wear, centric contacts are most often on opposing inclines and over embrasures and are difficult to reproduce, especially if carved directly in the mouth. If the centric contacts are incorrectly reproduced, the supporting tissues may be traumatized by imbalanced forces (Fig. 17-19B). Ramfjord and Ash suggest that it would be more practical "to place the centric stop for the opposing cusp on a flat surface in the bottom of the fossa" (Fig. 17-20).[12] This method allows for slight freedom of movement in

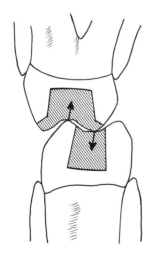

FIG. 17-20. *Alternative to reproducing reciprocally balanced contacts on inclined planes. Centric stops of restorations carved as a flat surface to accommodate the centric holding cusps.*

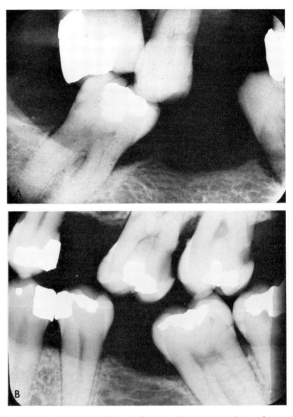

FIG. 17-21. *Posterior bite collapse. Note extrusion of unopposed teeth, mesial tilting of remaining molars, and interproximal caries. A. Right side. B. Left side.*

centric occlusion. There is little experimental evidence in favor of one method over the other; as long as the forces are axially directed and the centric holding cusp tips free from interferences during lateral and protrusive excursions, either method may be used.

Failure to restore proximal contacts adequately may result not only in food impaction but also in detrimental occlusal changes; teeth may tilt into new relationships, causing marginal-ridge discrepancies. Amalgam is adequate for contact areas, but if the space is too large, gold castings are preferable.

Another common cause of occlusal problems is failure to·replace an extracted first molar. This frequently results in posterior bite collapse that may place excessive stress on the anterior teeth, cause anterior tilting, and increase overjet and overbite (Fig. 17-21, 5-23). This is a most difficult occlusal problem to correct. Modern restorative techniques are available, so that there is no excuse for condemning grossly carious first molars out of hand, but if extraction is inevitable, the dentist should promptly prevent drifting and space closure by inserting either a space maintainer if the patient is very young or a fixed bridge if the age of the patient permits.

References

1. Abrams, L., and Coslet, J. G.: Occlusal adjustment by selective grinding. *In* Periodontal Therapy, 5th ed. H. M. Goldman and D. W. Cohen, Eds. St. Louis, C. V. Mosby, 1973.
2. Ahlgren, J., and Posselt, U.: Need of functional analysis and selective grinding in orthodontics: A clinical and electromyographic study. Acta Odontol. Scand., *21*:187, 1963.
3. Beyron, H. L.: Occlusal changes in adult dentition. J. Am. Dent. Assoc., *48*:674, 1954.
4. Glickman, I.: Inflammation and trauma from occlusion; Co-destructive factors in chronic periodontal disease. J. Periodontol., *34*:5, 1963.
5. Goldman, H. M., and Cohen, D. W.: Periodontal Therapy, 5th ed., St. Louis, C. V. Mosby, 1973.
6. Guichet, N. F.: Enameling of casts and occlusal adjustments. *In* Principles of Occlusion. R. W. Huffman, and J. W. Regenos, Eds. London, Ohio, H & R Press, 1973.
7. Halpert, L.: Occlusion in periodontal pathology and therapy. Alpha Omegan 25:130, 1967.
8. Lauritzen, A. G.: Atlas of Occlusal Analysis. Colorado Springs, HAH Publications, 1974.
9. Mühlemann, H. R., Herzog, H., and Rateitschak, K. H.: Qualitative evaluation of the therapeutic effect of selective grinding. J. Periodontol., *28*:11, 1957.
10. Prichard, J. R.: Advanced Periodontal Disease: Surgical and Prosthetic Management. Philadelphia, W. B. Saunders Co., 1965.
11. Ramfjord, S. P.: Dysfunctional temporomandibular joint and muscle pain. J. Prosthet. Dent., *11*:353, 1961.
12. Ramfjord, S. P., and Ash, M. M.: Occlusion. Philadelphia, W. B. Saunders Co., 1971.
13. Rhoads, J. E.: Repositioning of malposed teeth prior to oral rehabilitation. J. So. Cal. State Dent. Assoc., *31*:347, 1963.
14. Schuyler, C. H.: Correction of occlusal disharmony of the natural dentition. N.Y. State Dent. J., *13*:445, 1947.
15. Shore, N. A.: Occlusal Equilibration and Temporomandibular Joint Dysfunction. Philadelphia, J. B. Lippincott Co., 1959.
16. Stuart, C. E.: Occlusal Adjustments. *In* Principles of Occlusion. R. W. Huffman and J. W. Regenos, Eds. London, Ohio, H & R Press, 1973.

18

Temporary Stabilization— Removable and Fixed Splints

18

Temporary Stabilization- Removable and Fixed Splints

When teeth are seriously loosened by periodontal disturbances, stabilization by splinting is an extremely valuable adjunct before, during, and after corrective therapy. A splint is a device for holding the teeth together and is one of the oldest forms of aids to periodontal therapy. By redistribution of stress upon the affected teeth, the splint minimizes the effects caused by loss of support. When teeth are loosened, it is in most cases because functional loads have exceeded the resistance of the supporting structures. The prime objective of the many methods of temporary and long-term stabilization by splinting is to rest the affected structures and to redistribute functional and parafunctional forces and to reduce especially those that act in a horizontal direction. Since an axially inclined force is known to be the least traumatic, splinting provides for this by controlling excessive mobility and thus aids in the prevention of further breakdown of a weakened periodontium, tooth migration, and subsequent bite collapse.

Prolonged mobility often results from occlusal traumatism, with or without predisposing factors, and if the mobility is reduced or eliminated during periodontal therapy, the long-term prognosis will be greatly improved. Splinting transforms several individual teeth with varying degrees and patterns of mobility into a single functioning unit similar to a multirooted tooth, thereby improving the group's resistance to force and altering the area of application and the direction of force.[3]

The method to be used for stabilization is chosen after assessing the nature of the periodontal involvement, the nature of the destructive process, the extent of the damage, and the degree of resolution of the disease process that can be expected. Other factors to be considered are the crown-to-root ratio, the condition of the remaining teeth in the arch, and the mobility pattern of the teeth to be stabilized. More specifically, if there is reason to believe that the mobility is temporary, any form of stabilization should be conservative, and the teeth should not be altered by removal of tooth structure by operative procedures. However, if mobility is due to a permanent loss of support, the overall projected treatment plan must take long-term stabilization by permanent splinting into consideration, and a form of stabilization that is less conservative of tooth structure may be justified.

The purposes of splinting are:

1. To rest the affected tissues by stabilizing the vectors of force
2. To distribute the forces over a number of teeth so that individual teeth are not subjected to as much stress as before

3. To ensure that the stress upon a single tooth does not exceed the adaptive capacity of the surrounding tissues and that jiggling movements contributing to periodontal disease are prevented
4. To change the direction of the force, such that the transmission assumes a near-axial direction
5. To stabilize the proximal contacts

CLASSIFICATION OF STABILIZATION BY SPLINTING

There are several different methods of splinting teeth. Major classification is based on the length of time the splint is to be used and whether provisional or long-term splinting is contemplated in conjunction with the periodontal prosthetics decided upon. Minor classifications are based on whether the technique of splinting involves removal of coronal tooth structure or leaves the teeth unaltered.

For convenience, we have chosen and slightly modified the classification formulated by Ross, Weisgold, and Wright.[18]

A. Temporary Stabilization
   1. Extracoronal splints not requiring cavity preparation
      a. Removable
         i. Acrylic bite guards
         ii. Cast continuous clasp appliances
      b. Fixed
         i. Wire-and-acrylic splints
         ii. Wire-mesh-and-acrylic splints
         iii. Orthodontic bands soldered in series
   2. Intracoronal splints requiring cavity preparation
      a. Wire-and-acrylic splints
      b. Wire-and-amalgam splints
      c. Combination amalgam, wire, and acrylic splints
      d. Interproximal splints of acrylic or amalgam with friction or threaded pins
B. Provisional Stabilization
   1. Acrylic splints
   2. Gold-band-and-acrylic splints
C. Permanent or Long-Term Stabilization
   1. Removable splints
   2. Fixed splints
   3. Combination removable and fixed splints

Discussion in this chapter will be limited to temporary stabilization. Methods of provisional and permanent stabilization are described in Chapters 28 and 29.

INDICATIONS FOR TEMPORARY STABILIZATION

The term *temporary* is applied

1. To a splint that is used until such time that stabilization is no longer necessary, e.g., in cases of mobility caused by accidental or surgical trauma or occlusal traumatism, all of a reversible nature.
2. As a phase in the therapy being undertaken to determine whether hypermobility is resolvable by conservative methods or whether mobility is due to loss of support sufficient to create permanent hypermobility (as in occlusal traumatism associated with periodontitis), root resorption, or any extrinsic or intrinsic precipitating factors, as listed in Chapter 5.
3. When advanced periodontal disease dictates permanent fixation by extensive restorative methods, but this cannot be done either (a) for economic reasons or (b) because prognosis for all remaining teeth is extremely doubtful or (c) because poor health seriously affects the longevity of the dentition, or even the life of the patient, or (d) because the patient cannot emotionally accept the prolonged procedures of permanent fixation.

Prior to construction of any splint for periodontally involved dentitions, certain basic considerations should be applied whenever possible:

1. For most patients, splinting should be considered only after the preliminary phase of periodontal therapy has been completed, including the elimination of all local factors contributing to inflammation and occlusal adjustment by selective grinding. Exceptions to this are dentitions where mobility is so great that adequate occlusal adjustment is impossible. In these circumstances the teeth should be stabilized as early as possible and then the occlusion can be definitively adjusted.
2. The method of splinting is dictated by the etiology and degree of mobility, the coronal condition of the teeth to be incorporated in the splint, and evaluation of the state of hypermobility, whether temporary or permanent. If the coronal portions of the teeth are in relatively good condition, the extracoronal method of splinting should be used (Figs. 18-7, 18-8). If, however, the teeth obviously require extensive restorative therapy, as well as periodontal therapy, a form of intracoronal splinting is justified and preferable (Figs. 18-11, 18-12).
3. The extent of splinting is dictated primarily by

the number of teeth involved and their degree of mobility. In all cases a sufficient number of nonmobile teeth should be included in the splint. If all the teeth in a quadrant demonstrate hypermobility, splinting should be extensive enough to include the support of anterior teeth and, on occasion, teeth on the opposite side of the arch. For the same reasons, it is often necessary to include the support of posterior teeth when anterior segments are mobile.

4. If, in a case of occlusal traumatism associated with severe bone loss, all the teeth demonstrate hypermobility, cross-arch splinting is beneficial, because the pattern of mobility of some teeth is in a buccolingual direction and of others in a mesiodistal direction. With splinting, a group of single-rooted teeth in effect become a multi-rooted unit.[3]

5. The method of splinting should neither impede normal functions nor frustrate the oral hygiene and physiotherapeutic efforts of the patient. The splint must not irritate the gingival tissues and, whenever possible, it should be esthetically acceptable.

6. The patient must be informed that future restorative measures will usually be necessary if any form of intra- or circumcoronal splinting is to be used.

All methods of splinting have advantages and disadvantages. For temporary stabilization, a method should be chosen that is the simplest, least expensive, and time-consuming to construct, esthetically acceptable to the patient, and yet which meets the needs of the individual. Ironically, some methods of stabilization by splinting are so time-consuming and demanding in construction that they are most impractical and expensive.

REMOVABLE EXTRACORONAL SPLINTS

Sometimes stabilization is required for a period of time, and yet the appliance must be removed by the patient or dentist conveniently and easily for varying lengths of time. The most commonly used splints in this category are the acrylic bite guards and the continuous clasp appliances. These appliances are relatively economical to construct but do have limitations in their use.

Acrylic Bite Guards

A conservative and simple method of providing temporary stabilization for mobile teeth is to use an

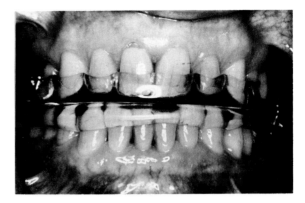

FIG. 18-1. *Acrylic bite guards for the maxillary and mandibular arches, a conservative method of stabilization of teeth pathologically mobile because of parafunctional habits.*

acrylic bite guard. Several varieties such as the hard-acrylic bite guard for upper and/or lower jaw, the resilient bite guard for upper or lower jaw, and a variation on the Hawley appliance, which gives the lower anterior teeth contact with the palatal surface of the upper acrylic plate are in common use.[17] The hard, clear, acrylic bite guard for the upper and lower jaw has been successfully used by the authors for several years and is the type described (Fig. 18-1).

A disadvantage of this form of stabilization is that the bite guards are usually worn only at night because they impede normal functions and are unesthetic. However, in cases of severe hypermobility caused by dysfunction or parafunction, both guards should be worn during the day as well, if some other form of stabilization cannot be substituted.

There are several indications for the use of the bite guard. For periodontal therapy, the removable bite guard is the treatment of choice when a full complement of teeth suffering from temporary hypermobility is in need of support. This appliance establishes a balanced articulation with the teeth in the opposing jaw and protects single or multiple teeth and their periodontia against occlusal overloads. Bite guards can also be used as retention appliances after minor or major orthodontics.

The bite guard is an important adjunct in the treatment of bruxism or the effects of bruxism. Bruxism is often treated by occlusal adjustment and/or occlusal reconstruction. Patients may continue to grind or clench in spite of treatment, however, resulting in wear and subsequent failure of the gold restorations. Since it has been established that these parafunctional jaw movements occur mostly during light sleep, bite guards worn at night can greatly reduce trauma to the temporomandibular joint and other supporting structures.

Bite guards can also be used for treating temporomandibular-joint dysfunction by correcting the condyle-fossa relationship and relieving muscular spasm and joint pain. By stretching muscles, the bite guard gives relief to the joints and painful muscles.[17] The construction of the bite guard in common use can be carried out by the dentist with the help of a trained technician and is described.

PROCEDURE FOR IMPRESSIONS AND WORKING CASTS

The accuracy of the bite-guard fit depends mainly on the quality of the impressions and working casts. Alginate impression material is sufficiently accurate, although any recognized elastic impression material may be used. It is imperative that the mouth be free from calculus and debris before taking the impression. If not, the teeth must first be scaled and polished.

The procedure for making impressions and working casts is exactly the same as that described in Chapter 12. Follow these instructions; then mount the casts on a semiadjustable articulator with the aid of a face-bow (Fig. 12-16). Take the lateral registration and set the articulator for greater functional accuracy in the finished waxing (Fig. 18-2). The waxing can be carried out by a trained technician or by the dentist.

PROCEDURE FOR WAXING

Increase the vertical separation of the occlusal surfaces of the teeth by separating the two members of the articulator to allow at least a 2-mm clearance of the anterior teeth during protrusive movements. Survey the height of contour (Fig. 18-2). During waxing, it is important not to extend the wax gingivally beyond the height of contour. Preferably, the wax should stay occlusal to this line to prevent unnecessary adjustment

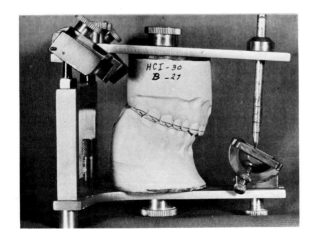

FIG. 18-2. *Surveyed casts mounted on a semiadjustable articulator in preparation for bite guard waxing.*

during insertion. For added strength, stainless steel wire may be luted over the occlusal surfaces of the posterior teeth and the lingual surfaces of the anterior teeth (Fig. 18-3A). Embrasure clasps may be used in selected areas for added retention if necessary (Fig. 18-3B).

The occlusal plane of the bite guards should approximate the patient's occlusal plane. With the aid of a template, wax the mandibular bite guard. Lubricate the occlusal portion of the waxed mandibular bite guard with petroleum jelly and obtain the plane of the maxillary bite guard by placing softened wax over the teeth, closing the articulator to the correct vertical dimension, and moving the upper member throughout all excursions while the wax is still soft. Trim off all excess wax. After completion of the waxing (Fig. 18-3C), flask the casts in regular denture flasks, boil the wax out, and process the bite guards in clear acrylic resin (Fig. 18-3D-F).

Carefully remove the processed bite guards and trim and polish them. Caution must be exercised, lest they be broken or warped during the finishing procedures.

PROCEDURE FOR INSERTION AND ADJUSTMENT

Check the bite guards for retention and stability. If a slight rocking motion is detected, reline them directly in the mouth with a quick-cure acrylic resin. Detect high spots with articulating ribbon and adjust the bite guards for maximum contact, in centric relation position and throughout all excursions of the mandible. Highly polish the occlusal surfaces of the bite guards, taking care to prevent warpage. Instruct the patient in their removal, insertion, and care, and advise him to wear both guards nightly. Make periodic checks to see if the patient is following instructions and check the bite guards for any necessary adjustment.

Continuous Clasp Appliances

Splinting with a removable continuous clasp appliance is a rapid and economical way of controlling hypermobility. Its main disadvantages are that if the anterior teeth must be included the appliances are unesthetic (Fig. 18-4) and that they will not effectively control intrusive movement of excessively mobile teeth unless designed in a manner that prevents or modifies their removal by the patient (Fig. 18-4D).

Because continuous clasp appliances are rigid castings of either gold or steel, they may be used for long-term stabilization if generally poor prognosis of the entire dentition or the financial limitations of the patient preclude the use of other types of splints. These

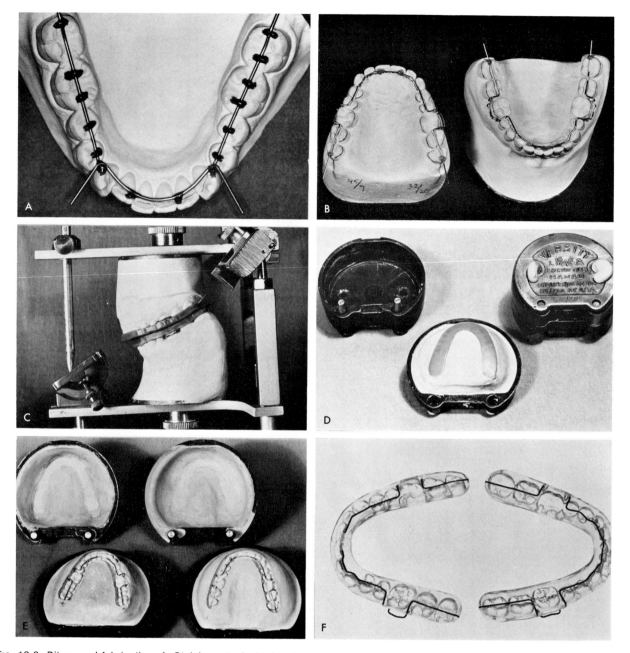

FIG. 18-3. *Bite guard fabrication. A. Stainless steel wire luted over occlusal and lingual surfaces to reinforce the acrylic guards. B. Embrasure clasps placed around the first molars to increase the retention. Note that the ends of the clasps are extended over the occlusal and/or lingual surfaces for reinforcement. C. Bite guards waxed in accordance with the articulator settings. D. Bite guards flasked. E. Wax removed (with boiling water). F. Processed maxillary and mandibular bite guards. (Courtesy W. Loew.)*

appliances offer the advantages of replacing missing teeth (Fig. 18-5) and of being either entirely tooth-supported or tooth-and-tissue-supported (Fig. 18-6). The continuous clasp appliance can be conveniently removed for cleaning purposes and for examination and adjustment. One useful variation suggested by Friedman is to eliminate the unesthetic characteristics by not clasping the labial aspects of the anterior teeth.[8] However, this modification necessitates securing the appliance by cementation or ligation, making its re-

moval by the patient for better oral hygiene impossible and its adjustment and repair by the dentist more difficult.

FIXED EXTRACORONAL SPLINTS NOT REQUIRING CAVITY PREPARATION

As with removable extracoronal splints, fixed splints offer the advantages of simplicity and economy, and

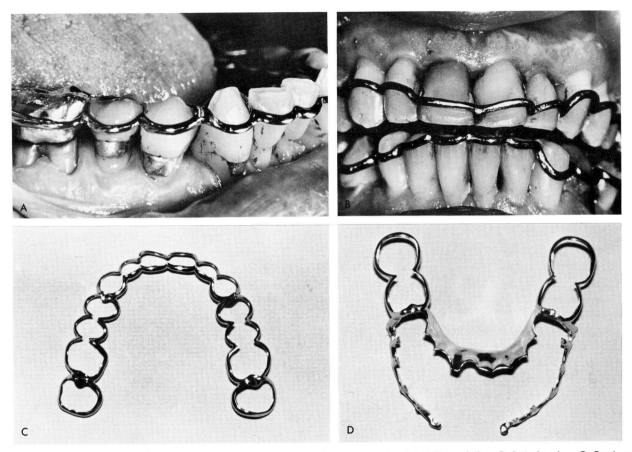

FIG. 18-4. *Continuous clasp appliance used as a removable form of extracoronal splint. A. Buccal view. B. Anterior view. C. Occlusal view of maxillary appliance removed. D. Occlusal view of mandibular appliance modified to engage labial undercuts to control intrusive forces. Modification is of the swing-lock variety.*

when they are no longer required, they can be readily removed by the dentist without need of replacement by restorative means. The fixed types of splints offer greater stability and the certainty that they are being worn constantly. Unfortunately, all fixed extracoronal splints have major inherent disadvantages. By their bulkiness they increase axial contours, thereby con-

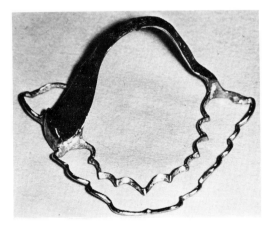

FIG. 18-5. *Tooth-supported continuous clasp appliance modified to replace missing molar as well as to improve cross-arch stabilization by incorporating a palatal strap.*

stricting interproximal embrasures, and thus promoting greater plaque and food retention. They often interfere with adequate oral hygiene and physiotherapeutic measures and are esthetically objectionable to many.

All these devices must be routinely removed by the dentist to prevent decalcification and caries. Once removed they have to be reapplied if stabilization is still necessary. There is no way of knowing if mobility has decreased unless they are removed. Except for the continuous-orthodontic-band splint, the application of this form of splinting is usually limited to the anterior segments.

Fixed extracoronal splints are usually indicated for dentitions with a higher probability that hypermobility is only temporary and can be resolved. Examples of conditions where hypermobility is significantly present or may arise during or after therapy and warrants consideration of this method of stabilization are as follows:

1. Severe occlusal traumatism with periodontal disturbances warranting surgical intervention
2. Temporary hypermobility due to accidental or surgical trauma

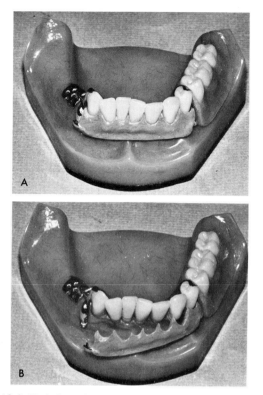

FIG. 18-6. *Variation of removable splint appliance modified to utilize tissue as well as tooth support (referred also as a swing-lock partial denture). A. Appliance in locked position. B. Appliance unlocked for removal (Courtesy Harrison Dental Laboratory, Seattle, Washington.)*

3. Patients requiring bone-reattachment procedures
4. Patients requiring combined periodontic and endodontic therapy
5. Patients requiring moderate osseous correction for which the need for long-term tooth stabilization after corrective surgery cannot be predicted
6. Any condition involving unexplained hypermobility
7. A dentition requiring temporary stabilization prior to partial coverage by three-quarter crowns or pin splints rather than full crowns

Extracoronal fixed splints provide an effective method of temporary stabilization, since they do not predestine the dentition to full-coverage fixation, but this method of stabilization is not indicated when permanent fixation by full coverage is a necessary part of the overall treatment plan. For such cases, it is preferable that the restorative dentist prepare the teeth for provisional acrylic splints, in the manner described in Chapter 28. This method is not indicated for teeth having a hopeless prognosis unless their extraction and replacement is economically or otherwise prohibitive. For such cases, early extraction and replacement with provisional bridges will expedite the therapy. Too often, attempts to save hopelessly involved teeth by prolonged and expensive therapy jeopardize approximating teeth.

Wire-and-Acrylic Splints

The most common and easiest method of fixed extracoronal splinting uses wire-and-acrylic splints.[7] In some cases only wire is used, but the acrylic resin offers the advantage of increased stability and improved esthetics, especially where diastemata are present. This method is commonly used to splint mandibular anterior teeth, but can also be used for maxillary anterior teeth if the patient does not object to the cosmetic disadvantages. Occasionally this technique can be adapted for splinting posterior teeth if the coronal form permits. However, other forms of splinting such as orthodontic bands or intracoronal occlusal wire, acrylic resin, and amalgam are more advantageously used for posterior teeth. Extracoronal wire-and-acrylic splints greatly exaggerate the axial contours of posterior teeth, promoting plaque retention and severely limiting the ability of the patient to carry out adequate plaque control procedures.

PROCEDURE

Prior to applying the splint, make certain that all subgingival and supragingival accretions have been removed by thorough root planing, scaling, and polishing. The use of the rubber dam will greatly facilitate the application of the wire and acrylic resin by maintaining a dry field, restraining the patient's tongue, and protecting the gingiva from any procedural trauma. It also affords a better opportunity to apply a topical fluoride to inhibit caries prior to application of the acrylic resin (Fig. 18-7).

Adapt a double strand of soft orthodontic ligature wire (0.010) as illustrated (Fig. 18-7A-B). Where diastemata are present, twist the labial and lingual wire to span the interproximal space and continue to include all teeth to be splinted (Fig. 18-8). Position the labial and lingual wire just apical to the interproximal contact areas, so that slipping is prevented and damage to the gingiva by the ligature is avoided. At this point in the procedure, secure the splint with interproximal ties, engaging the lingual and labial arch wires (Fig. 18-7A-B). Cut and carefully bend the twisted ends of the interproximal ties, making certain not to obliterate the interproximal embrasure spaces (Fig. 18-7C). Do not overtwist the interproximal wires or the teeth may separate. To avoid later confusion, twist all ties in the same direction.

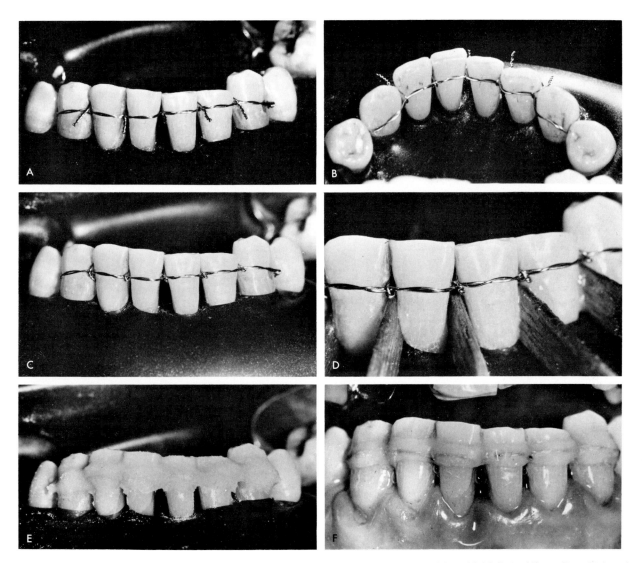

FIG. 18-7. *Application of extracoronal wire-and-acrylic splint. A. Labial view of wire positioned labially and lingually apical to the contact areas, but occlusally to the cingula. Note interproximal ties between each pair of teeth being splinted. B. Lingual view of wire in place. C. The cut ends of the twisted interproximal ties bent into the embrasure spaces. D. Lubricated soft wood wedges placed interproximally to prevent the flow of acrylic resin into the embrasures. E. Autopolymerizing acrylic resin applied after removal of wooden wedges. F. Occlusion refined and splint polished (Courtesy Dr. V. Jekkals.)*

When the wire is secure, place softwood interproximal wedges lubricated with petroleum jelly below each contact area (Stim-u-dents are suitable*) (Fig. 18-7D), and with a small brush apply enough autopolymerizing tooth-colored acrylic resin to the interproximal labial and lingual surfaces to cover and stabilize the wire (Fig. 18-7E). In addition to securing the ligature wire, the acrylic resin improves the esthetics. The wooden wedges will prevent the acrylic resin from flowing into and obliterating the interproximal embrasures. While the acrylic resin is still at the rubbery

* Stim-u-dent, Inc., Detroit

stage, remove the wedges, and with a sharp curet carefully trim away any excess acrylic resin that may have flowed over the limits. After the acrylic resin has finally set, trim it to proper contour, polish it, and remove the rubber dam (Fig. 18-7F).

Before dismissing the patient, examine the occlusion to ensure that the labial aspect of the splint does not interfere in centric relation occlusion or during lateral and protrusive excursions. In many cases of deep overbite where there is insufficient overjet, the labial surface of the acrylic and wire splint may have to be completely ground away so that there will be no interference. In such cases, the remaining interproximal and

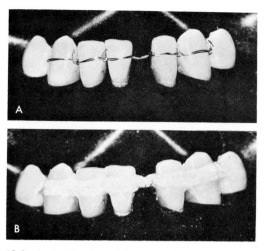

FIG. 18-8. *A. Application of ligature wire to span diastema. Note that the labial and lingual wires are twisted together. B. Acrylic resin to secure the ligature wire trimmed and polished.*

lingual acrylic and wire splints are usually sufficient to provide the necessary stabilization. This step may also be necessary for cosmetic reasons if the patient wishes.

Carefully instruct the patient in any necessary modification of home-care procedures. With splints of this type, greater effort is required to keep the dentition free from microbial plaque.

If the splint is to remain in place for a long time, the teeth should be examined periodically for signs of caries activity. It is advisable to reapply topical fluoride routinely during recall visits.

Wire-Mesh-and-Acrylic Splints

Wire-mesh-and-acrylic splints are especially appropriate for splinting posterior teeth. The band of wire mesh provides greater stabilization than does ligature wire. The greater stability is often necessary when posterior teeth, complicated by occlusal factors, are in need of surgical therapy. Splints of this type readily permit the joining of splinted anterior segments to posterior quadrants to provide cross-arch stabilization whenever necessary. Unfortunately, this technique has the same disadvantages and limitations as the extracoronal wire-and-acrylic method. Axial contours are often grossly increased to the degree that oral hygiene efforts are frustrated.

If this method of splinting is to be used, the procedures are similar to those described for extracoronal wire-and-acrylic ligation, except that a narrow strip of 80-gauge brass mesh is used in place of wire and is adapted to the buccal and lingual surfaces of the teeth to be included in the splint. Interproximal ties are made as described for wire-and-acrylic splints, and a thin veneer of autopolymerizing acrylic resin is ap-

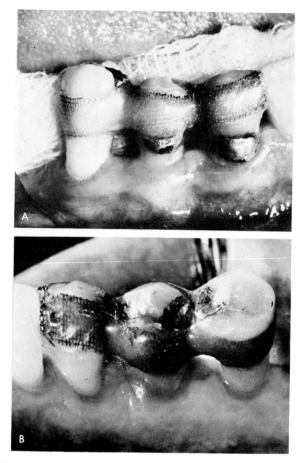

FIG. 18-9. *Extracoronal wire mesh-acrylic splint adapted for stabilization of posterior teeth. A. Buccal view. B. Lingual view.*

plied over the mesh (Fig. 18-9). The same procedures regarding care and maintenance apply.

Orthodontic Band Splint

Orthodontic bands welded in series can be used effectively for stabilizing both anterior and posterior teeth (Fig. 18-10). Cosmetic factors, however, limit their use. If adapted correctly they are preferable to wire mesh and acrylic resin because they only minimally increase the axial contours. Care must be taken during adaptation to trim carefully and adapt the gingival borders of the bands to prevent overextensions that impinge upon the tissues. Periodic examinations are necessary to guard against cement washouts. A modification substituting wire ligation for solder between the bands is described by Block.[6] This allows adjustments in tension to be made. This type of splint has the advantage of being removable at any time without undue damage to the splint. It is, therefore, reusable if the teeth require further stabilization. This is not possible with the wire or wire-mesh-and-acrylic ligation.

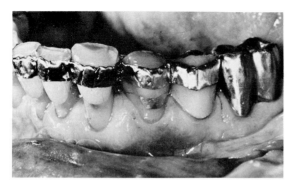

FIG. 18-10. *Orthodontic band splint.*

INTRACORONAL SPLINTS

The intracoronal type of temporary splint for mobile teeth has been used for many years.[15] It is an excellent method for stabilizing teeth with severe periodontal involvement and a questionable prognosis. The stabilization is therapeutic, especially during the surgical phase of periodontal therapy, as it eliminates the obstructive mobility patterns that contribute to further breakdown and retard healing.

Several methods of intracoronal splinting have been devised, using amalgam,[13] amalgam and wire,[2] acrylic resin and wire,[15] wire, threaded or friction-lock pins, and acrylic resin,[11] or a combination of amalgam, wire and acrylic resin especially adaptable to posterior quadrants.[21] In most circumstances intracoronal splinting is reserved for cases where the severity of periodontal disease makes future permanent stabilization by extreme restorative measures essential.

When the severity dictates this procedure, the patient must be informed that extensive restorative measures will still be necessary. This method of splinting is justifiable as a long-term splint in exceptional cases of financial hardship, for certain physical or emotional reasons, or for cases where periodontal involvement is so generalized that prognosis for all remaining teeth is extremely doubtful and permanent stabilization by costly restorative methods is impractical. For such patients, it is important to make it quite clear that this method of splinting is considered the intermediate step to a future removable prosthesis (Fig. 18-13). They must fully understand that intracoronal splints may have to be remade periodically because of recurrent caries or breakage.

Temporary intracoronal splinting has the following advantages:

1. It is more retentive and provides greater stabilization than do most other forms of temporary stabilization.
2. It is fixed, ensuring that the patient constantly wears it.

3. It lasts longer and can be considered in exceptional cases a long-term temporary splint.
4. It neither irritates the gingival tissues nor impedes home-care measures.
5. It is relatively simple to construct, requires less time and less tooth reduction, and is consequently less expensive than the conventional full-coverage provisional splint.
6. It is relatively simple to repair.
7. Most variations are esthetic.

Like most methods of temporary stabilization, intracoronal splinting has disadvantages. There are dangers of pulp injury during preparation, and the splint cannot appreciably alter or correct undesirable coronal contour or functional occlusal discrepancies, nor are some varieties, such as the wire-and-acrylic type, indicated for patients who have a high caries rate. Where these potentials apply, the all-acrylic or acrylic-and-gold-band provisional splint (described in Chapter 28) or, at least, the combination amalgam-wire-and-acrylic type is preferable.

Techniques for Posterior Teeth

The following variation for posterior teeth, modeled on that refined by Trachtenberg,[21] is the combination of amalgam, wire, and acrylic resin. Although it is more time-consuming, it has advantages over the wire-and-amalgam or wire-and-acrylic types that are described later in this chapter.

PROCEDURE

For obvious reasons, cavity preparation is best carried out with the advantages of a well-placed rubber dam. Cut mesioocclusodistal cavity preparations in the routine manner, ensuring that the occlusal depth of the preparation is sufficient to accept an adequate layer of amalgam, wire, and acrylic resin. This variation usually requires the occlusal portion of the cavity preparation to have greater dimensions buccolingually and occlusogingivally than are normally required for routine amalgam restorations (Fig. 18-11A).

After cavity preparation, paint the internal surfaces with a cavity varnish. Place well-condensed amalgams with the aid of a properly contoured and supported matrix band. All the principles of correct interproximal contour must be adhered to, ensuring that contours or poor margin adaptation do not contribute to plaque retention. Carve the occlusal anatomy of each tooth in such a way that centric holding areas are not in supraocclusion (Fig. 18-11B). Allow the amalgam to set for at least one day. At a subsequent appointment, replace the rubber dam, and with a #35 inverted-cone bur cut

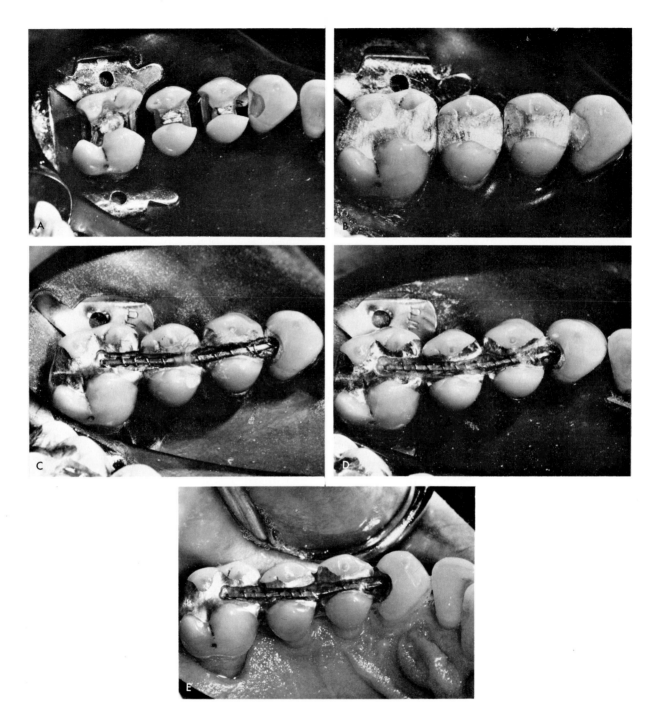

FIG. 18-11. *Application of intracoronal amalgam-wire-and-acrylic splint. A. Mesio-occlusodistal cavity preparations of sufficient depth and width to accept an adequate layer of amalgam, wire, and autopolymerizing acrylic resin. B. Cavity preparations, individually filled with amalgam. C. Wire placed in channel cut to extend mesiodistally and include all the teeth to be splinted. D. Channel filled with autopolymerizing acrylic resin. E. Occlusion refined to perfect centric relation contacts and to eliminate unnecessary contacts. (Courtesy Dr. S. Sapkos.)*

an occlusal groove, sufficiently wide and deep occlusogingivally and buccolingually to accept 0.027 wire and acrylic resin. It is desirable to contain the occlusal groove entirely within the amalgam (Fig. 18-11C). If there is perforation into the dentin of the pulpal or axial wall of the amalgam groove, the advantages of

the amalgam protection against acrylic percolation and subsequent caries are greatly reduced. Such perforations should be repaired with spot amalgam fillings if the splint is to remain in place for a long time.

Place lubricated interproximal softwood wedges (Stim-u-dents) between teeth to prevent the flow of acrylic resin into the interproximal embrasure. Wrap a sufficient length of 0.027 stainless-steel wire or orthodontic square-bracket wire around with 0.010 dead-soft ligature wire and place it in the depth of the prepared occlusal groove (Fig. 18-11C). Paint autopolymerizing clear acrylic resin into the preparation with the aid of a camel's-hair brush, so that the groove is completely filled (Fig. 18-11D). Allow the acrylic resin to set, trim the excess, remove the rubber dam, and check the occlusion (Fig. 18-11E). Trim high spots and build up any centric holding areas that lack contact by spot addition of more acrylic resin. Reduce broad centric holding areas to spot contacts. Bridge edentulous areas of one-tooth width or less, by adding extra acrylic resin and reducing it to the shape of a hygienic pontic (Fig. 18-12). The splint is then highly polished. A splint of this type constructed with care provides the adequate stabilization and caries protection required if the splint is to be considered a long-range temporary splint.

There are variations of this splint. The occlusal groove is often cut into the tooth structure without first putting in an amalgam filling (Fig. 18-13). This technique provides rapid stabilization and will be satisfac-

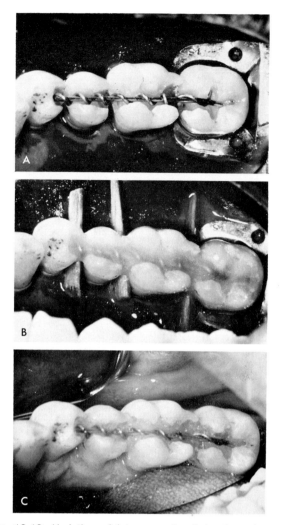

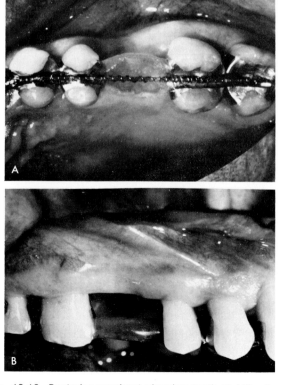

FIG. 18-12. *Posterior quadrant showing teeth stabilized and edentulous area bridged with an intracoronal amalgam-wire-and-acrylic splint. A. Occlusal view. B. Buccal view. (Courtesy Dr. C. Filipchuk.)*

FIG. 18-13. *Variation of intracoronal splint using wire and acrylic resin only, a simple method for rapid stabilization and a precursor to more durable long-term stabilization. Because the risk of caries is high, splints must be carefully checked during frequent recall visits. A. Channel cut and wire positioned. B. Interproximal wedges placed and acrylic applied. C. Occlusion refined and acrylic polished. (Courtesy Dr. R. L. Johnson.)*

tory if the splint is to be worn for a short time only as a precursor to more durable long-term stabilization. Its disadvantages are the danger of caries and tooth sensitivity caused by acrylic percolation. If this variation is used, it is imperative that clear acrylic resin be used so that recurrent carious activity and percolation can be readily detected on recall visits.

Another variation involves the use of amalgam and wire only (Fig. 18-14). This provides excellent stabilization but has the disadvantage of unpredictable amalgam fracture, especially if the splinting includes more than 2 or 3 teeth. With fracturing, the danger of recurrent caries is more imminent. The amalgam-wire-acrylic combination is the preferred type, since it

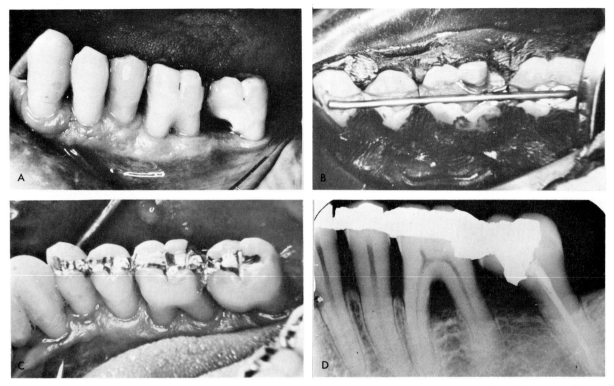

FIG. 18-14. *Another variation of an intracoronal splint, using wire and amalgam only. Higher risk of amalgam fracture and recurrent caries are disadvantages. A. Buccal view of quadrant requiring stabilization. B. Occlusal channel cut, wire positioned and compound matrix applied in preparation for condensation of amalgam. C. Completed wire-and-amalgam splint. D. Radiograph 10 years postoperatively.*

allows for slight movement of individual teeth with little likelihood of fracture.

Techniques for Anterior Teeth

As with intracoronal posterior splints, there are several variations of the anterior type. The indications for their use are the same as those given for the posterior type. Kessler describes a variation that provides excellent stabilization, has adequate retention, requires conservative removal of tooth structure, and yet in most cases preserves the original esthetics of the teeth, since the cavity preparation is limited to the lingual aspect of the tooth.[11]

PROCEDURE

The use of a rubber dam is recommended during the preparation of the teeth and placement of the acrylic resin. Starting at the junction of the upper and middle thirds, make grooves in each tooth to be splinted and undercut them with a $33\frac{1}{3}$ inverted-cone bur (Fig. 18-15A). Prepare a mesial or distal box 1 mm deep in the long axis of each tooth and make a 0.021 hole with a helical-twist drill for the insertion of a pin (Fig.

18-15B). Coat the cavity preparations with fluoride solution and cavity varnish; coat the pins with varnish and insert them. Either ligate the vertical pins internally with dead-soft stainless-steel wire (0.008 or 0.010) or bend them over 0.025 continuous horizontal wire connecting the teeth (Fig. 18-15C). Seal the preparations with the pins and wire in place with acrylic resin. Trim and polish the acrylic resin and adjust the occlusion (Fig. 18-15D-E-F).

Ross and his associates describe another variation that involves cutting a circumcoronal groove into each anterior tooth (Fig. 18-16).[18] Wire ligation is provided and acrylic resin is painted into each groove. This method provides for adequate stabilization without the use of embedded pins. However, after a period of time the acrylic resin becomes discolored from staining and percolation and is esthetically objectionable. Caries may recur unless the splint is remade frequently. This method also precludes the use of partial coverage pin-splinting as the final form of stabilization, which may have been the method of choice. The choice is now limited to the more radical full-coverage crown.

The circumferential intracoronal type described above is not recommended if the coronal condition of anterior teeth warrants full coverage. The teeth should

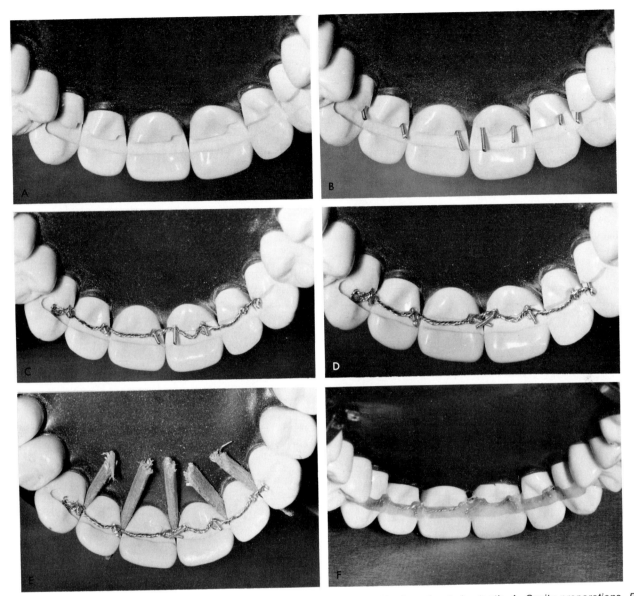

FIG. 18-15. *Esthetic modification of intracoronal splint for temporary stabilization of anterior teeth. A. Cavity preparations. B. Insertion of threaded pins. C. Ligation of pins. D. Pins bent into cavity preparations. E. Lubricated soft wood wedges placed interproximally to limit the flow of acrylic resin. F. Acrylic resin applied, occlusion refined, and acrylic resin polished. (After Kessler, M.: A variation of the A splint. J. Periodontol., 41:268, 1970.)*

be reduced and stabilized with the all acrylic or combination gold-band-and-acrylic provisional splint.

Regardless of the method, intracoronal stabilization allows the anterior segments to be readily joined to posterior segments and provides for cross-arch stabilization whenever needed.

References

1. Allen, D. L.: Accurate occlusal bite guards. Periodontics, 5:93, 1967.
2. Alloy, J., and Kato, M.: The amalgam splint. J. Am. Dent. Assoc., 65:381, 1962.
3. Amsterdam, M., and Abrams, L.: Periodontal prosthesis. *In Periodontal Therapy*, 4th ed. H. M. Goldman and D. W. Cohen, Eds. St. Louis, C. V. Mosby Co., 1968.
4. Ballavia, W., and Ciancio, S. G.: Pin-retained amalgam splints. J. Am. Dent. Assoc., 78:525, 1969.
5. Berliner, A.: Ligatures, Splints, Bite Planes and Pyramids. Philadelphia, J. B. Lippincott Co., 1964.
6. Block, P. L.: A wire-band splint for immobilizing loose posterior teeth. J. Periodontol., 39:17, 1968.
7. Clark, J. W., Weatherford, T. W., and Mann, W. V., Jr.: The wire ligature-acrylic splint. J. Periodontol., 40:371, 1969.
8. Friedman, N.: Temporary splinting: an adjunct in periodontal therapy. J. Periodontol., 24:229, 1953.

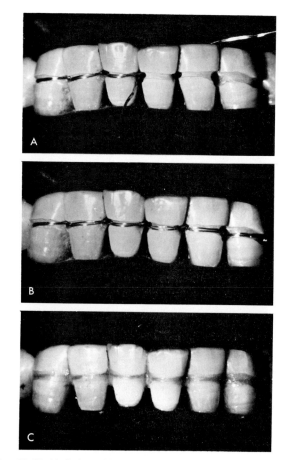

FIG. 18-16. *Variation of intracoronal temporary splint that provides excellent stabilization for anterior teeth. A. Circumcoronal grooves cut in all teeth to be included. Double-strand 0.010 ligature wire being positioned within grooves. B. Wire ligation completed. C. Acrylic resin applied, trimmed, and polished. Disadvantages include recurrence of caries unless the splint is remade frequently and predestining the splinted teeth to full-coverage restorations when partial coverage may have sufficed. (Courtesy Dr. L. Shelton.)*

9. Hampton, J. L.: Staple-type of fixed splint. Dent. Pract. Dent. Rec., *8:*22, 1957.
10. Johnson, W. N.: A new fixed temporary dental splint. Periodont. Abstracts, *14:*153, 1966.
11. Kessler, M.: A variation of the A splint. J. Periodontol., *41:*268, 1970.
12. Kothe, J., and Taatz, H.: Die intrakoronale Kunstoff-drahtschiene. D. D. Z., *18:*77, 1964.
13. Lloyd, R. S., and Baer, P. N.: Permanent fixed amalgam splint. J. Periodontol., *30:*163, 1959.
14. Liatukas, E.: The amalgam splints. J. Periodontol., *38:*392, 1967.
15. Obin, J., and Arvins, A.: The use of self-curing resin splints for the temporary stabilization of mobile teeth due to periodontal involvement. J. Am. Dent. Assoc., *42:*320, 1951.
16. Peery, W. S.: Removable periodontal prosthesis and temporary splints. North Carolina Dent. J., *48:*115, 1965.
17. Posselt, U.: The Physiology of Occlusion and Rehabilitation, 2nd ed. Philadelphia, F. A. Davis, 1968.
18. Ross, S. E., Weisgold, A., and Wright, W. H.: Temporary stabilization. *In* Periodontal Therapy, 4th ed. H. M. Goldman and D. W. Cohen, Eds. St. Louis, C. V. Mosby, 1968.
19. Shatzkin, E. H.: Semi-permanent splinting—an adjunct to restorative dentistry. J. Prosthet. Dent., *10:*946, 1960.
20. Stern, I. B.: Status of temporary fixed-splinting procedures in the treatment of periodontally involved teeth. J. Periodontol., *30:*217, 1960.
21. Trachtenberg, D. I.: A combined amalgam-wire-acrylic splint. J. Periodontol., *39:*255, 1968.
22. Wulff-Cochrane, V.: Splints in periodontal treatment. Leeds Dent. J., *6:*55, 1967.
23. Zamet, J. S.: Splints in periodontal therapy. Dental Health, *6:*57, 1967.

19

Minor Tooth Movement in Periodontal Therapy

19

Minor Tooth Movement in Periodontal Therapy

LEONARD HIRSCHFELD

There are many occasions when changing the position of one or several teeth is an essential part of periodontal treatment. Several of the important *causes* of periodontal disease can be corrected by moving teeth. Marked occlusal trauma can be relieved by uprighting tipped molars, correcting crossbites or deep overbites, or otherwise improving the axial inclinations of individual teeth. Selectively grinding the teeth would be completely inadequate for relieving the trauma in many of these cases.

Tooth crowding can lead to gingival enlargement and inflammation because of difficulty in maintaining satisfactory oral hygiene. Crowding also can cause deep interproximal crater formation because of insufficient interseptal bone. Such crowding can often be corrected, sometimes requiring removal of one of the teeth to obtain room for rearranging the others. Conversely, an open contact causes food impaction which can produce rapid destruction of the interproximal periodontal structures. Such open contacts are frequently corrected by making fillings or inlays, but moving a tooth to close the contact may reduce or eliminate the need for the restorative procedures.

Many *results* of periodontal disease also require minor tooth movement to restore the dentition to a tolerable esthetic and functional status. When periodontally involved teeth protrude and elongate and diastemata open, the teeth frequently can be moved back into alignment. In periodontal disease, alveolar bone is lost, and it may be necessary to undertake splinting. Teeth also may be lost and may have to be replaced. Abutment teeth and teeth that require splinting often are not sufficiently parallel to permit these procedures. Reorienting such teeth into better axial inclinations, or even moving them bodily for short distances, can make the splints or bridges possible.

In some periodontal patients, many teeth must be moved considerable distances to provide the desired results. In such cases, there may be incorrect relationships of one arch to another or of large segments of the dentition. Some teeth may be too large or too small for the jaws, or teeth may have erupted in an incorrect sequence. To treat most of these anomalies, major orthodontic therapy, with complex fixed appliances, must be used.

In many other cases, only one or a few teeth are malposed and must be moved only a few millimeters to be in acceptable positions. A number of simpler procedures can be used to accomplish these changes, often rapidly. The techniques for this minor tooth movement include the use of light latex elastics;[10] grass-line,[8] elastic thread,[7] and wire ligatures; and removable appliances such as Hawley retainers with active springs, bite planes,[9] split-plates,[17] and elastic positioners.[11] Fixed sectional arches and even simple full arches are also used for movement of a limited number of teeth.

TIPPING, BODILY MOVEMENT, AND TORQUING

Application of a force can tip a tooth or move it bodily. A tooth being *tipped* has its crown moving in one direction and the root apex in the opposite direction, with a fulcrum about at the junction of the apical and middle third of the intra-alveolar root (Fig. 19-1).[14] A periodontally involved tooth with reduced alveolar bone therefore has the fulcrum nearer to the apex and is tipped less than a tooth with normal periodontal support. When a tooth is moved *bodily*, the crown and root move in the same direction. When the mesio-incisal corner of the tooth is moved 3 millimeters bodily, 3 millimeters of bone mesial to the entire root surface must be resorbed and 3 millimeters of bone distal to the root must be built up. But when an incisor is being *tipped* mesially 3 millimeters, only 1 or 2 millimeters of bone need to be remodeled. This explains why tipping takes a much shorter time. Rotating a molar takes a very long time, since, in effect, the roots are being moved bodily through the bone as the crown rotates.

Torquing of teeth, in which the crowns remain in position but the roots are moved in order to achieve better axial inclinations, requires even longer time, since a great deal of remodeling is necessary.

Most malpositions requiring major orthodontic therapy are caused by genetic and developmental factors acting *before* or during the eruption of the permanent teeth. Most malpositions amenable to *minor* tooth movement are caused after eruption by periodontal disease, by extraction and nonreplacement of adjacent teeth, by occlusal forces, or by various habits. Since such forces usually *tip* the teeth out of position, they can be realigned by forces tipping in the opposite direction. Most of the techniques for minor tooth movement apply tipping forces, although sectional arches can be used for some of the cases requiring bodily movement or torquing.

EXAMINATION PROCEDURES

Procedures for minor tooth movement are gratifying when they succeed, but frustrating and disappointing when they fail. The most important factor in achieving success is the proper selection of cases. The most skilled technician is not likely to be successful with an unsuitable case. Selection, in turn, depends upon a thorough examination and understanding of the possibilities and limitations of the available methods.

After a brief discussion of the patient's medical background, the history of the malposition is obtained and recorded. The rapidity of migration may be an important factor in prognosis. The basic relationships of the jaws to each other and to the skull are observed and noted. There are several classifications, but the Angle classification into Classes I, II, and III with several divisions is most commonly used. The shape of the arches (such as square, oval, wide, or narrow) and the occlusal curve are noted. The degree of overbite and overjet are observed and the angle of incisal guidance is compared with the occlusal curve to see whether there is posterior interference in the protrusive excursions.

The axial inclinations of the tooth to be moved and the prospective anchor teeth are examined. The mobility of these teeth is recorded as are their periodontal and pulpal status. Crowded areas and open interproximal contacts are recorded. These notations are important for purposes of comparison as the treatment progresses.

The last part of the examination is concerned with functional and parafunctional movements. The physiologic rest position, the free-way space, and the path of closure are studied. Any premature contacts in closure, with resulting mandibular shifts, are observed, since the elimination of such a shift may make it possible to treat a case which would not be successful otherwise. Overloading of specific teeth in the protrusive or lateral excursions is recorded for further correction. Inquiries are made about habits that may contribute to malposition.

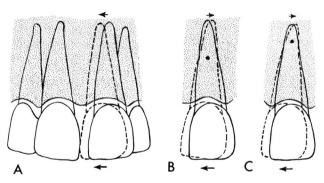

FIG. 19-1. *A. Bodily tooth movement with a fixed appliance, with crown and root moving in the same direction. B. Tipping force exerted when fulcrum is about two thirds of the way down the root from the alveolar crest. C. Reduction in tipping effect when the fulcrum is closer to the apex. (From Hirschfeld, L., and Jay, J: Minor tooth movement by means of rubber dam elastics. J. Am. Dent. Assoc., 50:282, 1955.)*

CRITERIA FOR
SELECTION OF CASES

Although individual tooth manifestations of major malocclusions can sometimes be treated by minor movement methods, the majority of successful cases are those with relatively normal basic relationships. In any case, four prerequisites must be met:

1. There must be enough room into which the tooth can be moved, or such room must be obtainable by stripping, moving adjacent teeth, or extraction.

2. It must be possible to prevent occlusal trauma to the tooth during and after the movement procedure. Grinding and bite plates may be used to reduce trauma during movement, but, unless extensive fixed splinting is to be used for retention, a tooth in its final position must have an acceptable balance of muscular forces acting upon it or it will relapse rapidly.

3. The axial inclination must be such that moving the tooth, with means practical for that case, will not cause it to be at a more unfavorable angle to the occlusal forces and the supporting structures. In other words, a mesially tilted tooth should not be tipped further mesially. It must be moved bodily or even torqued into an upright position.

4. All factors causing the malposition must be correctable. Some etiologic factors, such as tongue thrusts, are difficult to correct. In other cases, crowding may be caused by clenching and grinding habits, and the corrected teeth will buckle again unless the habit is controlled.

COMMON PROBLEMS IN MINOR TOOTH
MOVEMENT

The techniques of minor tooth movement mentioned at the beginning of this chapter can be used in coping with many abnormalities. A given technique may be the best for one problem but less effective for another. The best methods for treating several abnormalities often seen in periodontal patients will be described.

Closure of Anterior Diastemata
by Mesiodistal Movement

Diastemata may occur when anterior teeth migrate labially and form the arc of a larger circle. Because the mesiodistal widths of the individual units remain unchanged, spaces are produced.

Examination will show whether the diastema should be closed by moving one or several teeth mesiodistally or by moving the teeth lingually into the arc of a smaller circle. If the teeth have been fanned out

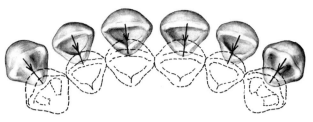

Fig. 19-2. *Closure of uniform small diastemata between all the teeth by moving teeth back labially.*

labially, it is most desirable to move them back palatally (Fig. 19-2), but not always possible to do so. The occlusion may be such that the lower teeth prevent the upper teeth from coming back. In such a case, the larger arc must be accepted, the diastemata must be closed by mesiodistal movement, and a pontic must be used to fill the remaining space.

An excellent method for moving incisors mesiodistally is the light latex or rubber dam elastic. To move two teeth together reciprocally, a ¼-inch diameter elastic is stretched between the fingers and placed around the two teeth. It is kept in the middle third of the crown by the anatomy of the cingulum (Fig. 19-3). The elastic is removed before meals and replaced afterwards with a new elastic. The elastics exert a safe, light force and are extremely esthetic, hygienic, and comfortable. However, they must be used under close observation because several cases have been reported in which elastics have slipped far up under the gingiva, causing extensive periodontal destruction. This can be prevented by looping a piece of 0.008-inch wire around the cervix of one of the teeth, twisting the ends enough times to reach the middle of the tooth, and then looping the wire incisally to the cingulum (Fig. 19-4). The resulting spur keeps the elastic in the proper

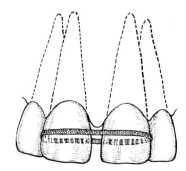

Fig. 19-3. *Moving the central incisors together with an elastic encircling them at the level of the middle third of the crown, incisally to the cingula and gingivally to the contact points. (Adapted from Hirschfeld, L., and Jay, J: Minor tooth movement by means of rubber dam elastics. J. Am. Dent. Assoc., 50:282, 1955.)*

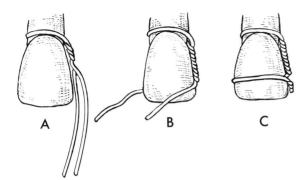

FIG. 19-4. *A. A loop of wire tightened apically to the cervix. B. Enough twists made to enable the strands to encircle the crown incisally to the cingulum. C. The second loop in place with the ends twisted together to act as a spur in the interproximal space. (Adapted from Hirschfeld, L., and Jay, J.: Minor tooth movement by means of rubber dam elastics. J. Am. Dent. Assoc., 50:282, 1955.)*

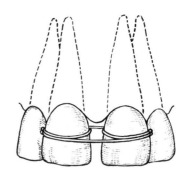

FIG. 19-5. *Using silk ligature to move two teeth together. (Adapted from Hirschfeld, L.: The use of wire and silk ligatures. J. Am. Dent. Assoc., 41:647, 1950.)*

position on both teeth. If the tooth is to be crowned later, a niche or groove can be made in it to keep the elastic in position. The patient is asked to come in weekly, and the occlusal surfaces of the tooth are ground if it has moved into a position where it is subjected to occlusal trauma. The desired movement usually takes 1 to 3 weeks, depending upon the distance and the amount of alveolar support.

If four incisors are to be moved together to close a diastema, one elastic is placed around both central incisors and the left lateral incisor, and another is placed around both central incisors and the right lateral incisor. This applies a mesially directed force to each tooth, and an efficient reciprocal system is set up.

To move one tooth toward another, the reciprocal force must be distributed on two or more teeth. This distribution will reduce the force on each of the anchor teeth below the level which would cause it to move. If two anchor teeth are close together, the elastic can encircle them and the tooth to be moved. However, if there are to be three anchor teeth, they should be ligated with an 0.010 wire ligature, and the elastic should encircle just the tooth being moved and the nearest anchor tooth.

For patients who lack the manual dexterity or discipline required for application of the elastics, there are two alternative methods—grass-line (contracting silk) and elastic thread ligatures. Unlike elastics, they can also be threaded under the solder joints of splints or bridges.

The length of a piece of grass-line contracts by about 20 percent when it becomes wet, as a result of swelling of the fibers.[1] The ligature applies a fairly heavy force for one day and little after that, but it is usually left in place from 4 to 7 days before the ligature is replaced to

obtain additional movement. While a grass-line ligature is being applied, the area is kept dry by cotton rolls and warm air. An 8-inch length of grass-line is cut from the spool and stretched briefly to remove the kinks to make it easier to handle. If two central incisors are to be moved together, the grass line is looped around one of them, incisally to the cingulum, and is knotted at the distal side (Fig. 19-5). The two ends are then passed labially and lingually to the distal side of the other central incisor, where they are knotted. The ligature then is looped around the same tooth and is knotted triply at the distal side. The ends are cut short and the cotton rolls are removed. The knots are made at the distal side in order to have longer contracting sections, which provide adequate force for the movement. In most cases, one or two applications of the ligature will be sufficient to accomplish the movement.

If one tooth is to be moved toward another, the anchor tooth must be tied to one or two adjacent teeth to prevent its movement by the reciprocal forces. Elastic thread is used in the same manner.[2] The main difference is that elastic thread exerts a lighter force, but one which continues as long as the ligature is in place.

When movement of a posterior tooth is going on simultaneously, mesiodistal movement of anterior teeth can be accomplished with loop springs soldered to the arch of a Hawley-type appliance. A more esthetic way is to use a finger spring soldered to a high labial arch (Fig. 19-6).

In order to move two teeth together bodily, with a minimum of tipping, it is necessary to use a small sectional arch. Bands are placed on the two teeth, with either brackets or tubes on the labial surface, according to the procedure being performed.

There are two main types of sectional arch appliance. In one, the arch wire acts as a track along which the teeth are moved by ligatures, elastics, or coil springs (Fig. 19-7). The wire runs through tubes welded

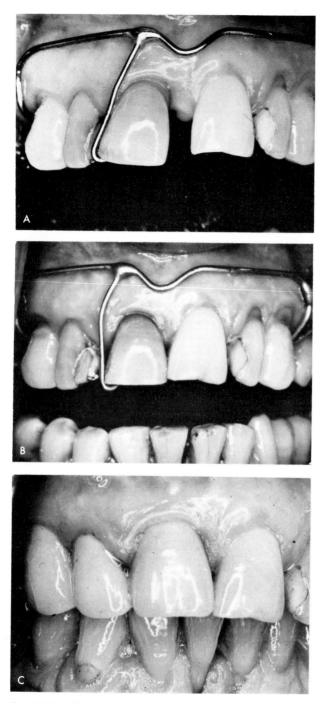

FIG. 19-6. *A. Finger spring from high labial arch moving upper right central incisor mesially. B. After movement. C. After splinting.*

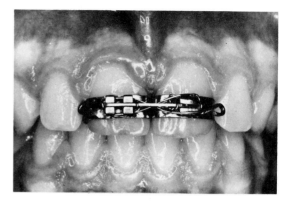

FIG. 19-7. *Sectional arch for moving upper central incisors together bodily.*

necessary to remove the arch wire to adjust it for further deflection.

In the last few years several systems have been developed for bonding plastic brackets directly to the enamel.[3,12] This provides great benefits in esthetics, speed of application, and hygiene (Fig. 19-8). It is not necessary to separate teeth to provide for the thickness of band material. The different methods have provided varying degrees of strength of the bond, but there has been consistent improvement.

Closure of Anterior Diastemata by Movement Lingually

In many instances a diastema is best closed by moving the teeth lingually into the arc of a smaller circle (Fig. 19-2). In such cases, one must be sure that it will be possible to eliminate excessive occlusal forces in the protrusive and lateral protrusive excursions in the position into which the teeth are being moved. There must be simultaneous contact between some posterior teeth during these excursions to prevent the occlusal traumatism. In cases with sufficient free-way space, it may be possible to obtain such posterior support by

to the bands. In the other type, the arch wire itself is shaped so that it is activated when it is placed into brackets on the bands. It is held in the brackets with wire ligatures or small circles of elastic which are stretched over the occlusal and gingival arms of the brackets. As the movement progresses, it is usually

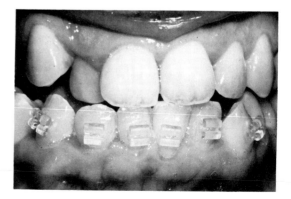

FIG. 19-8. *Plastic brackets bonded to enamel.*

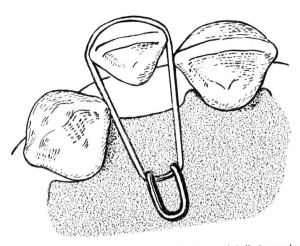

FIG. 19-9. *Light latex elastic moving incisor palatally towards a cleat embedded in acrylic appliance.*

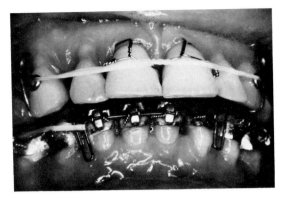

FIG. 19-10. *Light latex elastic used as arch to apply pressure to incisors. Wires have been placed on the upper central incisors to prevent elastic from sliding gingivally.*

building up the posterior teeth prosthetically or by using a bite plate to produce elongation of the posteriors. When those steps are not feasible, the teeth being moved lingually can be ground or even depressed to reduce trauma. Of course, there are many cases where all these steps will be inadequate, and then minor movement procedures should not be attempted.

If movement of one or two teeth in a lingual direction will close the diastema, the best method is to use a light latex elastic to move the tooth toward a cleat in an acrylic appliance. After the appliance is inserted, a ¼-inch elastic is placed around the tooth and then is slipped over the cleat which is embedded in the acrylic appliance at least ½ inch from the tooth (Fig. 19-9). The acrylic appliance is cut away on the lingual side of the tooth to permit it to move inwards. The appliance does not need a labial arch, and the elastics are almost invisible, so that the effect is most esthetic. The clasps are placed on the most distal teeth of the arch, so that there are no occlusal interference problems with the clasps.

A spring soldered to a Hawley arch wire or a high labial arch is also effective, but less esthetic. To move several teeth lingually, a Hawley-type arch wire can be adjusted to apply the necessary force to each tooth. The adjustment is made by closing the cuspid loops. The patient should feel some pressure, but no pain. One way of ascertaining pressure is to pass dental floss between the tooth and the arch wire. It should not pass through easily. Acrylic resin is cut away to permit the teeth to move in.

A variation of the Hawley arch is the use of elastic stretched between two hooks in the cuspid areas. This method provides a lighter force and a more esthetic appliance for moving groups of teeth lingually. A ⅝-inch light latex elastic is used. Because of the labial

tilt of the incisors, it is necessary to keep the elastic from sliding cervically in many cases (Fig. 19-10). A 0.010 inch wire is tightly looped around the cervix of one of the central incisors, and the twisted section is bent incisally to the gingivo-occlusal center of the crown. The ends then are looped around the tooth incisally to the cingulum and are twisted together. This wire will keep the elastic in the middle third of the tooth.

Crowded Teeth

There are three main reasons why teeth are crowded out of alignment:

1. The teeth are too large for the jaw.
2. Some of the teeth have erupted in a wrong sequence or position so that the later teeth must erupt bucally or lingually to their correct positions.
3. The teeth are forced out of line by the mesial pressures of the anterior component of the masticatory force.[18] This occurs *after* the eruption of the teeth and is most common in patients who clench and grind. After the teeth have been moved back into position, a night guard must be used to prevent relapse.

The prerequisite that is hardest to satisfy in cases of tooth crowding is adequate room. If the amount of extra space required is not too great and the teeth are bell-shaped and have adequate proximal enamel, they can be stripped to make room. If considerably more space is needed, a tooth sometimes can be extracted, and the remaining ones can be realigned.

The adjacent teeth are *never* used for anchorage, since the reciprocal forces might move them together slightly and valuable space would be lost. Therefore,

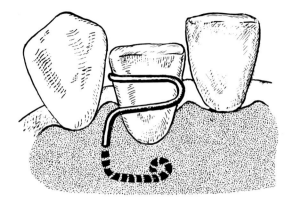

Fig. 19-11. *Recurved spring for moving incisor labially.*

the method of choice usually is an acrylic plate, clasping distant teeth and resting against the other teeth. Springs or elastics are used for power.

An excellent and esthetic way of moving a crowded anterior tooth lingually is with a ¼-inch light latex elastic and a cleat embedded in the acrylic plate (Fig. 19-9). An arch wire of a Hawley-type appliance or a finger spring from a high labial arch can also be used (Fig. 19-6).

For moving a crowded anterior or posterior tooth labially, a recurved spring is most effective (Fig. 19-11). In the case of an anterior tooth, the force must be applied near the gingival margin to prevent the reciprocal force from dislodging the appliance.

An easy way of applying a force in a labial direction is to incorporate a spring-loaded screw instead of a recurved spring in the acrylic plate. When the appliance is inserted, the screw is pushed into its housing, activating a small coil spring. As the tooth moves labially, the screw is lengthened by turning it in its threaded sleeve. The screws come in three interchangeable lengths, and as the procedure goes on, the pressure can be kept up by substituting a longer screw.

For moving a posterior tooth palatally, a recurved spring with a helical loop exerts a well-controlled force. The spring can be anchored in the acrylic plate, passing in back of the last tooth to avoid interference with the occlusion. Since it is a fairly long spring, it must be deflected a considerable distance to apply adequate pressure for moving a posterior tooth. Therefore, in activating the spring it is bent more than half the buccolingual diameter of the tooth and must be snapped into place when the appliance is inserted. For moving a bicuspid, the spring can be soldered to the cuspid loop of a Hawley appliance.

Anterior Crossbites

The first thing to do in case selection is to jiggle the patient's relaxed mandible back into the most retruded position—centric relation.[6] If there is still a noticeable crossbite, the case probably falls in the Angle Class III category. If the centric relation position is approximately end to end, correction of the premature contacts that have caused the mesial shift into a convenience position may be possible. After such correction, there may still be a slight crossbite relationship of one or several teeth that may be amenable to minor tooth movement procedures.

The next thing to observe is the axial inclinations of the teeth in the crossbite relationship. In many instances, the upper tooth is inclined too far palatally; in other instances the lower tooth is tipped labially and in some patients both teeth have incorrect inclinations. In general, the tooth that is furthest from the normal axial inclination is moved. The upper tooth can be moved labially by a recurved spring or a spring-loaded screw, as described earlier. A lower tooth is moved in lingually with an arch wire, a finger spring, or an elastic and cleat.

If there is crowding as well as crossbite, it may be necessary to strip the adjacent teeth to obtain room for the movement. It is desirable to prevent severe trauma to a tooth being jumped. For patients with a considerable overlap of the teeth, it is advisable to make the acrylic part of the appliance extend over the occlusal surfaces of the posterior teeth to open the bite. If the overlap is relatively small, just grinding the occlusal surfaces of both teeth may be sufficient. However, it is important to remember that the teeth eventually must be retained in place by their new position in the occlusion. If they are ground too much, they may be too short to be held by the opposing teeth.

After movement, the incisal edges are rebeveled (the palatal side of the upper teeth and the labial side of the lower) so that the occlusal forces will be applied in the proper directions. This usually is all that is necessary for retention.

Inclined planes[16] and tongue-depressors have been used for many years to correct localized anterior crossbites, especially in children. Occlusal forces provide the power for such techniques.

Posterior Crossbite and Buccoversion

The same approach is used for case selection in posterior crossbites. The axial inclinations are studied to see if a great deal of bodily movement is necessary. If the upper tooth is in complete buccoversion and is leaning buccally, with the lower tooth in a normal position, the upper tooth may be moved palatally by a spring which comes around the back of the last tooth. If an acrylic bite opener covering the occlusal surfaces of all the other teeth is being used to provide clearance for the movement, then a spring can come over the other teeth at any convenient place to provide clearance for the movement. In a posterior crossbite, a buccally tipped lower tooth is moved lingually in the same way.

When a lower tooth is in complete linguoversion, it can be moved labially by means of a recurved spring, or a spring with a helical loop, applying force to the lingual surface. A spring-loaded screw also is useful for this purpose. The same procedures are effective in tipping buccally an upper molar in crossbite, if it is tilted palatally. If more bodily movement is necessary to achieve the desired position, a full labial arch or a sectional arch can be used. Of course several teeth must be used for anchorage.

If the upper and lower teeth both have to be moved to correct a crossbite or buccoversion, cross elastics are attached to cleats on bands on both teeth to provide reciprocal forces (Fig. 19-12). If the upper tooth is in buccoversion, the elastic is stretched from a buccal cleat on the upper tooth to a lingual cleat on the lower. If the teeth are in crossbite, of course, the directions are reversed. Cross elastics can also be used to move just one of the teeth, by having the cleat on the other extend to adjacent teeth, providing three teeth for firm anchorage.

The elastics used are heavier than the rubber dam elastics and come in different sizes. To select the proper size, an elastic in its unstretched state is hooked around one cleat. It should extend about half the distance needed to attach it to the other cleat. The elastic should be changed twice daily. Unless a bite-opening appliance that provides occlusal clearance is being used, the patient is warned not to grind or clench the teeth even though the occlusion may feel strange. The elastic going over the occlusal surface helps to cushion the occlusal forces. As the movement proceeds and the teeth begin to achieve the correct relationship, the occlusal forces are received in beneficial directions.

Mesial or Distal Movement of Posterior Teeth

Mesial or distal movements are usually designed to facilitate prosthetic procedures. When a tooth has been extracted and adjacent teeth have drifted, it is often necessary to move the anterior tooth mesially and the posterior one distally. Sometimes only the posterior one must be moved, since the anterior component of the masticatory force has kept the anterior tooth in position.[18]

In a majority of cases, such drifted teeth may be moved back into position by tipping, since they have been tipped by occlusal forces into their malpositions. However, when the missing tooth is lost early, the adjacent teeth can erupt in fairly normal axial inclinations but in incorrect positions. In such cases, they will have to be moved bodily with fixed appliances.

A bicuspid can be tipped mesially by pulling or pushing it. It is pulled when the anchorage is in the cuspid area. The anterior teeth can be ligated or otherwise splinted into an anchor group, and the bicuspid is moved towards the group with elastic thread or grass line or a light latex elastic. Another way of doing it, with a removable appliance, is to use a helical loop spring. The spring is embedded in the cuspid area, goes over the occlusal surface, and has its helical loop buccal to the tooth being moved. It catches the distal surface of that tooth and is activated to provide pressure in a mesial direction. Such an appliance would be used if movement is being attempted in another area simultaneously.

A bicuspid can also be pushed mesially with a helical spring embedded in the molar area and exerting pressure on the distal surface. A bicuspid can be pulled distally with a similar spring designed so that it exerts pressure on the mesial surface. It is activated by adjusting it so that, in its passive position, it is in the middle of the tooth, and slipping it into its correct position on the mesial surface deflects the wire to apply the force.

A good way of pulling a bicuspid distally is to have a cleat embedded in acrylic about $\frac{3}{4}$-inch distally to the tooth. A $\frac{1}{4}$-inch light latex elastic is placed around the tooth and then is slipped over the cleat. The acrylic appliance is cut away just distally to the tooth to permit its movement. It is important to check the occlusion as the tooth is tipped distally to be sure there is no interference.

To push a molar distally, a helical loop spring can apply pressure on the mesial surface. However, if the tooth has a mesial inclination, the spring can slide gingivally. In such cases, a split plate is preferable and easier to adjust (Fig. 19-13). There are wire loops on the buccal and the lingual sides and the acrylic plate is split so that the ends of the wires are embedded in both sections. The distal part is bent out by finger pressure, and when the appliance is inserted it is deflected back towards the body of the appliance. This activates the wire loops and applies force in a distal direction against the tipped molar. The anchorage is distributed on all the other teeth of the arch. The patient can be taught how to activate the appliance by bending the distal part out when the pressure diminishes. A jackscrew also can be used between the two pieces of the split plate, but there are less flexibility and a heavier force.

An excellent way of uprighting a molar is to band it and two bicuspids. An arch wire with a helical loop is put into a tube on the molar and in its passive position should be below the gingival margin of the bicuspids.

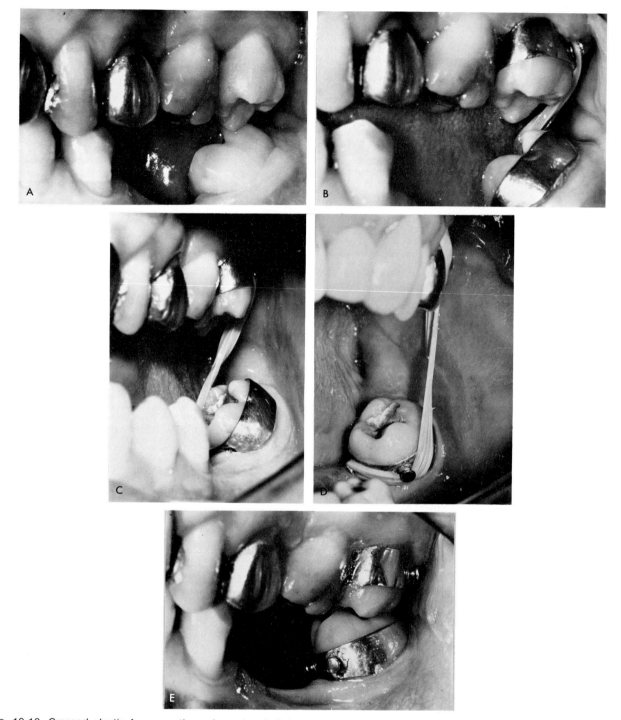

FIG. 19-12. *Crossed elastic for correcting a buccal malrelation of a maxillary molar. A. Precorrected condition. Note that the mandibular molar is rotated and positioned lingually. B. Bands with cleats and cross elastic to effect a buccolingual pull. C. Direction of pull of elastic during mandibular opening. D. Subsequent elastic applied to additional mesiolingual and mesiobuccal cleats to effect a rotation of force on the mandibular molar. E. Molar positions after correction. (Courtesy Dr. C. Carlson.)*

A distally tipped bicuspid can be uprighted in the same way (Fig. 19-14). When it is deflected upward and is slipped into the brackets on the bicuspids, an uprighting force is applied. The effect of the distal reactive force against the anchor molar is minimized by the lightness of the force applied.

When teeth with good axial inclinations have to be moved more than a millimeter or two, bodily movement is necessary. A sectional arch is usually the method of choice. The arch wire acts as a track, and compressed coil springs exert the force.

A miniature sectional arch can serve a special pur-

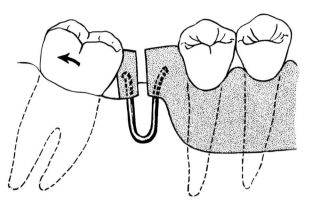

FIG. 19-13. *Appliance with a split block of acrylic over the ridge with springs between the two segments of acrylic.*

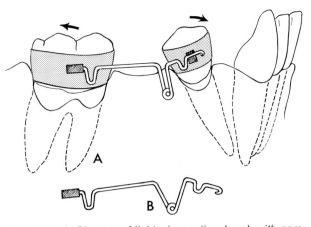

FIG. 19-14. *A. Diagram of light wire sectional arch with compressed helical spring to tip a bicuspid tooth mesially and correct its axial inclination. The ligature that fastens the arch into the bicuspid bracket has not yet been applied. B. The passive shape of the arch before activation.*

pose in periodontal therapy. A molar with a furcation involvement can be cut in half, and the two halves can be moved apart if an adjacent tooth is missing. Preformed bicuspid bands can be used on each half of the tooth, and a small arch wire is fitted into brackets or tubes on the buccal and lingual sides (Fig. 19-15). The force can be applied with coil springs or jackscrews, or the arch wire itself can have a loop built into it.

Rotation

Incisors can be rotated with removable appliances in one of two ways, depending upon the desired axis of rotation. If the mesial corner is rotated out of line and the distal corner is in the right place, a fulcrum is established with the acrylic appliance or a short rigid

wire at the distal corner (Fig. 19-16). Pressure is then applied to the mesiolabial line angle with an arch wire or a spring.

If the axis is to be in the center of the tooth, a force must also be applied against the distolingual surfaces. A recurved spring or a spring-loaded screw is used for that purpose.

Minor rotation of several incisors can be accomplished by using a rubber or elastic acrylic positioner.[11] To prepare the appliance, the rotated teeth are cut off a model and glued back in desired positions. The appliance is processed to fit the revised model and will

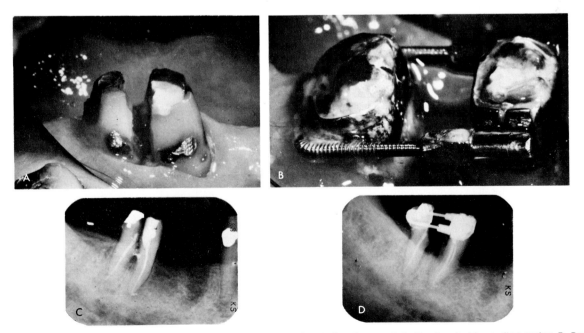

FIG. 19-15. *Prefabricated appliance for moving the halves of a hemisected molar apart. A. Hemisected lower first molar. B. Position of roots after two months. Note jackscrews used for power. C and D. Radiographs before and after movement.*

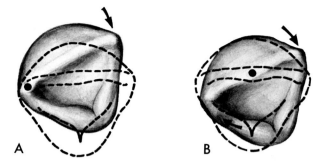

FIG. 19-16. *Determining the desired axis of rotation. A. If the axis is at one corner, the acrylic appliance may be used as a fulcrum, and the elastic or arch wire will exert pressure on the other corner. B. If the axis is to be in the center of the tooth, force from the lingual side is required, and the use of springs is necessary. (Adapted from Hirschfeld, L., and Jay, J.: Minor tooth movement by means of rubber dam elastics, J. Am. Dent. Assoc., 50:282, 1955.)*

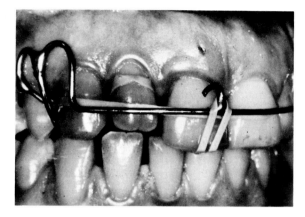

FIG. 19-17. *Light latex elastic depressing an upper central incisor. The elastic stretches from a hook on the arch to a cleat embedded in the acrylic appliance.*

not go into place when it is placed in the mouth. When the patient bites down, as he is trained to do, the appliance is forced down and the material is distorted, applying pressure at all the right places.

Unlike the incisor, a cuspid or bicuspid does not have flat surfaces against which forces can be applied. Therefore, they must have bands with hooks or spurs to obtain a grip on the tooth for rotation. If a tooth is to be crowned, a temporary crown can be made with spurs incorporated. In fact, under some circumstances, a pin can be screwed into a tooth to act as a spur, and then it can be cut off when movement is completed.

The anchorage for the elastics or ligatures that perform the movement is obtained on adjacent groups of teeth, or, better still, on a removable appliance.

It is difficult to rotate molars with minor movement appliances. In order to rotate the crown of a molar with two or three roots, the roots must be moved bodily through the bone. This takes a long time, since there is a large total alveolar area to be remodeled. Remodeling can be done slowly with bands and lever springs, but it is difficult.

Depression

Incisors often must be depressed as they are brought lingually. This can be done by means of a ¼-inch light latex elastic stretched from a hook on an arch wire over the incisal edge to a cleat on the palate (Fig. 19-17). A small nick may be made in the incisal edge to keep the elastic in place. It is a good idea to have clasps on the first bicuspids as well as on the molars to keep the appliance from being dislodged by the reciprocal forces.

Posterior teeth can be depressed slowly by using appliances that place all the occlusal pressure on those

teeth. If the tooth being depressed has extruded as a result of the loss of an opposing tooth, it is not in function and therefore can be depressed somewhat more easily than a tooth that is in function. The appliance used on the arch opposite the tooth being depressed is built up with elastic acrylic resin just at the point of occlusal contact. In that way, a force is applied each time the jaws are brought together, but the elastic acrylic cushion prevents excessive pressure, which could cause pericementitis. It takes several months to depress a molar. The tooth is also shortened by grinding as much as possible in order to reduce the amount of depression required.

Retention

The bone surrounding teeth that have just been moved is called transitional bone. It has not yet developed the structure of mature bone.[14] As a result, even light forces of the tongue and mastication can cause the tooth to move back into its malposition. For that reason, some form of stabilization usually is necessary. In most cases, this retention is only temporary, but in other instances permanent retention is required. Of course, many minor movement procedures are undertaken in order to make possible the use of a bridge or splint that will act as permanent retention.

Several forms of temporary retention are used:

1. Wire ligatures, often used after movement with elastics or grass-line or elastic thread ligatures.
2. The movement appliance itself, such as a Hawley retainer or a bite plate.
3. Acrylic night guards.
4. A-splints, in which troughs or dovetails are cut into adjacent teeth, knurled wire is laid in, and

then acrylic resin is painted in. Of course, such a procedure commits one to further restorations.

Temporary retention is usually necessary 24 hours a day for at least twice as long as the movement procedure required. Removable retainers can then be used only at night for a while and later can be withdrawn by degrees. Wire ligatures are used a little longer because they cannot be withdrawn by degrees.

Reitan wrote in 1953 that one of the reasons for relapse is that, although the intra-alveolar fibers of the periodontal ligament are replaced during tooth movement, the gingival, transverse, and circumferential fibers are not replaced.[15] They may be merely stretched. Edwards tattooed dots on the gingiva before tooth movement was started and found that the tissue was pulled in the direction of movement, indicating stretching of the gingival fibers.[4] This could cause relapse. For this reason, it has been suggested that any periodontal surgery contemplated should be delayed until after tooth movement in order to remove these supra-alveolar fibers. Ewen and Pasternak have cut all gingival and transverse fibers down to the bone after movement and have found that relapse was reduced.[5]

The most important requirement in the success of retention is the complete elimination of occlusal or muscular factors which would cause relapse—establishment of a balance of muscular forces acting on the teeth.

References

1. Berliner, A.: Ligatures, Splints, Bite Planes and Pyramids. Philadelphia, J. B. Lippincott Co., 1964.
2. Boise, L. R.: Increased stability of orthodontically rotated teeth following gingivectomy in Macaca nemestrina. Am. J. Orthod., 156:273, 1969.
3. Dietz, V. S.: A technique for direct bonding of orthodontic attachment. J. Clin. Orthod., 6:681, 1972.
4. Edwards, J. G.: A study of the periodontium during orthodontic rotation of teeth. Am. J. Orthod., 50:441, 1963.
5. Ewen, S. J., and Pasternak, R.: Periodontal surgery, an adjunct to orthodontic therapy. J. Am. Soc. Periodont., 2:162, 1964.
6. Glossary of prosthodontic terms. J. Prosthet. Dent., 6: 1956.
7. Goldstein, M. C.: Adult orthodontics and the general practitioner. J. Can. Dent. Assoc., 24:261, 1958.
8. Hirschfeld, L.: The use of wire and silk ligatures. J. Am. Dent. Assoc., 41:647, 1950.
9. Hirschfeld, L., and Geiger, A.: Minor tooth movement in general practice. St. Louis, C. V. Mosby, 1966.
10. Hirschfeld, L., and Jay, J.: Minor tooth movement by means of rubber dam elastics. J. Am. Dent. Assoc., 50:282, 1955.
11. Kesling, H. D.: Co-ordinating the predetermined pattern and tooth positioner with conventional treatment. Am. J. Orthod. Oral Surg., 32:285, 1946.
12. Mitchell, D. S.: Bandless orthodontic-bracket. J. Am. Dent. Assoc., 74:102, 1967.
13. Oppenheim, A.: The crisis in orthodontics. Int. J. Orthod., 19:1201, 1933.
14. Oppenheim, A.: A possibility for physiologic orthodontic movement. Am. J. Orthod. Oral Surg., 30:277, 1944.
15. Reitan, K.: Tissue changes following experimental tooth movement as related to the time factor. Dent. Rec., 73:559, 1953.
16. Rogers, A. P.: The use of inclined planes in the treatment and retention of amloclusion. Items Interest, 33:21, 1911.
17. Schwarz, A. M.: Denture appliances for tooth adjustment. Dtsch. Zahn. Mund. Kieferhsilkd., 5:192, 1938.
18. Stallard, H.: The anterior component of the force of mastication and its significance to the dental apparatus. Dental Cosmos, 65:467, 1923.

20

Reevaluation of Periodontal Tissues After Initial Therapy

Gingival Shrinkage and Pocket Depth

Reevaluation for Mobility

Temporary Stabilization

Minor Tooth Movement and its Results

Minor Tooth Movement and Root
Prominences

The Two-Phase Approach to Therapy

Reevaluation of the Physical Health Status
of the Patient

Recording of Revised Treatment Plan

20

Reevaluation

of

Periodontal

Tissues

After

Initial

Therapy

Periodontal therapy is constantly involved with tissue response to the various modalities applied. Constant reevaluation is therefore going on throughout the entire course of treatment. There are, however, certain periods in the treatment plan when a new and different method is applied. At such a time, a taking of stock and an evaluation of the efficacy of all the preceding treatment on the part of both the therapist and the patient are very much in order.

There are questions in future procedure to be determined which must, of necessity, be settled on the basis of tissue response to earlier effort. In this context, the evaluation of treatment already rendered is an important component of the treatment plan and cannot be separated from it. The first formally established treatment evaluation and assay is logically placed after initial therapy has been performed and enough time has elapsed to permit maximum tissue response.

GINGIVAL SHRINKAGE AND POCKET DEPTH

The standard response of gingiva to debridement is shrinkage. To expect shrinkage, however, the therapist must take for granted that the gingival response to the irritational effects of microbial plaque and calculus will be edema and enlargement. He also presumes that gingival fibrosis is not an important factor in the enlargement of the gingiva. These phenomena have been dealt with in Chapter 3.

This would not bear repetition at this point, except that at this moment in the treatment plan a decision must be made either to continue with repeated circuits of root curettage, to proceed with a projected series of flap reflections for open root curettage, or to attempt definitive pocket elimination through resective or inductive periodontal surgery or through a combination of several of these.

If shrinkage of the gingiva is sufficient to eliminate abnormal or excessive sulcular depth completely and to restore normal contour to the gingiva, then total response has been achieved and no further methods are required in the area or areas being evaluated. These decisions are easy to make.

More difficult to evaluate is the subtotal or partial response. The operator must decide whether further curettage will be rewarding to a patient whose initial treatment plan includes a surgical phase. Basic to any decision of this nature are a return to normal color and a resolution of exudate and of any residual inflammation. What periodontists are concerned with in reevaluation is normal form. The simple projection of sulcular depth alone may not provide a useful criterion for judgment.

In referring to the objectives of therapy it has been stated many times, and repeated in many contexts, that the primary objective is the creation of a milieu in which the teeth may be retained in health throughout the life of the individual. Reduced to purely periodontal terms, it means (1) that the attachment apparatus must be healthy, (2) that irritational factors can be eliminated by the patient on a daily basis, and (3) that the occlusal requirements are well within the ability of the tissue to withstand. Nowhere in this list is the total elimination of the pocket mentioned as an indispensable ingredient. The principal reason pocket elimination enjoys such a high position in the periodontist's list of secondary objectives is that it makes possible the highest level of patient achievement in tissue maintenance. The elimination of the sulcus and the reshaping of the tissues of the periodontium to provide access for brush, floss, stimulator, and toothpick are the rewards of successful periodontal surgery.

In determining how much or how little surgical intervention is necessary after initial therapy, the magnitude or degree of aberration is plotted against the performance level of the patient. Both factors are projected against the level of response of the tissues. In other words, a highly skilled patient who is well motivated toward self-administered therapy can and will compensate for much greater aberrations in form than will one who is less motivated.

Tissue response also enters here as a consideration. That same patient, well motivated and skilled, can accomplish wonders in therapy if the periodontal tissues are responsive to debridement techniques applied by the periodontist, and instruction in maintenance methodology is sufficient to cope with most situations. It is with such patients that some dentists deduce rather simplistic approaches to the periodontal problem.

In reevaluation particularly it must be borne in mind that there is no such thing as a standard patient with standard responses. The range of reaction of the tissues to therapy is wide, and it is by no means limited to a single response. Unfortunately, most patients have neither the total motivation nor the tissue responses to make shrinkage and a return to normal form as common as we are led to believe. These patients are the main concern in the first reevaluation.

REEVALUATION FOR MOBILITY

Reassessing the initial treatment plan must include the reassay of the originally recorded mobility of the teeth. The generally projected patterns of mobility should be downward. With the effect of the debridement techniques on the tissues of the supporting apparatus being rehabilitated added to the more direct result of occlusal adjustment, it should come as no great surprise that mobility, where it exists, should be decreased. Since mobility usually increases immediately after surgical procedures, the long-term gain in stability will have to be assayed at a later date.

Mobility, in concert with other signs and symptoms, must be plotted against the background of the amount of support remaining and the demands made on that support by bruxism, removable prostheses, and habit. Even a long-range evaluation of mobility must be made with these factors in mind. A low degree of mobility may be acceptable under certain circumstances. In many cases, mobility calls for temporary stabilization of some or all of the teeth in the presurgical phases of therapy.

TEMPORARY STABILIZATION

Temporary stabilization is a common expedient for the immobilization of loose teeth during periodontal therapy (Chapter 18). The appliances used for this objective are varied. Intracoronal splints of wire and acrylic resin or amalgam are commonly used. These are best inspected at the formal reevaluation. It is not rare by any means to find cracks and separations between the filling material and the enclosed wire or between the filling material and the tooth. Obviously, repairs will be needed quickly.

The more mobile the teeth, the more likely is fracture of some portion of the splint. Repairs are not difficult. It should be kept in mind that bruxism does not stop with occlusal adjustment followed by temporary stabilization. The fabrication and use of night guards to palliate the effects of bruxism is highly recommended to maintain the integrity of intracoronal splints.

MINOR TOOTH MOVEMENT AND ITS RESULTS

One of the neglected facets of tissue behavior is the changing of gingival contour in relation to altered tooth position. Although it is perfectly true that papillary height and recession of the marginal gingiva are repeatedly associated with tooth malposition, it is also true that the proliferation of gingiva under the protective roof of a tilted tooth has been generally overlooked. Pocket depth becomes greater in the interproximal area toward which the tooth is tilted. Molars are the commonest offenders, since failure to replace a first molar that has been extracted makes possible many mesially tilted second molars. These commonly reveal excessive mesial sulcular depth.

Much of the sulcular depth is just that and no more. It is bounded by the enamel of the mesial surface of the tooth, since the cementoenamel junction has been submerged by the tilt in the tooth so that it is deeper subgingivally than would be the case in a tooth in more normal position.

Many skilled clinicians place the correction of a number of malpositions in initial therapy. If this is done, the teeth must be reevaluated for sulcular depth. Teeth that have been uptilted to a more erect position commonly show a dramatic diminution of sulcular depth. There is, however, a disappointing proclivity toward an *increase* of sulcular depth on the distal side where there may have been little or none before. This new depth is unquestionably due to the piling up of gingiva behind the tooth as it is moved into an upright position. Whatever the cause, the abnormal sulcular depth must be taken into consideration and dealt with.

MINOR TOOTH MOVEMENT AND ROOT PROMINENCES

In tilting teeth and in bodily movement of teeth, roots are commonly moved into or out of a prominent position. These altered relationships of roots to alveolar processes have an important effect on position, width, and character of the gingiva as well as the bone. This will, in turn, qualify the nature and extent of alveolar and mucogingival repairs and alterations. Surgical procedures that appeared mandatory preoperatively may often require considerable alteration in character and scope.

In concert with shrinkage induced by debriding techniques, alterations in gingival and bone topography require reevaluation in the light of changed relationships. Pocket depth is frequently altered, and the surgical regimen originally established may no longer be germane. Heavy ledges of bone that once required reduction may no longer be present where they once were but may be on the opposite side of the alveolar process.

Although thin bony investment of roots precludes, by definition, heavy ledges of alveolar bone, the operator is frequently confronted by adjacent areas with thick buccal or lingual bone that must be thinned to achieve positive architecture. The specificity of approach required by such a clinical picture can only be solved by the judicious use of vertical releasing incisions of variable length so that relatively small flaps may be reflected. Clinical impressions of surgical management are best recorded at the time of reevaluation.

THE TWO-PHASE APPROACH TO THERAPY

Because of the interdependence of so many rather complex factors, a growing number of therapists establish an interregnum in the orderly progress of therapy at the end of the presurgical portion of the treatment plan. The reevaluation of the response of the tissues to therapy becomes a recurrent and periodic routine.

No one can quarrel with careful and meticulous assay of results up to this point, but it can be overdone so that definitive management is inordinately delayed. In many patients, this delay may be resorted to with relative impunity if the supervision and reexamination are rigid. In others, however, where a complex or extensive restorative treatment plan awaits the completion of periodontal treatment, such protracted delay is poorly advised unless the reasons for it are of overriding importance. Repeated reevaluations could become a refuge for the too busy therapist to delay further therapy.

REEVALUATION OF THE PHYSICAL HEALTH STATUS OF THE PATIENT

The end of the presurgical therapy is an excellent place to reassess the general health status of patients whose history raises problems in management at the outset. A careful review of consultative reports from other dentists and physicians and inquiry into the patient's status relative to other current therapy is in order. Especially useful is the investigation of allergies. The surgical phase of treatment now requires considerably more use of drugs than did earlier methods. Tranquilizers, both intravenous agents and those orally administered, are in common usage. Analgesic drugs for postoperative use are also commonly prescribed. Those contemplated for use should be checked out carefully so that no untoward response to them mars the postoperative course.

Physicians for patients who are on anticoagulant medication should be consulted to determine the advisability of interrupting anticoagulant therapy for the period of each surgical treatment. The importance of this is obvious.

It is also advisable to recheck carefully into the patient's experience with aspirin and bleeding episodes. These are becoming frequent enough so that aspirin and aspirin-containing drugs are withdrawn and prohibited by many periodontists during the entire surgical phase, beginning about two weeks prior to the first procedure.

RECORDING OF REVISED TREATMENT PLAN

As in all treatment plans, the careful revision of the initial plan should be recorded for easy reference. The revised plan is not the blueprint for progress into the surgical phase or into a reduced plan or into an altogether nonsurgical approach. In some patients who do extraordinarily well in the early stages of treatment, there is a falling off of motivation and a regression of maintenance effort and effectiveness. It should not surprise the operator too much to find his patient a candidate for a second, or even third, reevaluation. Nowhere is it more clearly shown that periodontal case management is a constant struggle with patient failure than in the formal reevaluation.

Recharting is a useful expedient. Many therapists routinely rechart the sulcular depth on the same diagram used in the original charting, either with a differently colored pen or with a special position of the numerical values used.

Recharting and reevaluation are especially useful in the complex case. In many advanced cases key teeth must be most carefully evaluated, and their response to initial therapy must be assayed. Prognosis for these teeth frequently determines the nature of the restorative treatment plan, and error in this situation may be costly to the patient. At the same time, a timid, overly conservative approach to the difficult case will fail to achieve optimum results for the patient. Lowered horizons and altered goals in treatment are acceptable if the clinical facts require them. If they are the result of timidity, then the therapist is not doing the most he can for his patient (and for many other patients as well).

We see, then, that reevaluation is the key to optimum therapy, and that is the ultimate objective.

21

Principles of Periodontal Surgery

21

Principles of Periodontal Surgery

The surgical approach to periodontal therapy has become a greater segment of management with each passing decade. In fact, a commonly expressed opinion is that periodontics is one of the surgical specialties in dentistry. This statement is not strictly true because of the rather elaborate preparatory steps that are commonly taken prior to the surgical phase—steps, in some cases, which obviate the need for surgery—and in the demanding postsurgical and parasurgical methods that are so integral a part of periodontics. Reference is made here to occlusal adjustment and to other adjunctive procedures. In spite of all these qualifying steps, however, surgery unquestionably occupies a major portion of total periodontal therapy. In more recent years, it has lost its basic simplicity of approach, so that periodontal surgery has become more complicated, and subtle differences in approach assume major importance as refinements are introduced and developed.

To return to basic considerations, however, we should refer to the aims and objectives of periodontal therapy and to the concept of cure which we have set up as a goal. Pocket elimination remains a basic objective, but other factors weigh quite heavily. Problems in tissue quality and texture, alterations in intraoral topography, and the establishment of physiologic form conducive to adequate maintenance are serious considerations to be dealt with. Periodontal surgery constitutes the major modality in the attainment of our therapeutic objectives. It is for this reason that it is so extensively discussed in this text.

RESECTIVE AND INDUCTIVE PERIODONTAL SURGERY

Periodontal surgery may be conveniently divided into two broad and general categories: (1) resective and (2) reconstructive or inductive. Resective surgery depends upon the creation of a selective recession to achieve pocket elimination. It involves reshaping of gingiva and of bone, where necessary, to attain this objective. Normal form may be created at a more apical level in the process, but this is not always the case.

Methods are available to regain lost attachment by the reconstitution of lost bone, cementum, and periodontal ligament in some special lesions. A number of techniques are available, some well-established, some frankly experimental. These will be described and evaluated. As in all methods, case selection is critically important. In the area of inductive surgery, however, the range of suitable cases is considerably narrower than in most periodontal methods. Vigorous efforts are being made to broaden that range.

Another area in periodontal surgery may be properly reparative or inductive—mucosal repairs. The objective of this kind of surgery is to establish, or reestablish, a favorable gingival and mucosal milieu in the mouth. This is essentially directed to marginal tissue, but its effects range far afield.

This brief and superficial view of the surgical aspects of periodontics serves only to establish the place of surgical procedures in the total treatment effort. There is a tendency to forget that many methods are blended in the treatment of every patient. Although the techniques are individually described in separate chapters, it must be remembered that they are usually performed in combination, even in a single limited region. This most important point will be emphasized in the discussion of surgical treatment planning in Chapter 22.

ANESTHESIA

Periodontal surgery is always preceded by anesthesia of one kind or another. Since the choice is most frequently a local anesthetic, some brief attention should be paid to its application.

Block anesthesia on lower quadrants and infiltration in upper areas are the general rule. No great elaboration is necessary here, except to take note of a certain amount of controversy existing in the field. Some periodontists perform their surgical procedures in hospital operatories under a general anesthesia. General anesthesia imposes certain difficulties. A mouth prop must be used which prevents access to the lingual aspects of the lower molars. In addition, the compulsion is strong to complete total surgery in a single operation. This may mean a 4- to 5-hour procedure in advanced cases. Other periodontists hospitalize patients after extensive surgery performed in their office operatories under local anesthesia. This latter practice appears to be a useful expedient, since the operation is performed by a team familiar with all the ramifications and nuances of the procedures involved. The patient's apprehension can be managed by intravenous premedication or by preoperative subcutaneous meperidine plus oral promethazine hydrochloride (Phenergan) and pentobarbital, particularly if the patient is to be hospitalized immediately after the surgery.

SEDATION

Preoperative sedation for periodontal surgery is resorted to often and on several levels. The most common is the self-administered tranquilizer, which the patient takes frequently without informing the periodontist. The operator should question the patient about medication he is taking and adjust the regimen accordingly. Before preoperative sedation is administered in the office operatory, certain precautions should be taken. If the patient is given a short-acting barbiturate such as pentobarbital and nothing else, then a recovery period after the surgical procedure need not exceed 30 minutes to an hour. Even so, the patient should have someone to accompany him to his home. With the use of some of the more powerful drugs, on the other hand, considerable care should be exercised in postoperative management of the patient. When a subcutaneous injection of 50 mg of meperidine is preceded by 1.5 gm pentobarbital, sometimes repeated later in the operation, the patient is in no condition to do anything for himself.

The control of anxiety in the patient sometimes makes the difference between the acceptance or rejection of periodontal surgery as part of the treatment. The use of drugs in this connection, as well as postsurgical analgesia, is a large and complex area in patient management. The therapist would do well to arm himself with three source books that have proved invaluable to the authors: (1) *Clinical Drug Therapy in Dental Practice* by Thomas J. Pallasch (Lea & Febiger, 1973); (2) *Physician's Desk Reference* published by the Medical Economics Company in Oradell, N. J.; and (3) *Accepted Dental Therapeutics*, published by the American Dental Association. The *Physician's Desk Reference* is published in annual editions and is, since 1962, carefully supervised by the Food and Drug Administration. It is an invaluable ready reference for drug identification, dosages, and indications. *Accepted Dental Therapeutics* is issued in a new edition every two years.

The more commonly administered operative relaxants are the following:

1. Diazepam (Valium) tablets: 2 mg to 5 mg; 2 to 3 times per day on the day of operation
2. Meprobamate (Equanil) tablets: 200 mg; 3 to 4 tablets per day on the appointment day
3. Chlordiazepoxide hydrochloride (Librium) tablets: 10 mg; 3 times per day on the day of surgery

For postsurgical analgesia: codeine in combination with acetaminophen (Tylenol). Tylenol #4 (30 mg codeine phosphate combined with 300 mg acetaminophen) is very effective.

Another effective postsurgical analgesic is meperidine hydrochloride (Demerol). It is supplied in 50 mg tablets to be taken for pain in a dosage of one tablet every 6 hours while the pain lasts.

The list of useful analgesics is a large one. It is important to avoid aspirin and aspirin-containing compounds such as the various Empirin numbered

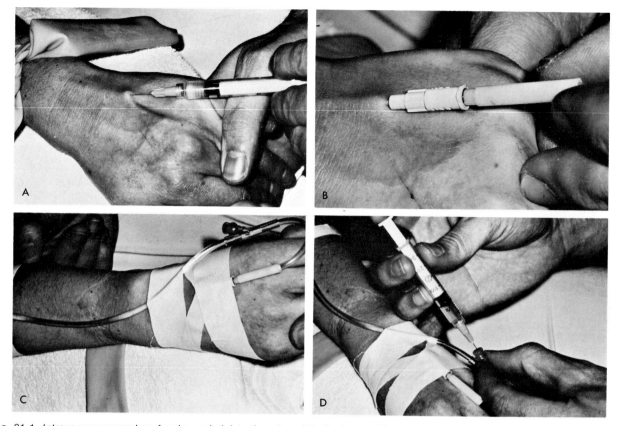

FIG. 21-1. *Intravenous procedure for drug administration. A and B. Finding and inserting an intravenous needle into a vein made prominent by the use of the rubber tourniquet. C. Adjusting the tubing and stabilizing the intravenous needle and tubing with adhesive tape. D. Adding one of various pharmacologic agents to the intravenous system.*

compounds, Percodan, Anacin, and many others. The hazards of aspirin are discussed later in the chapter.

It is good practice to give the patient a printed slip of preoperative and postoperative instructions. People under stress or moderately sedated are not too reliable in remembering verbal directions.

Many periodontists who use a full-mouth surgical approach administer intravenous sedation for the comfort and control of the patient. Some training in venipuncture is therefore essential before using this method on a patient. Intra-arterial and periarterial deposition of drugs is a serious hazard and is dangerous in the hands of the uninitiated.

The safest area for insertion of the needle is the dorsum of the hand, and the best needle to use is a scalp-vein infusion needle with continuous intravenous infusion during the operation. Having the infusion needle in position throughout the procedure is a distinct advantage, since repeated venipunctures are thus avoided and an effective avenue for the immediate injection of drugs in the event of an emergency is always available (Fig. 21-1).

The major drugs used in intravenous sedation are of four general classes:

1. Barbiturates (pentobarbital)
2. Narcotics (meperidine, morphine, alphaprodine)
3. Ataractics or tranquilizers such as promethazine (Phenergan), diazepam (Valium)
4. Anticholinergic agents such as scopolamine

Little more than this brief and superficial review is possible in this context. Training and supervised experience are necessary before the operator may safely administer these agents in intravenous infusions.

USEFUL PROCEDURAL RULES

There are no special principles of periodontal surgery. There are only general surgical practices that are applied to periodontics. Ignoring these basic surgical requirements may result in lost flaps, excessive marginal necrosis, delayed healing, aberrant healing patterns, or excessive postoperative complications.

INSTRUMENTS

The number of precepts about instruments are relatively few, and compliance is not difficult.

Instruments are best stored and used in a sterile pack or tray set-up. It is difficult to imagine how instruments can remain sterile in drawer storage. The difficulty of maintaining even cleanliness in open drawer storage is, however, so obvious that mere mention of it should be sufficient.

The number of instruments should be as low as is consistent with the operation. Large numbers of instruments needlessly clutter the tray at surgery and waste time in searching for a particular instrument during the procedure. It is possible to load a tray with a large number of special purpose instruments that are rarely used, but it is far better to use multipurpose instruments. They promote better operative habits. The constant rustle and search for just the proper instrument, frequently changing it for another, results in unnecessarily prolonged operations that could have been much shorter with better instrumentation.

The condition of instruments is a critical point. It is surprising how many otherwise careful operators fail to check the condition of an instrument—curet or blade—until a gross failure of function occurs during surgery. Instructions about maintenance when everyone should be concentrating on the surgical procedure are likely to be forgotten. It is far better to establish a maintenance routine which ensures that instruments are kept in optimum condition, so that curets and fixed blades are sharp, files are in biting condition, and the hinges of shears and needle holders are lubricated and easy to use.

With the more frequent use of disposable blades such as the Bard Parker and Beaver instruments, there is a tendency to rely upon their initial sharpness. Failure of these blades to be sharp at the outset is, unfortunately, not a rare occurrence. In addition, even if they are sharp to begin with, incisions against bone and root will dull even a sharp blade. It is good practice to have sterile spare blades of each type at the ready on the tray. It is surprising how often these are brought into use if they are available. The most basic of all surgical principles is the use of the sharpest blades possible for all incisions.

Gingivectomy Knives

Knives are basic instruments and are obtainable with both fixed and replaceable blades. In the fixed version the familiar kidney-shaped or heart-shaped knives are the most common. They are made in pairs so that a right or left approach is possible. This gives these knives flexibility that is particularly useful in posterior

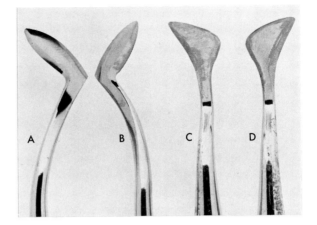

FIG. 21-2. *Fixed blade periodontal knives. A and B. Merrifield #3 and #4, excellent general purpose knives. C and D. Kirkland K15 and K16, gingivectomy knives.*

incisions and excisions. Examples of such knives are the Merrifield #3 and #4 and the Kirkland 15K and 16K (Fig. 21-2). The Kirkland knives, which are standard gingivectomy knives, have a wide application in gingival resection and flap thinning and are also useful as gingival scrapers in gingivoplasties. Many variant but similar knives are available, but none is useful interproximally.

Spear-shaped Knives

Examples of spear-shaped knives are the Goldman-Fox #8 (double ended), and the Orban #1 and #2. They are useful for interproximal incision. Merrifield #3 and #4 knives serve well as a combination and modification of both the kidney-shaped knife and spear-shaped knife so that they are useful on both the facial and lingual gingiva and interproximally as well. The authors find these instruments useful as all purpose knives for thinning poorly accessible areas of palatal flaps, emptying a tuberosity, sharply delimiting the apical extension of the secondary flap, or thinning an incision (Fig. 21-2A,B).

Knives with Disposable Blades

The familiar Bard Parker knives are useful. They enjoy the advantage of disposable blades which eliminate the need for constant sharpening. They are not well adapted to intraoral surgery because their blades are not angled, and their use presents certain awkward situations in tuberosity resections and in some palatal incisions. By the employment of some ingenuity, however, many operators find it easy to perform most incisions and excisions with them.

Several of the Bard Parker blades are more useful than others. The standard basic blade, #15, is most useful. The #12B, is a hook-shaped blade with a sharp edge on both leading and trailing edges. This knife is useful in flap thinning, especially in papillary thinning after initial scribing. Unfortunately, it has a sharp point at its tip which makes its use somewhat more restricted than would be the case if it were rounded. The #10A is a disk-shaped blade which has a cutting edge throughout its entire circumference. It is small enough to be useful in splitting flaps and thinning margins, as well as for initial incisions. (Fig. 21-3)

The Beaver sclerotome, an ophthalmic knife, is very sharp and therefore excellent for thinning palatal flaps. Its cost makes its use questionable. Beaver also makes a gingivectomy knife designed with an angled blade. Unfortunately the cutting edges become dull.

Tissue Forceps

Forceps constitute a small component in the armamentarium. The most important one is the Adson forceps, which are excellent instruments for holding a flap margin in place for the insertion of a suture needle. They are also excellent all-purpose forceps in the instrument set-up. They are often used for holding fine needles and for tying as in suturing free gingival grafts, or pedicle suturing. The most useful and convenient is the $4\frac{3}{4}$ inch size with carbide beaks (Fig. 21-4A).

Curved Allison forceps for grasping larger masses of tissue to be removed, such as a fibrous mass of tissue found in the tuberosity, are convenient but may be dispensed with (Fig. 21-4B).

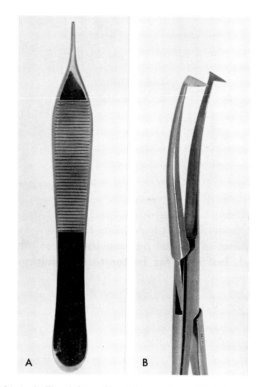

FIG. 21-4. *A. The Adson tissue forceps. B. The Allison curved tissue forceps.*

Some operators find special suture pliers useful in stabilizing a pedicle, especially for suturing. The Corn suturing pliers are well adapted for this purpose. They are fine tissue forceps with circular beaks with an open center and a small gap in the circle to permit extricating the suture after puncture (Fig. 21-5C,D). They are designed to stabilize thin flaps while the suturing needle is inserted through the notches in the edge of the beaks.

Needle Holders

There is an extremely wide choice in needle holders in length, shape of beaks, and general delicacy or sturdiness of the instruments (Fig. 21-5A). For periodontal surgery a 6-inch Ochsner or Crile-Wood model is a good all-purpose choice. The Mayo-Hegar is another. It is advisable for the operator to make the choice on a personal basis. Any of these in carbide-lined beaks provides excellent choices for general periodontal suturing. For the delicate suturing required in mucogingival surgery some operators prefer, in addition, more delicate needle holders usually used in eye surgery, such as a Castroviejo needle holder with carbide-lined beaks (Fig. 21-5B). It must be used with an extremely fine needle; a heavy gauge needle will distort the delicate beaks. These, however, are not used

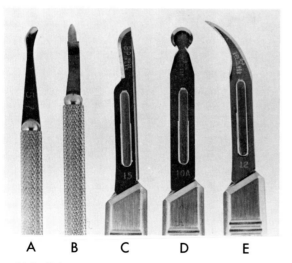

FIG. 21-3. *Knives with disposable blades. A. Beaver sclerotome. B. Beaver gingivectomy knife. C. Bard Parker #15. D. Bard Parker #10A. E. Bard Parker #12B.*

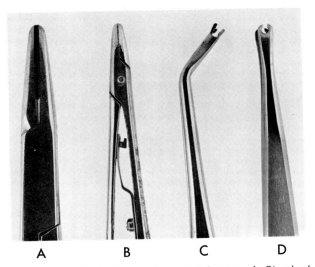

FIG. 21-5. *Needle holders and suturing forceps. A. Standard needle holder with carbide-lined beaks. B. The Castroviejo ophthalmic needle holder with carbide-lined beaks. C and D. Suturing forceps.*

widely enough in periodontics to justify their cost. The Adson needle holder and tissue forceps are excellent substitutes in fine suturing.

Scissors

The oversized tenotomy shears such as the Goldman-Fox serve well for general-purpose use, fine-tissue contouring, and tissue-tab removal. They are especially useful in gingivoplasties.

Chisels

A number of chisels are useful in periodontal surgery. For debridement of interproximal soft and hard tissues the Wiedelstadt is a serviceable instrument (Fig. 21-6A). The Hu-Friedy #29, a reverse chisel, is excellent for reducing thin line-angle peaks of bone with mesial and distal approaches (Fig. 21-6B). A general purpose chisel for bone reshaping is the Chandler #1 chisel (Fig. 21-6C).

The Ochsenbein chisels #1 and #2 are modifications of a broad standard chisel, which makes them far more useful for the periodontist in reshaping bone (Fig. 21-6D,E). A semicircular notch beveled to blade-edge sharpness on each side and immediately adjacent to the cutting edge of the chisel makes this instrument a valuable tool in ostectomy, particularly, since it can be used with a push and pull stroke. This makes it especially useful on thin plates of bone on distobuccal line angles. Many operators use it to excise gingiva as well.

A reverse chisel results from an ingenious use of

right and left wing scalers, instruments almost 100 years old. They are extremely effective for line angle ostectomy. The right and left instruments are the 43 and 44 scalers which are available in a double-ended cone-socket version, as well as in the standard models (Fig. 21-6F).

Files

Files are especially useful in interproximal crater reduction where space is constricted and a rotary instrument would be hazardous to use for fear of scoring the adjacent roots. A modification of the Buck interproximal trimmer, curved for better access and function and bent to a right or left approach, is most useful. They are called Schluger files by the manufacturer (Fig. 21-7). The #9 and #10 are designed for interproximal crater leveling and hemiseptal reduction. Although it does not have the applicability of a Schluger #9 file, the Schluger #1 is a coarser file useful in general spicule and ledge reduction.

Curets

The ubiquitous curet is indispensable in periodontal surgery as well as in most other aspects of therapy. The standard set of curets used in curettage and debridement is essential in the removal of adherent fibrous and granulomatous tissue from the necks of the teeth after incision. In addition to the standard curets, some oversized curets such as the Prichard surgical curets 1 and 2, made by Hu-Friedy, are most useful.

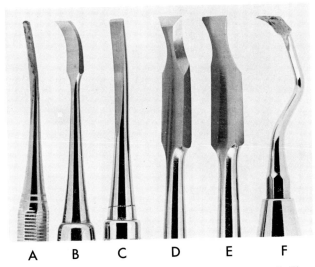

FIG. 21-6. *Chisels useful in periodontal bone surgery. A. The Wiedelstadt chisel. B. Reverse chisel Hu-Friedy #29. C. Chandler #1 chisel. D and E. Ochsenbein chisel #1. F. Wing scalers #43 and #44 used as a reverse bone chisel.*

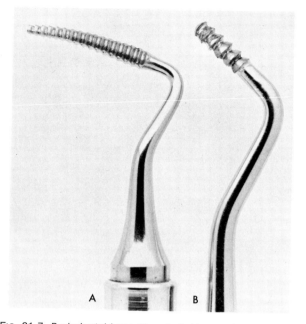

FIG. 21-7. *Periodontal bone files. A. Schluger file #9 and 10. B. Schluger file #1.*

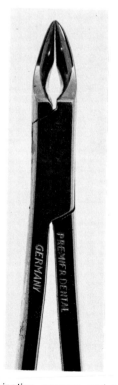

FIG. 21-8. *A combination rongeur and soft tissue nipper (Cleveland #5–Hu-Friedy) is applicable to heavy spicules of bone as well as soft fibrous tissue debridement.*

Ancillary Instruments

In addition to the instruments described, there is a mixed array of instruments:

Combination rongeur and soft tissue nipper for removing heavy spicules of bone and for debridement of soft tissue (Fig. 21-8).
#8 round long-shank angle surgical burs
#1, #2, and #3 coarse-grained Fox mounted diamond stones
Prichard #3 retractors
Michigan O probe
Mouth mirrors

INCISIONS

Little elaboration is needed here, other than to repeat that all incisions should be made definitely and without equivocation. Timid and tentative incisions make for "hashing."

In making an incision, control of the scalpel is of critical importance. Control of the blade is achieved by using (1) a sawing motion and (2) a stable rest.

The restricted, controlled sawing motion in initial incisions is an excellent method to maintain precise control over the direction of a long incision in both thin and thick tissue (Fig. 21-9). The splitting of the gingiva for the split-flap approach, for example, requires a precise incision that is quite difficult for the inexperienced. The palate, with its thick refractory tissue, is also difficult to incise exactly on a predetermined line and thickness with a free-hand traverse. Here, too, the sawing motion with a firm finger rest, which allows the incision of small dimension at each stroke, serves well for the initial incision. Once this is finished, a secondary incision may be made quite easily in the trace of the initial effort.

A stable rest is indispensable for adequate control. No matter how tenuous the rest, it is most important to establish it on the same jaw that is being treated. Patients commonly move the jaw to relax tired masticatory muscles.

There is a tendency in making internal bevel incisions on the palatal side to thin the flap excessively. While this produces a flap that is easy to place and manipulate, its margin is thin. Sometimes the margin is so thin that not enough lamina propria remains at the margin to survive—especially over bone not covered by a connective tissue bed. These sites commonly undergo necrosis and delayed healing marginally.

In order to thin the palatal flap, the operator may establish flap thickness in the initial incision so that the

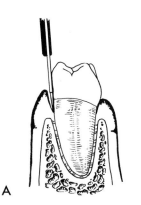

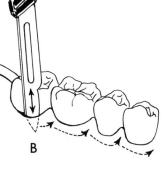

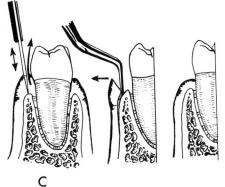

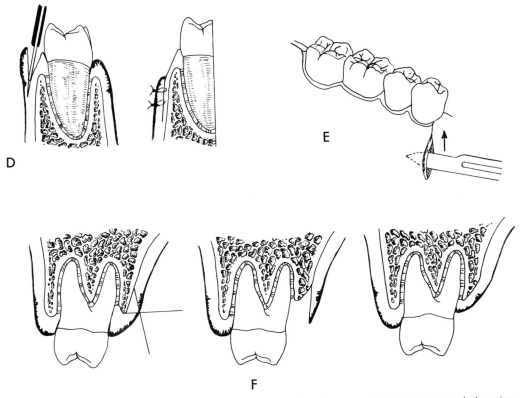

FIG. 21-9. *Various techniques of incision. A. The sulcus cut, used primarily in oral surgery. B. The recommended sawing motion for optimum control in making the initial incision. C. The crestal cut, flap reflection, and replacement at a slightly more apical level, a common incision in flap reflection. D. The split flap and its repositioning apically for added gingiva. E. The split flap made from an apical position in a marginal direction by the use of a vertical releasing incision and the separation of the alveolar mucosa from the underlying periosteum. F. Three stages of the ledge and wedge: the initial horizontal incision, secondary wedge incision, and placement of the resultant flap to cover marginal bone.*

lamina propria is split in the internal bevel (Fig. 21-10). The flap is then reflected, and the remaining connective tissue is removed from the bony surface of the palate. The underside of the palatal flap is tidied with fine iris shears or tenotomy shears and nippers.

Many skilled periodontists incise the internal bevel to the surface of the bone and reflect a full thickness flap on the palatal side to the extent required. Then they use a new razor-sharp replaceable blade to incise the inside of the palatal flap held in a stable position

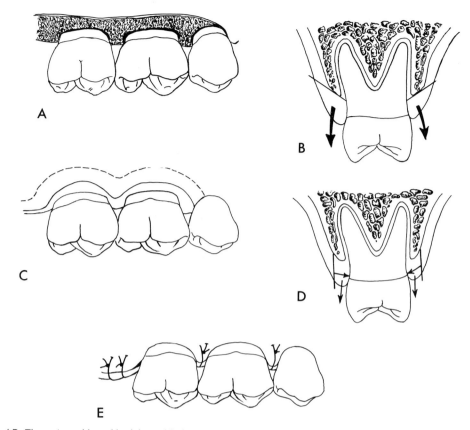

FIG. 21-10. *A and B. The external bevel incision with the arrows indicating the tissue to be removed and discarded. C and D. Internal bevel incisions. Note that the entire exposed area of the resultant flap is mature, keratinized masticatory mucosa. E. Closure of wound with interrupted sutures.*

with Adson forceps for splitting to the desired thickness, by incising the thick flap between the beaks of the Adson forceps. The marginal dimension can be corrected with fine shears.

The Ledge and Wedge

A useful expedient in managing the palatal flap is the ledge and wedge approach (Fig. 21-9F). This is performed in the following manner:

1. The marginal outline of the palatal mucosa is scribed to bone margin by an incision at a 90° angle, very much like the old gingivectomy. This technique leaves thick, blunt incised margins.
2. The remaining palatal marginal tissue is then thinned by an acutely angled internal bevel incision to the surface of the bone.
3. The flap is reflected and snipped clean of tabs and irregular tissue remnants.

This method is especially useful to beginning opera-

tors, although it is in wide use by mature and skillful operators as well.

Releasing Incisions

The extent of an incision is imprecise. It should be ample in length to provide clear and easy flap retraction without traumatizing the flap. While no one will defend an incision that is excessive in length, it is definitely better to have an incision that is a bit long than one that is a bit short. A short incision makes retraction difficult and necessitates constant tugging at the flap, not uncommonly causing tears. "Mouseholing," as operating with constricted access is called in vernacular, is poor procedure, designed to provide inadequate correction because poor visibility, as well as stormy postoperative courses because of tissue tears.

Retraction

Intimately tied to the extent of the incision is trauma from retraction. Flaps can be crushed and torn. Palatal flaps seem to be traumatized more than others because they require actual retraction rather than displacing apically during the surgical procedure. Flaps can be badly dehydrated by being tied in retraction with a suture tie. This practice is not recommended.

FLAPS AND FLAP CONTROL

Examples of flap control can be seen throughout the chapters on surgical procedures. Flap placement and control are particularly important when more than one procedure is to be used in a single quadrant and two levels of gingival margin are required, for example, a reattachment attempt on a single tooth requiring complete closure and protection in the same general operative field also requiring a repositioned flap with a slight marginal exposure (or a split-flap procedure). With the use of vertical releasing incisions and a careful specificity of approach in closure precisely directed to two levels of gingiva, this objective can be accomplished. Precise control of gingiva is the key.

The mucoperiosteal flap reflected to expose the alveolar process had its origin in antiquity. In its basic form, it was probably a simple apron of gingiva and mucosa delimited by two vertical releasing incisions and freed by marginal incision and papillary splitting and reflected. The instrument usually employed to loosen and disengage the gingiva from the underlying bony plate was a periosteal elevator which, in most cases, resembled a chisel. This sharp blade was useful in tearing the fiber apparatus binding the gingiva to the cortical plate of the alveolar process.

The flap approach has been used in all the surgical disciplines in dentistry, and periodontics is no exception. Flaps were used by periodontal therapists in the late nineteenth century, and curettage of the exposed lesions and bone was performed. This approach is used to this day by some of the most sophisticated operators.

The flap reflected for periodontal therapy differs in some ways from the standard flap commonly used in oral surgery. It is more often a dual flap, that is, a buccal and a lingual flap. Also, the flap is usually not returned to its preoperative position but is placed so that its edge is in a different position, often a more apical one. Furthermore, tight coaptation of both buccal and lingual flaps is not always the objective, although this is not the invariable rule. Control is often exercised by the use of sling suspensary sutures and a surgical cement to place the flap precisely where the operator desires (Fig. 21-11). Flaps of this kind are longer, taking in a quadrant or more in many cases. For this reason envelope flaps are more commonly used (these are flaps with no vertical releasing incisions),

since their length provides easy retractability by simple distension.

Flap release must be adequate to the clinical situation. Sutures will not hold if there is too much tension on the flap, and the flap will be displaced (Fig. 21-12).

The Initial Incision

Even the initial marginal incision differs from the simple splitting of the papillae and the sucular incision used so widely in simple flaps. Too often, the sulcular region is involved as pocket wall. It is helpful to remember that in periodontic surgery not only is the flap reflected to expose the underlying bone and roots, but frequently the flap itself is intimately involved both in the disease and in its treatment. For this reason alone, it seems best to begin with the basic flap, its creation by incision and reflection, special problems in its control in the desired position, and specific methods in coaptation and security against impingement (Fig. 21-13).

Establishing Flap Dimension

Another aspect to the initial incision is of far greater importance to the success of the operation. The level at which the incision is made is frequently the controlling factor in wound closure, gingival width, and in the length of postoperative healing time. When the initial incision is about to be made, the operator should carefully examine the field and give some serious consideration to closure of the surgical wound (Fig. 21-14).

For example, if there is a shortage of gingiva, the buccal incision should be as coronal as possible to preserve a maximal amount of this tissue so that any new gingiva induced will be *added* to the already existing width. If this precept is ignored and the incision is such that some of the existing gingiva is needlessly sacrificed, then the newly induced gingiva will merely serve to replace lost tissue. Once the initial incision is made, this particular operative result is irrevocable (Fig. 21-15).

In a similar situation, which differs merely in the choice of a vertical relaxing incision, it becomes the prudent approach to assume that because of other placement problems in the flap a slight gapping in the edges of the vertical incision is sometimes unavoidable. Since this gapping exposes bone, the location of that possible exposure should be decided upon early in field opening and should be made so that root prominences are scrupulously avoided and tuberosity areas are chosen instead.

Palatal incisions, on the other hand, are much more

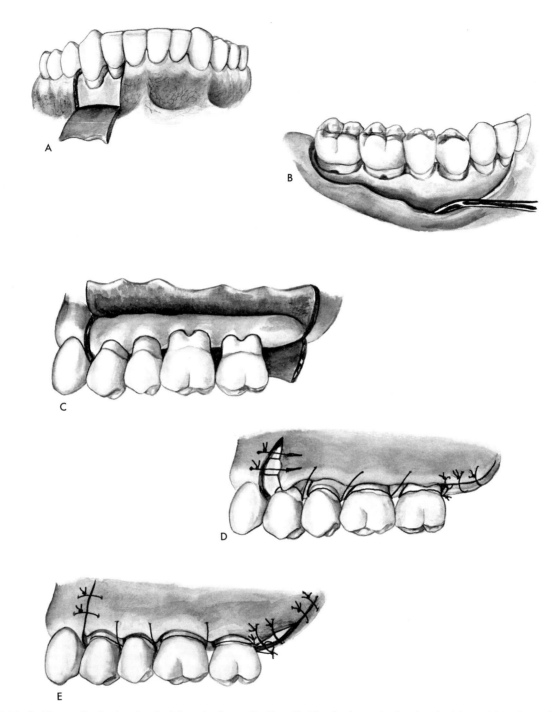

FIG. 21-11. *A. The vertical releasing incisions in flap reflection. B. The horizontal releasing incision which depends upon its mesiodistal length for its relaxation and retractability. C. Flap reflection with a vertical releasing incision distal to the canine and crestal on the tuberosity. D. Improper closure due in part to the initial suturing of the tuberosity incision (which often displaces the flap distally) causing a distal displacement of all the interproximal scribings plus a gaping deficiency distal to the canine. E. Proper closure to allow for snug approximation of the interproximal scribings with the deficiency in flap dimension at the expense of distal closure which is not especially destructive.*

routine in nature. Two factors operate to make them so. First, there is no deficiency of masticatory mucosa in this area; second, palatal tissue is relatively immobile. For these reasons, among others, the initial incision on the palatal side is carefully made to the margin of the alveolar bone in a horizontal cut. This is the ledge cut of the well-known ledge and wedge palatal approach described earlier.

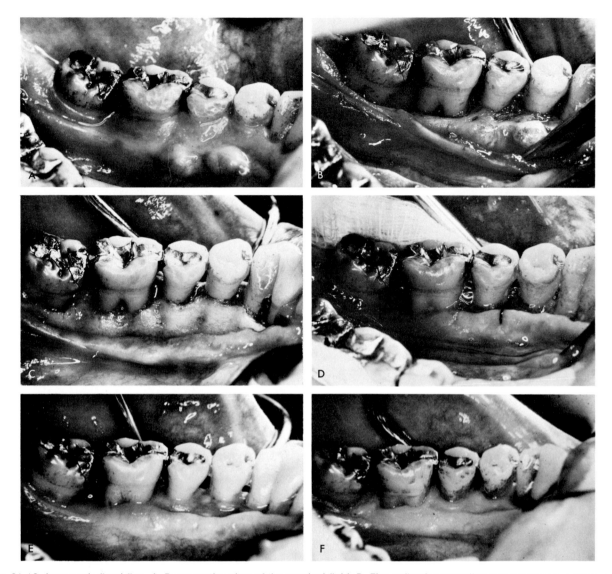

FIG. 21-12. *Insecurely fixed flap. A. Preoperative view of the surgical field. B. Flap reflection revealing two exostoses, craters, and circumferential funnel-shaped resorbtive lesions. C. Osseous correction within limits deemed desirable. D. One week postoperative. Note that the flap is displaced and the sutures have not held. E. Healing pattern one month postoperative. F. One year postoperative. The demarcation between old and new tissue is clearly visible. The pockets have been effectively eliminated, but the mucosal repair is not as good as it might have been with effective flap control. (Courtesy Dr. N. Bassaraba.)*

Flap Reflection

In reflecting any flap, the instrument of choice is a curet used with the toe or tip of the instrument riding along the crestal margin of the bone. A moderately fine curet may be used. This method of initial flap reflection has a distinct advantage over a periosteal elevator so commonly brought into play. The curet incises or tears the attachment of the gingiva to the underlying crestal bone by a direct assault on the fibers themselves. With a periosteal elevator, the tensile strength of the tissue itself is sometimes inadvertently used to tear the attachment. This tensile strength is frequently inadequate, and the flap tears instead of the attachment. The more fragile the gingiva, the more careful the operator should be in reflection. With the curet, it is rare to encounter a torn flap.

In flap reflection, the extent of release is most important. If a simple small envelope flap is to be used to approach the crestal margin, then access is the only desired result of reflection—especially when no apical repositioning is required. If, on the other hand, repositioning as well as access is desired, then release must be made apically beyond any attachment and well into the zone under alveolar mucosa. Only in this fashion

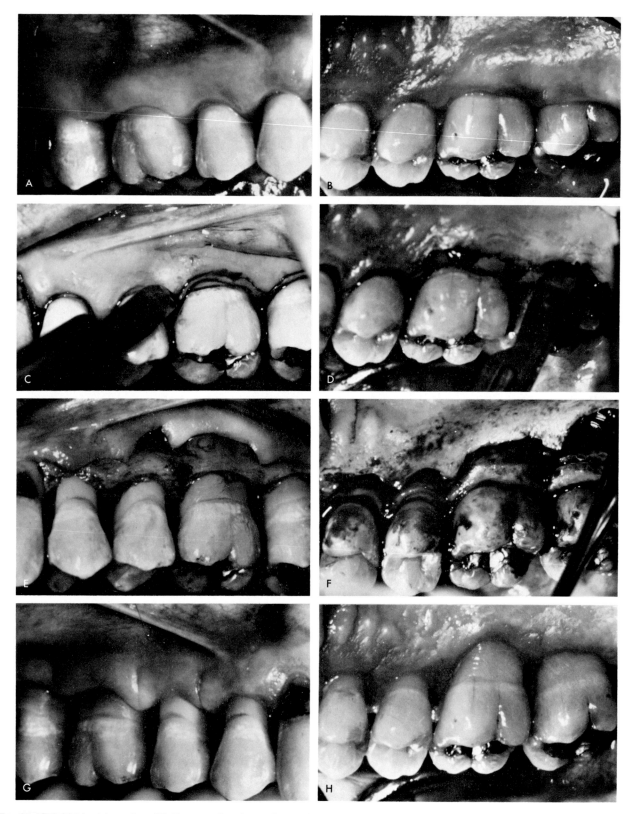

FIG. 21-13. *Initial incisions. A and B. Preoperative views of part of the surgical field. C and D. Buccal and palatal initial incisions. The buccal incision is just apical to the crest of the marginal gingiva, the palatal mucosa is scribed to marginal bone level. E and F. Reflection of both buccal and palatal flaps. G and H. Two weeks after surgery consisting of a buccal repositioned flap and a palatal replaced flap. (Courtesy Drs. W. F. Ammons and L. Schectman.)*

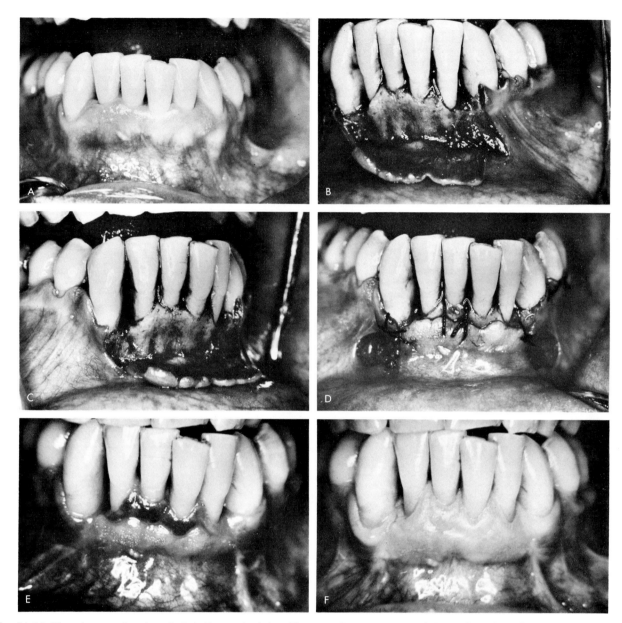

FIG. 21-14. *Flap placement and control. A. Presurgical view. There are bony craters mesial to both canines. B and C. Flap reflected and both craters ramped toward the facial aspect. D. Placement of the flap so that the margin of the flap is level with the facial crest of bone mesial to the canines. Since the bone level on the incisors is more coronal than that mesial to the canines, the margin was left denuded. E. Two weeks postoperative. Note the difference in healing pattern between the mesial of the canines and the incisors. Both are normal for the respective areas. F. One year postoperative. Note that the line of demarcation between old and new tissue over the incisors is still clearly visible. This minor flaw in an otherwise excellent result could have been avoided with vertical releasing incisions at the distal line angles of both lateral incisors so that two levels of flap placement could have been accomplished. (Courtesy Dr. W. Dahlberg.)*

will the flap be freely movable in an apical direction for repositioning.

In general, flaps may be precise and specific in dimension on the buccal side but not so much on the lingual. It is not at all unusual to place a vertical releasing incision in the buccal interfurca of an upper first molar, for example, because the mesial root appears suspiciously prominent and exposure is neither required nor desirable, but distal reflection is necessary. No such specificity is possible on the palatal aspects or the lingual surfaces of the lower arch—the upper because of the branches of the palatine artery plus the refractory nature of the tissue, and the lower because of the necessity to avoid vertical releasing incisions of any significant dimension so that the fascial planes under the floor of the mouth are not involved.

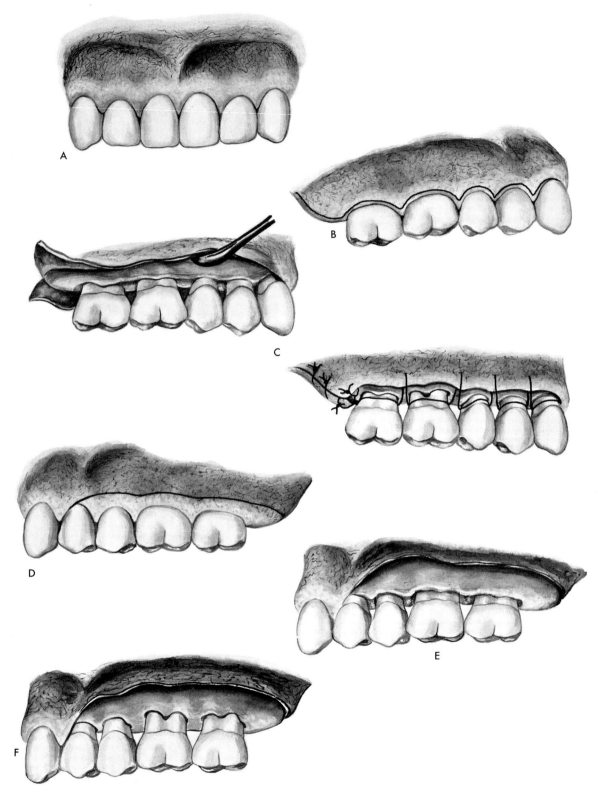

FIG. 21-15. *Flap incision and placement. A. Normal position of gingiva. B. The crestal cut. The initial incision is made on the crest of the marginal gingiva extending to the crest of marginal bone. C. Apically repositioned flap to expose some marginal bone postoperatively to gain new gingiva in addition to the preservation of the original gingiva. D. A mucogingival line cut removing all the original gingiva in the area so that a denudation results. E. Denudation with bony craters. F. Correction of bony resorptive patterns, an old-fashioned approach that is seldom indicated. Healing will be protracted and postoperative discomfort will be considerable. In addition, some marginal bone may be lost to marginal necrosis.*

Split-Thickness Flaps

The standard use of the split-thickness flap is usually reserved for pedicle tissue grafts and free gingival grafts. Some periodontists, however, use split flaps as a standard opening to the operative field. There are two general advantages to this procedure: (1) parts of the lamina propria and periosteum lie upon the bony cortical plate undisturbed by flap reflection, thus theoretically protecting it from bone loss and possible root exposure; and (2) in replacing the reflected flap to a more apical position it can be stabilized by sutures to the lamina propria.

While both these advantages are real, there are disadvantages as well: (1) marginal bone cannot be seen because the covering tissue masks, among other aberrations, circumferential bony wells; and (2) the healing pattern in the gingiva results in thick and irregular margins which almost always require a second-stage external bevel gingivoplasty for optimum results.

Some observers doubt the efficacy of the protection offered by the split flap to the underlying bone. They feel that the cover merely blocks visibility and is not thick enough to protect the bone from resorption by the acute inflammatory infiltrate common in surgical wounds. This lack of protection is especially true because the tissue covering the roots and bone is usually trimmed extremely thin.

There is sometimes in standard mucogingival procedures a need to use split-thickness flaps in closing all or part of the wound. Insertions into the marginal frenum in the midline of the lower anterior region can be treated in this fashion. Although repositioning a full-thickness flap is a method commonly used, there are advantages to be gained by using a split-thickness flap over thin labial plates or over fenestrations and dehiscences. This allows the labial plate to remain covered and inviolate. Corn used an interesting variation on a standard split flap reflection by perforating the periosteum lying upon the labial plate deep in the wound near the apices of the teeth. In healing, this area scars and is often bound firmly to the labial or buccal plate for a variable period and acts as a barrier to a possible reinsertion of the frenum marginally. Robinson introduced an almost identical method independently at approximately the same time.

The execution of the split flap is simplicity itself. In reality, only the gingiva is split in thickness. This is achieved by sharp dissection in a mesiodistal direction to the depth of the mucogingival junction. From this point apically, the fibrous periosteum is allowed to remain undisturbed on the labial plate, and the mucosa is easily separated from it and reflected. This is an easy task, since the mucosa is only loosely joined to its underlying periosteum. The initial cut is commonly made marginally, usually in the papillae, and is continued into the body of the gingiva in the proximal portion of the operative field. Once the gingiva is traversed in an apical direction and the areolar mucosa is reached, the blade of the scalpel is then reversed, and by pushing distally between the mucosa and the fibrous layer of the periosteum, the gingiva can be more easily split in an apical-to-marginal direction.

Another useful method is to make the proximal vertical releasing incision into the areolar mucosa. This apical portion of the incision gapes, so that the blade can be pushed into the wound distally, dividing the mucosa and splitting the gingiva from below, so to speak, and then incising in a marginal direction.

Split-flap entries are used in pedicle grafts. Both pedicle and free autogenous gingival grafts will be given somewhat more definitive description and discussion in Chapter 25.

CONTROL OF BLEEDING

General surgical principles must include the management of the occasional bleeding episode. Bleeding from causes inherent in the blood elements is discussed at the end of this chapter.

The disturbing fact is that the volume of blood lost in a single quadrant of periodontal surgery requiring flaps, thinning of tissue, tuberosity reduction, and some bone contouring approaches 300 to 350 ml. This volume approaches and even surpasses that in such general surgical procedures as hysterectomy, colostomy, and even cesarean section.

The reason is not difficult to understand. The general surgeon ties off his bleeders (vessels incised in the procedures) as he progresses—often even before he severs the vessel. The periodontal surgeon deals with large incised surfaces in which capillary bleeding is copious. Most often, he incises no sizable vessels at the time of operation. These may be eroded later. This gives rise to the wry joke that the periodontal surgeon ties off *his* bleeders 12 hours postoperatively.

Postoperative bleeding is not a common occurrence in periodontal surgery; neither is it rare. When it does occur, it is best to address the problem systematically. When the operator is confronted with a patient who is bleeding postoperatively, the patient feels a certain amount of apprehension. The periodontist's manner should be confident and reassuring.

First, all clots extruding from the wound are removed with a gauze sponge. This simple expedient sometimes reveals the source of bleeding, but since, for the most part, the blood emanates from under the flap, the true point of hemorrhage may be some distance from the apparent source.

Many topical agents have been used by many operators with generally poor results. The latest in a long list was topical thrombin. Whatever may be its effect upon capillary bleeding generally, it is certainly not effective in the kind of bleeding encountered postoperatively in periodontal surgery. Cellulose derivatives such as Gelfoam and Surgicell are effective in a minor way if only a small capillary bed is bleeding.

A local anesthetic injection will temporarily stop bleeding and for that reason is to be used with caution. Its use effectively masks bleeding sources and, after the effect of the epinephrine it contains wears off, the bleeding often resumes.

The most effective method of arresting other than minor hemorrhage is the classic method of tying off the offending vessels. Since in periodontal surgery blood vessels are rarely if ever resected and isolated, the tying off must be done by a suture noose. An effective way of determining the source of hemorrhage is to use the pressure of a blunt instrument handle in trial locations from whence the bleeding emanates. A knowledge of some rudimentary surgical anatomy of the oral cavity is helpful. After one or more trial pressure points are attempted and the results have been determined, the point where pressure caused bleeding to stop is encircled with a blind suture that is firmly tied. Knowledge of the point of origin of the principal vessels is an important aid in the placing of the suture. If the first attempt stops bleeding, no further effort is necessary. If it does not, then a second or even a third blind suture is taken along the course of the vessel. These usually suffice. The most common error in blind suturing is that of making the sutures too superficial to occlude the vessel properly. The suture noose should encircle the entire thickness of flap.

It is usually not necessary to disturb sutures or dressings (although often dressings are floated off by the hemorrhage). On rare occasions, however, it will be necessary to reflect flaps again to find the offending bleeder. The method of control is the same.

After the bleeding has stopped, it is good practice to place the patient in a recumbent position for 15 to 30 minutes to see whether the hemorrhage will recur. If it does not recur in that period, then the patient may be dismissed with the usual precautionary directions.

METHODS IN BONE RESHAPING

The reduction and reshaping of bone are simple matters in the hands of a dentist who is accustomed to reduction of enamel—a far more refractory and resistant substance. In fact, it is the relatively soft texture of bone that demands special precautions and extraordinary care. Overcutting is a real hazard.

Most operators use slow- or intermediate-speed handpieces because they give greater control. When a rotary instrument is used on bone in the neighborhood of roots, unnecessary damage is sometimes inflicted because of overcutting. The temptation to overcut is great because of the ease and speed with which the bone melts away.

There is a real question whether it is good to use air-driven turbines of any speed because the aerosol escaping has oil droplets in it and may cause emphysema in the tissues. It is true, however, that no such cases have been reported in the periodontal literature, although there have been some reports in oral surgery journals. Nonetheless, the danger exists and should be taken into account.

A bur is a more logical and less traumatic instrument than a diamond instrument, since the bur removes fragments of bone and generates far less heat than does a diamond abrasive instrument. A bur, however, has a strong tendency to gouge into the bone and cause little potholes in a surface that should be smooth and undulating. It is good practice to reduce large masses of bone with a bur and finish with a diamond rotary instrument. In this manner, both speed and finish are easily attained. Water coolant is standard with all rotary instruments.

Least irritating of all are the hand instruments—the file and chisel. These are available in several convenient shapes for bone reshaping. Because they are slow and require considerable digital manipulation, they are used where relatively small amounts of bone are to be removed. Commonly used in combination with rotary motor diamond instruments, the file and the chisel constitute finishing instruments where precise control is critical because of the proximity to the roots of the teeth.

SUTURES AND SUTURING

Suturing is basic in any approach to flap control and wound closure. It is not the only skill needed, but it is the one always used and so serves well to open this subject. It is a skill common to almost all surgical procedures, and time spent in developing facility yields dividends in rapid, uneventful healing, with good and pleasing contour resulting.

Conversely, slipshod suturing results in torn flaps, gaping wounds, and ugly healing patterns. While other factors are involved in wound healing on a gross clinical level, there is no doubt that suturing is an important one. It is the principal agency in flap control.

One of the cardinal rules in suturing is that placing

tension on the tissues being sutured to the extent of inducing blanching is to court almost certain necrosis of the sutured area and the subsequent loss of the suture entirely. Unfortunately this is a common occurrence. It is for areas in which some resistance to surgical approximation is encountered that the mattress suture is so useful. Both the vertical and horizontal mattress sutures are described, together with indications for the application of each.

The Interrupted Suture

The interrupted suture is the simplest and most basic of all sutures. It consists of the fixing and coaptating of two edges of an incision by passing a suture through both and tying a surgeon's knot, or square knot, so that both edges are in good approximation (Fig. 21-16).

The interrupted suture is used in linear incisions, split-flap fixation, interproximal papillary sutures—in fact, it is probably the most common suture in mucosal surgery. It is at its most useful when both edges are to be brought together in a simple closure. It is not effective when one or both flaps are to be repositioned. For repositioning in a full-thickness flap, enough slack must be left to allow the flap to be apically displaced precisely to the level decided upon by the operator. This slack is then taken up by a properly placed dressing which fixes the flap at the predetermined level. The dressing acts as a stent.

The interrupted suture is, of course, useful in simple linear closure such as is used in long tuberosity areas and elsewhere.

The Simple Sling Suture

The simple sling suture is a suspensary suture consisting of a two-tooth unit (Fig. 21-16D). The suture is passed interproximally through the embrasure, engaging the papilla, passed back through the same embrasure, engaging the next papilla, passed back through the same embrasure, engaging the next papilla, passed back through the same embrasure and tied to the tail at the original entry. This is a good suspensary device, variable in vertical dimension at the will of the operator, but limited to two adjacent papillae. Because of this limitation in extent, its use is relatively uncommon.

The Continuous Sling Suture

Directly adapted from the simple sling, the continuous sling overcomes the limitation of the former to two adjacent teeth (Fig. 21-16E). The continuous sling can be used to include as many teeth in a quadrant as

desired and has all the advantages of easy placement of the flap at precisely the level desired.

A loop suture is taken in the terminal papilla and is knotted securely, but the loop should not be so tight that the papilla is constricted to the embarrassment of its circulation. The suture is then passed interproximally through the embrasure of the papilla just engaged, the neck of the tooth is partly encircled, the suture is passed out again at the adjacent embrasure, the papilla is engaged by the needle and suture, the suture is passed back once again through the same embrasure, round the neck of the tooth. This procedure is repeated in as many interproximal embrasures as the surgical field contains until the other terminal embrasure is reached.

At the other terminal embrasure a slight variance is performed. A loose loop is allowed to remain in the penultimate embrasure and is then used as a tie for the last papillary suture passing through the terminal embrasure.

Although by no means the only suture used, the continuous sling suture is as close to a standard suture as periodontists are likely to come by. Used both on the buccal and the lingual aspects, it allows precise placement of the flap margin. By making several loops, pulled tight, surrounding the terminal tooth, the sling on one side is secured in length and tension. The other side, buccal or lingual as the case may be, can be looser or tighter as the clinical situation may require. This is the belaying principle used by sailors and mountain climbers. The suture is most often paired on both buccal and lingual sides, each one of the pair performing its special role—for example, a snug adaptation of the flap on the palatal side and a slack for repositioning on the facial—with no regard necessary for its opposite number, each being totally independent of the other.

The Vertical Mattress Suture

In performing either the simple sling or the continuous sling—or even the interrupted suture, for that matter—there is sometimes a need for additional control of one or more papillae. This is the case when the tissue is friable and delicate and a single puncture is likely to tear; too deep a bite of the suture needle would contract the flap into a horizontal fold and leave the papillary margin unsupported. In that contingency a double bite, one above the other, would furnish security and good control.

The vertical mattress suture is made by inserting the needle from the surface inward at the tip of the papilla, inside the papilla to the base, out again at the base, and back over the surface of the papilla through

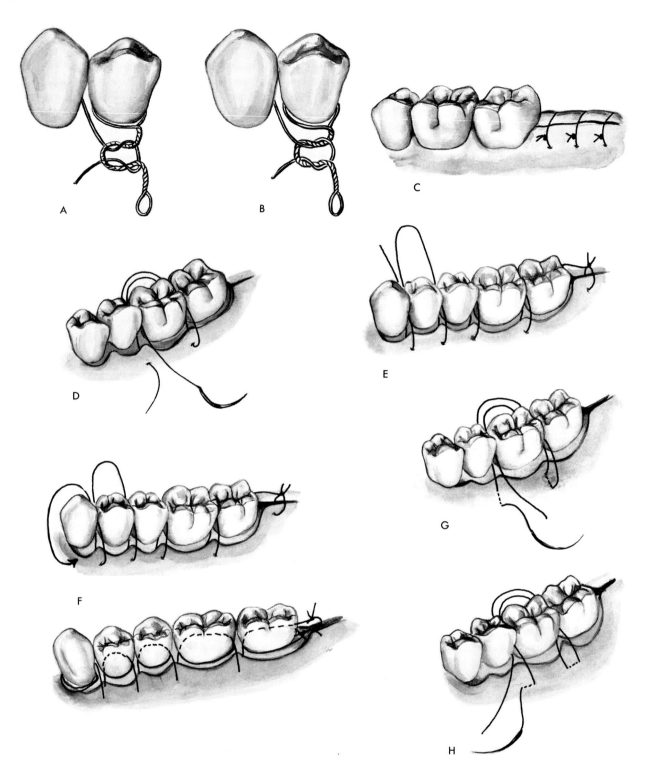

FIG. 21-16. *Various sutures and ligations. A. The square, or surgeon's knot. This is the standard knot for secure and dependable closure. B. The granny knot, which is an improperly tied square knot. Although this knot slips, it does so grudgingly and therefore is an excellent device to allow for precise placement of a flap margin, after which it can be secured from slippage by adding a third throw or tie. C. Interrupted suture—single sutures, each complete in itself. D. The simple sling. This tie is rarely used but forms the basis for the continuous sling ligature. E. The continuous sling suture. This suspensary ligature can extend for as long as the operator likes. F. The double continuous sling suture. By wrapping the ligature several times about the neck of the terminal tooth both buccal and lingual flaps can be secured—one replaced and the other repositioned. G. The vertical mattress suture—useful in securing fragile flaps by the double bite and fixing the edge of the scribed papilla firmly. H. The horizontal mattress suture. This suture makes it possible to fix the tip of the scribed papilla by straddling it.*

the embrasure to the opposite side (Fig. 21-16G). The papilla is firmly and securely fixed by this procedure.

The Horizontal Mattress Suture

The horizontal mattress suture is similarly designed to provide papillary control and fixation, except that in this expedient the concern is with the tips of the reflected papillae (Fig. 21-16H). In tying the suspensary or sling suture using the single puncture and passage of the suture through the papilla, a problem of control emerges. The tip of the papilla slips mesially or distally to the single strand of suture designed to hold it. Either position violates all our precepts of good flap control.

The horizontal mattress suture is designed to control the tip of the papilla. It consists of *double* parallel strands of suture straddling the papilla and holding it firmly in place. Some operators prefer the double strand crossed over the papilla for even firmer control, but that is a detail.

The horizontal mattress suture is produced by beginning the continuous sling in the usual manner with the terminal tie. At the first interproximal puncture of the suturing needle, it is inserted to one side of the midline of the base of the papilla, passed under the tissue and out again on the other side of the midline of the papilla and back through the embrasure. This provides the parallel strands of the horizontal mattress suture. This same procedure can be repeated in every interproximal space if desired.

SUTURE MATERIALS

In the closure of periodontal surgical wounds the choice of sutures is limited to three general types: (1) braided silk, (2) Dacron coated and thoroughly impregnated with Teflon, and (3) reasorbable collagen. All three types have some variants, but these form the basic group of the sutures generally used.

Braided Silk

Braided silk is the standard suture material. It has some important advantages in manipulation in that it is probably the most easily tied, remains securely tied with a surgeon's knot (square knot), is adjustable with a granny knot so that precise positioning is possible, and generally is well suited to periodontal wound closure.

Since it is braided, it suffers from an important disadvantage—capillarity. It will allow fluid from the oral cavity to enter the wound; indeed it will help these fluids with the accompanying sepsis to penetrate through the suture holes and into the deeper recesses of the wound under the flap.

The disadvantage has encouraged the manufacturers to seek materials or additives to behave like a monofilament (nonbraided) suture. The search for material which will be as dead-soft, inert, and easily tied as braided silk and yet be monofilamentous is a difficult one indeed.

Many expedients have been tried with natural and synthetic fibers. Most are either too stiff to be useful with the tissues encountered in the mouth or are impossible to tie securely because of slippage. One of the most successful of the innovations has been Dacron fiber boiled in Teflon.

Dacron and Teflon

Dacron impregnated with Teflon provides a great improvement over silk in that it is totally inert within the tissues through which it passes. In valvular and vascular surgery, for which it was developed, no giant-cell response has been demonstrated after even years of remaining in the tissues sutured. It behaves like a monofilament because of the filling of the fiber interstices with Teflon, it permits minimal capillarity, and it is soft and easily managed—with a single exception. It is subject to slippage unless carefully and securely tied with a *double* square knot—four throws, each drawn tight with even tension on each of the two legs or strands and with somewhat longish ears of about $^3/_{16}''$ allowed to remain. Secured in this fashion, it will remain tied.

As might be expected, this material is quite costly and is not necessary for routine suturing. A good case for its use can be made, however, in flap closure in inductive procedures such as in classic new attachment procedures and autogenous grafts of various kinds to help prevent infection and to help provide optimum conditions for a successful take.

Collagen

The various resorbable sutures are quite useful to those therapists who find it difficult to see their patients for suture removal because of great distances. As a general rule in standard procedures the collagen suture is used in inaccessible areas such as deep into the vestibular trough where labial flaps were formerly secured in some procedures. When a fiber suture is used in these inaccessible areas, removal is most difficult at times, and sutures are often missed altogether and remain to be exfoliated after necrosis. Theoretically, the resorbable suture will solve this problem. In actual practice, however, resorbable sutures do not always resorb as quickly and completely as they are supposed to. Small knots and pieces remain embedded in the tissue for longer periods than one would wish, and healing is uneven and leaves ugly nodules of scar tissue in the deep recesses of the mouth.

It must be kept in mind that collagen sutures are the most irritating and among those eliciting the greatest giant-cell response. Overlong retention is irritating indeed. We are left, then, with the only indication for using them for standard closure being in patients who cannot return for more normal management. This is a real advantage that outweighs some of the shortcomings of this material in periodontal surgery.

Suture Gauge

The size of the suture used, of whatever material, is a matter of preference and of the requirements of the closure. Obviously, some tissues are coarse and thick and must be secured under some slight tension. Other tissues are thin, delicate mucosa that should be coapted or placed under no tension whatever. In the former, a heavier suture is required for two reasons: (1) strength of material and (2) less likelihood of cutting through the flap to be secured.

On the other hand, suture material that is too thin will have a tendency to cut and pull through the flap. This is particularly true in the apically repositioned flap that is maintained in position by sutures which establish the limits of apical displacement and the surgical cement which does the apical displacing to the limits imposed by the sutures. Injudicious pressure in placing the cement will pull the suture through the margin of the flap.

The objection to thin sutures can be met to a degree by taking a larger bite with the suture needle, so that the puncture will be somewhat apical to the margin. There is a limit to this expedient, however, since the mucogingival line is soon met, and when the puncture is made in mucosa there is a bunching of the tissue under the suture. A vertical mattress suture can be resorted to when a thinner suture material is used.

The unfortunate aspect of tearing the suture through the flap in pushing the cement into place is that the tear is not visible to the operator because of the covering cement until some days have passed and healing has begun. When flaps are thus torn, the resultant wounds are ugly and healing is inordinately delayed. Frequently, a follow-up gingivoplasty is required to repair the thick, knobby marginal tissue with several zones of new and old gingiva apparent.

Basic principles of surgery have a way of pervading all areas of periodontal surgery. Even the length of the suture material may be a difficulty. What would be the point of using sterile instruments if the long looped strand inadvertently brushes the sleeve of the patient, or even his face? Long sutures are useful and economical, but they must be carefully watched in use.

Vigilance and care in all aspects of surgery are best reduced to routine so that specific attention need not be paid to every punctilio in every procedure.

References

1. Ariaudo, A., and Tyrell, H.: Repositioning and increasing the zone of attached gingiva. J. Periodontol., 28:106, 1957.
2. Berdon, J. W.: Blood loss during gingival surgery. J. Periodontol., 36:102, 1965.
3. Carranza, F. A. Jr., et al.: The effect of periosteal fenestration in gingival extension operations. J. Periodontol., 37:335, 1966.
4. Corn, H.: Classification of periodontal flaps. Presented to the American Society of Periodontists, Chicago, 1966.
5. Corn, H.: Periosteal separation, its clinical significance. J. Periodontol., 33:140, 1962.
6. Dahlberg, W.: Consideration of periodontal flap design and management. Presented to the American Society of Periodontists. Chicago, 1966.
7. Donnenfeld, O., Marks, R., and Glickman, I.: The apically repositioned flap—a clinical study. J. Periodontol., 35:381, 1964.
8. Kohler, C., and Ramfjord, S.: Healing of gingival muco-periosteal flaps. Oral Surg., 13:89, 1960.
9. Luebke, R. G., and Ingle, J. I.: Geometric nomenclature for muco-periosteal flaps. Periodontics, 2:301, 1964.
10. Malamud, E. H.: A technique of suturing flaps in periodontal surgery. Periodontics, 1:207, 1963.
11. Morris, M. L.: Suturing technique in periodontal surgery. Periodontics, 3:84, 1965.
12. Nabers, C. L.: Repositioning the attached gingiva. J. Periodontol., 25:38, 1954.
13. Pfeifer, J. S.: The growth of gingival tissue over denuded bone. J. Periodontol., 34:10, 1963.
14. Robinson, R. E.: The distal wedge operation. Periodontics, 4:256, 1966.
15. Robinson, R. E.: Periosteal fenestration in muco-gingival surgery. Periodont. Abstracts, 9:107, 1961.
16. Tauber, R.: Basic Surgical Skills—A Manual with Appropriate Exercises. Philadelphia, W. B. Saunders Company, 1955.
17. Wade, A. B.: The flap operation. J. Periodontol., 37:95, 1966.
18. Widman, L.: The operative treatment of alveolar pyorrhea. Br. Dent. J., 37:105, 1917.

21A

Aspirin and Blood Coagulation

21A

The Effect of Aspirin and Related Compounds on Blood Coagulation

GOTTFRIED SCHMER

Numerous publications have appeared in the past few years dealing with the problem of drug interference with the coagulation mechanism. Aspirin (acetylsalicylic acid), for many years thought to be a safe drug, became one of the centers of interest. This section describes briefly the impact of aspirin and other salicylates on blood coagulation, the clinical and biochemical effects, the dangers, and safe substitute analgesics. It should be emphasized that hundreds of publications have appeared on aspirin alone and that this section describes only the most important developments.

THE COAGULATION MECHANISM

When vascular injury occurs and blood comes in contact with tissue, blood platelets, the cellular elements of hemostasis, adhere to the exposed collagen (adhesion). The next step is referred to as release reaction, where intrinsic adenosine diphosphate (ADP), platelet factor 3, and other chemicals are released. The released ADP causes the platelets to aggregate (aggregation) and to form the initial platelet plug, which by itself has a hemostyptic capacity. Platelet factor 3 is a phospholipid, which is required for the interaction of clotting factors.

A modern concept of coagulation chemistry has been described,[1] but the principle of a cascade or waterfall mechanism is still valid as a simplified scheme of blood clotting.[2] Clotting factors are mostly enzymes that are present in blood as inactive proenzymes. When clotting is initiated by the so-called contact factors, a waterfall-like sequence of proenzyme-enzyme conversion occurs, resulting in a magnification effect, which finally leads to the formation of a visible fibrin clot. In healthy individuals the activation of the blood-clotting factors and the formation of the platelet plug occur simultaneously.

Of special interest regarding the interference of aspirin and related compounds on the clotting mechanism are the so-called vitamin K-dependent clotting factors II, VII, IX, and X, which, with the exception of IX, are measured by the one stage prothrombin time.[3] These factors are severely decreased by the use of anti-vitamin K (Coumadin) to treat or to prevent thrombotic states.

PLATELET FUNCTION TESTS

Platelet function *in vivo* is checked by the bleeding time. An artificial wound is set by a lancet or a blade, and the time elapsed before clotting occurs is referred to as bleeding time (BT). Different methods are in use.[4,5,6] We prefer in our laboratory the standardized

Ivy bleeding time of Mielke et al.,[7] which gives reliable, reproducible results. Two parallel cuts made in the forearm with a standardized blade will yield a BT of 4 to 8 minutes in normals. A defect in the formation of the initial platelet plug results in a prolongation of the BT, which therefore reflects the physiologic or pathologic behavior of the platelets.

An excellent study of the bleeding time as a screening test for evaluating platelet function has been published by Harker and Slichter.[8] The reliability of the bleeding time is shown by the fact that it correlates well with a platelet count between 10,000 and 100,000 platelets per μ1, if the platelet function per se remains normal.

Much less significant for clinical evaluation are the *in vitro* assays of blood platelets. The *in vivo* adhesion of platelets can be simulated by adsorption to glass.[9,10] Aggregation can be triggered *in vitro* by collagen, ADP, and epinephrine, which first leads to a primary aggregation, followed by a secondary aggregation caused by a release of intrinsic ADP. These aggregation processes can be followed spectrophotometrically by registering an increased intensity of light passing through a cell of platelet-rich plasma the moment platelet aggregation occurs.[11] The applicability of *in vitro* assays for clinical situations is still contended and should not be given priority over the standardized BT at the present state.

STUDIES OF THE EFFECTS OF ASPIRIN

Aspirin can act at two different levels in coagulation by exhibiting a Coumadin-like effect, resulting in a decrease of vitamin K-dependent factors, and by interfering with normal platelet functions, resulting in a prolonged bleeding time.

The Coumadin-like effect of aspirin and other salicylates has been known for a long time.[12,13,14] This effect occurs only after prolonged treatment with high doses of salicylates as in long term therapy of rheumatoid arthritis. No decrease of vitamin K-dependent factors has been found after administration of a single dose. The increase of the one-stage prothrombin time can be excessive. Recently we had the opportunity to investigate four patients with chronic rheumatoid arthritis on symptomatic long-term therapy with sodium salicylate. The patients showed an apparent bleeding tendency with large bruises occurring spontaneously or after minimal trauma. The one-stage prothrombin time was greatly prolonged, and the concentration of factors II, VII, IX and X was between 5 and 10 percent of normal. Termination of the salicylate therapy led to a return of the factors to normal. In these cases salicylates exert a Coumadin-like effect, which can be counteracted by the administration of vitamin K.[15]

The occurrence of this event is relatively rare when compared to the effect of aspirin on the platelet function. A large number of publications have described the effect of aspirin on the bleeding time.[7,16,17,18,19] A thorough description of the bleeding time in 60 normals is given by Mielke et al.,[7] using their standardized Ivy BT. The average BT was 5 minutes with a range of 2 minutes 30 seconds to 10 minutes. After a single dose of 1 gm aspirin a mean BT of 9 minutes 30 seconds (range 4 minutes to 21 minutes) could be found in 30 persons 2 hours after the ingestion of the drug. Practically identical results have been obtained by Blatrix.[16] It is interesting in this connection that the effect of aspirin on the platelets takes place as fast as 5 to 10 minutes after ingestion.[20] It must be emphasized that normals do not respond to aspirin as a single population,[7] but show a large variability in the change of BT from insignificant to quite large increases. This is in contrast to the hemophilic population which shows quite a uniform and large increase in BT after aspirin ingestion.[21] Similar results were found in Von Willebrand's disease, a hereditary bleeding disorder with a low factor VIII and a prolonged BT in the classic case.[19]

Although it is generally agreed that aspirin causes only a moderate prolongation of the bleeding time in normals and that spontaneous bleeding is not observed, other authors have published clinical reports of bleeding after salicylate ingestion and have expressed warnings.[22,23,24]

A highly interesting study was published by Sutor et al.,[18] who developed a semiautomatic quantitative BT, which not only measured the time but also the pattern and the intensity of the bleeding from a skin puncture. Within 70 minutes after the ingestion of aspirin all 15 healthy volunteers of this study showed an increase of BT and most significantly an increased blood loss in 75 percent of the cases of at least four times of normal. This important fact has to be kept in mind when the influence of aspirin on the hemostatic mechanism is evaluated under surgical conditions.

Especially in the case of biopsies, which include the tonsillectomy, a normal BT is paramount, except in bone marrow biopsy. All cases of prolonged BT should be excluded from the biopsies until the reason for this prolongation is clear and the defect has been corrected. We recently observed heavy bleeding after a gastric biopsy in a volunteer who had taken aspirin the previous day and was not subjected to a BT. The bleeding time turned out to be 21 minutes, and massive blood transfusions were necessary.

On numerous occasions we could observe a tendency

to excessive bleeding after periodontic surgery and aspirin ingestion. The BT was prolonged, although in no instance was blood transfusion required and the bleeding could be controlled by mechanical pressure.

DURATION OF THE ASPIRIN EFFECT

The effect of aspirin on the platelets is thought to be dose independent besides the initial critical concentration of 150 to 300 mg as a single dose.[25] The clinical effect of aspirin can be found up to 4 days after the uptake of the drug.

BIOCHEMICAL EFFECT OF ASPIRIN ON THE PLATELETS

There is general agreement that aspirin causes a loss of secondary aggregation of platelets in response to extrinsic ADP, epinephrine, or collagen by blocking the mechanism of intrinsic ADP release.[7,26,27,28,29,30]

Mielke et al.[7] were unable to evaluate the effect of aspirin on *in vivo* adhesiveness according to the method of Borchgrevink,[31] while Stuart[25] and Beaumont et al.[32] found a decreased platelet adhesiveness in vitro. Aspirinated platelets were shown to have a decrease in platelet factor 3 release.[26] Aspirin might interact with the platelet membrane[33] and exert an influence on the membrane permeability.[29,30]

The effect of aspirin on the platelets is certainly complex, and the biomolecular mechanisms leading to these effects are still unknown. Impaired glycolysis has been described in aspirinated platelets.[34] It is thought that the acetyl group in aspirin is responsible for the changes in platelet physiology, since similar in vitro effects can be produced by other acetylating agents like acetic anhydride.[26]

ANALGESICS AND TRANQUILIZERS NOT INTERFERING WITH PLATELET FUNCTIONS

Presently there are not too many reports published dealing with this question. Sutor et al. found that sodium salicylate had no effect on hemostasis and that acetaminophen did not prolong the bleeding time in 14 out of 15 normal cases.[18] A comparative study between aspirin and acetaminophen after tonsillectomy showed that acetaminophen should be given preference.[5] This analgesic seems also to be safe in hemophilia.[35,36] Another oral analgesic with no effects on the platelets is dextropropoxyphene hydrochloride.[19] Chlordiazepoxide HCl (Librium), which is still often used preoperatively, did not show any effect on the coagulation, especially on the bleeding time, so that it can be safely prescribed.[37]

References

1. Coagulation. G. Schmer and P. E. Strandjord, Eds. New York, Academic Press, 1973.
2. Davie, E. W., and Ratnoff, O. D.: Science, 145:1310, 1964.
3. Quick, A. J.: J. Biol. Chem., 109:73, 1935.
4. Duke, W. W.: Arch. Intern. Med., 10:445, 1912.
5. Ivy, A. C., Sapiro, P. F., and Melnick, P.: Surg. Gynecol. Obstet., 60:781, 1935.
6. Borchgrevink, C. F., and Waaler, B. A.: Acta Med. Scand., 162:361, 1958.
7. Mielke, C. H., Jr., et al.: Blood, 34:204, 1969.
8. Harker, L. A. and Slichter, Sh., J.: N. Engl. J. Med., 287:155, 1972.
9. Hellem, A. J.: Thesis. Scand. J. Clin. Lab. Invest., 12(Suppl. 51): 1960.
10. Salzman, E. W.: J. Lab. Clin. Med., 62:724, 1963.
11. Born, B. U. R.: Nature, 194:927, 1962.
12. Rapaport, S., Wing, M., and Guest, G. M.: Proc. Soc. Exp. Biol., 53:40, 1943.
13. Meyer, O. O., and Howard, B.: Proc. Soc. Exp. Biol., 53:234, 1943.
14. Shapiro, S., Redish, M. H., and Campbell, H. A.: Proc. Exp. Biol. Med., 53:251, 1943.
15. Shapiro, S.: JAMA, 125:546, 1944.
16. Blatrix, C. H.: Nouv. Rev. Fr. Hematol., 3:346, 1963.
17. Quick, A. J.: Am. J. Med. Sci., 252:265, 1966.
18. Sutor, A. H., Bowie, E. J. W., and Owen, Ch. A., Jr.: Mayo Clinic Proc., 46:178, 1971.
19. Sahud, M. A., and Cohen, R. M.: Calif. Med., 115:10, 1971.
20. Okonkwo, P.: Thromb. Diath. Haemorrh., 25:279, 1971.
21. Quick, A. J.: Am. J. Med. Sci., 254:392, 1967.
22. Bowie, E. J. W., and Owen, Ch. A., Jr.: Circulation, 40:757, 1969.
23. Muir, A.: Salicylates: An International Symposium. A.S.S. Dixon, et al., Eds. Boston, Little, Brown & Company, 1963, p. 230.
24. Muir, A., and Cossar, I. A.: Br. Med. J., 2:7, 1955.
25. Stuart, R. K.: J. Lab. Clin. Med., 75:463, 1970.
26. Al-Mondhiry, H.: Proc. Soc. Exp. Biol. Med., 133:632, 1970.
27. Weiss, H. J., and Aledort, L. M.: Lancet 2:495, 1967.
28. Zucker, M. B., and Peterson, J.: Proc. Soc. Exp. Biol. Med., 127:547, 1958.
29. O'Brien, J. R.: Lancet, 1:779, 1968.
30. Weiss, H. J., Aledort, L. M., and Kochwa, S.: J. Clin. Invest., 47:2169, 1968.
31. Borchgrevink, C. F.: Acta Med. Scand., 168:157, 1960.
32. Beaumont, J. L., Willie, A., and Lenegre, J.: Bull. Soc. Med. Hop. Paris, 71:1077, 1955.
33. O'Brien, J. R.: Br. J. Haemat., 17:610, 1969.
34. Doery, J. C., Hirsh, J., and de Grouchy, E. C.: Science, 165:65, 1968.
35. Reuter, S. H., and Montgomery, W. W.: Arch. Otolaryng. (Chicago), 80:214, 1964.
36. Mielke, C. H., Jr., and Britten, A. F.: N. Engl. J. Med., 282:1270, 1970.
37. Lackner, H., and Hunt, V. E.: Am. J. Med. Sci., 256:368, 1969.

22

Resective Periodontal Surgery in Pocket Elimination

22

Resective Periodontal Surgery in Pocket Elimination

Resective periodontal surgery is, as its name implies, the creation of a morphologically normal periodontium at the expense of the remaining tissue. This tissue may be within normal limits at the time of surgery. In fact, most presurgical procedures are directed toward achieving in the periodontal tissues a state as close to normal as possible. The form and relationships of these tissues, however, make them prone to breakdown and to the development of periodontal lesions. Reshaping them offers an expedient to more efficient and effective maintenance by both the patient and the periodontist.

The objectives are obviously to improve morphology, and to evaluate methods one must weigh the objectives against the permanence of the expected results. Long-term pocket elimination is the goal, either by gingivectomy or osseous resection. The names of the procedures are derived from the tissues to be resected.

STANDARD GINGIVECTOMY

Gingivectomy is essentially an excision of gingiva. The earliest attempts at gingivectomy were made to eliminate persistent refractory sulcular depth and represented, perhaps, the first expression of the importance of restoring normal contour to the gingiva. The objective of its successful performance was pocket elimination. Gingivectomy was the first excursion into periodontal surgery to attain almost universal acceptance. Since the procedure of A. W. Ward in this country,[66] there have been several methods for eliminating pockets, all of which were rather elaborate approaches to an essentially simple operation. Today, the Black procedure is most prevalently used, probably because it is the simplest and most direct method with the fewest flourishes.[5] Those who are interested in some of the older approaches to gingivectomy should read descriptions of the Ward, Crane-Kaplan, and Kirkland procedures.[10,29,66]

The Black Procedure

After presurgical curettage has been completed, and the gingivae no longer reveal gross signs of inflammation and edema, the operative site is carefully probed to establish the degree of pocket depth. Using the same probe, the pocket depth is measured on the outside, and a series of bleeding points are made on the surface of the gingiva to reflect the depth and dimension of the pockets in the area to be treated (Fig. 22-1).

In essence, the operation consists of making an incision along the bleeding points, using them as a guide, and the subsequent excision and removal of the gingiva

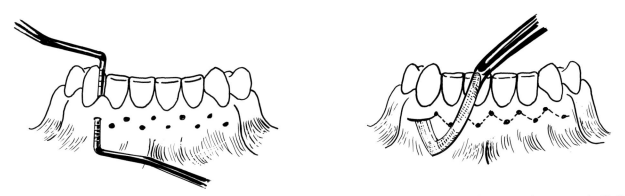

FIG. 22-1. *The Black procedure for gingivectomy. The depth on the facial and lingual surfaces of the gingiva is measured with the probe after it was used for measuring pocket depth. The bleeding points serve as a guide for incision.*

forming the outer wall of the pocket (Fig. 22-2). There are a number of other conditions, however, that must be met:

1. The initial traverse of the scalpel must be firm and controlled, so that repeated incision is not necessary. Failure to observe this precept frequently makes repeated passages of the scalpel necessary, with resulting hashing of tissue, leaving tabs and remnants of gingiva that are difficult to remove because of their small size.

2. The mesial and distal ends of the incision should be blended into the adjacent gingiva where possible, so that a sharp demarcation in gingival level is avoided.

3. An external bevel is traditionally imparted to the incised edge of the remaining gingiva. This necessitates angling the scalpel, so that the incision *ends* at the bleeding points in the inner wall of the gingival pocket. It follows that the thicker the gingival wall, the steeper is the required bevel. An extremely thin gingival wall requires little or no bevel, but, on the palatal aspect of an involved area where the gingiva is thick, it is occasionally difficult to achieve the required degree of beveling. There are ways to overcome this: for instance, if beveling cannot be made by incision because of a low palate, it can sometimes be made by scraping and by rotary abrasives on the thick gingival ledge of the palatal tissue (Fig. 22-3).

4. A pair of spear-shaped knives (right and left) are particularly useful in the performance of standard gingivectomy in severing the interproximal tissue clearly and completely. Interproximal tabs leave ragged edges and poor operative habits of this kind should not be encouraged.

5. If all incisions through the tissues are bold and definitive, removal of the excised gingiva should be quite easy. It is, however, no exaggeration to state that more time is spent in removal of tissue and in tidying the area than in all the other steps combined. Much of

the difficulty can be by-passed by avoiding indecisive hashing incisions.

6. After the gingivectomy has been completed and bleeding is controlled, a dressing, consisting usually of a medicated cement, is applied. Various types of dressing, are available, each having its own special virtue. These will be considered separately. In applying any dressing, a mass of cement adequate to cover the incised area is used. Commonly the total amount is divided into (1) rather large pellets, sufficient to fill each interproximal embrasure in the surgical field completely, and (2) two rolls, long enough to provide the buccal and lingual flanges for the area requiring protection. The pellets are inserted into the interproximal embrasures throughout the extent of the gingivectomy. The rolls of dressing are then placed on the buccal and lingual surfaces of the incision and pressed into proper form. The interproximal wedges serve to lock the dressing into place, since it will not adhere to the underlying tissue. Only the necks of the teeth should be covered with cement; overextension should be avoided both apically and occlusally. Care should be taken not to extend the pack over the occlusal surface or incisal edges, since it will fracture on setting if the patient bites on it. In addition, patients should be cautioned not to drink hot fluids for about 3 hours after surgery until the final set of cement occurs.

Generally speaking, the smaller and thinner the dressing, the more comfortable it is, and muscle trimming and smoothing can be done, at least on the buccal side, by lip and cheek manipulation. The tongue helps on the lingual side especially in avoiding overextension. An overextended dressing causes pain to the tissue upon which it impinges. The ordinary cement dressing may be left in place for from 5 to 7 days. More often it needs no replacement, since healing progresses more rapidly after the initial period of protection with no artificial aids.

7. A precaution to keep constantly in mind is that the standard gingivectomy must be confined to the

gingiva. The alveolar mucosa will not readily adapt itself to become marginal tissue. When it is forced to assume a role for which it is unsuited, it responds by retraction and usually manifests a thick, rolled margin which is fragile and hyperemic.

The Periodontal Cement Dressing

A number of periodontal cements and dressings are available, each with certain advantages and disadvantages. It must be stated at the outset that no pack, regardless of ingredients, promotes healing. Originally, the only purpose for the postgingivectomy pack was to protect the rather broad incised surfaces on the gingiva from oral irritants. Since flaps have become so common, the pack has been used as a stent in flap control rather than as a protective device.

The basic pack was a zinc oxide-eugenol cement with certain additives incorporated for their special properties.

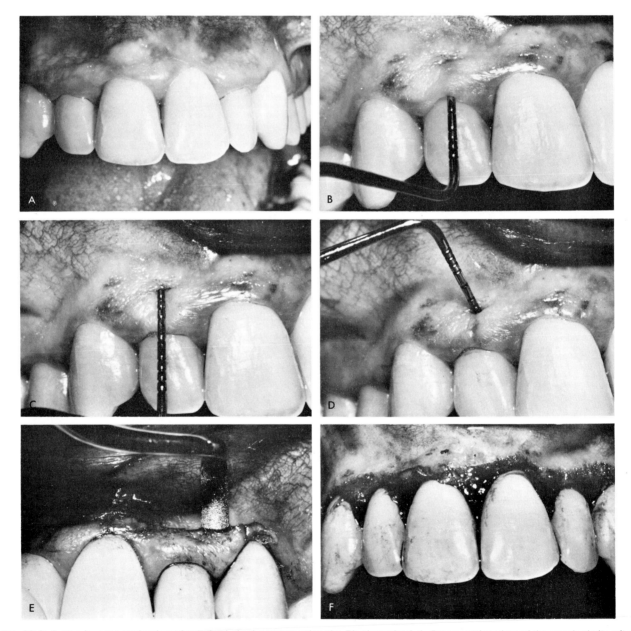

Fig. 22-2. A step-by-step projection of standard gingivectomy using the Black method. A. Preoperative view of the surgical site after curettage. B. Measuring the depth of the sulcus. C. Establishing sulcular depth on the labial surface of the gingiva. D. Puncturing the gingiva at the base of the sulcus to delineate the deepest point of detachment. When the entire operative site interproximally, labially and lingually has been outlined with these bleeding points, the area is ready for incision. E. Incision for making an external bevel using the bleeding points as a guide. F. After completion of the initial incision and with the tissue removed.

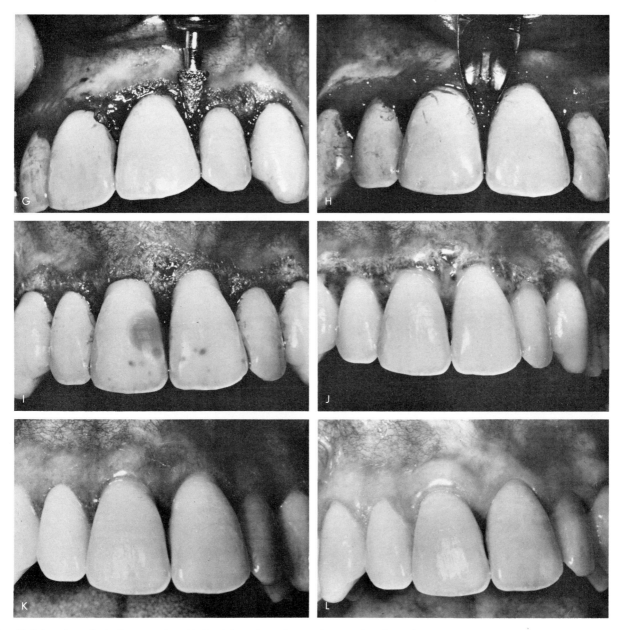

FIG. 22-2 (continued). *G. Refining the initial incision with a diamond rotary abrasive point. H. Removing the shreds of tissue from the surgical site with nippers. I. Immediate postoperative view of gingivectomy and gingivoplastic refinement. J. Seven days postoperative. K. Twenty-one days postoperative. L. Two-hundred-ten days postoperative. (Treated by Dr. R. Lamb.)*

There is no definitive data on the superiority of one pack over another except patient comfort, ease of removal, and similar characteristics.

THE KIRKLAND FORMULA

Powder: | Zinc oxide | 150.0 gm |
| Tannic acid | 14.0 gm |
| Powdered rosin | 198.5 gm |

Liquid: | Lump rosin | 70.0 gm |
| Sweet almond oil | 29.5 cc |
| Eugenol | 59.0 cc |

Sig. Melt the lump rosin in the eugenol and add to the sweet almond oil. Mix powder to a thick puttylike consistency and apply.

This basic pack has been extensively modified by the addition of asbestos fibers or cotton fibers in small amounts to minimize fracture of the cement during the 5 to 7 days it is in place. The liquid was modified by the substitution of peanut oil or olive oil for the sweet almond oil. Antibiotic properties were added by the incorporation of traces of bacitracin and/or polymyxin powder to the cement powder. There are other variations, too, for commercial purposes.

THE BAER FORMULA

Powder:

Rosin	0.52 gm
Zinc oxide	0.41 gm
Bacitracin	3,000 U

Liquid:

Zinc oxide	5%	of the amount
Hydrogenated fat	95%	necessary to make a mix of puttylike consistency.

This pack sets to a rubbery consistency.

THE COE PAK FORMULA

Tube 1   Metallic oxides
          Bithionol (Lorothidol)

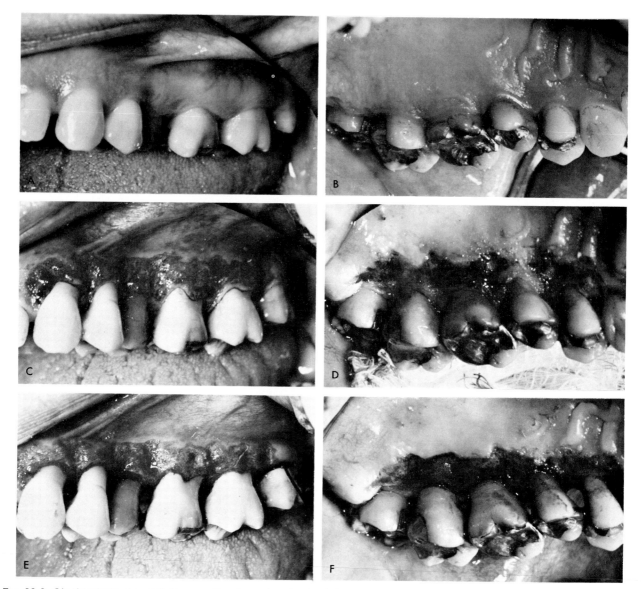

FIG. 22-3. Gingivoplasty. A and B. Preoperative, buccal and palatal views. C and D. Immediately after incision, buccal and palatal views. E and F. After rotary abrasion, buccal and palatal views.

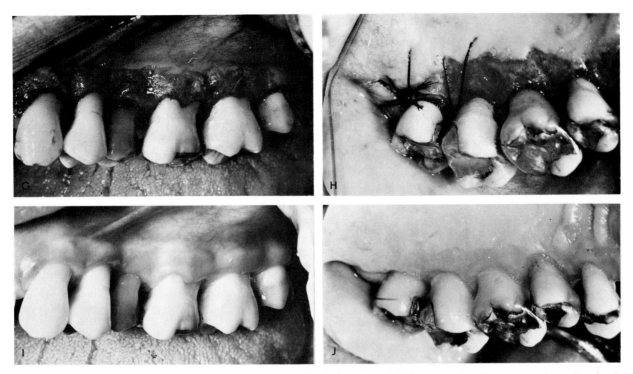

FIG. 22-3 (continued). *G and H. Postoperative, buccal and palatal views. I and J. Seven weeks after surgery, buccal and palatal views. (Treated by Dr. H. Selipsky.)*

Tube 2 Nonionizing carboxylic acids
Chlorothymol

Sig. Mix about 1 to 2 inches of tube 1 and tube 2 to proper rubbery consistency and apply. This pack is not always consistent in its behavior. It varies somewhat from batch to batch but is well received by both patients and periodontists because of its ease of removal.

N-BUTYL CYANOACRYLATE

N-butyl cyanoacrylate is a liquid not yet released for standard professional use by the Food and Drug Administration. It sets on contact with tissue. Clinicians who have access to this agent find it most useful in flap control in concave zones such as furcal area fluting. No deleterious results have as yet been reported except for an occasional excessive amount of exuberant granulomatous tissue.

INTERNAL-BEVEL GINGIVECTOMY

There are a number of clinical conditions for which standard gingivectomy is uncomfortable for the patient in spite of its relative simplicity. It was therefore inevitable that some refinement would be introduced. Internal, or inverse-bevel gingivectomy, is just such an improvement. The excision of redundant gingiva is essentially the same with the important exception that little or no raw gingival surface is exposed. This is accomplished by an internal bevel—the opposite of the long-exposed bevel used in standard gingivectomy.

Technique for Internal-Bevel Gingivectomy

The internal-bevel gingivectomy is somewhat more difficult than is the standard method because of the necessity to project precisely the margin of the incised bevels, particularly on the crestal aspect where it will coincide precisely with the crestal margin of bone. It consists essentially of incision and the reflection of flaps. Since at least one surface is immovable, in the context of the operation, incisions on the palatal side must be precise and the margin must be outlined in the initial cut.

There are two general approaches to achieving this requirement on the palatal surface: (1) the so-called ledge-and-wedge approach and (2) a freehand initial cut that establishes the bevel and the margin. It should be clear that the other surfaces of the gingiva (other than palatal) are not incised in the same manner when using either of these approaches, for the simple reason that with a flap reflection the flap on the facial and lower lingual becomes freely movable and can be precisely placed marginally. With palatal mucosa, for which this internal-bevel technique is used quite often, there is no need to conserve gingiva and the remaining tissue is apically fixed.

On the palatal side, both the ledge-and-wedge approach and the freehand incision method offer two choices: (1) a carefully scribed palatal mucosal margin cut to the bone margin with a scalloped edge simulating papillae and (2) a straight line incision to the crestal bone margin. In both, the flap is thinned as a part of its reflection. Most practicing periodontists use the straight or undulating line palatal incision, since it is more expeditiously done and suffers no great disad-

vantage in healing when compared with the scribed scalloped palatal margin. The patient does not seem to suffer either pain or delayed healing when the straight or undulating line incision is used. For the buccal flap, which is easily scribed, the straight line incision is never used.

The ledge-and-wedge approach is simplicity itself (Fig. 22-4). Pocket depth is delineated with bleeding points in the same manner as is done in standard gingivectomy. A horizontal gingivectomy is then performed throughout the field. This results in a blunt thick ledge of palatal tissue. It should be mentioned that the ledge incision is made to follow dental con-

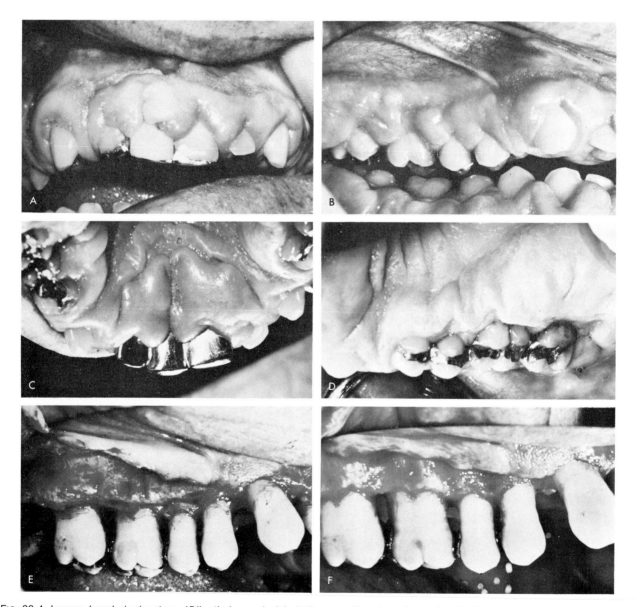

FIG. 22-4. *Inverse bevel gingivectomy (Dilantin hyperplasia). A. Preoperative view of anterior gingiva. B. Preoperative buccal view. C. Preoperative anterior palatal view. D. Preoperative posterior palatal view. E. Internal-bevel gingivectomy, buccal flap thinned and reflected. F. After osseous reshaping.*

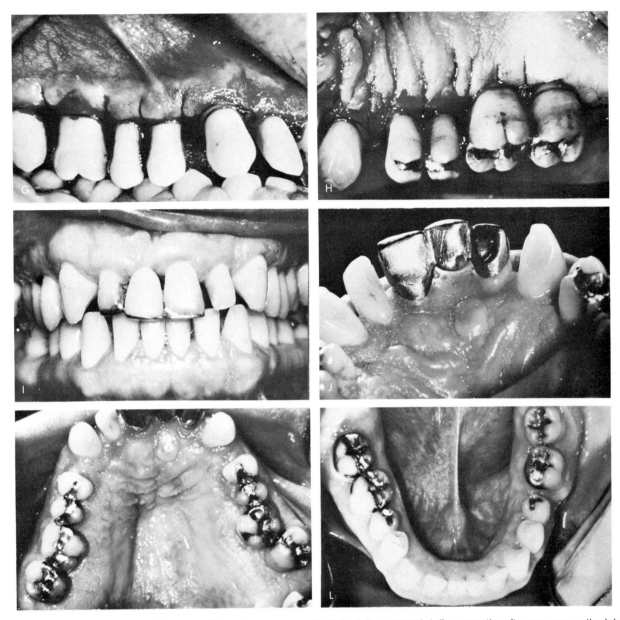

Fig. 22-4 (continued). *G. Buccal flap repositioned and sutured. H. Palatal flap sutured. I. Four months after surgery on the labial aspect of the upper anterior teeth. J. Four months after surgery on the palatal aspect of the anterior teeth. K. Panoramic view of the upper arch 4 months after surgery. L. Panoramic view of the lower arch 4 months after surgery. (Treated by Dr. S. Sapkos.)*

tour, with newly created papillae. It is, however, thick everywhere. Next, a #15 or a #12B Bard Parker blade is used to excise a wedge of tissue marginally, by cutting the internal bevel and thinning the palatal ledge. This is the classic internal-bevel gingivectomy, since no flap is retracted.

A similar procedure without the ledge and wedge can be used on the buccal gingiva, which is thinned and beveled internally in the same way, without the reflection of a flap if it is not indicated. Interrupted sutures or continuous sling sutures are then used for the final snug approximation. Many therapists do not apply

a dressing after the sutures are placed, since it is not needed in either wound protection or flap control.

In the second, or freehand, internal-bevel gingivectomy, the incision is made in the palatal tissue after the bleeding points have been made delineating pocket depth throughout the field (Fig. 22-5). Using the bleeding points as a guide and with a Bard Parker #15 blade, the operator creates the marginal incision and bevel, with a careful stroke and a deliberate, controlled, sawing motion. The scalpel is directed at such an angle as to create a rather steep bevel. The incision is repeated, this time using a smooth stroke and made

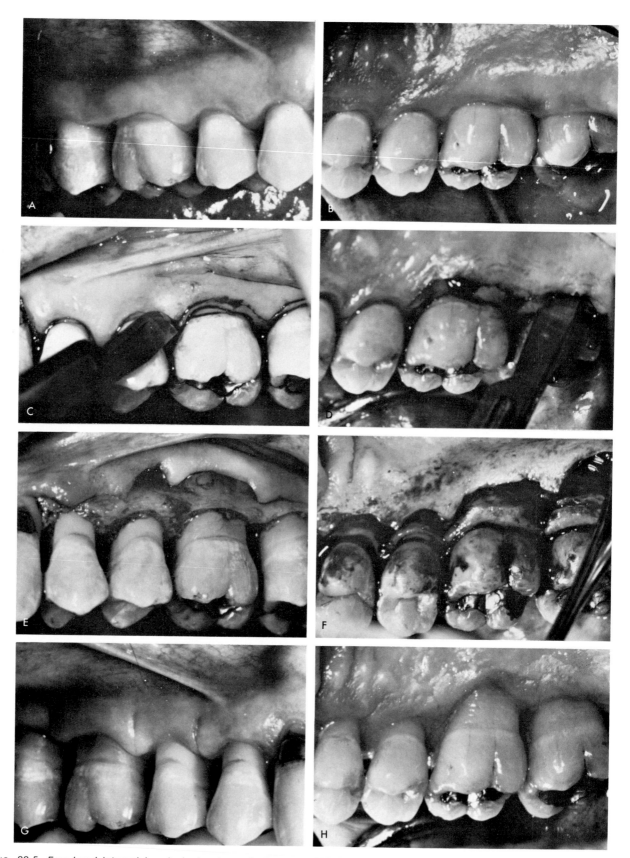

FIG. 22-5. *Free-hand internal bevel gingivectomy. A. Preoperative view, buccal aspect. B. Preoperative view, palatal aspect. C. Primary buccal incision. D. Primary palatal incision. E. Buccal flap reflection. F. Palatal flap reflection. G. Buccal view 2 weeks after surgery. H. Palatal view 3 weeks after surgery.*

firmly to reach bone everywhere, so that the marginal tissue may be cleanly removed with a minimum of tags. Interproximal areas are especially vulnerable to careless incising technique.

It might be inferred that the second method is more expeditiously made by more experienced operators. This is true. Some prior experience with the ledge-and-wedge technique is most helpful in the quicker, more direct method of incision. Two considerations should be kept in mind.

1. The thicker the tissue incised, the longer will be the bevel. Caution should be used when incising palatal gingiva. This is an area commonly treated with an internal bevel in both gingivectomy and flap retraction. Because of the presence of a number of small branches of the palatine artery, which come off the principal branch vertically along the lateral border of the palate, severing these branches is common. Bleeding from these vessels can be troublesome.

2. When incising an internal bevel, there is a tendency to make that incision almost vertical so that the remaining tissue has a long and extremely thin bevel. This confers two apparent advantages in flap handling: (1) the long and thin margin is easily adapted to the cervical margins of the wound, and (2) immediate postoperative form is apparently superior to what would be the case in a somewhat blunter bevel.

Both these advantages are more apparent than real. In the first place, it is an error to consider that, since the surface of the flap consists of mature keratinized tissue, marginal necrosis of the flap would be minimal. The thinner the flap at the expense of the lamina propria, the greater the marginal tissue loss through necrosis. The precision of the marginal flap control is illusory.

The handsome immediate postoperative appearance of the margin is transitory. The loss of proximal and marginal edges of the flap through necrosis of the flap edge leaves rather ugly gingival ledges and craters. Fortunately, these are temporary and respond well to stimulation and cleansing.

Management of Tuberosity and Retromolar Areas

Distal problems are solved in stride with the routine surgical management of the quadrant under treatment. Their somewhat special consideration is not to be construed as a separate excursion.

In the diagnosis and in the recording of pockets in the initial and reevaluative examinations, the therapist is sometimes in a quandary when measuring distal sulci of the distal teeth as to whether he is dealing with a pocket or a normal anatomic feature. In this connection, it might be helpful to reiterate that a pocket is not measured in terms of depth alone, but is judged essentially on its dynamic nature as a lesion in a state of active retrogression.

Simple recorded depth alone is not necessarily a sign of disease in these distal zones. In fact, when a distal tooth requiring a large restoration is needed for an abutment tooth, the clinical crown is often surgically extended by tuberosity reduction in order to permit preparation and proper finishing. In distal zones, it is not unusual, however, to find anatomic configurations that are clearly pathologic and encourage tissue pileup. Bone resorption, exuberant tissue proliferation, and copious bleeding on probing are signs that should alert the operator to the need for correction.

Another factor to keep in mind is that the distal areas, both tuberosity and retromolar pad, are commonly incised mesiodistally along the crest of the ridge to provide good reflection for flaps anterior to them, and without reduction necessarily in mind. Long experience proves that these crestal incisions, as releasing incisions, are more satisfactory by far than are vertical or sloping incisions for retraction. Bleeding problems are common in these areas with vertical or sloping incisions. They are far less frequent with crestal incisions for retraction.

There is a distinct temptation to empty the tuberosity and retromolar areas that require incision. The tuberosity particularly is commonly reduced. It is composed, just under a thin covering of mucosa, of dense, white, tough collagenous tissue. Under its mucosa the retromolar pad consists of loose tissue and is not nearly as discrete as is the tuberosity. Also, it has a strong tendency to return to its original level after surgery. The tuberosity remains quite flat after surgery properly performed.

Reduction of both areas is achieved by essentially similar procedures. With the tuberosity reduction, the hard mass of tissue is usually removed with part of the palatal wedge, since the tissue is contiguous and similar in texture. There are several good methods.

TECHNIQUE FOR TUBEROSITY REDUCTION

Two nearly parallel crestal incisions in a mesiodistal direction are made on the crestal surface of the tuberosity, about 2 mm apart and converging at the distal end (Fig. 22-6). Care should be taken not to end the distal ends of the incisions too soon. They should just traverse the bulge of the tuberosity. The incisions need not be deep, since the covering mucosa here is rather thin. The mucosa is carefully resected away from the tough collagenous mass under it, and the first reflection

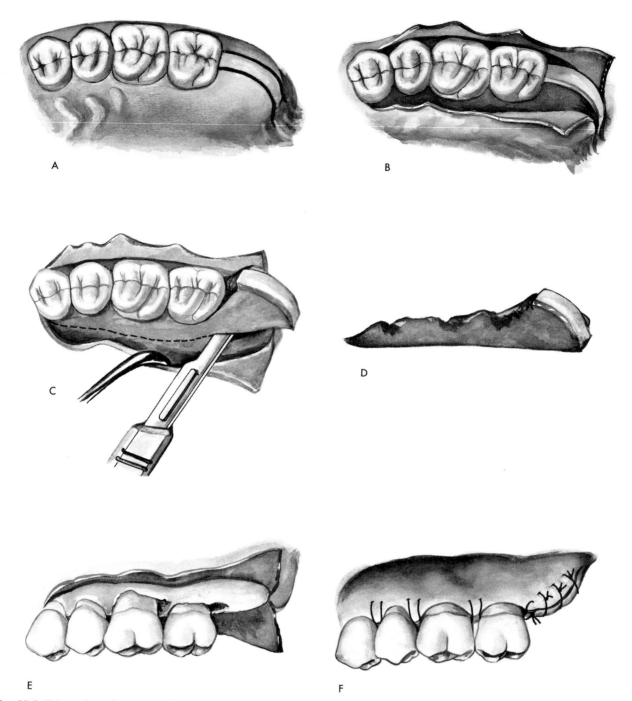

FIG. 22-6. *Tuberosity reduction. A. Initial incisions, delineating one approach to tuberosity reduction. B. Flap reflection. C. Removal of incised connective tissue attached to bone and root. D. Soft tissue, including the tuberosity removed from palate. E. Surgical field debrided of soft tissue. F. Replaced flap with a horizontal mattress sutures.*

is blended into the buccal inverse bevel of the buccal flap.

The palatal aspect of the tuberosity is similarly exposed by careful resection, blending the flap into that of the palatal surgical field (Fig. 22-7). This exposes the tough, white collagenous inner mass of the tuberosity, leaving the narrow longitudinal strip of mucosa in the center intact. Careful resection is performed throughout its entire extent, taking particular care to free any attachment distal to the distal tooth. The large mass may be grasped with tissue forceps for better resection. Many operators extend the resection of the tuberosity mass into the palatal wedge, since the tissues are somewhat similar.

Complete removal of the soft tissue of the tuberosity should expose the bony base. Careful inspection will reveal whether bone correction is necessary. Resorptive lesions on the distal aspects of the distal teeth are certainly not uncommon and, when present, should be leveled, if feasible. What may escape the notice of the inexperienced operator is the broad flat form that this area commonly assumes. Since the operation is performed with the prime objective of letting the distal tooth (usually the second molar) stand unencumbered by redundant gingiva, it will be found that reducing the broad bony table from the buccal and palatal surfaces will expedite the achievement of prominence for the molar with extremely shallow sulci, since it will throw the distobuccal and distolingual line angles into prominence.

A good part of the postoperative result will depend upon closure of the operative site. The removal of the large mass of submucosal tissue from the tuberosity region leaves an empty sac of mucosa, the sides of which are continuous with the buccal and lingual flaps of the quadrant being operated upon. It will be found that trial closure will reveal redundant mucosa that would overlap unless it is trimmed to a good fit. In

addition, it will frequently be found that it is advantageous to make short vertical incisions of perhaps 3 mm from the margin of the flap, precisely at the distobuccal and distolingual line angles of the distal molar. When the tuberosity flap is properly sutured, these little vertical incisions permit the mucosa to sit flat and snug on the bony base and against the distal surface of the molar. There is no gaping of the flap around the distal corners of the molar because of poor fit.

Care must be taken on closure not to displace the entire flap distally, because it will compromise the accurate positioning of the carefully incised papillae throughout the quadrant being treated. The little vertical incisions help here, too, in orienting the sutures accurately for closure.

Many operators prefer to use the interrupted suture in the tuberosity area if more than a single pair of sutures is required. On the whole, this type of suture works well. Usually two or three sutures are enough to close the area. Some therapists, on the other hand, choose a figure-8 closing suture, because they feel that the cross-lacing effect holds down the incised margins somewhat flatter.

The retromolar pad is reduced in much the same

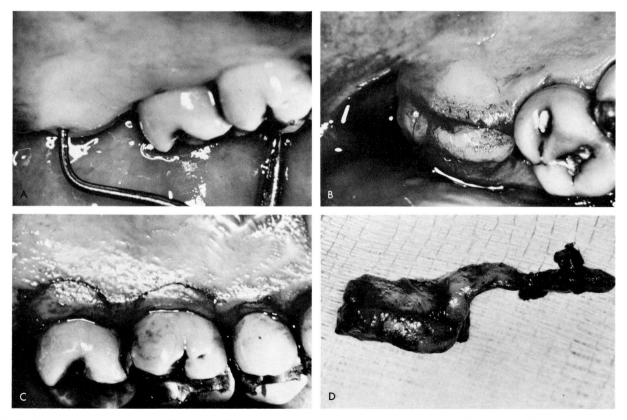

FIG. 22-7. *Tuberosity reduction. A. Sounding with a periodontal probe into the tuberosity to establish the level of underlying bone. B. Two parallel incisions extending back over the curve of the tuberosity. C. Palatal ledge and wedge incisions. D. Tuberosity contents removed together with the palatal wedge.*

way except that the quality of the submucosal content of the pad is different. It is looser and more difficult to handle; also, its tendency to regenerate is somewhat greater. Suturing the lower pad area is exactly the same as for the upper tuberosity area.

Postoperative sequellae in both areas are remarkably mild. Closure by suture is so successful that the protective dressing is not required, although it is sometimes used as a stent.

Reduction of the tuberosity and retromolar pad constitutes merely an addendum to the internal-bevel gingivectomy, since it is a continuum of incision and suturing techniques. In many cases, the tuberosity and retromolar pad do not require reduction, but they are opened with a releasing incision to provide access to deeper structures.

Advantages of Internal-Bevel Gingivectomy

1. Obvious advantages in patient comfort are that the internal-bevel gingivectomy exposes no incised tissue after closure. This is particularly welcome on palatal tissue where the gingiva is thick (requiring a broad incision) and constitutes an area of active lingual participation in speech, eating, and simple curiosity because of its unfamiliar contour.
2. Superficial healing is quite rapid, so that dressings are required for relatively little time. In fact, many skilled periodontists dispense with a postoperative dressing altogether and achieve excellent healing and patient comfort.
3. Removable partial dentures and night guards may be used normally, with little interruption.

Disadvantages of Internal-Bevel Gingivectomy

As with every method, there are certain disadvantages to be weighed against the benefits expected. The internal-bevel gingivectomy is no exception.

1. During healing, the resultant trench created by the internal bevel must be eliminated by securely placing the incised tissue around the cervical areas of the teeth in the field. This is the so-called snug-up and requires much care and attention. Most often, the margin is secured by sutures and slings (note the section on flap placement and control in Chapter 21). On occasion, it is possible to eliminate the gaping margin with a dressing, but this method used alone is not reliable. In most cases, dressings are soft and yielding for a consid-

erable time after they are placed, and the displacement and distortion of the margin frequently occurs without being visible to the operator until the dressing is removed, revealing thick, ugly margins that stand well away from the necks of the roots. Aside from food entrapment and difficulty in maintenance, the thickened margin may require further reshaping by gingivoplasty.
2. The time and skill required for the performance of the internal-bevel gingivectomy is considerably more than for a simple external-bevel gingivectomy. The precise scribing of the flaps, suturing, and general flap control are all time-consuming.
3. Postoperative bleeding problems are more common than in simple gingivectomy. These, however, present no problem.

Dressings for the Internal-Bevel Gingivectomy

Dressings for the internal-bevel gingivectomy are of minimal importance, since no tissue protection is required and the dressing becomes merely an agency in flap adaptation. The flap is usually firmly established and fixed in place in up to 7 days. Most therapists remove the dressing after 7 days. Many achieve flap control by means of sutures alone and dispense with the dressing altogether when a stent is not required for repositioning.

It is obvious that, although the actual application of the dressing is a simple matter, the indications for its application are fraught with objectives and with the uses to which the dressing is to be put. For example, should the flap be a long one to be held firmly against the root of a tooth, it becomes plain that simple apposition is not enough. Some firm pressure constantly exerted upon the flap against the root is required. If properly applied, an acrylic premixed cement that will maintain pressure after it has set will achieve this end.

If, on the other hand, the flap is to be short and will have some appreciable marginal exposure, then the dressing is protective in the real sense of covering the exposed interproximal and marginal tissues. If sling sutures are to be placed, with some slack to allow for apical displacement, the cement pack aids the apical repositioning by exerting an apical push or stenting and reinforcing the limited displacement.

Postoperative Management

Postoperative management of internal-bevel gingivectomy is extremely short and simple. The comfort of the patient is the rule, so that there must be no exposed incised bevels to be tender to touch and to condiments. Sutures and dressings can be easily dispensed with after 7 or 10 days. Initial healing does not mean complete healing, but recovery at 10 days has progressed to the point that the tissues require no special protection.

In postoperative follow-up, the relatively inexperienced operator is likely to experience some disappointment with the form of the tissues as healing progresses. It must be remembered that all internally beveled flaps with flap margins ending in a feather edge have some marginal necrosis where the tissue is too thin to survive. Because of this common phenomenon, the gingival margins appear thick, interproximal gingival craters are revealed where none existed preoperatively, and both show new granulation tissue emanating as cervical collaring from the periodontal space. These double contours do not persist long. They yield to maintenance and stimulation, so that in 4 or 5 weeks the new marginal tissue blends with the old to make a pleasing normal contour. Should they fail to heal properly, simple gingivoplasty that can be performed in a few minutes corrects marginal discrepancies. Many periodontists routinely perform these corrective gingivoplasties 2 weeks postoperatively.

Some periodontal surgeons avoid or minimize marginal necrosis by making a horizontal cut of approximately 1 mm before beginning the internal beveling incision. This procedure avoids the feather edge margins of the flap and tends to minimize marginal necrosis.

Flap Adaptation

Postoperative gingival craters and aberrant contours can be minimized if meticulous care is taken with the initial incision. Firstly, the cervical contour of the roots must be precisely scribed, if this method is used, so that the fit is accurate, with no gaping spaces for granulation tissue to proliferate. Secondly, the gingiva must be skillfully thinned internally so that control is easily attainable. Thirdly, suturing must be carefully done to achieve precise apposition. When an incision for reduction of a tuberosity or retromolar pad is first closed, there is a tendency to suture the incision so tightly as to displace the entire flap distally. This means that each carefully scribed papilla will be displaced distally just enough to make an accurate fit impossible, with resulting loss of the chance of a good postoperative course. This may be avoided by suturing distal areas last after papillary fit in the whole field has been insured.

Periodontists who do not scribe palatal flaps do not avoid the necessity to establish good tissue adaptation. The same care in suturing is required to avoid blanch-ing around sutures, to ensure a snug closure in a flat, stable flap, and to make certain that no dressing impinges under the flap. One of the most widely used dressings remains in a plastic state for several hours after placement, and its flow can invade through even a minor gaping of the flap. This commonly occurs and results in an ugly healing pattern. Although such a result is correctable, it is not good surgical practice to allow it to happen.

OPEN OR FLAP CURETTAGE
(The Modified Widman Procedure)

Flap curettage occupies an interesting position in periodontal methodology, lying as it does between curettage on the one side and resective techniques on another and having some slender connection with inductive methods on yet another aspect. Such a therapeutic approach does not lend itself to easy classification. Although it is basically related most intimately with subgingival curettage, it surely cannot be classified with initial therapy. It was decided, more for convenience than for logic, to discuss flap curettage with other surgical modalities because of its concern with flap design, flap adaptation, and flap control (Fig. 22-8).

The most active protagonist for flap curettage, or the modified Widman flap, as he calls it, is Ramfjord. In a recent publication with Nissle he describes in detail the "crestal cut," the "sulcus cut," and the standard internal-bevel incision. The internal-bevel incision is used on the palatal aspect to thin the flap as an aid to flap management.

The sulcus incision is commonly used to provide a flap long enough to cover the field completely. Many operators find the crestal cut preferable to the sulcus cut in the presence of deep pockets. In the sulcus cut the scalpel drops into the recesses of the pocket, making flap release difficult. Retreat and reincision are then necessary.

Critical to the success of flap curettage are (1) careful and complete debridement and (2) flap adaptation and coaptation so that healing by the first intention occurs. Flap reflection is kept to a minimum apically, to provide access for curettage only. This is done to avoid possible bone resorption in wound healing which may occur under reflected flaps. Readaptation, then, is not too difficult, since displacement has been minimal (Fig. 22-9).

Debridement of the surgical field is done with knives when possible, and curettage is reserved for bony areas involved with the periodontal lesion. The bone in the pockets is curetted vigorously to remove all adhering

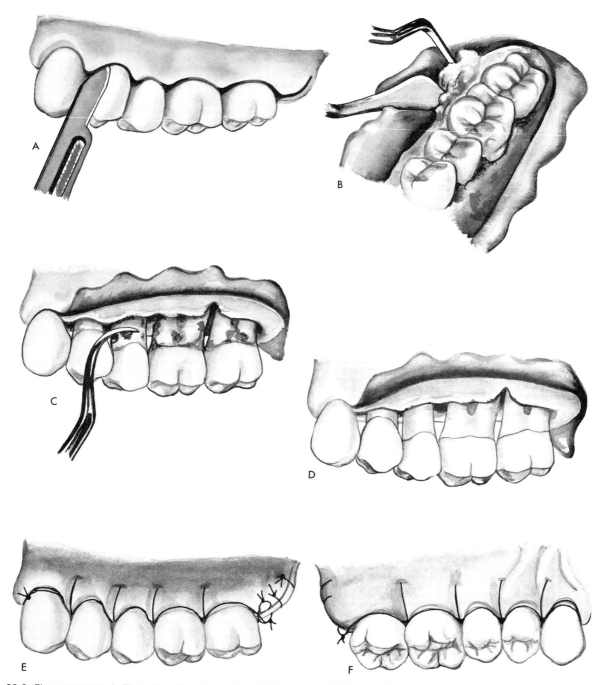

FIG. 22-8. *Flap curettage. A. The sulcus incision as the initial traverse. B. Thinning the palatal flap and tuberosity and removing the thick, fibrous lining tissue. C. Debriding the operative field of granulation tissue, calculus accretions on the roots, and generally tidying the area short of osseous resection. D. The debrided operative zone. E and F. Closure of buccal and palatal flap and tuberosity to the original gingival position. This is of some importance in this procedure because good approximation of the flap makes possible healing by first intention and in some cases pocket closure.*

soft tissue tabs. The root surface in the pocket is curetted to remove all accretions.

After the open curettage has been performed, the flaps are carefully readapted to the roots and bone and are stabilized with interrupted sutures throughout the operative field. Careful and precise flap stabilization

and suturing are required so that favorable healing takes place. If healing by first intention fails to occur, the chances for pocket elimination by a long epithelial attachment are sharply reduced. Great care is used in conserving as much of the flap as possible, since re-adaptation of the flap to its original position is desired.

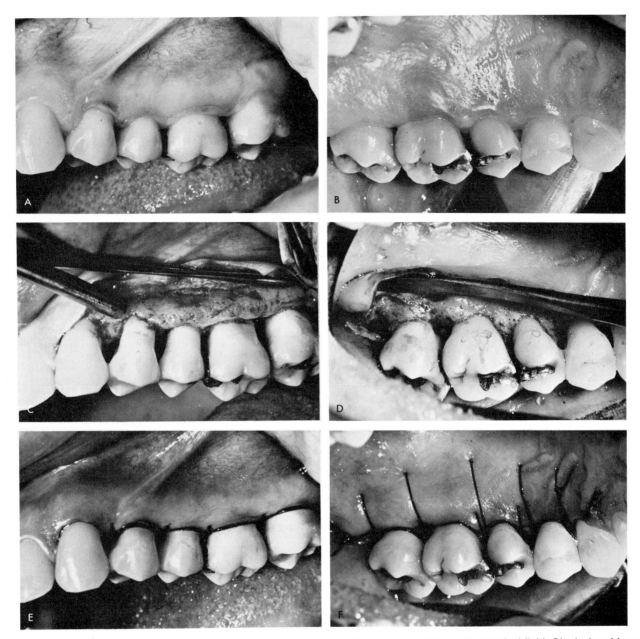

FIG. 22-9. *Flap curettage (the modified Widman procedure). A and B. Preoperative views of the surgical field. Gingival and bony craters can be probed. C and D. Flaps reflected and the area thoroughly debrided. Note the heavy ledges and interproximal crater-shaped resorptive patterns. E and F. Buccal and palatal views of suturing. Note that on the buccal side the suture engages the papilla near the tip so that it folds into the interproximal space precisely. In order to avoid tearing through the gingival papilla by the suture, the flap must be passive and should not require tension for control. On the palatal flap the vertical mattress is used to advantage.*

Even bone reduction was suggested by Widman to insure close flap coaptation. Preservation of the flap involves scribing the interproximal tissue into as long papillae as possible to make good approximation of buccal and palatal or lingual flaps with no intervening space interproximally (Fig. 22-10).

The reason for the attention to interdental tissue approximation is that reattachment to root surfaces is hoped for. Although not always forthcoming, it sometimes does occur either by a long epithelial attachment or by adhesion. For the most part, however, while flap curettage makes debridement of affected roots efficient and, in some cases possible, pocket elimination is not the usual reward for good flap curettage. When pockets are not eliminated, the postoperative course is the same as that for standard subgingival curettage.

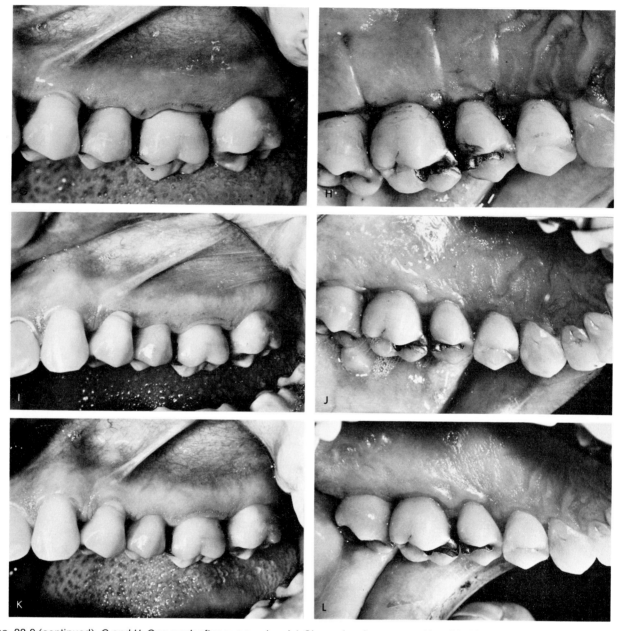

FIG. 22-9 (continued). *G and H. One week after surgery. I and J. Six weeks after surgery. K and L. Eighteen weeks after surgery. At this time careful probing reveals normal sulcular depth. Experience in long time lapses after therapy (one to several years) reveals regression in many cases to greater sulcular depth. The areas treated then become similar to those treated with definitive curettage. Reference is made to areas that do not undergo extensive gingival recession. (Treated by Dr. D. Smith.)*

Indications for Flap Curettage

In deep lesions for which resective techniques are not feasible, flap curettage is ideal. The entire approach is almost identical to that of definitive curettage. The same criteria apply, and in the opinion of the authors the same results are attained with the exception that open curettage conveys advantages in access and visibility not possible with closed curettage.

In a number of patients suffering from juvenile periodontitis, flap curettage has proved to be singularly successful. This is especially true in attaining root attachment or adhesion by the replaced flaps. Whether this is true because of the condition of the cementum on the roots in younger patients or is due to some other factor is not known.

The esthetic factor is definitely important in the anterior segments of the mouth. Many operators who use resective methods elsewhere to achieve pocket elimination use flaps in the anterior region for esthetic reasons and accept a deep sulcus postoperatively.

Contraindications for Flap Curettage

Flap curettage is not indicated, in the opinion of the authors, where resective methods can eliminate the deep sulcus to advantage. The question of pocket elimination versus the retention of deep sulci enters here once again. Accessibility for maintenance is still the rule.

OSSEOUS RESECTION

In the section on gingivectomy-gingivoplasty both long external-bevel (standard) and internal-bevel approaches have been described in conjunction with soft tissue excision. Bone management, where necessary, follows naturally in its wake.

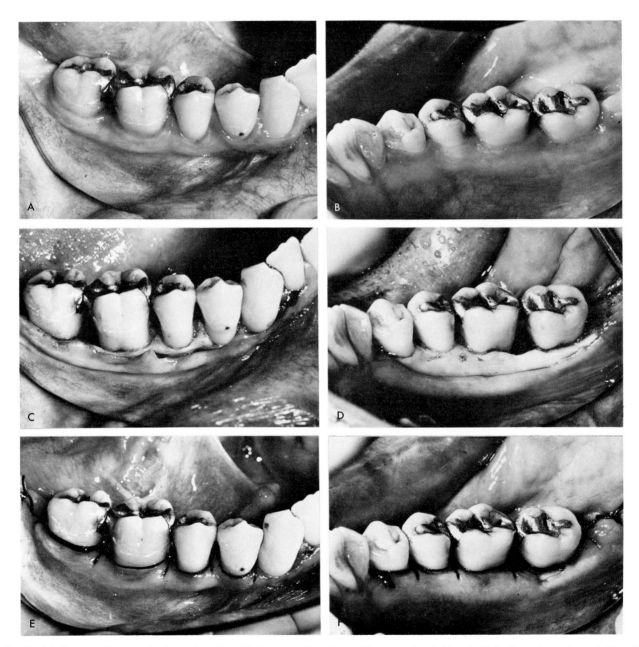

FIG. 22-10. *Flap curettage on the lower jaw. A and B. Preoperative views of the operative field on both the buccal and lingual sides. C and D. Flaps reflected on both the buccal and lingual sides. Note the deep crater interproximally between the first and second molars and the narrow hemiseptum on the distal of the first premolar. Neither of these aberrations is corrected. Only debridement is performed. E and F. Flap control and suturing after debridement. Note the close coaptation achieved.*

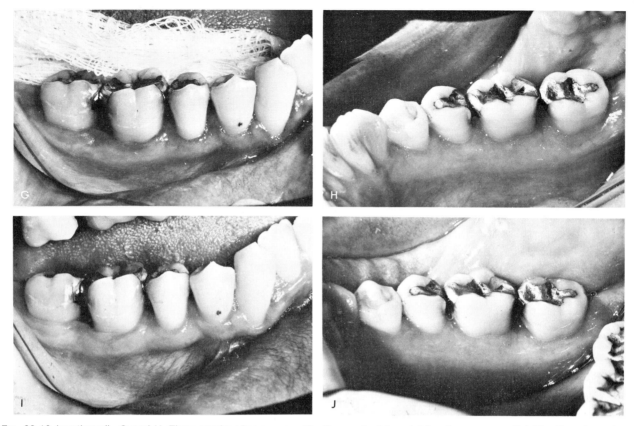

FIG. 22-10 (continued). *G and H. Three weeks after surgery. Healing up to this point has been uneventful. The flaps have been successfully coapted so that no interproximal necrosis of the tips of the papillae has occurred. I and J. Twelve weeks after surgery. Flap coaptation has been successful. The sulci can be probed only to normal dimension. The pockets seem to have been successfully closed. (Treated by Dr. D. Smith.)*

In reexamining the response of the tissues to inflammation on a gross clinical level the following observations can be made: (1) The usual response of gingiva to inflammation is enlargement because of edema. (2) The bone in proximity to inflammation resorbs.

The therapist is then confronted with a complex of soft and hard tissues which in health are adjacent to each other in space and are consistent with each other in form. In disease their behavior becomes disparate, gingiva enlarges, and bone resorbs. This inconsistency would be more easily managed if alveolar bone retreated in apical direction but maintained its basic outline. This, however, does not occur. Since most pockets and inflammation are found interproximally, most resorption occurs in this region. Bony architecture is then reversed in disease. Craters occur interproximally in significant numbers. Interproximal resorptive lesions and all possible variations are encountered. Thick ledges occur because of marginal resorption. Since the number of possible variants is endless, it is unrewarding to attempt a point-by-point description of correction of specific lesions. Aberrant architecture as an etiologic factor in periodontal disease is almost as common as aberrant architecture as a result of periodontal disease. Broad general principles of correction can easily be adapted to specific problems.

In the surgical management of periodontal disease, the overriding considerations are lesion form and tissue consistency. Stated differently, one pocket is pathologically much like any other, no matter what its topography or form. The only reason for the introduction of the several techniques for pocket elimination is that pockets vary in form and that the pathologic changes in the supporting tissues are progressive, causing a change in consistency. Of these two factors, form is the more easily overlooked and is usually ignored in standard treatment, however sophisticated. A few observations on form are given here which, it is hoped, will illustrate the spectrum of changes and aid in varying the technique to fit the case.

Since the only way in which the periodontist can treat the inflammatory lesion directly is by subgingival root and gingival curettage, periodontal surgery is designed to correct aberrations in form resulting from disease. Thus, it follows logically that tissue consistency and form assume considerable importance in any surgical approach. Surgical objectives have been described variously as plastic repair, or as the establishment of a selective recession or by other similar designations. It has been clear for some time that the morphologic approach is the only one that allows resective periodontal surgery to assume a rationale in the management of common lesions in the present state of the art.

Examination to Determine Lesion Form

The aging lesion with its accompanying process of fibrosis cannot be expected to respond to effective curettage with shrinkage. This fact has long been recognized and has been countered by the use of the gingivectomy-gingivoplasty which imposes shrinkage.

Bone has no simple pattern of response to periodontal disease. It is resorbed in the presence of inflammation. Interproximal craters, hemisepta, circumferential funnel-shaped patterns, and mushroom-shaped areas of resorption are commonly found by the therapist. It is for this reason that certain principles were enunciated in an effort to an orderly approach to this problem. The literature on the subject lays down certain principles for recognizing these forms and, though not complete, they are ample for the most part (Fig. 22-11).

One approach to the effect of periodontal disease on bone is to regard it from the standpoint of bone volume and configuration before the onset of disease and the predictability of the type and shape of the resorptive lesion that will result from periodontal destruction in a given region. The reason this approach may prove to be useful is that the response of bone to inflammation is well-documented and is characterized by resorption whenever an inflammatory infiltrate is present nearby. The presence of the invested root and its relationship to the volume and shape of bone surrounding it are, however, the determining factors in lesion form. It is obvious that the same type of infiltrate will, given two widely differing bone volumes and relationships, cause two lesions of distinctly different shapes. The involved root with a heavy volume of bone will give rise to a funnel-shaped resorption pattern, but that with a thin layer of bone over the root surface may, with the same involvement, result in a dehiscence.

Alveolar Bone Topography

Certain configurations of alveolar bone occur as anatomic norms. The presence of the root of a tooth in an alveolar socket presents no problem in health. In periodontal disease, however, normal anatomic features may create difficulties in soft-tissue recontouring. Several examples come to mind (Fig. 22-12).

THE INTERPROXIMAL BONY CRATER

Possibly the most ubiquitous of all resorptive bone lesions are interproximal bony craters. These are saucer-shaped depressions, and their common occurrence is due to the anatomic arrangement of the circulation relative to bone mass (Fig. 22-13).

Consider the bony septum between two adjacent molars. Examination of any number of skulls with normal bone topography will reveal that bone septa in the molar region are *flat* and are not peaks of bone such as found in the anterior region. Even the buccal and lingual marginal contours are relatively flat, although there is a gentle festoon to be seen at times.

The anatomy of the flat interproximal septum is further characterized buccolingually by a midplane lumen in the bone, which contains the vasculature serving the alveolus on either side and which continues through the crest of the bone septum and arborizes into capillaries to the interproximal gingival papilla. It is generally accepted that the patterns of pocket formation and the resultant bone resorption are due both to the resorption of bone in the proximity of inflammation and to the distribution of the blood vessels in the region (Fig. 22-12). A principally midplane distribution will result in midplane resorption.

When the papilla becomes inflamed, the infiltrate involves the capillary tree it contains. If inflammation extends at all, it will do so via the perivascular channel so that the crestal bone is resorbed in midplane. The transseptal ligament is no protection from deeper penetration because it is pierced by the lumen of the vasculature (Fig. 22-14).

With buccal and lingual plates affected to a far lesser degree, if at all, a saucer-shaped resorption results. Since the buccolingual dimension is far greater than is the mesiodistal one, a bone crater results.

BUCCAL AND LINGUAL RESORPTIONS

Buccally and lingually the bone and gingival configurations are different. There is no solid block of bone from buccal to lingual as exists interproximally. The roots of the teeth intervene. In addition, the blood supply is a different type, the area being served by a circulatory bed or vascular network instead of by a central complex of nutrient vessels.

For this reason, the pattern of resorption is a random one. Narrow deep penetrating lesions interradicularly and circumferential funnel-shaped or well-shaped le-

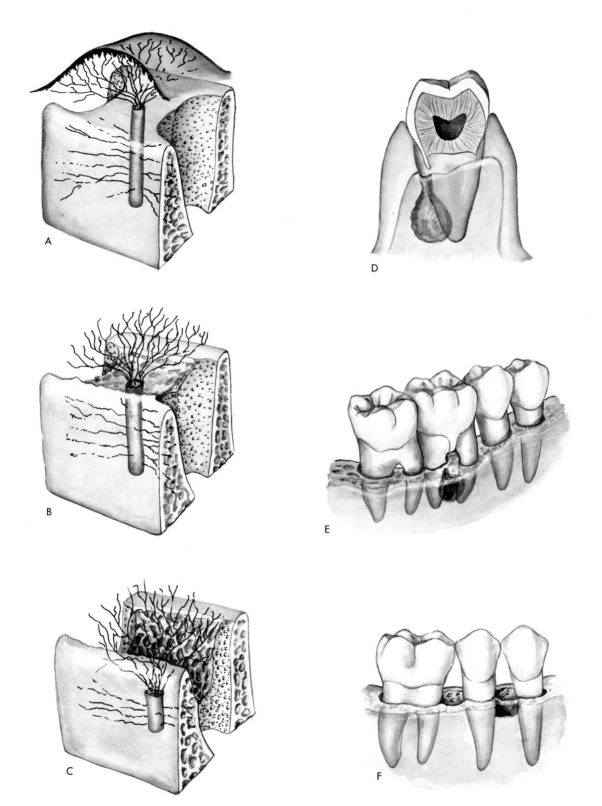

Fig. 22-11. *Lesion form. A. Schema of adjacent alveoli with the gingival papilla lying over the interproximal septum and with the interseptal blood supply represented as a single vessel lying within the lumen in the bone. B. In this drawing the interproximal papilla has been deleted. The proximity of the inflammatory elements to the capillary tree over the crest of the bone and within the perivascular channels within the bone septa enhances the resorptive lesion in midplane buccolingually, thus initiating the interproximal bony crater. C. A further extension of the resorptive lesion causing deeper midplane craters with less marginal resorption on the buccal or lingual edges. D. A cross-section schema of a common buccal resorptive lesion showing no predictable form because the vascular bed here has no sharply delimited circulatory channel as is the case interproximally. E. A lower segment showing a first molar with an enamel projection interradicularly initiating an enormous mushroom-shaped interradicular lesion. F. Interproximal bony craters with little or no marginal resorption.*

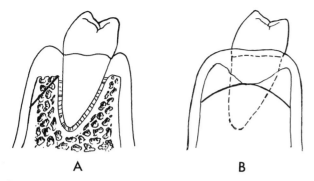

FIG. 22-12. *Bony craters and ledges. A. A thick ledge and its projected correction. B. An interproximal bone crater and its correction.*

sions are possible and commonly occur in these regions. The resorption still follows the pathway of inflammation, but that pathway is different.

Since no standard prototypical patient is possible, the variations are many. The pattern of resorption is clearly dependent on the mass of bone available in the region. If the root of the tooth is invested in a thin sleeve of bone—and this is by no means a rare occurrence when the alveolar process is slender or the roots large or both—thick ledges of bone marginally are not a factor. In fact, these areas are subject to gingival recession because the roots are often in dehiscence under the gingiva. This dehiscence is sometimes caused by marginal gingival inflammation which initiates the resorption that destroys the entire labial plate marginally over the root prominences.

In other anatomic contexts where there is a thick alveolar process and the same marginal inflammation on the buccal or lingual margins, the resultant pattern of resorption would very likely be a circumferential trench or well. This variable results from a single phenomenon. It will be noted in the drawing that the form of the gingiva gives no hint of what the bone form is beneath it.

Although our attention is directed to gingival behavior in general, it might be useful to note that in Figure 22-13 there is a difference between a cone-shaped septum in bone and a saddle area in a similar situation but with the roots separated.

Similarly, hemisepta also fail to be reflected in the gingival form (Fig. 22-13). Bone craters interproximally do not cause a loss in papillary height. A carefully examined problem area might prove revealing to the student.

Prichard in 1960 wrote of the common problems of a deep pocket and a resorptive lesion occurring on the mesial side of the lower canine tooth. The reason that these resorptions assume a deeply cratered form lies with the large labiolingual dimension of the canine and the much smaller size of the adjacent lateral incisor, plus the relative arrangement of these teeth, in addition to a low-contact point in many of them.

In many patients the canine is quite prominent labially relative to the lateral incisor. In fact, in a surprising number of such patients the lateral incisor and canine roots lie in close proximity because of slight malposition of the lateral incisor which may escape casual notice. The contact relationship between these teeth is frequently a long one and not effective as a contact should be. The interproximal anatomy is such that the sudden reduction in root volume from the canine to the lateral incisor is not reflected in the bone topography. Frequently a thick margin of bone is labial to the lateral incisor and may be adjacent to a thin one over the canine. This arrangement, coupled with the inefficient contact relationship, is most conducive to pocket formation. Because of the relative root proximity in this region, there is an extremely constricted mesiodistal dimension to the interproximal bone. This leads to deep craters in the interproximal bone with thin labial walls. These craters present a multiple problem in elimination: (1) they are usually quite deep, and leveling may require more bone reduction over the labial and lingual surfaces than the therapist is prepared to accept; (2) in most of these patients the incisors are relatively undamaged, and the operator is faced with an extreme disparity in bone levels in a constricted area; and (3) these bone craters must usually be leveled at the expense of the labial plate by ramping it only toward the labial side. The reason is that it is most difficult to achieve a selective recession on the concave curve presented by the lingual surfaces of teeth and alveolus of the area.

Because the location of the blood supply in the interproximal septa varies, there is a wide variation in the form and configuration of the septal walls. Ochsenbein has made a searching report and classification of form in bone craters of periodontal origin.

Another normal anatomic arrangement is found on the palatal margin of bone investing the upper second molar areas. It is common to find a flat shelflike bony excrescence extending from the mesial side of the second molar to the tuberosity. Lower molars commonly have the mylohyoid ridge on their lingual aspect. Both upper and lower molars are prone to funnel-shaped resorptive lesions in these areas.

There are, of course, buccal exostoses involved with pockets as well and, as a general rule, these are managed similarly. A torus and an exostosis are similar in that both are deviations from the norm. Later, when the thick margin is considered from the standpoint of therapy it makes little difference whether the aberration is natural or acquired. If pocket elimination is the

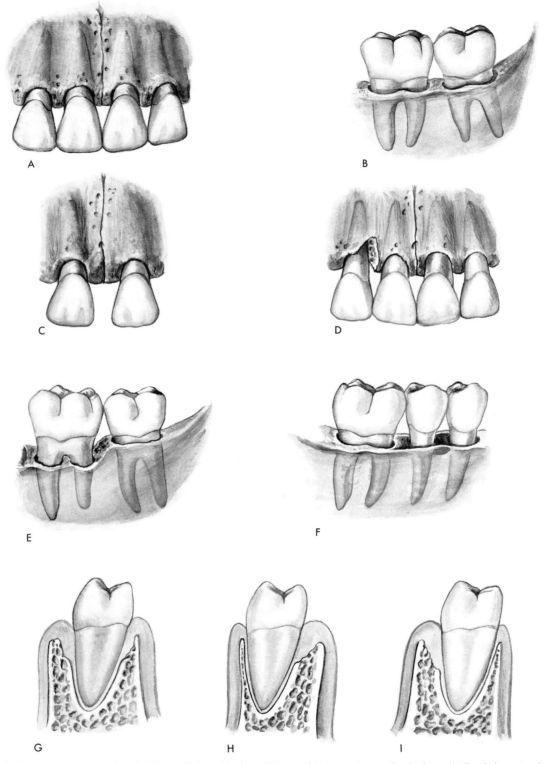

Fig. 22-13. *Some common responses in bone form to tooth position and to some resorptive lesions. A. Teeth in normal contact in periodontal health. The interproximal bone septa are pyramidal or cone-shaped. The overlying gingiva reflects this form. B. Normal posterior bone configuration. Note the flap contour in bone that is reflected in the covering gingiva. Buccal, lingual, and inter-proximal contours in gingiva are also flat. C. Periodontally healthy upper anterior incisors with wide diastema interproximally. Note the flat saddle area interproximally in place of the pyramidal or cone-shaped interproximal septum. The gingiva reflects this form in health. D. Chronic inflammatory periodontal disease on a line angle of an anterior tooth. The labial plate, being thin, has been completely eroded. The interproximal bone, being thicker, shows hemiseptal resorption. E. Hemiseptal resorption on a lower molar. The example illustrated has not been initiated by a cementoenamel junction (CEJ) discrepancy in adjacent teeth, but many hemisepta are related to CEJ discrepancies. F. Crater formation in bone interproximally caused by midplane inflammation buccolingually in a relatively broad alveolar process. G, H, and I. Three common resorptive lesions in bone. Both the bone and the overlying gingiva are shown in proper position. Note in G there is a broad alveolar process buccolingually and so a marginal inflammatory resorption adjacent to the tooth will create funnel-shaped or well-shaped resorptive lesions in bone. In H only the lingual process is broad enough for a well-shaped defect. Should the inflammatory resorption occur on the buccal side, it would create a dehiscence because of the complete destruction of the buccal plate. I shows the reverse situation.*

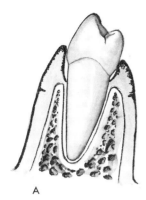

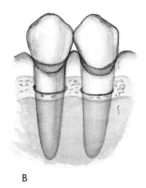

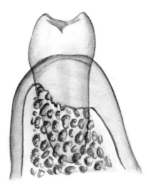

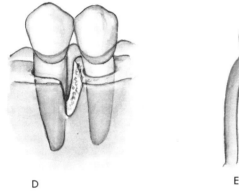

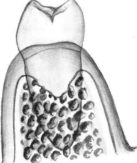

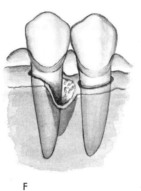

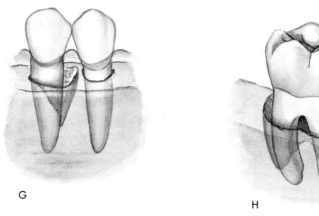

FIG. 22-14. *Some common anatomic and pathologic combinations in bone and gingiva in periodontal pocket formation. A. Gingival pocket due to gingival proliferation or incomplete eruption. B. Relative greater interproximal papillary height due to adjacent root proximity. The bone crest provides merely the baseline for the gingiva. It is for this reason that much pocket depth is due to papillary height. To lower the height it would be necessary to lower the baseline (which means removal of facial and lingual bone and not interproximal bone). C. A one-walled interproximal bony pocket with only the buccal or facial wall coronal to the epithelial attachment. D. A hemiseptal one-walled interproximal bony pocket. E. An interproximal bony crater. A common two-walled intrabony pocket with only a buccal or facial and lingual wall of bone. F. A combined lesion where the deeper recesses of the interproximal pocket are three-walled, but as the bone margin is approached the facial plate is partially resorbed making the crestal portion of the lesion two-walled (proximal and lingual walls only). G. A three-walled resorptive lesion in a single-rooted tooth. H. A three-walled lesion in a multirooted tooth, illustrating that each root may have an individual circumferential lesion. It is not rare to find a multirooted tooth with a single desperately involved root and the others practically normal. All intermediate invasions are possible.*

objective, certain basic requirements must be met in relation to the form of the tissues and their relationship to each other.

Areas of resorption of every possible variation in shape are also occasionally encountered on a single multirooted tooth. It is not rare to observe two completely disparate lesions on one tooth. For example, a rotated molar may reveal a dehiscence on a mesial root and a thick ledge showing a funnel-shaped resorptive pattern of the distal root. This is far from an uncommon finding.

The volume requirements for the interproximal crater are easily met, since the mass of bone is solid from buccal to lingual areas and the pattern of the inflammatory infiltrate is predictable. In the posterior interproximal zones, where the buccolingual contour of the bony crest is flat in health, a crater results rather quickly from an inflammatory infiltrate in midplane. Once the crestal cortical plate has been resorbed, formation of the bone crater is fairly rapid for a chronic lesion.

In the interproximal bony septa between the anterior teeth, on the other hand, the volume and configuration of the bone are different, as is the topographic arrangement. Here a peak is a frequent feature and results from several factors. Firstly, the labial and lingual marginal bone forms an arc of a shorter radius than is the case posteriorly. This alone is sufficient to establish a peaked interproximal septum. Secondly, the labiolingual dimension is much smaller than the posterior dimension. Volumes of both bone and invested root are much less, and the alveolar process is far thinner in the anterior region. This factor, too, contributes to the conical or pyramidal form of the anterior septa. With this form, the interproximal and labial and lingual resorptive patterns differ considerably from those found posteriorly. In the anterior region, craters are less frequent and dehiscences are not rare. This is not to say that the standard response is dehiscence and no crater. What is implied is that the therapist is frequently confronted with a different configuration in the anterior region than in the posterior.

It would appear that in some circumstances the resorptive process would correct itself, in a manner of speaking, in that the normal anatomic configuration would be preserved but at a more apical level. This is not a frequent finding. When it does occur, however, it is due to the slenderness of the bone in relation to the root volume and the distribution of bone available in root investment.

The bone lesions described here are not limited to the anterior region. Dehiscences and their thin bony veneers are found in the posterior region as well, and because of them the normal festooning may be exaggerated. Figure 22-13G,H,I, shows the persistence of normal looking gingiva in various bony configurations.

SOUNDING

Knowledge of the bone topography to be dealt with is useful before surgical entry is made. There are some important therapeutic procedural decisions to be made before surgical entry. Bone loss due to exposure has been mentioned earlier and will be more fully discussed. It is enough for our purposes here to make clear that it does occur. The buccal and lingual bony plates are of variable thickness, depending upon location. It may be assumed, however, that interproximal areas have relatively more bone and that on root prominences the bone coverage is relatively less. It is our aim to avoid needless flap reflection. Where the bone is too thin to allow further loss without permanent damage, it is logical to direct procedural acumen to the root prominences *before* flap reflection.

Even the most skilled therapist cannot see through tissue any better than can the merest neophyte. He can and does, however, assay the situation with a practical and practiced eye. He also uses some real aids in coming to a conclusion that it is safe to enter the area. This was discussed in Chapter 13.

Palpation of the area yields some general information, but such information is admittedly imprecise. Visual assay is also useful, but requires a large background of experience to evaluate it advantageously.

After the anesthetic has been administered, there is no good reason why a periodontal probe should not be inserted through the gingiva close to where the bony crest is thought to be and the margin of bone carefully sought out and delineated throughout its buccal contour over the root prominence. Such evidence is, of course, not conclusive. It is true that the thickness of marginal bone can be felt by skillful horizontal probing along the crestal margin after the initial insertion, but there is no assurance that what is being felt is only the isthmus of bone crestal to a fenestration; nevertheless, the value of immediate preoperative sounding should not be underestimated. It is a useful diagnostic method in determining the possible contingencies of reflection. Palpation, visual assay, and periodontal probing must be used to reinforce one another. What appears to be a thick buccal plate may in reality be an area of fibrotic gingiva.

Exposure of Bone

The inflammatory lesion is not the sole contingency with which the therapist deals. An inevitable price is paid for therapy in terms of bone resorption for other reasons. Whenever an area of bone is exposed, there is resorption of the cortical plate in the area of exposure. Although this has not been incontrovertibly established, it appears from extensive observation that just so long as the resorbed cortical plate is supported by marrow or cancellous bone, repair and reconstitution of the lost tissues ensues. If, on the other hand, the exposed bony veneer is too thin to contain a marrow bone reinforcement to the cortical plate, then the resorption, when and where it occurs, will not be reconstituted by new bone. These phenomena have been observed many times. It is rather obvious that the bone over the root prominences is thinnest, if it is there at all. It also follows that unreconstituted bone will result in dehiscence and fenestration. The dehiscence, particularly, will exaggerate the usual scalloped marginal curvature in the bone and leave the interproximal bone in a relatively extreme coronal position. This does not seem to be too difficult to maintain, if the gingiva is correctly formed.

What has not been definitely established is a quantitative factor in this phenomenon of bone resorption. The idea has been offered that the simple reflection of the mucoperiosteal flap is one of the basic causes of the resorption because of circulatory disruption. This can be corroborated from many sources.

It also becomes obvious that cortical plate resorption is a necessary precursor to the reinsertion of the attachment apparatus between gingiva and bone when any flap is replaced and allowed to heal. In other words, the therapist need not be disturbed about the resorption phenomenon. It is the repair of the resorption that is of definite concern. Certain important questions intrude here. Since the initial resorption process is set in motion by reflection of the flap, is it aggravated by long exposure of the bony plate? And in what way? By dehydration? By reshaping procedures? By the dressing? It can be seen that these questions are of great importance to periodontists, and the answers to them are of even greater importance.

Some of the work attendant upon answering these questions has been begun, but the burning need here is for a sophisticated approach supported by sound clinical research in a single team, and this combination is difficult to come by. One publication suggests that the resorption of the buccal and lingual spines of a crater and the leveling of that particular aberration is a more natural approach than is reshaping by bur, stone, or chisel. Correction by ventilation is an entirely novel approach. Obviously no help lies in this direction, since the method suggested is totally random and uncontrolled. We should, however, know how much and where bone is lost under varying procedures and for how long.

Applying a dry rubber wheel to bone (as has been done), or some other unusual tissue insult is of doubtful clinical value. There must be a concerted effort on the part of workers in the field to solve problems of bone exposure. This points up a need which is far from new—that of clinical research of a high order in periodontal surgery, certainly not only for the purpose of answering questions and meeting problems so that techniques can be standardized, although this is important, but rather to generate new questions and new problems on a more sophisticated and more knowledgeable level.

Several important points must be established at the outset. Since osseous resection (including osteoplasty and ostectomy) is an excisional technique, there is a limitation in the depth of the lesion that is conducive to reshaping. Only moderately deep resorptive lesions are practical material for osseous resection. For example, a deep bony resorptive lesion will require such an extreme amount of bone removal to produce a level or consistent bone contour as to remove critical support from adjacent teeth that may not be so seriously involved or which may not be involved at all. It is certainly conceivable that poorly planned and excessive bone removal can create a Class II tooth mobility. Surely this violates every precept of sound therapy. There are, of course, always exceptions, but generally only moderate bone resorption is prime material for ostectomy. Osteoplasty, on the other hand, is much more widely applicable.

Osteoplasty

Osteoplasty is a term introduced by Friedman in 1955 to describe the reshaping of bone in an effort to achieve more normal form without removing alveolar bone from the supporting apparatus of the root. It is analogous to the use and performance of gingivoplasty as distinct from gingivectomy in soft tissue management. Much of osseous resection is osteoplastic, in that it consists of the thinning of thick marginal ledges of bone and of establishing an undulating buccal contour by interradicular grooving (Fig. 22-15). The leveling of bony craters, the reduction of hemisepta, and the elimination of circumferential wells in bone sometimes require the cutting away of some supporting bone, but it is often mainly an osteoplastic procedure.

Osteoplasty and ostectomy are frequently combined in practice. When they are, the osteoplastic portion is usually performed with rotary instruments and the ostectomy with hand instruments.

Tori and exostoses constitute the classic aberrations when considerable quantities of bone are to be removed by osteoplasty. Techniques for the removal of

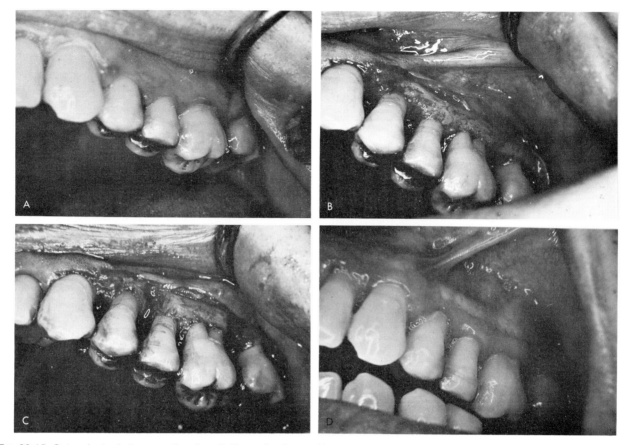

FIG. 22-15. *Osteoplasty. A. Preoperative view. B. Flap reflection and bone exposure. C. Recontouring of bone by osteoplasty. Little or no alveolar bone is removed. D. One year postoperative view.*

massive quantities of bone are described in the section on bone reshaping. Much easier is the standard removal of bone to achieve acceptably thin margins, flat septa, correctly shaped interfurcas and properly managed interproximal bone craters.

Ostectomy

Leveling bone profiles is one of the basic stages in pocket elimination. It is obvious that mucosa, both alveolar and masticatory, will always cover bone in healing. Mucosa will not, however, faithfully follow bone profiles under all circumstances. Gingiva will pile up interproximally into a papilla. In fact, the height to which the papilla ascends depends far more upon the relative proximity of adjacent roots than upon the height of the interproximal bone septum under it. Careful observation of the tissues with which we deal in management of periodontal disease will reveal over and over again that the gingiva is one of the most refractory of tissues. Its patterns of behavior and response appear to be inexorable, and bone reshaping is an attempt to match bone form once again within the

limits of variation of gingival form in a given clinical situation (Fig. 22-16).

First, the bony craters are reduced so that no thin spines remain unleveled at the line angles of a root to provide even a temporary base from which the gingiva will establish itself, and then the thick ledges are thinned marginally by osteoplasty. For example, sharply varying levels in bone in adjacent teeth in close proximity cannot be followed precisely and accommodated by the gingiva. Any failure to make this precise accommodation results in recurring pockets, proportional to the degree of failure to follow the contour of the bone. This means that the general bone profile in an area must be leveled or nearly leveled if the pocket is to be eliminated. Compromise usually results in some residual pocket depth. The operator than becomes enmeshed in the rather dubious exercise of determining whether a 5-mm pocket is better than the 8-mm pocket that he set out originally to eliminate.

Of course, it is possible in some instances to hold back resurgent gingival tissue by heroic maintenance procedures. This is usually expressed as "making demands on the patient proportional to the extent of the

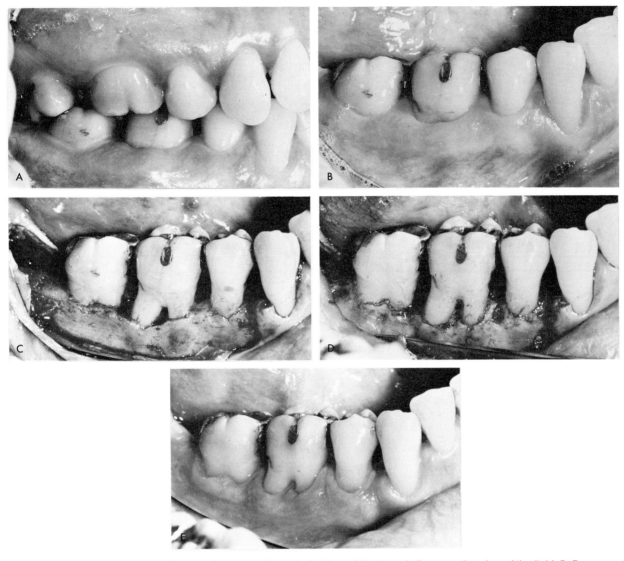

FIG. 22-16. *Ostectomy combined with osteoplasty to achieve desirable architecture. A. Preoperative view of the field. B. Response to curettage. Shrinkage reduced pocket depth but did not eliminate it. C. Flap reflected and area debrided. Note the inconsistent bony margin around the first molar in addition to the interproximal crater between the first and second molars. D. After surgery. Ostectomy over the mesiobuccal root of both second and first molars plus osteoplastic thinning and grooving the marginal bone. E. Six months after surgery. Pocket depth has been eliminated and contours have been established that can be maintained permanently. (Treated by Dr. H. Selipsky.)*

compromise." Since the entire surgical gambit is taken to permit normal maintenance by the patient and the dentist, the extent of failure becomes apparent, not only in the degree of danger to tooth retention in health but in the effort required to maintain relative health. After all, it is possible to maintain a dentition fairly well with definitive curettage plus exceptional maintenance on the part of the patient. Surgery is a solution to this problem only insofar as it makes maintenance easier.

The dilemma is best expressed by an extreme example for illustration (Fig. 22-17). Let us suppose that a resorptive lesion measures 9 to 10 mm interproximally.

Such a pocket has been found to be a suprabony defect and would not be conducive to bone and new attachment repair. The teeth adjacent have little or no pockets. The therapist is then confronted with a hard choice. Should he attempt to eliminate the pocket, he must level the bone profile in the entire region encompassing several teeth. Such a leveling would require that several adjacent teeth be denuded of bone to the level of the deepest point of resorption. The only other alternatives are (1) maintenance with definitive curettage and avoiding surgery altogether or (2) extraction of the teeth involved with the deep lesion.

Ineffective surgery is not a good solution. Effective

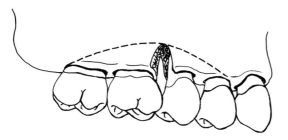

FIG. 22-17. *Drawing of a deep precipitous resorptive lesion and an indication by the dotted line of the amount of bone that would have to be removed if pocket elimination by resection was contemplated. The requirement of a gradual rise and fall is illustrated here.*

surgery is too destructive and self-defeating to be considered. Either maintenance or extraction remain as possible choices, depending on many factors, some rather complex, but certainly bone reshaping is not an acceptable solution.

Moderately deep resorptive patterns are a different matter altogether. The interproximal bony crater, usually a saucer-shaped interproximal lesion that ranges from a shallow depression to all possible variations, is prime material for osseous resection. Certain procedural requirements must be met for a successful result.

Correction of the Interproximal Crater

Probably the most common aberration in bone form due to periodontal disease is the interproximal crater (Fig. 22-18). This is a resorptive lesion of characteristic pattern and of ubiquitous nature, and the special problems attendant upon its correction merit some attention.

Leveling the crater is in itself a relatively simple procedure (Fig. 22-19). It merely involves reducing the buccal and lingual walls forming the crater so that the base of the original depression is now extended to become a fairly level floor of interproximal bone. If the lesion is too deep, several complications immediately intrude other than excessive denuding of bone.

1. One wall may be thin and the other thick. In this case the interproximal floor may be sloped toward the thin wall. In other words, the thin wall is leveled, and the thick wall is merely sloped. The solution, however, introduces possible complications in turn. The simple act of leveling a crater interproximally commonly involves carving interproximal notches in the buccal and lingual plates between each tooth in the operative field. This introduces reversed architecture into the picture. Instead of a level interproximal septum, bone excisions are geometric. The remedy for this is to level the bone over the buccal and/or lingual surfaces of the

tooth along with the interproximal bone to eliminate the discrepancy and the notches.

2. A common error is made in leveling a crater and in the reduction of the buccal and lingual plate to conform with the new level. The line angles of the roots seem to blind the critical eye of the operator, so that he leaves small peaks of bone on these line angles. These thin and altogether insignificant spicules (peaks of bone) are resorbed, but not before the healing epithelial attachment has regenerated and become coronal to them. These coronal insertions act as curtain rods holding the gingiva in a craterlike pattern after the crater has been leveled. The result of these holding attachments is the failure to achieve pocket elimination.

3. There are other hazards to be considered. Some buccal or lingual leveling may create a therapeutic invasion of a furca. This means that leveling a crater on one side or the other will depend upon more than the simple natural slope or the random location of a thin wall. This one feature has given rise to the adoption of a palatal approach in crater leveling in upper molar areas, because of the ability of the operator to level palatally (and even festoon) without running into the danger of invading a furca.

In lower-molar areas, a lingual approach to major leveling may be taken to avoid a possibly troublesome excursion into an inadequate vestibular trough that may promise meager or disappointing results.

4. Because of convergent roots, crater reduction can engender difficulties in providing room for an interproximal papilla. This is particularly true in the upper first and second molars. The distobuccal root of the upper first molar, with its extreme distal flare, is a common offender. Second molars, both upper and lower, have more or less vertical roots, close together, with constricted interradicular room. Here again is reason for a palatal leveling on upper molars. These principles have been clearly described by Ochsenbein and Bohannan, who observed that the mesial and distal furcal flutings in upper molars are well-oriented palatally so that a palatal approach will make these furcas more readily available to maintenance by the patient than would otherwise be the case.

5. The tendency to convert slopes into long bevels must be carefully avoided. A long bevel for correction of undue and excessive reverse architecture, directed toward one side or the other, brings in its wake a deeper notch interproximally with its greater cost in buccal or lingual bone (Fig. 22-20).

Interradicular Grooving

Even a casual observation of tissue behavior in the mouth reveals that the more prominent a root in the

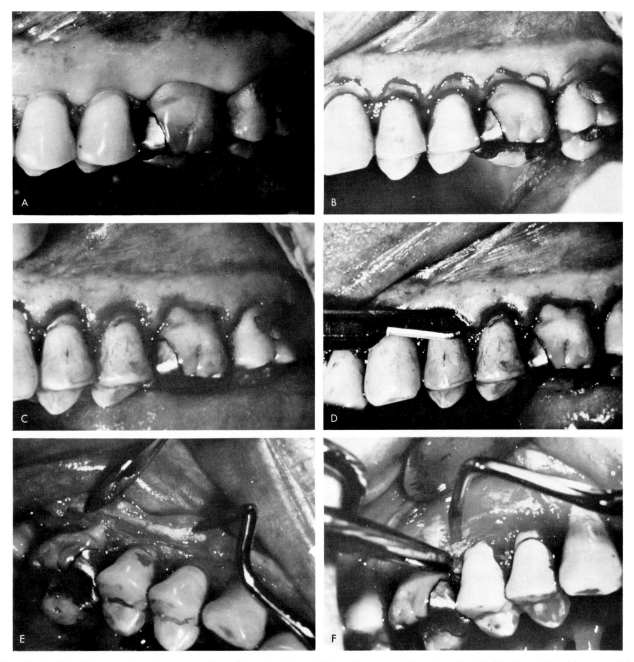

FIG. 22-18. *The ledge-and-wedge approach to flap reflection. A. Buccal preoperative view. B. Initial horizontal incision carefully scribing the tissue, buccal aspect. C. Incised tissue debrided. D. Secondary incision imparting an internal bevel to the buccal flap. E. Reflection of the buccal flap. F. Debriding the exposed buccal aspect of the surgical field.*

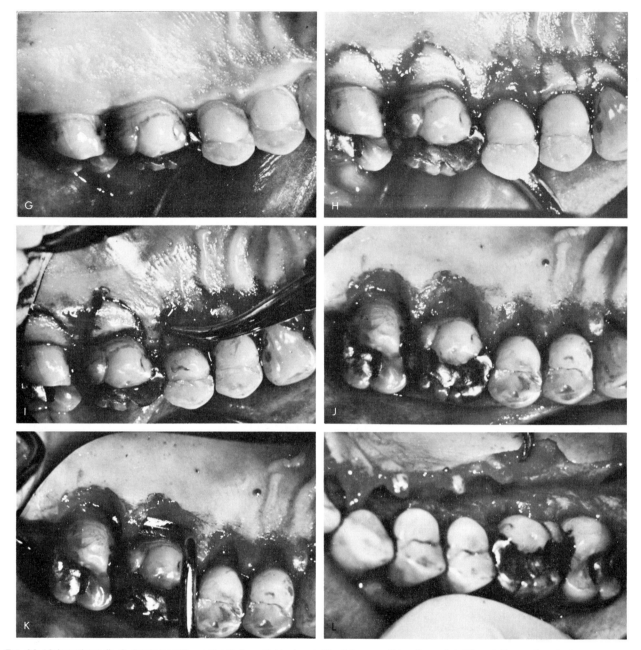

FIG. 22-18 (continued). *G. Postoperative palatal view. H. Horizontal incisions scribing the palatal flap. I. Removing the incised tissue. J. Excised tissue removed completely (revealing the ledge). K. Thinning the ledge. L. Reflecting the internally beveled palatal flap.*

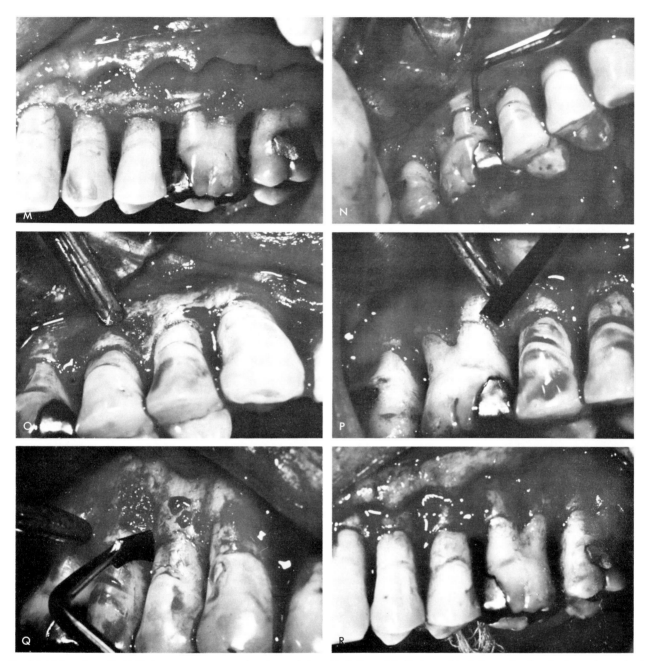

FIG. 22-18 (continued). *M. Before osseous resection, buccal view. N, O, P, and Q. Various chisels for reshaping the buccal marginal bone. R. After osseous resection, buccal view.*

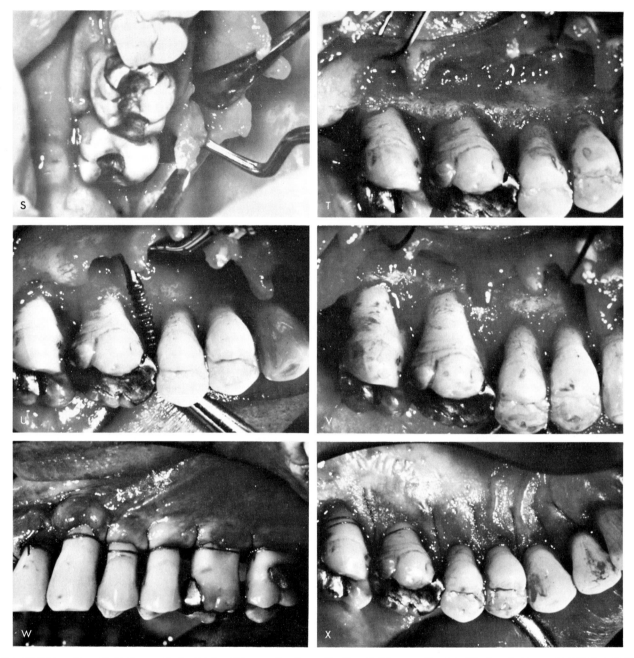

Fɪɢ. 22-18 (continued). *S. Removal of palatal soft tissue after flap reflection. T. After curettage and before osseous resection, palatal view. U. Use of interproximal files in crater leveling. (A surgical bur has been used previously to thin the heavy palatal ledges, establish a consistent marginal profile, and generally produce a bone topography resembling the normal). V. After osseous resection. W. Buccal flap placement and suturing. X. Palatal flap control and wound closure. (Treated by Dr. S. Sapkos.)*

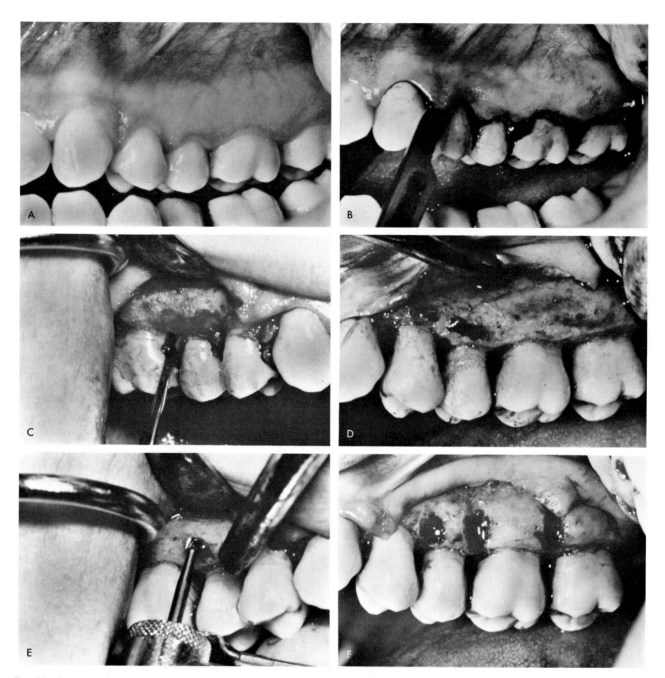

FIG. 22-19. *A step-by-step procedure in flap reflection and preparation followed by osseous resection for the correction of bone defects. A. Presurgical view of the facial aspect of the surgical field. B. Initial incision imparting an internal bevel in the facial flap. C. Facial flap reflected and interproximal soft tissue debridement initiated by a chisel. D. Bone is debrided and craters and ledges exposed to view. E. Interradicular grooving of bone with a long-shank surgical. F. Initial cut for interradicular grooves. The operator would be well advised to level the craters and perform the necessary ostectomy before grooving interradicularly.*

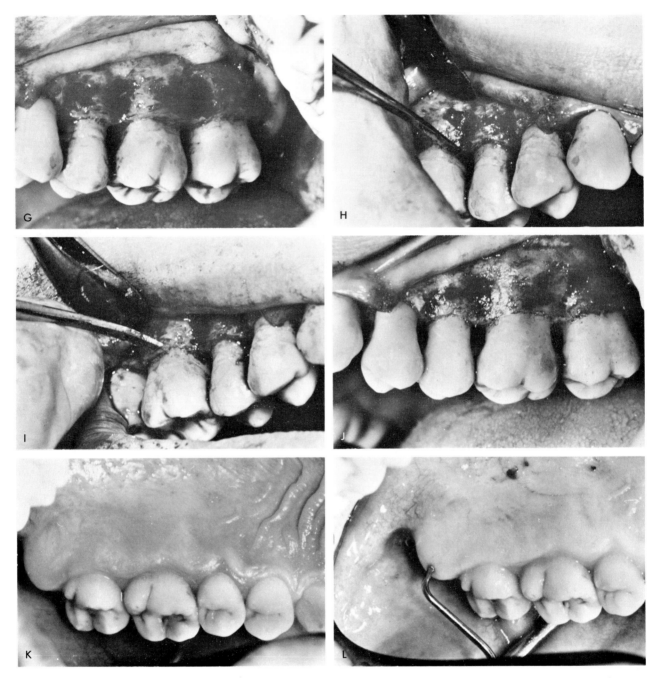

FIG. 22-19 (continued). *G. Facial ledges thinned and blended into the interradicular grooves facial view. H. Interproximal craters being leveled and finishing touches being imparted by a chisel. I. Facial ostectomy performed with a chisel after the ledges have been thinned with a bur. This makes final finishing with hand instruments easier. J. Bone reshaping completed on the facial side. K. Presurgical view of the palatal aspect of the surgical field. L. Sounding the tuberosity area for depth and bone configuration.*

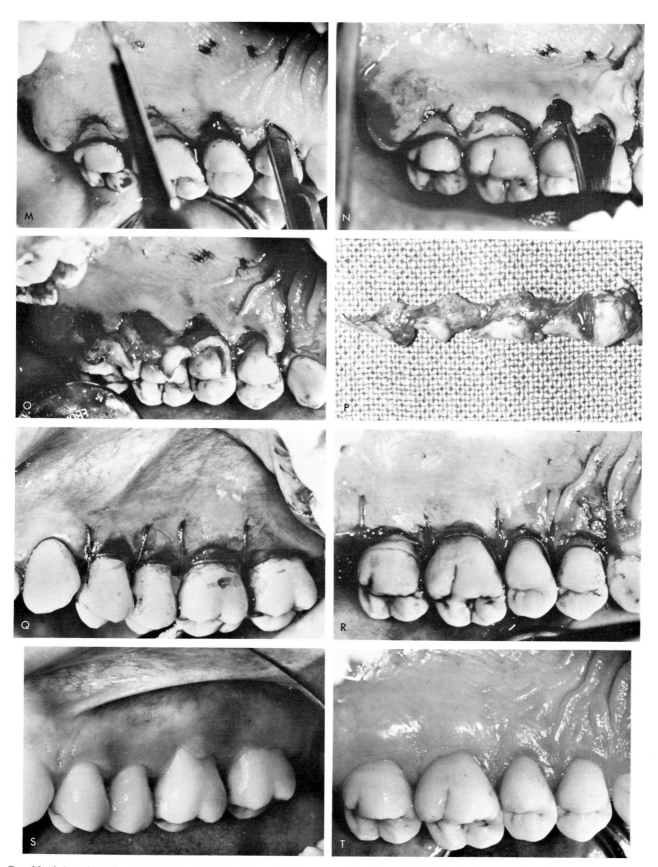

FIG. 22-19 (continued). *M. After careful delineation of the bone crest on the palatal side the festooned, scribed palatal incision imparting an internal bevel, is made with a #15 BP blade throughout the entire surgical field. N. Note the tuberosity pad incisions preparatory to resecting the dense fibrous mass of tissue from this area. O. Debriding the incised tissue from the surgical field. Note the short vertical releasing incision between the 1st premolar and the canine. P. The excised tuberosity pad continuous with palatal wedge of tissue. Q. Wound closure and suturing on the facial aspect. R. Wound closure and suturing, palatal side and the tuberosity region. S and T. Six months after surgery. (Treated by Dr. M. Dragoo.)*

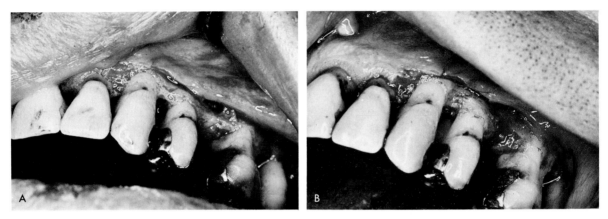

FIG. 22-20. *A. Bony crater revealed between the canine and the first premolar. B. The crater leveled on the buccal aspect and opening up the interproximal for maintenance in the fluting so common on first premolar roots.*

arch, the more apical is the gingival margin. One of the prime objectives of periodontal surgery is the substitution of a gingival recession (a selective recession) for a pocket. The creation of vertical grooves in the bone between adjacent roots has the effect of throwing the root into relative prominence, with the result that a gingival recession is nicely maintained. Great caution must be maintained not to angle these grooves so that they become long bevels. They must be consistently vertical.

A great deal of misunderstanding exists in regard to interradicular grooves. Easy to overdo and easier to mismanage in certain areas, they warrant some discussion. It should be clear at the outset that grooving is a refinement in method, designed to take advantage of a punctilio in gingival behavior over bone and root prominence in certain configurations. The advantages gained must be weighed against cost in tissue and time (Fig. 22-21).

Grooving is most effectively used where there are

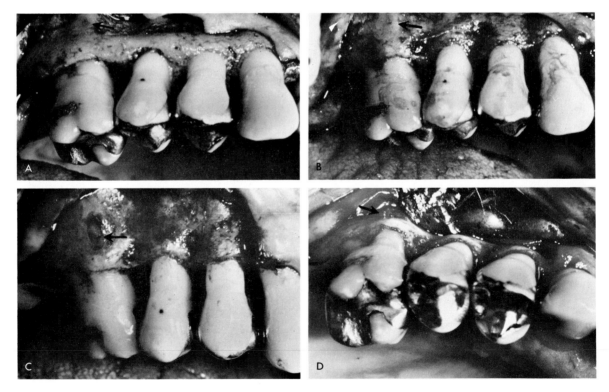

FIG. 22-21. *Interradicular grooving. A. Before surgery: buccal view. Note fenestration over the mesiobuccal root of the first molar (arrow). B. After interradicular grooving. C. Reentry 282 days postoperative. Note the persistence of the interradicular grooves; fenestration is only slightly enlarged. D. Occlusal view of C. (Treated by Dr. R. Lamb.)*

sharply differing bone levels and three or four teeth in rather tight quarters. In this situation the behavior pattern of gingiva over a root prominence affords considerable help. It enables the operator to perform minimal ostectomy to achieve only a fairly consistent bone profile and yet attain a maximum of gingival recession. This is a classic example of osteoplasty minimizing ostectomy.

It is obviously redundant to groove routinely, especially where the bone profile is fairly level and consistent even though heavily involved with generalized pocket formation. Grooving is contraindicated in the intraproximal bone between most upper first and second molars because of the sharp distal flare of the distobuccal root of the upper first molars. Interradicular grooving in such an area exposes the root and creates more problems than it solves.

The rule, then, is to groove where necessary and where advantageous, and to groove deeply enough to be effective. Groove nowhere else.

Correction of Thick Bony Margin

Almost as common as the crater is the heavy ledge of marginal bone that makes a deflective gingival margin difficult to achieve, if not impossible. These thick margins take several forms. There are the flat tablelike bony excrescences that may occur anywhere but are most common in molar regions of the lower arch, and the standard type of torus is not uncommonly involved in a deeper extension of a periodontal pocket. Then there are marginal bony beads, which consist of a discrete marginal enlargement, commonly thought to be a response to heavy functional demands. Whether this is true is of little importance in therapy. If bone is involved in any way with the periodontal lesion, it should be reshaped just as any other bone is reshaped. After all, tori, exostoses, and other bony enlargements are composed of normal bone. It is the *form* and not the origin that is at fault, and it is the form that must be corrected.

The reduction of thick marginal bone is a relatively simple matter (Figs. 22-22, 22-23). Form requirements are rather obvious and demand several important precautions.

1. In the creation of normal labial or lingual festooning, there is a tendency to remove too much bone and leave the margins too thin. It must be kept in mind that even when immediately covered with a flap, an additional 0.5 mm or so of the marginal bone is lost through continued osteoclastic activity within the bone. Too thin a bone

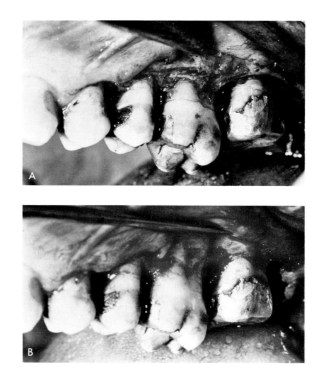

FIG. 22-22. *Correction by osteoplasty of the circumferential funnel-shaped resorptive pattern plus ostectomy to achieve a consistent bone margin. A. Ostectomy on the buccal margin of the first molar to achieve a consistent marginal level of bone. B. After surgery. Note that the bone level has been lowered over the distobuccal line-angle of the first molar incident to the leveling of the interproximal crater. This constitutes ostectomy. The thinning and leveling of the funnel-shaped defect in the second molar region consisted mainly of osteoplasty.* (*Treated by Dr. H. Selipsky.*)

plate means unnecessary fenestrations and dehiscences.

2. Exaggerated contours may not be well maintained by the overlying gingiva, and the postoperative result may often be a number of thick, rolled festoons. These are extremely persistent and are commonly found in overcontoured margins. Some simple observation of normal gingival contour in the various areas of the mouth is extremely helpful in the execution of all periodontal surgery, and bone reshaping is no exception. It is a serious error to attempt to improve upon nature. The rule, is "do not overcontour."

3. Remember, a thick, beaded margin may draw attention away from a possible fenestration apical to it.

4. It is false conservatism to reflect tight inadequate flaps (mouseholing). It reflects not so much conservatism as timidity. Many serious errors are committed in the name of conservatism that is not conservatism at all. The first rule in any sur-

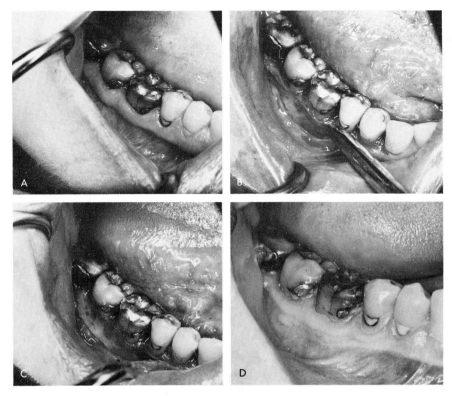

FIG. 22-23. *Reduction of a thick bony margin. A. Preoperative view. It is sometimes difficult to determine whether the operator is dealing with gingival fibrosis or an underlying thick ledge of bone. B. Bony margin exposed. C. Correction by osteoplasty of the thick margin. D. Five years after surgery.*

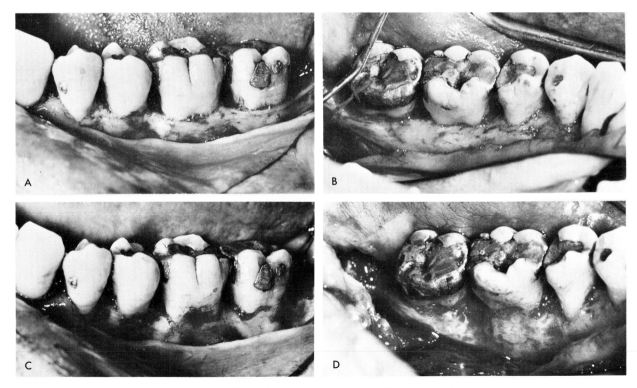

FIG. 22-24. *Crater leveling from both buccal and lingual sides. A. Buccal view of interproximal craters with flaps reflected. B. Lingual view of the same area. C. Craters leveled by ostectomy and osteoplasty. Buccal view after bone correction. D. Lingual view after surgery to correct bony craters interproximally. (Treated by Dr. H. Selipsky.)*

gical procedure is to provide adequate room for proper observation and performance.

Malposed teeth frequently result in heavy buccal plates adjacent to teeth with little or no plate at all. This is valuable information to have when the decision for a vertical releasing incision is to be made. It may just be that the exposure of a root with fenestrations or dehiscence is indicated, in spite of the usual penalties that may be forthcoming. These penalties should not, however, come as a surprise to the skilled therapist. Consideration of malposed teeth should enter into the surgical treatment plan.

Objectives of Osseous Resection

To recapitulate, osseous resection, both osteoplasty and ostectomy, consists essentially of leveling interproximal craters, reducing bony craters that are not conducive to repair because of a wide orifice, shallow topography, or for other reasons, and the thinning of thick, heavy marginal bone (Fig. 22-24). In general, it is directed toward establishing normal form in the bone where it did not exist before. The objective is to present a sound and solid base for the gingiva to rest upon, without generating excessive sulcular depth. Essentially, it is to eliminate pockets and is to be judged on that basis. Permanence of results is the hallmark of success. Techniques in themselves are of little interest, except insofar as they affect the result. In this instance, a selective recession is the reward.

POCKET ELIMINATION IN PERIODONTAL THERAPY

The question of pocket elimination as a justifiable therapeutic objective has a long and troubled history. While great numbers of periodontal surgeons publish and show many cases of long-term survival in health after extensive periodontal surgery, there is no linear study proving incontrovertibly that the dentitions of patients with deep pockets survive longer after periodontal surgical procedures than they would with curettage alone and with similar postoperative maintenance.

In fact, the absence of such a study serves to point up the enormous difficulty in clinical research in establishing controls of any sort. We are, therefore, forced to rely on clinical impressions of knowledgeable and reliable therapists. Although this reliance results in considerable imprecision, the mass of opinion holds that generally a tooth with little sulcular depth is easier to maintain than is a tooth with a deep sulcus.

There are, of course, exceptions. In some cases it is impossible to eliminate pockets without inflicting enormous damage. In others, the therapist must pause because of a high level of caries. Other exceptions are mentioned in Chapters 13 and 14. What should concern the periodontist is the permanence of pocket elimination after it has been achieved. If pocket elimination is a temporary phenomenon, then it is obviously not too rewarding.

Figure 22-25 provides a clinical case that clearly illustrates some of the critical factors involved in pocket elimination. The patient was a highly motivated male who had practiced meticulous maintenance from postadolescence into middle age.

At the time of the initial examination the dentition was obviously failing. The lower left posterior segment is a fair and accurate sample of what was happening throughout the entire dentition. In Figure 22-25, A and B reveal handsome and apparently healthy gingiva on both the buccal and lingual aspects of the area under discussion. C, which is a lingual view, shows fairly clearly the deep intrabony pockets that have formed throughout the molar region, with hemisepta on the mesial side of both second and first molars and a deep intrabony resorptive lesion on the distal side of the second molar. C and D show the bone reshaping that was done to achieve the maximum possible architectural correction. Some compromises had to be accepted in the hope that the excellent plaque control practiced by the patient preoperatively would, if continued postoperatively, maintain shallow sulci in spite of some reverse architecture. The follow-up photographs, G through L, demonstrate that this patient did do far better in plaque control and maintenance with shallow sulci than with the preoperative normal gingival arrangement. Reference is made to the failing of the dentition preoperatively and the arrest of the downhill course of the tissues postoperatively. Homeostasis appears to have been established.

This is the kind of clinical evidence that supports the contention that shallow sulci are more conducive to health than are deep ones. While such cases are not scientific proof of the opinion offered, they offer strong presumptive evidence upon which the case for resective surgery for pocket elimination is based.

Correction of Hemisepta

Hemisepta that are formed by deep pockets immediately adjacent in the same interproximal space are not always suitable material for resective surgery. When the hemisepta are deep, the tooth involved with the pocket may be lost. Shallow hemisepta, on the other hand, lend themselves to resection. This is especially true when the teeth have bell-shaped crowns

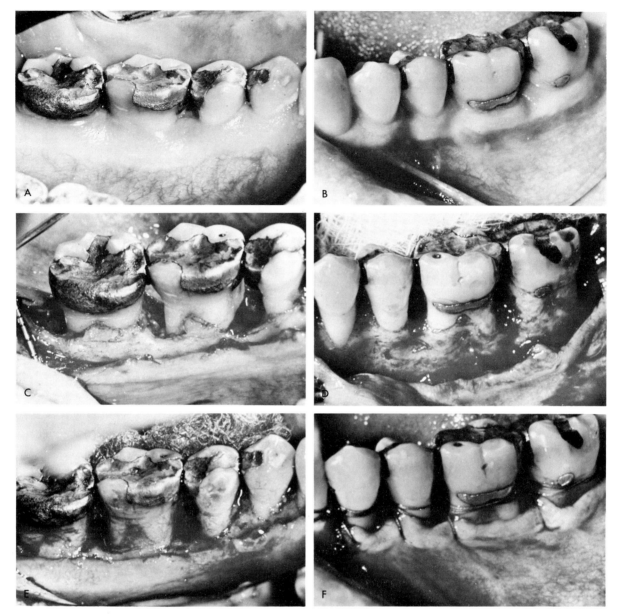

FIG. 22-25. *Osseous resection for pocket elimination. A and B. Preoperative lingual and buccal views of the area under discussion. C. View with flaps reflected to reveal lesions. D. After osseous resection. Note the compromise in leveling the hemiseptum between the first and second molars. E. After osseous resection on the lingual side. F. Sutures. Note slight flap displacement distally.*

that naturally create wide interproximal embrasures.

The reduction is, of course, an ostectomy, but the simple resection of the hemiseptum is usually not enough. Some osteoplastic finishing is required to blend the buccal and lingual bone margins into the pattern of the surrounding bone. Particular care must be taken to level all line-angle spines of bone which are commonly left in hemiseptum reduction.

Chisels and hand files are the instruments of choice in resecting the thin, easily cut bony hemiseptum. Rotary instruments are hazardous to use on so small amount of bone in so small a space.

Correction of Circumferential Bony Lesion

Surprising numbers of bone resorptive patterns yield to simple osteoplastic reduction. Here again the periodontist is confronted with a clinical situation in which shallow lesions are good material for resection, but deep pockets of the same form must be treated with inductive methods if they are to be treated at all. The discussion will be limited to the shallow to moderately deep circumferential bony lesion. In order for such a lesion to exist at all, the width of the alveolar process

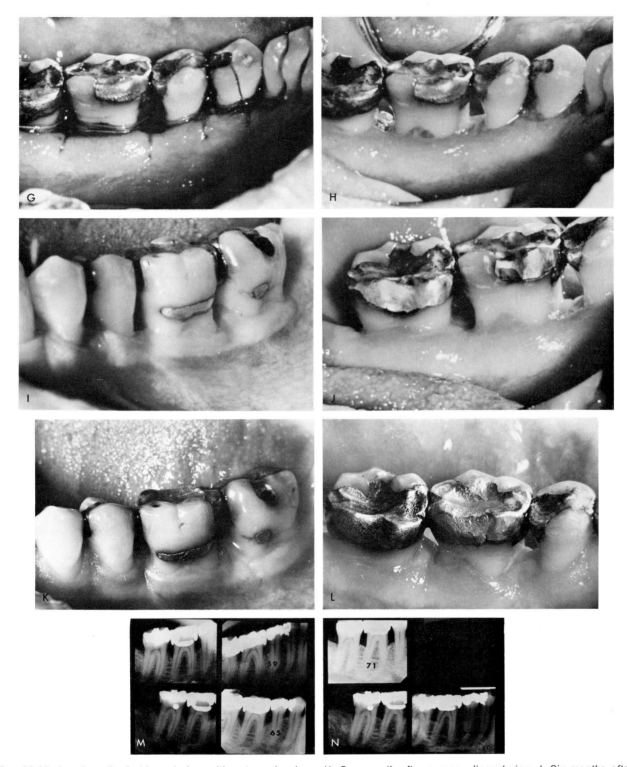

FIG. 22-25. (continued). *G. Lingual view with sutures in place. H. One month after surgery—lingual view. I. Six months after surgery—buccal view. J. One year after surgery—lingual view. K. Four years after surgery—buccal view. L. Four years after surgery—lingual view. M and N. Radiographic records of the area in 1959, 1965, 1971 (2 years after surgery) and 1973 (4 years after surgery). (Treated by Dr. R. L. Johnson.)*

must be considerable. A thin process in such a location would be completely destroyed to the extent of the resorption.

The reason this point is made is that leveling the area of bone resorption surrounding the tooth reveals a thick ledge at the base that must then be thinned and blended into adjacent architecture. The success with which these funnel-shaped lesions can be converted to acceptable positive architecture is always a pleasant surprise. It must be kept in mind that the mesial and distal portions of the circumferential lesion constitute hemisepta. These must be corrected in routine fashion of the common lesion previously described.

WOUND HEALING AFTER OSSEOUS SURGERY

It becomes obvious that, in order to reshape bone, to level craters, and thin out heavy ledges, the bone itself must be exposed with the instrument of choice. A number of procedures, reparative and excisional, have come into wide use in the last decade.

Bone used to be uncovered by excising and discarding the attached gingiva lying over it to the entire extent of the operative field. Since the mucosa apical to the mucogingival line is thin and vascular and contains elastic fibers in its stroma, reflection causes it immediately to shrink and to a considerable extent. This immediate shrinkage effectively exposes ample bony plate, particularly on the buccal aspect, so that any reshaping that was required could be done uninhibited by lack of operating room.

The postoperative dressing was applied over naked bone up to and beyond the mucosal margin of the wound. Little attention was paid at the outset to the consequences of bone exposure and of the postoperative course of wound healing. Long before these effects were studied, better surgical methods were introduced for field exposure and surgical wound closure—a flap approach generally with ample mucosa left to cover the exposed bone adequately.

The source of the elements of healing was of great interest to the clinicians. It was soon established that the early proliferating granulation tissue emanated from the periodontal space. This can be demonstrated in almost every healing area treated by denudation of the alveolar bone, by merely observing the week-by-week healing record. Collaring of proliferating granulating tissue circumferentially about the cervical portion of root at the level of investment in the alveolus at its crestal margin was usually observed as an irregular delicate band approximately 1 to 2 mm in extent. Subsequent weeks would reveal that proliferation continued from this single source in an apical direction and

slowly covered the exposed plate of bone. This process seemed to continue for a sufficient number of weeks to allow for about 5 to 6 mm of bone margin to be covered. After that point, speculation suggested that necrosis of bone surface brought other factors into the wound-healing picture.

It is interesting to note that, following the denudation of bone, the crestal 5 to 6 mm will, to a considerable extent, be covered with attached gingiva. However, in spite of the denudation of a far greater area than 5 to 6 mm—even to the extent of 15 mm—only a maximum of 5 to 6 mm would be covered in alveolar mucosa.

Unlike healing of other similar wounds in this particular type of surgical wound, healing is *not* peripheral until possibly its late stages. Certainly, in the initial phases, healing arises crestally and proliferates apically.

Some animal studies were made by Wilderman, Wentz, and others on the fate of marginal bone and of cortical plate in the denuded area. Their results were all in essential agreement. There appeared to be considerable crestal bone loss in areas where the bony plate was thin. In areas where the bone was thick enough to be backed by cancellous bone, there was surface necrosis of the cortical plate, but repair occurred.

Not clearly recognized in the animal studies was that results gleaned from animals with no periodontal disease could not, without serious modification, be transposed to human beings with marginal periodontal disease. There was no question that cortical plate resorption takes place when a flap is raised and the continuity of the tissue is broken, if only momentarily. Considering the way gingiva is attached to the cortical plate (insertion of Sharpey's fibers), it is clear that reattachment of the detached flap can occur only after the removal by resorption or necrosis of the old cortical plate. This involves the laying down of new fibers from the gingiva, and the reconstitution of a new cortical plate imbedding the new fibers. This loss occurs in any exposure of surface bone in the alveolar process. It is part of the repair mechanism.

Friedman and Levine in 1964 observed that in human material the marginal loss of bone adjacent to a tooth averages 0.55 mm—an insignificant amount—if the operative field is covered postoperatively by a replaced or repositioned flap. Their explanation for the relatively slight loss of marginal bone was that only teeth affected with periodontal disease were used in the study, and such teeth regularly show thicker marginal bone because the disease has caused crestal resorption. A most important factor, too, is the relatively benign effect that mucosal cover has on the bone during healing. It is far quicker than would be the case with a denudation and the long periods of bone exposure under dressings waiting for proliferating granulation tissue to cover the field.

These observations are probably sound and seem to have been corroborated by the clinical behavior of the various tissues. Certain patterns emerge, however, in the management of bone and gingiva. If the resorbed bone plate covers cancellous bone, healing occurs. On the other hand, when the cortical plate is backed by the cortical bone of the alveolus (with no cancellous bone intervening), no repair seems to follow and the loss of bone is permanent.

THE THIN PERIODONTIUM

In areas of thin buccal or lingual plate, the thinnest bone is in a rather narrow zone vertically over the root prominences. This is the area in which the greatest care must be taken in a flap reflection. In all other areas, a variable mass of bone covers the root and the interproximal areas (where a solid block extends from the buccal side to the lingual). In such areas, flap reflection presents few problems in bone repair. In areas where the bone plate covering the invested root is extremely thin over the root prominences, the danger of root fenestrations or dehiscences is great when this bone is exposed by flap reflection.

The advantages in knowing in advance whether the operator will encounter paper-thin bone covering the root prominences is obvious. The problem becomes one of diagnosis. The roentgenogram offers little help, since it reveals the interproximal bone only, and even there it is notoriously unreliable.

Some experience is helpful in determining the form and thickness of the margin of alveolar bone. This experience is quickly gained with application. Assay and delineation of the margin will give no definite information on fenestrations of the root more apically through the bone plate. Although no area is immune to chance fenestrations because of random variations in root form, a thin crestal margin will give cause for some caution. This is particularly true over distobuccal roots of upper first molars, mesiobuccal line angles over lower first molars, and over all four cuspids. When the crestal isthmus of bone is thin, it is almost inevitable that the fenestration will result in a dehiscence when the isthmus is lost.

Such irretrievable losses in bone bring up some interesting considerations in therapeutic judgment. Far too often these resorptions have served to frighten timid therapists into a false conservatism. The pains to determine submucosal anatomy and bone configuration should create a cautious and knowledgeable approach

in the operator. This means a weighing of relative advantages and disadvantages of exposure against possible costs to the patient in terms of lost tissue. It does not mean automatic retreat. Once again the old question of pocket elimination is brought into prominence. The question should be whether pocket elimination or maintenance of deep sulci with curettage will best serve the patient. One of the alternatives should *not* be inadequate surgical procedures to achieve some linear reduction of pocket depth with no definitive result.

Compromise is good if all alternatives are considered sagaciously. The possible loss of some marginal bone over a root prominence may be a fair price to pay for pocket elimination in an area where it would confer considerable advantage—for example, where there will be a periodontal prosthesis, and where risks should possibly not be taken on exacerbating an inflammatory lesion.

To the charge that this sort of treatment planning and such a surgical approach calls for complicated, many-faceted decisions we can only plead guilty. Simple approaches are for general averages that seem to exist only in the aggregate and never in the specific case.

THICK VERSUS THIN PERIODONTIUM

After many years of observation by many knowledgeable therapists, the conclusion is slowly achieving ascendancy that there is an inherent form to the bony investment of the teeth. Patients with thick-necked teeth, large, thick roots, and blocky crowns apparently have a rather thick periodontium with a tendency to revert to this form if any deviation from it is imposed artificially. Conversely, the patient with bell-shaped teeth with relatively slender roots will most likely have a thinner periodontium with more pronounced marginal scalloping and festooning. If this observation is valid, the surgical reshaping of bone, especially, must take into account the relative configuration of the tissues and of the tooth itself and must project a corrected anatomy of supporting and investing tissues to conform to that morphology.

This precept is consistent with the basis of bone reshaping in respect to the creation of bony architecture to which the overlying soft tissue can adapt. It carries this precept a step farther, however. The concern is not only with bone and ligament and tooth arrangement but with which of these can be violated only at the expense of the objective.

Illustrative of the principle is the case illustrated in Figures 22-26 and 22-27. The patient had a rather square or thick periodontium and a similar degree and pattern of periodontal destruction on both the upper

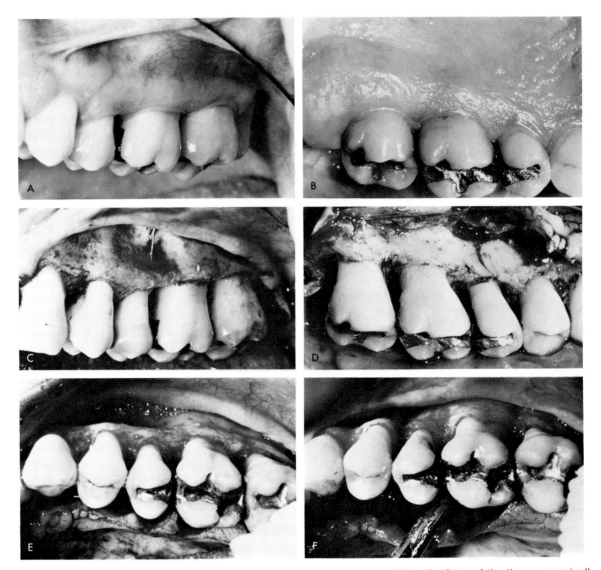

FIG. 22-26. *Osseous resection. A. Preoperative view of upper right buccal aspect. Note the form of the tissues marginally. The gingival margin is relatively flat. B. Palatal view of A. These gingival margins are similarly flat with only minimal festooning. C. Flap retraction and debridement revealing buccal bony contour. Note the flat bony contours. D. Palatal view of C. Bone profile is relatively flat. E. Occlusal view of the right side before osseous reshaping. F. The right side undergoing osseous reshaping.*

right (Fig. 22-26) and upper left (Fig. 22-27) posterior segments. By standard osseous resection in reshaping the bone on the upper left side, a thin periodontium was imposed with exaggerated marginal festooning and extremely thin investing bone. On the right side, on the other hand, a heavier bone plate was permitted to remain on the buccal side with more conservative festooning and more modified interradicular grooving.

The healing response on both sides was watched and recorded. Of particular interest was the response of the gingiva to two differing corrective approaches, both correcting pocket-generating inconsistencies in bone. On the left side was imposed an exaggerated configu-

ration with an anterior anatomy of investing bone on an area that had apparently originally had a much flatter bone profile and less festooning; on the right side the anatomy imposed was that which was thought to have existed before periodontitis had altered the bone profile.

Examination of the postoperative views at 9 weeks (Fig. 22-26K,L) and at 8 months (Fig. 22-27M,N) shows that inexorably the gingival arrangement resumes what, for it, was normal form. Pocket depth is returning to the area (the left side) that was reshaped by thinning. Overcorrection endangers the result it was designed to achieve.

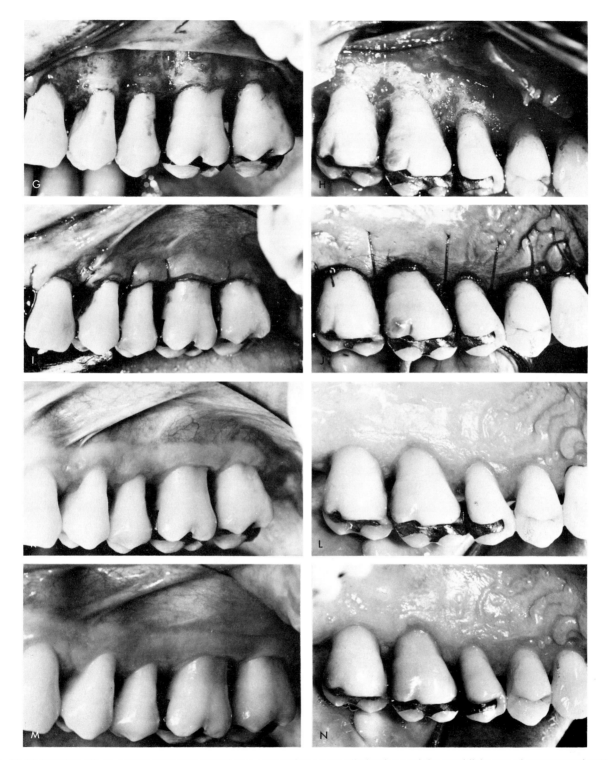

FIG. 22-26 (continued). *G. Upper right side after bone contouring crater elimination and the establishment of contour and pattern conducive to pocket elimination but avoiding pronounced festooning. H. After osseous resection. Palatal view. I. Flap sutured on the buccal side. The relatively flat contour is maintained in the flap margin which is carefully placed to coincide with the bone margin. J. Palatal flap sutured into proper position. K and L. Nine weeks after surgery; buccal and palatal views. Note the excellent sulcular control. M and N. Eight months postoperative views. (Treated by Dr. J. Jerome.)*

METHODS OF BONE RESHAPING

The actual methods used in the reduction and reshaping of bone are quite simple. Bone is a relatively soft material, as hard tissues go, and is not nearly so resistant to the bur as is enamel. For this reason, most inexperienced operators prefer slow to moderate speed in a turbine or belt-driven rotary instrument.

Care should be used when roots are approached to avoid nicking and scratching their surfaces, which will cause sensitivity and other operative complications. When the amount of bone to be reshaped is relatively thin, hand instruments are by far the most satisfactory

approach to the problem. Thin rasps and chisels are most effective in leveling craters and in carving marginal bone that is not too thick.

With heavier ledges of bone, the bur at moderate speed will serve well if used with care. The crude reduction can be made in crater correction until the roots are approached, when the procedure can be finished with hand instruments. Interradicular grooving can be finished with a rotary instrument. Hand instruments are not too efficient in heavy masses of cortical plate.

In the reduction of heavy masses of bone, such as is found in tori or in other bony excrescences, the high

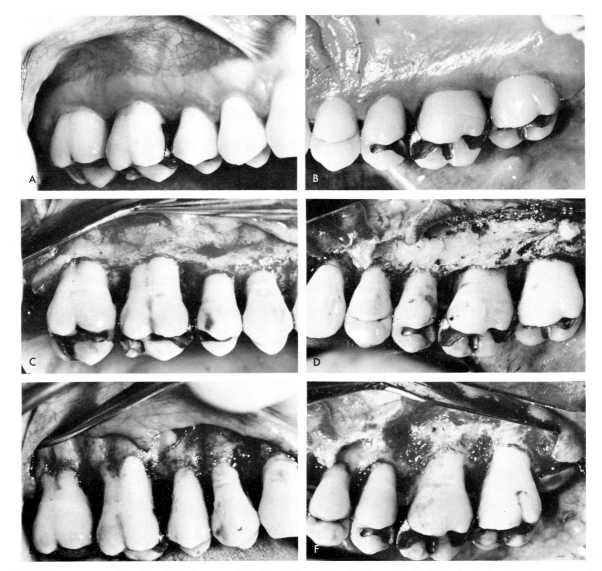

FIG. 22-27. Osseous resection. A and B. The upper left side of the patient in Figure 22-26. The gingival contours and margins are similar to those on the right side. They present a relatively flat contour. The crowns of the teeth are square and thick-necked. C and D. Buccal and palatal flaps reflected and the underlying bone debrided. Note the same flat profile as is exhibited by the overlying tissue. E and F. Buccal and palatal views after exaggerated bone contouring. Note the deep interradicular grooves, the artificially emphasized marginal festoons, and the extremely thin investing plates of bone.

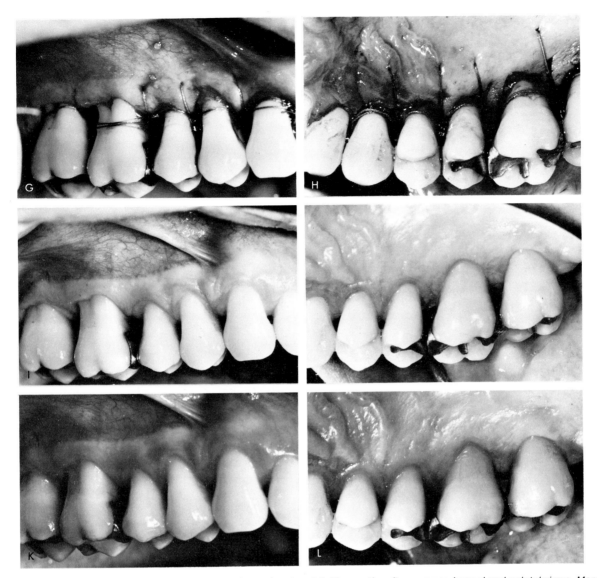

FIG. 22-27 (continued). *G and H. Flap adaptation and suturing. I and J. Six months after surgery, buccal and palatal views. Marginal gingival proliferation can already be noted, especially in the premolar region, both buccally and lingually. K and L. Seventeen months after surgery. Note continued marginal proliferation. (Treated by Dr. J. Jerome.)*

speed turbine is quite safe to use if ordinary care is taken. Again, it should never be used in bone adjacent to roots, since the slightest error in judgment can result in a major accident. Many operators prefer to use vertical and horizontal grooving to the depth desired in removal and to finish the procedure with a chisel and a controlled mallet.

When root proximity is a clinical problem, hand instrumentation is the only expedient that can be used. Even so, great care must be used in manipulation adjacent to roots. Root damage is certainly not impossible with hand instrumentation. While it is true that some bone files and rasps are safe-sided, they are not so safe that a tilt in the angle of use does not present the possibility of inflicting a scratch or a gouge in roots.

The greatest danger inherent in the resort to rotary instruments at high or even at moderate speed is that of overcorrection. The bone melts away with such ease under the bur that the tendency to idealize the architecture of the area is great. All too frequently, areas with investing bone over root prominences have been thinned to such a degree that resorption and dehiscences are inevitable.

In choosing a rotary instrument, whether it be a bur or an abrasive point, it is wise to choose the largest size suitable. Small points or burs have a tendency to make small pits in the surface to be corrected that are difficult to make smooth and level. It is not a rare occurrence to invade a nutrient canal with a small bur when invasion could have been avoided with a large one.

This is particularly true of the necessarily small rotary instruments in a high speed turbine. Great care must be taken to use feather-light brushing movements. Even then the task is a difficult one that usually must be followed by another instrument for finishing.

RESECTIVE SURGERY AND ITS PLACE IN THERAPY

Since the entire range of periodontal surgery constitutes plastic repair and is not definitive therapy for inflammatory lesions, the results must be evaluated and judged on the basis of making the maintenance of the natural dentition easier and more successful and practicable. A better case can be made for reconstructive surgery, since some of it, at least, results in a recapture of lost attachment. Insofar as it is successful, it constitutes a reversal of the destructive process and creates a greater quantum of attachment and support.

Standard techniques of resection can make no such claims. Their success, to be sure, is predictable to a far greater degree and, because of this, they have been incorporated into standard methodology. Since they are performed at the expense of bone and gingiva, the scope of their value is limited by the amount of these tissues available for reshaping. This must always be kept in mind. This means that moderate resorptive lesions are best suited to all resective methods. This point has been made before, but its repetition here serves to point up that no single method is the universal choice for a standard lesion. Neither such a choice nor such a lesion exists.

Bibliography

1. Barkann, L.: A conservative surgical technique. J. Am. Dent. Assoc., 26:61, 1939.
2. Berdon, J. W.: Blood loss during gingival surgery. J. Periodontol., 36:102, 1965.
3. Beube, F. E.: Periodontology. New York, Macmillan, 1953.
4. Bernier, J., and Kaplan, H.: The repair of gingival tissue after surgical intervention. J. Am. Dent. Assoc., 35:697, 1947.
5. Black, G. V.: A Work on Special Dental Pathology Devoted to the Diseases and Treatment of the Investing Tissues of the Teeth and Dental Pulp. Chicago, Medico-Dental Publishing Co., 1915.
6. Burch, J. G., et al.: Tooth mobility following gingivectomy. A study of gingival support of the teeth. J. Am. Soc. Periodont., 6:90, 1968.
7. Chace, R.: The surgical approach in periodontal treatment. J. Am. Dent. Assoc., 52:709, 1956.
8. Chaikin, B. S.: Newer concepts in periodontal therapy. N.Y. J. Dent., 25:300, 1955.
9. Coolidge, E. D.: Elimination of the periodontal pocket in the treatment of pyorrhea. J. Am. Dent. Assoc., 25:1627, 1938.
10. Crane, A. B., and Kaplan, H.: The Crane-Kaplan operation for prompt elimination of pyorrhea alveolaris. Dental Cosmos, 73:643, 1931.
11. Deib, E.: The use of rotary abrasives in gingivoplasty. Dental Survey, 33:31, 1957.
12. Dement, R. L.: The surgical treatment of periodontoclasia. J. Am. Dent. Assoc., 20:993, 1933.
13. Donnenfeld, O. W.: A biometric study of the effects of gingivectomy. J. Periodontol., 37:446, 1966.
14. Everett, F. G., Waerhaug, J., and Widman, A.: Leonard Widman: Surgical treatment of pyorrhea alveolaris. J. Periodontol., 42:571, 1971.
15. Fox, L.: Rotating abrasives in the management of periodontal soft and hard tissue. Oral Surg., 8:1134, 1955.
16. Friedman, N.: Periodontal osseous surgery: osteoplasty and ostectomy. J. Periodontol., 26:257, 1955.
17. Friedman, N.: The anatomy of the periodontium. Rocky Mountain Dental Seminar, Glenwood Springs, Colo., 1959.
18. Gilson, C. M.: Surgical treatment of periodontal disease. J. Am. Dent. Assoc., 44:733, 1952.
19. Glickman, I.: Hypertrophic gingivitis, its diagnosis and treatment. J. Dent. Med., 3:32, 1948.
20. Glickman, I.: The results obtained with the unembellished gingivectomy technique in a clinical study in humans. J. Periodontol., 27:247, 1956.
21. Glickman, I.: Complete mouth gingivectomy—a hospital procedure. Dent. Clin. North Am., 3:13, 1960.
22. Goldman, H. M.: Gingivectomy, indications, contraindications and method. Am. J. Orthod. Oral Surg., 32:323, 1946.
23. Goldman, H. M.: The development of physiologic gingival contours by gingivoplasty. Oral Surg., 3:879, 1950.
24. Goldman, H. M., and Cohen, W. D.: Periodontal Therapy, 4th Ed., St. Louis, The C. V. Mosby Co., 1968.
25. Gottsegen, R.: Should the teeth be scaled prior to surgery? J. Periodontol., 32:27, 1961.
26. Heins, P. J.: Osseous surgery: an evaluation after twenty-five years. Dent. Clin. North Am., Jan., 1969, p. 75.
27. Johnson, R.: Gingivectomy in the treatment of suppurative periodontoclasia. J. Am. Dent. Assoc., 18:1455, 1931.
28. Kaplan, H., and Nulobsky, L.: A surgical procedure for periodontal pocket technique. Oral Surg., Oral Med., Oral Path., 4:456, 1951.
29. Kirkland, O.: Surgical flap and semiflap technique in periodontal surgery. Dent. Dig., 42:125, 1936.
30. Kohn, J. D., and Kramer, G. M.: The use of ultraspeed rotary instruments in periodontal therapy. J. Am. Soc. Periodont., 1:73, 1963.
31. Korn, N. A., and Schaffer, E. M.: A comparison of the postoperative bacteremia induced following different periodontal procedures. J. Periodontol., 33:226, 1962.
32. Kramer, G. M.: Is the simple gingivectomy obsolete? Periodont. Abstracts, 13:63, 1965.

33. Kronfeld, R.: Condition of alveolar bone underlying periodontal pockets. J. Periodontol., 6:22, 1935.

34. Levine, S.: Failures with gingivectomy. Dent. Pract., 17:182, 1967.

35. Löe, H.: Chemical gingivectomy, effect of potassium hydroxide on periodontal tissues. Acta Odontol. Scand., 19:417, 1961.

36. Morris, M.: The removal of pocket and attachment epithelium in humans: a histologic study. J. Periodontol., 25:7, 1954.

37. Nabers, C. L., Spear, G. R., and Beckham, L. C.: Alveolar dehiscence. Tex. Dent. J., 98:4, 1960.

38. Ochsenbein, C.: Osseous resection in periodontal surgery., J. Periodontol., 29:15, 1958.

39. Ochsenbein, C.: Rationale for periodontal osseous surgery., Dent. Clin. North Am., March, 1960, p. 27.

40. Ochsenbein, C., and Bohannan, H. M.: Palatal approach to osseous surgery. I. Rationale. J. Periodontol., 34:60, 1963.

41. Ochsenbein, C., and Bohannan, H. M.: The palatal approach to osseous surgery. II. Clinical application. J. Periodontol., 35:54, 1964.

42. Ochsenbein, C., and Ross, S. E.: A reevaluation of osseous surgery. Dent. Clin. North Am., Jan., 1969, p. 87.

43. Orban, B.: To what extent should the tissues be excised in gingivectomy? J. Periodontol., 12:93, 1941.

44. Orban, B.: Indications, technique, and postoperative management of gingivectomy in the treatment of periodontal pockets. J. Periodontol., 12:89, 1941.

45. Orban, B., and Archer, E. A.: Dynamics of wound healing following elimination of gingival pockets. Am. J. Orthod. Oral Surg., 31:40, 1965.

46. Powell, R. N.: Treatment of periodontal disease: The eradication of soft tissue deformities. Br. Dent. J., 120:61, 1966.

47. Prichard, J. F.: A technique for treating intrabony pockets based on alveolar process morphology. Dent. Clin. North Am., March, 1960, p. 85.

48. Prichard, J. F.: Changing concepts in periodontal therapy. Tex. Dent. J., 79:4, 1961.

49. Prichard, J. F.: Gingivectomy, gingivoplasty and osseous surgery. J. Periodontol., 32:257, 1961.

50. Prichard, J. F.: Philosophy of practice. Periodontics, 3:32, 1965.

51. Prichard, J. F.: Management of soft tissue in periodontal surgery. Bull. Acad. Gen. Dent., Dec., 1967.

52. Ramfjord, S., and Costich, E. R.: Healing after simple gingivectomy. J. Periodontol., 34:401, 1963.

53. Ramfjord, S., and Kiester, G.: The gingival sulcus and the periodontal pocket immediately following scaling of the teeth. J. Periodontol., 25:167, 1954.

54. Ramfjord, S.: Gingivectomy—its place in periodontal therapy. J. Periodontol., 23:30, 1952.

55. Ramfjord, S.: Clinical trials of therapeutic measures in periodontics. Int. Dent. J., 21:16, 1971.

56. Ramfjord, S. P., et al.: Longitudinal study of periodontal therapy. J. Periodontol., 44:66, 1973.

57. Ramfjord, S. P., and Nissle, R. R.: The modified Widman flap. J. Periodontol., 45:8, 1974.

58. Schaffer, E. M.: Use of rotary diamond instruments in gingivoplasty. Acad. Rev., 10:84, 1962.

59. Schluger, S.: Osseous resection—a basic principle in periodontal surgery. Oral Surg., 2:316, 1949.

60. Schluger, S.: Surgical techniques in pocket elimination. Tex. Dent. J., 70:246, 1952.

61. Scopp, I. W.: Hematologic analysis after gingivectomy. J. Am. Dent. Assoc., 70:1422, 1965.

62. Stern, I. B., Everett, F., and Robicsek, K.: S. Robicsek—a pioneer in the surgical treatment of periodontal disease. J. Periodontol., 36:165, 1965.

63. Swenson, H. M.: Success or failure in periodontal surgery. J. Am. Dent. Assoc., 67:193, 1963.

64. Waerhaug, J., and Loe, H.: Tissue reaction to the gingivectomy pack. Oral Surg., 10:923, 1967.

65. Wade, A. B.: Where gingivectomy fails. J. Periodontol., 25:189, 1954.

66. Ward, A. W.: The surgical eradication of pyorrhea. J. Am. Dent. Assoc., 15:2196, 1928.

67. Weinmann, J. P.: Progress of gingival inflammation into the supporting structures of the teeth. J. Periodontol., 12:71, 1941.

68. Widman, L.: The operative treatment of pyorrhea alveolaris. A new surgical method. Sven. Tandlak. Tidskr., Dec., 1918.

69. Williams, C. H. M.: Rationalization of periodontal pocket therapy. J. Periodontol., 14:67, 1943.

70. World Workshop in Periodontics, 1966.

71. Zamet, J. S.: The limitations of gingivectomy. Dent. Pract., 17:182, 1967.

72. Zamet, J. S.: A comparison of "unembellished gingivectomy" with the inverse bevel flap procedure incorporating osseous recontouring. Dent. Pract., 17:387, 1967.

73. Zemsky, J. L.: Surgical treatment of periodontal disease with the author's open view operation for advanced cases of dental periclasia. Dent. Cosmos, 68:465, 1926.

74. Zentler, A.: Suppurative gingivitis with alveolar involvement. A new surgical procedure. J.A.M.A., 71:1530, 1918.

23

Elimination of Periodontal Pocket Inductive Methods

23

Elimination

of

Periodontal

Pocket

Inductive

Methods

Reconstructive surgery has been one of the two most dynamic therapeutic procedures in periodontics in the past decade. The attraction of recapturing lost periodontal attachment has been an old one. Prichard and Goldman and Cohen have been most successful in efforts to achieve reconstitution of lost periodontal attachment, but successful attempts occurred much earlier by Younger and many others. In 1957 Prichard established incontrovertibly that success was a clinical fact and that it was, in certain circumstances, predictable. His reentry procedures provided definite proof that new bone and new attachment had indeed been gained. His conclusions were confirmed shortly by Goldman and Cohen.

The interest with which this accomplishment is regarded is underlined by the fact, repeated several times in varying contexts, that resective techniques in pocket elimination have serious limitations in extremely deep defects. Reattachment, the reconstitution of lost bone and ligament, has no such limitations if other special requirements are met.

Unfortunately, the application of methods of reconstituted attachment do require special topographic features to be successful. While intrabony pockets are by no means rare, they are not nearly so common as are other periodontal resorptive lesions. They are common enough, however, to constitute a sizable minority of periodontal lesions.

TOPOGRAPHY

In surgery so completely identified with plastic repair it is not surprising that topography should play so important a role. It is certainly well understood that the pathology of a pocket is the same everywhere, no matter what its form. Other factors dictate the shape of the resorptive lesions. Aside from the age of the lesion and its severity, it is principally the mass of bone investing the root that will determine the form the defect will take.

In Chapter 22 the topographic requirements for lesion form were dealt with in some detail. Some discussion of topography is in order in the context of the intrabony pocket. Certain areas naturally lend themselves to intrabony pockets. The mass and configuration of bone in which the roots are invested are critical to lesion form.

A good example is the mylohyoid ridge of the mandible. A resorptive lesion adjacent to the root of the tooth will unavoidably assume an intrabony form in this area. The same is true in areas adjacent to the external oblique ridge. It is impossible for it to be otherwise. Tori near the crest of the alveolar process fall into the same category as do all bony excrescences that are marginal to the process.

Some thick bony margins are due to muscle insertions. Whether the enlargement of bone is a physiologic response to function or a pathologic manifestation, however mild, makes little difference in the course of periodontal destruction. Once again it must be stated that the form a lesion takes depends upon the mass and distribution of bone in which the affected root exists. This fact becomes central to therapy in a great number of cases.

The intrabony pocket has many forms. There are hemisepta, funnel-shaped patterns, two-walled intrabony pockets in the form of bony craters, a two-walled pattern in the shape of a hemiseptum with a proximal wall plus a buccal or lingual wall, and, finally, a three-walled intrabony pocket. Then all the variants come into the picture: the three-walled lesion in the deep recesses of the defect which becomes two-walled and even one-walled crestally as one or another wall is lost.

A number of methods have been introduced having the objective of inducing bone, cementum, and ligament to regenerate so that the defect will be obliterated in whole or part by a reconstituted attachment apparatus. The most successful induction of new epithelial attachment has been routinely attained in deep, narrow cryptlike intrabony pockets having three bony walls. A number of methods were introduced to induce new attachment in intrabony lesions not so well endowed. Wide, shallow three-walled lesions, two-walled lesions, and hemisepta are examples of topographic resorptions that showed little or no repair with standard methods and constituted a challenge for imaginative operators.

The response to the challenge consisted of the introduction of insertions and additives of various substances into the bony defect. Autogenous ground bone, bone chips, bone and marrow, and plaster are some of the substances used with varying success; swaging of hemisepta or other solitary bony walls into the lesion is another expedient.

In all cases the method to be applied depends upon the task to be accomplished. Whether a classic reattachment approach is used or whether a so-called swaging procedure is to be applied obviously depends upon the topography and the availability of bone, marrow, and linear dimension of periodontal tissue, and upon the application of these factors to the solution chosen for the clinical problem.

The particular form of the lesion is most important in all periodontal case management but nowhere as critical as in inductive methods. If any proof were needed, one need only examine the careful pairing of method and lesion form in every projection of technique.

THE THREE-WALLED INTRABONY LESION

Induction of new attachment to replace that destroyed by chronic destructive periodontal disease has, until recently, been proved incontrovertibly only in the three-walled bony crypt adjacent to the affected root. For this reason, the treatment of the three-walled lesion has been called the classic intrabony therapy. Of course there is nothing classic about it. The deep, narrow, three-walled bony lesion merely lends itself to successful therapy on a predictable basis. This has been shown by Prichard so many times as to have established the results beyond cavil.[35]

The question might be asked "Why does this particular result require so much proving?" The answer to this reasonable question lies in the long history of reattachment. Over the years there have been many apparently sincere claims of reattachment. These have all been based upon radiographic and subjective probing evidence. It must be understood that the results were random—no clear list for the requirements for success was ever drawn. An occasional pair of radiographs (the preoperative and postoperative films) seemed to reveal a healed intrabony lesion by a bone-fill (Fig. 23-1).

It was not long before the unreliability of radiographic evidence was brought to light. It is not surprising that, considering the vague criteria for therapy and

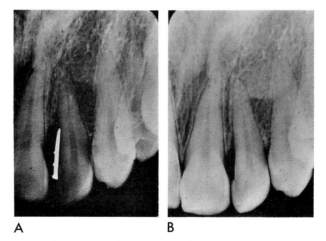

A   B

FIG. 23-1. *Radiographic evidence of an intrabony fill or of a partial reconstitution of lost periodontal attachment. A. Preoperative view with a Hirschfeld silver point in the pocket scored to indicate that an 8-mm lesion was measured from the gingival margin. B. Two years after intrabony pocket therapy the pocket cannot be probed by any means.*

the questionable dependability of the medium of proof of success, that some doubt was thrown over the entire effort. Many therapists were frankly skeptical of all proof of success. No one before Prichard had offered direct visual proof both before and after treatment. It was perfectly reasonable to doubt the evidence when it consisted only of radiographic films plus the mere statement of the therapist that the lesion could not be probed. The failure of other therapists to eliminate pockets by the means described was another factor in the widespread skepticism with which these results were held.

The question is often raised, "Why is success in the three-walled intrabony pocket relatively predictable?" There is really no mystery in this when it is considered that the only known and established source for osteogenetic elements and multipotential primitive mesenchymal tissue generally lies in the periodontal space. It seems obvious that the greater the quantity of these elements available relative to the magnitude of the defect to be repaired, the greater the chance for success. These conditions are best met in the long, narrow,

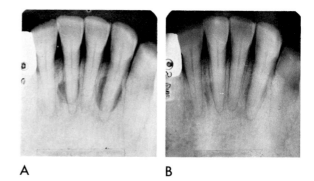

A   **B**

FIG. 23-3. *A rather unusual topographic configuration of bone resorption of an intrabony nature. The pocket aperture is in the lingual marginal gingiva. There were no habit patterns to which the lesions might be attributable.*

constricted three-walled cryptlike defect; which has the maximum amount of the necessary tissue and minimal amounts of space to be filled and repaired (Fig. 23-2).

On the other hand, a shallow, wide-mouthed, broad intrabony defect presents far greater volume of defect with far less availability of repairing tissue in the comparatively short linear dimension of periodontal space bordering the lesion. All the variants between these two extremes will respond proportionally to the availability of multipotential tissue in relation to the volume of the defect (Fig. 23-3).

If this is true, then all the mystery of the relative success in the cryptlike defect disappears. The two-walled defect, such as the bony crater or other configurations, and the one-walled lesion, such as the hemiseptum, all require enormous volumes of repaired tissues relative to the meager amount of multipotential tissue available. It becomes easier to understand why these last have meager success, if any, and why the search for inductive aids has been so active.

These inductive aids have been several. Allografts and autografts of various kinds have been used with variable success. So-called swaging has been attempted in suitable sites. The success rate has not been spectacular. None of these latter inductive methods can be said to have achieved the status of standard methods as yet.

Even the successful postoperative results in pocket repair in these methods using inductive aids have a disturbing tendency to break down after a period of months or several years. There is a growing tendency to avoid using teeth showing a successful repair as key abutments in prostheses. Some outstanding restorative specialists require information on the method used in achieving pocket closure. They consider only the deep, narrow, three-walled lesion with a definite bone fill to be reliable for restorative purposes.

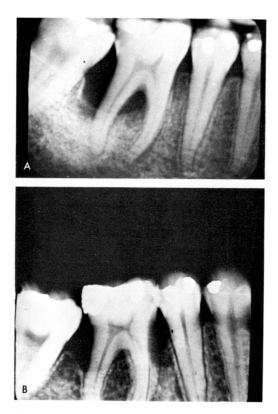

FIG. 23-2. *Radiographic evidence of new attachment induction in a lower first molar. A. Before treatment. The lower molar has a deep intrabony resorptive lesion on its distal aspect which has apparently involved the interfurcal bone and epithelial attachment as well. B. Four years after treatment. The distal and interfurcal lesions can no longer be probed.*

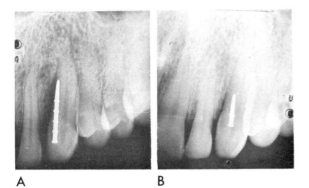

FIG. 23-4. *Radiographic evidence of successful new attachment in an uncontrolled diabetic. A. Before treatment. Therapy consisted of simple curettage of the root and the three-walled bony crypt after flap reflection and field exposure. B. One year after treatment. Note that the opaque point cannot be inserted on the mesiopalatal line angle after therapy but was deflected to the midpalatal surface of the canine.*

At the present writing the two most promising methods of induction of new attachment are the iliac crest bone and marrow grafts and, more recently, scleral grafts. Not much is known about scleral inserts except that in some cases closure is achieved. Reentry reveals that the scleral graft is apparently intact and unchanged. The iliac crest bone and marrow graft, on the other hand, undergo certain interesting changes, some of which are discussed later in the chapter.

Field Exposure

In all methods designed to induce new epithelial attachment, whether by the so-called classic approach, or by grafts or inductive agents, the requirements for field exposure are identical. Full-thickness flap reflection is the rule in these areas, since the bony margins of the lesion should be thoroughly exposed and carefully debrided. There are exceptions to the rule when the labial plate is suspected of being very thin. In such a contingency only the margin of bone is exposed, leaving the remainder of the labial plate covered with much of the lamina propria of a split-thickness flap.

The mesiodistal extent of exposure should be at least one tooth on either side of the defect. Usually the attempt for new attachment in a single lesion is made as part of routine treatment for an entire quadrant. If, however, the intrabony pocket is a single lesion in the entire quadrant, then the full-thickness flap reflection applies (Fig. 23-4).

Flap Design for New Attachment Procedures

In flap design for an intrabony approach the wisest course is to ensure that the flaps are long enough to

adequately cover the treated area so that the margins are well coapted to seal the mouth of the lesion. In ensuring such a secure and adequate cover the flaps may be somewhat long. These flaps are usually closed in too coronal a position. This means that postoperatively there will be some redundant tissue that will require gingivoplastic repair. This is of little consequence, considering the advantage gained.

OPERATIVE TECHNIQUE

A vertical releasing incision will permit flexibility in the management of the various types of resorptive lesions (Fig. 23-5). Cryptlike lesions may be treated by curettage and induction of an additive such as bone marrow, osseous coagulum, or sclera, whereas shallow craters are best reshaped by osseous resection. Both methods may be used if principles of flap management are observed. The cuspid region may require a crestal approximation, but the posterior region should usually have an apically repositioned flap.

Suturing may be by either continuous sling or interrupted suture, depending upon the requirements of the individual area. Obviously the isolated intrabony pocket would require interrupted sutures for closure. Where suspensary sling sutures are used, care must be taken to ensure adequate flap coverage in the intrabony area. This sometimes means that the flap will be carefully tailored to meet two or more differing mucosal repair situations, complete coverage in one area with vertical releasing incisions to permit repositioning in others.

If cement dressings are used, the sutured flap should be covered with foil to avoid impingement of the dressing into the treated pocket. Some operators also cover the cement with foil.

POSTOPERATIVE MANAGEMENT

Postoperative probing may not be safely done earlier than 3 months. Perforation of the healing tissue is likely earlier. Reentry for bony reshaping is not advisable earlier than at least 6 months after surgery.

Objectives of Treatment

The objective in the treatment of the three-walled intrabony defect is essentially one of debridement of the root surface within the pocket confines with curets, plus the removal of all soft tissue covering the bony walls. The epithelial attachment must also be completely removed to expose the periodontal space.

Prichard contends that excessive curettage of the root surfaces is easy to do and that it is his distinct

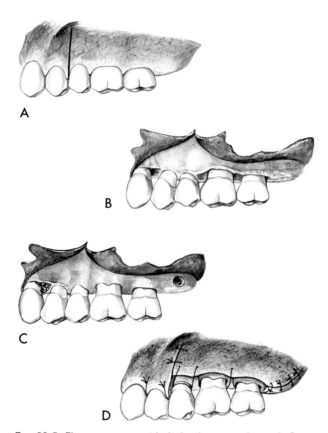

A

B

C

D

FIG. 23-5. *Flap management in inductive procedures. A. Sample segment representing the operative field. The heavy vertical line divides the canine and first premolar from the second premolar and first and second molars. It also represents the site of the vertical releasing incision and permits different modes of management of different resorptive lesions. B. Flaps reflected at the line of the releasing incision, revealing a three-walled intrabony lesion on the distal side of the canine, which requires an attempt at induction. Distal to that area, in the interproximal bone of the second premolar and the first and second molars are bony craters, which are best treated by reshaping by resection. Induction and resection can both be used if principles of flap management are observed. C. After treatment of the intrabony lesion with curettage and the insertion of bone marrow. The distal lesions were reduced by osseous resection. The trephine aperture in the tuberosity region illustrates an expedient in obtaining bone marrow intraorally. D. Wound closure, following principles of flap management. Note the snug closure in the region of the intrabony lesion where induction of new epithelial attachment was attempted. The apically repositioned flap in the distal segment of the area seems to expose marginal bone. This approach is not commonly used but is illustrated here for contrast.*

impression, shared by others, that the chances for success diminish with extensive curettage of root surface. The conclusion drawn must be that cementum on the root contributes something to successful induction of new attachment. It appears that new cementum is laid down much more readily over old cementum than would be the case if it were removed by curettage.

This proscription does not apply to the bony walls of

the crypt. Not only should they be curetted with meticulous care to remove every shred of ligament or other soft tissue adhering, but many skilled clinicians perforate the bony walls with a bur. For some reason this procedure is referred to as decortication.

Great care must be exercised in curettage of the bone within the lesion to reach all the recesses of the pocket. It is easy to miss the edges of the crypt because of extremely constricted quarters. Small sharp instruments are a prime necessity for the removal of the epithelial attachment. A fine sharp-pointed scaler is useful, although by no means indispensable; a fine curet would do as well. The tip of the instrument is used as a gouge to remove the epithelial attachment and to expose the periodontal space. Care must be exercised to traverse the entire extent of the pocket. The bony walls of the pocket must be carefully examined under a good light to make certain the bone has been completely debrided.

Decortication

In all intrabony lesions many therapists use a #$\frac{1}{2}$ round bur to perforate the bony wall at 2-mm to 3-mm intervals within the crypt or defect to expose cancellous bone. The designation of the procedure as decortication is not, strictly speaking, an accurate one, since it is not cortical bone that is being perforated. However, the term is widely used and is universally understood in periodontal circles (Fig. 23-6).

Just what these perforations accomplish is difficult to state with certainty. It is generally accepted that cancellous bone is far superior to cortical plate as source material for bone induction, but the bony wall itself is cancellous bone. The possible availability of

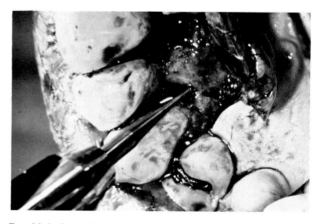

FIG. 23-6. *Decortication with a #$\frac{1}{2}$ round bur within the confines of the bony resorptive lesion. In this illustration the bony wall of the pocket is being perforated at 2 to 3 mm intervals after removal of all vestiges of soft tissue remnants. The purpose of the perforations opening into marrow spaces is to make available granulation tissue with osteogenetic potential.*

osteogenetic tissue in cancellous bone does not provide a rationale for the repeated perforation of the bony wall of the pocket.

Decortication is only one of the expedients used in the hope of a take. It is, however, the only one that does not require an additive. Any fill that occurs is therefore totally endogenous, as it were, and not attributable to any extraneous material.

Antibiotic Therapy

The use of antibiotics in therapy for the intrabony pocket is more or less standard procedure with most clinicians. The reason for this practice is completely empirical. It seems to be effective as a preventive of sepsis in the healing wound. Whether antibiotic therapy is a necessity in successful treatment has not been established on a rational or scientific basis, but antibiotic coverage is almost universally used in the usual manner, i.e., one day preoperatively and for 5 to 6 days after that so that any surgical procedure for inducing new attachment is performed under the protective effect of the drug of choice. These include the tetracycline, erythromycin stearates, or penicillin in proper dosage and administration.

THE WIDE-MOUTHED SHALLOW INTRABONY POCKET

Some topographic features are not favorable to the formation of new attachment. One of these lesions is the three-walled intrabony pocket that is wide, or even cavernous, but shallow. Using the rationale of the availability of multipotential tissue for repair on a volumetric basis, it can be seen that such a funnel-shaped pocket presents a distinctly unfavorable prospect for success. In this respect the bony crater, the hemiseptum, and other two- and one-walled infrabony resorptive lesions present similar unfavorable topographic features for repair by the standard intrabony treatment of curettage of root, bony crypt, and epithelial attachment. It is for this reason that these topographic aberrations stimulated a search for inductive methods or materials designed to overcome the unfavorable repair factors. Additives to help induce a fill and reconstitution of new attachment have included bone chips, granulating tissue, and bone coagulum.

Bone Chips

Bone chips taken from an area some variable distance from the lesion site have been used for some time. Nabers and O'Leary reported successful takes using bone chips.[30] The method of application is rather a straightforward one. The bony defect is prepared to receive the graft in precisely the manner used in the deep narrow bony crypt. The root is adequately curetted, although not overcuretted, the bony walls are meticulously freed from all fibrous shreds, and the epithelial attachment is removed with the tip of the instrument (Fig. 23-7).

The bone chips are packed into the defect firmly and are incorporated with some extravasated blood from the area. The flap is carefully coapted and closure by interrupted suture is accomplished.

The procurement of the bone chips presents some features that should be taken into account. The picture is by no means clear on the relative merits of cancellous bone over cortical plate as grafting material. This is not to be confused with osteogenetic tissue. The grafting material provides a scaffold upon which osteogenetic tissue lays down new bone. It is commonly held that cancellous bone in small chips, or even powder, is superior to cortical bone in larger fragments. This position does not seem to be supported by the facts as currently understood. Cortical bone in larger fragments, consistent with the size of the lesion, is at the moment preferred by some sophisticated operators.

Practical procedure requires that the donor site be somewhat adjacent to the operative field. Since the results of these grafts are far from predictable, heroic methods in procurement are hardly indicated.

Granulation Tissue

Occasionally a donor site can be developed from a recent extraction site. Developing granulation tissue within a healing socket provides excellent material to be used in a graft for bone induction. Such a transfer provides an ample graft but must be carefully planned in treatment sequence. In other words, the extraction must be performed precisely 6 to 8 weeks before the lesion is reconstructed so that properly aged granulating tissue is available in suitable amounts on demand.

Opening into the intrabony lesion and closure postoperatively is precisely like the opening and closure for any intrabony approach to induce new attachment. The flaps should have long interproximal papillae so that the mouth of the lesion may be effectively closed with tissue to ensure a fairly good seal. Even under optimum conditions some of the graft is usually lost through the gingival margin of the lesion.

Bone Coagulum

Everyone who has reshaped bone with a rotary instrument has noticed ground bone powder—some-

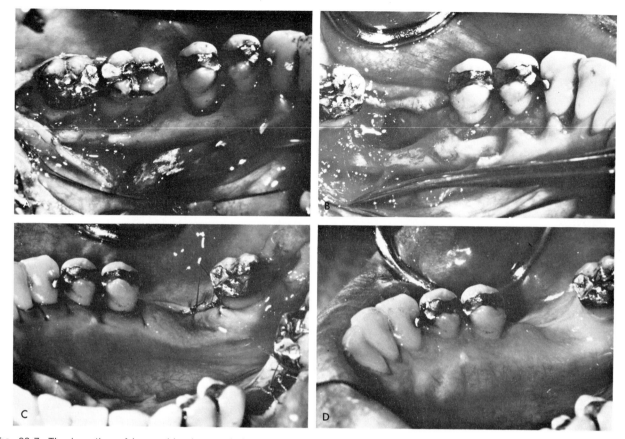

FIG. 23-7. *The insertion of bone chips into periodontal defects. The bone chips were procured from the extraction site of the hopelessly involved first molar. A. Flaps reflected and the operative field exposed. B. The first molar has been removed, and the bone chips have been procured from the resultant socket margins and have been packed into the lesions lingual to the premolars. C. The flaps sutured and the extraction partially closed. The apparent reversal is due to the use of a mirror for the last two photographic exposures. D. Three months after surgery. Probing reveals minimal depth at this time. (Treated by Dr. D. Engen.)*

times mixed with blood—which accumulates in variable quantities on retractors and mouth mirrors. Robinson has collected this material in a dappen dish and has reserved it for immediate use in filling a bony defect due to periodontal disease.[39,40] It is used in precisely the same indications as bone chips. In fact it is often used in combination with bone chips when either chips or bone dust is in short supply. Aside from the vagaries of a take, which is not reliably predictable, the difficulty with this method lies in procuring the grafting material. Donor sites are sometimes present and sometimes not. Careful planning will provide a donor site where it might have been overlooked by a routine approach.

In inserting a coagulum graft it is well not to overfill the defect, since excess grafting material is lost in any case through the margins even though they be well closed (Fig. 23-8). The gradual extrusion and exfoliation of chips and coagulum continues for a number of weeks even when the area is not overfilled.

THE TWO-WALLED AND ONE-WALLED INTRABONY LESIONS

Up to this point the principal focus of interest has been on the three-walled intrabony lesion or, more correctly, on the intrabony lesion leaving a three-walled component as a portion of its extent. It is no secret that the most common lesions are the two-walled and single-walled intrabony resorptive patterns. Many of these are craters and hemisepta.

A significant portion of the effort to find inductive aids has been for the reason that these two-walled and one-walled defects are so common. For the most part additives such as bone chips, osseous coagulum, and iliac crest marrow on bone implants are used precisely as they are in the more fortunately endowed three-walled defects. The lack of response in this clinical context has been discouraging. The only exception to this finding has been the response in Dragoo's experience with bone marrow.[12-14]

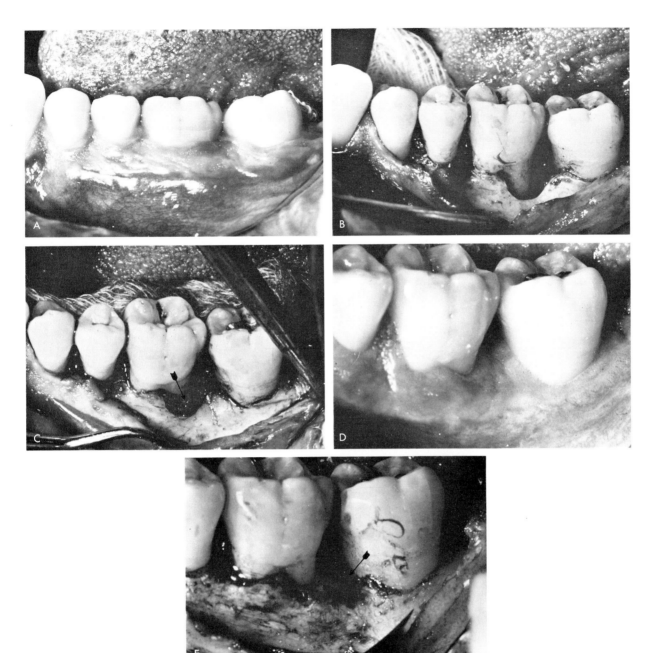

FIG. 23-8. *Coagulum insert in new attachment induction. The use of ground autogenous bone in a wide-mouthed intrabony lesion with a portion of the resorptive pattern with less than three bony walls. A. The operative site before entry. On probing the lower first molar a deep distal lesion is revealed which extends to the buccal aspect of the distal root. The septal bone on the mesial of the second molar is undisturbed and intact when probed. B. Flaps reflected and the operative site revealed showing an extensive lesion more or less confirming the impression gained by probing. C. Bone coagulum or ground autogenous bone dust mixed with extravasated blood inserted into the lesion up to the bone margin but not coronal to it. The arrow is directed to the coagulum insert. D. The operative site one year after surgery. Probing reveals minimal sulcular depth throughout the operative site. E. Reentry into the operative site showing new attachment and bone to about the level of the coagulum insert. (Treated by Dr. H. Selipsky.)*

Swaging

The one method that seems designed specifically to treat one- and two-walled craters and hemisepta is bone swaging. It consists of bending and breaking thin bony walls *into* the periodontal defect. The rationalization that these fractured spines and unsupported walls behave like greenstick fractures in long bones in young individuals is totally unsupported by any sound data. Some of the results obtained are equivocal and can be evaluated only by admittedly imprecise clinical impression. Some successes appear to have been due to new attachment rather than shrinkage. Swaging does not always concern itself with thin walls that lend themselves to bending and partial fracture to move them into the periodontal defect. One such case is shown in Figure 23-9 in which a deep cavernous *three*-walled defect on the mesial side of a second molar is treated by cutting a wedge of bone in the

saddle area just mesial to the defect and swaging the wedge of bone into the defect and in close approximation to the mesial surface of the root. The flaps are then sutured.

The so-called swaging method is designed to induce the filling of an intrabony defect with new bone and attachment. It is performed by carefully undermining the bony wall or walls comprising the intrabony defect. Care must be exercised not to completely separate the

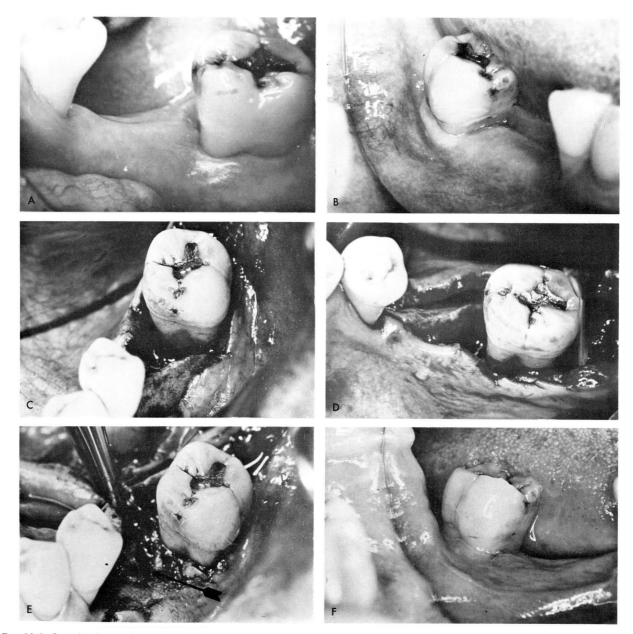

FIG. 23-9. *Swaging by cutting a block of bone with a three-sided cut on the buccal, lingual, and proximal sides to the depth of the defect with a fissure bur. A. Preoperative view of the molar from the lingual side. B. Preoperative view from the buccal side. C. Flaps reflected and the lesion exposed. D. Lateral view of the resorptive crypt in bone. E. The bone of the saddle area mesial to the molar has been cut in a U-shaped block and pushed into the defect and against the root. This opened a space mesial to the block of bone (arrow). F. Eight months after surgery. The site of the pocket can be probed only to normal depth. (Treated by Dr. L. Pearson.)*

bony wall from its base, since it is felt that some of the potential for a bone fill will have been lost if this happens. The actual undermining is best done with a narrow tapering fissure bur. The cut in bone is made at the base of the bony walls to facilitate bending the wall into the defect. The cut is not made quite through the entire base, however. After this is completed, the undermined wall is pushed into the defect. The method of accomplishing this is quite straightforward. A number of operators use an amalgam plugger as a useful instrument. The serrated face of the instrument engages the bone to be swaged firmly so that either hand pressure, if that is sufficient, or a light blow from the mallet will move it into the defect.

After the bony wall has been swaged into the previously prepared and debrided defect, the flaps are tightly closed with interrupted sutures. It should be kept in mind in reflecting flaps for all the procedures destined for autogenous bone grafts that they need all the gingiva available, since tight closure is paramount. It is for this reason that a sulcus cut is the rule in marginal flap design.

Swaging is useful in one-walled or hemiseptal defects. Craters with extremely thin buccal or lingual walls are other defects which have been treated in this fashion. Success in these attempts is difficult to evaluate. It is well known that mere exposure will cause thin processes and spicules of bone to resorb. This will occur even more readily if these thin walls are bent and broken into a defect. It is for this reason that all reports of crater filling or hemiseptum repairing must be viewed with skepticism. The question must be asked, "Did the defect heal from the bottom or did it resorb from the peripheral walls delimiting the lesion?" The mere shallowing of a crater is not enough. Incontrovertible evidence has never been offered.

Skepticism alone, however, will heal no pockets. Although it is useful to maintain balance, it should not be used to discourage innovation. There is a success rate to these procedures. They are, however, not standard methods with clearly predictable results. For that reason they are used in lesions not manageable by any other means. Gaping wide-mouthed resorptive lesions, hemisepta, and deep craters with thin buccal and lingual walls that cannot be leveled without mortally damaging the support for the adjacent teeth, these are the prime indications for autogenous bone grafts of all kinds. It is true that the success rate is low in most. For this reason their inclusion into a routine treatment plan must await further developments and a higher ratio of success to failure.

The alternative is to accept reverse architecture, often practically impossible to maintain, or extraction of the involved teeth. It is true, of course, that the corollary to a low success rate is the resort to these alternatives only as a last resort. When these alternatives must be resorted to, it is important that the operator does not delude himself and his patient with false hopes. In some of the apparent successes with swaging, the pockets regress after 6 months to a year postoperatively. This result is also true of other autogenous procedures as well. For this reason it is best to take a rather pessimistic view of these lesions in prognosis. Unscheduled and unpromised success is easy to explain to a patient who has been prepared to accept failure.

Autogenous Marrow and Bone Grafts

The use of red marrow and bone of various kinds for the induction of bone is not new. Orthopedists have been using this material for a long time. Hematologists routinely take biopsy cores from the sternum and ilium. It remained for Schallhorn, however, to apply these tissues to grafting to induce new attachment in defects caused by periodontal destruction.[46]

Generally the marrow grafts are of two general types: (1) marrow and bone from the tuberosity, or from some other alveolar process site, and (2) marrow from the posterior or anterior iliac crest. The iliac crest can yield far more marrow and cancellous bone than can the tuberosity. In fact, some tuberosities yield little or none, whereas orthopedists may remove the anterior cortical plate and literally use a cupful of marrow to aid in the repair of large defects in bone. Such quantities are not necessary for repair of periodontal lesions in bone, however. The use of the Westerman-Jensen biopsy needle or the Turkell biopsy needle for obtaining small cores provides enough marrow and bone for most periodontal purposes. These cores, about 1 cm long with a diameter of 2 to 3 mm, pack nicely into bony defects. Usually as many as three cores may be obtained from a single puncture of the posterior iliac crest, and many more (12 to 15) from the anterior crest. The use of the posterior iliac crest for entry yields a meager amount of bone and marrow for use in large cavernous defects. In using this entry an occasional second puncture is required. This is not the case when using the much larger Turkell needle in the anterior crest.

The defect should be filled to the marginal lip of bone, not overfilled, and firmly packed. The wound is closed in the usual manner. The flaps are best coapted with interrupted sutures throughout. A cement dressing can be placed over the sutured flaps although many therapists dispense with this step. Most allow the sutures to remain for 8 to 10 days.

These hip marrow grafts are quite successful in

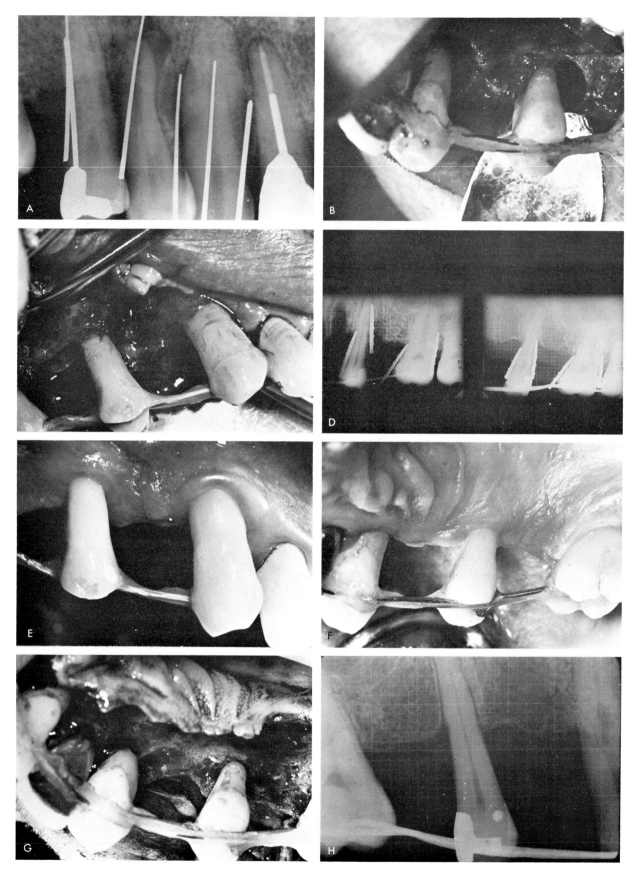

FIG. 23-10. *Iliac crest bone marrow and bone grafts in new attachment induction procedure. A. Preoperative radiographs with radiopaque points inserted into the periodontal pockets of the upper left quadrant. The "hopelessly involved" teeth were then extracted. B. Palatal view 5 months after the extraction in A with the operative site exposed by the reflection of full thickness flaps*

selected cases when given half a chance. Too many marrow grafts have been placed in hopeless situations about teeth that were doomed under any circumstances. Wide-mouthed three-walled infrabony pockets, some craters, and even narrow, deep hemisepta have some interesting successes to show.

The connotation of success should be clearly established before claims are made or disputed. In a recent study by Dragoo and Sullivan using block sections of preoperatively scored roots of teeth treated with fresh bone and marrow, it has been shown that 2 to 3 mm gain in new epithelial attachment was a definitely attainable result in properly selected cases.[13] The occasional and random spectacular fill is certainly not a common result, but the occasional brilliant success illustrated in Figure 23-10 should stimulate more and better clinical research. Even with reentry procedures recorded photographically, too much depends on angles of view, illusion, and altered relationships to make quantitative assay practical. Properly scored roots in block sections are another matter, however. On the basis of such an assay 2 to 3 mm constitutes a successful take.

One disturbing factor, however, has been the predilection to root resorption in many of the successful results. This means that, if resorption is not arrested, the root will eventually be resorbed. Several explanations have been offered for this phenomenon. One has been overscaling the root so that most, if not all, the cementum has been removed. Just how this has been determined is not clear. Another reason offered is that fresh, newly obtained marrow is altogether too active an osteogenetic tissue and that it attacks the root and replaces it with bone. The opinion is that frozen marrow is reduced just enough in viability to make bone regeneration possible without destroying the root. This reasoning, too, is highly conjectural with no solid evidence to support it. The area of root resorption is not adjacent to the graft. It seems to be coronal to the lesion area and is commonly supracrestal (Fig. 23-11).

The pattern of root resorption is worthy of note. The resorptive bays are supracrestal. The connection between a successful take and root resorption is certainly not clear. The picture of hyperactive osteogenetic tissue destroying the root does not seem to be as simple and straightforward as it once seemed, since the supracrestal location of resorption places all earlier explanations in doubt. Marginal gingivitis is ubiquitous enough to have established a clear relationship with root resorption if any existed. The possibility that the impending root resorption results in a marginal gingivitis is a distinct possibility. This possibility, too, has not been established.

In an interesting series of photographs of a patient treated by Dragoo and Sullivan in 1972 an iliac crest bone and marrow graft was evidently successful (Fig. 23-12).[13,14] Closure of the wound was followed by a gingival hyperemia and hyperplasia. Root resorption resulted and progressed to an alarming degree. Vigorous and repeated root curettage reinforced by improved maintenance by the patient resulted in a reversal of the root resorption and an apparent remineralization of the root.

It is too early at the present writing to give consideration to autogenous iliac crest grafts as a standard method. It is certain that many are being done. Most are failing at the moment, but failure may be due to poor technique, poorly chosen cases, an inherent weakness in the material, or possibly a combination of two or all three of these. Work going forward at the moment should provide more definitive information.

All new procedures are attractive and present interesting alternatives in treatment. None is more exciting than the induction of new periodontal attachment. It is unquestionably in this direction that the horizons of therapy lie.

---

and debridement of the area. Note the cavernous lesions involving the canine and second premolar. C. Buccal view immediately before the insertion of the bone and marrow grafts. D. Radiographs of the operative site before graft insertion and 8 months after insertion of bone and marrow grafts with Hirschfeld points inserted in both radiographs. E. Eight months after the graft insertion: buccal view. Temporary stabilization was achieved by the use of a wire and acrylic splint. F. Palatal view of the area shown in E 8 months after surgery. G. Reentry into the operative site 8 months after surgery. H. Eight months postoperative radiograph of the site. (Treated by Dr. M. Dragoo.)

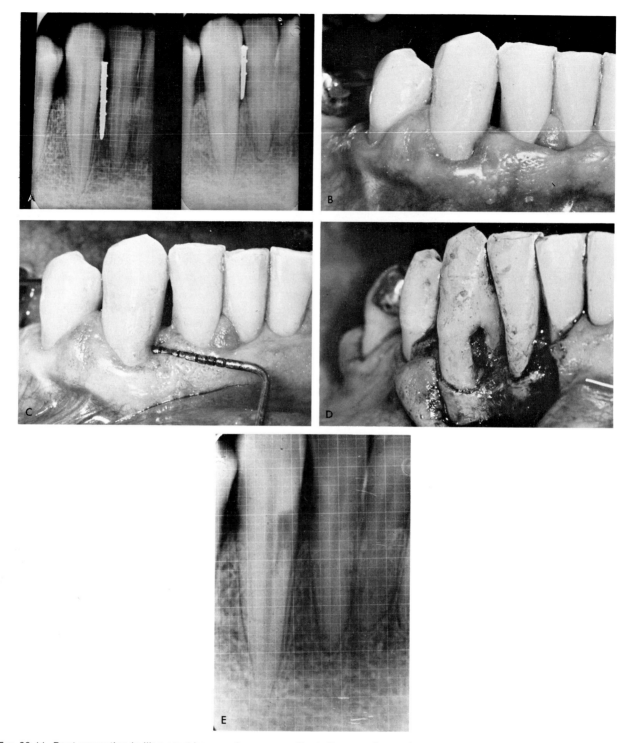

FIG. 23-11. Root resorption in iliac crest bone and marrow grafts. A. Preoperative and postoperative radiographs of an autogenous bone and marrow graft on the mesial side of the lower left canine. The postoperative radiograph was taken 8 months after the insertion of the graft. B. Photograph of the canine region 8 months after the graft insertion. Note the marginal hyperemia and hyperplasia. The postoperative history revealed poor maintenance on the part of the patient and a resultant persistent gingivitis. C. Probe inserted into the resorption lesion in the root. The lesion is clearly supracrestal to the bone margin. D. Flap reflected from the teeth and bone in the resorptive area. E. Eight month postoperative radiograph. The depth and extent of the resorption is close to the pulp. The tooth was eventually lost. (Treated by Dr. M. Dragoo.)

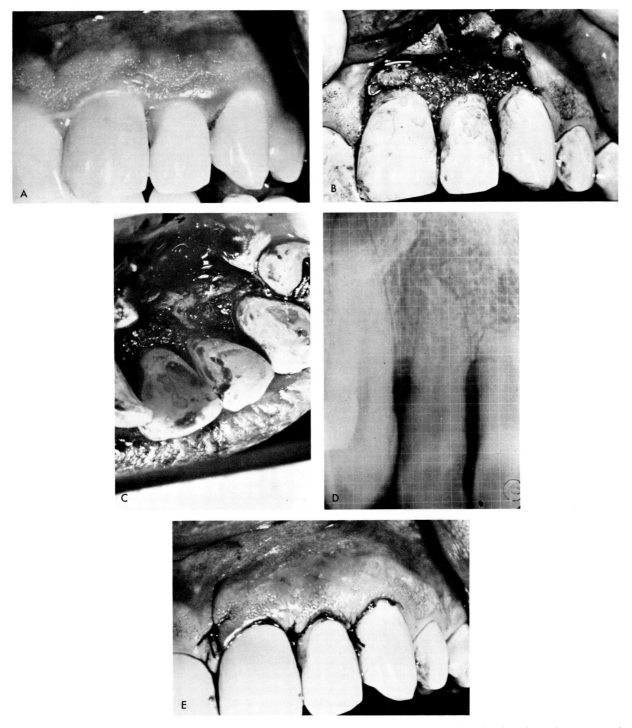

FIG. 23-12. *Iliac crest bone and marrow graft in an upper left lateral incisor which began to show alarming signs of root resorption (once again supracrestally) associated with marginal gingival hyperemia and hyperplasia. A. Preoperative view of the area to be treated. B. Labial flap reflected and the large defect filled with an iliac crest bone and marrow graft. C. Palatal view of the surgical field with flap reflected and the circumferential defect filled with iliac crest bone and marrow graft material. D. Radiograph of the area at the time of surgery. Root resorption has apparently begun. E. Area closed and flaps sutured with good coaptation.*

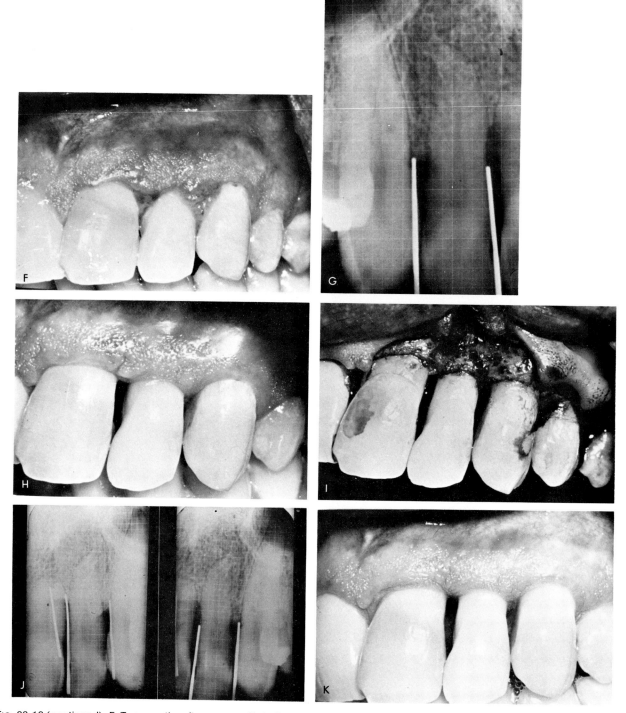

FIG. 23-12 (continued). *F. Two months after surgery. Note that marginal gingivitis and enlargement have recurred. G. Radiograph of the area with opaque points inserted. H. Gingival response to repeated subgingival curettage. I. Reentry into the operative field revealing a good take of the graft. Resorption has stopped, and the root has apparently remineralized and repaired itself. J. Preoperative and 8-month postoperative radiographs. K. Final postoperative view of the area 2 months after reentry. The root is sound and has apparently recovered from the resorptive onslaught. (Treated by Dr. M. Dragoo.)*

References

1. Burnette, E. W.: Limitations of the roentgenograph in periodontal diagnosis. J. Periodontol., *42:*293, 1971.
2. Carranza, F. A.: A technique for reattachment. J. Periodontol., *25:*272, 1954.
3. Carranza, F. A., Jr., and Glickman, I.: Some observations on the microscopic features of infrabony pockets. J. Periodontol., *28:*33, 1957.
4. Carranza, F. S., and Carranza, F. A., Jr.: The management of the alveolar bone in the treatment of the periodontal pocket. J. Periodontol., *27:*29, 1956.
5. Carranza, F. S., Carranza, F. A., Jr., and Carraro, J. P.: Paradontal disease: local therapy. Int. Dent. J., *7:*209, 1957.
6. Cohen, B. M.: Antibiotics and intraoral bone grafts. J. Oral Surg., *13:*34, 1955.
7. Cohen, B.: Pathology of the interdental tissues. Dent. Pract. Dent. Rec., *9:*167, 1959.
8. Cross, W. G.: Bone grafts in periodontal disease. Dent. Pract. Dent. Rec., *6:*3, 1955.
9. Cross, W. G.: Reattachment following curettage. Dent. Pract. Dent. Rec., *7:*2, 1956.
10. Cross, W. G.: The use of bone implants in the treatment of periodontal pockets. Dent. Clin. North Am., Mar, 1960, p. 107.
11. Cushing, M.: Review of literature. Autogenous red marrow grafts: their potential for induction of osteogenesis. J. Periodontol., *40:*492, 1969.
12. Dragoo, M. R., and Irwin, R. K.: A method of procuring cancellous iliac bone utilizing a trephine needle. J. Periodontol., *43:*82, 1972.
13. Dragoo, M. R., and Sullivan, H. C.: A clinical and histologic evaluation of autogenous iliac bone grafts in humans. I. Wound healing, 2–8 months. J. Periodontol., *44:*599, 1973.
14. Dragoo, M. R., and Sullivan, H. C.: A clinical and histologic evaluation of autogenous iliac bone grafts in humans. II. External root resorption. J. Periodontol., *44:*614, 1973.
15. Ewen, S. J.: Bone swaging. J. Periodontol., *36:*57, 1965.
16. Forsberg, H.: Transplantation of ospurum and bone chips in the surgical treatment of periodontal disease. Acta Odont. Scand., *13:*235, 1955.
17. Friedman, N.: Reattachment and roentgenograms. J. Periodontol., *29:*98, 1958.
18. Goldman, H. M.: The relationship of the epithelial attachment to the adjacent fibers of the periodontal membrane. J. Dent. Res., *23:*117, 1944.
19. Goldman, H. M.: A rationale for the treatment of the intrabony pocket. J. Periodontol., *20:*83, 1949.
20. Goldman, H. M., and Cohen, D. W.: The infrabony pocket: classification and treatment. J. Periodontol., *29:*272, 1958.
21. Halliday, D. G.: The grafting of newly formed autogenous bone in the treatment of osseous defects. J. Periodontol., *40:*511, 1969.
22. Ham, A. W., and Harris, W. R.: Repair and transplantation of bone. *In* The Biochemistry and Physiology of Bone. G. H. Bourne, Ed. New York, Academic Press, 1956.
23. Hiatt, W. H.: Regeneration of the periodontium after endodontic therapy and flap operation. Oral Surg., *12:*1471, 1959.
24. Klingsberg, J.: Periodontal scleral grafts and combined grafts of sclera and bone: two year appraisal, J. Periodontol., *45:*262, 1974.
25. Mann, W. V.: Autogenous transplant in the treatment of an infrabony pocket. Case Report. J.A.S.P., *2:*205, 1964.
26. Morris, M. L.: Healing of human periodontal tissues following surgical detachment from non-vital teeth. J. Periodontol., *28:*222, 1957.
27. Morris, M. L.: Healing of human periodontal tissues following surgical detachment. Periodontics, *1:*147, 1963.
28. Morris, M. L.: Periodontal healing in man. N.Y. Dent. J., *35:*333, 1969.
29. Morris, M. L.: The implantation of human dentin and cementum with an autogenous bone and red marrow into the subcutaneous tissues of the rat. J. Periodontol., *40:*259, 1969.
30. Nabers, C. L., and O'Leary, T. J.: Autogenous bone transplants in the treatment of osseous defects. U.S.A.F., S.A.M., T.D.S., 64-30, May, 1964.
31. Nabers, C. L., and O'Leary, T. J.: Autogenous bone grafts: case report. Periodontics, *5:*251, 1967.
32. Pfeifer, J. S.: The present status of bone grafts in periodontal therapy. Dent. Clin. North Am., *13:*1969.
33. Prichard, J. F.: Management of the periodontal abscess. Oral Surg., *6:*474, 1953.
34. Prichard, J. F.: The regeneration of bone following periodontal therapy. Oral Surg., *10:*247, 1957.
35. Prichard, J. F.: The infrabony technique as a predictable procedure. J. Periodontol., *28:*202, 1957.
36. Prichard, J. F.: Treatment of infrabony pockets based on alveolar process morphology. Dent. Clin. North Am., March, 1960, p. 85.
37. Prichard, J. F.: Criteria for verifying topographical changes in alveolar process after surgical intervention. Periodontics, *4:*71, 1966.
38. Prichard, J. F.: The etiology, diagnosis and treatment of the infrabony defect. J. Periodontol., *38:*455, 1967.
39. Robinson, R. E.: Osseous coagulum for bone induction. J. Periodontol., *40:*503, 1969.
40. Robinson, R. E.: The osseous coagulum for bone induction technique: a review. J. Cal. Dent. Assoc., *46:*1, 1970.
41. Rosenberg, M. M.: Free osseous tissue autografts as a predictable procedure. J. Periodontol., *42:*195, 1971.
42. Ross, S. E., and Cohen, D. W.: The fate of a free osseous tissue autograft. A clinical and histologic case report. Periodontics, *6:*145, 1968.
43. Ross, S. E., Malamud, E. H., and Amsterdam, M.: The contiguous autogenous transplant—its rationale, indications, and technique. Periodontics, *4:*246, 1966.
44. Schaffer, E. M.: The new attachment operation in subcrestal pockets. Oral Surg., *11:*253, 1958.
45. Schallhorn, R. G.: Eradication of bifurcation defects

utilizing frozen autogenous hip marrow implants. Periodont. Abstracts, *15*:101, 1967.

46. Schallhorn, R. G.: The use of autogenous hip marrow biopsy implants for bony creater defects. J. Periodontol., *39*:145, 1968.

47. Schreiber, H. P.: Management of vertical bone resorption in periodontal disease. Oral Surg., *17*:161, 1964.

48. Seltzer, S., Bender, I. B., and Ziontz, M.: The interrelationship of pulp and periodontal disease. Oral Surg., *16*:1474, 1963.

49. Sternlicht, H. C.: Bone regeneration following periodontal treatment. J. Tex. Dent. Assoc., *88*:12, 1970.

50. Younger, W. J.: Some of the latest phases in implantation and other operations. Dental Cosmos, *35*:102, 1893.

24

Furcation Invasions

24

Furcation

Invasions

NEIL BASARABA

Chronic marginal periodontitis is characterized by resorption of the marginal bone of the alveolar process with accompanying loss of the attachment of the gingival and periodontal fibers. As the loss of the periodontium progresses apically, the regions of the bifurcations and trifurcations of multirooted teeth are invaded. The lesions of marginal periodontitis develop as a sequel to chronic marginal gingivitis and have essentially the same etiologic agents, i.e., plaque, calculus, food impaction, overextended and inadequate margins of restorations, and other iatrogenic factors. These give rise to areas of chronic local inflammation.

In a dentition invaded by inflammatory periodontal disease, it is inevitable that in some cases progressively deepening pockets will invade one or more furcae to varying degrees (Fig. 24-1). When added to the topographic and anatomic problems normally encountered, the involvement of a furca brings into play an altogether different series of factors.[7,10] Not only is the degree of detachment important in that it affects alveolar support, but furcal anatomy is in many cases equally important.[9,23] Plaque is most poorly removed from and usually accumulates in greatest abundance in the interproximal regions and together with calculus is responsible for the perpetuation of the inflammatory disease (Fig. 24-2). The response of the alveolar bone to the inflammation results in the formation of interproximal craters. Overhanging margins of restorations contribute to the problem of plaque and food retention. The proximal furcae of maxillary molars and birooted first bicuspids may be invaded rather early in the progression of marginal periodontitis. Invasion of the furcae in mandibular molars occurs later because of their buccal and lingual position; however, invasion

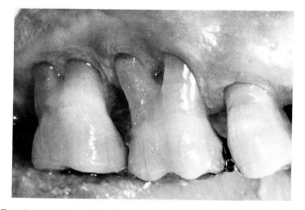

FIG. 24-1. *Molars showing extensive furcal invasion following alveolar bone resorption and accompanying gingival recession typical of chronic marginal periodontitis. Communication is complete from the buccal side to both mesial and distal furcas and poses a difficult therapeutic and maintenance problem.*

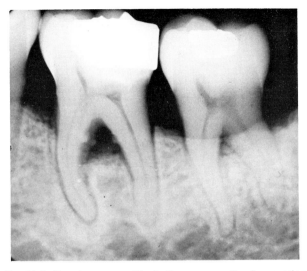

FIG. 24-2. *Roentgenogram illustrating a generalized resorption of the alveolar crest involving the interfurcal regions of both molars. A widened periodontal ligament space (often seen as evidence of occlusal traumatism) and calculus suggest a long-standing involvement with chronic marginal periodontitis.*

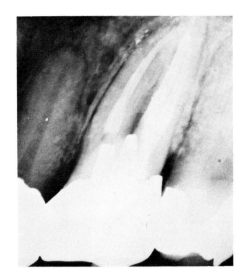

FIG. 24-4. *Roentgenogram showing the inadvertent perforation of the pulpal floor during the placement of a dowel restoration into an endodontically treated maxillary molar. A recurring periodontal abscess resulted in extensive loss of bone and attachment in the furcal region.*

may be earlier if gingival restorations have overhangs or extend into the fluting between the roots (Figs. 24-3; 24-4). The topographic characteristics of the resulting defects of the soft and hard tissues vary greatly as to their vertical and horizontal extensions, especially when they involve multirooted molars and bicuspids.

Masters in 1964 observed in many multirooted teeth a slender enamel projection extending from the enamel of the crown into the furca for a variable distance.[21] It is obvious that no fiber attachment is possible into an enamel surface of one of these projections (Fig. 24-5); hence it was suspected that such an aberration is a strong predisposing factor in the initial breakdown

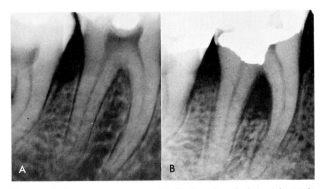

FIG. 24-3. *Roentgenograms of a first molar. A. Intact bone is seen in the furcal region. Beginning loss of crestal density is apparent in the distal interproximal region. B. Extensive rarefaction has occurred in the bifurcation region following the placement and presence for some time of an overhanging buccal amalgam restoration. Loss of crestal bone in the distal interproximal space is minimal during the same time interval.*

where it is present.[14,19] Figure 24-6A,B of a mandibular first molar with pocket depth into the furcal area shows evidence of progressive radiolucency in the furcal region. Surgical exposure revealed an extended enamel projection into the region of the furca (Fig. 24-6C). The extent of bone resorption in the interproximal regions was minimal. Enamel projections are not found in every furcal invasion, however; many are due to simple deepening pockets into a furca.

Pulpal pathosis relative to furcal invasion is of great concern.[16,18,24,28,31] Accessory canals may extend into the furcal area and provide access to this area for the products of pulpal necrosis, resulting in resorption of the interradicular bone (Fig. 24-7A). A fistula may appear lateral to this area without destroying the gingival and periodontal complex, but it is not unusual for communication to extend from the aperture of the accessory canal, along the root surface, and out through the gingival crevice or pocket, if such exists (Fig. 24-7B). Pulp death resulting in periapical periodontitis may also progress to establish a communication with the oral cavity by extending coronally along the periodontal ligament and out through the gingival sulcus or through a deepening pocket coincident to periodontitis. In this way furcae of multirooted teeth with pulpal pathosis, free of acute symptoms, are vulnerable to destruction of the periodontium in the furcal region.[30] Subsequent linking of the periapical and marginal periodontal lesions is a common result.[18] Clinical experience has shown that the extent of the resolution of the resulting periodontal lesion following endodontic therapy is inversely related to the duration

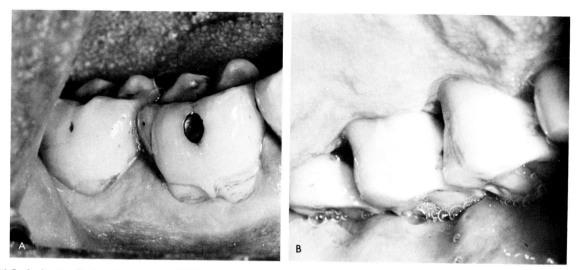

Fig. 24-5. *A. A mandibular first molar exhibiting a well-defined enamel projection extending well into the interradicular area. A projection of the enamel, though somewhat less prominent, is nevertheless present in the second molar. B. A four-rooted maxillary second molar also showing an enamel projection.*

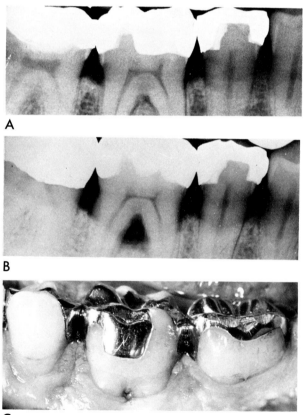

Fig. 24-6. *A. Roentgenogram of a molar, illustrating beginning radiolucency in the furcal region. B. Roentgenogram of same molar, illustrating extensive radiolucency in the furcal region. Interproximal involvement is not relatively as great in progression. C. Clinical view, illustrating projection of enamel into the bifurcations of both molars. The second molar projection is less extensive (mirror view).*

of the pulpal contribution to the inflammatory involvement.

Occlusal traumatism with resulting mobility and widening of the ligament space as a result of lateral bone resorption can exaggerate the extent of vertical bone loss due to inflammation (Fig. 24-8). This may result in the earlier involvement of the furca. Occlusal traumatism as a contributory etiologic factor cannot be ignored.[36]

Although a multirooted tooth enjoys advantages in mechanical support over a single-rooted tooth, furcal invasion presents problems not simply because it causes loss of support but because the furca has a complicated structure. Some of the problems are due to the peculiar nature of periodontal destruction in these sheltered areas.[12] Others are due to the topogra-

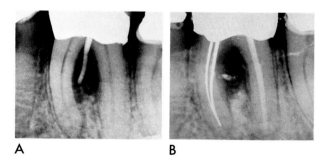

Fig. 24-7. *Roentgenogram illustrating the termination of a gutta percha point introduced into a buccal pocket of a molar plagued by repeated periodontal abscesses. B. Roentgenogram illustrating the molar treated endodontically, with evidence of extruded cement passing through an accessory canal into the furcal region. Healing of the gingival fibers was uneventful.*

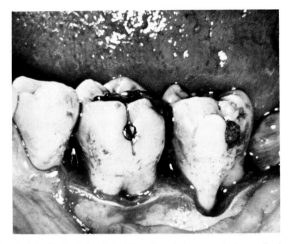

FIG. 24-8. *Surgical exposure of molars reveals bone lesions with extension into the bifurcations. Both molars were subjected to severe balancing interferences. The thick ledge of buccal bone discouraged recession and deep vertical and lateral defects developed into the furcal regions. Note the enamel projection in the first molar. This is a clinical view of the roentgenogram shown as Figure 24-2.*

phy of the furca and the number of roots forming it.[9] Still others are distinctive because of the direction from which the furca has been entered—distal invasion, for example, in contrast to buccal invasion.

Since anatomic considerations are of such importance, it might be advisable to review some salient features of the multirooted tooth in the areas of furcation. First, in most of these teeth fluting in the root surface blends into the actual furca. Second, the furca itself presents an altogether singular form if it is formed by two rather than three roots. Third, the furca's shape varies widely with the relative spread of the roots forming it. Usually, the more vertical the roots, the more constricted is the furcal zone and the more acute is their angle of junction.

The buccolingual dimension of the alveolar process and the depth of the overlying gingival tissues influence the nature of the defect and its extent into the furca as a result of the apical regression of the bone and soft tissue attachment. The presence of thick buccal and lingual ledges of bone and also of tori does not permit soft-tissue recession. The result is the formation of deep vertical and horizontal pockets and intrabony lesions surrounding the furcal regions (Figs. 24-8, 24-14).

Conversely, narrow buccolingual alveolar processes are usually accompanied by individual root prominences, and loss of crestal bone height is commonly accompanied by gingival recession. The subsequent exposure of the furcal area is less of a problem in management for the patient and therapist because recession of the gingival tissues leaves less pocket

depth and is not usually associated with development of buccal or lingual lesions (Fig. 24-9). An individual misaligned tooth, because of its buccal or lingual position within the alveolar process, may present such a problem. The position of the bifurcation or trifurcation relative to the entire tooth length is vital. A furca near the cementoenamel junction is invaded early in the course of marginal periodontitis. Conversely, an apically situated furca will be less vulnerable in the initial stages of marginal periodontitis, but once involved will have a more guarded prognosis because of diminished alveolar bone support. These anatomic variations have an important bearing upon the behavior of the furca in exposure and invasion. Teeth with constricted furcal areas are prone to exacerbated periodontitis as well as to caries.

Successful periodontal therapy is based on the initial elimination and subsequent control of recurring etiologic factors. The subsequent management and maintenance of any permanent alteration to the architecture of the periodontium is subject to a combined

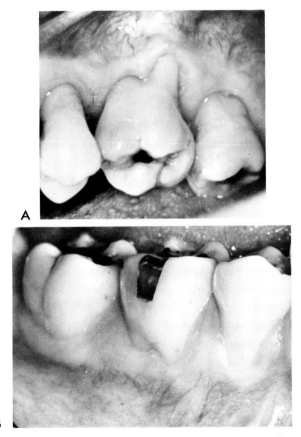

FIG. 24-9. *A. Recession of gingival tissues following resorption of alveolar bone initially eliminating the development of furcal pocket depth. B. Slight furcal invasion of molars rendered accessible to oral hygiene methods because of generalized recession of delicate gingival tissues.*

program on the part of the patient and dentist (or auxiliary) to eliminate inflammation. If the nature and extent of the persisting defect created by this inflammation defies the patient's best efforts at care, it becomes obvious and necessary for the dentist to participate more frequently in the elimination of local factors through root planing and curettage. It is also necessary that all pulpal, restorative, and occlusal etiologic factors be eliminated. Should the patient undergoing initial therapy (maintenance) demonstrate a progression of furcal invasion, i.e., increasing pocket depth or increasing radiographic radiolucency with or without periodontal abscess formation, it becomes necessary to extend active therapy to include the alteration of the periodontal lesion to make it more accessible and available to the patient's best efforts at care. After a thorough examination and exploration of the furcal

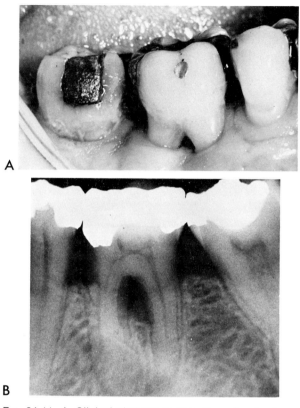

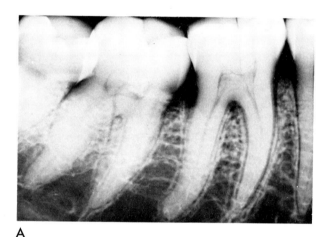

A

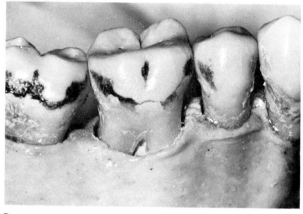

B

FIG. 24-10. *A. Roentgenogram of a dry skull illustrating a slight radiolucency in the furca of a first molar, suggesting very minimal invasion (Class I). B. Dry-skull picture of same jaw as in A, revealing loss of bone into the furcal area and emphasizing the shortcomings of using roentgenographic evidence for primary diagnosis. This example would certainly qualify as a Class II invasion.*

FIG. 24-11. *A. Clinical photograph showing extensive loss of the periodontium in the first molar as a result of chronic marginal periodontitis. Mirror view of a Class III or "through-and-through" bifurcation involvement. B. Roentgenogram of the same first molar suggests extensive loss of interradicular bone.*

defect (invasion), the severity of the problem must be assessed, and an appropriate treatment plan must be developed.

Furcal invasion may vary in horizontal and vertical depth according to existing anatomic features—namely, root form, buccal and lingual contours of alveolar bone, tori, root diversions or proximities, restoration contours, and extent of the attached gingival tissues. It is necessary to obtain a correctly angled radiograph showing the furcal area clearly and defining the presence or absence of a continuous periodontal ligament. Figure 24-10 demonstrates an example of an improperly angled radiograph that can result in misdiagnosis of a furcal invasion. Figure 24-11A is correctly angled, showing the interfurcal lesion and suggesting the surgical course to be taken (Figs. 24-11B, 24-12). Exploration of the extent of loss of attachment (pocket depth) and bone resorption is best accomplished with curved explorers or fine curets. The extent of soft-tissue attachment loss and bone resorption is recorded and categorized according to a classification previously developed.

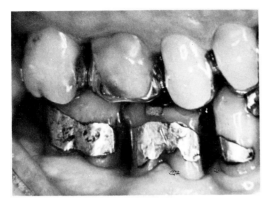

FIG. 24-12. *Odontoplasty of the first molar and to a lesser extent of the second molar is done to accentuate root prominence and decrease the depth, both horizontal and vertical, of the tissue in the interradicular region. This exposes the furcal invasion to a greater degree.*

CLASSIFICATION

Invasion may be a simple matter, but the resulting configuration is often complex. In the past, attempts to describe the nature of each lesion were cumbersome and imprecise. A classification was clearly called for and two were introduced. They were similar, though not identical. Easley and Drennan used a numerical system of three classes,[8] whereas Heins and Canter used a verbal descriptive system,[15] also with three general classes of invasion. Concerned not only with the mechanics of invasion, but with the shape and condition of the bordering roots and with the arch, both systems described the lesion and directed attention to other features of the furca that might have a bearing on therapy. Both classifications were made on the basis of the severity of the lesion and on the extent of the invasion. They are straightforward morphologic classifications. They have no pathologic implications, but many therapeutic ones.

Class I: The Incipient Furcal Invasion

The incipient furcal invasion develops by moderate and uniform horizontal bone loss with a soft-tissue lesion or pocket extending into the furcal region (Fig. 24-13). The incipient invasion is, as its name implies, a beginning lesion. It may not be particularly serious. It may even be an exaggerated terminal of a deep interradicular fluting that has been slightly exposed. Diagnosis of the Class I invasion is simple, since the incipient lesion is marginal and can be quite easily discovered with a circumferential traverse of the probe. The probe will sink into the shallow V-shaped notch in the crestal outline. There is no intrabony lesion.

Class II: The Patent Furcal Invasion

A Class II furcal invasion is, as its name implies, an open (and even gaping) penetration by the resorptive lesion. This type of invasion creates deep pockets and varying degrees of bone destruction, extending into the region of the furca. The defect may occur on any surface of the tooth, or on more than one. There is no through-and-through communication. The path of the destruction into the furca in a horizontal direction often extends for several millimeters and creates a definite space with an arched roof created by the furca and bordered by roots and bone (Fig. 24-10). It may extend for a variable distance and is frequently involved in a cavernous lesion that may doom the tooth. This type of lesion is quite easily discovered on the buccal and lingual surfaces in routine probing. Even when sequestered in a deep pocket, the open furca is accessible to the probe in even a casual circumferential traverse.

Interproximal furcal invasions, on the other hand, require a searching probe to reveal them to the exam-

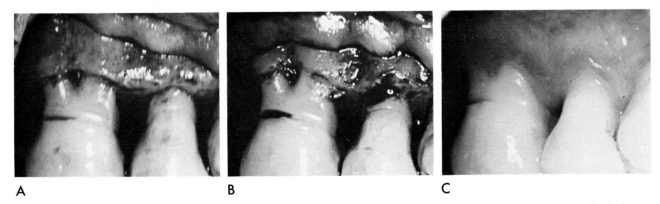

A   B   C

FIG. 24-13. *A. Surgically exposed Class I furcal invasion. B. Minor ostectomy and vertical grooving performed interradicularly and interproximally to eliminate bone defect. C. Healing following apical positioning of the mucoperiosteal flap at the level of the new crestal bone, yielding a pocket-free gingival architecture and exposing the incipient furcal invasion.*

iner. Frequently the standard periodontal probe is not too effective because of anatomic barriers to its insertion to the deepest extent of the penetration. A slender curet is commonly used for probing an interproximal furca, although some operators prefer an explorer. The objection to the use of the bayonet explorer is mainly that it is not so conducive to irregular probing of the bone surface as is the periodontal probe. It is too prone to catch and trip. The curet, on the other hand, is a good instrument for probing interproximal furcae. The toe of the curet easily slips interproximally into the patent invasion area, and some idea can be gleaned of the extent of the invasion.

Class III: Communicating Furcal Invasion

The Class III furcal invasion is a patent exposure that communicates with a second or third furcal opening. For example, a buccal furcal invasion of a mandibular molar that extends through to a lingual exposure is a communicating lesion. In maxillary molars, examples would be invasions from the buccal side through a distal exposure or mesial exposure.

When the resorptive periodontal lesion invades the furca so extensively that two or more furcae are open and communicate with each other, the clinical situation of the tooth is grave and considerable care must be taken to gain every discernible piece of information on the status of the roots and of the form and extent of the investing bone around each root (Fig. 24-11).

The discovery of a communicating furcal invasion in a mandibular molar is a simple matter in routine probing. What is not so simple is the determination of the extent of the furcal damage and resorption. It is always a surprise to the examiner to stumble into an area of cavernous resorption in the interradicular space. Often the resorptive cavern is so large that only mesial and distal bone and attachment maintain the tooth in the arch.

The etiology of some of these lesions is not so obscure as it once was. The barely discernible enamel projection into the furca is surely more common than was once thought (Figs. 24-6C, 24-8). One thing sometimes overlooked is that the ease with which such a furca is entered suggests that retention of debris and impingement occur in these areas, just as extensive penetration into the furcal area from the buccal aspect of maxillary molars implicates both mesial and distal furcae by association and immediately makes the extent of their invasions suspect. The mesial furca is approached with a cow-horn explorer or fine curet from the palatal side, using a circumferential buccal-to-lingual sweep to map the extent of invasion into the

furcal area. It is not unusual for the mesial furca to be situated more lingually than one would believe. Distal furcas of maxillary molars are somewhat less accessible and at times may defy accurate assessment. Proximity of the adjacent mesiobuccal and distobuccal roots may impede exploration from the buccal side. The extent of a horizontal extension of an apically positioned furca may also be difficult to ascertain.

TREATMENT OF CLASS I FURCAL INVASIONS

Management of the furcal invasion is a special problem that is complicated by other problems. This creates an interesting and challenging exercise in treatment planning. Even the occlusal factor is different when a tooth with furcal invasion is involved. That particular problem will be enlarged upon and fully discussed in Chapter 25.

All the skills and methods of periodontal therapy are called into play in furcal management. Aside from the standard methods of pocket elimination, special techniques are needed when furcae are involved.

Therapy for Class I furcal invasions is limited to reducing pocket depth; there are few if any bone defects. Horizontal bone resorption may have occurred uniformly, but will not yet have penetrated the furcal region. Management of this type of defect is often confined to oral hygiene instruction in the use of a soft toothbrush and the Bass technique, but careful debridement of the area by root planing and curettage is also part of the treatment. In this way, excessive contours of the existing restorations are eliminated and the tooth is reshaped, if necessary. This rather simple method consists of reshaping the furcae, especially the coronal prefurcal anatomy, with a rotary instrument. This is particularly useful on the buccal aspect of maxillary molars and both buccal and lingual surfaces of the mandibular molars (Fig. 24-12).

Odontoplasty has its most useful application in incipient or Class I furcal invasions. It is in these that reduction of the anatomic undulation in coronal topography has the greatest effect upon gingival form. In an incipient furcal invasion, the gingival margin dips into the depression or into the fluting leading to the furca. The distinct papilla that forms in this area often juts out and becomes traumatized. Commonly, the result is an enlarged, fibrotic papilla for which gingivoplasty is futile. An effective expedient, however, is the reduction of the anatomic feature that makes the furcal papilla possible. Flattening the surface so as to eliminate all features is effective. The reduction is made at the expense of the crown surface adjacent to the fluting on both sides. This eliminates the fluting altogether, with its resulting gingival enlargement and pocket depth. The gingival margin of a successfully reshaped crown is a single curve unbroken by an intermediate papilla. The degree to which the anatomy of a tooth can be altered by grinding is sharply limited because the amount of enamel is limited. The possibility for routine use of odontoplasty simply does not exist. That is not to say, however, that it is not a useful method where feasible.

Surgical elimination of significant pocket depth, if present, is usually accomplished by means of the flap approach. Gingivoplasty or gingivectomy may be used, but these neither provide a visual confirmation as to the extent of the bone deformity nor leave minimal zones of attached gingiva.[13] When marginal periodontitis progresses to the extent that furcal invasions appear, significant interproximal pocket depth involving several teeth or an entire segment may also be present. Surgical treatment is subsequently devoted to the elimination of all pocket depth by the apical positioning of mucoperiosteal flaps (Fig. 24-13). Isolated furcal invasions requiring surgical treatment, such as those from the buccal or lingual side of a molar, may respond well to localized gingivectomy or gingivoplasty or to limited flap exposure. The surgical procedure is followed by suture placement and appropriate dressing application. Healing is usually uneventful and is followed by a review of oral hygiene procedures.

TREATMENT OF CLASS II FURCAL INVASIONS

Class II furcal invasions present significant pocket depth and varying amounts of bone resorption, both horizontal and vertical. The lesions may appear on any aspect of the tooth, but do not extend sufficiently into the furca to communicate with any invasions on the opposite side of the tooth, as is the case with mandibular molars or with a lesion on an adjacent interproximal surface as in three- and four-rooted maxillary molars. The Class II invasion is an extension of the Class I lesion, and in most patients, because of its deeper progression, it is frequently not responsive to initial therapy alone. The definitive treatment of this class of invasion requires surgery, including bone recontouring (Fig. 24-14). Serious attention must be given to interradicular bone before entry.[33]

The roentgenogram sometimes reveals more of Class II lesions than of other periodontal resorptions, but it is far from definitive diagnostic evidence. Heavy buccal and lingual cortical plates commonly mask cavernous resorption areas. Frequently, affected molars are only minimally invested in bone at the apices of the roots, and the rest of the roots sit in a funnel-

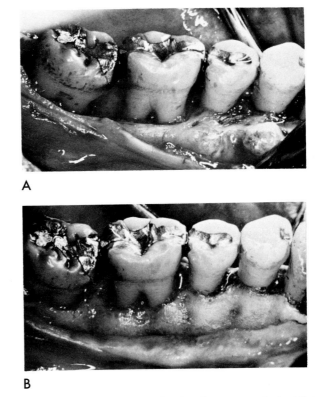

A

B

FIG. 24-14. *Surgical exposure by elevating mucoperiosteal flap on the lingual sides reveals extensive bone lesions, bifurcation invasions, and tori. B. Bone resection and recontouring expose the furcas to the depth of their invasion and create a bone architecture that will aid in supporting a pocket-free gingival contour amenable to hygiene maintenance.*

shaped surrounding wall of bone that provides no support. Roentgenographically, these teeth may appear to be only minimally involved. Great care must be taken to avoid the surprise of finding extensive resorption after beginning therapy. Figure 24-10 illustrates the shortcomings of roentgenographic evidence of the extent of invasion.

Access is achieved by the reflection of mucoperiosteal flaps. The soft tissue in the interproximal area and in the furcal regions is curetted, and any remaining calcarious deposits or irregularities of the root surfaces are removed. This removal is accomplished with a hand instrument or by ultrasonic debridement. The bone is recontoured to achieve an architecture free of lesions and interproximal craters (Fig. 24-14). The contours achieved comply with the principles of bone surgery and are designed to encourage and support normal gingival contour. An effort is always made (and generally exaggerated) in interradicular vertical grooving to decrease the tendency toward high or broad gingival-margin regeneration. The mucoperiosteal flaps usually involve the entire segment, but may be confined to one or two teeth. Apical positioning of

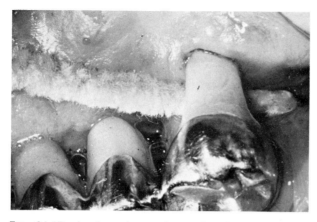

FIG. 24-15. *A pipe cleaner is employed to maintain a "through-and-through" involvement free of plaque.*

the flaps is necessary. Odontoplasty is done to accentuate the root prominence and enhance the vertical grooving of the interradicular bone, in an effort to decrease the bulk of soft-tissue regeneration in the furcal region.

On rare occasions, Class II furcal invasions may extend to become through-and-through or Class III invasions. The approach to the lesion is gained by buccal and lingual flaps, and the bone surgery completes the removal of the interradicular bone and thereby completes the communication. The selection of therapeutic extension of a furcal invasion is usually based on anatomic variations in crown, root, and alveolar bone form that do not limit the surgical exposure of the furcal region to make it more accessible for oral physiotherapy and maintenance. Theoretically, the creation of a through-and-through communication out of a patent or Class II lesion was intended to enable the patient to exercise better plaque control via pipe cleaners and irrigation (Figs. 24-15, 24-16, 24-17). However that may be, all maintenance

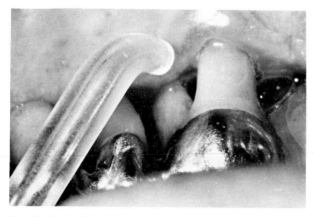

FIG. 24-16. *An irrigating device can be an aid in cleansing a Class II furcal area.*

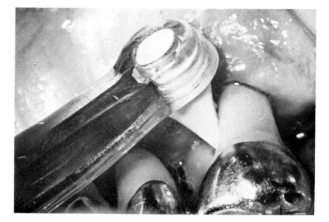

FIG. 24-17. *A rubber or plastic tip forcefully applied discourages soft-tissue proliferation that would obscure the patent communication established surgically. The lesion may have been a Class III invasion or a Class II invasion extended to complete the communication.*

devices have some shortcomings. Even if the gingival floor of the area is well maintained, there is always the danger of caries in the sharply angled vault of the furca formed by the roots. This area is by no means easy to clean and is commonly found to retain debris. Caries is an everpresent danger. The popularity of this solution to Class II invasions has greatly waned following long-range observations revealing shortcomings in the control of caries and the retention of pulp vitality.

A limited number of Class II furcal invasions are also treated by root amputation. The decision to do this is influenced by the potential for an acceptable surgical result and dictated and influenced by local anatomic features. The subsequent need for an extensive restorative treatment plan involving periodontal prosthesis usually demands the definitive treatment of defects and elimination of potential sites of progressive inflammatory disease. Such areas of progression may arise if the patient is unable to eliminate daily all plaque deposition and food retention. A postsurgical environment must be created so as to be amenable to reasonable efforts at oral hygiene. The potential for breakdown in such an environment is inversely proportional to the ease with which maintenance—free of local irritants—can be accomplished.

TREATMENT OF CLASS III FURCAL INVASIONS

A Class III furcal invasion is characterized by loss of soft-tissue attachment and bone in the interradicular region, to the extent that a through-and-through communication exists—either buccal-to-lingual or mesial-to-distal or from the buccal to either or both of the interproximal surfaces (as may be the case in maxillary molars). Class III furcal invasions are usually found in cases of well-advanced chronic marginal periodontitis. Teeth may be missing, others may have a hopeless prognosis, and the potential of the remaining teeth as individual functioning units or abutments may not be resolved until all are subjected to the multiple disciplines of dentistry. Ultimately, treatment may include extraction, surgery, endodontic treatment, and fabrication of a fixed or removable prosthesis to restore the dentition to a useful degree of function. A comprehensive treatment plan must be formulated.[29]

Once the periodontal lesion has invaded the furcal zone of a multirooted tooth, several responses by the tooth are possible:

1. Such teeth are prone to formation of periodontal abscesses because the marginal orifice to the pocket is constricted and the lesion in the furca is relatively large.
2. Teeth so involved frequently suffer cavernous resorptions without marginal evidence. Even the radiograph is unreliable where there is a heavy buccal or lingual cortical plate or where other superimposition occurs.
3. Aberrant root canals sometimes occur in the furca, so that even a narrow furcal invasion results in pulpal exposure with pulpal pain, which confuses the inexperienced therapist.
4. Root caries is all too common in furcal exposures. Frequently, the tooth is decimated before the carious lesion is noticed.
5. Furcal lesions may provide a nidus for pocket formation, thereby enveloping adjacent roots in funnel-shaped resorptive lesions.

No discussion of furcal invasion can be quite complete without a fairly extensive discussion of root amputations. In many extreme cases, the resection and removal of one or more roots of a molar are the only recourse for eliminating a lesion that owes its pernicious form and its refractory response to therapy to its inaccessibility to maintenance by the patient.

The alternative to root amputation is frequently the sacrifice of the offending tooth. If there is a sound terminal abutment somewhere else in the segment, extraction may be the treatment choice. If all the remaining teeth are weakened, however, even a single sound root may be of use, but it is impossible to draw hard-and-fast rules in planning treatment for these cases. If the invasion is definite but not too extensive into the central furcal region, then root amputation is too radical an approach. If, on the other hand, only a thin layer of bone remains in the buccal furca and the buccal roots are exposed or very thinly covered, then a root amputation may rationally be considered. This treatment is especially recommended if root proximity is a problem on the distal side.

The extent of the furcal invasion is the main factor in choosing extraction, amputation, or definitive curettage and maintenance with no amputations as the solution. The therapist makes his ultimate decision on the basis of (1) the critical case for tooth retention, (2) anatomic arrangement that might make possible easy access to ensure prolonged successful maintenance, and (3) the performance level of the patient in maintenance procedures.[4]

Teeth with furcal invasions have to be evaluated for their strategic position in the overall treatment plan. Once it has been decided that a tooth or teeth with furcal invasion are vital to the restorative treatment plan, certain things must be established. Accurate clinical assessment of the extent of periodontal destruction is vital for the correct application of the root amputation or hemisection technique. Although the extent of bone loss in the furcal region cannot be assessed from roentgenograms alone, taking several views from different angles can be valuable. Together with careful exploration using probes and fine curets, a more accurate assessment of the extent of the lesion can be determined. The amount of bone to be retained over the roots must be sufficient to resist occlusal stresses. Splinting to overcome occlusal traumatism must be feasible, if required, as part of the restorative treatment plan.

Endodontic therapy of the remaining roots must be possible, and the roots intended for retention should be judged for accessibility to endodontic therapy.[34] If any doubt exists, the canal should be prepared ahead of time, and the decision as to which roots are to be retained should be made preoperatively. Endodontic therapy on these roots is usually completed prior to amputation.[12] The possibility of acute pulpitis developing in the remaining roots is thereby avoided, as is the unintentional retention of endodontically inoperable canals. When amputation or hemisection is contemplated and no decision has been reached prior to surgery regarding which roots to retain, acute pain from pulpal injury can be avoided by first removing the pulp and treating the canal(s) with medication. When doubt exists whether pulpal pathosis has contributed to the periodontal lesion, an extended healing period should follow endodontic therapy. When nonvital pulp is largely contributory to the lesion, it greatly influences the lesion as a whole and, in consequence, the treatment plan. Hiatt in his discussion of pocket elimination by combined endodontic-periodontal therapy, illustrates this well.

Thorough and complete clinical roentgenographic examination, including an assessment of the patient's maintenance skills and potential for a restorative treatment plan, set the stage for considering root amputation and hemisection.[2]

Indications for Root Amputation and Hemisection in Class III Furcal Invasions

1. Severe vertical bone loss involving only one root of a mandibular molar or one or two buccal roots or a palatal root of a maxillary molar that has resulted in an inaccessible furcal invasion. Sufficient bone must surround any roots to be retained (Fig. 24-18).
2. Exposed roots too close together as a result of

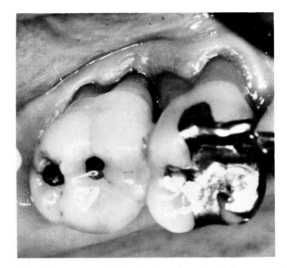

FIG. 24-19. *Close proximity of buccal roots of two maxillary molars prevents maintenance access to proximal furca.*

interproximal bone resorption, to the extent that maintenance of Class I or II interproximal invasion is impossible (Fig. 24-19).
3. Furcas exposed through caries or bone resorption to the extent that subsequent surgical and restorative results would defy adequate maintenance.
4. Abutments or piers within a fixed bridge or splint with a hopeless prognosis because of periodontal disease.[3,32]
5. Multirooted teeth with individual root fracture
6. Inadequacy of mucogingival surgery to restore attachment and replace an adequate zone of attached gingiva.
7. Single roots of nonvital teeth that cannot be treated by conventional root-canal therapy or retrograde techniques because of the presence of lateral canals, partial calcification, dilaceration, pulp stones, perforations, or broken instruments.

Contraindications for Root Amputation and Hemisection in Class III Furcal Invasion

1. Inadequate bone support on the roots intended for retention despite splinting to withstand occlusal stress.
2. Fusion of the roots apical to the area of invasion.
3. Inoperable canals of roots selected for retention and not amenable to treatment by retrograde filling.
4. Lack of good form or position of any of the roots.
5. Ill health, economics, or medical reasons that contraindicate extensive and prolonged endodontic, periodontic, and restorative treatment.
6. Position of the furca relative to the root apex that defies the surgical creation of a minimal amount

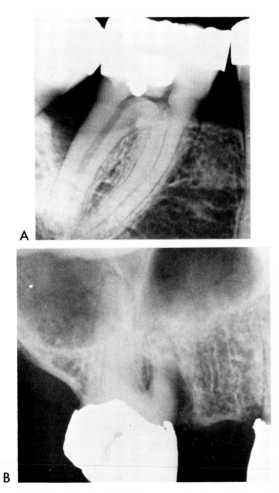

FIG. 24-18. *A. Molar with distal one-walled bone lesion that is not amenable to correction by osteoplasty or reattachment procedures. This tooth has a long, well-formed mesial root. B. A maxillary molar with severe bone loss around the mesiobuccal root and an extensive buccal and mesial furcal invasion.*

of reverse architecture or would jeopardize the support to the remaining roots and adjacent teeth.

7. Patient's oral hygiene performance inadequate for plaque control.

It is highly appropriate to make some basic procedural decisions before amputation or hemisection. If root removal is decided upon preoperatively, it is best to arrange for the endodontic procedures to be done first. This plan eliminates the surprise and disappointment of encounters with inoperable canals and lateral canals that cannot be obliterated. One should not discount the retrograde approach to salvage roots with canals that cannot be instrumented to their entire length. The endodontist should be asked to insert amalgam into the canal of the root to be removed to a level beyond the point of amputation (Fig. 24-29). Teeth to be hemisected should have the entire pulp chamber filled with amalgam.

If the etiology of furcal invasion implicates a nonvital pulp, it is highly desirable to complete endodontic therapy on all roots (including those considered for amputation). Healing of a contributory periapical lesion may well lead to the reestablishment of periodontal structures to the extent that root amputation is no longer required (Fig. 24-7). It is not uncommon for reattachment to eliminate a communicating oral-apical tract that has been incorrectly diagnosed as a deep periodontal pocket. The best solution to the pulp question is to arrange for the endodontic treatment to be done first.[22] Then the resection can be done under optimum conditions. Many therapists use this approach. It requires, however, a definite commitment to resection in advance, and in many situations this cannot be done. It is by no means rare to make a therapeutic decision during surgery under optimum visibility and access.

The surgical approach to an involved tooth or teeth is gained by elevating mucoperiosteal flaps on both buccal and lingual aspects (Fig. 24-20). The exposure is usually extended to involve the entire segment or quadrant if pocket elimination and bone recontouring are also deemed necessary (Fig. 24-21). The chronic inflammatory and/or fibrotic tissue is curetted from the interproximal and furcal regions to complete the exposure of the bone contours and the extent of the furcal invasion. At this time, examination of root size, position, residual bone support, and extent of resorption and the potential for an acceptable postsurgical bone architecture will confirm the choice of roots to be retained.[6]

When the entire coronal portion of the tooth is to be retained, removal of the buccal or lingual alveolar

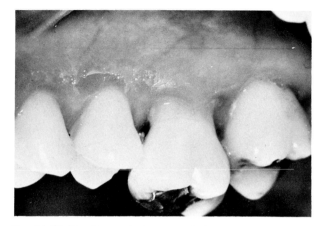

FIG. 24-20. *The first molar has extruded to the extent that the distal furca has been invaded rather early in the progression of periodontal disease. Recurring periodontal abscesses in this area necessitate definitive resolution of this uncontrollable invasion.*

bone over the amputated root will facilitate its removal. Frequently the resorptive lesion will create a dehiscence, and further bone removal will be minimal (Fig. 24-21). Most roots of mandibular molars and buccal roots of maxillary molars will be removed from the buccal side and pose less of a trial than does the removal of a palatal root.

Bone is removed to expose the most coronal extent of the furca. The root is then severed from the rest of the tooth (Fig. 24-22), using a long fissure bur or a diamond stone. Some general precautions should be taken when resecting a root. The most basic is the actual cut itself. It is highly desirable that the cut severing the root from the rest of the tooth be made as close to the point of furcation as possible. It may not

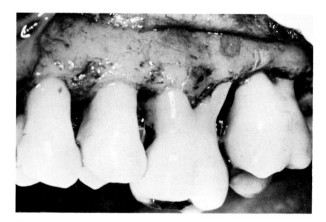

FIG. 24-21. *Access to Class III furcal invasion is gained by reflecting a mucoperiosteal flap. A fenestration of the distobuccal root is exposed. All chronic inflammatory and interproximal soft tissue is removed to reveal the depth of the invasion and adjacent bone contours. Note the Class I invasion of the buccal furca of the second molar.*

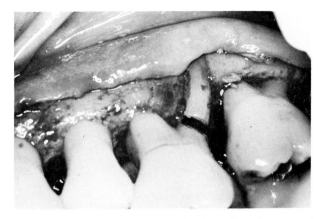

FIG. 24-22. *The bone covering the distobuccal root is removed and the root is severed.*

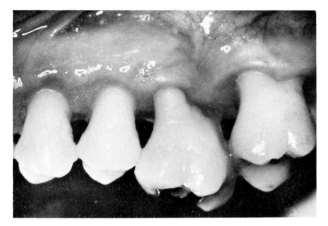

FIG. 24-24. *After healing. Gingival contours and interproximal embrasure spaces are easily accessible for plaque removal.*

always be possible to sever the root with the initial cut so that no remnant of the furca remains, but the attempt should be made. The remnant of the furca left after failure to observe this precaution encourages retention of plaque and creates an area difficult to maintain. Irrigation with saline during the cutting procedure enhances visibility and debrides the area. Whether separation is complete is ascertained by gentle prying to establish that the root moves independently of the crown.

The amputated root is then removed with elevators, curets, or forceps. Sectioning the amputated root into smaller segments often facilitates its removal. This is particularly true in the case of palatal roots and mandibular molar roots when the corresponding crown portion is retained. The furcal area is curetted free of soft tissue, and any calculus on the remaining root is removed. If the amputation involves a vital tooth, the

exposed pulp is partially removed with a small round bur and the remainder is covered by a dressing of zinc oxide and eugenol. If pulp removal has been done prior to amputation, the pulp chamber and portion of the canal should have been filled with amalgam. The bone is reshaped to eliminate contours that would preclude gingival healing, free of reverse architecture and pseudopockets (Fig. 24-23).

If the initial cut has been judiciously made, little recontouring of furcal area and crown is necessary or should be done at this time. Subsequent removal of projecting root remnants or contours is difficult if not impossible without anesthesia and flap elevation. Figure 24-23 also shows that the initial buccal furcal invasion of the second molar has been treated by ostectomy and osteoplasty. The flaps are repositioned or apically positioned to ensure pocket elimination and are secured by continuous or interrupted sling sutures. A vertical incision through the flap extending into the alveolar mucosa may facilitate the placement of the

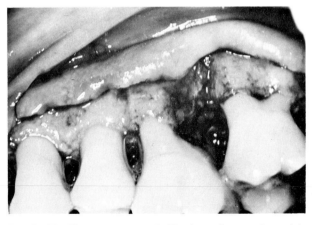

FIG. 24-23. *The root removed. The bone is recontoured to allow the soft-tissue flap to be repositioned uniformly. The slight furcal invasion of the second molar has been treated by ostectomy and osteoplasty.*

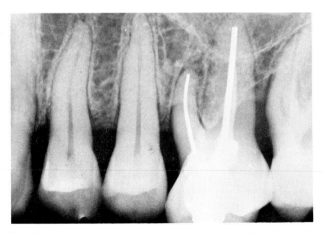

FIG. 24-25. *Roentgenogram showing completed endodontic therapy on remaining two roots of the first molar.*

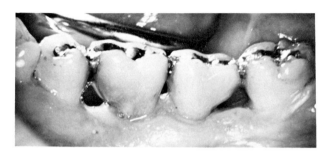

FIG. 24-26. *An intracoronal amalgam-and-wire temporary splint created to stabilize the remaining distal root of the first molar and mesial root of the second molar to the second bicuspid and third molar.*

flap into the depression created by the removal of the root and by subsequent bone reshaping. A suitable surgical dressing is applied and the patient is instructed in postsurgical care. Healing is usually uneventful (Figs. 24-24, 24-25).

Postsurgical mobility and susceptibility to occlusal traumatism are important considerations when one contemplates root amputation or hemisection. All lateral stresses due to cross-arch and cross-tooth balancing contacts or working contacts should be eliminated by selective grinding and, if necessary, by occlusal narrowing. The careful reshaping of mandibular lingual cusps and maxillary buccal cusps without the obliteration of the cusp-to-fossa relationship in centric relation is generally accepted.

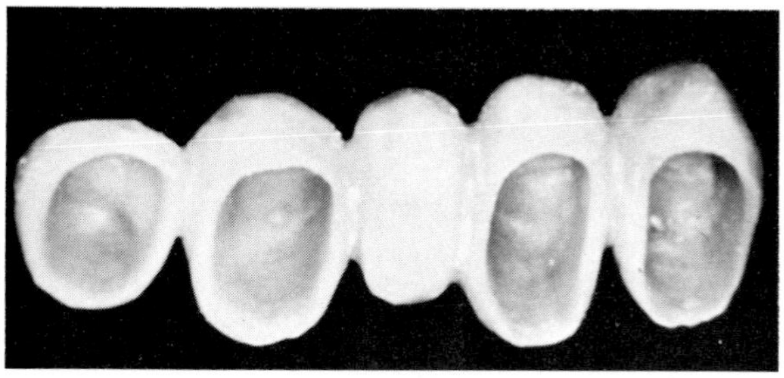

Temporary stabilization may be employed to avoid occlusal traumatism due to lesser root and bone support (Sternlicht 1969). Increased support from adjacent teeth can be achieved by splinting with wire and acrylic resin, orthodontic bands, or reinforced amalgam (Fig. 24-26). Occlusal splints (bite guards) may be used immediately after hemisection. Acrylic provisional splints can be used to provide a satisfactory degree of immobilization (Fig. 24-27).

Therapy for the Mandibular Molar Furca

As in all furcal invasions, the basic objective in therapy remains the exposure of all marginal gingiva to maintenance efforts. In most cases this means interradicular grooving of bone, crater leveling, and the elimination of hemisepta, where possible, by leveling the shallow ones or by inducing bone fill in the deeper lesions. In other words, basic principles of pocket elimination apply here just as they do everywhere else. Sometimes this is not possible and root resection and the alteration of basic root structure must be resorted to.[1,20,25] In root resection, as in other situations, the variations are many (Fig. 24-28; 24-29).

The Hemisection of Mandibular Molars, Retaining Both Segments

In a significant number of mandibular molars with furcal invasion there is ample bone to maintain both roots individually in the fashion of two adjacent premolars. The furca must be located relatively near to the crown, and the roots must be divergent to allow for as much interradicular bone as possible. The principal advantage gained by splitting the crown vertically and separating the root lies in the potential for modifying

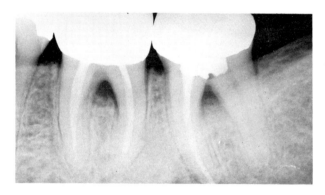

FIG. 24-28. *Roentgenogram illustrating endodontically treated molars in preparation for hemisection. The first molar will be hemisected, and both roots will be retained and restored to simulate bicuspids. Only the mesial root of the hemisected second molar will be retained. Splinting of the three roots will be accomplished with a full-coverage fixed prosthesis.*

A

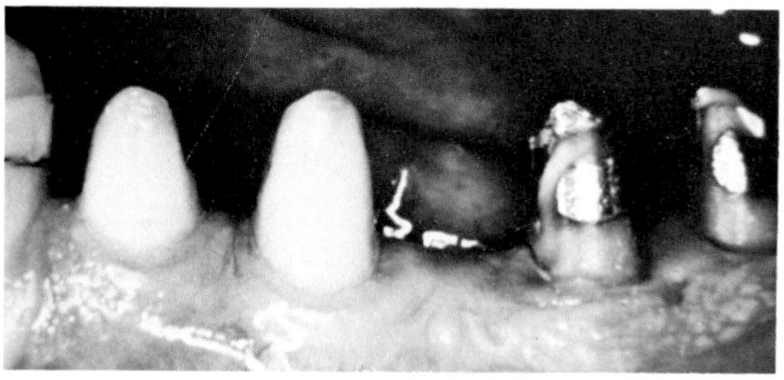

B

FIG. 24-27. *A. The shell of an acrylic provisional splint to be used to stabilize remaining roots of hemisected molars to bicuspids. B. The bicuspids and molar roots are prepared to accept the provisional splint.*

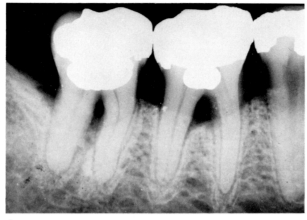

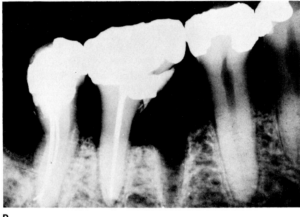

A

B

FIG. 24-29. *A. Roentgenogram illustrates extensive loss of periodontal tissues, and clinical examination corroborates Class III invasions of both molars. B. The mesial root of the second molar and distal root of the first molar are treated endodontically and temporarily splinted with amalgam. The mesial half of the crown of the first molar is retained to facilitate splinting and is not intended to be retained permanently.*

the furca itself. The hemisected coronal portion of the tooth is subsequently restored by two individual full crowns with a simple contact and marginal-ridge relationship. The inaccessible furcal area is thus converted into a simulated interproximal space, accessible to flossing and protected from caries by virtue of the full coverage. If restorative principles require splinting of the separated roots, the solder joint should be placed as near to the occlusal surface as possible to facilitate cleansing of the remodeled furcal region. This approach to the problem may be a sequel to the creation of a through-and-through furcal communication, where the therapeutic plan has been to provide access and ease of maintenance, but resulting carious breakdown with or without pulpal involvement has necessitated a more comprehensive approach. The extensive endodontic and restorative therapy would only be

justified by a favorable periodontal prognosis, and this by now would have been established.

Hemisection of a Mandibular Molar in Which One Root is Extracted

A fairly common pattern of resorption is that in which the mesial or distal root of a mandibular molar is involved with an overwhelming lesion that seems to have little effect on the other root. These lesions are usually seen roentgenographically as a limited area of radiolucency involving one root completely from apex to margin (Fig. 24-29). Probing is easy. Commonly, the probe may circumscribe the entire root; yet the adjacent root of the same tooth appears undamaged and untouched by disease. The furca may show little if any invasion, and the clinical crown-root ratio will not be jeopardized. Careful examination often corroborates the roentgenographic evidence.

These catastrophic root involvements bear careful examination and probing. Sometimes the circumferential resorptive lesion is narrow and lined with bone throughout its entire area. Even the interradicular bone stands at its normal height or nearly so. This type of lesion may respond to techniques for inducing a new attachment; this is obviously the best solution by far. Successes are not common, unfortunately, and these teeth commonly face root resection or hemisection.

The mandibular molar crown raises problems which, in our opinion, are commonly overlooked. The cantilevered crown supported by the single remaining root is a common result of root resection (Fig. 24-30).

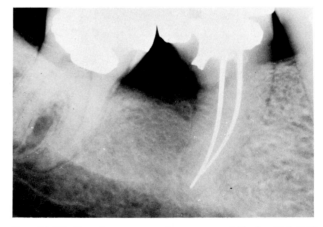

FIG. 24-30. *Roentgenogram of a successfully treated first molar. The root has been amputated below the distal cantilevered portion of the crown which was retained and splinted to the second molar. Initially intended to be temporary, it was later found to serve and function satisfactorily on a permanent basis. This illustrates an exception rather than a rule. Note the amalgam plug in the distal canal.*

The usual excuse that it is only a temporary expedient is a rather weak one. The single mandibular molar root, even if completely invested in bone, is rarely as efficient a retentive device as is a premolar root. Even if it were as effective, no sagacious operator would cantilever another premolar pontic from it, especially immediately postoperatively when mobility is greatest. A mandibular molar whose entire crown has been retained following a root resection may function satisfactorily for a considerable time, but only if it is splinted to the adjacent teeth with at least an intracoronal form of splint such as an amalgam-and-wire or a wire-and-acrylic splint. However, definitive treatment should take the form of a fixed prosthesis that gains stability through union with adjacent teeth. It follows then that the safe procedure to follow is to hemisect the tooth and reshape each half of the crown to simulate a premolar (Fig. 24-31A).

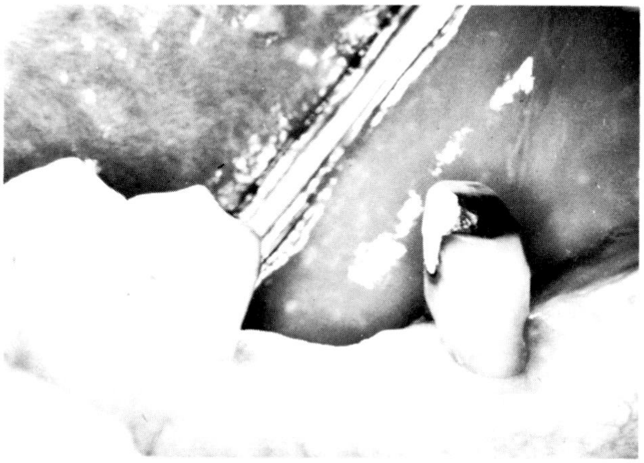

The position of the retained root in respect to other teeth in the quadrant will dictate the method of temporary stabilization to be employed immediately pre- or postoperatively. Temporary stabilization is easily accomplished with amalgam, wire-and-acrylic splints, or welded orthodontic bands (Fig. 24-31B). An acrylic provisional splint can be used for a considerable time if the prognosis for the teeth is guarded to the extent that placement of a permanent splint is considered premature.

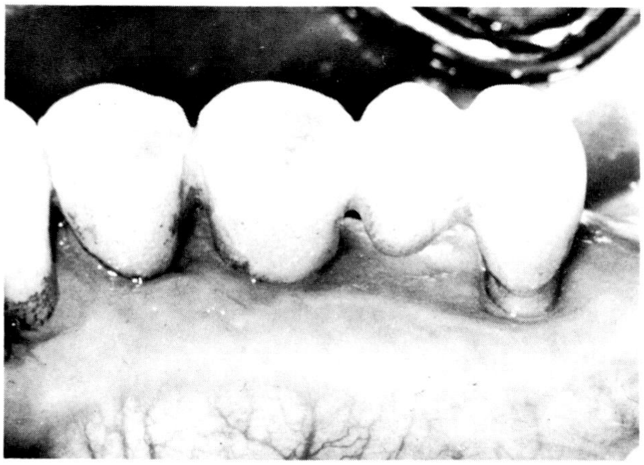

Maxillary Molar Root Resections

The maxillary molars with their rather complex root arrangements present more variations of approach than do mandibular molars (Figs. 24-32, 24-33, 24-34, 24-35, 24-36). The problems are somewhat complicated by the difficulty of determining the status of the interradicular bone. This area becomes critical in the treatment of furcal lesions. The furcal invasion itself becomes more tortuous because of the root arrangement and configuration.

Probing the lesions is not too difficult, particularly on the buccal side. The proximal furcae must be subjected to a more searching probing. Great care must be taken here to differentiate clearly between an incipient (Class I) and a patent (Class II) invasion. Merely hooking the toe of the curet into the furca will not give sufficient information for planning therapy. Not only is it important to explore the furca as far into the central zone as possible, but some attempt should be made to delineate the topography of the interradicular bone. This is at best a highly imprecise procedure, but in planning therapy each bit of information is important.

All too often the precise anatomy and bone topography of the furcal region is revealed only when flaps are retracted at the time of corrective surgery. Unpleasant surprises are by no means rare, but they can be made

FIG. 24-31. A. A single root of a molar retained to serve as a terminal abutment. B. The single root incorporated into a four-unit provisional splint that satisfies the requirements of stabilization and function until the prognosis warrants definitive restoration.

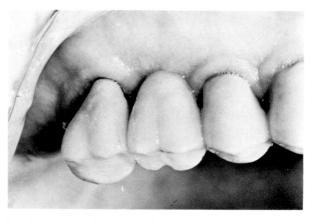

FIG. 24-32. A maxillary second molar with its distobuccal root amputated serves as a terminal abutment for a fixed bridge.

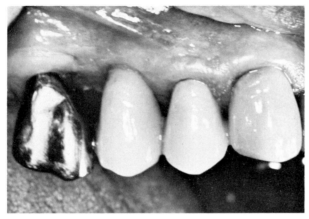

A

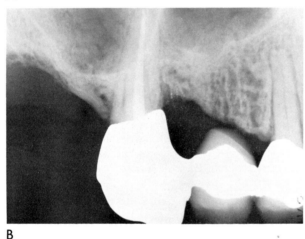

B

FIG. 24-33. *A. A first molar with its mesiobuccal root amputated serves as a terminal abutment for a fixed bridge. B. Roentgenogram showing the completed root-canal therapy and restoration.*

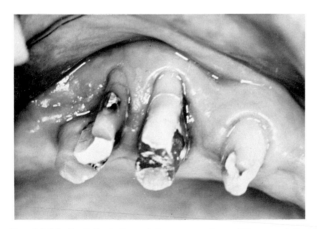

FIG. 24-34. *A clinical view of the preparation of the remaining crown portions of the second molar with its distobuccal root amputated and the first molar with its mesiobuccal root amputated. It is important to reduce totally the portion of the crown that was once situated over the root now missing.*

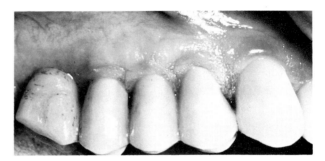

FIG. 24-35. *The mesiobuccal root is the sole survivor of a first molar and serves as the terminal abutment for an extensive fixed restoration. A molar pontic is cantilevered off the multiple splinted abutments.*

more infrequent by obtaining more and more bits of information during diagnostic probing. Sometimes all three roots are seriously undermined, and the removal of one root only removes support. Root resection presumes that the remaining roots will have adequate investment to support the crown of a maxillary molar in some kind of function (Figs. 24-32). The maxillary molar does not lend itself to splitting as does the mandibular molar. Some reshaping of the crown is in order, but not nearly to the extent required for the mandibular molar.

The factors upon which a treatment plan for such a tooth is determined are not always obvious; however, several questions keep recurring. The answers to these are sometimes helpful and should be recorded.

1. How extensive is the bone loss in the interradicular zone?
2. Is the distobuccal root invested with bone on its buccal aspect?
3. Is the distobuccal root of the maxillary first molar

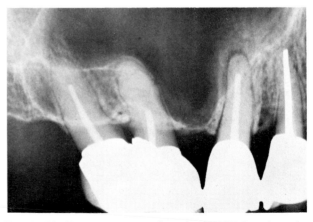

FIG. 24-36. *Roentgenogram of retained palatal and mesiobuccal roots of a rotated first molar. The two roots were separated and prepared to accept copings and splinted telescopic crowns as part of a fixed splint extending to the anterior teeth.*

flared distally? Is the root vertical? Is it bowed, with a possible fusion at the apex? (It should be stated categorically that the roots of the maxillary first molar have a sharp distal flare, often coming dangerously close to the mesiobuccal root of the second molar. The buccal roots of the maxillary second molar, on the other hand, are usually more vertical, and the furca is tight and acutely angled.)

4. When the root is resected, will a socket remain or has the buccal wall of bone formerly over the root been removed, requiring a specially placed vertical releasing incision to allow covering of the thin remaining bone in the defect to minimize postoperative resorption?

5. What are the positions of the mesial and distal furcae relative to the bone levels on adjacent teeth and where are they situated relative to the entire tooth length?

Variations on the Standard Single-Root Resection of the Maxillary Molar

There are variations in every method used in periodontal therapy, and the resection of roots is no exception. Some clinical situations would seem to require the removal of both buccal roots or of the palatal root alone (Fig. 24-37). The odds against survival of such a tooth are high, but the alternative may be even more unfavorable to the preservation of the integrity of the arch. Fortunately, such situations are rare; but they exist.

It naturally follows that the fewer the number of roots remaining after root surgery, the more critical is the investing support remaining to those roots. For this reason, the decision should be made to resect more than a single buccal root in a maxillary molar, with flaps retracted and the surgical area well debrided of soft tissue. Then the amount of remaining support can be truly and critically evaluated.

The palatal root, because of its shape, presents most resistance to displacement in a mesiodistal direction and does not do nearly so well with torquing forces in a buccolingual direction without the stabilizing influence of even a single buccal root.

The distobuccal root of maxillary molars is the most likely candidate for amputation (Figs. 24-32, 24-33, 24-34, 24-35, 24-36). Its proximity to the second molar, its usual thin spindly form, its confluence with the palatal root in a difficult interproximal space, and its affinity for bone fenestrations prejudices its prolonged survival in an environment of advanced marginal periodontitis. The mesiobuccal root, with its greater

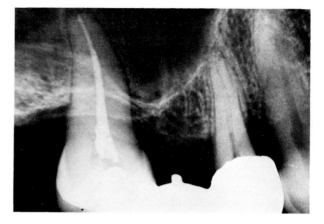

FIG. 24-37. *Roentgenogram of a maxillary molar with both buccal roots removed. For additional stability the fixed bridge was replaced with a restoration extending to the cuspid.*

buccolingual width and more lingually placed furca, usually survives longer and on occasion may indeed be the sole survivor of a maxillary first molar to serve as a useful abutment (Fig. 24-35).

Both buccal roots may be retained if a Class III invasion is from the mesial to the distal surface and if the destruction is severe on the lingual side of the palatal root. The therapist should be prepared to be confronted with an extensive resorptive lesion in the furcal region upon removal of the palatal root. He then must make a careful assessment of the prospect of a favorable postsurgical result to justify the continuance of the amputation procedure, with all its implications of endodontic treatment and restoration.

Buccal roots without the palatal root must have good buccal plate covering. They are almost always spindly and are not sturdy enough to provide too useful an abutment, except in special cases.

The greatest difficulty encountered with these teeth is not in the corrective surgery but in the resulting anatomy of the finished case. It is virtually impossible to remove both buccal roots and salvage the palatal root or, conversely, to remove the palatal root to save the buccal roots without creating serious problems in the restoration of these teeth. These problems, together with others of similar nature in less extensive root surgery, will be dealt with in Chapter 29 (Fig. 24-34).

The final disposition of teeth treated by root amputation or hemisection involves a completion of endodontic therapy, placement of the fixed prosthesis, and detailed instruction in the home-care procedures to ensure freedom from progressive inflammatory periodontal disease. This ensures a life expectancy of sufficient duration to warrant the effort involved in this aspect of periodontal, endodontic, and restorative therapy.[26,27]

References

1. Amen, C. R.: Hemisection and root amputation. Periodontics, 4:197, 1966.
2. Amsterdam, M., and Rossman, S. R.: Technique of hemisection of multirooted teeth. Alpha Omegan, 53:4, 1960.
3. Arvins, A. N.: Technique for root resection of periodontally hopeless teeth included in multiple splint bridges. J. Dent. Med., 12:79, 1957.
4. Arvins, A. N.: Changing concepts in periodontal prognosis. J. Dent. Med., 16:133, 1961.
5. Basaraba, N.: Root amputation and hemisection. Bull. Can. Acad. Periodontol., 2:2, 1958.
6. Basaraba, N.: Root amputation and tooth hemisection. Dent. Clin. North Am., 13:121, 1969.
7. Black, G. U.: Special Dental Pathology, 1st ed. Chicago, Medico-Dental Publishing Co., 1915.
8. Easley, J. R., and Drennan, G. A.: Morphological classification of the furca. J. Can. Dent. Assoc., 35:2, 1969.
9. Everett, F. G.: The intermediate bifurcation ridge: a study of the morphology of the bifurcation of the lower first molar. J. Dent. Res., 37:162, 1958.
10. Farrar, J. N.: Radical and heroic treatment of alveolar abscess by amputation of roots and teeth. Dental Cosmos, 26:79, 1884.
11. Glickman, I.: Bifurcation involvement in periodontal disease. J. Am. Dent. Assoc., 40:528, 1950.
12. Glickman, I.: Clinical Periodontology. Philadelphia, W. B. Saunders Co., 1964, p. 603.
13. Goldman, H. M.: Therapy of the incipient bifurcation involvement. J. Periodontol., 29:112, 1958.
14. Grewe, J. M.: Cervical enamel projections: prevalence, location, and extent; with associated periodontal implications. J. Periodontol., 36:460, 1965.
15. Heins, P. J., and Canter, S. R.: Furca involvement: a classification of bony deformities. Periodontics, 6:84, 1968.
16. Hiatt, W. H.: Periodontal pocket elimination by combined endodontic-periodontic therapy. Periodontics, 1:152, 1963.
17. Hiatt, W. H.: Regeneration via flap operation and pulpal periodontal lesion. Periodontics, 4:205, 1966.
18. Hiatt, W. H., and Amen, C. R.: Periodontal pocket elimination by combined therapy. Dent. Clin. North Am., 8:133, 1964.
19. Leib, A. M.: Furcation involvements correlated with enamel projections from the cemento-enamel junction. J. Periodontol., 38:330, 1967.
20. Lloyd, R. S., and Baer, P. N.: Periodontal therapy by root resection. J. Prosthet. Dent., 10:362, 1960.
21. Masters, D. H.: Projection of cervical enamel into molar furcation. J. Periodontol., 35:49, 1964.
22. Messinger, T. F., and Orban, B. J.: Elimination of periodontal pockets by root amputation. J. Periodontol., 26:213, 1954.
23. Orban, B.: The development of the bifurcation of multirooted teeth. J. Am. Dent. Assoc., 16:297, 1929.
24. Orban, B., and Johnston, H. B.: Interradicular pathology as related to accessory root canals. J. Endodont., 3:21, 1948.
25. Pearson, H. H.: Hemisection of a lower molar: A case report. Dental Digest, June, 1955.
26. Rosen, H., and Gitnick, P. J.: Integrating restorative procedures into the treatment of periodontal disease. J. Prosthet. Dent., 14:343, 1964.
27. Rosen, H., and Gitnick, P. J.: Separation and splinting of the roots of multirooted teeth. J. Prosthet. Dent., 21:34, 1969.
28. Rossman, S. R., Kaplowitz, B., and Baldinger, R. S.: Treatment of periodontally and endodontically involved teeth. Oral Surg., March, 1960.
29. Saxe, S., and Carmen, D.: Removal or retention of molar teeth: the problem of the furcation. Dent. Clin. North Am., 13:783, 1969.
30. Seltzer, S., Bender, I. B., and Zionetz, M.: The interrelationship of pulp and periodontal disease. Oral Surg., 16:1474, 1963.
31. Simon, P., and Jacobs, D.: The so-called combined periodontal-pulpal problem. Dent. Clin. North Am., 13:45, 1969.
32. Sorrin, S.: Bridgework and periodontal treatment: A report of a case. J. Am. Dent. Assoc., 37:607, 1948.
33. Staffileno, H. J.: Surgical management of furca invasion. Dent. Clin. North Am., 13:103, 1969.
34. Steiner, J. C.: Guidelines for selecting teeth to be treated with endodontic therapy. Dent. Clin. North Am., 13:769, 1969.
35. Sternlicht, H. C.: Principles and techniques for the stabilization of loose teeth. Dent. Clin. North Am., 13:213, 1969.
36. Yuodelis, R. A., and Mann, W. V.: The prevalence and possible role of nonworking contacts in periodontal disease. Periodontics, 3:5, 1965.

25

Mucosal Reparative Surgery

25

Mucosal

Reparative

Surgery

Up to this point in periodontal case management the principal concern had been the elimination or control of the periodontal lesion and the preservation or restoration of the periodontal attachment apparatus and its environs. It soon became apparent to periodontists that pocket elimination was not enough. The periodontium exists in a definite milieu or climate in which certain anatomic arrangements are more or less critical to periodontal health, if not survival, and which exert a powerful influence upon its integrity.

GINGIVAL AND VESTIBULAR PROBLEMS

The gingiva is the marginal tissue of the oral cavity. The free gingiva is not the major concern in reparative procedures, but the attached gingiva is of overriding importance, since it furnishes the only useful arrangement for marginal tissue to the investing structures of the teeth. The attached gingiva also provides a barrier preventing the musculature of expression and lip and cheek mobility from retracting the free gingival margin.

Because of this property, the width of gingiva becomes of major concern in almost every pocket-eliminating procedure. At one time the total arena for pocket elimination was limited to the gingiva, since to traverse it into areolar mucosa was to expose a tissue totally inadequate for marginal use. Those days have passed, primarily because of the introduction of newer methods of treatment and of conservation of gingiva through apically displaced flaps and the use of autogenous free gingival grafts and pedicle grafts for gingival reconstitution and extension, when deficient.

Distribution of Gingiva

Generally the zone of gingiva on the facial surfaces of both upper and lower arches is widest in the incisor regions, with the dimension gradually decreasing toward the molars. This is not a hard and fast rule, of course, since considerable variation is possible. These variations occur most frequently over the canines and premolars where there is sometimes as little as 1 mm of gingiva other than the free margin.

It is interesting to note how stable the zone of gingiva is throughout the life of the individual. The width of gingiva is established in the newborn when the entire alveolar process is covered by this tissue. As the alveolar process grows and enlarges, the original bank of gingiva is no longer sufficient to cover the process alone, so that the adult vestibular fornix is lined with areolar mucosa and the tougher, more resistant tissue is crestal and lingual for a variable distance, beginning at the mucogingival line.

With the eruption of the teeth, many new factors are introduced. The gingival sulcus with its free gingival margin, root form, and position enters the picture as a serious factor in gingival position and location. In another context it was pointed out that root position and root relationship exert a considerable influence upon the gingival level.

Tooth Position and the Gingiva

It is widely observed that the more prominent the root in the orderly regular alignment, the more apical is the gingival margin. This is true on the lingual as well as on the labial side. It is true, however, that most of our problems with gingival recession are on the labial side, but lingual recessions are by no means uncommon. The resultant recession is always at the expense of the original band of gingiva. Gingival recession is one of the most common phenomena observed in marginal contour. Since it represents to a variable extent a loss of periodontium, it may properly be called a periodontal disease or, at the least, periodontal atrophy. However it is called, gingival recession gives rise to environmental problems.

Function of the Gingiva

Gingiva performs an indispensable function. It is the first soft tissue to encounter the thrust of the bolus and the searching probing of a semiliquid mass under certain hydraulic pressures. It not only must resist abrasion, but it must deflect invasive forces separating it from the underlying hard tissues. Gingival tissue is tough and, when healthy, is firmly anchored to the root and bone it envelops and covers. Its attachment is aided by a complex fiber arrangement of ingenious design; but anchors are never tougher than the tissues they are designed to fix and render immobile. Although gingiva serves admirably, the areolar mucosa is poorly endowed for such a role.

Gingival Recession

Since gingival recession is at the expense of gingiva, it is obvious that extensive recession will have destroyed the entire zone of gingiva in a given area as the gingival margin approaches the mucogingival line. If recession is allowed to progress, the result is an ugly thick rolled margin that continually retracts and is extremely refractory to conservative therapy (Fig. 25-1). In seeking a remedy, the therapist is offered three alternatives, all of them surgical.

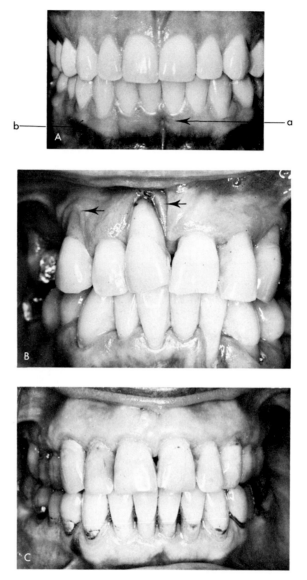

FIG. 25-1. Gingival survey. A. Normal gingiva (a); mucogingival line (b). B. Gingival recession traversing the mucogingival line with thick, rolled gingival margins (arrows). C. Gingival recession with a flat outline. This type poses no threat to gingival integrity.

The Shallow Vestibular Trough

There is another soft-tissue sequel to gingival recession. The vestibular trough is diminished by the migration of the gingival margin apically. This is a relatively minor problem in most cases, but any dentist who is faced with the establishment of a crown margin at or near the fundus of the vestibular fornix will appreciate that it can create serious problems that are anything but minor. The fortunate aspect of vestibular trough problems is that they are resolved concomitantly with gingival corrections in most cases.

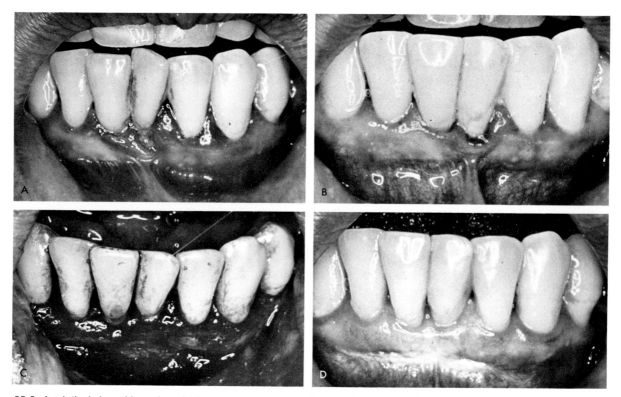

FIG. 25-2. *A relatively broad insertion of a lower midline frenum showing distension and retraction of the gingival margin when the lip is stretched. In addition, the lower left central incisor is rotated so that an unesthetic situation exists in the region. A. Preoperative view showing the frenum insertion and the accumulation of plaque and calculus in the area. B. After curettage plus the reshaping of the lower left central incisor on its incisal and labial and lingual surfaces to create a somewhat more normal appearance. C. Denudation of the labial plate of bone from first premolar to first premolar after reshaping the interproximal papillae with gingivoplasty. D. Five years after surgery. Note the scar throughout the extent of the denudation. The scar remained firmly fixed to bone.*

Frena

Points of insertion of frena usually become troublesome where the gingival margin is approached. Sometimes this occurs because of an unusually high frenal insertion or in other clinical situations a gingival recession destroys the marginal gingiva to the extent that any remaining gingiva meets an otherwise normal insertion of the frenum. Frenal insertions sometimes distend and retract the marginal gingiva and interproximal papilla where the lip is stretched. These distensions and retractions occur most frequently in the lower midline region.

The phenomenon generates several questions on etiology and functional aberrations. First the question on etiology: did the frenum cause the gingival recession with which it is associated? There is no clear answer to this, since there are many high frenal insertions where the gingiva does not recede. Yet papillary and gingival retraction may occur with lip distension. It is safer to suggest that the lower midline frenum is sometimes associated with gingival recession and, at times, with gingival retraction in a normal or receded position.

Functionally it was believed that an abnormal insertion of the frenum prevented proper brushing and cleansing, thus explaining the calculus commonly found on the tooth at the point of insertion. This is probably not exactly true, but there is some logic to the opinion.

Frenum insertions occur in various forms: long, narrow insertions; broad, flat insertions; and all the variants in between. Upper midline frena are usually more prone to be long and narrow, and lower midline frena have a tendency to be broad and flat. These frena have been regarded by some as sharply localized shallow vestibules (Fig. 25-2). This opinion is especially true for broad frenum insertions rather more common in lower midline regions.

DENUDATION PROCEDURES

As little as 20 years ago, mucogingival problems were solved by rather heroic methods. Reference is made to the various denudation procedures in use at that time. The approach was simplicity itself. All the corrective procedures were begun by resecting the entire ribbon of the facial gingiva from the operative field and discarding it. The remaining alveolar mucosa retracted, leaving large areas of cortical plate exposed. After the various bone alterations (if any) and treatment were completed, the area was covered with a standard surgical cement. Since there was no longer any gingiva to cover the bone, the surgical cement was placed directly upon cortical plate of the bone of the buccal surface of the operative field. There were two separate procedures—really two variations of a single method, since everything but the dressings was identical and those not too radically different from each other.

Gingival Induction with Denudation

One technique for gingival induction, described by Goldman and his colleagues and called the push-back in the vernacular, consisted of placing the surgical cement over the exposed cortical plate and extending it to the margin of the retracted alveolar mucosa.[17] Placement of such a dressing was designed to induce new gingiva to form under the cement. This objective was realized routinely. New gingiva resulted from the proliferation of granulation tissue that emanated from the periodontal space (Fig. 25-3). In a study on gingival induction in a somewhat different context, Bohannan observed that the pattern of healing was consistent after every denudation procedure.[3] The periodontal space was the source of the granulation tissue that later matured into gingiva firmly attached to the cortical plate. However, no matter how extensive apically was the denudation, he found that new gingiva would extend only 5 to 6 mm in an apical direction. This growth was found even when the denudation extended apically as much as 15 mm. The newly formed gingiva in these denudations proved to be smooth and without a blemish or irregularity. There were no lines of demarcation between new and old gingiva and no cervical irregularities; as a result, no gingivoplasties were required for repairs.

There were, however, two great drawbacks to denudation: (1) the postoperative course was routinely stormy, with a protracted period of healing that often exceeded 3 to 4 weeks, and (2) the permanent loss of bone from the exposed cortical plate was excessive and too high a price to pay for the handsome postoperative gingiva. It was for the reasons cited that the denudation procedures are no longer used routinely. In unusual situations, they are occasionally used today, but they are definitely out of the mainstream of therapy.

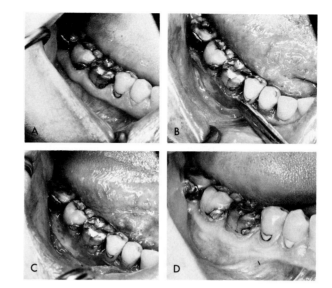

Fig. 25-3. *Gingival induction with denudation. A. Preoperative view of the lower molar facial surface. What appeared to be a fibrotic marginal gingiva turned out to be a thin marginal enlargement in bone. B. The operative field denuded. All the gingiva was excised and discarded. C. Marginal osteoplasty on the bone. After this step was completed, periodontal dressing was placed against the bone. D. Two years after surgery. New gingiva has formed.*

Vestibular Trough Extension with Denudation

The extension of the depth of the vestibular trough is a fairly common objective in periodontal therapy. The vestibular fornix is sometimes shallow in the lower arch, particularly in the anterior region. The shallow vestibule is almost always associated with the narrow or almost absent zone of attached gingiva.

Experience showed that denudation of the labial plate by blunt dissection and reflection of the marginal gingiva and alveolar mucosa would yield a deepened vestibular trough in addition to a broad zone of attached gingiva if, after completion of the surgical procedure, the surgical cement was inserted deeply into the cavernous space *apical* to the margin of the wound. Stated differently: after the operative field had been entered in the usual manner for denudation of that area, a total gingivectomy consisting of resection of the entire gingival ribbon marginal to the operative field was performed. From the line of resection, dissection was used to reflect the mucosa and to create the denudation to a depth of 12 to 15 mm from the margin of the alveolar plate. The cement dressing was then pushed into this 12 to 15 mm space and beyond. The healing response was exactly the same as that in the procedure for gingival extension denudation. The only discernible differences were that the healing period was longer and more painful and the postoperative vestibular trough was considerably deeper.

The clinical report by Bohannan in 1961 was the definitive evaluation of the effectiveness of this procedure in extending the depth of the vestibular fornix on a long-term basis.[3] There was no question of the effectiveness of the operation. The reasons for its relegation to limbo were its painful postoperative course and the excessive loss of crestal bone through exposure of thin labial bone to the cement dressing.

It should be noted that in the most successful postoperative results the extension of the shallow vestibular trough was limited to the anterior region. The most refractory in management is the shallow vestibular trough encompassing an entire arch.

It must be kept in mind that other factors make extension of the vestibular trough difficult. Muscle insertions, mandibular anatomy, and overall mouth volume all operate to establish the given vestibular trough. Any invasion of this terrain involves alterations that may or may not be tolerated. The topography of the bone is practically unalterable. Flared oblique ridges and prominent genial tubercles can be slightly modified, but spectacular alterations are neither possible nor even desirable. For example, in a patient with a horizontally flared external oblique ridge forming the buccal wall of a buccal pocket on a lower second molar, any attempt to achieve a significant reduction of this mass of bone has only a slight chance for success. Obviously, such a procedure is quite traumatic. The postoperative edema and mucosal distortion incident to it usually result in the gingiva and mucosa becoming thick and flabby and completely obliterating any vertical gain in gingival topography.

FLAP DESIGN AND CONTROL AS A MUCOGINGIVAL PROCEDURE

The earliest attempt in recent times to palliate the postoperative effects of the old denudation procedures was by reflection of the full-thickness flap for entry into the operative field and its replacement at the new bone margin. The flap was secured by several interproximal interrupted sutures and reinforced by a surgical cement dressing. This approach was introduced by Claude Nabers in 1954.[28]

Full-Thickness Flaps

Entry via the full-thickness flap is an old and well-tried approach to underlying structures in several branches of dentistry, periodontics among them. In the more modern flap entries, some unusual operations are performed while the flap is reflected. Procedures to induce bone and new gingival attachment and to reshape bone are the most common operations requiring flap reflection, but instead of simple replacement of the flap, several variations in flap positioning have been introduced.

Early marginal flap design consisted of two straight line incisions at the crest of the buccal and lingual bone margins in the surgical area. The incisions were made with an internal bevel, so that thinning was done at the expense of the lamina propria, leaving a keratinized flap preserved to cover the operative field. Flaps in that era were rather thick, particularly on the palatal side. Sutures were interrupted and simple, with an occasional mattress suture stabilizing a fragile flap.

By displacing the full-thickness flap apically for several millimeters and by stabilizing it in that position, the effect of marginal denudation was realized without the penalty of noticeable bone loss incident to an extensive denudation. Stabilization of the flap is discussed in Chapter 23. Since the source of new gingiva in the denudation procedures is the periodontal space, the marginal collaring about the neck of the tooth is usually enough to cover the exposed marginal bone. This procedure is used to induce a new marginal gingiva that ends in a knife-edge. At one period this method fell out of favor, but it has been gaining new adherents in recent years.

As methods are introduced, they are commonly taken up with considerable enthusiasm because they are usually designed to accomplish a given objective currently deemed desirable. Sometimes in the adoption of new techniques advantages are gained at the expense of others lost in the discarded method. So it was that when the margin of the flap was replaced coronally to the margin of the bone, the course of healing most often resulted in thick margins. This was due to necrosis of the beveled edges of the soft tissues. The problem was so common that many careful operators performed a gingivoplasty as a routinely scheduled repair 2 or 3 weeks after the initial surgery. The marginal necrosis due to knife-edged margins in the internally beveled flaps can be avoided by making a 1 to 2 mm horizontal cut in marginal flap outline *before* beginning the internal bevel. Many operators do this.

When the flap is placed 2 to 3 millimeters apically to the bone margin, the new marginal gingiva granulates into a knife-edged margin, just as the old denudations used to do. Of course, this advantage is gained at the cost of quicker healing that occurs when the flap is placed precisely at the bone margin.

The full-thickness flap is an opening gambit to the principal procedure to be performed. It might precede any one of five operations:

1. Open or flap curettage
2. Internal-bevel gingivectomy with repositioned flaps
3. Osseous reshaping to eliminate morphologic aberrations
4. Induction procedures for new attachment
5. Mucogingival induction procedures

Flaps and flap control were discussed in Chapter 21 No attempt will be made to repeat these descriptions other than to enumerate the implications for mucogingival repair. These include the various pedicle flaps and the apically positioned flaps combined with marginal denudation for the induction of additional gingiva.

The Partial or Split-Thickness Flap

The split-thickness flap has been described in Chapter 21. Its relevance in the current context of mucosal repairs is that of an induction technique for the extension of gingiva. Its principal application is in splitting the gingival thickness so that, by placing the movable segment just apical to the split segment, the whole width of the gingival zone is left undisturbed and its width is effectively doubled.

The claims that the paper-thin bed of split gingiva and periosteum prevents some cortical plate resorption and by so doing prevents crestal loss of bone are totally unsupported by anything save opinion. However, these controversies are best discussed elsewhere. Whatever studies have been done seem to point to more resorption, not less, than would occur under a full-thickness flap. Gingival gain, however, is incontrovertible when the procedure is done (Fig. 25-4).

The Pedicle Flap Used as a Graft

The pedicle flap is one of the most widely used methods in plastic and reconstructive surgery. By definition, it is a flap of tissue connected with its origin by a stalk. Although the width of this stalk is not specified in periodontal surgery, it is considerably wider than one would suppose. Even the basic flap, both full-thickness and partial-thickness, may be considered a pedicle flap with a broad connecting stalk. It is widely used in plastic surgery, in skin grafting.

It is common knowledge that survival of tissue that has been resected from its original locus depends upon the availability of fluid interchange. The free graft will survive only if it lies upon a bed of tissue vascular enough to provide, through diffusion, fluid exchange of the minimal metabolite requirements and the waste

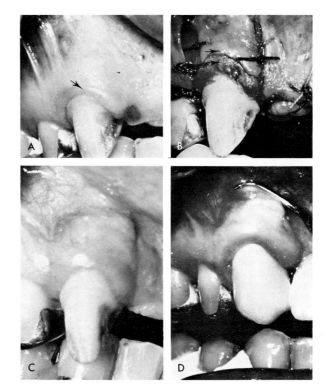

FIG. 25-4. An apically positioned split-thickness flap for inducing additional gingiva. A. Preoperative view. Note that almost all the remaining gingiva is free gingiva. A crown is to be placed on the canine. B. Split-thickness pedicle is mobilized and apically positioned so that the zone of gingiva remaining is placed just apical to the undisturbed split zone of gingiva. C. Postoperative view of the gain in gingiva. D. Full crown restoration in place with the margin under an adequate zone of gingiva. (Treated by Dr. W. P. Ammons.)

products. It follows, then, that a free graft requires a carefully prepared vascular bed.

Clinically, when such a bed is missing or faulty, the pedicle graft is a useful expedient, since the connecting stalk provides for the circulatory needs of the tissue being grafted. There are the inevitable advantages and disadvantages. The most obvious disadvantage is that the pedicle flap is sharply limited in mobility by the stalk. The donor site can never be far removed from the recipient site. Therefore, the right type of tissue, in the quantity required, must be present near the area of deficiency. This limits the application of pedicle grafts.

On the other hand, root denudations can be covered with gingiva, firmly attached, in no other way on a predictable basis. Free grafts over denuded roots depend upon a widely extended bed so that the circulatory requirements are met by cantilevering, so to speak, for short distances on either side of the recession. Therefore, when the tissue can be found in an adjacent saddle area or from an interproximal segment of gingiva, the pedicle graft becomes practicable.

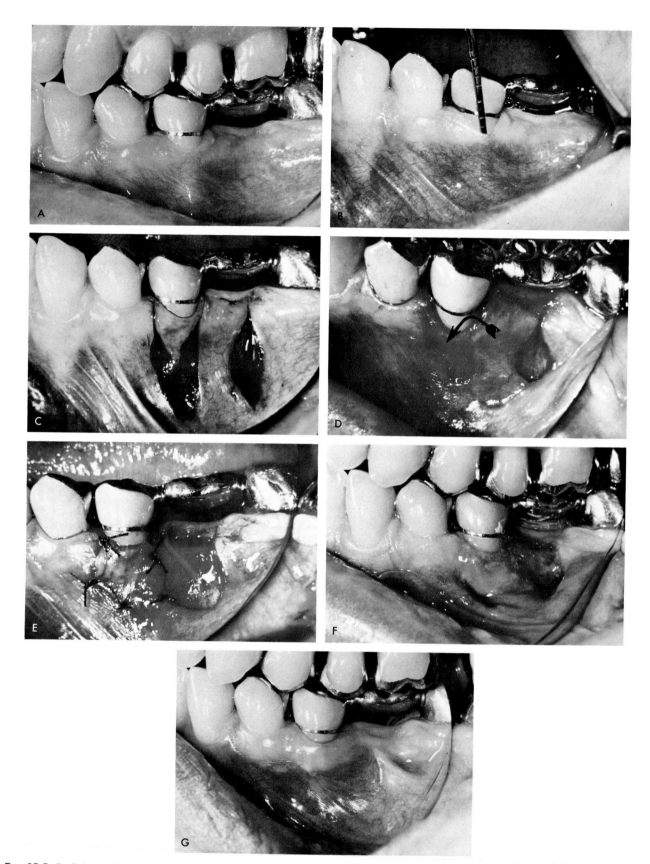

FIG. 25-5. *Pedicle grafts from adjacent saddle area. In this patient gingival recession occurred after a fixed bridge replacing the lower left first molar was inserted. A. Preoperative view of the operative field. Note the lack of gingiva on the facial side of the premolar abutment. B. Probe inserted into the sulcus revealing that there was no attached gingiva. C. Incisions for the bed preparation and pedicle design. D. Bed preparation of the recipient site and mobilization of the pedicle. The arrow points to the margin of gingiva created by the pedicle graft. E. Suturing of the pedicle in position over the premolar root. F. Nine days after surgery. G. One year after surgery. The gingiva seems to be extending coronally. (Treated by Dr. S. Sapkos.)*

The size of the pedicle flap becomes practicable when gingiva is available immediately adjacent to the area requiring it; in other words, the recipient site and the donor site are side by side. This means, in most cases, that the tooth requiring the graft is adjacent to a saddle area of variable length (Fig. 25-5).

If the saddle area has enough gingiva on its labial aspect to supply all the clinical requirements, then the pedicle flap design can be carried out by beginning the crestal incision at or near the crest of the ridge. Some saddle areas, however, do not have enough keratinized masticatory mucosa on the labial aspect alone. Grafts for these areas must be raised by incision from the lingual aspect of the alveolar ridge and continued over the crest and in an apical direction on the labial side on approaching the vestibular trough.

In designing the shape and length of the pedicle, certain principles must be kept in mind, and objectives must be clearly visualized. First, an attempt must be made to raise and mobilize a flap of tissue to be rotated mesially or distally, as the situation requires, to cover a defect in the gingiva (Fig. 25-6). Second, if the flap is to survive as a pedicle, it must be kept in mind that its base or stalk should not be too narrow. Although no hard and fast rule is possible, a length-to-base proportion of four to one is safe. Full-thickness pedicles can more safely tolerate a narrow stalk than can partial-thickness flaps. This precaution ensures that circulation to the pedicle will be adequate to the demands made upon it. Strangulation of the stalk of the pedicle is to be avoided so that circulation to the graft is not cut off. Encroachment on the vital vasculature at its base may doom the entire pedicle to necrosis. Third, before making *any* incisions, certain measurements should be taken to make the proper design possible. This, in turn, ensures the fit of the rotated pedicle to the projected bed, without stretching or pinching the base and embarassing the circulation.

The third factor will need some elaboration, since its requirements are at once critical but not obvious. In rotating a pedicle, it will be noted that an adequate vertical linear dimension in the flap is quite short when rotated to a diagonal position. The safest procedure to ensure an adequate length of pedicle is to establish the base of the flap directly apically to the area to which the pedicle is to be rotated. In this way the design of the flap with its two more or less vertical incisions will be slanted toward a point in the vestibule directly apical to the deficient area. Rotation is no problem, and an inadvertent shortage in length is highly unlikely (Fig. 25-7). Pinching or constriction of the base is not a factor in such a flap design. In 1964 Corn suggested that small cutback incisions be made at the base of the pedicle to facilitate rotation without constriction at

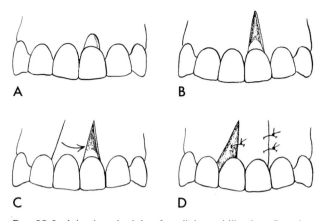

FIG. 25-6. *A basic principle of pedicle mobilization. Drawing illustrating the proper angle of incisions in designing a pedicle to be moved laterally. A. The problem area with gingival recession on the labial of the upper left central incisor. B. Bed preparation of the recipient site. C. Releasing incisions with the angle of incision correctly made in the direction toward which the flap will be rotated so that the base of the pedicle is apical to the recipient site. D. Pedicle rotated into position and sutured.*

the base, but these are rarely necessary if the outline incisions are angled toward the base of the deficiency to be corrected.

SUTURING THE PEDICLE

In positioning the pedicle upon the exposed root and its bordering vascular bed, it is common to place the graft a few millimeters coronally to the cemento-enamel junction. Suturing to the bed of lamina propria remaining is not difficult; two or three sutures on each side of the cleft suffice. A cervical sling about the neck of the tooth is enough to suspend the flap in good position upon the root.

Postoperative dressing may be used or dispensed with, depending on the stability established by the sutures and suspensory sling.

The sutures are allowed to remain for 9 to 10 days postoperatively before removal. Caution should be exercised not to remove the sutures too early, since healing may not have progressed sufficiently for the graft to stabilize. Stabilization first is the rule in the early postoperative course (Fig. 25-8).

THE LATERALLY POSITIONED SLIDING FLAP

Grupe and Warren in 1956 reported on the successful correction of gingival recession over a single tooth by mobilizing adjacent tissue covering the process over two or three teeth and displacing it laterally over the defect. These defects were primarily gingival recession

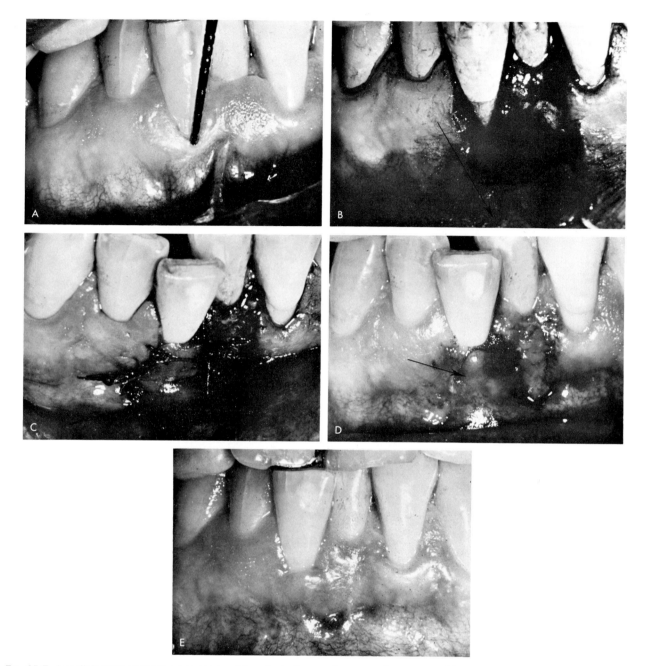

FIG. 25-7. *A pedicle graft of gingiva used to treat the gingival recession over a lower central incisor which is prominent in the arch. A. Preoperative view of the gingiva with a probe inserted traversing the entire narrow zone of free gingiva (which constitutes all the available gingiva over that tooth). The donor site is obviously the adjacent central incisor gingiva which has ample dimension. B. The split-thickness pedicle raised and lying in the fundus of the vestibular trough (arrow). C. The properly designed pedicle rotated and sutured into position. D. One week after surgery. The arrow points to the tissue gain marginally. E. Twenty days after surgery. There is only normal (2 mm) sulcular depth on midlabial probing. (Treated by Dr. L. Tibbetts.)*

associated with aberrant frenal tension. This lateral sliding flap is no more or less than a pedicle graft with a broad base. It requires a healthy and adequate labial plate of bone covering the teeth to be involved in the flap. The design of the flap is such that a heavy plate of bone over the root is exposed by the lateral displacement of the flap.

This procedure has a limited application because of the special requirements in the adjacent donor area. Pedicle flaps in general are more complicated than are free autogenous gingival grafts. They are complicated by the restrictions imposed by the donor area on size and mobility of the graft. Pedicle grafts are, however, more successful over gingival recessions than are free gingival grafts and for this reason are used when applicable (Fig. 25-9).

The technique used for the lateral sliding flap is the same as that used for any other pedicle graft. The same excision of 1 to 2 mm of the marginal gingiva bordering the recession is made. The incision is extended apically from the most apical point of the marginal gingiva into the vestibule, to the extent necessary to provide the proximal margin of the flap to be mobilized. The marginal incision of the flap is now made as far crestal to the marginal gingiva as is possible and on the distal side, extending along the margin of the tissue to be moved. The distal vertical releasing incision may be made at this time or may be deferred until the flap has been freed, the partial-thickness flap by incision from the lamina propria or the full-thickness one by blunt dissection from the labial plate.

Whenever it is made, the lateral sliding flap is raised and moved the dimension of one tooth into the defect so that the proximal line of incision may be approximated to the remaining incised margin bordering the

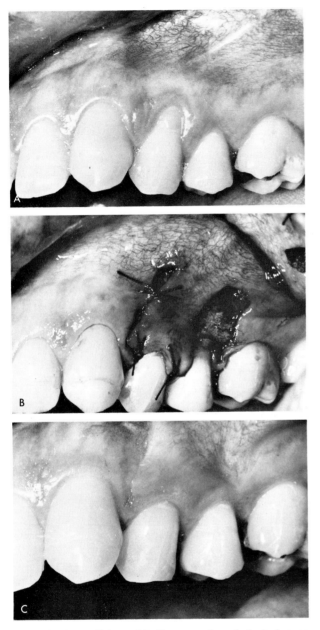

FIG. 25-8. The pedicle graft in the correction of gingival recession. A. Gingival recession of 4 mm on the facial surface of the first premolar partially exposes the root. The margin of the gingiva is thick, rolled, and hyperemic. B. A split-thickness pedicle has been raised from the facial surface of the second premolar and rotated and sutured on its medial aspect as well as in the interproximal papillary area on the distal. C. Clinical view one year after surgery reveals a normal gingival position as well as a resolution of inflammation. (Treated by Dr. D. Mathews.)

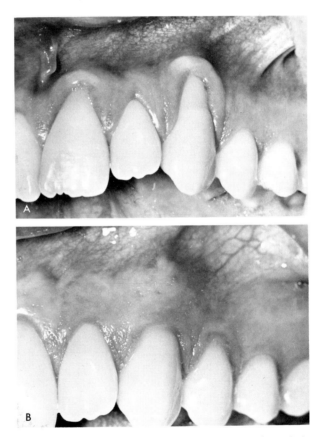

FIG. 25-9. Full-thickness pedicle graft. A. A portion of the upper arch with thin gingiva and gingival recession over the canine as well as over the central incisor. B. One year after a full thickness pedicle from the distal side was raised and rotated mesially to cover the root of the canine. The pedicle was sutured and stabilized and the area packed with a cement dressing. Note that the first premolar shows slightly more recession than it did preoperatively but that is not a high price to pay for the improvement in the canine. (Treated by Dr. D. Mathews.)

It should not be assumed that pedicle grafts are uniformly successful over gingival recessions. There are failures, sometimes many months after the operator congratulates himself and his patient on success. They have, however, a better record of success over recessions than do free grafts.

recession. The line of juncture is fixed with several sutures, so that the entire flap has been moved laterally to the extent of the area of the denuded root.

Other stabilizing sutures are made where required to stabilize the graft, either by a suspensory sling or into the remnants of the interproximal papillae. Exerting gentle unremitting pressure on the graft with a moist sponge for 5 to 6 minutes will ensure that extravasated blood does not pool under the graft.

A surgical cement dressing may now be applied, and the patient may be dismissed with the usual precautionary instructions on postoperative care. The sutures should not be removed for 7 to 10 days postoperatively, as is the case with other grafts.

THE DOUBLE-PAPILLA PEDICLE GRAFT

The double-papilla pedicle graft is used on occasion to cover a root denuded by gingival recession. It is a useful expedient when ample gingival tissue is present in the interproximal papillae but there is a lack of gingiva over the midfacial surfaces of adjacent teeth or a suspicion of dehiscence under gingiva. It consists of using the papillae on both sides of the denuded root for donor gingiva. These grafts are used in both full-thickness and split-thickness versions with varying success. Generally, the full-thickness papillary pedicles have a higher success rate. Figure 25-10 illustrates a clinical situation favorable to the use of the double papilla graft.

The difficulty with the papillary pedicle graft lies in that two papillary segments are brought together to be sutured over the naked root. When these grafts fail, it is at the suture line. Failure is manifested as a cleft that later breaks down completely.

There are successes, however. The procedure is not an arduous one for either the operator or the patient, nor is failure costly in terms of lost supporting bone or gingiva. Taking these considerations into account, the double-papilla pedicle graft is a logical trial procedure in covering portions of roots exposed by gingival recessions (Fig. 25-11).

Problems in pedicle-flap mobilization in double pa-

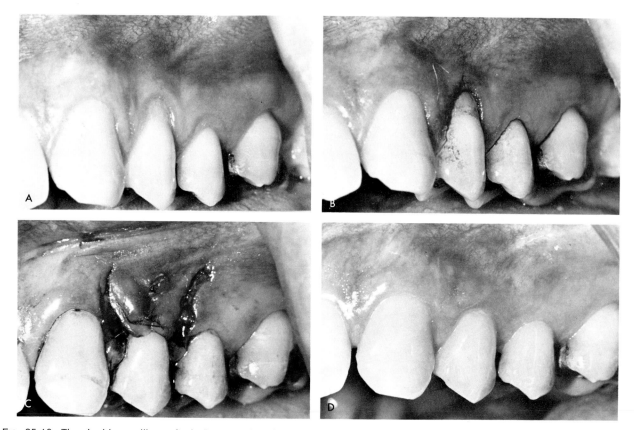

FIG. 25-10. *The double papilla graft. A. Preoperative view of an upper first premolar with gingival recession. The immediately adjacent papillary areas are relatively broad and well endowed with gingiva. B. The initial internal beveling incisions. These are made so that there are no butt joints over the denuded root but area overlapping lines of junction. C. Mobilization and rotation of the adjacent papillae and suturing over the junctional line over the root. D. Two years after a successful surgical "take" of the double papilla graft. (Treated by Dr. D. Mathews.)*

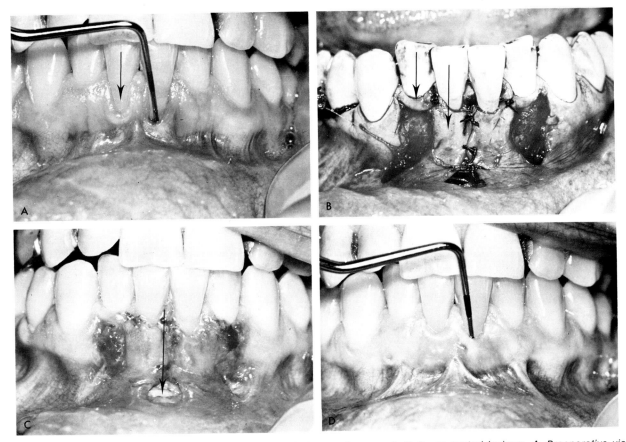

FIG. 25-11. *A double pedicle gingival graft to palliate gingival recession over both lower central incisors. A. Preoperative view revealing gingival recession over the lower central incisors (arrows). The probe in position reveals that whatever gingiva remains is free. B. Both pedicles are raised and mobilized and sutured into position. The pedicles are split thickness. C. Ten days after surgery. Healing is satisfactory except for the aperture in the mucosa in the fundus of the vestibular trough (arrow). This aperture persisted for 8 weeks. D. Fifteen months after surgery. Note the broad band of gingiva and the gain in gingival level. (Treated by Dr. L. Tibbetts.)*

pilla pedicle procedures are minimal. The distance of movement is so small that the releasing procedures helpful in a normal pedicle do not apply.

After the flap has been stabilized, it is further immobilized by a surgical cement dressing. The sutures are allowed to remain for 7 to 10 days postoperatively before they are removed.

Failure, if it occurs, will always be at the suture line lying upon the root. It is unfortunate that the essentially conservative nature of the procedure makes the midroot suture unavoidable, but once a more broadly based pedicle is raised, the special character of the double-papilla pedicle graft is lost and the procedure becomes something else.

THE FREE AUTOGENOUS GINGIVAL GRAFT

The free autogenous gingival graft has become the most commonly used procedure for the induction of new gingiva. Its ease of performance and its wide application have made for its development into a standard procedure. In 1968 Sulivan and Adkins did most of the basic work on autogenous free gingival grafts.[42,43] They have discussed feasibility, healing patterns, and applicability to the practice of periodontics.[44] Although their procedure has been refined, it has never been superseded.

Early on, grafts had a tendency to be thick, small, oversutured, and overstabilized, if such a thing is possible, so that wire extrusions, acrylic stents, and sutures about the entire circumference of the graft, including the apical margin deep in the vestibular trough, were features of the standard technique to be performed. Since then, grafts have become thinner and larger mesiodistally and have been positioned with sutures only crestally, with an occasional stabilizing suture on vertical margins. An apical suture has become a rarity (Fig. 25-11). Stabilization has been achieved by the fibrin clot. It has been recognized that, at best, the vestibular sutures were not necessary. At worst, they encouraged ballooning of the central portion of the graft due to the entrapment of blood, with resultant failure of the graft.

The greatest hazard to a successful take is the formation of a space between graft and bed. Usually blood collects in this space and interposes a barrier to diffusion of metabolites so critical to the survival of the graft. It is for this reason that only crestal or superior margin sutures are taken and the graft is draped or suspended from them. Gentle and constant pressure for 5 to 6 minutes against the bed of the graft with a gauze sponge moistened with normal saline solution, until the initial clot has formed, binds the graft down to its bed.

Preparation of the Bed for a Free Graft

The bed of the recipient site is an important consideration in the entire grafting procedure. It delineates the shape and size of the projected graft, but that is by no means its only property. It is of utmost importance that the remnants of the lamina propria and periosteum be trimmed to extremely thin dimensions. This trimming is best done with fine iris shears or tenotomy scissors or by small sharp nippers—or all three.

INITIAL INCISION

The initial incision for preparing the bed is a splitting incision of the marginal gingiva beyond the projected length of the graft. It is made with a #15 Bard Parker blade or with a #10A Bard Parker blade. It should be recalled that the objective of the graft is to extend and increase the zone of gingiva, so it may be assumed that the preoperative band of gingiva is a narrow one. This splitting incision will therefore be a shallow one before the mucogingival line is reached. From this line apically, only mucosa will be split from its underlying periosteum. When sufficient depth is attained, ordinarily about one and one-half times the extent of the graft apically unless a frenum is encountered, it will be noted that the elastic fibers in the alveolar mucosa will cause retraction if the area is long enough mesiodistally to permit it.

TRIMMING THE BED

The resultant untrimmed bed will have numerous shreds and lumps of tissue on its surface and will bleed fairly copiously. Snipping with shears, scissors, and nippers will reduce the surface to a smoother, thinner bed of incised tissue that will bleed little, if at all. At this point, the operator is approaching a good bed for a graft. Further thinning of the tissues of the bed is done

just short of perforation and exposing significant areas of labial plate.

The reason for this careful thinning of the periosteum and adhering shreds of lamina propria is based on observations of the fate of successful grafts months and even years postoperatively. It was noted that some grafts were apparently successful after tissue maturation, except that the newly induced gingiva was freely movable. If for any reason a flap had to be reflected consisting of one of these movable grafts, the marginal incision released the entire flap. In other words, there was no Sharpey's fiber attachment of the gingiva into the labial plate of the underlying bone.

Many skilled observers associated movable gingival grafts with thick beds. The thick bed composed of periosteum and some corium is effectively interposed between graft and bone. Since the periosteum itself is only tenuously attached to the labial plate, the successful graft sits upon it and is itself movable.

Careful thinning of the bed apparently leaves a base with enough remaining capacity for fluid exchange with the overlying graft but not enough to prevent resorption of the labial plate under it. It will be adaptable to reinsertion of a new Sharpey's fiber apparatus. Whatever the mechanism, thin beds induce firmly attached, immobile grafts (Fig. 25-12).

Choice of Donor Site

Practically all free autografts originate as palatal mucosa. The palate is a particularly ample source of keratinized tissue, usable for transposition to alveolar margins. Buccal gingiva is a meager source of graft material. The palate, on the other hand, offers an extensive area of gingiva for autografts and is the only area with enough surface for large grafts.

Even in the raising of a thin superficial layer of mucosa, design is important at a number of levels. The outline is the easiest requirement of design to satisfy. The use of tinfoil for a template is practically universal with neophytes. After the bed has been prepared and the bleeding has been well controlled, the proposed outline of the graft is made in foil that is tried over the recipient site. Usually the foil template is cut amply so that try-ons result in trimming the foil to size.

The corrected template is then placed on the palate as close to the marginal gingiva as possible without actually encroaching on it, and the outline of the foil is scribed on the palate with a #15 Bard Parker blade to incise the outline of the graft. (The palatal mucosa has been anesthetized prior to the procedure, of course.)

If the graft is to be large and will exceed the dimension of the palate without encroaching on rugae or soft palate, then the foil can be cut longitudinally in half,

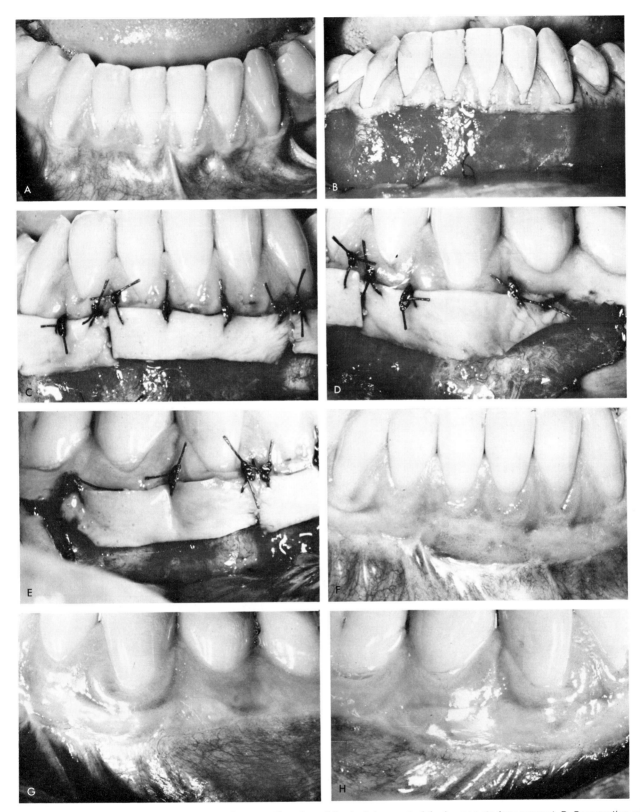

FIG. 25-12. *Free autogenous gingival graft. A. Preoperative view of the facial aspect of the lower anterior segment. B. Preparation of connective bed throughout the recipient site. C, D, E. Sections of the free graft from the donor site in the palate sutured in position. Note that only the superior edge of the graft is sutured so that the graft is suspended over the graft site. Stabilization of the graft is accomplished by the fibrin clot. F. One hundred two days after surgery. G and H. One-hundred-two days after surgery. An effective barrier of gingiva has been established which will, it is hoped, stop further recession of the marginal gingiva. (Treated by Dr. R. Lamb.)*

and one half can be added to the other half in width so that an outline is scribed twice as wide and half as long. The resultant graft is then cut in half anteroposteriorly just as the foil was and the two pieces of tissue are placed side by side on the recipient site and sutured in place as two adjacent grafts (Figs. 25-13; 25-14).

A useful practice when using this expedient is to leave a narrow isthmus of undisturbed palatal mucosa (about 2 mm) between the two halves of the graft (Fig. 25-13C; 25-14C). The healing of the wide palatal donor site is far more rapid than would be the case with a large square surface wound.

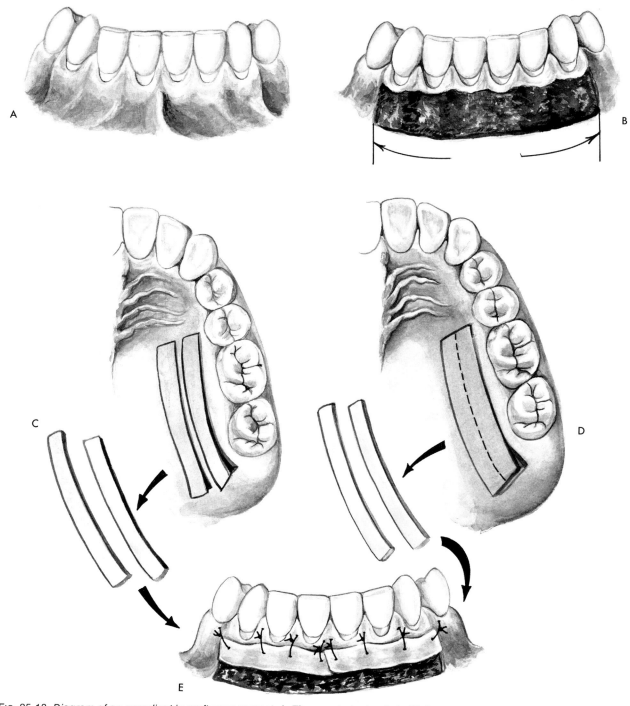

FIG. 25-13. *Diagram of an expedient in graft procurement. A. The area to be treated with free autogenous gingival graft. B. Diagram of the bed preparation. C. Divided graft, leaving an isthmus of palatal mucosa. The donor site will heal more rapidly. D. Use of an undivided graft cut in half to cover a large area of gingival deficiency. E. Placement of either graft.*

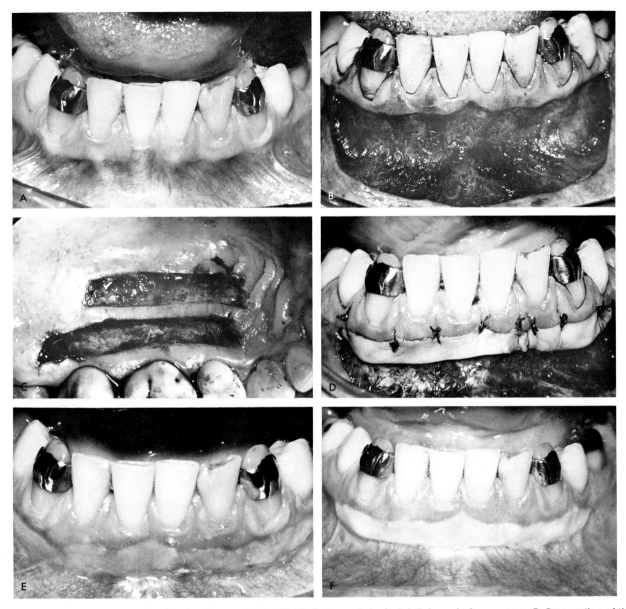

FIG. 25-14. *A clinical case replicating the diagram in Fig. 25-13. A. Area of gingival deficiency before surgery. B. Preparation of the connective tissue bed to receive the free autogenous gingival graft. C. The palatal donor site divided by an isthmus. D. The placement of the graft in two pieces. E. Two weeks after surgery. F. Six months after surgery. (Treated by Dr. G. Douglass.)*

However the design is executed, the resection of the graft takes considerable patience. The operator should make every effort to incise the graft evenly, about 1 mm thick or thinner throughout. Hashed and hacked incised surfaces must be smoothed after the graft is detached from the donor site. Careless overthinning results in perforations and, though not automatically fatal to a take, is poor technique. Thick, lumpy zones on the incised areas of the graft contain numerous fat cells that are easily identified visually by their yellow color. These must be removed and the graft must be leveled by snipping and incision. Scraping with a

Kirkland #15 or #16 blade or a Bard Parker #15 blade sometimes serves to thin and level any irregular surface.

Deep gouges into the palate incident to making these thick lumpy incised surfaces frequently invade one of the vessels in the palatal vasculature, particularly in the anterior border of the graft, and somewhat refractory bleeding may occur from the palate. This sometimes occurs several days postoperatively and can be annoying to both patient and operator. Patience and care pay great dividends in saving time and trouble.

A gauze sponge soaked in normal saline solution is useful as a repository for the newly raised graft. The incised surface should be carefully inspected under the strongest available light for fat and irregular areas for possible correction. After any necessary correction or alteration, the thin graft may be placed on the soaked sponge and set aside while the recipient site is inspected for bleeding. The bed should be ready to receive the graft.

Suturing the Graft

The graft may be placed on the bed in the position it is to be sutured, and the suturing is begun. To facilitate the suturing, some operators find it helpful to make all the prospective needle holes with the needle at the outset, since these holes can be easily seen.

The needle used in graft suturing should be a fine one. Cardiovascular needles or some of the larger oph-

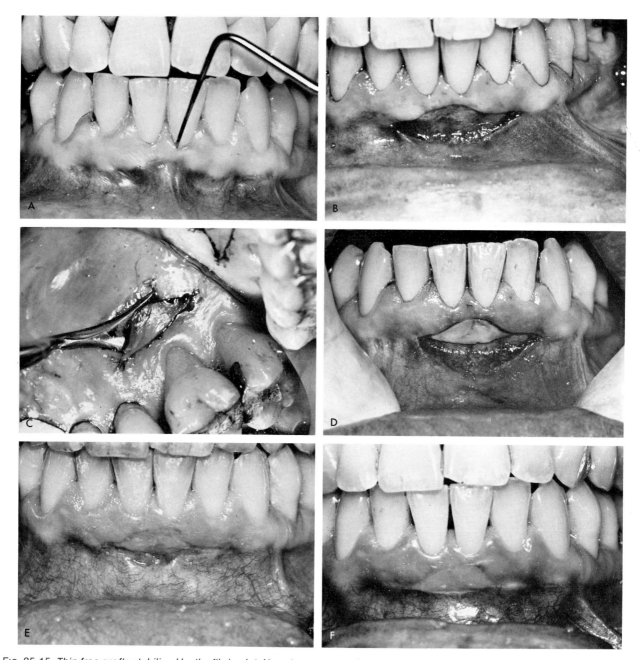

FIG. 25-15. *Thin free grafts stabilized by the fibrin clot. No sutures are used. A. The lower anterior segment revealing a localized lack of gingiva. B. Bed preparation of the recipient site. C. The taking of the extremely thin free autogenous graft from the palate. D. Graft placement on the recipient site. D. Seven days after surgery. F. Six months after surgery. (Treated by Dr. S. Sapkos.)*

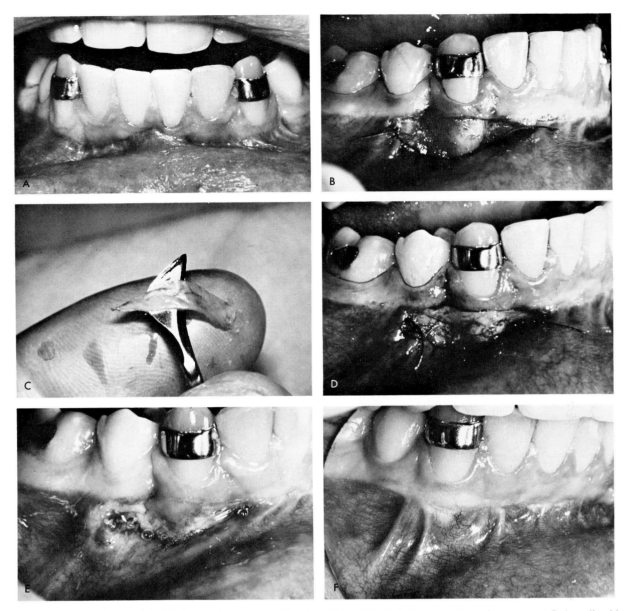

FIG. 25-16. *The use of extremely thin free autogenous grafts of small dimension. A. The lower anterior segment. B. Localized bed preparation over the lower right canine. C. The free autogenous graft taken from the palate. Note how thin it is. D. Placement of the graft in the recipient site bed and stabilized by the fibrin in the clot. No sutures or dressing is used. E. Five days after surgery. F. Ten months after surgery. (Treated by Dr. S. Sapkos.)*

thalmic needles with a 5–0 suture will serve well. Cutting needles generally are best avoided by the beginner. They have an annoying tendency of cutting through the thin graft and slitting it from needle puncture to graft margin.

The suturing need only secure the coronal margin. Great care should be exercised not to suture the vertical margins if by doing so the center of the graft may balloon away from the graft bed and allow the intervening space to fill with extravasated blood. Some years ago it was common practice to suture the apical margin to the periosteum in the fundus of the trough.

This practice was abandoned when it was realized that these sutures contributed nothing to the stability of the graft but, on the contrary, constituted a hazard to its success. In fact, a small but growing group of operators have been making the graft so thin that it can be so thoroughly fixed by the fibrin clot that no sutures at all are required (Fig. 25-15).

Dressings are sometimes dispensed with after suturing has been completed, although this is not a universal rule. Many operators feel that the dressing contributes little or nothing and delays cleansing the area by use of Perio-aids, toothbrush, and floss (Fig. 25-16).

Postoperative Care

Postsurgical care is a relatively simple matter as far as the graft itself is concerned. Suture removal after the ninth to tenth postoperative day is standard. No subsequent dressing is used. In fact, the entire graft site is remarkably comfortable. Whatever discomfort there is seems concentrated in the donor site. It is here that postoperative pain and bleeding occur if they occur at all.

If the graft is a large one, the use of a palatal stent is a useful expedient. A stent is quickly and easily made of fast-curing acrylic resin, and no clasps or other retaining devices are needed other than a fair fit against the palatal contour of the teeth. Palatal stents are useful in the control of pain and bleeding until healing is well advanced. They are used primarily when large areas are exposed to the action of the tongue and of the impingement of food.

The graft will heal and steadily mature, week after week. In three months, healing may be considered to be fairly complete as far as the outer surface is concerned. It is not completely healed, however, for at least 4 months. Many a graft that at first seems to be an unqualified success turns out to be movable later. Claims for success had best be modest until the graft is definitively bound down to the underlying bone plate (Fig. 25-17).

Shrinkage of the free autogenous gingival graft is common when the graft is thick. Thin grafts do much better in this respect. Any effort expended in this direction is well spent.

A carelessly trimmed bed margin peripherally can result in a bright red border of alveolar mucosa intervening between new and old gingiva. Careful attention to beveling the margin of the bed—especially the gingival portion—will allow a slight overlap of the margin of the graft, and the red line of demarcation is thus avoided.

Results

Gingival induction had a tremendous vogue in therapy when initially introduced. It is not a difficult technique to master, and the predictability of success is extremely high. It is an attractive method to both operator and patient. All these attributes are still true,

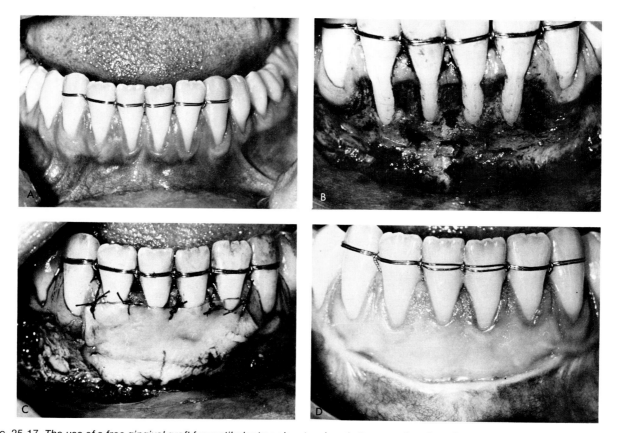

FIG. 25-17. *The use of a free gingival graft for vestibular trough extension. A. Preoperative view of a lower anterior segment deficient not only in gingiva but also in vestibular depth. B. Preparation of the bed to receive the free autogenous gingival graft. C. Suturing of an extremely wide but thin free graft obtained from the palate. D. A greatly extended depth of vestibular trough 18 months after surgery. (Treated by Dr. D. Mathews.)*

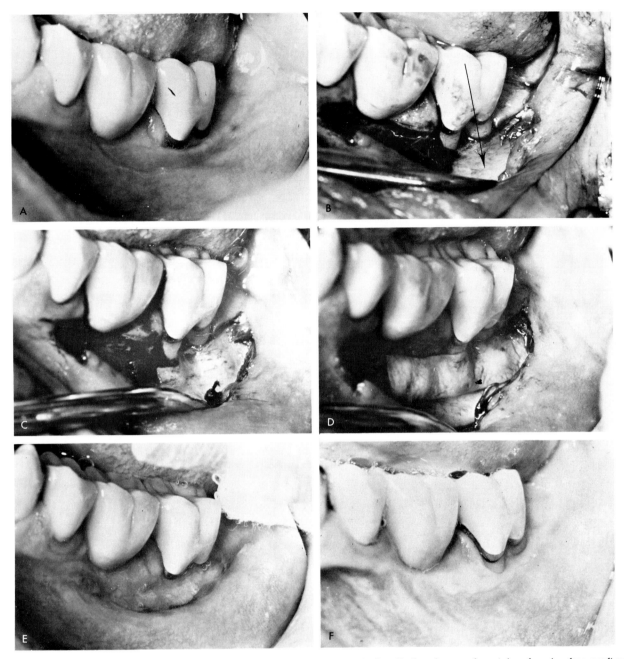

FIG. 25-18. *Free autogenous gingival graft over an area of denuded bone. Ordinarily the chances for a take of such a free graft are not good. A. Preoperative view of a lower left second molar abutment. Gingival recession had begun after seating of the bridge. B. In the bed preparation a thick marginal ledge of bone was found with an extremely unfavorable furcal milieu because of the bony margin. C. Osteoplasty of the buccal bone adjacent to the furca. D. Placement of the free autogenous gingival graft procured from the palate. E. Two weeks after surgery. F. One year after surgery. (Treated by Dr. M. Dragoo.)*

but good judgment and more conservative evaluation reduce the need for grafting, and when done it is on better grounds and for sounder requirements. An ample number of indications for grafting stand up under critical evaluation. The mere existence of a narrow margin of gingiva in an otherwise normal, healthy periodontium is no longer an indication for surgical intervention.

Some overtreatment is probably inevitable because of incomplete data and hastily conceived treatment plans. Constant self-evaluation and case evaluation are critical to rational therapy.

Free grafts are occasionally used in areas and in situations that do not promise success but do succeed in spite of unfavorable circumstances, for example, over an area of denuded bone (Fig. 25-18). These should be regarded for what they are—unusual results due to factors unknown to us. They do, however, stimulate study and clinical effort to extend therapeutic horizons. It is obvious that not all the factors are understood.

References

1. Ariaudo, A. A., and Tyrrell, H. A.: Repositioning and increasing the zone of attached gingiva. J. Periodontol., 28:106, 1957.
2. Becker, N. G.: A full gingival graft utilizing a pre-suturing technique. Periodontics, 4:194, 1967.
3. Bohannan, H. M.: Preliminary investigation into the results obtained from the vestibular fornix extention operation. Master's Thesis, University of Pennsylvania, 1961.
4. Bohannan, H. M.: The fixed long labial mucosal flap in vestibular alteration. Periodontics, 1:13, 1963.
5. Carranza, F. A.: Mucogingival techniques in periodontal surgery. J. Periodontol., 41:294, 1970.
6. Chacker, F. M., and Cohen, D. W.: A clinical and histologic study of healing following resection of the attached gingiva and reflection of the alveolar mucosa in monkeys. Presentation before the American Academy of Periodontology, Los Angeles, 1960.
7. Clark, J. W.: Mucogingival surgical techniques: an appraisal. J. Periodontol., 34:158, 1963.
8. Cohen, D. W., and Ross, S. E.: The double papilla positioned flap in periodontal therapy. J. Periodontol., 39:65, 1968.
9. Corn, H.: Periosteal separation—its clinical significance. J. Periodontol., 33:140, 1962.
10. Corn, H.: Technique for repositioning the frenum in periodontal problems. Dent. Clin. North Am., March, 1964.
11. Corn, H.: Edentulous area pedicle grafts in mucogingival surgery. Periodontics, 2:229, 1964.
12. Dahlberg, W. H.: Incisions and suturing: some basic considerations about each in periodontal flap surgery. Dent. Clin. North Am., 13:149, 1969.
13. Friedman, N.: Mucogingival surgery. Tex. Dent. J., 75:358, 1957.
14. Friedman, N.: Mucogingival surgery: the apically repositioned flap. J. Periodontol., 33:328, 1962.
15. Friedman, N., and Levine, H. L.: Mucogingival surgery; current status. J. Periodontol., 35:5, 1964.
16. Gargiulo, H. W., and Arrocha R.: Histo-clinical evaluation of free gingival grafts. Periodontics, 5:285, 1967.
17. Goldman, H. M., Schluger, S., and Fox, L.: Periodontal Therapy. St. Louis, The C. V. Mosby Co., 1956.
18. Gordon, H. P., Sullivan, H. C., and Adkins, J. H.: Free autogenous gingival grafts. II. Supplemental findings—histology of the graft side. Periodontics, 6:130, 1968.
19. Gottsegen, R.: Frenum position and vestibule depth in relation to gingival health. Oral Surg., 7:1069, 1959.
20. Grupe, H. E.: Horizontal sliding flap operation. Dent. Clin. North Am., March, 1960.
21. Hattler, A. B.: Mucogingival surgery—utilization of interdental gingiva as attached gingiva by surgical displacement. Periodontics, 5:126, 1967.
22. Hawley, C. E.: Clinical evaluation of free gingival grafts in periodontal surgery. J. Periodontol., 41:105, 1970.
23. Hileman, A. C.: Surgical repositioning of vestibule and frenums in periodontal disease. J. Am. Dent. Assoc., 55:676, 1957.
24. Janson, W.: Development of the blood supply to split thickness free gingival autografts. J. Periodontol., 40:34, 1969.
25. Kohler, C. A., and Ramfjord, S. P.: Healing of gingival mucoperiosteal flaps. Oral Surg., 13:89, 1960.
26. Marfino, N. R., Orban, B. J., and Wentz, F. M.: Repair of dento-gingiva junction following surgical intervention. J. Periodontol., 30:180, 1959.
27. McFall, W. T.: The laterally repositioned flap—criteria for success. Periodontics, 5:89, 1967.
28. Nabers, C. L.: Repositioning the attached gingiva. J. Periodontol., 25:38, 1954.
29. Nabers, J. M.: Extension of the vestibular fornix utilizing a gingival graft—case history. Periodontics, 4:77, 1966.
30. Nabers, J. M.: Free gingival grafts. Periodontics, 4:243, 1966.
31. Ochsenbein, C.: Newer concepts of muco-gingival surgery. J. Periodontol., 31:175, 1960.
32. Ochsenbein, C.: The double flap procedure. Periodontics., 1:17, 1963.
33. Oliver, R. C., Loe, H., and Karring, T.: Microscopic evaluation of the healing and revascularization of free gingival grafts. J. Periodontol., 3:84, 1968.
34. Oliver, R. C., and Woofser, C.: Healing and revascularization of free mucosal grafts over roots. I.A.D.R., Abst. #469, 1971.
35. Pennel, B. M., et al.: Free masticatory mucosa graft. J. Periodontol., 40:162, 1969.
36. Pfeifer, J. S.: The reaction of alveolar bone to flap procedures in man. Periodontics, 3:135, 1965.
37. Prichard, J. F.: Changing concepts in periodontal therapy. Tex. Dent. J., 79:4, 1961.
38. Prichard, J. F.: Periodontal surgery. Practical Dental Monographs, Nov., 1961.
39. Ramfjord, S. F., and Costich, E. R.: Healing after exposure of periosteum on the alveolar process. J. Periodontol., 39:199, 1968.
40. Stern, I. B.: The use of Telfa as a periodontal surgical dressing. N.Y. Dent. J., 24:260, 1958.
41. Sugarman, E. F.: A clinical and histologic study of the attachment of grafted tissue to bone and teeth. J. Periodontol., 40:381, 1969.
42. Sullivan, H. C., and Adkins, J. H.: Free autogenous gingival grafts. I. Principles of successful grafting. Periodontics, 6:121, 1968.
43. Sullivan, H. C., and Adkins, J. H.: Free autogenous gingival grafts. III. Utilization of grafts in the treatment of gingival recessions. Periodontics, 6:152, 1968.
44. Sullivan, H. C., and Adkins, J. H.: The role of free

gingival grafts in periodontal therapy. Dent. Clin. North Am., *13:*133, 1969.

45. Sullivan, H. C., Carman, D., and Dinner, D.: Histological evaluation of laterally positioned flap. I.A.D.R., Abstr. #467, 1971.

46. Tisot, R. J., and Sullivan, H. C.: Evaluation of the survival of partial thickness and full thickness flaps. I.A.D.R., Abstr. #470, 1971.

47. West, T. L., and Bloom, A.: A histologic study of wound healing following mucogingival surgery. J. Dent. Res., *40:*675, 1961.

48. Wilderman, M. N.: Exposure of bone in periodontal surgery. Dent. Clin. North Am., March, 1964.

49. Wilderman, M. N.: Repair after a periosteal retention procedure. J. Periodontol., *34:*487, 1963.

50. Wilderman, M. N., Wentz, F. M., and Orban, B. J.: Histogenesis of repair after mucogingival surgery. J. Periodontol., *31:*283, 1960.

Section III
Occlusal and Restorative Interrelationships

26

Basic Procedures in Dental Therapy That Affect the Periodontium

26

Basic
Procedures
in Dental
Therapy
That
Affect the
Periodontium

It is universally accepted that for a natural dentition to function optimally the supporting tissues must be in a state of health. The dentist should therefore strive to recognize and to eliminate as many existing pathologic factors as possible before undertaking any therapeutic procedures, whether basically operative, prosthodontic, exodontic, orthodontic, or endodontic in nature. If an existing oral disease is unrecognized or disregarded prior to the start of dental therapy, it may be aggravated by the therapeutic procedure itself.

It is also recognized that the etiology of periodontal disease can be iatrogenic in nature. The purpose of this chapter is to discuss and to illustrate those injuries that are the result of injudicious or careless therapy and those that initiate or aggravate an already existing periodontal condition.

FACTORS CONTRIBUTING TO PERIODONTAL DISTURBANCES

Microbial dental plaque is the single most important factor associated with the causing of dental pathology, whether caries or periodontal disease.

The co-destructive relationship of abnormal occlusal stress and plaque and periodontal disturbances is thoroughly emphasized in Chapter 5. In addition to occlusal stress, there are many other factors that further the destructive nature of microbial plaque, and it is common to find several of these factors interacting.

In treating dental diseases it must always be borne in mind that the dentist is attempting to restore the oral structures to health as a functional unit and that no matter how precise his work in one region of the mouth, it will be worthless if in other parts of the mouth conditions are permitted to exist that adversely affect the total structure. Major contributing factors calculated to upset the equilibrium are tooth drifting, which is commonly the result of failing to replace or restore strategic teeth, injudiciously executed restorative and surgical procedures, and the placement of faulty prostheses, either fixed or removable.

The Need for Preliminary Periodontal Care

It has been emphasized that prior to any dental procedure, with the exception of treatment of acute carious lesions that involve or threaten the health of the pulp, existing pathologic conditions of the supportive structures must be recognized and treated in order to set up a healthy environment. Restoring the periodontium to health is a basic necessity prior to other dental therapy. This stage of treatment includes the removal of gingival irritants, correction of functional occlusal interferences, treatment of morphologic and pathologic gingival conditions, and correction of bony deformities of the supporting structures. The recognition of the various factors and the manner of their correction are referred to in other parts of this book and are emphasized in Chapter 27, especially as they relate to restorative procedures.

This period of restoring health to the periodontium requires the cooperation of the patient and should be beneficially employed in educating him in the correct routines for oral hygiene. Without the patient's early attention to maintenance of his own mouth, any attempt on the part of the dentist to restore the dentition will be of little avail. The restorations, no matter how carefully performed, will be short-lived, and eventual loss of teeth can be predicted.

Nonreplacement of Strategic Teeth

Dental caries and periodontal disease are contributory one to the other.[3] Dental caries contributes to periodontal disease by destroying proximal contacts and breaking up smooth surfaces, trapping food and inducing accumulation and retention of microbial plaque, by encouraging tooth drift which results in root proximity and bite collapse, by disturbing natural chewing and cleansing habits, by causing premature loss of teeth and by introducing iatrogenic factors that alter form and function. Periodontal disease promotes the incidence of caries by increasing the amount of microbial plaque, by providing extra surfaces conducive to bacterial culture, and by changing root sensitivity and hence altering natural chewing and cleansing habits. The most serious sequela of these factors is the loss of strategic teeth.

To avoid both morphologic and functional disarrangements in the occlusion, missing teeth should be replaced as soon as possible in order to maintain arch integrity. Otherwise, changes will occur that will upset the masticatory system, such as extrusion of the teeth opposing edentulous areas, along with their alveolar housing, their supporting tissues, and ultimately the maxillary sinus. Concurrently with the extrusion, shifting of the interproximal contacts and migration of the adjacent teeth occur, impairing function and causing disharmony. Good oral health cannot be achieved when changes in tooth position alter coronal contour and the occlusion and interfere with mutual support. Further changes take place as a result, such as changes of form in the papillae and embrasures, encouraging food impaction and retention, so frequently the forerunners of osseous defects.

Posterior-bite collapse is a most serious sequela of loss of arch integrity. In fact, it has been stated that 95 percent of all patients requiring complex periodontal prosthetic therapy have posterior-bite collapse.[3]

The majority of these dental casualties are initiated by the extraction of posterior teeth, usually the first permanent molar, without replacement. This most frequently allows the accelerated drift of the adjacent teeth into the edentulous space. In consequence, the stabilizing support of the posterior teeth is lost, and an excessive load is shifted to the anterior teeth, negating the natural protection normally provided by the posterior teeth (Fig. 5-23).

RESTORATIVE DENTAL PROCEDURES AND PERIODONTAL HEALTH

The marginal periodontium is where the fields of restorative dentistry and periodontics overlap. In order to understand this interdependence, it is essential that there be agreement upon what constitutes a healthy marginal periodontium and how a pathologic condition can be corrected or prevented. Any restorative dental procedure must be carefully executed. This especially applies to dentitions with preexisting periodontal disease, since these patients often have an exaggerated response to the slightest tissue insults (Fig. 26-5). Conversely, close attention should be paid to the response of the periodontium to the irritants arising from careless techniques, which can initiate or add to existing gingival inflammation. This in turn can lead to loss of periodontal support and to subsequent tooth loss, if the condition is not recognized and treated in its early stages.

The dentist performing restorative dentistry is almost certain to be fully aware of the consequences and effect of his work upon the dental pulp; but it is of equal importance that he should not lack a thorough understanding of the nature and degree of the response to be expected in the periodontal tissues to the procedures carried out. Diseased pulps and missing tooth structure are routinely replaced with inert materials, but at our present state of knowledge no material can substitute for a lost periodontal ligament. Therefore, the total environment, internal and external, of the tooth must be considered as one field of operation.[16]

Properly designed and created dental restorations provide functional stimulation and contribute to and are supportive of the periodontium. Conversely, the healthy periodontium is essential to the proper function of the restoration.

Application of the Rubber Dam

During routine operative procedures, the rubber dam is an extremely useful aid in protecting the sur-

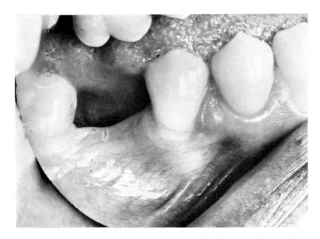

FIG. 26-1. *A poor environment for a cervical restoration or for a full crown because of lack of attached gingival tissue on the buccal aspect of the second premolar. Care must be taken not to injure the epithelial attachment during cavity or crown preparation.*

rounding gingival tissues. It affords protection against gingival abrasion and keeps the area free from contamination by saliva or debris, thus helping to ensure well-placed restorations. Another advantage of the rubber dam is that it slightly retracts the free gingival margin. This retraction may aid in subgingival margin placement, impression making, finishing of the gingival margins of restorations, and after the restorations have been cemented, in removal of excess cement and loose debris.

It is not always possible to use a rubber dam during crown preparation, since it often interferes with adequate subgingival margin extension, if this is required. For such cases, precautions must be taken to prevent excessive gingival abrasion with stones or burs. This is especially important where the zone of attached gingiva is insufficient or if the surrounding gingival tissue is thin and delicate (Fig. 26-1).

In correctly placing the rubber dam clamp, care must be exercised to ensure that it is firmly seated on the hard tissues of the tooth. The clamp should not be forced subgingivally to such a degree that it causes stripping of the epithelial attachment, nor should it be placed in such a way or for such a length of time as to cause ischemia to the degree that tissue sloughing and subsequent recession result. A mobile clamp may cause similar damage to the epithelial attachment and must often be stabilized with compound to prevent its migration in an apical direction (Fig. 26-2).

Cavity and Crown Preparation

Care must be exercised not to injure the gingival tissues unduly during cavity or crown preparation.

Slight abrasions usually heal rapidly, but even minor procedural trauma must be avoided in regions where the attached gingiva is minimal (Fig. 26-3A). Such injuries may cause recessions, depleting the entire zone of attached gingiva and hastening its recession (Fig. 26-3B). If the margins must be placed subgingivally, this procedure must be cautiously executed so as not to disturb the epithelial attachment. The epithelial attachment is the most vulnerable of all the supporting structures to periodontal disease, and procedural trauma can initiate its apical migration and result in periodontitis or recession.

The marginal gingiva and its attachment can be protected during the placement of subgingival margins by using a rubber dam (Fig. 26-4A). Some dentists,

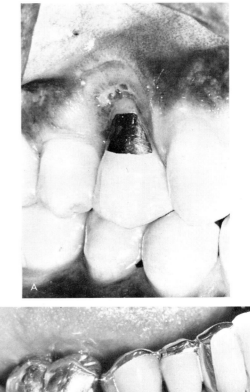

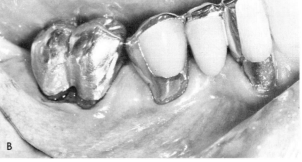

FIG. 26-2. *Effects of injudicious restoration procedures. A. Soft-tissue damage and recession induced by unstable rubber dam clamp. B. Progressive recession of minimal delicate zone of attached gingiva following multiple restorative procedures and improper brushing technique (See correction in Fig. 27-12.)*

prior to placing a subgingival finish line, retract the marginal gingiva either by electrosurgery,[41,42] or else by using retraction cord. Use of a thin blunted instrument to retract the free gingival margin during the subgingival placement of the finish line helps to avoid damaging the epithelial attachment, should the use of a rubber dam be impractical (Fig. 26-4B).

Location of the Gingival Margins of the Restoration

Where to place the gingival termination of the restorations relative to the free margin of the gingiva is a matter of controversy. The location of the restoration margin depends greatly upon a number of factors. Some of the more important are:

1. Esthetics
2. Need for additional retention of the restoration
3. Degree of personal oral hygiene
4. Susceptibility of the individual to caries

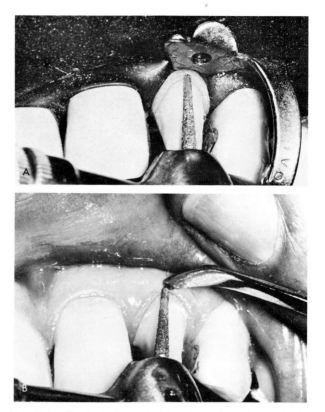

Fig. 26-4. *Methods for retracting free gingival margin for subgingival extension of coronal preparation. A. Use of a rubber dam and clamp. B. Use of a thin, blunted instrument.*

5. Susceptibility of the marginal gingiva to irritants
6. Morphologic characteristics of the marginal gingiva
7. Degree of gingival recession

These factors are often interdependent and must all be considered in each individual case before a decision is reached.

If one is to accept only the traditional approach, then the gingival margins of all restorations should end subgingivally.[8,44] Black's theory of "extension for prevention" of caries and sensitivity has influenced the practice of restorative dentistry for well over 50 years. He advocated the extension of all smooth-surface cavities into the sulcular area, and the facial and lingual margins into the embrasure, where he maintained that the friction of mastication would provide self-cleansing. Now, after more than half a century, it is becoming increasingly accepted that this theory has been overemphasized and that not only can extension of the cavity be wasteful of healthy tooth structure but caries is not prevented by extension (Figs. 26-18, 20). Currently, more emphasis is placed on caries prevention by plaque control and by systemic and topical application of caries inhibitors rather than on extension for

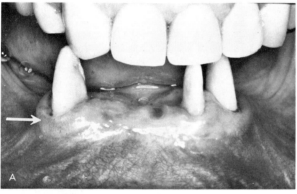

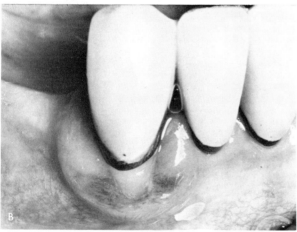

Fig. 26-3. *Traumatized free gingival margin and epithelial attachment of mandibular cuspid (arrow) created during extension of subgingival margin. A. Immediately after coronal reduction. B. Two months after restoration, showing severe recession and loss of entire zone of attached gingiva.*

prevention. There is no evidence that mastication has effective self-cleansing properties.

If one accepts only the biologic approach, the gingival termination of all restorations should be placed well coronally to the edge of the free gingiva. The reason for this is that it is most difficult to finish a subgingival margin in such a way that it does not act as a source of irritation,[4,31,51] and in addition the gingival line provides a place where food can be retained and plaque can accumulate, making this region more susceptible to caries.

There are obvious arguments for extension of both subgingival and supragingival margins. Each has advantages and disadvantages. Probably more important, regardless of where the margin is placed, are factors such as the degree of accuracy of fit, the surface finish, the type of material that will be in contact with the periodontal tissues, and the gingival contour of the restoration. In creating and finishing the gingival portion of the restoration, the dentist must not only reproduce the predamaged configuration of the external anatomy of the tooth as nearly as possible, but if necessary he should endeavor to improve upon it. This procedure will reduce the degree to which microbial plaque, which is often the cause of the original lesion, will accumulate.

Supragingival placement of the margin reduces the probability of irritation of the gingiva by the restoration, but may be unesthetic. On the other hand, subgingival placement brings the epithelium of the gingival sulcus into contact with the filling material, which may induce inflammation (Fig. 26-5). However, if the restoration is of an inert material, smooth and correctly contoured, and its margins are accurately adapted, the irritation will be minimal, and bacteria are unlikely to accumulate unmanageably if proper oral hygiene is

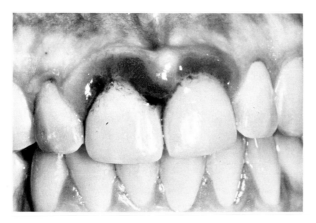

FIG. 26-5. *Exaggerated response of the marginal gingiva possibly related to subgingival placement of margins and overcontoured porcelain jacket crowns.*

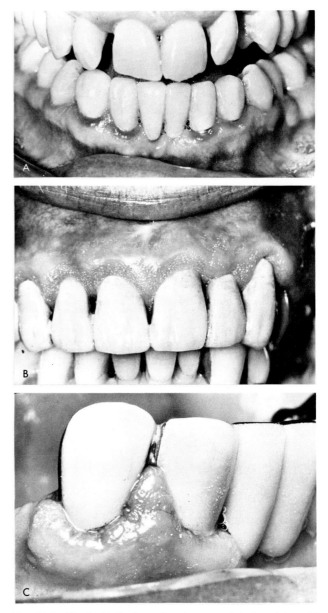

FIG. 26-6. *Gingival irritation related to porcelain-fused-to-gold restorations. A. Inflammation due to poor subgingival margins and inadequate embrasure space, which encouraged plaque retention. B. Gingival changes resulting from poorly glazed porcelain extending into the gingival sulcus, further aggravated by mouth breathing. C. Hyperplasia due to tissue trauma during coronal reduction, poor subgingival margins, and clasp impingement. Note also edematous papilla between cuspid and lateral incisor, resulting from lack of embrasure space.*

observed. Carelessly adapted margins or inaccurate veneering of gold crowns may bring dental cements, acrylic resin, or porcelain into contact with the sulcular epithelium (Fig. 26-6). These materials may be rough and porous so that they are physically and/or chemically irritating.

There are instances when the indications to place

margins subgingivally are obvious. In anterior segments of the mouth, crowns should end subgingivally for esthetic reasons. Special care should be taken during tooth reduction to place the finish line with as little trauma as possible, especially where the gingival tissue is thin and delicate or where there is an inadequate zone of attached gingiva. Unnecessary trauma will most likely result in gingival recession, exposing the margin and having an unpleasing cosmetic appearance. Occasionally, in spite of excellent fit, proper contour, and smooth polish, gingival tissues react adversely to the porcelain-faced anterior crowns, and the crowns cause a marginal gingivitis such as is observed in response to certain hormones related to pregnancy and puberty. The reasons for this reaction are not clearly understood.

Another indication for placing margins subgingivally is to increase the retention of the restoration, should this be required. Often the presence of existing restorations dictates subgingival extension.

Modification of the axial contour of the restoration to any appreciable degree also requires subgingival extension of the margins. This is especially true when there is some recession around the teeth requiring restorations as a result of periodontal therapy (Fig. 26-20), toothbrush trauma, or slight furcation involvement (Fig. 26-21). If contours in the gingival regions are not smoothed, there is a great tendency for plaque accumulation and retention. The effect of contour on plaque retention is further discussed later in this chapter.

There are also important indications for ending margins supragingivally. Unless caries or cosmetic needs dictate otherwise, margins should be left supragingival in regions where the zone of attached gingiva is inadequate in width or thickness or where the clinical crown is excessively long, subsequent to periodontal therapy (Figs. 26-1; 26-7).

In summary, the choice between supragingival and subgingival placement of the margin should be based upon evaluation of the needs of each patient and of each tooth. This should be considered before deciding upon the best marginal depth. If the sulcus can predictably be kept irritant-free by accurate margin adaptation, smooth surfaces, and proper contour, termination below the gingival margin but clear of the epithelial attachment is feasible and desirable. However, the margin should not end so far subgingivally as to make it impossible to gain a good impression or properly finish the restoration in this region.

An acceptable, healthy gingival sulcus is 1 to 3 mm in depth in most regions of the mouth, and subgingival margins should finish at least 0.5 mm short of the epithelial attachment. A good way to estimate is to place

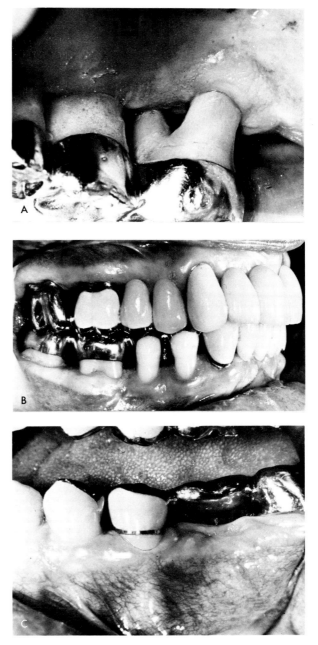

FIG. 26-7. Indications for supragingival placement of margins. A. Long clinical crowns with furcation involvements where subgingival extension would necessitate excessive tooth reduction. B. Long clinical crowns and low caries activity. C. Delicate and/or minimal attached gingiva.

the margin halfway into the sulcus if the sulcus is of normal depth. If the sulcular depth is greater than 3 mm, serious consideration should be given to reducing this depth by surgical means before starting the restorative phase of the therapy. Exceptions to this apply to the tuberosity and the retromolar pad, where greater depths are considered normal. In most instances the deeper the subgingival extension, the greater is the risk of irritation to the epithelial attachment.

If the margin is to be supragingival, the question is where exactly should it be placed? Preferably, the margin should be located in enamel, where it can be accurately finished and polished, and in such cases it should be placed at least 2 to 3 mm supragingivally. This placement is not possible, as stated, in cases of severe recession, and the margin may even have to end in root structure.

Some studies indicate that it is preferable to end a restoration above the gingival margin or level with the gingival crest.[24,26] It has been the experience of the author that the gingival crest area is where there is greatest plaque accumulation and that termination at that level tends to increase rather than decrease the incidence of caries and inflammation (Fig. 26-18).

Following periodontal surgery, the sulcus often has virtually no depth at all. If subgingival margin placement is necessary in such cases, it is advisable to wait until a free gingival margin develops before attempting crown preparations; otherwise the relationship of the free gingival margins to the finish lines may be inaccurate. This period of regeneration takes from 6 weeks to several months.[37]

Placing the Matrix

After cavity preparation, a properly designed and contoured matrix should be placed in such a manner that it does not injure the epithelial attachment, yet can be accurately adapted to the margins. In the case of Class II restorations, this necessitates the careful placement of well-contoured interproximal wedges, often further supported by compound. The matrix must be rigid and well-contoured in order to reproduce proper form and to prevent subgingival overhangs. Improperly contoured interproximal restorations including such faults as excessively broad contact areas, insufficient or absent interproximal contacts, interproximal undercontour or overcontour at the gingival third, and gingival overhangs (Fig. 26-8) account for such problems as interproximal food impaction and exaggerated accumulation and retention of microbial plaque, which will result in recurrent caries and/or periodontal breakdown.

Though *interproximal wedges* are often necessary to restrain the interdental tissues, their placement should be done with care to avoid injury to the attachment in this vulnerable region. Injudicious separation of anterior teeth for Class III restorations will also cause similar injury to the periodontal ligaments. It should be borne in mind that separation should always be minimal and should not exceed the width of the periodontal ligament. Any separating device should be removed as soon as possible.

Impressions

Whenever margins are placed subgingivally, it is more difficult to obtain impressions of these teeth because some manner of displacing the free gingival tissues becomes necessary. The injudicious use of gingival-retraction techniques can often injure the soft tissues and cause permanent alterations such as recessions; but with careful consideration for the tissues during crown preparation and impression making, any unavoidable small injury will disappear without permanent alteration within a few days.

If tube impressions are made, the individual tubes must be carefully adapted to the preparation and their length must accurately relate to the gingival line. Excessive digital force should not be used during im-

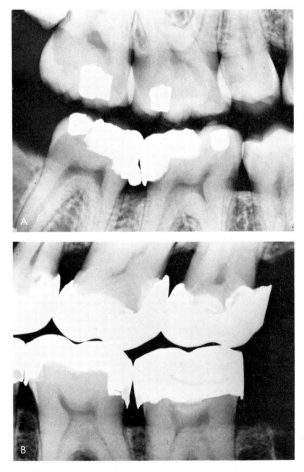

FIG. 26-8. *Improperly contoured interproximal restorations, resulting from careless adaptation of matrix band prior to amalgam condensation. B. Interproximal overhang of gold restorations, the result of careless impression and waxing technique.*

pression making, in order to avoid stripping off the epithelial attachment.

Gingival retraction cords, widely used during impression procedures, can be used with relative safety. Precautions must be taken not to use too much or to use cord of excessive diameter in the sulcular space. Undue force in cord placement will cause damage to the attachment. Special precautions must be exercised in retracting thin and delicate free gingival tissue and in cases where the attached gingiva is inadequate. Undue insult in such cases usually causes rapid recession.

Electrosurgical retraction is currently accepted as a means of creating a trough surrounding the subgingival finish line. If carefully used, this method greatly facilitates accurate impression taking. Electrosurgical retraction is not indicated, however, in regions of inflammation or extremely thin gingival tissue, since it will usually result in recession.

Temporary Coverage

Temporary coverage made in haste and without consideration for the periodontium can cause disturbances that may result in permanent damage. Examples of factors that may embarrass the periodontium are the following:

1. *Overextended temporary crowns* that may result in permanent gingival alterations in the interdental region or in facial and lingual marginal regions. The result may be gingival hyperplasia (Fig. 26-9) or recession if the epithelial attachment has been severely injured. The effects of overcontouring are thoroughly discussed later in this chapter.
2. *Underextended temporary crowns* which, although not as serious as overextension, may contribute to hypersensitivity by interfering with adequate oral hygiene measures.
3. *Poor proximal-contact relationships* that contribute to food impaction and retention and to drifting of the approximating teeth.

If the finishing of the temporary coverage is uniformly poor, the patient is often frustrated in his attempts to maintain good oral hygiene, and plaque will accumulate.

In temporary coverage, the aim is to protect the prepared teeth and to promote gingival healing. The marginal fit is important. It should be as accurate as possible, especially if there is a long delay between temporary coverage and final restoration. If the period of transition is relatively short (less than one week) it is

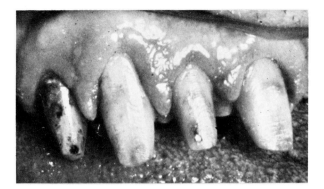

FIG. 26-9. *Gingival pathology resulting from poorly designed temporary crowns. Note excessive col formation and gingival hyperplasia arising from inadequate interproximal embrasures.*

far better to protect a prepared tooth or several teeth with a periodontal pack preparation rather than with carelessly made temporary crowns. One of the authors (R.A.Y.) has on many occasions used a freshly mixed periodontal pack (Coe-pak) to cement temporary acrylic crowns that are purposely underextended. The inherent qualities of this material serve admirably to protect both the hard and the soft tissues, and it also helps to stabilize the proximal relationships of the teeth. This method is advocated only when the temporary crowns are used for less than a week. If the transition period is extended, it is important to remove the old pack and reset the temporary crowns with a new mix.

Placement and Finishing of the Restoration

It is unfortunately common to find a slight but progressive destruction of the periodontium in the proximity of fillings and crowns. This may be initiated by the materials used in restoration, but it is not so much their innate properties as their potential destructive capacities after the restoration has been completed that should be feared and anticipated. The dangers to be avoided by all means possible are marginal discrepancies between the preparation and the restoration, such as deficiencies or overhangs and surface roughness. Extreme care must be exercised, therefore, to finish a restoration correctly, particularly below the gingival margin where removal of overhangs is much more of a problem than is the removal of subgingival calculus.

An area of intervening cement will incite physical and chemical irritation and, furthermore, will be exposed to erosion by oral fluids, with consequent cavitation and creation of rough areas. It is imperative to smooth and contour the area of restoration so that it duplicates or improves upon the original. Rough areas and overhangs not only cause irritation subgingivally, but being always covered with microbial plaque they soon become areas for the generation and accumulation of microorganisms and their destructive secretions.

After completing such restorations, the interproximal-contact relationship should be carefully checked with dental floss for the correct degree of contact. Subgingival marginal adaptation should be carefully examined, and any excess filling material should be carefully removed with instruments especially designed for this purpose. If the restoration is a gold inlay or crown, care should be taken not to cement it until proper marginal and interproximal relationships are ensured.

MORPHOLOGIC CHARACTERISTICS OF THE RESTORATION AND PERIODONTAL HEALTH

A restoration must be considered from the point of view of contour, occlusal anatomy, margins, proximal contacts, esthetics, and function. Furthermore, the tooth must be looked upon as a harmonious part of the whole dentition.

The restored contours of teeth uncomplicated by recession should be those of the original anatomy of the teeth, and bulbous curvatures and overhangs must be eliminated by adequate interproximal finishing. There must also be no interdental impingement to cause irritation and pressure on the gingival tissues and lead to their breakdown, because it is often difficult for the

patient to gain access to these areas for cleansing purposes and a potential for a chronic periodontal lesion is thereby set up, with resulting inflammation. In addition, microbial plaque is established and remains undisturbed upon the restoration.

Microbial plaque, especially that which is in or nearly in contact with the free gingival margin, is the principal etiologic factor in both caries and periodontal disease. Clinically it is evident that plaque retention is greatest in regions that are relatively inaccessible to routine oral hygiene measures. These regions are the interproximal and the facial and lingual cervical areas of the teeth. To maintain these vulnerable regions in a plaque-free state, the close relationship between the morphologic characteristics of the clinical crown and the degree of accessibility must be realized and remembered. The correct external morphology of all restorations is important, but this in particular must be borne in mind during dental procedures involving full-coverage restorations.

It is the full-crown restoration that most taxes the dentist's ability to recreate the original anatomy. For this reason, the following discussion on coronal morphologic characteristics will be directed to the full-coverage restoration, and its morphology will be discussed from all aspects. This will include the restoration of crowns with and without the complication of gingival recession and loss of supporting bone, because crowns complicated by recession present unusual problems related to their restoration, which in turn is closely related to accessibility for plaque control. These characteristics will be covered from the standpoint of occlusal morphology, proximal-contact relationships, and facial and lingual contours.

Contours of Full-Crown Restorations of Teeth Uncomplicated by Recession

OCCLUSAL MORPHOLOGY

Since the desirable aspects of functional occlusal morphology have already been covered in Chapter 12, the following discussion will be limited to the width of the occlusal table. Excessive occlusal wear results in a widening of the occlusal table, and it has long been considered desirable to reduce the buccolingual width of such teeth, especially when restoring them (Fig. 26-10). Why is this necessary and how narrow should this width be?

One explanation given is that less axial stress is transmitted to the periodontium during mastication with narrow occlusal tables than with wide ones. In our opinion this result is doubtful. More important is that the narrower the occlusal table the greater control

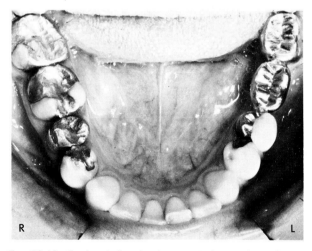

FIG. 26-10. Occlusal view to show posterior teeth on the patient's left side restored to correctly narrowed occlusal width as compared with posterior teeth on the right side that are in need of similar treatment.

there is for the dentist in recreating a functional occlusion free of interferences. The occlusion should be free from abnormal stresses during lateral mandibular excursions, whether they be functional or parafunctional excursions.

For protective reasons, the overbite and overjet relations of the cuspids should, whenever possible, be such that there is disclusion of the posterior teeth during lateral excursive movements. This slight disclusion is difficult to attain unless the width of the occlusal table is within normal limits. The wider the occlusal table, the greater is the incidence of cross-arch and cross-tooth balancing interferences during lateral excursive movements of the mandible. It is the stress created by these contacts that is undesirable, especially since the stresses are not axially inclined.

The buccolingual width of the occlusal table should not exceed that which was normal for the dentition prior to any wear or breakdown. In the case of pontics, it is unnecessary to have the occlusal tables buccolingually narrower than those of the abutment teeth.

PROXIMAL-CONTACT RELATIONSHIPS

It is most important to consider the characteristics of the proximal contacts, because improper management will jeopardize the interdental soft tissues, which are most vulnerable to periodontal breakdown. It is the proximal contacts that determine marginal-ridge relationships, occlusal embrasure form, and buccal and lingual embrasure form, which in turn greatly affect the health of the interdental tissues.

Tilting will cause discrepancies in the marginal ridges. *Marginal ridges* of unequal height or of improper contour will encourage food impaction and retention and contribute to the breakdown of interdental tissues and subsequently to interproximal bone loss (Fig. 26-11). The same will result from contacts that are located too far occlusally; in addition, this type of contact relationship will also tend to eliminate the marginal ridge (Fig. 26-12).

Proximal-contact areas should be as near as possible to normal. A common error is to make the contact areas too broad faciolingually and/or occlusocervically (Fig. 26-13A–C). The broadened contact will result in serious morphologic and pathologic changes of the interdental papilla, which takes on the shape of a col. The col is then changed in contour in such a way that the slight saddle-shaped area is broadened and exaggerated, and the epithelium of the col, nonkeratinized like that of the lining of the gingival sulcus, becomes more prone to breakdown (Fig. 26-13D–F). The tissue in this region must have sufficient space to remain free of disease. Occlusogingivally and faciolingually broad-

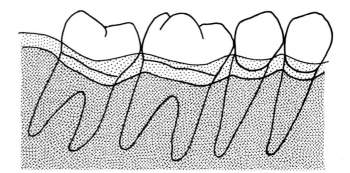

FIG. 26-11. *Effect of tilting which causes marginal ridge discrepancies and creates undesirable proximal contact relationships and interseptal bone morphology.*

ened proximal contacts prevent this by constricting both occlusal and interproximal embrasures (Fig. 26-14). The patient is less able to clean the interdental areas, and characteristic changes of the interdental tissues occur. Because of lack of space, there is a facial and lingual hyperplasia of the affected interdental papillae which causes exaggerated col formation and exposes this vulnerable region to microbial invasion, inflammation, edema, and subsequently to osseous involvement (Fig. 26-6C). Correct faciolingual and occlusocervical proximal-contact relationships will allow sufficient stimulation of the interdental papillae through normal functions and oral hygiene. Excessively narrow proximal contacts, as well as lack of contact, will promote food impaction and retention. In addition, lack of contact will allow tooth drifting.

It is important to adhere to creating correct contours when shaping coronal interproximal surfaces cer-

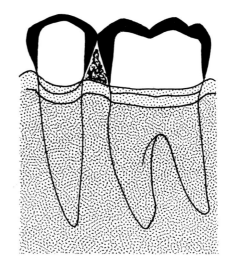

FIG. 26-12. *Proximal contacts of restorations placed too high occlusally and lacking sufficient area of contact, encouraging food impaction.*

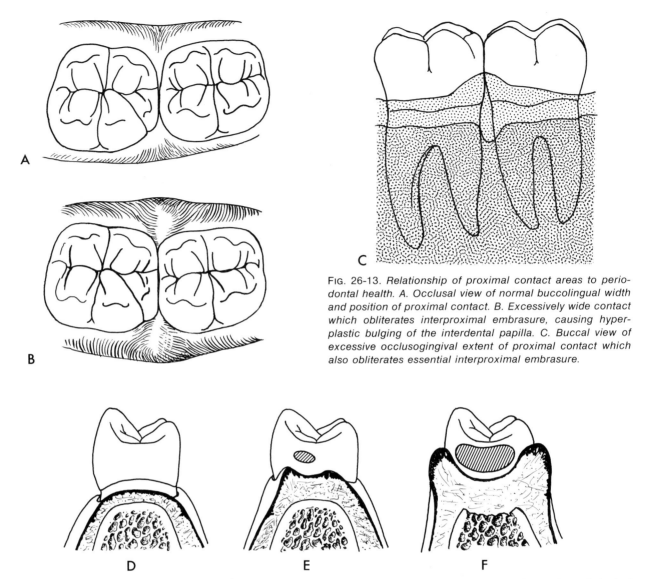

FIG. 26-13. *Relationship of proximal contact areas to periodontal health. A. Occlusal view of normal buccolingual width and position of proximal contact. B. Excessively wide contact which obliterates interproximal embrasure, causing hyperplastic bulging of the interdental papilla. C. Buccal view of excessive occlusogingival extent of proximal contact which also obliterates essential interproximal embrasure.*

FIG. 26-13 (continued). *D. Proximal view of tissue morphology related to lack of approximating tooth. Note that surface of gingival tissues assumes a convex form. This form is desirable and should be maintained, if possible (See Fig. 26-24). E. Interproximal view of normal position and size of proximal contact and morphology of interproximal gingiva, creating a slight col, which is normal for posterior regions. F. Interproximal view of tissue morphology related to abnormally widened proximal contact, resulting in exaggerated col formation that is subject to breakdown.*

vical to the contact area.[3] The region directly gingival to the contact area is always slightly concave. This also is true, to a lesser degree, in the transitional region where the interproximal surface meets the facial and lingual surfaces. This slight concavity leaves adequate space for the soft tissues (Fig. 26-15).

FACIAL AND LINGUAL CONTOURS

Not infrequently it has been stated by authorities that the purpose of the facial and lingual enamel bulge of human teeth is to protect the free gingival margin from the traumatic effects of mastication. Mention

should also be made of the supposed importance of muscle molding and of tissue contact from lips, cheeks, and tongue in offsetting food impaction.[27] Although there is no way of refuting this hypothesis, there is equally no way of proving its validity. The enamel bulge is said to deflect food over the gingival sulcus and onto the keratinized gingival tissues, which are better able to withstand the impact of the food. This theory has long been perpetrated in many textbooks and has not been seriously challenged. Overcontouring, ostensibly to protect the gingival sulcus from food particles passing down over the tooth surface, in fact encourages the accumulation of particulate and micro-

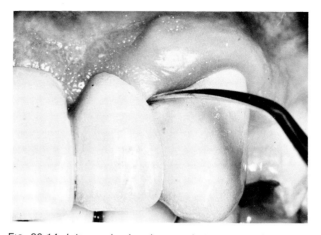

FIG. 26-14. *Interproximal embrasure between cuspid and lateral incisor obliterated by porcelain to the degree that it is difficult to pass a curet tip through. Note characteristic hyperplasia of interproximal papilla.*

bial matter in an area inaccessible to the patient. Undercontouring, on the other hand, eliminates this created space between gingiva and tooth. It is, in fact, doubtful that the gingival sulcus itself is in need of extra protection for the following reasons:

1. There is little in our modern diets that could injure the free gingival margin except accidentally or when, for some reason, the proprioceptive senses are impaired.
2. Proprioceptive response usually provides adequate protection for the free gingiva during mastication of hard foods.
3. The potential impact of food as the crushed bolus passes over the axial contour of the teeth is usually dissipated by the time the food reaches the gingiva.

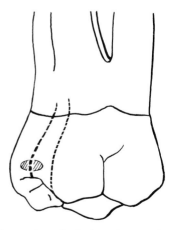

FIG. 26-15. *The occlusogingival contour at the proximal and transitional line-angle regions. Both should assume a flattened or slightly concave appearance gingival to the contact area.*

4. Most of the crushed bolus never reaches the gingiva, since it is directed by the cheeks, lips, tongue and other parts of the mouth into a position for deglutition.
5. Most human dentitions have little if any clinical bulge and yet show no deleterious effects from mastication.
   a. The facial bulges of deciduous and adolescent dentitions are below tissue, and yet these tissues do not suffer trauma from mastication.
   b. The slight bulge in the buccal sides of mandibular posterior teeth becomes ineffective for food deflection because these teeth are in most cases lingually inclined (Figs. 26-16A, C). Conversely, this same inclination exaggerates the lingual height of convexity and causes almost the entire lingual surface of the crown to become an area of stagnation.[45]
   c. Dentitions suffering from such abnormalities as enamel hypoplasia or peg-shaped lateral incisors do not have cervical bulges and yet demonstrate normal gingival tissue (Fig. 26-16B).
6. The dentitions of lower species of animals do not provide this hypothetical protection, since buccal and lingual bulges, if present at all, are usually subgingival (Fig. 26-17). The diets of the lower animals include foods that are much coarser than those in human diets and that are potentially traumatic to the gingiva, and yet it is difficult to demonstrate traumatic effects of mastication. Absence of trauma is obvious when watching a dog chew on bones and demonstrates that proprioceptive response is more important than tooth morphology.

In an experiment to ascertain how tooth contours affect the gingiva, Perel remodeled the mandibular teeth of full-grown mongrel dogs by removing tooth structure from either buccal, labial, or lingual surfaces.[28] Overcontouring of the buccal surfaces was done with self-curing resin, which was not in contact with the gingiva.

Results showed that undercontouring caused no apparent gingival pathoses, whereas overcontouring gave rise first to inflammation and later to the collection of debris, hyperplasia and engorgement of the marginal gingiva, scant keratization, and deterioration of the fibers of the gingival collar. The unhealthy state of the gingiva 4 weeks after overcontouring revealed that the so-called protective convexity not only served as a food trap but also prevented massage of the gingival margin.

In our opinion, the so-called protective cervical

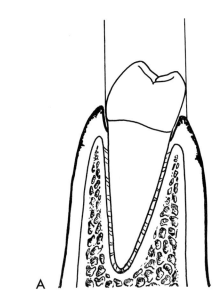

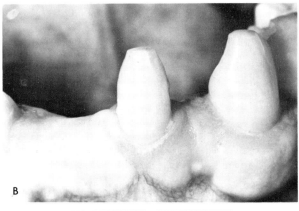

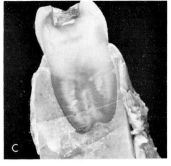

FIG. 26-16. *Facial and lingual contours. A. Slight bulges on buccal aspect of mandibular teeth that are ineffective for food deflection because of lingual inclination of crown. B. Peg-shaped mandibular incisor and cuspid lack protective bulge, but supporting tissues show no signs of periodontal disease. C. Frontal section of human mandibular first molar and alveolar process to show relationship of buccal and lingual contours to the gingival margins. Note lack of excessive buccal bulge at gingival third.*

bulge that hypothetically protects the human gingival crevice protects nothing but the microbial plaque. This is based on the following observations:

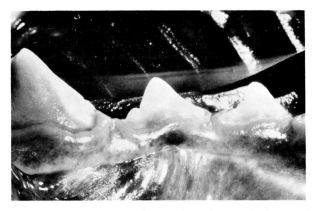

FIG. 26-17. *Dentition of a dog to show that cervical enamel bulges are usually subgingival and offer no protection to marginal gingiva during mastication.*

1. Plaque accumulation initiates, and its retention is greatest, in the cervical region of the tooth gingival to the height of contour. This can be demonstrated readily by using disclosing solution.

2. The greater the degree of facial and lingual bulge, the more plaque is retained in the cervical region (Fig. 26-18). The flatter the contour, the less plaque is retained. The explanation for this lies in the accessibility to oral hygiene. It is easier to keep the portion of the tooth occlusal to the height of contour plaque-free than the cervical region gingival to the height of contour. Most patients, unless they receive special instructions in brushing and use of floss or such devices as Stim-u-dents and Perio-Aids, which are specifically designed to remove plaque in the cervical region, will miss the plaque in the cervical region that is gingival to the height of contour. This is because of the overprotection given to this region by the height of contour and the free gingival margin. On many occasions we have observed the response of the gingiva to

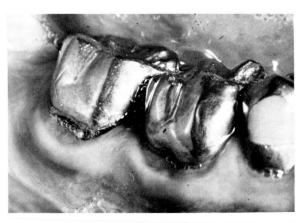

FIG. 26-18. *Clinical example to show the effects of excessive buccal overcontouring which promoted plaque accumulation, resulting in cervical caries and gingival inflammation.*

posterior teeth that have been prepared for full crowns and have lost their temporary crowns for periods as long as two years (Fig. 26-19). In all instances, the free gingival margin remained healthy, and the cervical regions of such teeth demonstrated little plaque retention compared with that of approximating unprepared teeth.

We have never observed teeth with little or no facial or lingual curvature that demonstrated a free gingival margin that has been stripped or pushed apically because of lack of protection and consequent overstimulation. We have, however, observed many teeth with excessively bulky contours that demonstrated disturbances attributable to the overprotection of the free gingival margin and which in consequence retained microbial plaque because the patients were unable to reach the areas by routine oral hygiene (Fig. 26-20).

For these reasons, we endeavor to flatten the facial

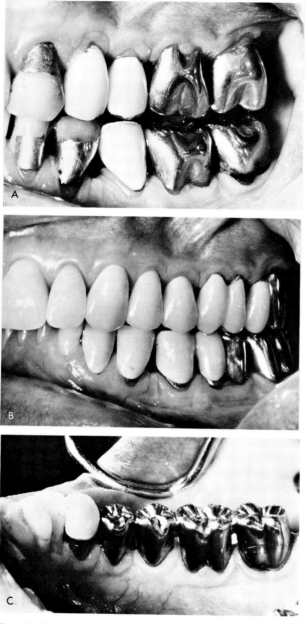

FIG. 26-20. *Facial and lingual contours of restored teeth, complicated by varying degrees of recession. A. Posterior teeth to be included in periodontal-prosthodontic reconstruction. Recession is due to surgical correction of generalized periodontal defects. Note overcontoured crowns and cervical caries. B. Buccal view to show occlusogingivally flattened contours and fluted contour in midbuccal and lingual regions of molars which greatly aid in ease of plaque removal. C. Lingual view to show same flattening. Note excellent gingival tone. (Courtesy of Dr. J. Weaver.)*

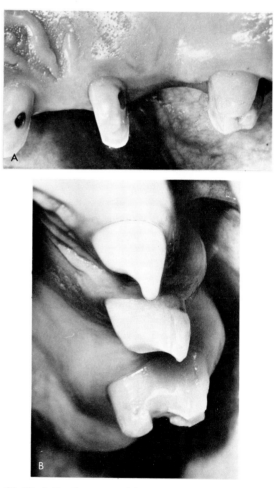

FIG. 26-19. *A. Teeth prepared for restoration and unprotected by temporary crowns for a period of approximately two years. Note lack of any cervical bulge and yet excellent tissue health. B. View to show lack of any lingual cervical bulge.*

and lingual contours of restorations and have observed excellent gingival response, most probably because the cervical region is made more accessible for routine home care. This is especially obvious where recession is present. The greater the degree of recession, the more difficult it becomes to clean the teeth adequately. Recession often exposes furcations and root flutings. These are especially difficult areas to keep plaque-free and may become impossible to clean if the coronal contours of restorations do not remain at least within the confines of the original tooth structure.

Contours of Full-Crown Restorations of Teeth Complicated by Recession

After periodontal therapy that involves osseous resective procedures, clinical crowns are often longer than normal. Surgically lengthened clinical crowns in need of full-coverage restorations are more difficult to restore than are crowns of normal clinical length. The increased length may cause pulpal complications during crown reduction, resulting from the need to remove much more coronal tooth structure in order to gain sufficient convergence. In fact, occasionally it becomes necessary to extirpate vital pulps from teeth that require splinting if convergence cannot be achieved in any other way than by tooth reduction.

Anatomic variation of the clinical crown poses other problems related to contours. The exposed portions of the roots are usually fluted buccolingually in the interproximal regions and mesiodistally in the furcation regions. These fluted regions require the most disciplined oral-hygiene efforts to keep them plaque-free. If plaque is allowed to accumulate for long periods of time, demineralization of the cemental surfaces will rapidly cause increased sensitivity and root caries. If root portions need to be covered by full-crown restorations, the contours of the gold castings should not be such that they frustrate the oral-hygiene efforts of the patient. If recession is excessive and there is little evidence of caries, it is often better to exclude the root portion from the preparation and depend on the oral-hygiene efforts of the patient and topical application of caries-inhibiting solutions to control sensitivity and root caries (Fig. 26-7).

When it is necessary to cover the root portion, it is advisable to modify only the contours of the original anatomic crown and to recreate the original contours of the root portion as closely as possible. The modification of the anatomic coronal form entails reduction of unnecessary bulges in order to create additional accessibility to the gingival third portion of the fluted regions of the restoration for the removal of accumulations of microbial plaque. Management of the occlusal morphology for such crowns does not differ in any manner from that described for normal crowns. The width of the occlusal table should be narrowed if the width prior to restoration has been increased through wear or faulty restorations (Fig. 26-10). The cuspal height should be reduced as much as possible, and the marginal ridges should be carefully created in accordance with correct interproximal-contact relationship. Because of the increased space for the interproximal soft tissue, the contact area can be broadened slightly, in an occlusogingival direction. However, widening must never be done to the extent that it impedes interproximal cleansing. Attempts should be made to flatten as much as possible, both facially and lingually, the original cervical bulge immediately occlusal to the cementoenamel junction in an occlusogingival direction (Fig. 26-20). This flattening will greatly enhance removal of plaque accumulations.

MANAGEMENT OF FURCATION REGIONS

If the exposed furcation regions of root structures must be covered by the full-crown restoration, care must be taken not to overcontour this region. It is this region and the interproximal fluted areas that are the most vulnerable to plaque accumulation and periodontal breakdown and are the most difficult to cleanse.

To maintain original contours in the furcation region after restoration, one must be prepared to remove adequate tooth structure during crown preparation. The preparation must be fluted occlusogingivally for the full length of the anatomic crown (Fig. 26-21). The waxing procedures must not recreate the original contours of the clinical crown, but must follow the furcation fluting of the prepared crown (Fig. 26-20). This technique will eliminate the triangular region that is created by the roots and the cervical bulge (Fig. 26-22). This area is most difficult to maintain plaque-free with normal brushing.

MANAGEMENT OF INTERPROXIMAL REGIONS

After periodontal surgery, the interproximal gingiva is keratinized and in most cases assumes a triangular instead of a col shape. A triangular papilla is ideally shaped for oral physiotherapy and attempts should be made to preserve it. Improper management of coronal contours that unnecessarily constrict interproximal embrasures will frustrate oral-hygiene and physiotherapeutic procedures and will result in a reversion of the interproximal tissues to a col-shaped configuration (Fig. 26-9). Although the col configuration is not necessarily an indication of a diseased papilla, most diseased papillae tend to be col-shaped. Reversion of the triangular papilla to col shape will encourage microorganisms and their by-products to accumulate in the middle portion of the col which is devoid of keratin (Fig. 26-13). Therefore, the interproximal region should be left large enough to accommodate the tissues

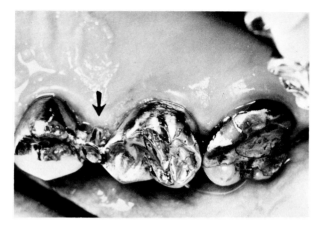

FIG. 26-34. *Improper pontic design for decreased space* (*arrow*).

righted orthodontically or by proximal reduction (Fig. 26-35E).

IMPROPERLY DESIGNED REMOVABLE PARTIAL DENTURES

Wherever possible teeth should support removable partial dentures. This method necessitates careful assessment of the abutments with respect to their periodontal environment. Teeth that lack sufficient support should be splinted to other teeth by means of soldered crowns. If strategic abutment teeth are missing or are in a weakened condition, it is often necessary to rely on tissue support as well as tooth support. In such cases, unless the partial denture is carefully constructed, it may exert a cantilevering effect on the abutment teeth, resulting in occlusal traumatism. Patients with removable partial dentures must be routinely examined to assess the degree of morphologic tissue changes that result from progressive alveolar resorption and to determine whether the base requires relining.

Improperly designed clasps also have damaging effects on abutment teeth (Fig. 5-8) by continuously causing excessive stresses, with resulting occlusal traumatism. During the settling of a posterior partial denture, the arms of the clasp may impinge upon the marginal tissue of the abutment tooth unless the denture is adequately supported on occlusal rests (Fig. 26-36).

The Effects of Claspless Partial Dentures

Wherever possible, it is preferable to construct fixed partial dentures rather than removable partial dentures. Economically, however, this is not always possible. Patients with removable partial dentures should be made aware that good oral hygiene is extremely important to prevent periodontal breakdown. The one-tooth or two-tooth removable partial denture, solely tissue-supported, is commonly seen as a prosthetic replacement for teeth removed for reasons of caries or trauma. This is often the only treatment that can be provided because of the age of the patient or the severity of the injury. Patients should be made to realize that these are only temporary and should be replaced with a fixed prosthesis in due time.

It is quite common for a tissue-supported partial denture to initiate inflammation within a few days (Fig. 26-37). The degree of inflammation may be slight and innocuous in appearance and thus be disregarded by the patient. It should be borne in mind that all periodontitis, even in its severest form, once started with the minimal lesion. The most common reaction of patients ignorant of proper oral hygiene is to neglect brushing an area that bleeds easily. The further accumulation of microbial plaque, with subsequent increase in inflammation, may lead to periodontitis (Fig. 26-38). Eventual settling of such partial dentures superimposed on plaque and calculus will cause apical migration of the epithelial attachment. The effects of these insults must be corrected prior to restoration with a fixed prosthesis. If the damage is slight, curettage and instructions for home care may suffice. If these insults have given rise to a gingival hyperplasia, however, ridgeplasty may be necessary (Figs. 26-39, 26-40). If the outcome is periodontitis with bone involvement, flap surgery may be necessary to correct the defects. Surgical intervention to correct such defects may undesirably alter the tissue form, but nevertheless it is still necessary prior to undertaking fixed-prosthetic therapy. The methods for surgical correction of such ridges are described in Chapter 27.

EXODONTIC PROCEDURES THAT AFFECT THE PERIODONTIUM

Not infrequently, because of severe caries, periodontal involvement, or crowding, selected extraction of teeth is necessary. Injudicious tooth removal can often initiate periodontal disease or aggravate an existing pathosis in the vicinity of the extraction. In tooth extraction, some common errors in technique may adversely affect the periodontium:

1. Manner in which facial and lingual flaps are raised
2. Manner in which the teeth are luxated and elevated
3. Degree of postextraction debridement
4. Way in which the wound is closed

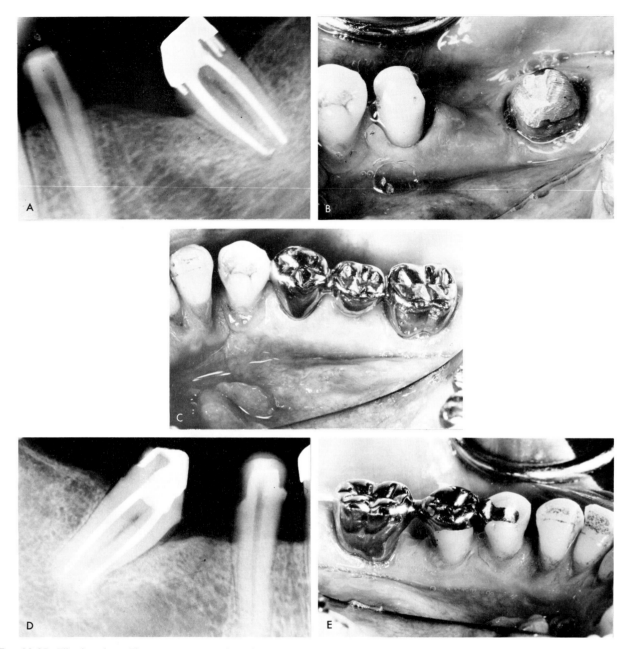

FIG. 26-35. *Tilted molars. The crown preparations have been modified to compensate for lack of orthodonic uprighting and to provide a normal environment for pontic adaptation and oral hygiene. Both molar abutments required endodontic therapy prior to coronal reduction because of extensive carious involvement. A. Right mandibular quadrant. Note reduction of mesial aspect of molar abutment. B. Lingual view of prepared teeth. C. Lingual view of fixed prosthesis. Note excellent tissue tone. D. Left mandibular quadrant, showing mesial reduction, E. Lingual view of restoration in place showing design of solder joint to compensate for lack of pontic. Note mesial contour of molar designed to create environment conducive to tissue health. Soft-tissue ridgeplasty was performed to eliminate excessive pseudopocketing on mesial aspects of both molars, a condition characteristically associated with tilted teeth. Tooth has been uprighted by proximal reduction to prevent regeneration of hyperplastic tissue.*

Apart from surgically releasing the cervical epithelium and connective-tissue attachment of the tooth, the creation of flaps is in many cases unnecessary for the purpose of extraction. Not uncommonly, however, flaps are necessary to expose the alveolar supporting bone for its reduction, to simplify removal of the tooth, or to correct morphologic or pathologic aberrations of the hard and/or soft tissues concomitantly with the extraction. In such cases, all the principles of flap management, debridement, and flap closure, as outlined in Chapter 22, are equally as important in exodontics as in periodontal surgery.

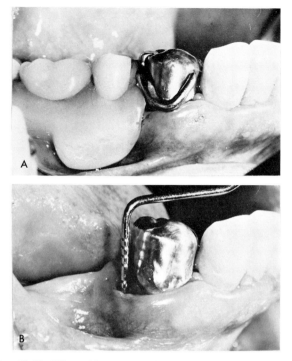

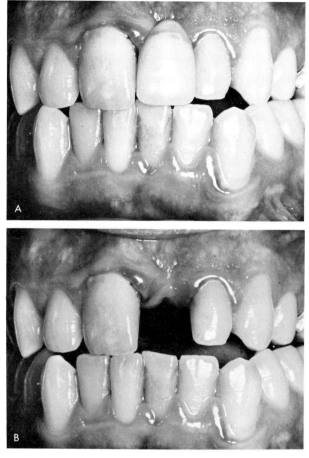

FIG. 26-36. *Effect of improperly designed clasp that impinged on the gingival tissues. A. Buccal view to show proximity of clasp to gingival margins. B. Probe in place to show extent of damage.*

If the width and thickness of the band of attached gingiva are normal, gingiva should be preserved and accurately repositioned in its original site and stabilized by careful suturing. The practice of tightly suturing flaps to achieve hemostasis without regard for flap position may result in their being positioned too far occlusally. Since connective tissue does not attach to

FIG. 26-38. *Localized periodontitis caused by settling of tissue-borne removable partial denture and inadequate plaque control. A. Note difference in incisal level between central incisors, indicating amount of settling. B. Note tissue damage on the mesial aspects of both central and lateral incisors.*

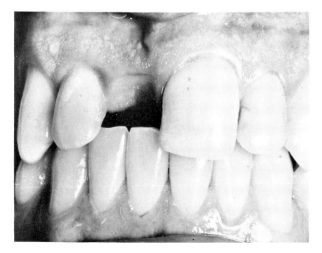

FIG. 26-37. *Characteristic signs of inflammation three days after insertion of tissue-supported removable partial denture (mesial aspects of lateral and central incisors).*

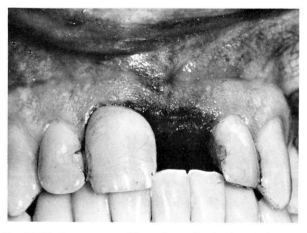

FIG. 26-39. *Appearance of tissue immediately after ridgeplasty procedure. Intention was to eliminate unnecessary hyperplastic tissue before replacing missing tooth with a fixed prosthesis.*

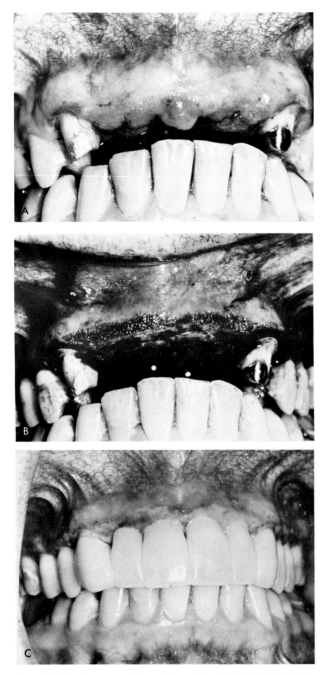

FIG. 26-40. *Case requiring ridgeplasty to eliminate hyperplastic tissue which resulted from poorly fitting removable partial denture. A. Presurgical appearance. B. Postsurgical appearance. C. One week after surgery, at time of placing temporary acrylic bridge.*

the enamel surface, not only will pseudopockets result, but also the incorrectly positioned band of gingiva will become afunctional, since it will have lost part or all of its attachment and become an exaggerated free gingival margin (Fig. 26-41). This is especially serious if the original zone of attached gingiva in the vicinity of the

extraction is minimal or nonexistent. When such is the case, the flaps should be apically positioned after the extraction rather than repositioned into their original site, in order to allow for exposure of sufficient alveolar bone. Formation of granulation tissue in this zone of exposed bone will give rise to a wider zone of firmly attached gingiva, which will greatly improve the environment of both the approximating teeth and the edentulous ridge for pontic adaptation, if a fixed prosthesis is necessary.

If the zone of attached gingiva is more than adequate or if it is thicker than normal, it may not be necessary to preserve the entire width of this band while raising the flap. In such cases the internally beveled flap procedure described in Chapter 22 can be advantageously applied. If properly executed, this procedure will result in a uniformly thinned flap that will improve the soft-tissue characteristics surrounding the extraction site.

Where selected extraction is required because of periodontal involvement, internally beveled flaps are in most cases a necessary part of the extraction procedure. This will permit surgical curettage of any diseased sulcular and interproximal soft tissue to expose the alveolar bone for correction of any associated morphologic or pathologic osseous aberrations. Associated soft-tissue and osseous defects should be corrected concomitantly with the extraction (Fig. 26-42). If neglected, such pathologic conditions will be perpetuated and can only increase in severity.

Partially impacted third molars are not infrequently complicated by periodontal breakdown of the approximating tooth. Removal of the impacted tooth should always be followed by treatment of the periodontal lesion. This should include soft-tissue debridement, correction of any osseous defects, and judicious soft-tissue replacement and stabilization by careful suturing to avoid perpetuating the periodontal pathology or creating new periodontal disturbances where none previously existed.

Injudicious use of the forceps or elevators during luxation, elevation, and extraction may result in crushing injuries to the alveolar bone. Elevators should therefore be used carefully, so as not to loosen the approximating teeth or crush the radicular bone of these teeth. If, in spite of precautions, fracture of segments of alveolar cortical bone inadvertently does occur, the fractured segments should be carefully repositioned and stabilized with properly placed sutures. In many cases, such bone segments will remain viable and reattach.

Occasionally, close root proximity associated with periodontal involvement obviates either selected extraction or root amputation. Attempts to correct inter-

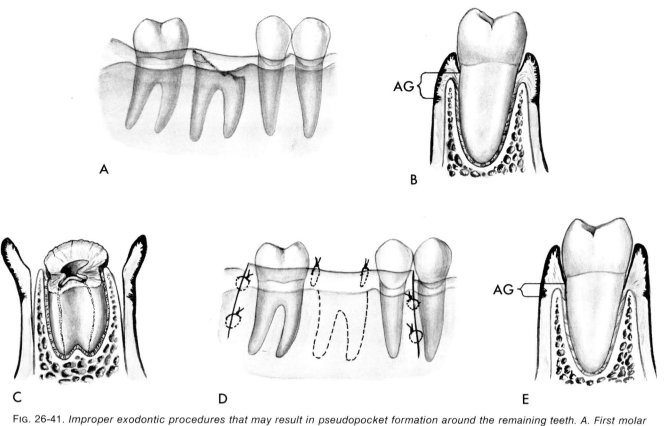

FIG. 26-41. *Improper exodontic procedures that may result in pseudopocket formation around the remaining teeth. A. First molar before extraction. Note position of gingival margin relative to clinical crown. B. View of molar adjacent to condemned tooth showing amount and level of functional attached gingiva (AG) prior to exodontic procedure. C. Buccal and lingual flaps raised to expose condemned molar and surrounding alveolar bone. D. After extraction, showing flap positioned too high coronally. E. View of molar adjacent to extraction site showing that by improper positioning of the flap most of the original zone of functional attached gingiva has lost its usefulness and has become part of the free gingival margin, thereby creating a pseudopocket.*

proximal osseous defects and to restore teeth that have close root proximity usually result in undesirable hard- and soft-tissue contours (reverse architecture) (Fig. 26-43). The practice of heroically attempting to save every tooth in every mouth is often met with frustration and failure. Our goal in dentistry should be to save dentitions, and often selective extraction of seriously involved teeth with subsequent replacement is the most expedient and economical manner in which this can be accomplished.

ORTHODONTIC THERAPY AS IT RELATES TO OCCLUSAL TRAUMATISM AND PERIODONTAL DISEASE

In orthodontic treatment, teeth are moved into new positions and relationships, and soft tissues and underlying bone are altered in order to accommodate changes in esthetics and function. Of the two objectives, function is the more important. The patient, to whom esthetics are of major concern, must be made to realize that orthodontic intervention that leaves him with functional disturbances will in time fail.

Periodontal disease can be briefly described as the process by which tooth support is lost as a result of bone resorption and apical migration of the attachment apparatus. It is important to note that even though the major causative factors of the disease and the necessary steps in treatment to slow or stop its progress are known, not enough is known about what occurs at the molecular level. Until the exact sequence of events at the most basic structural level is learned, the etiologic factors can only be ascertained from clinical observation and from experience with empirical treatment. Some of the less obvious factors contributing to the etiology of periodontal disease have not been fully investigated, mainly because of difficulties of investigation and documentation. The long-term effects of orthodontic treatment may fall into this category. It is important to understand that all therapy exacts a price for benefits bestowed. Irritational factors such as ill-fitting band margins, variable form and

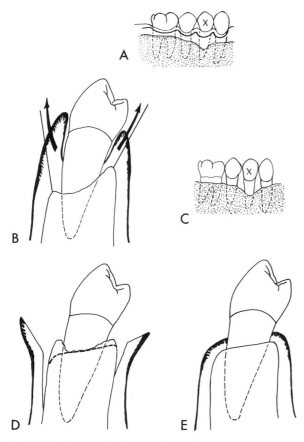

FIG. 26-42. *Concomitant correction of osseous defects surrounding teeth adjacent to extraction site of a hopelessly involved tooth. A. Buccal view showing anteroposterior extent of internal-beveled incision (thick line). This will expose alveolar bone surrounding the condemned first premolar (X). B. Proximal view of condemned premolar, showing that an adequate amount of attached gingiva must be preserved. The sulcular epithelium and excess attached gingiva is removed with curets. C. The alveolar bone with its defects exposed. D. Proximal view of second premolar adjacent to extraction site with mesial interproximal crater and amount of bone that must be removed. E. Apically positioned flaps that will be stabilized with sutures.*

dimension of the embrasure during movement, and tooth movement itself—all exact a toll.

Occlusal traumatism has been dealt with at great length earlier in this text. Although much agreement exists among investigators, some divergence of opinion remains, and so for the purpose of discussion reference will be made to the points that are accepted as true by the majority. Four significant points in regard to occlusal traumatism should be reemphasized:

1. Occlusal traumatism by itself does not cause pocket formation or gingivitis.
2. Occlusal traumatism can by itself cause tooth mobility, bone resorption, and widening of periodontal space.
3. Local irritants, microbial plaque, and environmental conditions that harbor plaque can cause pocket formation, apical migration of the epithelial attachment, and bone loss.
4. A combination of local irritants and occlusal traumatism will cause more rapid destruction than will local factors by themselves.

It is, therefore, important to keep these relationships to local factors in mind when evaluating occlusal traumatism. A brief consideration should be given to the anatomic stage at which these forces are encountered when the periodontitis first appears.

Arnim and Hagerman demonstrated the existence of a band of dense collagenous connective-tissue fibers encircling each tooth.[5] According to them, these fibers play an important part in keeping particulate matter out of the sulcus. Disruption of this apparatus permits further insult to the attachment and the spread of inflammation into the deeper tissues, permitting occlusal traumatism to influence the rate of apical migration. This system is the first to be damaged by the disease process, particularly in the interproximal areas, which are more vulnerable because the fibers there are fewer in number. Fish also pointed out that the interproximal epithelium, which is thought to be a vestigial remnant of the epithelial attachment, is not keratinized and hence is more vulnerable.[14]

From the foregoing, the importance of occlusal traumatism in connection with orthodontic treatment can be seen. How occlusal traumatism differs in these patients from occlusal traumatism in patients who have not undergone orthodontic treatment will be considered in three phases.

Circumstances before Therapy

The patients who present themselves to the orthodontist are for the most part in the age group from 12 to 15 years. They are seeking treatment because of some type of malocclusion that manifests itself in unsatisfactory esthetics or because they have been referred by other dentists. By virtue of this malocclusion, they have a higher-than-average incidence of periodontal disease.[35] This is probably because malpositioned teeth are more difficult to keep clean. Ahlgren and Posselt showed that of a group of 120 children requiring orthodontic treatment, 55 percent had severe cuspal interferences, either balancing contacts or a deflecting slide from CRO to CO—factors that contribute to occlusal traumatism.[1] Direct anterior slides of 1 mm or less were not considered traumatic. The study also disclosed that no specific malocclusion was associated with any specific cuspal interferences. In fact, the Angle Class I group showed the highest number of interferences.

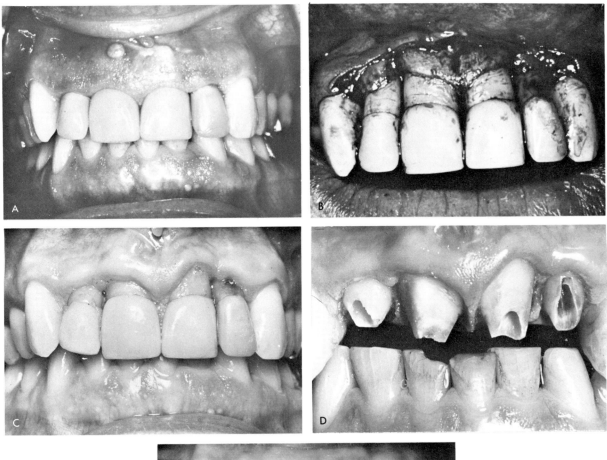

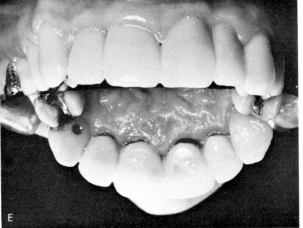

FIG. 26-43. *Improper management of teeth with close root proximities and in need of periodontal, endodontic, and restorative therapy. A. Before surgery. Note hyperplastic gingiva and fistula above central incisor. B. During surgery, showing unsatisfactory attempt to correct osseous craters between the central and lateral incisors. Reverse osseous architecture has resulted because of close root proximity. C. After healing, showing reverse architectural form of soft tissues which followed the form of the underlying bone. D. Teeth prepared for post crowns. Note interproximal soft tissue cratering between the lateral and central incisors on either side, due to lack of sufficient space. E. After restoration, showing facial and lingual obliteration of interproximal embrasures that will aggravate existing interproximal cols. Extraction of the lateral incisors to alleviate the root proximities and replacement with a fixed prosthesis would have been preferable to attempting to save all the anterior teeth.*

Of importance also is the incidence of periodontal disease in children. There have been a number of reports on the percentage of incidence in certain age groups. In analyzing these reports, Goose and his asso-

ciates found considerable variations between groups and considerable differences in data obtained because some authors included all children showing any signs of gingivitis and others included only well-established cases.[15] They also noted that an individual mouth can vary in its manifestations of periodontal disease with the season and over time. The overall incidence was in the neighborhood of 60 percent and increased with age.

Circumstances Arising during Therapy

Several factors introduced during therapy influence the state of health of the tissues in regard to inflammation. The placement of tooth-separating appliances causes inflammation to the interdental tissues and risks causing movement of teeth into positions subject to cuspal interferences. The placement of bands in subgingival areas alters the environment within the sulcus.[46] It is impossible not to have bands below the crest of the interproximal gingiva. Waerhaug has shown that materials placed in the sulcus do not of themselves cause irritation unless they provide a means for plaque to accumulate[50] Stainless steel is an inert substance.

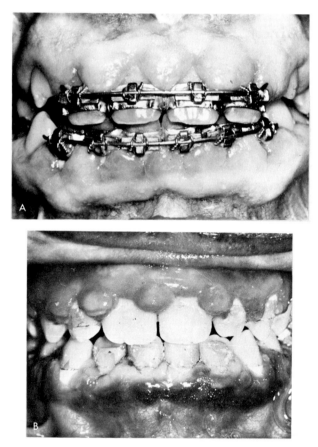

FIG. 26-44. *Alteration in tissue form related to orthodontic therapy. A. Impingement of appliance on tissues and plaque accumulation resulted in exaggerated hyperplasia and inflammation. B. Another case with bands removed showing similar response.*

However, studies relating to cements show that they readily retain microbial plaque.[49] The ability to fit bands perfectly in this area is questionable because of the concavity of the tooth surfaces. Phillips and Schwartz demonstrated the microbial retention *in vitro* by rough enamel surfaces and the inability to clean these surfaces mechanically.[29] This is a factor to consider when teeth are stripped to gain space. Oral hygiene is hampered by the amount of hardware present, and conventional use of floss is prevented by arch wires (Fig. 26-44A). Alterations have to be made in methods of home care. At the age of the patients being treated, difficulties are encountered from the standpoint of motivation.[5] Special attention must be paid to this matter. Direct trauma from appliances can occur if they impinge on the soft tissues (Fig. 26-44B).

Occlusal alterations occurring during any type of dental therapy can create conditions that may affect the health of the periodontium. While teeth are being orthodontically moved, a form of occlusal traumatism is unavoidably created. What effects such trauma may have on the young patient remain unclear. Obviously the supporting structures are altered by the orthodontic movement, and the histologic picture is similar to that in occlusal traumatism. However, this may be more tolerable since the teeth are supported by the splinting effects of the bands and arch wires. Unfortunately other irritating factors such as microbial plaque, prematurities, root resorption, and parafunctions enter into the picture.

Throughout orthodontic therapy new prematurities are unavoidably introduced. If carefully controlled, these may not result in irreversible damage, but they may cause muscle strain and lead to spasm and increased parafunctional activity.[34] This result has been shown to be true at any age. Parafunctions, unlike normal functions, are not self-protected, and even under normal conditions may evoke tissue destruction, especially during sleep.[13]

Root resorption is a phenomenon that occurs often during orthodontic treatment. Henry and Weinmann showed that in a random sample cemental resorption takes place in 90 percent of teeth.[19] Trauma appears to be the most important factor in producing cemental resorption. Although it has been shown that predisposition to root resorption is likely to exist in any individual, orthodontic treatment has been seen to accelerate this process (Fig. 5-14). Root resorption may or may not be significant, depending upon the degree of trauma or disease encountered by the individual later in life, but a tooth with a shortened root is less satisfactory as an abutment tooth, because it provides less support if periodontal disease progress to advanced stages.

Circumstances Arising after Therapy

At the completion of orthodontic therapy, there are often several morphologic entities that may be deleterious to the resistance of the individual to occlusal traumatism and other periodontal diseases. Root proximity is often the result of either stripping or tilting the teeth, and an unfavorable interproximal area for the soft tissue is established. From the standpoint of periodontal surgery, should it become necessary to eliminate craters, the situation may be irredeemable or may require root amputation. In cases involving stripping, the interproximal contact areas are usually too wide buccolingually. This, in conjunction with the increased plaque retention on roughened enamel surfaces, is a predisposing factor in periodontal disease.

Another situation encountered as a result of some types of orthodontic treatment is the movement of the roots outside the confines of the alveolar process (Fig. 26-45). The resulting dehiscences or fenestrations may be of no consequence unless trauma or periodontal disease occurs in the area at a later date. With the present incidence of caries and periodontal disease and the manner of treatment available for these conditions, the probability of eventual damage is high. For example, in the treatment of caries, the manipulation of the soft tissues during operative procedures jeopardizes the maintenance of the attached gingiva, which is minimal in mandibular premolars and cuspids, the same areas often affected by fenestration or dehiscence. The loss of attached gingiva enhances loss of soft-tissue root coverage, a situation difficult or impossible to correct with periodontal surgery to any satisfactory degree. The same difficulty arises if periodontitis creates the need for surgery. Overzealous or improper brushing procedures by themselves may result in dehiscences.

Posttreatment Occlusal Status

Arguments exist as to the need for postorthodontic occlusal adjustment. Before this can be discussed, it is necessary to investigate the type of occlusion sought in orthodontic treatment. Ideas on desirable occlusion vary, but most practitioners agree upon several points.

It is desirable to have CRO coincide with CO or at least to have freedom of movement from one to the other on the same occlusal plane. A cuspid rise or group function should exist on the working side without balancing interferences.[39,54] For the sake of stability, the cusp-to-fossa relationship should be adopted where possible. This removes wedging forces from the occlusion, directs forces in a more axial direction, and provides the dentition with greater stability. Beyron advocates the provision for smooth, multidirectional

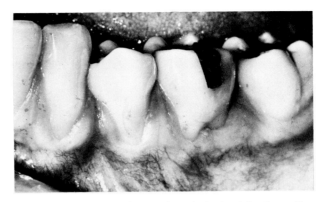

FIG. 26-45. *Clefting and recession of gingiva following orthodontic movement of teeth and further aggravated by improper brushing.*

gliding movements in order that the inevitable occlusal changes will not be unfavorable.[7] Careful attention must be given to incisal guidance, which, according to Schuyler, is the most important factor in controlling favorable or unfavorable function in eccentric position.[38] The dentition that has these qualities will be the one least likely to fall into parafunction.[36]

Does an ideal relationship exist in the completed orthodontic case? Several studies indicate that few dentitions are free from occlusal traumatism. Ahlgren and Posselt screened 23 postorthodontics patients and found interferences in 14 of them.[1] Cohen's extensive investigation showed interferences in 90 percent of postorthodontics cases.[12] Of 10 cases studied by Heide and Thorpe all showed anterior shifts from CRO to CO.[17]

There are other reasons for occlusal adjustment. Tooth surfaces are rarely equilibrated with each other through natural functions. Selective grinding is usually necessary to eliminate interferences and fit cusps properly into fossae. This will create better retention and greater stability. In addition, a tooth moved because its relationships have been changed will seldom function in harmony with others right away. Wear will adapt it to a certain extent, but movement of the tooth will probably occur before wear takes place. If interferences exist, it is unlikely that occlusal wear will adjust the dentition.

A good outline for integrating occlusal adjustment by selective grinding with orthodontic treatment was prepared by Heimlich.[18] He divided the procedures into five phases:

1. Reshaping teeth to normal before treatment. This entails the correction of restorations and reshaping of teeth for esthetic reasons.
2. Orthodontic treatment, with minor reshaping during treatment, if desirable.

3. Removal of gross prematurities after initial settling. Interferences placed in the paths of function as a result of treatment should be eliminated to prevent occlusal traumatism and drifting. Definitive occlusal adjustment should not be considered at this stage because some drifting may still occur.

4. Refinement. After from 9 months to 1 year in retention, fine adjustments are made to compensate for any drifting and to complete the occlusal adjustment.

5. Resolution of any third-molar problem.

He states that "the orthodontist is in a unique position for placing the dentition in its ideal relationship. We should strive to take advantage of the opportunity."

Effects of Orthodontic Therapy

The overall effect of orthodontic treatment upon the supporting structures of the teeth is dependent upon several factors. In some cases, pathologic conditions arising from orthodontics can be pointed out as being attributable to specific factors. In general, however, little immediate postorthodontic damage is evident. Few long-term studies have been made.

Baxter showed loss of interproximal-crestal bone of less than 0.5 mm in 76 orthodontic cases.[6] Tirk and his associates reported in their study a higher percentage of alveolar bone and cemental resorption than had formerly been reported.[43] They mentioned that the vee-ing of alveolar crests is perhaps the beginning of destructive resorption. Their observations were that when resorption begins in these areas, it tends to progress unabated, even though the force of the original insult is lessened. Clinical evidence from many cases warrants further study of the long-term effect on the periodontium of orthodontic therapy. Whether damage can be attributed exclusively to the occlusion that is developed following orthodontic treatment remains to be seen. Some latent factors that could predispose the periodontium to easier breakdown cannot be discounted.

In summary, it can be seen that irritational factors coexist during and after orthodontic treatment and that these can be affected by occlusal traumatism. However, the degree of damage that can be attributed to orthodontic treatment remains to be discovered.[21]

References

1. Ahlgren, J., and Posselt, U.: A need of functional analysis and selective grinding in orthodontics. Acta Odontol. Scand., 21:187, 1963.

2. Allison, J. R., and Bhatia, H. K.: Tissue changes under acrylic and porcelain pontics. J. Dent. Res., 37:66, 1958 (Abstract).

3. Amsterdam, M., and Abrams, L.: Periodontal prosthesis. In Periodontal Therapy, 5th ed. H. M. Goldman and D. W. Cohen, Eds. St. Louis, C. V. Mosby Co., 1973.

4. App, G. R.: Effect of silicate, amalgam, and cast gold on the gingiva. J. Prosthet. Dent., 11:522, 1961.

5. Arnim, S., and Hagerman, D. A.: The connective tissue fibers of the marginal gingiva. J. Am. Dent. Assoc., 47:271, 1953.

6. Baxter, D. H.: The effect of orthodontic treatment on the alveolar bone adjacent to the cemento-enamel junction. Angle Orthod., 37:35, 1967.

7. Beyron, H. G.: Characteristics of functionally optimum occlusion and principles of occlusal rehabilitation. J. Am. Dent. Assoc., 48:648, 1954.

8. Black, G. V.: Operative Dentistry, vol. I. Chicago, Medico-Dental, 1908.

9. Bowles, R. O.: Fixed bridges with special reference to tissue contact pontics and inlay abutments. J. Am. Dent. Assoc., 18:1521, 1931.

10. Burwasser, P., and Hill, T. J.: The effect of hard and soft diets on the gingival tissues of dogs. J. Dent. Res., 18:389, 1939.

11. Christensen, G.: Marginal fit of gold inlay castings. J. Prosthet. Dent., 16:297, 1966.

12. Cohen, W. E.: A study of occlusal interferences in orthodontically treated occlusions and untreated occlusions. A. J. Orthod., 51:647, 1965.

13. Drum, W.: Paradentose als Autodestruktionsvorgang und Hinweise für die Prophylaxe. Ber. Ärztebl., 71:300, 1958.

14. Fish, W.: Etiology and prevention of periodontal breakdown. Dent. Progress, 1:235, 1961.

15. Goose, D. H., et al.: Periodontal disease in children. Dent. Pract., 17:279, 1967.

16. Hazen, S. P., and Osborne, J. W.: Relationship of operative dentistry to periodontal health. Dent. Clin. North Am., Mar., 1967, p. 245.

17. Heide, M., and Thorpe, C. W.: The necessity for post-orthodontic precision grinding for balanced occlusion. Angle Orthod., 35:113, 1965.

18. Heimlich, A. C.: Occlusal equilibration in relation to orthodontic treatment. Dent. Clin. North Am., Nov. 1960, p. 807.

19. Henry, J., and Weinmann, J. P.: The pattern of resorption and repair of human cementum. J. Am. Dent. Assoc., 42:270, 1951.

20. Herlands, R. E., Lucca, J. J., and Morris, M. L.: Forms, contours and extensions of the full coverage restorations in occlusal reconstruction. Dent. Clin. North Am., Mar., 1962, p. 147.

21. Jekkals, V., and Yuodelis, R. A.: Periodontal and occlusal status of ten year post-orthodontic patients. Dissertation for M.S. in Dentistry degree, U. of Washington School of Dentistry, Seattle, Washington, 1969.

22. Kornfeld, M.: Mouth Rehabilitation, vol. I. St. Louis, C. V. Mosby Co., 1967.

23. Kraus, B. S., Jordan, R. E., and Abrams, L.: Dental Anatomy and Occlusion. Baltimore, Williams and Wilkins, 1969.

24. Larato, D. C.: The effect of crown margin extension on gingival inflammation. J. So. Cal. Dent. Assoc., 37:476, 1969.

25. Löe, H.: Reactions of marginal periodontal tissues to restorative procedures. Int. Dent. J., 18:759, 1968.

26. Marcum, J. S.: The effect of crown marginal depth upon gingival tissue. J. Prosthet. Dent., 17:479, 1967.

27. Morris, M. L.: Artificial crown contours and gingival health. J. Prosthet. Dent., 12:1146, 1962.

28. Perel, M. L.: Axial crown contours. J. Prosthet. Dent., 25:642, 1971.

29. Phillips, S., and Schwartz, M.: Comparison of bacterial accumulation on smooth and rough enamel surfaces. J. Periodontol., 28:304, 1957.

30. Pine, B. L.: Pontics for gold-acrylic resin fixed partial dentures. J. Prosthet. Dent., 12:347, 1962.

31. Pini, C. E.: Co-report: Hygienic considerations in crown and bridge prosthesis. Int. Dent. J., 8:357, 1958.

32. Podshadley, A. G.: Rat connective tissue response to pontic materials. J. Prosthet. Dent., 16:110, 1966.

33. Podshadley, A. G.: Gingival response to pontics. J. Prosthet. Dent., 19:51, 1968.

34. Posselt, U., and Emslie, P.: Occlusal disharmonies and their effect on periodontal disease. Int. Dent. J., 9:367, 1959.

35. Poulton, D., and Aaronson, S. A.: The relationship between occlusion and periodontal status. Am. J. Orthod., 47:690, 1961.

36. Ramfjord, S. P., and Ash, M. M.: Occlusion, 2nd ed. Philadelphia, W. B. Saunders Co., 1971.

37. Rosen, H., and Gitnick, P. J.: Integrating restorative procedures into the treatment of periodontal disease. J. Prosthet. Dent., 14:343, 1964.

38. Schuyler, C.: Factors contributing to traumatic occlusion. J. Prosthet. Dent., 11:708, 1961.

39. Stallard, H.: Dental articulation as an orthodontic aim. J. Am. Dent. Assoc., 24:347, 1937.

40. Stein, R. S.: Pontic-residual ridge relationship: A research report. J. Prosthet. Dent., 16:251, 1966.

41. Stein, R. S., and Glickman, I.: Prosthetic consideration essential for gingival health. Dent. Clin. North Am., Mar., 1960, p. 177.

42. Stein, R. S., and Sozio, R.: Personal Communication, 1971.

43. Tirk, T. M., Guzman, C. A., and Nalchajian, R.: Periodontal tissue response to orthodontic treatment studied by panoramix. Angle Orthod., 37:94, 1967.

44. Tylman, S. D.: Theory and Practice in Crown and Bridge Prosthodontics, 6th ed. St. Louis, C. V. Mosby Co., 1970.

45. Veldcamp, D. F.: The relationship between tooth form and gingival health. Dent. Pract., 14:158, 1963.

46. Waerhaug, J.: The presence or absence of bacteria in gingival pockets and the reaction in healthy pockets to certain pure cultures. Odont. Tidskr. Suppl., 1952.

47. Waerhaug, J.: Tissue reactions around artificial crowns. J. Periodontol., 24:172, 1953.

48. Waerhaug, J.: Effect of rough surfaces upon gingival tissues. J. Dent. Res., 35:323, 1956.

49. Waerhaug, J.: Effect of zinc phosphate cement fillings on gingival tissue. J. Periodontol., 27:284, 1956.

50. Waerhaug, J.: Tissue reaction to metal wires in healthy gingival pockets. J. Periodontol., 28:239, 1957.

51. Waerhaug, J., and Zander, H. A.: Reaction of gingival tissue to self-curing acrylic restorations. J. Am. Dent. Assoc., 54:760, 1957.

52. Wheeler, R. C.: Complete crown form and the periodontium. J. Prosthet. Dent., 11:722, 1961.

53. Wheeler, R. C.: Normal tooth form and dental maintenance. J. So. Cal. Dent. Assoc., 31:382, 1963.

54. Yuodelis, R. A., and Mann, W. V., Jr.: The prevalence of non-working contacts in periodontal disease. Periodontics, 3:219, 1965.

27

Initial Corrective Phase of
Oral Rehabilitation

27

Initial

Corrective

Phase

of

Oral

Rehabilitation

Before embarking on any restorative procedures, all existing pathologic conditions of the periodontium, such as gingivitis and periodontitis, and morphologic aberrations of the soft and hard tissues must be recognized and if possible treated. If this step is neglected, the restorative procedure, no matter how well performed, may in itself contribute to the aggravation of the disease.

Many of the minor periodontal problems should be seen as integral parts of the practice of general dentistry and it will be in everyone's interest when the day comes for the general practitioner to accept the treatment of many periodontal problems as a matter of routine. Because the demand for periodontal care is rapidly gaining momentum, it is only natural for the periodontist to confine his practice to the more severe problems, since these patients need help the most. It is not only impractical, but impossible for the periodontal specialist to treat all the minor periodontal problems that the general practitioner encounters every day. For one thing, there are not enough periodontists to handle them.

IMPORTANCE OF INITIAL DISEASE CONTROL

Since it is imperative to eliminate all pathologic conditions that could seriously compromise the longevity of the restorative work, therapy must begin with making the patient aware of the etiologic factors that have led to his present oral condition. In the majority of cases requiring extensive rehabilitation, the prolonged accumulation of excessive microbial plaque has played a major role in causing the existing oral pathology, whether caries or periodontitis. Early in the treatment oral-hygiene measures must be instituted and the patient must cooperate in carrying these out. The patient who will not cooperate before or during therapy most certainly cannot be expected to continue maintenance after treatment, and efforts at restoration will be short-lived, no matter how well they have been executed or how much they have cost the patient.

An effective method of dramatizing the etiologic effects of irritants on periodontal breakdown is to allow the patient to experience the rapid tissue response that follows removal of such irritants. Consequently, initial therapy should always consist of scaling and polishing the crown and root surfaces and giving the patient initial home-care instructions (Fig. 27-1).

The patient should then be allowed a reasonable period of time to prove that he is aware of his responsibilities and is willing to cooperate. Only after this should the practitioner concern himself with treatment

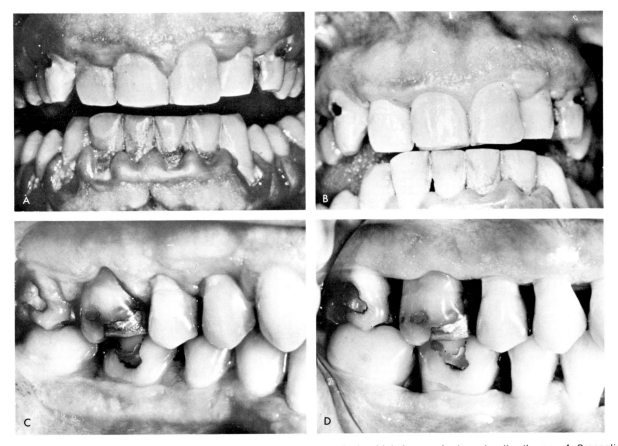

FIG. 27-1. *The effectiveness of disease control by removal of irritants and microbial plaque prior to restorative therapy. A. Prescaling of supra- and subgingival calculus. B. Ten days after scaling but with no microbial plaque control. Note that some signs of inflammation still exist. C. Before initiation of disease control. D. After initiation of disease control that included curettage, root planing, and microbial plaque control. Note reverse gingival architecture, a sign usually associated with interproximal bone craters that will also require correction prior to restorative therapy.*

of morphologic or pathologic soft-tissue and hard-tissue aberrations that have resulted from the prolonged effects of various etiologic factors. The remainder of this chapter will be concerned mainly with the recognition and correction of such periodontal factors as may seriously affect both the prognosis for the periodontium and the longevity of the restorations.

CORRECTION OF GINGIVAL ABNORMALITIES SURROUNDING PROSPECTIVE ABUTMENT TEETH

During examination of the periodontium prior to restorative therapy the dentist should note the quality and quantity of the zone of attached gingiva, especially in the vicinity of the abutment teeth and the edentulous ridges approximating them. Ideally, the qualities of the gingiva can be summarized as follows (Fig. 27-2):

1. The gingival margin should be free from any sign of inflammation and sharply demarcated.
2. It should be keratinized, stippled, and firmly attached.
3. There should be a definite demarcation between the uniformly lighter attached gingiva and the darker alveolar mucosa.
4. The band of attached gingiva should be adequate in width (at least 3 mm in addition to the free gingival margin).

In cases of long-standing periodontal disease, fibrosis may occur, stippling may return, and the color may look normal. This is not a return to health, but a scarring that is symptomatic of chronicity and that can be confirmed by the presence of deep pockets (Fig. 27-3).

Because the gingiva is keratinized and firmly attached to alveolar bone, an adequate gingival band can

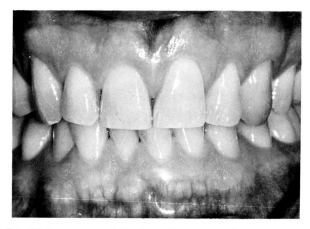

FIG. 27-2. *Example of ideal quality and quantity of attached gingiva.*

withstand inadvertent trauma associated with operative procedures such as tooth preparation, making impressions, cementation, and routine oral hygiene much more favorable than can gingival tissue lacking in quantity or quality. Also, an adequate zone of at-

tached gingiva protects the free gingival margin from the pulling effects of muscle attachments and frena.

Management of Teeth with Inadequate Attached Gingiva

If the zone of attached gingiva surrounding prospective abutments is inadequate or of a thin and delicate nature, the appearance may be one of almost translucence (Fig. 27-4). Often the roots of such teeth are in a buccally prominent position, indicating either an inadequate thickness or a complete lack of alveolar cortical bone covering these roots (Fig. 27-5). Inadvertent traumatization from restorative procedures can easily disrupt the free gingival margin and epithelial attachment in such cases, with the result that the rapid loss of the remaining attached gingiva gives rise to local clefts or to a generalized recession (Figs. 27-6; 26-3).

If the zone of attached gingiva is somewhat less than adequate and it is not deemed necessary to increase it, margins of restorations should be kept supragingival wherever possible. Care should be taken not to traum-

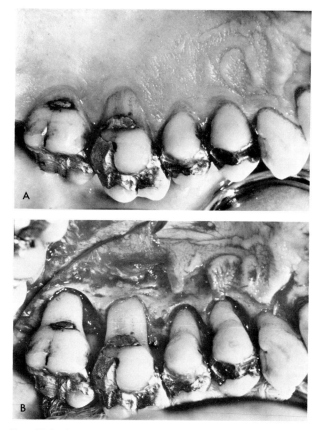

FIG. 27-3. *Appearance of soft tissue of a patient with long-standing periodontitis. A. Presurgical appearance. The color appears normal and no signs of inflammation are evident. B. Evidence of osseous cratering upon exposure of the alveolar bone. (Courtesy Dr. S. Sapkos.)*

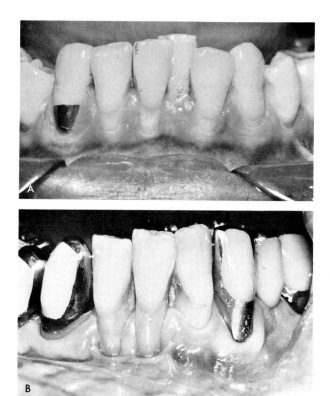

FIG. 27-4. *Undesirable characteristics of attached gingiva. A. Minimal zone of thin and delicate gingiva that will rapidly recede if injured during restorative procedures. B. Recession of a minimal delicate zone of attached gingiva following prolonged use of hard toothbrush and repeated restorative procedures.*

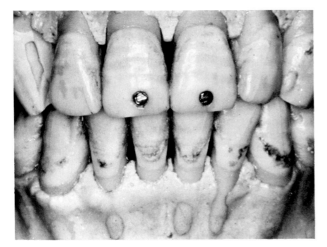

FIG. 27-5. *Characteristics of alveolar bone showing root fenestrations and dehiscences often associated with root prominence and thin attached gingiva.*

atize the soft tissue with gingival clamps (Fig. 26-2A), tooth reduction, impression making, and placement of filling material (Fig. 26-2B).

Increasing the Zone of Attached Gingiva

If margins must be extended to or below the gingival margin for reasons of management of existing caries, old restorations, esthetics, or simply because there is a need to increase the retentive qualities of the restorations, a minimal zone of attached gingiva may be increased by employing one of several recognized mucogingival surgical procedures. The most predictable of the techniques are the denuding of a sufficient width of crestal alveolar bone to allow regrowth of gingival tissue and the use of one of several soft-tissue grafting procedures.

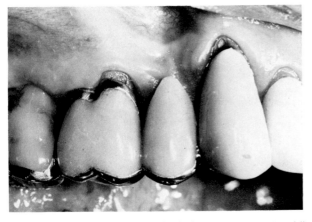

FIG. 27-6. *Case requiring mucogingival surgery to create additional zone of attached gingiva prior to full-mouth reconstruction.*

It is important to reemphasize that no periodontal surgical procedures other than limited soft-tissue curettage should be performed in the presence of gross acute inflammation caused by local irritants (Fig. 27-1) or by systemic factors. In the presence of gross inflammation, it is difficult to assess the amount of attached gingiva present and consequently how much more is required or how much may be removed.

DENUDATION OF CRESTAL BONE

Denudation of crestal bone should be used only if a slight increase in attached gingiva is needed (approximately 1 to 3 mm). If the area lacks attached gingiva entirely, one of the grafting procedures should be used instead.

At the outset, it must be emphatically stated that the quality and quantity of the radicular bone must be ideal before this procedure can be used. Injudicious exposures of fenestrations or dehiscences by full-thickness flaps can disrupt the connective-tissue attachment to the cementum and result in an anatomic defect. Also, exposure of radicular bone where the cortical plate is thin and lacking in underlying medullary bone may result in its partial or complete resorption. Another disadvantage of exposing bone is the prolonged healing that usually ensues. For these reasons, if this procedure is to be considered, the quantity of the radicular bone should be carefully predetermined by diagnostic sounding methods. If it is sufficient in thickness and there is no evidence of dehiscences or fenestrations, then the procedure of crestal denudation can be safely employed to gain additional attached gingiva.

The basic design of the full-thickness flap should be planned to conserve all of the existing attached gingival tissue. This necessitates a scalloped type of incision to release the flap from its attachment to the bone and cementum (Figs. 27-7, 27-8). The flap is carefully positioned at the desired level and securely immobilized

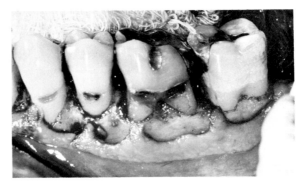

FIG. 27-7. *Scalloped internally beveled incision designed to expose the alveolar bone as well as to preserve all of the existing attached gingiva.*

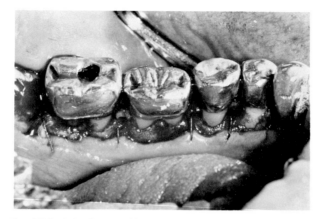

FIG. 27-8. *Apically repositioned internally beveled flap secured by sutures in a manner that allows a small amount of crestal bone to remain exposed for the purpose of increasing the zone of attached gingiva.*

with sutures and a surgical dressing. The level at which the flap is apically positioned is dependent upon the amount of additional attached gingiva that is required. During healing, the exposed crestal bone is covered by granulation tissue, which matures to form attached gingiva and when added to the original gingiva results in a total increase (Fig. 27-9).

SOFT-TISSUE GRAFTING

Grafts of soft tissues are more sophisticated mucogingival surgical procedures designed to relocate gingival tissue or gingiva-like tissue for the purpose of correcting anatomic defects such as radicular clefts and inadequate attached gingiva. These techniques are usually desirable to remedy either or both conditions. In comparison with the difficulty of complex osseous surgery or restorative therapy, gingival-grafting procedures are relatively easy and if judiciously performed are predictable, conserve the underlying attachment apparatus, and greatly improve the gingival environment of teeth in need of restoration.

There are essentially two main categories of soft-tissue grafting: the pedicle graft (often referred to as the laterally positioned flap) and the autogenous free soft-tissue graft (also referred to as the free gingival graft). Mucogingival procedures such as the double-papilla graft and the edentulous-area pedical graft are both variations of the pedicle graft. Detailed description and instrumentation of these procedures are presented in Chapter 25, and the reader is advised to review this section prior to attempting such procedures, since successful results or failures greatly depend on case selection and precise technique.

PEDICLE GRAFT

The pedicle-grafting procedure was introduced by Grupe and Warren and later modified by Corn and by Cohen and Ross.[2,4,5] As a general rule, the procedure can be applied when the need for additional attached gingiva is confined to one or two teeth and when there

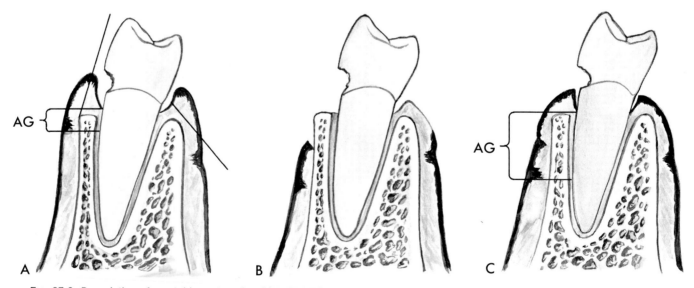

FIG. 27-9. *Denudation of crestal bone to gain wider zone of attached gingiva (AG). A. Illustration showing need to reduce pocket depth, expose more clinical crown, and gain additional gingiva on the buccal aspect. The direction of the buccal incision is designed to preserve the existing gingiva. An externally beveled incision is adequate on the lingual side since a sufficient zone of attached gingiva will remain. B. Buccal full-thickness flap positioned apically to expose some crestal bone. Later this is stabilized with sutures and surgical pack. C. Post-healing, showing the increased zone of attached gingiva (AG) and exposure of additional clinical crown.*

is both adequate vestibular depth and adequate donor tissue in the immediate vicinity. The donor tissue can be either gingiva surrounding adjacent teeth or gingiva from an adjacent edentulous area (as for the edentulous-area pedicle graft). This procedure should not be considered if there is unhealthy or insufficient adjacent tissue, or if there is concern over the quality or quan-

tity of the underlying alveolar bone of the donor site. The pedicle graft can be partial-thickness or full-thickness. However, if there is concern over the quality or quantity of the underlying radicular bone and dehiscences or fenestrations are suspected, the partial-thickness procedure should be used.

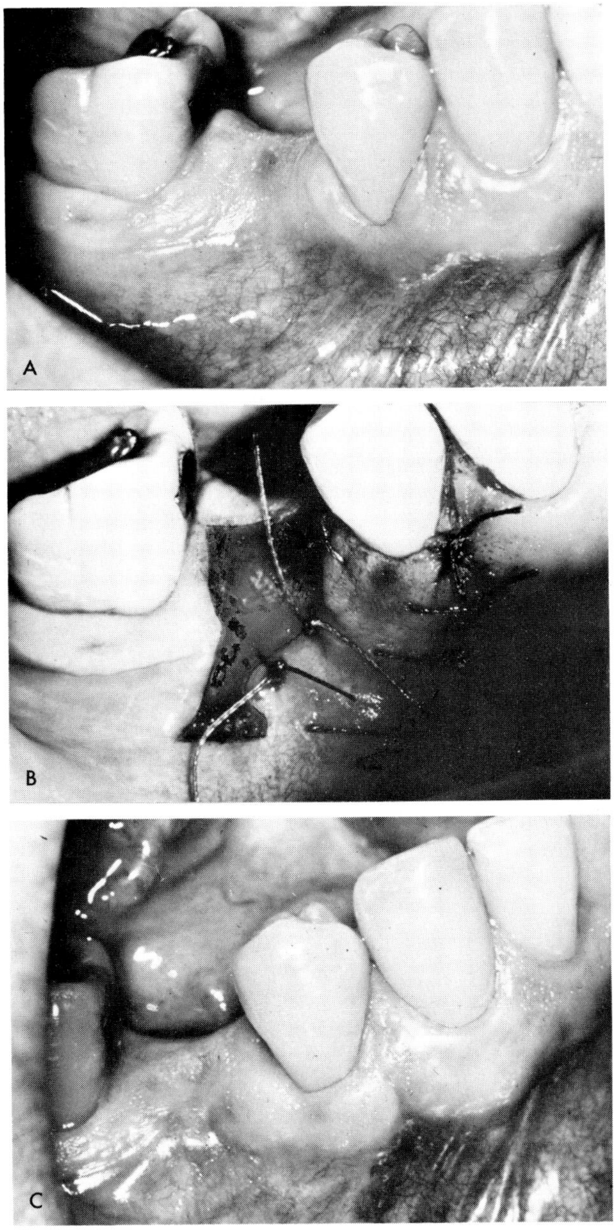

The recipient site should be prepared in such a manner that a thin layer of connective tissue would be left covering the radicular bone (Fig. 25-5). Ideally, there should be no perforations exposing the bone. The pedicle graft must not be used in regions where the vestibule is shallow or where the frena or muscle attachments intervene, since these factors will cause movement of the graft on its recipient connective-tissue base, regardless of whether the flap is of full or partial thickness, and failure will result. Failure to secure the graft adequately during initial healing disrupts revascularization and results in complete or partial necrosis of the graft. For this reason, the incisions should be designed in such a way that the graft can initially be mobile enough to be readily positioned into its new site without any tension (Fig. 27-10).

The double-papilla graft is essentially a double pedicle graft and was first introduced by Cohen and Ross.[2] This procedure is indicated where lack of attached gingiva is the result of localized clefting and the adjacent donor site is devoid of sufficient gingiva to reposition a single lateral flap. It is used to regain the original amount of attached gingiva (prior to clefting) and at the same time and to a limited degree to cover the denuded part of the root (Fig. 27-11). In such situations the adjacent interdental papillae are the source of gingival tissue. In order for this procedure to be successful, the gingival cleft must not be excessively wide.

A pedicle is raised on each side of the cleft (Fig.

FIG. 27-10. Pedicle soft-tissue graft as a means of increasing the zone of attached gingiva. A. Presurgical view, showing lack of sufficient attached gingiva over the premolar. B. Pedicle graft laterally positioned and sutured over a previously prepared connective-tissue bed on the buccal aspect of the premolar. C. Post-healing, showing additional zone of attached gingiva. (Courtesy Dr. J. Rudd.)

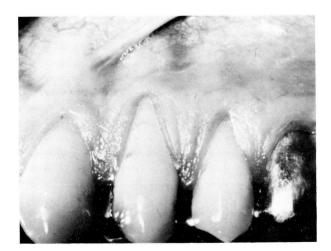

FIG. 27-11. Example of type of gingival clefting that can be repaired by a double papilla graft.

25-10), and the two pedicles are rotated to approximate each other over a carefully prepared base. They are then stabilized with sutures and a surgical dressing. Because of the delicate nature of this procedure, it should not be used where a single laterally positioned pedicle graft would correct the problem.

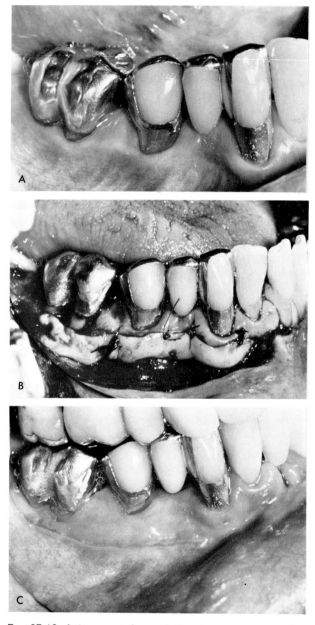

FIG. 27-12. *Autogenous, free soft-tissue graft to increase the zone of attached gingiva and the depth of the vestibule. A. Before surgery, showing need for additional zone of attached gingiva as well as for vestibular extension. B. Graft positioned and stabilized with sutures over a previously prepared connective-tissue base. C. Post-healing, showing increased zone of attached gingiva as well as vestibular extension. (Courtesy Dr. M. Dragoo.)*

AUTOGENOUS FREE SOFT-TISSUE GRAFT

The autogenous free soft-tissue graft was first introduced as a periodontal corrective procedure by King and Pennel and by Nabors.[6,7] It can be applied to most patients in need of additional attached gingiva, but it is especially appropriate for areas with shallow vestibules, since preparation of the recipient connective-tissue bed will result in the desired increased vestibular depth (Fig. 27-12).

It is also indicated for areas where there is a generalized lack of attached gingiva around several teeth. This procedure is not indicated if there is a concomitant need for osseous correction in the vicinity of the graft, since successful revascularization greatly depends upon a carefully prepared connective-tissue bed, preferably with no alveolar bone exposed.[8]

The source of gingiva can be the edentulous ridges or that part of the palate lying posterior to the rugae. The recipient site must be meticulously prepared to leave a thin layer of connective tissue, preferably with no perforations exposing the bone. If the connective-tissue layer is too thick and is mobile, the graft will not be firmly tied down to its base and will itself be mobile. In most cases, few sutures are needed to secure the graft (Fig. 27-12B). In fact, if the graft is extremely thin, sutures are often not required (Fig. 27-13).

The placement of a surgical dressing usually is not indicated. However, if one is required, extreme care must be exercised in its placement, so as not to disturb the initial fibrin clot that bonds the graft to its site.

When carefully executed, the autogenous free soft-tissue graft is a highly successful means of increasing the zone of attached gingiva.

CORRECTION OF GINGIVAL AND OSSEOUS ABNORMALITIES SURROUNDING PROSPECTIVE ABUTMENT TEETH

Sometimes initial therapy, including scaling, oral-hygiene instructions, soft-tissue and hard-tissue curettage, and the elimination of parafunctional habits, still leaves a favorable prognosis in doubt. This is because excessive pocket depth, resulting from tissue hyperplasia and/or bone involvement, demands a surgical correction. In addition, the restorative dentist is often faced with the need for exposing additional coronal tooth structure (crown lengthening) to facilitate removal of subgingival caries and/or to increase the retention of subsequent restorations. Without surgical crown lengthening, it is difficult to place adequate margins subgingivally in sound tooth structure and it is difficult to make an accurate impression because of

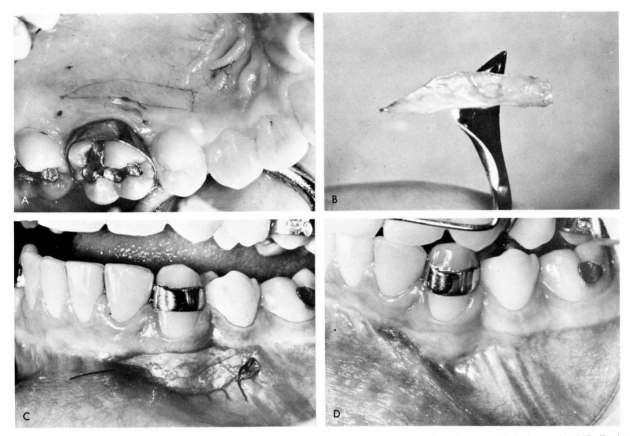

FIG. 27-13. *Free soft-tissue graft to increase zone of attached gingiva. A. Donor site and outline of graft to be excised. B. Excised graft to show its thinness. C. Graft site to show graft positioned over the connective-tissue bed. Graft is thin enough that suturing for its stabilization is not necessary; however, mucosa was sutured to periosteum to reduce hemorrhage. D. Post-healing, showing increased zone of attached gingiva. (Courtesy Dr. S. Sapkos.)*

excessive pocket depth. The procedures adopted to accomplish this corrective surgery vary, depending mainly upon the amount of attached gingiva present and the associated need, if any, for osseous correction.

EXTERNAL-BEVEL GINGIVECTOMY

When there is more-than-adequate attached gingiva and no bone involvement, one method of eliminating excessive pocket depth and/or of exposing additional coronal tooth structure is by external-bevel gingivectomy. This procedure requires little special training, and the results are predictable. However, it must never be used when there is need for concomitant ostectomy or osteoplasty or when the procedure would leave an inadequate zone of attached gingiva.

The incision is made in such a way as to eliminate the pocket and expose additional coronal structure and yet ideally not to expose any alveolar bone (Fig. 27-14). The amount of tissue to be removed is dictated by the depth of the pockets or by the desired amount of root to be exposed.

INTERNAL-BEVEL GINGIVECTOMY

Reduction of excessive pocket depth and exposure of additional coronal tooth structure in the absence of a sufficient zone of attached gingiva with or without the need for correction of osseous abnormalities requires a different surgical procedure (Fig. 27-15). In such cases, the external-bevel gingivectomy would remove all or most of the attached gingiva, leaving nothing but alveolar mucosa (Fig. 27-16). If correction of osseous pathology is needed, the flap must always be internally beveled so as to expose the supporting alveolar bone. Current refinements of the internally beveled flap ideally allow for a scalloped incision in order to cover maximally all supporting bone during suturing (Figs. 27-7, 27-8).

Since flap design is important for the success of this procedure, it is essential that the operator be familiar with the basic principles of flap design and reflection and with osseous resection. These procedures should not be attempted by the untrained. The details of the basic surgical technique are discussed and extensively illustrated in Chapter 22.

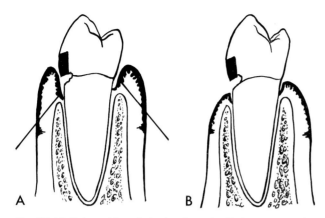

FIG. 27-14. *External-bevel gingivectomy to eliminate excessive pseudopocketing and to expose more of the clinical crown. A. Correct direction of incisions to preserve adequate attached gingiva. B. Post-healing, showing reduction of pockets and preservation of sufficient attached gingiva.*

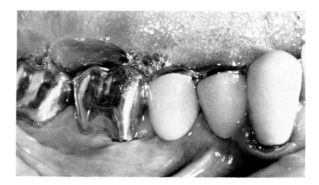

FIG. 27-16. *Restored quadrant, showing lack of attached gingiva over the buccal aspects of molars and cuspid as well as in pontic regions. This resulted from the incorrect application of the external-bevel gingivectomy in an attempt to eliminate pocketing. The internal-bevel gingivectomy should have been used.*

To release an internally beveled flap, the length of the incision is first decided upon. Then with a sharp periodontal knife or scalpel the incision is begun at a level that will preserve most of the attached gingiva or, if this zone is more than adequate, will leave as much as is desirable. The incision is directed toward the crest of the alveolar plate in a manner that will result in a uniformly thin flap that is ideally suited for suturing. Once the bone has been reached by the incision along its full length, a full-thickness flap is reflected with periosteal elevators, exposing the bone (Fig. 27-15C). Where there is concomitant need for osseous correction, this should next be performed. The flap is then apically repositioned to the desired level, preferably to cover the bone maximally, and is carefully stabilized with sutures and a surgical dressing.

Restoration of mouths with rampant carious involvement and requiring reconstruction can be greatly facilitated by removing excessive gingival tissue and exposing additional coronal tooth structure before treating the carious lesions. Many of these patients require extensive restoration, not so much because of periodontal involvement, but because of the need to replace many existing restorations that are literally crumbling or have little coronal tooth structure because of extreme carious involvement. In the presence of old restorations, it is difficult to detect the extent of recurrent caries, and since all caries must be removed, this difficulty necessitates, in most cases, the removal of all existing restorations in the areas under reconstruction. Commonly, by the time all restorations and caries have been removed, insufficient coronal tooth structure remains for the adequate retention of final restorations.

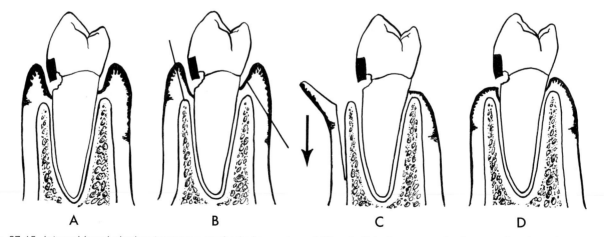

FIG. 27-15. *Internal-bevel gingivectomy as a method of exposing additional clinical crown and yet preserving the existing zone of attached gingiva. A. Illustration showing minimal zone of attached gingiva on the buccal side and more-than-adequate zone on the lingual side. B. Correct direction of incisions for the buccal and lingual aspects. C. Buccal flap apically positioned. D. Post-healing, showing adequate attached gingiva on the buccal and lingual sides.*

This may still be true even after these crowns are built up with pin-amalgam restorations. For such patients it is far more expedient to raise buccal and lingual flaps, in the manner described for internal-bevel gingivectomy in Chapter 22. This will expose the supporting bone and eliminate a sufficient amount of redundant soft tissue, thereby lengthening the crown to the desired amount. If there is a concomitant need for osseous correction, this can be done.

Besides soft-tissue reduction, a small amount of crestal bone may also have to be removed to facilitate removal of root caries, place margins in sound tooth structure, and increase the retentive qualities of the restorations. In some instances, the operative or crown-reduction procedures can be completed while the flaps are reflected. The flaps can then be positioned to the desired level and carefully sutured. Where there is need to create additional attached gingiva, the flap can be repositioned apically, allowing some crestal bone to be exposed, equal to the desired amount of additional gingiva that is required (Figs. 27-8, 27-9). The apically repositioned flap should be precisely stabilized with carefully placed sutures and a surgical dressing. The slight amount of exposed bone will soon be covered with epithelialized tissue that will mature to simulate attached gingival tissue (Fig. 27-9C). The results of this technique of gaining additional attached tissue are predictable, but it should be used only in regions having an adequate thickness of cortical bone covering the roots and not in areas of fenestration and dehiscence.

If dehiscence, fenestration, or an extremely thin cortical plate of bone is suspected over roots that require additional exposure, a full-thickness flap would be inappropriate. Instead, only a partial-thickness flap should be reflected,[3] allowing a connective-tissue covering to remain to protect the remaining bone. The technique of reflecting such a flap is described in Chapter 25. The desired amount of root structure can be exposed by carefully dissecting the fibrous tissue away with a sharp curet. The partial-thickness flap may than be repositioned to the desired level as determined by the additional amount of gingiva required, sutured to the periosteal bed, and stabilized with a surgical dressing.

MODIFICATION OF TUBEROSITY AND RETROMOLAR AREAS

When pronounced tuberosities or retromolar pads are next to the teeth to be restored or to be used as abutments, their management requires special consideration. Pocket depth in these areas is normally greater than in others. This does not mean that the sulci are pathologic. The geography of these regions is conducive to tissue hyperplasia and as a result the sulci are excessively deep. The soft-tissue excess interferes in restorative procedures. Distal abutment teeth are often needed to help support long spans of pontics. Consequently, such abutments require maximum exposure of the clinical crown for adequate extension of the distal wall of the preparation to gain sufficient retention (Fig. 27-17). In addition, surgical reduction of these areas greatly facilitates crown preparation, impression making, the finishing of the restoration, and the oral-hygiene efforts of the patient (Fig. 27-18). Bridges have commonly failed because the distal walls of crowns next to excessive tuberosities or retromolar areas could not be extended subgingivally sufficiently to gain the required retention (Fig. 27-19).

Several excellent methods currently are used for reducing the tuberosity and retromolar pad.[1] The standard approach is thoroughly described and illustrated in Chapter 22 and should be reviewed prior to attempting such a procedure.

As with most therapeutic procedures in dentistry there is a price to pay. The same applies especially to tuberosity reductions. If the prognosis for a distal abutment tooth, such as a molar with furcation or with complex pulpal involvement in addition to advanced occlusal traumatism, remains in serious doubt in spite of correction of soft-tissue and hard-tissue defects, the benefits of treating such a tooth should be weighed against losing it shortly thereafter. The elimination of pocket depth for such teeth necessitates gross soft-tissue excision, which will result in loss of most of the morphologic characteristics of a normal tuberosity. Such a dentition may not be retained long, and the normal tuberosity is often necessary for the retention of a full denture. Whenever there is doubt about saving a second or third molar for at least a reasonable length of time, and it jeopardizes the tooth next to it, maintenance by curettage or selective extraction of such a tooth should be considered.

MODIFICATION OF EDENTULOUS RIDGES FOR IMPROVED PONTIC ADAPTATION

The establishment of an ideal pontic relationship with an edentulous ridge is dependent upon the ridge contour and the availability of vertical space for the pontic. The availability of vertical space may depend upon the thickness of the soft tissue covering the edentulous region. Whenever modification of the ridge is feasible, it is often preferable to prepare the ridge to accept the pontic rather than to reduce the pontic in order to fit the edentulous ridge.

Irregular morphology of the edentulous ridge is not

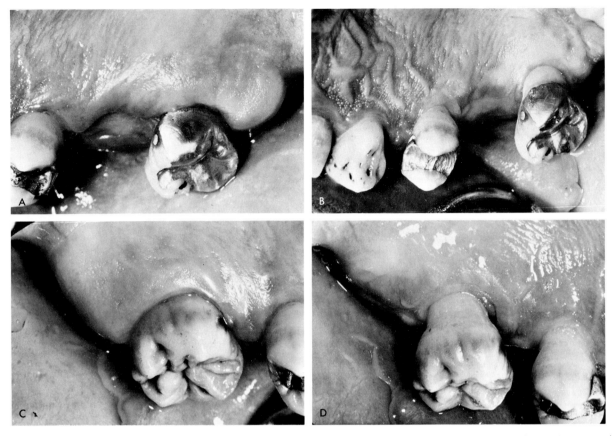

FIG. 27-17. Reduction of tuberosity to expose additional clinical crown for properly designed bridge retainers. A. Presurgical view of right side after pin-amalgam build-up of molar. B. After surgery, showing exposure of additional clinical crown. C. Presurgical view of left side. D. After surgery. (Courtesy Dr. J. Jerome.)

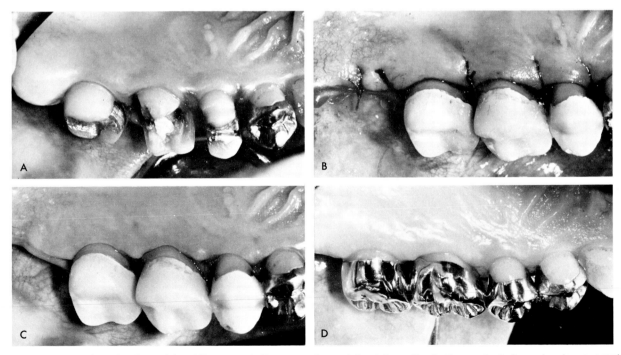

FIG. 27-18. Reduction of soft- and hard-tissue pocketing as well as of the tuberosity. A. Presurgical view, showing excessive tuberosity and interproximal soft-tissue craters. B. Sutured flaps after tuberosity reduction, elimination of interproximal defects, and placement of temporary restorations. C. One week after surgery, showing excellent healing of well-designed and sutured flaps. D. Postrestorative view showing design of interproximal embrasures and lack of fibrous tuberosity. (Courtesy Dr. C. Filipchuk.)

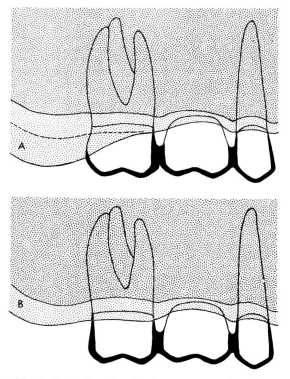

FIG. 27-19. *Illustration showing how an excessive tuberosity can interfere with extension of a subgingival margin to ensure adequate retention of a bridge retainer. A. Distal gingival margin of molar lacks sufficient extension because of excessively large tuberosity. B. After reduction of tuberosity distal wall of molar retainer can be extended to ensure adequate retention.*

uncommonly a response to ill-fitting removable partial dentures. The effects of such prosthetic appliances can range from soft-tissue hyperplasia (Figs. 26-28, 26-37, 26-38) to the initiation of periodontitis. Soft-tissue hyperplasia is commonly seen adjacent to the artificial teeth and assumes the characteristics of an exaggerated col. These cols are susceptible to breakdown and, with further settling of the partial denture, accumulation of microbial plaque, and neglect of adequate oral hygiene, the result will be an apical migration of the epithelial attachment of these prospective abutment teeth. Surgical correction of the edentulous ridge must always be performed prior to construction of a fixed prosthesis. If this is neglected, the bizarre contours of the edentulous region (Fig. 26-28) will interfere with correct pontic adaptation and desirable esthetics, and when the restoration is completed it will interfere with adequate oral-hygiene maintenance. The corrective measures will depend upon the extent of damage to the supporting bone.

There are essentially two methods of surgical modification for creating additional vertical space for pontics. The choice of method depends primarily upon availability of sufficient attached gingival tissue and secondly upon any need to modify the bone architecture underlying the soft tissue. If correction is limited to the gingiva, simple ridgeplasty procedures can be performed either conventionally by sharp resection or by reduction with coarse diamond stones or electrosurgically. If the supporting bone is involved or if the gingival tissue is minimal, internally beveled flaps must be made to expose the bone for correction (Fig. 27-23).

Any of these procedures, if skillfully performed, will improve the topography of an edentulous ridge for pontic adaptation and will also result in a healthier environment for routine maintenance of the restored areas.

Modification of Ridges with Sufficient Attached Gingiva and No Bone Involvement

The first procedure is one that may be used for reducing excessive thickness of fibrous tissue when there are an adequate band of attached gingiva and no evidence of any bone defects. If there is an excess of attached gingival tissue, the ridge can be modified easily by means of a technique similar to the external-bevel gingivectomy.

With a sharp scalpel or a periodontal knife, the desired amount of fibrous tissue is excised from the crestal surface (Fig. 27-20). Ideally, the depth of the incision should stop slightly short of the underlying alveolar bone. The remaining portion of the excess fibrous tissue can then be excised from the buccal and lingual aspects of the ridge. After correction, more space and a slight increase in the coronal height of the abutment teeth will aid in the retention of the bridge.

Modification of Ridges with Insufficient Attached Gingiva and No Bone Involvement

When there is insufficient attached gingival tissue and reduction of fibrous ridges is necessary, a different surgical procedure is needed in order to preserve the remaining attached gingiva. A wedge of tissue is first removed, giving a clear indication of the thickness throughout the length of the edentulous ridge (Figs. 27-21, 27-22). The width of the wedge must be gauged carefully, according to its thickness, which may be determined prior to surgery by sounding with a probe (Fig. 27-22C). Between 4 and 5 mm are not an uncommon thickness. Next, both the buccal and the lingual aspects of the fibrous ridge can be thinned out, as in the internal-bevel procedure (Fig. 27-21E). If the width of the initial wedge has been accurately gauged, the flaps can be approximated and sutured to cover the alveolar

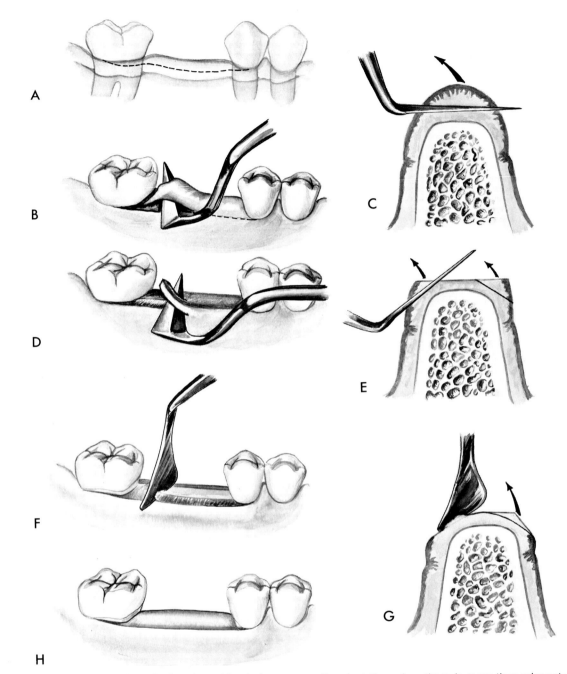

FIG. 27-20. *Soft tissue reduction of edentulous ridge to improve pontic adaptation when there is more-than-adequate attached gingiva, adequate vestibular depth, and normal osseous morphology. A. Amount of reduction necessary (broken line). B and C. Initial incision, showing manner of excision and amount of soft tissue to be removed. D and E. Beveling incisions to reduce sharp angles. F and G. Further trimming with Kirkland knife to round all sharp tissue angles. H. Postsurgical view.*

bone (Fig. 27-21G). Excessive width of the initial wedge will prevent close approximation of the tissue flaps and will result in exposure of bone. Approximately 2 to 3 weeks after surgical correction, any soft-tissue irregularities can be removed with a sharp periodontal knife in order to improve the contour of the ridge for better pontic adaptation (Fig. 27-22).

Reduction of Edentulous Ridges Needing Osseous Reshaping

Occasionally, the excessive dimensions of an edentulous ridge are due not only to too much soft tissue but also to the bulkiness of the underlying alveolar bone. Here surgical correction of the bone contour is also required.

To reshape the underlying bone, an initial wedge of tissue is removed, and the facial and lingual flaps are thinned and reflected to expose the bone, which can then be reduced to the desired amount (Fig. 27-23). The flaps are repositioned and sutured following osteoplasty. A preformed acrylic bridge can be adapted and temporarily set if esthetics require this, either immediately after surgical reduction or after initial healing (Figs. 27-23F, 26-40).

Care should be taken not to reduce anterior ridges excessively; this especially applies to maxillary anterior ridges. Overreduction can create an undesirable cos-

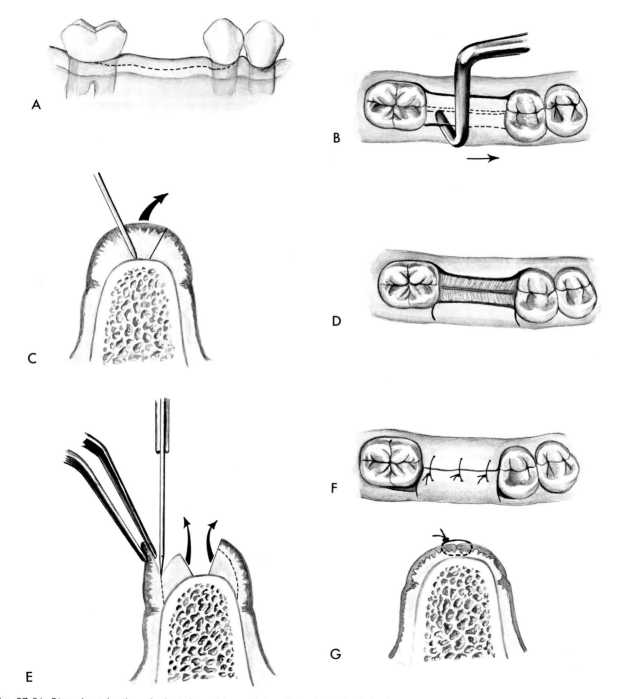

FIG. 27-21. *Steps in reduction of edentulous ridge with insufficient attached gingiva with or without bone involvement. A. Amount of reduction necessary (broken line). B. Initial wedge of fibrous tissue removed to expose bone. C. Sectional view, showing initial wedge. D. Occlusal view with initial wedge removed. E. Internal-beveled incision to reduce thickness of buccal and lingual flaps. F and G. Occlusal and sectional view of flaps repositioned and sutures in place.*

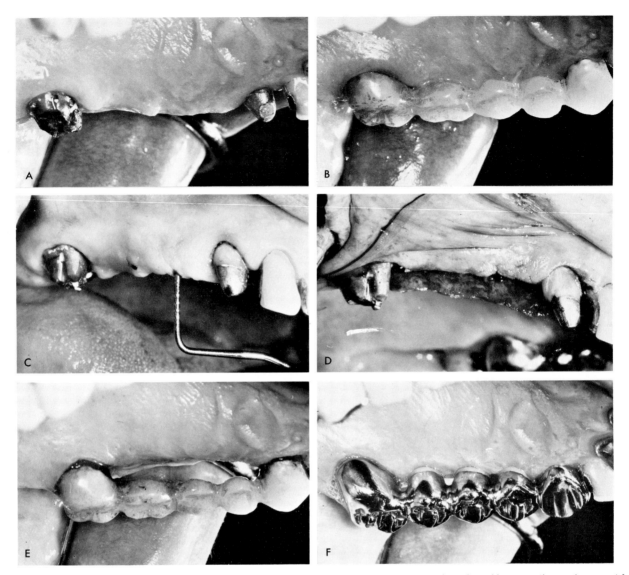

FIG. 27-22. *Clinical views of reduction of edentulous ridge and tuberosity to increase crown length and improve the environment for pontic adaptation. A. View showing excessively fibrous ridge over a long span between abutments of inadequate length—all factors that caused several of this patient's bridges to fail. B. Temporary acrylic fixed partial denture in place, showing inadequate occlusogingival thickness of pontics because of lack of space. C. Soft-tissue probing to determine thickness and estimate width of initial soft-tissue wedge. D. Initial wedge removed and flaps thinned. E. After healing, showing increased vertical space. F. After restoration, showing how ridge reduction allows for strong metal framework and good interproximal embrasures. (Courtesy Dr. H. Colman.)*

metic effect. The pontics must then be excessively long, and the interproximal spaces will appear black (Fig. 27-24B). In reducing the maxillary ridges, the incision should be slanted to allow for greater reduction on the facial aspect and less on the palatal aspect of the ridge (Fig. 27-24).

The pontics can now be adapted in such a manner that their interproximal embrasures will be superimposed to a large degree over the facial aspect of the edentulous ridge. This adaptation creates a desirable illusion of a normal interdental papilla.

Another way that excessive pontic space can be inadvertently created is in attempting to eliminate deep pockets of hopelessly involved anterior teeth by surgical resection. The restorative dentist is now faced with grotesquely elongated teeth that are extremely mobile from lack of support (Fig. 5-22). It is important to reemphasize that pocket elimination is not the sole aim in periodontal therapy. Hopelessly involved teeth should be diagnosed as such early in the treatment and extracted. This will preserve a structurally normal ridge contour and facilitate esthetic pontic adaptation.

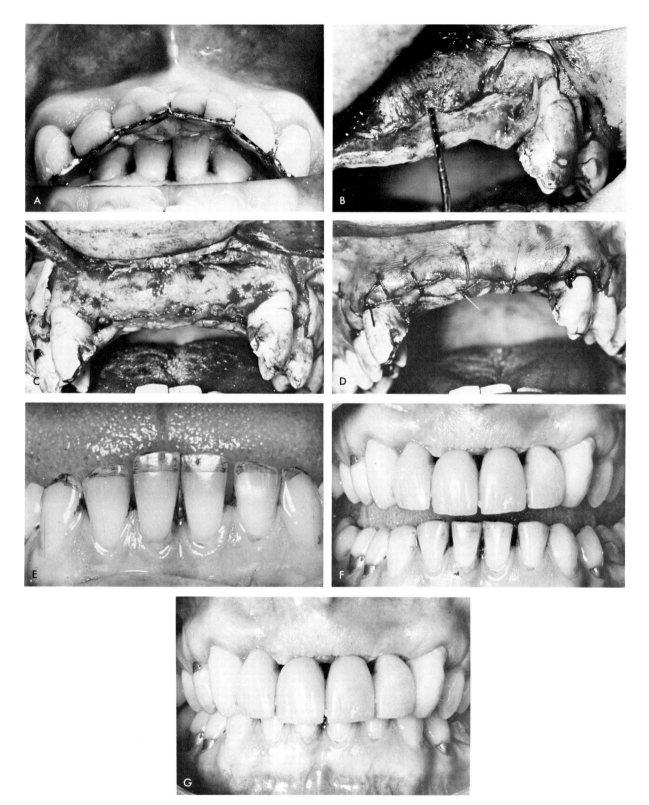

FIG. 27-23. *Reduction of edentulous ridge in need of osseous reshaping. A. Occlusal view showing excessive overlap and overbite. Pontics of bridge to be replaced were not positioned ideally because of excessively prominent alveolar process. B. Thinned buccal flap to expose bone. Note thickness of soft tissue which decreases towards midline. C. Thinned palatal flap and reduction of bony prominence. D. Flaps sutured. E. Amount of mandibular incisal reduction necessary to improve occlusal plane for protrusive function. F. Temporary acrylic bridge placed two weeks after surgery. Note reduced mandibular incisors. G. Mandibular teeth in occlusion with temporary bridge, showing reduction of procumbency, overlap, and overbite of the anterior teeth for improved functional occlusion and esthetics. (Courtesy Dr. T. Merchant.)*

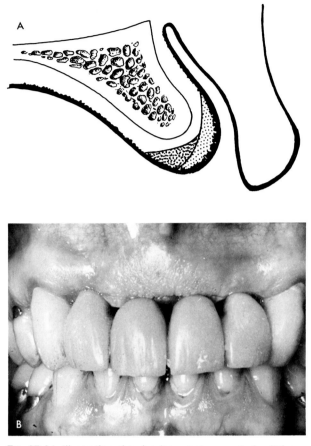

FIG. 27-24. *Illustration showing incorrect amount of soft tissue reduction (total stippled area) which will result in esthetically poor pontics because of dark embrasures. Correct amount of reduction (area lightly stippled) will provide a background to simulate interdental papillae and thus eliminate excessively open and dark embrasures. B. Clinical example of ridge that has been overreduced, resulting in black spaces.*

It is impossible to recreate normal esthetics if the ridge has been grossly excised.

Tissue Response to Ill-Fitting Removable Partial Dentures

Irregular morphology of the edentulous ridge is not uncommonly a response to ill-fitting removable partial dentures. The effects of such prosthetic appliances can range from soft-tissue hyperplasia (Figs. 26-28, 26-38) to the initiation of periodontitis. Soft-tissue hyperplasia is commonly seen adjacent to the artificial teeth and

assumes the characteristics of an exaggerated col. These cols are susceptible to breakdown, and with further settling of the partial denture, accumulation of microbial plaque, and neglect of adequate oral hygiene the result will be an apical migration of the epithelial attachment of these prospective abutment teeth. Surgical correction of the edentulous ridge must always be performed prior to construction of a fixed prosthesis. If this is neglected, the bizarre contours of the edentulous region (Figs. 26-28, 26-38, 26-40) will interfere with correct pontic adaptation and desirable esthetics, and when the restoration is completed all these will interfere with maintenance of adequate oral hygiene.

The corrective measures will depend upon the extent of damage to the supporting bone. If correction is limited to the gingiva, simple gingivoplasty can be performed either conventionally by sharp resection (Figs. 26-28, 26-39) or by reduction with coarse diamond stones or electrosurgically. If the supporting bone is involved or if the gingival tissue is minimal, internal-beveled flaps must be made, to expose the bone for correction. Any of these procedures, if skillfully performed, will improve the topography of an edentulous ridge for pontic adaptapion and will also result in a healthier environment for routine maintenance of the restored areas.

References

1. Braden, B.: Deep distal pockets adjacent to terminal teeth. Dent. Clin. North Am., *13*:161, 1969.
2. Cohen, D. W., and Ross, S. E.: The double papillae repositioned flap in periodontal therapy. J. Periodontol., *39*:65, 1968.
3. Corn, H.: Periosteal separation—its clinical significance. J. Periodontol., *33*:140, 1962.
4. Corn, H.: Edentulous area pedicle grafts in mucogingival surgery. Periodontics, *2*:229, 1964.
5. Grupe, H. E., and Warren, R. F.: Repair of gingival defects by a sliding flap operation. J. Periodontol., *27*:92, 1956.
6. King, K., and Pennel, B. M.: Evaluation of attempts to increase the width of attached gingiva. Presented to the Philadelphia Society of Periodontology, 1964.
7. Nabors, J. M.: Free gingival grafts. Periodontics, *4*:243, 1966.
8. Sullivan, H. C., and Atkins, J. H.: The role of free gingival grafts in periodontal therapy. Dent. Clin. North Am., *13*:133, 1969.

28

Provisional Stabilization

When it has been determined that generalized loss of bone support has reached the point at which pathologic tooth mobility is permanent, some form of long-term stabilization by periodontal prosthetic means is needed in order to prolong the life of the dentition. Frequently, generalized tooth mobility is complicated by factors such as existing periodontal soft-tissue and hard-tissue defects, missing teeth, posterior-bite collapse, migrated teeth, caries, and questionable restorations associated with pulpal problems, all of which may contribute to a guarded prognosis for several or all of the teeth in question. If all or many of these factors exist, current clinical thinking is directed toward total reconstruction procedures that may include full-coverage or partial-coverage multiple splinting. When such is the case, provisional splinting becomes necessary preliminary to the overall treatment plan. Without some form of provisional stabilization, too often the prognosis may shift from guarded to hopeless.

OBJECTIVES OF PROVISIONAL SPLINTING

The provisional splint not only serves as a transitional fixed appliance to protect the prepared teeth until the final restorations are inserted, but also serves several other important functions that are most necessary if periodontal prosthetic therapy is to be successful. Although the main objectives of the provisional splint are to reduce pathologic mobility and protect the dental pulp from irritation following tooth preparation, it also affords us the opportunity to determine the correct esthetic, phonetic, and functional occlusal qualities necessary for each individual patient. Many patients whose dentitions require reconstruction exhibit such bizarre morphologic and functional abnormalities that to disregard the provisional splinting phase prior to construction of the final restoration is to court disaster. If the desired esthetic, phonetic, and functional occlusal qualities in addition to achieving stabilization can be realized during the provisional splinting phase, the operator can proceed with confidence, knowing that it is possible to attain these same qualities in the final reconstruction.[1]

FULL-COVERAGE ACRYLIC PROVISIONAL SPLINTING

There are several methods of provisionally splinting teeth prior to long-term stabilization. The method chosen is dictated mainly by whether the final splint will be of the partial-coverage or the full-coverage type, and by how long the provisional splint is to be used.

28
Provisional
Stabilization

In cases requiring long-term stabilization with multiple-splinted, partial-coverage restorations such as three-quarter crowns or parallel vertical-pin-ledged restorations, the multi-unit acrylic provisional splint has its limitations. If, for reasons of evaluating the prognosis of questionable teeth after periodontal or endodontic therapy, such teeth require provisional stabilization for a long period of time prior to final restoration, methods other than multi-unit acrylic provisional splinting should be considered. Multi-unit acrylic splints used for partial-coverage restorations are not retentive enough and are notorious for working loose, which may result in migration of teeth as well as in hypersensitivity, recurrent caries, and even pulpal death. Extracoronal wire-and-acrylic splints or occlusal intracoronal wire-and-acrylic splints, as described in Chapter 18, are more dependable (Figs. 18-7, 18-13). The patient can wear this type of splint until such time as a favorable prognosis for the final, long-term splinting phase has been reached. The patient will still require acrylic multi-unit partial-coverage splints, but only to fulfill the functions of protecting the prepared abutment teeth and preventing tooth migration. This period lasts only until the final restorations are completed and should be relatively short.

The methods of provisional stabilization described are generally reserved for the comprehensively involved case in need of full-coverage long-term stabilization. It must be emphasized that in planning the type of final restoration, full-coverage restorations are needed not only because of coronal breakdown but also because of generalized severe mobility in the Class II to III range of the remaining teeth to be saved. We have frequently observed failures in such cases where splinting by partial-coverage restorations was used. The most common reason for failure is that one or several of the retainers loosen and caries recurs. That is why full-coverage restorations, which give more adequate retention, are recommended in such cases.

Exceptional cases for which partial-coverage provisional splinting may be used are those having the coronal portions of the abutment teeth large and long, relatively free from caries or large restorations, and having few teeth missing.

There are essentially two types of full-coverage provisional splints, the all-acrylic and the combination gold-band-and-acrylic. The advantages, fabrication, and application of both of these will be discussed.

Regardless of the type, the major phases of fabrication and application of the provisional splint are:

1. Functional analysis of the articulated casts
2. Diagnostic waxing
3. Fabrication of the shell of the provisional splint

4. Tooth preparation
5. Application of the provisional splint

Following the placing of the provisional splint, there should be several periods of re-evaluation.

Functional Analysis of the Articulated Casts

The fabrication of the provisional splint, regardless of whether it is all-acrylic or a combination gold-band-and-acrylic, must begin with the functional analysis of accurate stone casts, mounted with the aid of a face-bow in centric relation on an articulator that is at least semiadjustable (Fig. 28-1). In restoring dentitions that require concomitant therapy for temporomandibular-joint dysfunction or severe bruxism, accurate reproductions of the functional maxillomandibular relationships may be of great benefit. This information can be obtained by precisely locating the hinge axis, recording the border movements with a pantograph, and using these records to set a fully adjustable articulator. In most cases, however, the use of a semiadjustable articulator is sufficiently accurate for the construction of provisional splints, since the acrylic splints are of limited accuracy and final corrections must be made directly in the mouth. However, if a fully adjustable articulator is to be used for the final reconstruction, for most cases it is advisable that it also be used during the functional analysis of the patient's articulated casts. It is easier to obtain the necessary registration of the hinge axis for the face-bow mounting of the maxillary cast and the pantographic tracings if the teeth have not been reduced. Once the instrument has been set, it is not necessary to repantograph the mandibular movements and reset the instrument after tooth preparation unless there is some doubt as to the accuracy of the first tracings or unless changes in temporomandibular-joint and neuromuscular relationships are suspected.

The articulated casts allow the therapist to correlate his findings with radiographic and other clinical evidence gathered during history-taking, examination, and charting. It is imperative that the same preciseness be maintained during this phase of the oral-rehabilitation procedure as is described in Chapter 12 for functional analysis in the treatment of occlusal traumatism.

The articulated casts will clearly show any discrepancy between CRO and CO and how this may affect the treatment plan. Because the adjusted articulator will closely reproduce the patient's mandibular border movements, the eccentric relations can be carefully studied. The effect of cross-arch balancing interferences can be evaluated, as can the guidance and func-

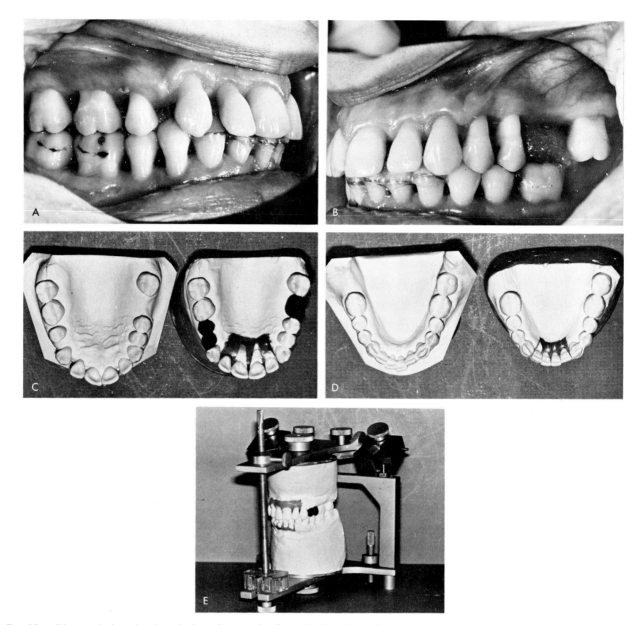

Fɪɢ. 28-1. *Diagnostic functional analysis and prewaxing for periodontal prosthetic reconstruction with only slight occlusal changes. A. Right side before restoration. B. Left side before restoration. C. Maxillary study casts before and after waxing. All maxillary incisors and the right second premolar will be extracted because of severe periodontal involvement. D. Mandibular study casts before and after waxing. All mandibular incisors are planned for extraction because of periodontal involvement. E. Articulated waxed study casts prepared for occlusal refinement and construction of shell of provisional splint. (Courtesy Dr. C. Filipchuk.)*

tion of the anterior teeth. The cuspid relation can be analyzed, and a decision can be made as to whether a cuspid-protected occlusion is desirable. The degree or effect of posterior-bite collapse, anterior and posterior tooth migration, and any extrusions may be evaluated, and a decision can be made as to whether minor or major tooth movement must precede provisional splinting or can be done concurrently with provisional splinting. Careful analysis of all these factors may indicate either an increase or a decrease of vertical

dimension. It is well to reemphasize that selected extraction of severely involved (Fig. 5-22) or malposed teeth may prove to be far more expedient than would heroic efforts to save them and include them in the rehabilitation program (Fig. 26-30A).

All of this information allows the practitioner to determine the type of preparations required to properly restore good function. The esthetic possibilities can be envisioned, but making such decisions without the aid of accurately articulated casts can have disastrous effects on the final restoration. It can result in needless or insufficient tooth reduction and perhaps necessitate remaking part or all of the restorations.

All salient information should be carefully documented and thoroughly studied before deciding how it will affect the final restoration. With this information, the patient's mouth may now be reexamined, and doubtful areas should be reevaluated. The diagnostic findings and treatment plan can be explained to the patient, and, based on the evidence to this point, the sequence of therapy, approximate costs, time involved, and a probable prognosis can be given.

It must be emphasized, however, that the patient must be made aware that it is not always possible to predict the exact course of treatment or outcome of the therapy. Many factors that could affect the final outcome may become evident only as the various steps in rehabilitation are reached, such as during tooth preparation, fabrication of the provisional splint, application of provisional splints, periodontal surgery, final tooth preparation, and final waxing. The patient should be allowed sufficient time to consider the treatment plan and arrive at a decision. Once the recommended therapy has been accepted, a diagnostic waxing of the articulated casts can be made.

Diagnostic Waxing

The waxing of the articulated casts should simulate as closely as possible the functional occlusal and morphologic characteristics of the final restoration, because from this waxing the shell stage of the provisional splint is fabricated. The degree of time and precision required for each patient depends upon the severity of the functional and morphologic anomalies of the individual patient. For patients with few missing teeth, little or no bite collapse, and a good esthetic arrangement of the teeth, little waxing will be required (Fig. 28-1). More involved cases may require either a total occlusal waxing or coronal reduction of the stone teeth to simulate final tooth preparations (Fig. 28-2A–C). This is followed with a complete diagnostic waxing to simulate coronal and functional occlusion (Fig. 28-2D–F).

Frequently the occlusal and morphologic characteristics of patients in need of periodontal prosthetic reconstruction are so bizarre that it is impossible to determine the degree of tooth reduction required unless this is predetermined on the articulated casts from a total functional waxing closely simulating the final restoration. Such a waxing should not be considered a waste of time, but essential in determining the following:

1. The best possible functional occlusal characteristics for each patient
2. The esthetic potential of the dentition
3. Whether full-coverage or partial-coverage restorations should be used
4. Whether major or minor orthodontic procedure is necessary
5. Whether the vital pulp of malposed teeth should be removed if no orthodontic repositioning is planned for them
6. Whether it is preferable to extract selectively the badly malposed teeth if these teeth are clinically expendable

Once the diagnostic waxing of the articulated casts has been completed, hard-stone duplicates are made (Fig. 28-3A–C). The maxillary stone cast is checked for any discrepancies and bubbles, and if acceptable it is occluded to the diagnostic mandibular waxing and secured with plaster to the upper member of the articulator. The stone reproduction of the mandibular waxing is next occluded to the mounted stone reproduction of the maxillary waxing and secured with plaster to the lower member of the articulator. This step gives a sturdy reproduction of the articulated diagnostic waxing casts that can be set aside for future reference. These stone casts are used first for the construction of the shell stage of the provisional splints and later as valuable time-saving aids in the functional waxing procedures for the final restorations.

Fabrication of the Shell of the Provisional Splint

There are several methods of fabricating the shell of the provisional splint. The method described here, with minor changes, simulates the procedures taught by Amsterdam and Fox for the construction of the combination gold-band-and-acrylic provisional splint.[1] With the advent of vacuum devices for fabricating acrylic matrices for trays, copings, and mouth guards, a vacuum device can also be used in a simplified technique for constructing provisional splints.

ARMAMENTARIUM

Duplicated stone casts of diagnostic waxing
Inlay wax
Wax-carving instruments
Alginate
Rim-lock trays
Spatula
Rubber bowl
Autopolymerizing acrylic powder, incisal shades

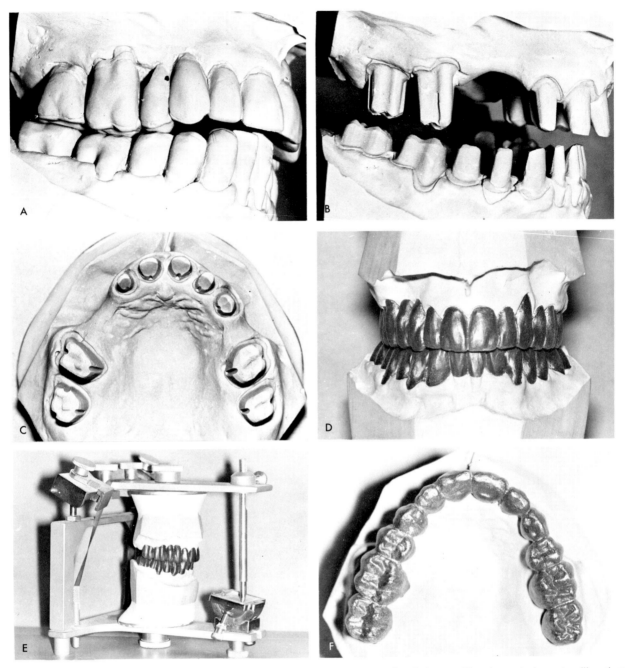

FIG. 28-2. *Diagnostic functional analysis for reconstruction with considerable occlusal change. The stone study casts will undergo coronal reduction of all abutment teeth to simulate final tooth preparation. This is then followed with a complete diagnostic waxing to simulate final functional occlusion. A. Articulated study casts in centric relation occlusion to show faulty occlusion. B. Lateral view of diagnostic coronal reduction to simulate final tooth preparation. C. Occlusal view of reduced maxillary teeth. D. Anterior view showing diagnostic functional waxing. E. Lateral view of waxing. F. Occlusal view of maxillary waxing.*

Autopolymerizing acrylic powder, gingival shades
Autopolymerizing acrylic monomer
Camel's-hair brushes, No. 00 and No. 2
Dappen dishes
Stainless-steel wire of appropriate gauge
Vibrator
Pressure pot

Long handpiece
Laboratory carbide burs for handpiece, round (Buffalo Dental Co.)
Steel bur, No. 8, round
Mounted separating disk
Mounted Burlew polishing wheels
Lathe

Polishing brushes
Pumice
Acrylic-polishing compound
Ultrasonic cleaner

PROCEDURE

Examine the cervical line of both maxillary and mandibular casts for imperfections, such as bubbles. Remove these and other imperfections and accurately

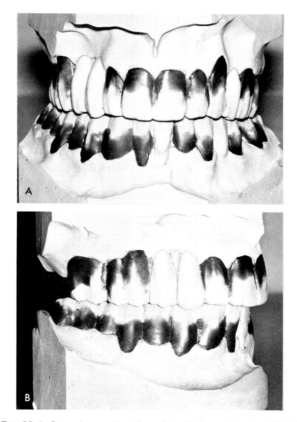

FIG. 28-4. *Steps in construction of shell of provisional splint. A. Anterior view of stone duplicate casts, with additional wax added to the gingival third of all prospective abutment teeth. B. Lateral view.*

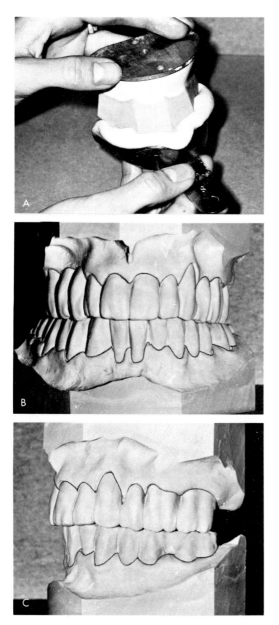

FIG. 28-3. *Steps in duplicating diagnostic waxings and articulating the hard stone duplicates. A. Alginate impressions taken of diagnostic waxings. B. Anterior view of hard stone duplicates with gingival margins precisely demarcated. C. Lateral view of articulated stone duplicates.*

pencil in the free gingival junction (Fig. 28-3B, C). Apply a layer of inlay wax approximately 1 mm thick to the cervical third of the crown, being careful not to extend the wax apically beyond the penciled gingival line (Fig. 28-4). This will allow for and result in a slightly greater diameter in the cervical third of the shell splint and facilitate the try-in of the splint after tooth preparation. The excessive diameter can be reduced and polished back to the original dimensions of the tooth after the relining phase of the provisional splint is completed. Soak the casts in water for a few minutes and make accurate alginate impressions of the casts.

If the splint needs additional reinforcement, appropriate lengths of 0.027 stainless steel wire may be placed midocclusally through the posterior quadrants and midlingually through the anterior segment of the arch. These reinforcing wires can be secured at each end with acrylic resin which is allowed to set (Fig. 28-5A). The reinforcing wire will reduce the incidence of fracture of the provisional splint for the duration of its use in the patient's mouth.

Place a small amount of incisal powder of the de-

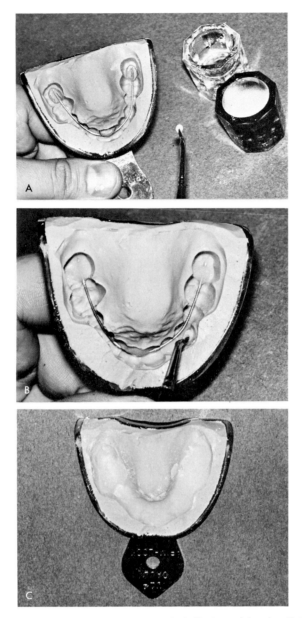

FIG. 28-5. *Steps in construction of shell of provisional splint (continued). A. Placing stainless steel wire in impression for additional reinforcement and securing its position with acrylic resin. B. Adding incisal-shade acrylic resin. C. Gingival-shade acrylic resin poured to fill remainder of impressions of the crowns slightly beyond the gingival line.*

sired shade and a small amount of autopolymerizing monomer in separate dappen dishes. Heat one of the impressions in hot water and lightly dry.

Wet the tip of a No. 2 camel's-hair brush with monomer. Dip the brush into the powder in order to pick up some acrylic resin and flow the desired amount onto the facial aspect of each tooth in the impression (Fig. 28-5B). The impression should be held at approximately a 45-degree angle to control the flow of acrylic

resin, so that a greater thickness of acrylic resin reaches into the incisal and occlusal thirds of the impression and gradually feathers out at the cervical third. The impression should be warm enough for the acrylic resin to gel in a few seconds. This gives better control over the thickness. Do the same for the other impression and allow the incisal acrylic resin to reach at least the gel stage.

Mix enough autopolymerizing acrylic resin of the desired gingival shade for both impressions. With a brush, wet the inside of the coronal portions of the impression with monomer and, with the aid of a vibrator, pour the liquefied acrylic resin into the coronal portions of the impressions up to and slightly beyond the cervical line (Fig. 28-5C).

Immediately place the poured impressions into a pressure pot containing warm water and raise the pressure to 20 to 25 p.s.i. This will produce a much denser acrylic impression. Allow the acrylic resin to set for a few minutes and remove it from the impression (Fig. 28-6A). Trim precisely to the penciled gingival line with the round laboratory carbide bur (Fig. 28-6B). With the aid of the separating disk and carbide burs, accurately create the interproximal embrasure forms, being careful to estimate adequate allowance for the cervical mesiodistal dimension of the prepared abutment teeth (Fig. 28-6C–E). Remove any imperfections on the occlusal surface with the steel burs and polish the entire splint with Burlew wheels, pumice, and polishing compound (Fig. 28-6F), being careful not to overheat the splint, as overheating may warp it.

As the last step after polishing, sufficiently grind out the coronal portions of the prospective abutment teeth with the round laboratory carbide acrylic-trimming bur (Fig. 28-7A, B). Smaller round steel burs are necessary for anterior teeth. Store the shell in a damp place until required.

Tooth Preparation

It is important to reemphasize that treatment of all deep carious lesions and replacement of questionable restorations should have been accomplished prior to tooth preparation.

In patients who suffer from generalized advanced periodontitis and require full-coverage tooth reconstruction it is often more expedient to prepare the tooth and adapt and set the provisional splint before treating the periodontal condition. Many of these cases demonstrate generalized pathologic mobility from loss of supporting bone. If mobility that results from severe bone loss combined with occlusal traumatism is present prior to surgical correction, it will most certainly increase severely immediately after surgery and during

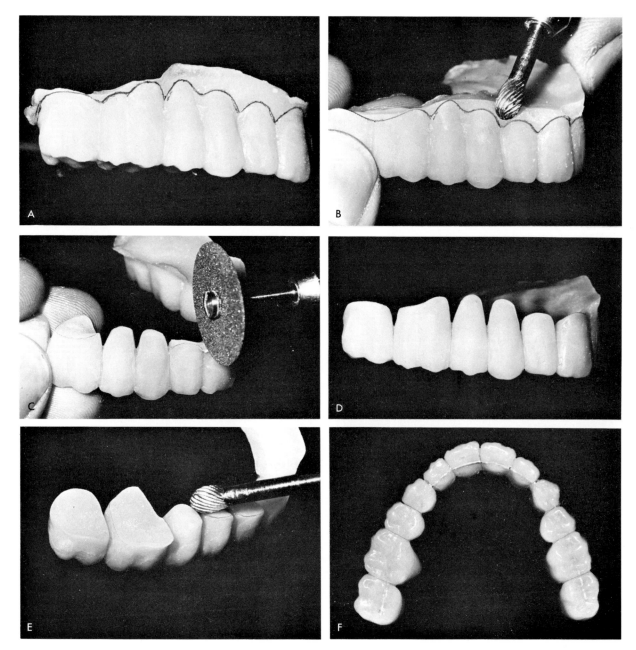

FIG. 28-6. *Steps in construction of provisional splint shell (continued). A. Untrimmed splint retrieved from impression and gingival margin pencilled. B. Splint partly trimmed to gingival line. C, D, and E. Interproximal embrasures and coronal dimensions of gingival third of the teeth formed. F. Splint polished.*

the healing period. It is our opinion that pathologic mobility in the Class II to III range can adversely affect normal healing. Since at the outset the plan is to splint such teeth anyway, splinting is best done prior to surgical correction. Not only will the provisional splint provide the necessary stabilization, but it also has another advantage. Reduction of the coronal surfaces will eliminate contacts and facial and lingual contours that impede periodontic surgical procedures (Fig. 28-8). This reduction exposes the soft tissues surrounding

the abutment teeth and facilitates the carving of precisely scalloped and uniformly thin soft-tissue flaps. It makes easier removal of the soft tissue surrounding the teeth after the flaps are raised. It also greatly facilitates osteoplasty and ostectomy and the subsequent precise positioning and stabilization of the flaps with sutures. Of course, resective procedures usually cause a recession (Fig. 28-8D), and this will necessitate finishing the preparations and relining the provisional splint. This is, however, a small inconvenience relative to the advan-

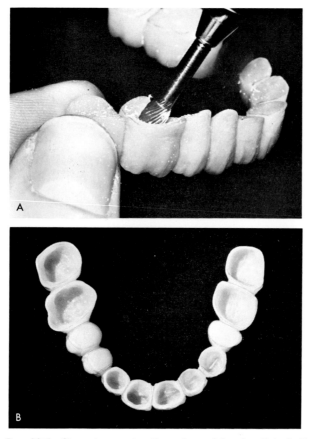

FIG. 28-7. *Steps in construction of provisional splint shell* (*continued*). *A and B. Intracoronal portions of acrylic crowns of prospective abutment teeth sufficiently reduced* (*Photos for Figs. 28-2, 3, 4, 5, 6, and 7 courtesy Dr. D. Smith.*)

tages of preliminary tooth preparation and provisional splinting prior to periodontal surgery.

It is not within the scope of this book to describe the details of tooth preparation. It is sufficient to say that the preliminary tooth preparations should end just short of the free gingival margin. There is no need at this time to extend them subgingivally, since preparations must be finished to extend the margins subgingivally after healing and maturation of the supporting tissues are complete unless, of course, supragingivally placed margins are desired.

If gold bands are to be used in conjunction with adapting the provisional splint, the preparation of choice is either a slice type of finish line or one that is slightly chamfered. It is more difficult to adapt gold bands accurately to shoulder-type or to heavily chamfered gingival finish lines.

If the dentition's original vertical dimension is to be retained, it is wise to prepare the teeth of only part of an arch and adapt the provisional splint to that segment, using the teeth on the opposite side as guides. All hopelessly involved teeth designated for extraction

should be extracted after preparation of the abutment teeth and just prior to the try-in stage of the provisional splint shell. Not only does this timing prevent unnecessary interference from hemorrhage, but these teeth can serve as a guide as to how much coronal reduction is necessary in the approximating teeth (Fig. 28-9). Care must be taken not to overheat the teeth during coronal reduction, as overheating may cause unnecessary hypersensitivity or even pulpal death. Immediately after each tooth is prepared, Metimyd° is painted over the prepared surfaces with a cotton pledget. The tooth is then dried (but not desiccated) with air and glazed with a cavity varnish (Copalite†). This will protect the exposed dentin when the provisional splint is relined with acrylic resin.

Application of the Provisional Splint

The method of application of the provisional splint depends on the type of the splint. The techniques for the gold-band-and-acrylic and the all-acrylic types are described.

GOLD-BAND-AND-ACRYLIC TYPE

If the provisional splint is to serve the patient for more than 6 months, it is advisable to use the gold-band-and-acrylic provisional splinting technique described by Amsterdam and Fox.[1] They cite the following advantages of this type of splint over the all-acrylic splint:

1. Ease of construction and maintenance
2. Accurate marginal fit and knifelike margins with good gingival contour
3. Optimal embrasure pattern
4. Increased strength
5. Facilitation of carving
6. Ability to be removed and reset with minimal disturbance of relationships
7. Ease of maintenance of periodontal environment before, during, and after periodontal surgery
8. Marginal protection against cervical sensitivity
9. Ease of repair

In addition, these splints are much more retentive than the all-acrylic splints and hence offer greater protection against dissolution of the temporary cement. The bands best adapted to this procedure are Ney's Zephyr‡ gold bands. They come in a variety of

° Metimyd Ophthalmic Suspension, Shering Corp.
† Getz Corporation, Chicago, Ill.
‡ J. M. Ney Co., Hartford, Conn.

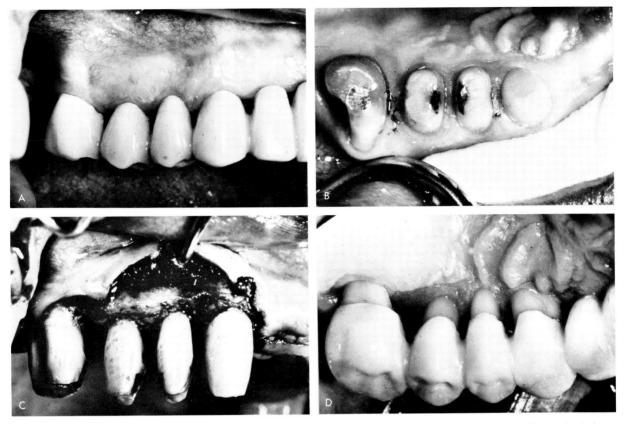

FIG. 28-8. *Applying provisional splint prior to periodontal surgical procedures to improve access and simplify surgical phase. A. Quadrant of splint in place. B. Presurgical occlusal view of quadrant to show how reduction of teeth improves access for surgery. Distobuccal root of molar was amputated at time of provisional splinting. C. Alveolar bone exposed for correction of defects. D. Surgical recession, two weeks after resection. Gingival extension of margins of coronal preparations will in most cases be necessary. (Courtesy Dr. G. Ronning.)*

sizes and are serrated. The steps in adaptation are as follows:

Choose a slightly undersized band and try the fit over the prepared tooth (Fig. 28-10A, B). Carefully festoon the band to follow the contour of the gingival line. Fluted molar or premolar preparations will require careful burnishing to the finish line (Fig. 28-10C). If the margins of the band are short of the finish line after festooning, rock the band in several directions while applying digital force in an apical direction. The gold is soft enough to conform to the finish line. Cut the band circumferentially, so that it extends to approximately the midpoint occlusogingivally. Serrate the occlusal rim of the band and try it in again to verify the fit (Fig. 28-10A–C). Adapt the axial walls of the band as closely as possible to the axial walls of the tooth and mark the facial side of each band for future reference. In the same manner, adapt bands for the remaining teeth and set all bands aside in a designated order.

Once the bands have been adapted to all the prepared abutments and set aside, the teeth destined for extraction are removed. The following steps are taken to reline the provisional splint shell:

Try the preformed splint shell over the prepared teeth and check for interferences. Remove the splint shell. If necessary, reduce the interferences by further hollow-grinding the shell, trimming the interproximal or gingival border of the shell, or if necessary by further occlusal reduction of the teeth.

Brush a thin layer of petroleum jelly over the prepared teeth and the immediately surrounding gingival tissue. Place all the gold bands on the respective teeth.

Try the splint shell over the bands and adjust the bands or splint as necessary. Check the vertical opening by guiding the patient's jaw into centric relation occlusion. See whether the remaining unprepared teeth on the opposite side occlude or whether other landmark registrations of vertical dimension correspond. If they do, then the shell is ready for relining.

Carefully remove the splint shell and paint the inside with autopolymerizing monomer. Check to ensure that all the bands are securely in position. Mix an adequate amount of autopolymerizing acrylic resin of

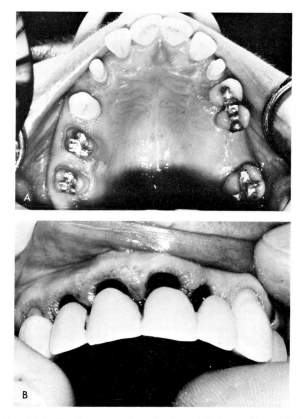

FIG. 28-9. *Tooth preparation. A. Completed cuspid and left molar preparations. The maxillary incisors and left second premolar are to be extracted because of severe periodontal involvement. The remaining teeth will be prepared at another appointment. B. Teeth extracted and anterior shell of provisional splint tried in, to prepare for relining.*

the desired shade and allow it to set to a doughy stage. Place sufficient acrylic resin into the splint to fill the shell of each prospective abutment tooth. Wet the surface with monomer to ensure adherence to the gold bands and place the splint over the banded teeth.

Guide the patient's jaw into centric relation occlusion and ask him to close to the desired vertical dimension. With a sharp explorer trim the gingival excess of acrylic resin. Instruct the patient to continue biting in centric relation and allow the acrylic resin to set for approximately 60 seconds or until it begins to harden. Before the acrylic resin gets too hard, remove the splint and rinse both the splint and the prepared teeth with cold water to remove excess monomer.

Repaint the teeth with petroleum jelly and replace the splint. Tell the patient to close his jaws and hold them together until the acrylic resin is set.

Tap off the splint and make any necessary additions to the gingival margins by the brush-on technique, so that all exposed margins of the gold bands are covered (Fig. 28-10D, E). Check the gingival and embrasure

contours for proper form (Fig. 28-11). All the principles of correct contours, as outlined in Chapter 26, must be observed. Any necessary occlusal corrections can be made to the opposing natural teeth, since these will be reduced later.

Set the provisional splint with zinc oxide-eugenol cement or a calcium-hydroxide-based temporary cement. Prepare the opposing teeth and adapt the provisional splint in the same way.

ALL-ACRYLIC TYPE

As stated earlier, the use of gold bands in the construction of provisional splints is not always necessary. All-acrylic splints can be used if it is fairly certain that the final restorations will be inserted in a relatively short time (up to 6 months) after the provisional splinting phase. After this period of time, the gingival margins of the provisional splint usually demonstrate progressive deterioration, mainly because of the chemical action of the temporary cement. Such deterioration contributes to plaque retention and cervical sensitivity and if allowed to progress will result in gingival disturbances and even root caries. In addition, the entire splint in general becomes weakened and is frequently subject to fracture.

The all-acrylic type of provisional splint is appropriate for the following conditions:

1. When periodontal surgery prior to splinting is not required
2. When all periodontal surgical correction and extraction of hopelessly involved teeth is completed prior to provisional splinting
3. When a favorable prognosis makes the periods between periodontal and/or endodontic therapy and final restorations short (less than 6 months)
4. When the treatment plan includes no minor orthodontic tooth movement, since minor tooth movement necessarily prolongs the total time of rehabilitation

The steps in the construction and application of the all-acrylic splint are similar to those for the construction and application of the gold-band-and-acrylic splint except that no gold bands are involved in fitting the splint shell to the prepared teeth. However, greater care is needed to ensure good marginal adaptation of the acrylic gingival margins. This is especially important if the coronal tooth preparations have been completed. Poor marginal adaptation will seriously affect the health of the gingiva and may result in recurring caries.

Regardless of whether the tooth preparations are

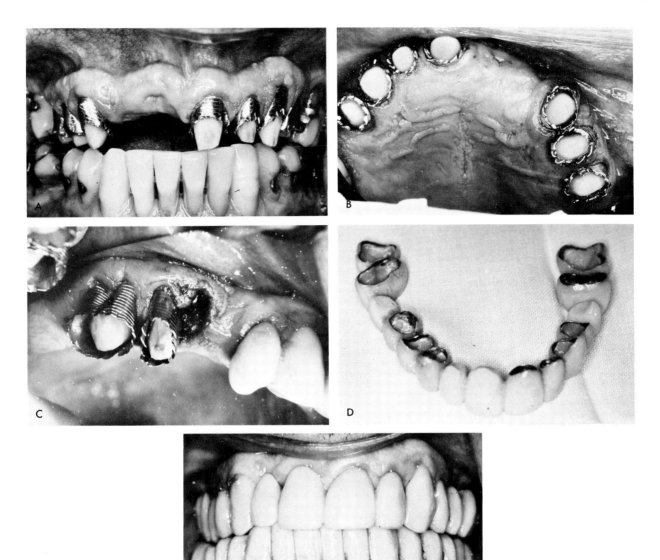

FIG. 28-10. *Construction of gold-band-and-acrylic provisional splint. A. Anterior view of adapted gold bands in place. B. Occlusal view. C. Lateral view of molar bands in place. Mesiobuccal root was amputated because of periodontal involvement. Note how band is contoured to follow fluting of second molar preparation. D. Completed maxillary splint to show margins of gold bands. E. Temporarily set maxillary and mandibular provisional splints.*

preliminary or final, adequate coronal tooth structure should be removed to ensure that normal interproximal, facial, and lingual contours can be produced in the provisional splint. After completion of coronal reduction, the shell splint is tried in as described earlier. If it is satisfactory, the teeth are coated with Metimyd, Copalite, and petroleum jelly in that order, and the shell splint is relined to fit the prepared teeth. Upon completion of the setting of the acrylic resin, the splint is removed and the margins are delineated with a pencil (Fig. 28-12A). With separating disks, stones, and pumice-impregnated rubber wheels, the margins are

trimmed to the desired amount and thickness (Fig. 28-12B, C).

The splint is again tried in place to check for overextensions or deficiencies. The overextensions and all axial contours are carefully reduced by the desired amount. The submarginal deficiencies are corrected by the brush-on technique as follows:

Place small amounts of autopolymerizing acrylic powder and monomer in separate dappen dishes. Carefully isolate and dry with air the area of the crown to which additional acrylic resin is to be applied. With a No. 00 camel's-hair brush, slightly wet this area with

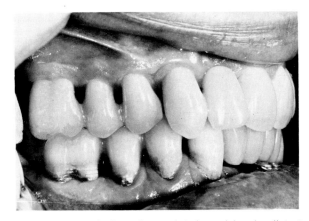

FIG. 28-11. *Lateral view of completed provisional splints to show coronal form, size of embrasures, and degree of polish necessary to promote tissue health and ease of oral hygiene. Maxillary splint is all-acrylic and mandibular splint is gold-band-and-acrylic. (Courtesy Dr. C. Filipchuk.)*

monomer. Dip the tip of the brush in monomer and pick up a small amount of powder (Fig. 28-13). If the brush is not excessively wet with monomer, a small bead of acrylic resin will cling to the brush tip. Apply this bead to the submarginal area, which it will rapidly flow over and cover. Do the same to any area that requires additional acrylic resin. In order to hasten setting, spray warm water over these additions. Spraying will also wash away the free monomer from the tissues.

After sufficient time, remove the splints and with small pumice-impregnated wheels (Burlew polishing wheels) carefully trim away any excess. With a little experience the quantity of the marginal additions can be controlled so that only minimal trimming is necessary to ensure an accurate fit.

Polish all segments of the splint to a high glaze with acrylic polish and thoroughly clean the splint with the aid of an ultrasonic cleaner and detergent. If surgical corrections to the periodontium are not necessary or planned for a later date, set the splint with the desired type of temporary cement in the manner described later in this chapter.

INTEGRATION OF PERIODONTAL AND ENDODONTIC THERAPY WITH PROVISIONAL SPLINTING

Surgical correction of periodontally involved regions and endodontic therapy may both be performed before the provisional splint is cemented into place. However, if these phases of therapy are to be referred to specialists, it is wise to set the provisional splint with a temporary cement that is modified with petroleum jelly. This will facilitate its removal and reduce the inci-

dence of accidental fractures of the splint or the teeth.

Procedures such as gingivectomy, gingivoplasty, mucogingival surgery, osteoplasty, ostectomy, reattachment, root amputation, crown lengthening, and endodontic treatment are easier to perform in less time and with greater accuracy if the splint is removed prior to these corrective procedures. Removal of the splint will expose all interproximal regions for easy access (Fig. 28-8), since all interproximal contacts and all facial and lingual contours of the teeth have been reduced. After the corrections have been made, the splint can be reset with a temporary cement.

Frequently, patients requiring periodontal prosthetic reconstruction have shortened clinical crowns because of broken restorations, gross caries, or gingival

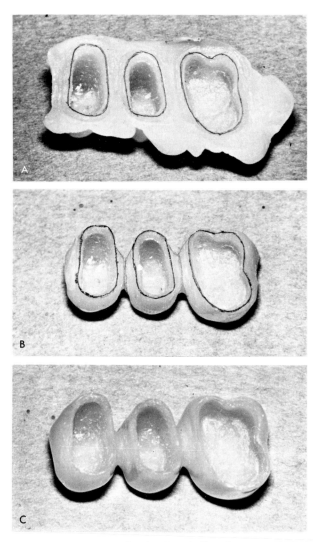

FIG. 28-12. *Trimming relined splint shell to fit prepared abutments. A. Relined quadrant of provisional splint showing gingival margins delineated with a pencil. B. Excess acrylic resin trimmed to delineated margins and interproximal embrasures formed. C. Polished splint.*

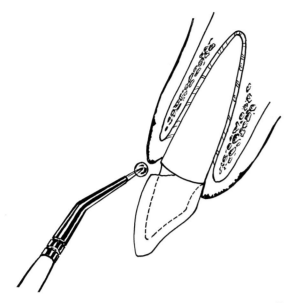

FIG. 28-13. *Correction of marginal discrepancies of relined acrylic provisional splint. Applying bead of acrylic resin that was formed by dipping small camel's-hair brush in monomer and then in polymer to deficient margin.*

hyperplasia (Fig. 28-14A). Their teeth usually require additional crown lengthening to increase retention. For these patients, the sequence of steps during the provisional splinting phase may be advantageously altered. Instead of preliminary crown preparation and the provisional splint relining, which are usually done prior to periodontal surgery, the following sequence of therapy is carried out.

1. The teeth are reduced for full-coverage crowns up to the gingival margin (Fig. 28-14B).
2. The alveolar process is exposed both buccally and lingually, using the internally beveled-flap technique (Fig. 28-14B, C).
3. All soft tissue surrounding the necks of the teeth is removed (Fig. 28-14C).
4. Craters are eliminated by ostectomy or osteoplasty, as required, and crowns are lengthened to the desired amount (Fig. 28-14C).
5. Full-crown reductions are extended to a level approximately 2 mm coronal to the crestal bone (Fig. 28-14C).
6. Gold bands are adapted to the prepared teeth (Fig. 28-14C).
7. The prefabricated shell of the provisional splint is relined, trimmed, and finished as completely as hemorrhage will allow (Fig. 28-14D).
8. The provisional splint is cemented in place with a weakened mix of temporary cement, and a surgical pack is placed, if necessary.
9. After one week, the splint, pack, and sutures are

removed, and any marginal discrepancies between the splint and the prepared teeth can be corrected.

This alteration in the sequence is greatly advantageous, in that it results in a much-needed increase in the retention of the provisional splint. The use of gold bands will reduce the degree of exposure of the soft tissue and bone to the soft acrylic resin during the relining and will result in a more accurate marginal fit and in greater retention. At the surgical phase, the acrylic lining should be purposely left short of the margins and should be added to at the same time that the pack and sutures are removed, by brushing acrylic resin around the exposed margins of the gold bands.

TEMPORARY CEMENTATION OF PROVISIONAL SPLINTS

Most temporary cements are of the zinc oxide and eugenol variety or are calcium-hydroxide based. These types of cement have the advantages of pulpal sedation, insulation to thermal changes, and minimal pulpal reaction, and, in the case of the calcium hydroxide cements, they stimulate the formation of secondary dentin.

The zinc oxide and eugenol temporary cements can be used full strength or may be modified with the addition of a varied amount of petroleum jelly to decrease their retentive qualities. In the author's experience, the calcium-hydroxide-based cements offer greater retention if this is needed, but have less working time. The zinc oxide and eugenol cements, however, have the disadvantage of attacking the acrylic resin after a period of time, causing discoloration, and they also tend to wash out more readily.

The type of cement and degree to which it is modified depend upon the length of time the provisional splint is to remain in place and the retentive qualities of the crown preparations. Regardless of the cement chosen, it should be applied properly.

PROCEDURE FOR CEMENTATION

Clean and dry, and brush the external surfaces of all segments of the splint with a thin coating of petroleum jelly. Clean and dry the abutment teeth and surrounding tissue. Paint the teeth with Metimyd unless done previously. If desired, glaze the teeth with a cavity varnish, dry, and isolate them with cotton rolls or gauze.

Mix the cement as suggested by the manufacturer and add modifier, if needed. Some prefer at this time to

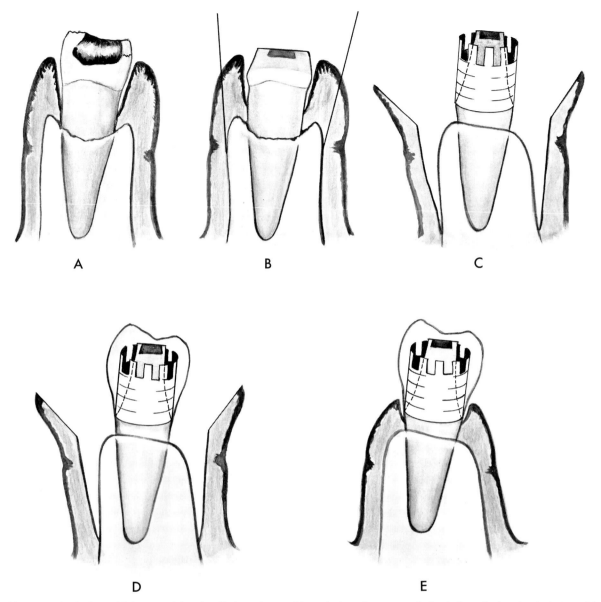

FIG. 28-14. *Method of combining provisional splinting phase with periodontal surgery. A. Periodontally involved abutment tooth before surgical correction. B. Coronal reduction to the approximate level of gingival margin and inverse-beveled incisions to expose alveolar process. C. Osseous correction performed, margins of crown preparation extended 2 mm above crestal bone and gold band adapted. D. Acrylic shell of provisional splint relined to incorporate adapted gold band. E. After healing and development of free gingival margin.*

incorporate into the mix a mixture of Mysteclin F° and aureomycin surgical powder to act as antibacterial and antifungicidal agents and offer greater protection to the teeth, in the event that the provisional splint loosens.[4]

Apply the mixed cement to the shell of each abutment tooth of the splint and firmly seat in place. Ask the patient to bite with it firmly on a soft orangewood stick or cotton roll until the cement has set. Setting can

° E. R. Squibb, Princeton, N.J.

be hastened by flowing warm water over the excess cement. Remove the excess cement carefully and completely with explorers and curets. Cement particles allowed to remain subgingivally will always result in gingival inflammation. Remove traces of excess cement from the coronal acrylic surfaces with orange solvent. If the splint is in several segments, join the segments if this is necessary, first cleaning, drying, and isolating each joint and flowing a slight amount of acrylic resin over it, using the brush-on technique and allowing it to set. If additional strength is required, an occlusal groove may be cut between the segments to be joined, a length of stainless steel wire may be placed in the base of the groove, and acrylic resin may be brushed in to fill the groove.

PROCEDURE FOR REMOVAL AND RECEMENTATION

Before completion of the final restoration, the provisional splint may have to be removed several times. If it is not removed carefully, the splint may be fractured or, what is more serious, the abutment teeth may be fractured (especially if it is necessary also to remove the more retentive gold-band-and-acrylic type).

For removal, a back-action crown remover or a straight chisel and mallet may be used. In either case, the direction of force must be as nearly parallel to the line of withdrawal of the splint as possible in order to reduce the force needed to remove the splint. The use of a straight chisel and mallet is preferable.

Loosen the endmost acrylic crown of the splint first by placing the chisel interproximally as nearly parallel as possible to the line of withdrawal and have the assistant tap gently at first and then with increasing force until the acrylic crown begins to loosen from the prepared abutment teeth. Repeat the tapping at each interproximal joint until the splint is visibly loosened from each prepared tooth.

After removal, clean the splint with an ultrasonic cleaner and appropriate solution to eliminate the old cement. If marginal repair or any additions have to be made to the acrylic splint, freshen the surface of the acrylic material with a stone or bur, paint this area with liquid acrylic monomer, and paint on any additions, using the brush-on technique. Perform necessary work on the teeth or soft tissue and reset the splint in a similar manner as that previously described.

REEVALUATION PERIODS

Provisional stabilization, as stated earlier, is therapeutic in nature and must not be regarded as only a means of temporary coverage. Several periods of reevaluation may be necessary before the tooth preparations are completed, the impression is made, and the final prosthesis is constructed. To disregard the reevaluations and proceed with the final restoration is to court disaster.

The first reevaluation should be within one month of the initial insertion of the provisional splint. Prior to removal of the splint, the effectiveness of the patient's oral-hygiene measures should be carefully reviewed and reinforced if necessary. All inflammation of the marginal gingiva should be checked to see if it is caused by plaque retention, marginal discrepancies, overcontouring, or a combination of any or all of these factors.

The mobility of the splinted segments should be evaluated, and the need for additional cross-arch stabilization should be assessed. The esthetic, phonetic, and functional qualities should be checked to determine whether they are satisfactory or need modification. Any improvements in vertical dimension, occlusal plane, tooth length, and width are noted for correction. The corrections that can be performed prior to removal of the splint should be undertaken at this point. The splint is then removed, and the functional and morphologic modifications are completed.

The interproximal and sulcular soft tissue is next examined for any inflammation, hypertrophy, or exaggerated col formation. Usually such signs can be related to plaque retention, overcontouring of the axial and proximal surfaces of the acrylic crowns, or excessive pontic pressure against the ridge (Fig. 28-15). Modification of axial occlusal morphology, such as thinning of gingival margins, opening of embrasures, and narrowing of the occlusal table is performed and the surfaces are repolished prior to recementation. Necessary soft-tissue corrections are made either by surgical excision or by electrosurgery.

Assessment is now made of the therapeutic response of each tooth to the periodontal surgical procedures it has undergone, such as soft-tissue and hard-tissue corrections, reattachment attempts, hemisection, and root amputations, and the need for any additional therapy is decided upon at this point.

The mobility of each tooth should be noted and compared with the mobility readings at the initial visit. Any tooth or roots of teeth deemed hopeless or jeopardizing key abutment teeth should be removed as early as possible.

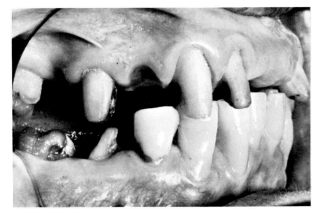

FIG. 28-15. *Effects of excessive pontic pressure and lack of sufficient interproximal embrasure space of an acrylic provisional fixed partial denture. Note hyperplastic papillae and inflamed ridge between maxillary cuspid, premolar, and molar.*

The endodontic environment should be carefully assessed and treated if necessary. It is wise to provide root-canal therapy for all teeth requiring this prior to the final impression stage.

During these periods of reevaluation, the treatment plan for the final restorations is carefully determined.

The degree of splinting, need for copings, need for reinforcement of endodontically treated teeth, additional pin-and-amalgam buildups, additional tooth reduction, and the need for minor tooth movement are assessed, and adjustments are made, if necessary. The dentist should be reasonably certain of the prognosis

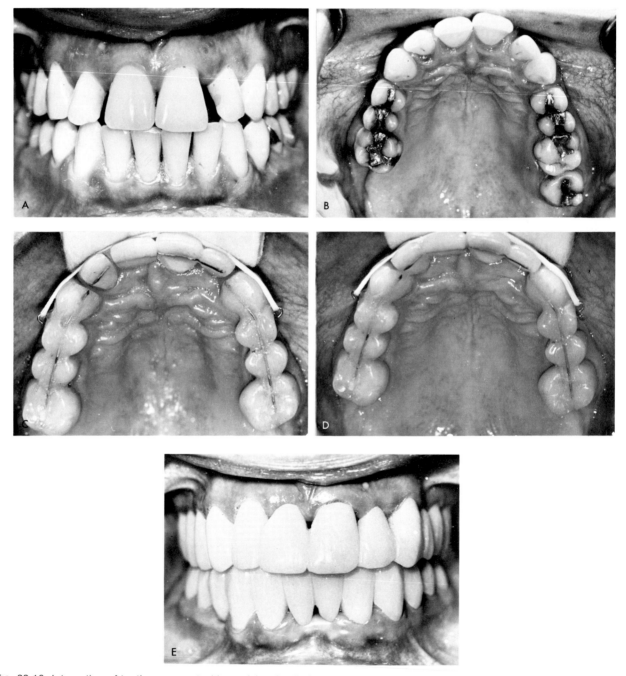

FIG. 28-16. *Integration of tooth movement with provisional splinting. A. Anterior view of teeth requiring repositioning. B. Occlusal view showing migrated anterior teeth. C. Provisional splint adapted and showing anterior segment separated from posterior segments. Stainless-steel hooks incorporated in buccal interproximal region of cuspid and premolars on both sides. Elastics are engaged to retract the anterior segment. D. Occlusal view, showing anterior segment retracted and joined to posterior segment. E. Anterior view, showing realigned anterior segment. (Courtesy Dr. E. Stang.)*

for each tooth before starting on the final restoration. If this is impossible for every tooth, the patient is made fully aware of this, and a revised evaluation of possible changes in the treatment plan is made.

All the information gathered during each reevaluation is accurately recorded and explained to the patient, in order to prevent misunderstanding.

Following therapy, certain conditions must be fulfilled before proceeding to the final stage:[1]

1. Mobility should decrease.
2. Soft tissues should appear healthy.
3. Osseous support should be free of pathologic conditions.
4. Mucogingival environment should be normal.
5. Widened periodontal ligament space should approach a normal dimension and a well-defined lamina dura should be roentgenographically evident.
6. Periapical areas of teeth treated endodontically should show signs of healing.

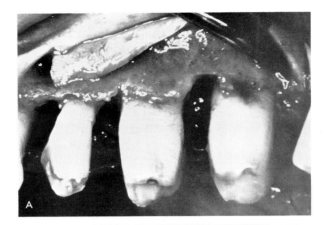
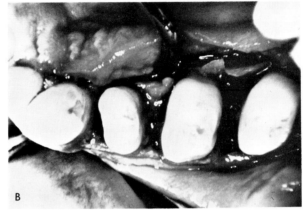

FIG. 28-18. *Premature surgical exposure for correction of periodontal defects in an adult patient, six months after orthodontic therapy. A. Buccal view, showing lack of interproximal bone and inadvertent curettage of interproximal soft tissue which appeared similar to granulation tissue but was in effect unmineralized osteogenic tissue. B. Occlusal view, showing resulting deep interproximal craters.*

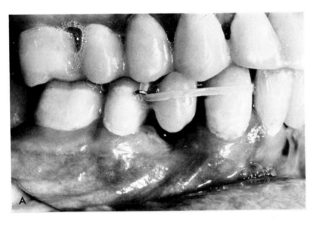
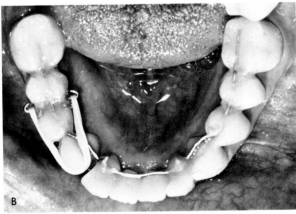

FIG. 28-17. *A. Buccal view of posterior quadrant of same patient as seen in Figure 28-16 showing distal movement of mandibular cuspid. B. Occlusal view of A, showing position of hooks and elastic.*

7. The patient should have no feelings of discomfort.
8. Esthetic, phonetic, and functional qualities should be satisfactory to the patient and to the dentist.
9. No symptoms of temporomandibular-joint dysfunction should be present.

INTEGRATION OF MINOR TOOTH MOVEMENT WITH PROVISIONAL-SPLINTING PROCEDURES

There are many types of minor tooth movement that can be integrated with the provisional-splinting phase.[1] Excessive procumbency of the anterior teeth that is the result of collapse of the posterior bite may be corrected, and the teeth may be stabilized. Diastemata can be closed and root proximities can be corrected. Such tooth movement is done only after the correct vertical dimension has been established and CRO has been determined for the posterior quadrants.

If the anterior teeth are in need of repositioning, one method is to provisionally splint the posterior quadrants at the correct centric relation and vertical dimension. Stainless steel hooks are incorporated into a convenient region, and with orthodontic elastics, the teeth to be moved are engaged and repositioned. Once they are repositioned, they are prepared for splinting and stabilized by joining the anterior segments to the posterior segments with acrylic resin and wire.

Another method is to splint the posterior segments as described and use a Hawley appliance to retract or move the teeth and subsequently splint and join this segment to the posterior segments.

Yet another method is to incorporate the malposed teeth in the provisional splint in their original positions (Figs. 28-16, 28-17). These teeth can then be separated from the splint and, with elastic bands engaged to strategically placed hooks, moved to the desired positions. Interproximal and occlusal relief must be made to ensure that there is no impediment to tooth movement. Once in position these teeth may be secured to the segments that are used for anchorage by painting acrylic resin in the interproximal regions, allowing the resin to set and polishing the joints.

If minor tooth movement is performed, it is preferable to complete this prior to surgical correction of osseous defects. A sufficient period of time must be allowed before exposing the alveolar process, so as to ensure recalcification or maturation of osteogenic tissue surrounding the teeth that have been moved. Failure to do this may have disastrous results. Excessively wide ligament spaces are common following orthodontic movement (Fig. 28-18). Exposing the alveolar process too soon after tooth movement will interfere with recalcification, and unnecessary resorption may occur. In addition, the soft tissue within the excessively widened ligament space may be mistaken for granulation tissue and may be inadvertently curetted.

If major orthodontic therapy is part of the comprehensive treatment plan, an intervening period of at least one year of retention is advocated, preferably sustained by provisional splinting. After this, correction of the remaining osseous defects can proceed, followed later by the full-coverage restoration.

References

1. Amsterdam, M., and Fox, L.: Provisional splinting-principles and technics. Dent. Clin. North Am., Mar. 1959, p. 73.
2. Cohn, L. A.: Integrating treatment procedures in occluso-rehabilitation. J. Prosthet. Dent., 7:511, 1957.
3. Kornfeld, M.: Mouth Rehabilitation, Vol. I. St. Louis, C. V. Mosby Co., 1967.
4. Thomas, P. K.: Personal communication, 1969.

29

Long-term Stabilization

Successful restorative dentistry, whether in the form of restoration of carious or missing teeth or as a phase of treatment of periodontally involved mouths, must be based on an understanding and appreciation of the many basic principles that have been developed over the years in all fields of dentistry. Numerous concepts of oral rehabilitation have evolved, some worthwhile, others questionable, most of which are based more on empirical evidence than on scientific evidence. For this reason, what appears to be a clinically successful application of a concept in oral rehabilitation must not be misconstrued as proof that it is the only acceptable concept. Clinical success in oral rehabilitation means that the patient, at least for the present, appears to tolerate the prescribed therapy. However, it may also mean that any of several different approaches to therapy could have evoked an equally good response. Dentists must have a working knowledge of the recognized methods of oral rehabilitation so that they do not stereotype diagnosis and treatment to fit one concept. Only with this philosophy can they choose a form of therapy that will work best for each individual diagnosis.

PERIODONTAL PROSTHETICS

The practice of periodontal prosthetics incorporates all restorative and replacement procedures essential in the treatment of advanced periodontal disease. There are concepts of principles and techniques in periodontal prosthetics that have greatly contributed to the field of restorative dentistry. The mouth requiring periodontal prosthetic therapy taxes the talents of the therapist to the highest degree. If favorable results can be gained by applying the principles, concepts, and techniques of periodontal prosthetics to advanced cases, no less can be expected when these same principles are applied to the less advanced condition.

Objectives of Periodontal Prosthetics

The major objective of periodontal prosthetics is to restore the dentition to a state of health in which it can safely resist the stresses of normal functions and also be better equipped to resist parafunctional forces. Permanent pathologic tooth mobility is common to all cases requiring periodontal prosthetics, and in order to reach the objective of restoring function to a dentition or to a group of teeth, the mobile teeth must be stabilized. The manner in which this is accomplished will greatly influence realization of the remaining objectives of periodontal prosthetics which are to replace missing strategic teeth, to enhance the patient's cosmetic appearance, and to improve phonetics. Ideally, these

29
Long-Term
Stabilization

objectives must be reached so that the procedures involved are biologically compatible with the hard and soft tissues of the mouth and so that the results will optimally afford protection to the periodontium against further deterioration of its supporting qualities.

The form that the prosthetics will take will in large part determine whether the objectives can be reached. Many patients requiring this difficult and costly service attach more importance to cosmetic and phonetic qualities than to good function. Patients must be made to realize that pleasing esthetics and improved phonetics are short-lived unless the basic biologic principles of stabilization, functional occlusion, and the physiologic form are strictly adhered to. For these reasons the theme of this chapter will adhere strictly to the basic principles necessary to obtain proper form as it relates to function and health.

The dentist who truly practices the discipline of periodontal prosthetics must not only be a trained prosthodontist, but must also have a deep insight into periodontics, endodontics, and orthodontics. This does not imply that he must be capable of performing all necessary procedures in the related disciplines, but he has a decided advantage if he can. More importantly, a theoretical knowledge in these disciplines is necessary if sequential integration of the various therapeutic procedures, usually necessary in the planned treatment of the comprehensively involved patient in need of periodontal prosthetics, is to be successfully carried out.

It has been clearly emphasized in Chapter 28 that for the most part the objectives of stabilization, function, esthetics, and phonetics should be realized during the provisional splinting phase of therapy. Procedures for long-term stabilization should not begin until these objectives have been met or until it is clear that they can be met during the final phase of periodontal prosthetics. Once this is ensured, the major concern is to carry out the following steps:

1. Assessing the type and extent of splinting needed
2. Finishing the tooth preparations
3. Making the impressions, casts, and dies
4. Articulating and recording functional characteristics of master casts
5. Designing and fabricating the prostheses
6. Cementing the prostheses

ASSESSING THE EXTENT OF SPLINTING

Assessing the extent of splinting must be done prior to finalization of the preparations, since the method and extent of splinting will often determine the degree of tooth reduction necessary for certain teeth, especially if precision attachments or telescoped crowns are planned. In order to determine the extent of splinting required, the provisional splints must be removed, and the remaining abutment teeth must be carefully examined for pattern and degree of mobility. The extent of splinting is dictated primarily by the number of teeth involved in the reconstruction, their position in the arch, and their degree of mobility.

Since the primary purpose of splinting is to stabilize segments or all of the dentition by distributing and optimally directing functional and parafunctional forces whenever possible, a sufficient number of nonmobile teeth must be included in the splint. Splinting of any type can be unilateral or bilateral.

Unilateral Splinting

Unilateral splinting involves the joining of teeth in the same segment of the arch and is applied only if there are a sufficient number of adequately supported teeth in the same segment to lend support to the mobile teeth. This manner of splinting has severe limitations if all the teeth in the segment are mobile to some degree, since little resistance is offered to forces in a buccolingual direction. It is true that splinting a segment of loose teeth may decrease the mobility, since in most cases the pattern and degree of mobility vary from tooth to tooth and, if several are splinted together, each will contribute to the stabilization of the others. However, this may be insufficient to provide resistance to the stresses over the years, and the entire splinted segment may become excessively mobile. Unless provision has been made to extend the splint to include adjacent segments of the same arch, the original splint may have to be remade. Whenever unilateral splints can be used, provision should be made for the incorporation of adjacent segments if the need arises. This can be accomplished by the use of semiprecision or precision attachments (Fig. 29-1), or by the use of telescoping crowns (Fig. 29-2).

Figure 29-1A illustrates unilateral splints that have been permanently set for a periodontally treated mandibular arch. At this time there is no indication of the need to splint bilaterally, since it is felt that these segments appear to be capable of resisting stress. In addition, the anterior segment is perfectly aligned and requires no restorations. However, milled dove-tailed grooves are incorporated into the mesial aspects of both first premolars so that if the need arises any or all of the anterior teeth can be splinted and indirectly attached to the posterior segments in a simple fashion without disturbing the posterior segments.

In Figure 29-2, the same principle is applied, with

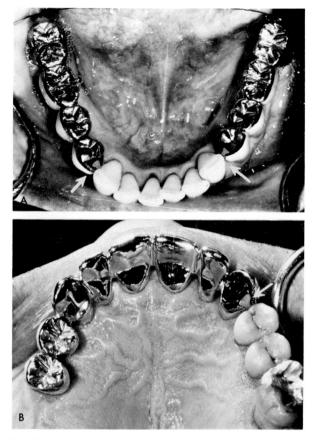

FIG. 29-1. *Dove-tailed semiprecision grooves incorporated into segment splints and filled with acrylic resin as a means of linking adjacent segments of teeth if they require future splinting. A. Splinted posterior segments with dove-tailed grooves (arrows) in mesial aspects of first premolars. B. Maxillary splint with dove-tailed groove (arrow) in distal aspect of right cuspid, which will allow linkage of right posterior segment should need arise.*

the use of precisely designed copings that are soldered to a splinted segment with individual telescoped crowns that are temporarily cemented to the copings. Whenever the unilateral splints require joining or the anterior segment requires stabilization, the anterior teeth can be prepared, and crowns can be constructed and soldered to the removable telescoped crown and set with a permanent cement.

Bilateral or Cross-Arch Splinting

If all the teeth in a posterior segment demonstrate hypermobility or if it can be ascertained that mobility is likely to increase in time, splinting should be extensive enough to include the support of the anterior segment and in some cases even the opposite quadrant. For similar reasons it may be necessary to include the support of sturdy posterior teeth when anterior segments are in need of splinting. It is disconcerting to see

an entire anterior segment of splinted teeth migrate anteriorly after a period of time because of failure to include a sufficient number of nonmobile teeth in adjacent quadrants.

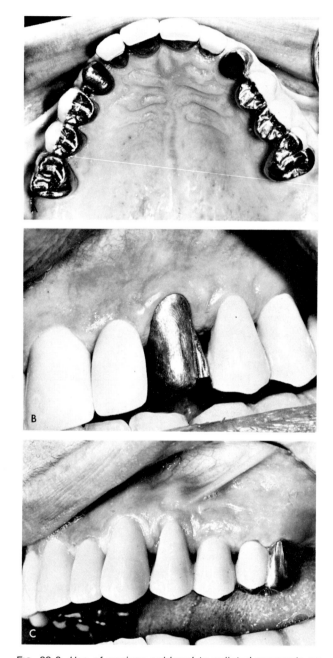

FIG. 29-2. *Use of copings soldered to splinted segments as another means of linking adjacent segments. A. Occlusal view of a maxillary reconstruction, showing the cuspid copings that are soldered to the splinted posterior segments. The incisors are not splinted. B. Lateral view of coping, prior to temporary cementation of telescoped cuspid porcelain-faced crown. Note that solder joint between coping and posterior splint does not obliterate the interproximal embrasure. C. Lateral view with telescoped cuspid restoration cemented with temporary cement.*

When all the remaining abutment teeth are mobile, bilateral or cross-arch splinting is mandatory, as this will provide additional resistance to stress in all directions. Since the pattern and degree of mobility are different for each tooth, mobile teeth can lend support to each other. The pattern of mobility in some of these teeth is in a buccolingual direction; in others it is in a mesiodistal direction. Cross-arch splinting of a group of such teeth in effect creates a single multirooted unit (Fig. 29-3).[1]

Occasionally, both maxillary posterior segments require stabilization, but the anterior teeth are in excellent condition from both the periodontal and coronal point of view and do not require splinting or restoration. Cross-arch stabilization for this condition can be obtained by incorporating a removable palatal strap (Fig. 29-4). This technique involves the milling of dove-tailed slots or incorporating precision attachments into the crowns or pontics in the molar region.

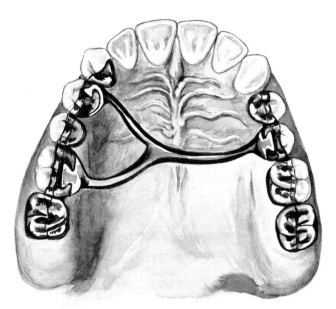

FIG. 29-4. *Method of cross-arch splinting with a precisely designed removable palatal strap that is keyed into premolar and molar pontics. This method can be used when the anterior teeth do not require splinting or restoration.*

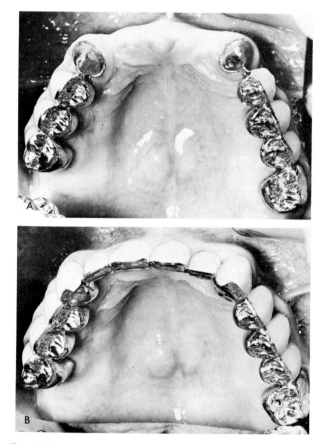

FIG. 29-3. *Method of cross-arch splinting by segmented cross-linked splints. A. Maxillary reconstruction showing cuspid copings that are joined to permanently cemented posterior segments. B. Separate anterior splint in place and set temporarily. This will allow for removal of the anterior segment for re-veneering or repairing if the need arises.*

FINISHING THE TOOTH PREPARATIONS

The final preparation of the abutment teeth is generally reserved until the supporting endodontic therapy is complete. There are five important factors to consider prior to finishing the preparations:

1. Protection of gingival and pulpal tissues during crown preparation (Fig. 26-4)
2. Location of the gingival margins of the restoration (Fig. 26-7)
3. Type of coverage to be used, partial or full
4. Amount of tooth reduction necessary and type of gingival finish line
5. Management of endodontically treated teeth

The first two factors were discussed in Chapter 26. The important point to stress is that patients requiring periodontal prosthetic therapy have an exaggerated response to the slightest tissue insults. Care must be exercised not to injure the gingival tissues unduly during the final abutment preparations. Such injuries may cause recessions, especially if the epithelial attachment has been disturbed (Fig. 26-2). Rosen and Gitnick describe a procedure for finishing crown preparation just after epithelialization of the attached gingiva has taken place (usually about 6 to 8 weeks after periodontal surgical intervention) (Fig. 29-5A, B).[10] At this time the free gingival margin has not yet developed, and insuf-

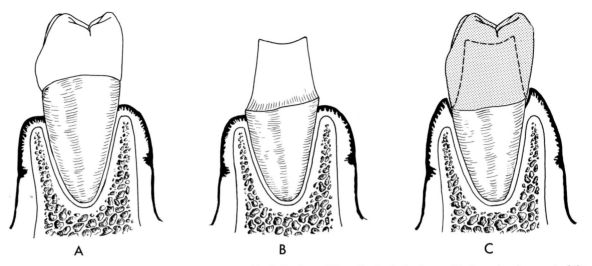

FIG. 29-5. *Finishing the coronal preparation just after epithelialization of the attached gingiva and before development of the free gingival margin of teeth that have undergone periodontic surgery (after Rosen and Gitnick). A. Six to eight weeks after surgery, showing lack of gingival sulcus. B. Immediately after coronal preparation with supragingivally placed margin. C. After development of a free gingival margin and sulcus. As a result, the crown margins will be covered.*

ficient sulcus depth prevents establishment of a subgingival margin. The margin is kept just above the gingival tissue line, and impressions are made without the need of gingival retraction. As the gingival tissues mature, a free gingival margin develops and covers the margin of the restoration, so that in most cases the supragingival margin becomes subgingival (Fig. 29-5C). Occasionally, however, there is further recession, so that on maturation of the free gingival margin the gingival margins of the restoration remain in a supragingival position. If it is imperative to keep the margin subgingival for reasons of esthetics, sensitivity, or a high caries index, it is best to wait for a period of approximately 6 months after periodontal surgery to ensure a stable gingival margin.

Partial versus Full Coverage

The decision as to whether partial or full coverage should be used is usually made at the time of provisional stabilization. Occasionally, however, because of unexpected endodontic therapy or because for some other reason three-quarter crowns or pin-ledged restorations prove insufficient, conversion to full-coverage crowns must be made in order to provide the needed retention. The use of full-coverage or partial-coverage crowns should depend upon the patient's need and not upon the dentist's preference for one type over another. Factors such as adequate tooth and arch alignment, sufficient periodontal support, and minimal coronal breakdown are usually indications for partial coverage (Figs. 29-6, 7E), whereas a high incidence of caries, permanent mobility from loss of bone support,

loss of strategically positioned abutments, long edentulous spans (Fig. 29-7A–D), minimal retention resulting from coronal breakdown or short crowns, and poor tooth and arch alignment all call for the use of full coverage. In addition, advanced cases of periodontal disease requiring periodontal therapeutic procedures that include extensive ostectomy and mucogingival surgery may result in severe recession. As a result, coronal contours that were once subgingival are now supragingival and are no longer physiologic. The management of such factors is best accomplished by full-coverage restorations (Fig. 26-20). Other factors in deciding whether full coverage or partial coverage should be used are discussed in Chapter 28.

Amount of Tooth Reduction and Type of Gingival Finish Line

The amount of tooth to be reduced and the type of gingival finish line is chiefly influenced by whether the crowns are to be acrylic-veneered or porcelain-veneered and whether copings are to be used, as in telescope reconstructions.

All too often many full-crown preparations are underreduced at the gingival third and overreduced at the occlusal third. This reduction usually results in excessively overcontoured crowns that have inadequate retention. The problems related to overcontouring have been stressed in Chapter 26. As a general rule, sufficient tooth reduction must be made so that the final restoration remains within the original confines of the tooth at the gingival third section. If the treatment plan calls for porcelain or acrylic veneering and for copings (Fig. 29-8), much more reduction of the facial and interproximal surfaces will be needed, especially at the gingival third of the tooth, than would normally be required for a full gold crown.

After resective procedures to eliminate periodontal pockets, many teeth have increased crown length and, in the case of multirooted teeth, exaggerated flutings in furcation regions. Vital pulp extirpation may be necessary in order to adequately reduce such crowns so that the final restoration is not overcontoured. Extirpation of vital pulp should not be a substitute for careful crown preparation, but when indicated it is an extremely useful procedure in reaching some objectives in periodontal prosthetic reconstruction.

Many dentitions require reorientation of the occlusal plane or sufficient reduction to gain parallelism of the individual crown with respect to other abutments (Fig. 26-35).

Following periodontal therapy, many problems in abutment preparation are magnified because of increased clinical-crown length, which may make parallelism impossible unless the pulps are extirpated or copings are used (Fig. 29-9). Bohannan and Abrams state that, "no tooth, or component of a tooth, should be regarded as sacred if the prognosis of the remaining dentition is improved by its sacrifice. Regard for the preservation of tooth structure becomes false conservation if, through this preservation, the prognosis of the entire masticatory mechanism is endangered."[3] We concur with this philosophy, but caution against the danger of overrationalizing in cases where a little care in crown preparation would preserve a healthy pulp.

Malaligned teeth and extensively long crowns create obstacles in full-arch splinting. Frequently parallelism is impossible to attain unless the pulp is removed. However, it should be removed only as a last resort, and only if minor tooth movement or the use of the telescoping principle is insufficient to solve the problem.

Coronal Preparation of Teeth with Root Amputations or Hemisected Teeth

It is not uncommon, when splinting teeth, to include the support of teeth that have undergone hemisection or root amputation in periodontal prosthetic cases.

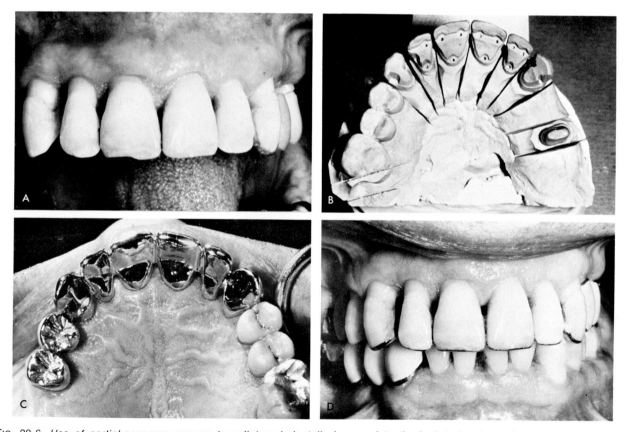

FIG. 29-6. *Use of partial-coverage crowns to splint periodontally loosened teeth. A. Anterior view, showing lack of coronal breakdown and good alignment, important factors if partial-coverage splinting is considered. B. View of stone dies of prepared teeth. C. Splint in place (Right posterior quadrant did not require splinting). D. Anterior view of permanently set splint. (Courtesy Dr. J. Weaver)*

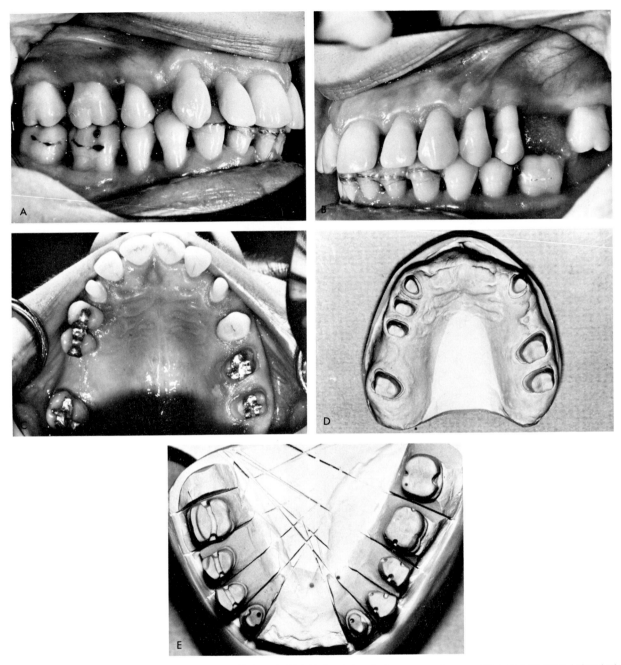

FIG. 29-7. *Use of both partial- and full-coverage splinting. A. Right lateral view before coronal preparation. B. Left lateral view before coronal preparation. C. Occlusal view of maxillary teeth at time of coronal preparation. All the incisors and right second premolar will be extracted because of severe periodontal involvement. D. Cast of prepared maxillary teeth, showing full coverage preparations of all teeth. Full coverage was decided upon because of generalized mobility and loss of too many periodontally involved teeth. E. Cast of prepared mandibular teeth, showing combinations of partial- and full-coverage preparations. All incisors also required extraction because of severe periodontal involvement (Courtesy Dr. C. Filipchuk.)*

Generally speaking, however, we recommend that such teeth should not be considered for use if approximating teeth are well supported and are sufficient in number to provide the stabilization required for the dentition undergoing treatment. Not uncommonly and sometimes for unexplainable reasons, the remaining bone support of some hemisected teeth and teeth with root amputations continues to deteriorate in spite of all efforts to stop deterioration. It is not always possible to predict which teeth may suffer deterioration, and if such teeth are contemplated for use, the risks must be considered. The advantages of including them must

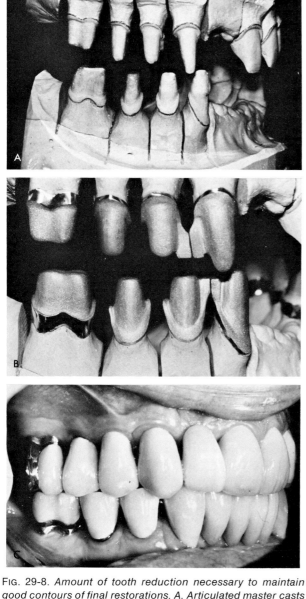

Fig. 29-8. *Amount of tooth reduction necessary to maintain good contours of final restorations. A. Articulated master casts of prepared teeth, showing amount of coronal reduction that is necessary if copings with telescoped reconstruction are planned. B. Cast copings in place, showing design to maintain contour and provide retention for superstructure. C. Telescoped reconstruction set to copings with temporary cement, showing good contours that were possible because of sufficient coronal reduction in (A). (Courtesy Dr. C. Filipchuk.)*

be weighed against the problems encountered when they fail. If there is no choice and they must be used because they are the only ones available and extraction obviates the fabrication of a removable partial denture, provision should be made to make simple alterations to the prosthesis so that it can function adequately when removal of such teeth becomes necessary.

Whenever there is a choice of which root to amputate to correct a periodontal lesion, the root that is most amenable to endodontic therapy and subsequent restoration should be the one preserved. Regardless of the bone support, the morphology of certain roots accounts for many difficulties in using them for abutments. An example of this type of root is the mesial root of the lower molars (Fig. 29-10). Usually these roots are narrow mesiodistally as well as fluted, and they also have two tortuous root canals that cannot be adequately prepared to accept dowels, which are usually necessary for anchoring the coping or retainer. If there is a choice for such teeth, the distal root of lower molars is morphologically better suited as an abutment, since it is bulkier, straighter, and has one canal.

There are rare occasions when both roots of a mandibular molar can be used as abutments after hemisection. In these instances, it is important that the roots be widely divergent and that they have approximately equal amounts of supporting bone. In such cases, the birooted molar is converted into single-rooted abutments (Fig. 29-11).

When such teeth are used as abutments, their coronal preparation requires special consideration. During the reduction procedures, the entire portion of the crown that was a direct extension of the amputated root should be cut away (Fig. 29-12). The coronal preparation is incomplete if any part of the amputated root is allowed to remain intact (Figs. 29-13, 14). This would only encourage plaque retention, frustrate oral-hygienic measures, and usually result in caries and gingival irritation. Typical preparations for maxillary and mandibular teeth that have undergone root amputations, and the manner in which such teeth are restored are shown in Figure 29-15 and throughout the text.

MAKING THE IMPRESSIONS, CASTS, AND DIES

A number of new materials that have been developed in recent years to aid the dentist in making precise reproductions of prepared teeth and their surrounding tissues maintain this dimensional accuracy during impression removal and cast pouring. This difficult phase of periodontal prosthetics has thereby been greatly simplified.

There are many recognized techniques for making impressions, casts, and dies, and several excellent texts to which the reader is referred.[5,6,7] Only those aspects of this phase of periodontal prosthetics that pertain to the supporting tissues will be discussed in detail here.

Of the impression materials, the reversible hydrocolloids, rubber, and silicone are the simplest to use. They do, however, require the retraction of the free

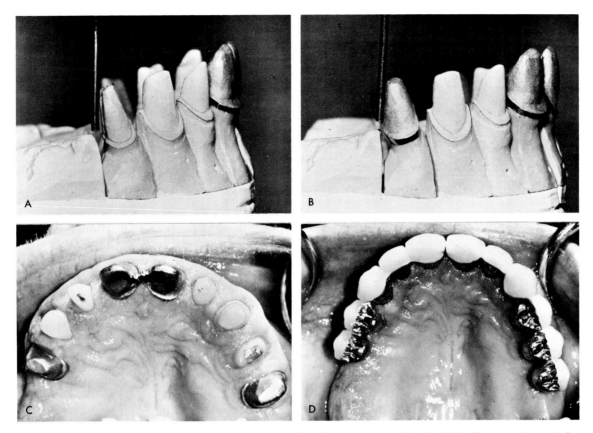

FIG. 29-9. *Method of overcoming lack of parallelism with the use of copings on selected teeth. A. Maxillary master cast of prepared teeth being surveyed to show amount of undercut. Further reduction of premolar would have necessitated pulp extirpation. B. Coping being surveyed to show parallelism with coping on central incisors. The coping was designed to eliminate the undercut. C. Occlusal view of copings in place. Copings on central incisors were joined by soldering to allow segmentation of maxillary splint into two parts while achieving cross-arch stabilization. D. Right and left splints in place. Premolar pontics were cantilevered on each side to provide for additional occlusal function.*

gingiva in order to expose any subgingivally placed margins, since none of these materials can adequately displace soft tissues. The manner in which retraction of the free gingiva is accomplished will greatly influence both the degree of accuracy of the impressions and the condition of the gingival tissues following the procedure.

Retraction of the Free Gingival Margin

The two most common methods, displacement with chemically impregnated retraction cords and electrosurgery, have been discussed in Chapter 26. Regardless of the choice of technique, meticulous care must be exercised to avoid damaging the gingival tissues.

Tissue-displacement procedures must never be undertaken if the tissues are in any degree swollen or hemorrhagic. Whichever of the two procedures is used, it will cause further insult to the gingiva and may bring about gingival recession (Fig. 26-3). A healthy gingival sulcus is usually one that is no deeper than 1 to 3 mm.

Any greater depth is highly suspicious and needs periodontal evaluation prior to extension of a subgingival margin or starting an impression procedure. Retraction procedures must be exercised with great care where thin and delicate or minimal zones of attached gingival tissue exist. Undue trauma will commonly result in recession or cleft formation.

PROCEDURE FOR USING RETRACTION CORDS

Most gingival retraction cords can be used with relative safety, though some should be avoided. The retraction can be by mechanical displacement or by combined mechanical and chemical means. However, precautions must be taken when using cords impregnated with 8 percent epinephrine solution while making full-arch impressions. The collective effect of so much epinephrine may evoke a pathologic response, which is sometimes severe in patients with cardiac involvement, hyperthyroidism, hypertension, or with inflamed or lacerated tissues. With such patients it is

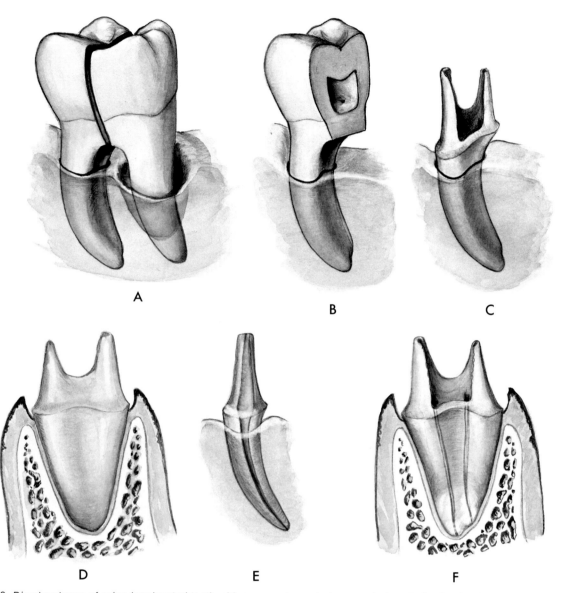

A

B

C

D

E

F

FIG. 29-10. *Disadvantages of using hemisected teeth with poor root morphology as abutments for fixed splints. A. Molar abutment requiring hemisection of severely involved distal root. B. View of remaining mesial portion showing poor morphology of root. C. Amount of reduction usually necessary to attain taper. This, unfortunately, often results in perforations to the pulp chamber which seriously decrease the retentive qualities of the abutment. D. Mesial view of prepared mesial portion of tooth to show amount of perforation into pulp chamber. E. Buccal view of preparation. F. Distal view of prepared mesial portion of molar to show lack of sufficient remaining tooth structure. Note also that the two canals are characteristically narrow and tortuous, preventing the use of endodontic posts to gain retention.*

better to use a plain cord in combination with a small amount of a hemostatic agent such as Hemodent° in order to obtain tissue displacement and hemorrhage control. Caution should be exercised in the excessive use of astringent agents in combination with retraction cords, since this may easily cause gingival sloughing and result in recession if the cord remains in position too long. There is no reason for the cord to remain in the sulcus longer than 10 to 15 minutes.

Excessive salivation should be controlled. This is not usually a problem in retraction and impression procedures in the maxillary arch and can be easily controlled with gauze or cotton rolls. However, salivation is not so easily controlled during mandibular procedures, and an antisialagogue such as Banthine° may have to be prescribed (50 to 100 mg one hour prior to procedure).

Remove the provisional splints and thoroughly clean the prepared teeth and gingival sulcus of all traces of

° Premier Dental Products, Philadelphia, Pa.

° Searle & Co., Chicago, Ill.

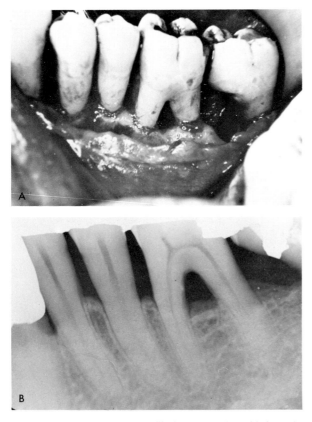

FIG. 29-11. *Example of a mandibular first molar with furcation involvement but where both roots may be used as abutments since the roots are sufficiently divergent. A. Surgical correction of osseous defect. Note that roots have equal amount of supporting bone. B. Radiograph to show wide divergence of mesial and distal roots.*

temporary cement. If zinc oxide and eugenol is the cement used, cotton pledgets soaked in orange solvent will adequately clean the teeth. Remove any stubborn stains or remnants of cement with prophylactic paste. Thoroughly rinse, dry, and inspect the teeth to ensure that all traces of cement and stain have been removed.

Isolate the teeth with gauze or cotton rolls. In the case of the mandibular arch a device such as a Svedopter† is greatly beneficial, not only to remove saliva but also to retract the tongue.

Dry the prepared teeth lightly, but do not dry them out completely. Choose a retraction cord suitable to serve the needs of each tooth individually. The nature of the tissue (delicate or fibrotic) and the depth of the sulcus will determine the choice of cord thickness. Precaution must be taken not to use too much or to use a cord of excessive diameter, since this will require undue force in placement and may cause damage to the attachment.

Cut a length of cord slightly greater than is needed

†Svedia Dental Industri, Enköping, Sweden

to encircle the tooth. An unduly long piece of cord will interfere with its placement. Soak the cord in Hemodent and blot it with gauze to remove the excess. The use of two packing instruments is recommended, one to tuck the cord into the sulcus and the other to hold securely that portion of the cord that has been tucked in. In this way, the cord is not dislodged by the packing procedure.

Position one end of the cord in an interproximal region, and with a tucking motion pack the cord into the gingival sulcus, to a depth that just barely exposes the gingival margin of the prepared crown. Carry the packing around on the lingual side and then into the other interproximal area. At approximately 5-mm intervals, hold the cord that has been tucked into the sulcus securely with a second packing instrument while

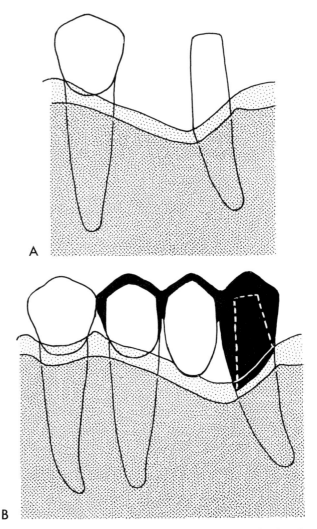

FIG. 29-12. *Typical preparation of distal portion of a hemisected mandibular molar to be used as an abutment. A. Preparation showing sufficient tooth reduction to extend margins subgingivally and to gain taper. B. Fixed partial denture in place.*

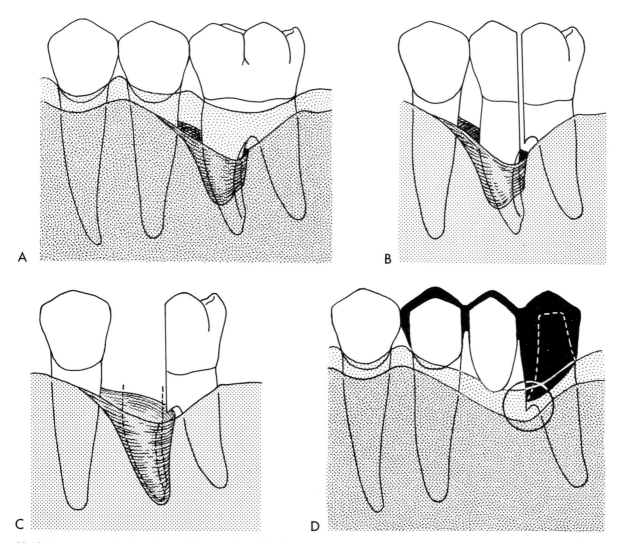

FIG. 29-13. *Improper reduction of remaining portion of hemisected molar. A. View showing periodontally involved mandibular first molar. B. Hemisected molar. C. Condemned mesial portion extracted. D. Insufficient reduction of remaining distal portion, leaving portion of amputated mesial root in bifurcation region. This will encourage plaque retention, frustrate oral hygiene, and result in caries and periodontal breakdown.*

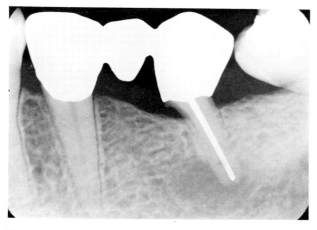

FIG. 29-14. *Radiograph of improperly reduced hemisected molar used as an abutment for a fixed partial denture as described in Fig. 29-13.*

continuing the packing procedure (Fig. 29-16). This will prevent the cord that has already been tucked into the sulcus from being dislodged by the packing motion.

Never overlap the free ends in the gingival sulcus on the facial aspect, since in most cases the free gingival margin in this region is less fibrous and is more vulnerable to trauma from the packing procedure. Overlap the free ends interproximally, leaving a small length of the end of the cord exposed (Fig. 29-16C). This will facilitate its rapid removal prior to injecting the impression material into the sulcus. Continue in this manner until the sulci of all the prepared teeth have been packed. If the gingival tissue is fibrotic, pack a second strand carefully into the gingival sulcus to a depth that is at or slightly coronal to the gingival margin of the prepared abutment. The sole purpose of the second strand is to displace the fibrotic free gingival margin so as to accommodate additional impression material. There will be less likelihood of the impression tearing in this region upon removal if this is done.

ALTERNATIVE METHODS OF TISSUE DISPLACEMENT

Another way of displacing the free gingival margin is to use a periodontal surgical dressing instead of the zinc oxide-eugenol cement when placing a provisional splint. This is especially recommended if there is insufficient time after the preparations have been finished to make the impression and reline the provisional splint. A thin mix of periodontal dressing such as Coe-

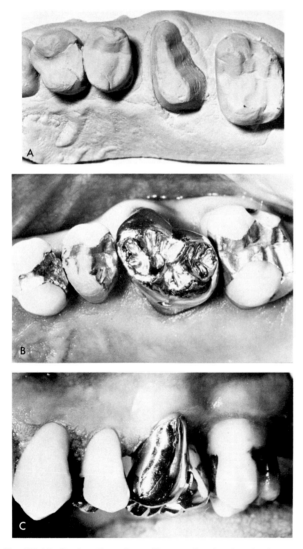

FIG. 29-15. *Restoration of maxillary molar that has had a root amputated. A. Stone die of prepared tooth showing altered form of coronal reduction required because of missing disto-buccal root. B. Occlusal view of restoration showing suggested occlusal form. C. Buccal view of restoration showing altered contour to eliminate excessive convexity that would interfere with plaque removal. (Courtesy Dr. J. Townsend.)*

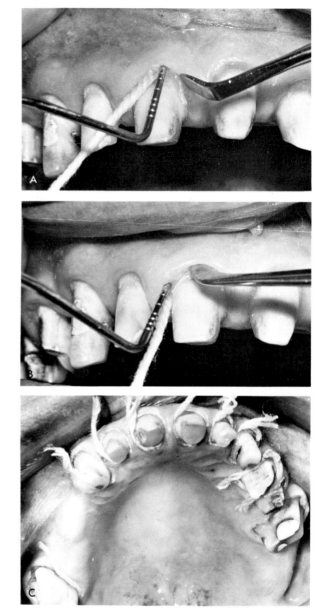

FIG. 29-16. *Procedure for gingival retraction. A. End of retraction cord properly positioned interproximally where the gingiva is usually firmer and less likely to be damaged during initiation of the tucking procedure and is more likely to hold the cord in position. B. Cord that has been tucked subgingivally being held in position by a second instrument to prevent its dislodgement while continuing the packing procedure. C. Free ends of cord are overlapped slightly in interproximal region.*

Pak° is made and quickly placed in the crowns of the provisional splint. If a firm biting pressure is maintained while it sets, the gingival sulcus will usually fill with the dressing and any excess can be molded interproximally, facially, and lingually (Fig. 29-17). At a subsequent appointment (preferably within 2 to 3 days

° Coe Laboratories, Inc., Chicago, Ill.

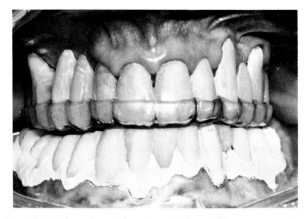

FIG. 29-17. *Use of periodontal pack (Coe-Pak) as a cementing medium to accomplish some of the retraction prior to making the impression.*

and never more than a week later), the splint is removed and the teeth and gingival sulcus are carefully cleared of any remnants of the surgical pack. In most cases all the margins of the preparations will be exposed. If, however, additional retraction is required in some regions, cord or electrosurgery may be used to complete the procedure.

Retraction by electrosurgery is rapidly gaining popularity. With care, the gingival sulcus can be widened electrosurgically to facilitate either the placement of the gingival finish line and/or the free flow of the impression material during making of the impression. This method is not recommended in regions of inflammation or to retract extremely thin gingival tissue, since the results will be a recession and a decrease or loss of the zone of attached gingival tissue.

If electrosurgery is done with skill and great care, a subgingival trough can be created, of a desired width and depth, prior to extending the subgingival margin of the coronal preparation. The preparation can now be precisely cut to the proper depth without any interference from the gingival tissue. This often results in much less abrasion of the sulcular epithelium. The impression can then be made in a routine manner without the need for further tissue displacement. Postretraction hemorrhage is eliminated, since the capillaries are sealed off during the creation of the trough.

Immediately following electrosurgical retraction, a water spray containing a 3 percent hydrogen peroxide solution is used to debride the area completely. This debridement leaves an area free of all charred pieces of tissue that were originally attached to tooth structure. The area is then dried with air, and the impression of choice is made. If this technique is carefully executed, impressions with precise definition are readily obtained.

Making the Impressions

If cords have been used to displace the tissues, the manner in which they should be removed depends upon the type of impression material used.

PROCEDURES

When reversible hydrocolloid is the material of choice, remove all the cords one minute prior to injection of the impression material. Following cord removal, spray the prepared teeth and gingival tissues with a 3 percent hydrogen peroxide solution and rinse thoroughly. This will irrigate the sulcular region, rid it of all particulate matter, control hemorrhage, and dissolve excessive saliva. Suction off excessive saliva, but do not attempt to dry the teeth. Inject the hydrocolloid material into the gingival sulcus, being careful not to tear the soft tissue with the fine tip of the syringe, since tearing may cause bleeding. It is not necessary to position the tip in the base of the sulcus. Keep the tip close to the finish line and keep the flow of hydrocolloid continuous. When all the prepared teeth have been covered, place the tray filled with the heavier-bodied hydrocolloid in position over the teeth and remove it after sufficient time has elapsed for the material to gel (usually 5 minutes). If satisfactory, wash the impression gently in water at room temperature and place it in 2 percent potassium sulfate solution for a maximum of 10 minutes before pouring in a suspension of hard stone-die mix.

If rubber impression material is used, have the assistant remove the retraction cords one at a time and immediately inject the material into the sulcus after each cord is removed. Complete the impression in a routine manner; remove and pour in the stone mix as soon as possible.

Carefully inspect each gingival sulcus for tears and remnants of impression material. Traces of impression material, especially of rubber impression material, carelessly neglected and allowed to remain in the gingival sulcus, will cause severe inflammation and, if allowed to remain long enough, tissue sloughing and permanent alteration of the supporting tissues.

Provisional-Splint Relining

If the impressions are made on the same day that the preparations are finished, the provisional splint will have to be relined with autopolymerizing acrylic resin, in order to protect any freshly cut portion of the abutment teeth. Failure to do this will result in hypersensitivity, promote retention of plaque and particulate matter, discourage adequate oral-hygiene measures, and promote rapid dissolution of the temporary cement. All of these factors will seriously affect the health of the supporting and pulpal tissues.

PROCEDURE

Clean the provisional splint with the aid of an ultrasonic cleaner and an appropriate cleaning solution. With round burs, freshen the inside of each abutment crown to remove any traces of temporary cement. Cut away approximately 2 mm of the gingival margin of each acrylic crown and serrate slightly the freshly cut margin. In addition, freshen the gingival third of the exterior surface of each acrylic crown.

Lightly dry the prepared abutment teeth, repaint with Metimyd° followed by cavity varnish, and reline the provisional splint in a similar manner as is described in Chapter 28 for relining the shell of the provisional splint. Carefully polish the splint, check for occlusal and gingival margin discrepancies, and, if satisfactory, reset the provisional splint over the prepared teeth, but do not cement in place. Reexamine the functional occlusion and correct any discrepancies, making sure that there is no discrepancy between CRO and CO; these should be coincidental. Polish and reset with petroleum jelly. Obtain accurate alginate or reversible-hydrocolloid impressions of the maxillary and mandibular provisional restorations. Pour these with a mix of hard stone. Allow sufficient time for setting; separate, trim, and carefully check. Remove any bubbles from the occlusal surfaces. Reset the provisional splints with temporary cement.

Preparation of Master Working Casts and Dies

A hard artificial die stone is recommended for the master working casts and dies. The impressions of the abutment teeth are poured, using an accurately proportioned mix of die stone, with dowel pins precisely positioned into the soft stone of each abutment. When this first pour has set sufficiently, the stone base by each pin is keyed with a round bur (Fig. 29-18). The stone base and dowel pins are lubricated with a separating medium, and the remainder of the impression is poured with a hard stone of a different color to form the base of the working cast. One hour should be allowed for setting of the stone before separating the cast from the impression. The dies are then separated and carefully trimmed to clearly expose all margins (Fig. 29-19).

At a subsequent appointment, the necessary registrations are obtained for transferring the working casts

° Shering Corp.

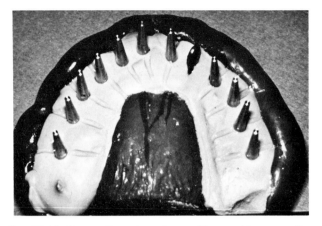

FIG. 29-18. *Preparation of master working cast incorporating removable dies. Note that stone base by each dowel pin is keyed before the base of the cast is poured.*

to an articulator of the dentist's choice. It is preferable to make these registrations and articulate the casts during the same appointment. This allows the dentist to verify the accuracy of the mounting by comparing the static and functional contact relationships of the

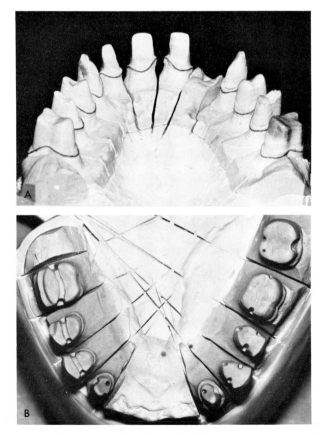

FIG. 29-19. *Dies separated for individual removal from base of master working cast, and carefully trimmed to expose clearly all margins which are then penciled in preparation for waxing. A. Maxillary master working cast. B. Mandibular master working cast.*

articulated master casts with those of the patient's prepared teeth.

ARTICULATING AND RECORDING FUNCTIONAL CHARACTERISTICS OF MASTER CASTS

The articulator that best serves the needs of the patient must be selected from among the many models that have been developed to complement the differing concepts of oral rehabilitation. The dentist is often perplexed by the need to select the right model, since designs have of recent years become specialized. Success in the complex discipline of oral rehabilitation cannot be ensured solely by virtue of the dentist choosing to use an intricately designed, fully adjustable articulator that is capable of copying the border movement of each patient. In any science or art an instrument is only as good as its operator. The knowledge and skill of the dentist and his technician are far more important in determining the quality of the results obtained, regardless of the concepts or instrumentation used.

Concepts of Occlusion in Oral Rehabilitation

Most of the emphasis of the more recent concepts in oral rehabilitation is centered on dental occlusion. Functional occlusion is only one important factor in achieving a successful result. Other factors—marginal fit, embrasures, coronal contours, and extent of splinting—must also be recognized. However, of paramount importance is the state of health of the periodontium before, during, and after oral rehabilitation. It behooves the dentist first to recognize morphologic aberrations and destructive factors that may affect the outcome of rehabilitation and to compensate for or correct these conditions, and second to train the patient to maintain his mouth in an optimal state of health. Therefore, the patient must be provided with the necessary knowledge so that he may adequately fulfill this important responsibility.

The morphologic characteristics of restorations as they may affect periodontal health have been reviewed in Chapter 26. It is comparatively easy to accept or reject concepts regarding morphology and periodontal health because results are readily measured. Variations in morphologic characteristics can either contribute to plaque retention and frustrate its removal or they can simplify its removal by the patient. Similarly, the degree of periodontal health or of support loss is easily measured. The long-term effects of the application of varying concepts of correct functional occlusion in oral

rehabilitation are more difficult to measure. Many of these concepts are controversial and probably will never be unanimously accepted. There are three reasons for this:

1. Much knowledge of occlusion is empirically rather than scientifically based.
2. Because of the great physiologic variation in different mouths, the fact that application of one concept may appear successful for one patient need not mean that it would be successful for all.
3. The individual dentist is an enormously variable factor, as are the standards by which he evaluates his therapy.

There is no simple solution to occlusal problems. The dentist should abide by the principles of what is accepted as a physiologically functional occlusion as it pertains to each individual patient. The same principles that are widely accepted as being functional and physiologic in natural dentitions, or what the end result of an occlusal adjustment should be, are also applicable to oral rehabilitation.

Some of the more commonly accepted methods of oral rehabilitation, among them the gnathologic concept (cusp-to-fossa, mutually protected occlusions),[12,13] and the Pankey-Mann-Schyler philosophy (long centric, incisal guidance, functionally generated group function),[8,11] all embrace the commonly accepted principles of what constitutes a normal physiologic occlusion. This fact helps to explain why proponents of differing concepts can claim success. To reiterate, certain principles of functional occlusion are widely accepted as being the most important in achieving a successful result in oral rehabilitation:

1. There should be maximum simultaneous contact of all centric holding areas in the CRO position.
2. Centric relation occlusal position should be a stable position with only a narrow range of cuspal noninterference before anterior guidance prevails.
3. Centric relation occlusion and centric occlusion should coincide.
4. There should be a stable cusp-to-fossa relationship whenever possible, rather than a cusp-to-marginal-ridge relationship.
5. Cusps should be shaped in such a way as to make contact as closely as possible with the centers of the fossae. In this way the horizontal forces will be directed axially.
6. There should be contact between the centric holding cusp tips (rather than a broad surface) and a flat horizontal area in the centers of the

fossae. There should be no cusp contact on inclined planes, except on the lingual surfaces of the maxillary anterior teeth or with a reciprocal contact on a balancing inclined plane. In unworn dentitions, cusp tips often do not reach the bases of the fossae; here multiple-point contacts on the balanced reciprocally inclined planes are stable and desirable.

7. A slight cuspid disclusion of the posterior teeth during lateral excursions is desirable except when (a) the cuspid is worn and there is an existing group function with no evidence of trauma or (b) the cuspid is malposed or periodontally weakened. In these cases posterior group function must be provided.

8. There should be no cross-arch and cross-tooth balancing contacts or deflective interferences.

9. There should be no deflective central or lateral incisor contacts that prevent cuspid function during lateral excursions.

10. Contact during protrusive excursions should be evenly distributed over as many anterior teeth as possible, with no posterior interference, except for the mesial slope of the buccal cusp of the mandibular first premolars, if these are within practical range.

It is obvious that these principles are not derived from a single concept, but from several. Many of our currently recognized concepts of rehabilitation have certain advantages and disadvantages. The choice depends greatly on the dentist's capabilities. Therefore, each dentist who wishes to perform such therapy should well understand his limitations and choose a method accordingly. Once he has mastered the basic techniques of less difficult procedures, he may then progress to treatment of more difficult cases that require the intricate knowledge and skills of the more sophisticated techniques of rehabilitation. It is unwise to attempt the complex procedures associated with oral rehabilitation before acquiring the basic talent and knowledge and the mastery of the skills of less complicated procedures in restorative dentistry.

Role of the Articulator in Periodontal Prosthetics

The type of articulator that the dentist chooses should depend on his ability to master the procedures associated with its use. The most sophisticated articulator can do no more than a simple hinge articulator unless the dentist is capable of accurately programming such an articulator to copy mandibular border movements.

It is obvious that the more complex, fully adjustable articulators, if properly programmed, will aid in achieving more intricate occlusal patterns. It is impossible to judge, however, whether the patient really requires such accuracy as can be offered by the gnathologic approach or if a less complex pattern of occlusion would be equally successful.

The principles of the fully adjustable articulator were conceived in an era when a fully balanced occlusion was erroneously thought to be ideal. If the fully balanced concept had proven to be the correct one, then such instrumentation would indeed be useful, since fully balanced occlusion would be most difficult, if not impossible, to attain without the aid of such an instrument. With the advent of the concept of mutually protected occlusions such accuracy becomes less significant. This is not to say that complex instruments have no place in oral rehabilitation. Indeed, the mastery of such instrumentation greatly helps to achieve precise functional occlusion, which is required for patients with little tolerance for occlusal discrepancies. It is for these patients that sophisticated instrumentation can be of great help, but only if the dentist has mastered the necessary skills to manage the complexities of its programming. If he is unwilling to do so, then it is far better for him not to undertake the treatment of complex cases, but to limit himself to the treatment of less involved cases.

Transfer of Master Casts to an Articulator

The accurate transfer of the master casts to the articulator of the dentist's choice is absolutely essential to the success of oral rehabilitation. The results of many hours of technical work depend primarily upon this phase. It behooves the dentist to master the procedures necessary to achieve accurate articulation of the master casts. He should never proceed with the laboratory phase of waxing unless he is certain of this accuracy.

As stated earlier (Chapter 28), it is usual for the choice of articulator to be made at the time of functional analysis and diagnostic waxing of the patient's study casts. In some cases, the articulator will also have been programmed to copy the patient's border movements. The information will come from the pantograph when a fully adjustable articulator has been chosen and from the lateral and protrusive wax records when semiadjustable instruments have been used. These registrations need not be repeated after articulating the master casts unless there is some doubt as to the accuracy of either the original registrations or the programming or a change in temporomandibular-joint and neuromuscular relationships is suspected. Thus, all that is needed to transfer the master casts is a kinematic face-bow and centric relation mounting for both the master casts of the provisional restoration or the stone duplicates of the diagnostic waxings, whichever is decided best to use, and the master working casts of the prepared abutment teeth.

It is imperative to make the spacial relationship of the articulation relative to the hinge axis the same in the master casts of the provisional restorations as in the master working casts. The reasons for this will become evident during the waxing of the prosthesis and will be discussed later. The steps and manner in which these transfers are made are described below.

PROCEDURE

The following instructions are applicable when diagnostic waxings and the shells of the provisional splints have been made from study casts mounted on a semiadjustable articulator with the aid of a kinematic face-bow transfer (see Figures 28-2 through 28-7). The technique is especially designed to ensure that the master casts of the provisional restorations and the master casts of the prepared teeth are articulated in the same spacial relationship relative to the hinge axis of the articulator.*

Locate the hinge axis (Fig. 29-20); obtain kinematic face-bow registration of the maxillary provisional restorations and use this for positioning the maxillary master cast of the provisional restorations when securing it with quick-setting plaster to the upper member of the articulator (Fig. 29-21A, B). Hand-occlude the mandibular master cast of the provisional restoration in centric relation to the mounted maxillary cast and secure it to the lower member of the articulator (Fig. 29-21C). A centric relation wax registration is not required for this step if the correct functional occlusion of the provisional restoration has already been established. There should be only one precise CRO interdigitation of the two casts.

Remove the maxillary provisional prosthesis and obtain a centric relation wax registration at the proper vertical dimension of the prepared abutment teeth and the mandibular provisional prosthesis (Fig. 29-22A). The manner of obtaining this is similar to that described for functional analysis (Chapter 12).

* The authors are greatly indebted to Drs. Dennis Smith and John Townsend for their assistance in the documentation and the treatment of the cases illustrated in Figs. 29-20 to 29-23 and Figs. 29-32 to 29-53. These cases were chosen specifically to represent the techniques of periodontal prosthetic therapy taught by the graduate division of fixed prosthetics at the University of Washington.

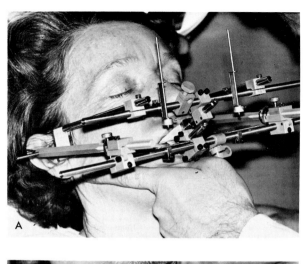

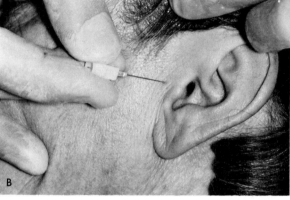

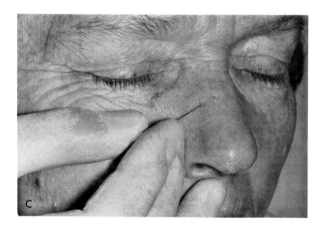

FIG. 29-20. *Location of hinge axis in preparation for kinematic face-bow transfer of the maxillary master working casts. A. Hinge-axis locator assembled. B. Permanent hinge-axis reference point tattooed. C. Third point of reference tattooed.*

With the aid of the centric relation registration, secure the maxillary master working cast to the upper member of the articulator (Fig. 29-22B). Check the accuracy of the mounting by comparing the point(s) of initial contact in the mouth, to see if these are located at precisely the same positions on the articulated casts.

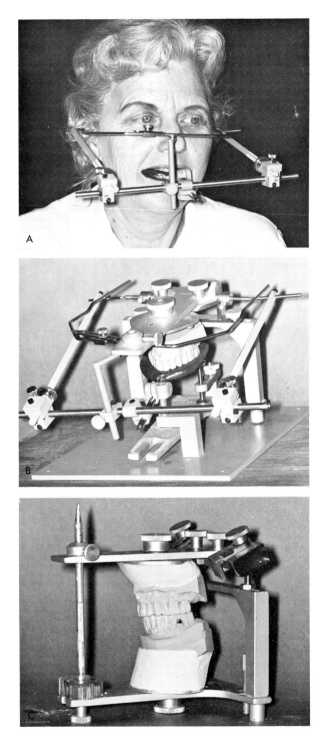

FIG. 29-21. *A. Kinematic face-bow registration of the maxillary provisional restoration. B. Face-bow transfer of maxillary cast of provisional restoration. C. Mandibular cast of provisional restoration hand-articulated in CRO and secured to lower member of articulator.*

If they are, then proceed to the next step, which is to obtain a centric relation registration of the maxillary and mandibular abutment preparations (Fig. 29-23).

There are many recognized methods of obtaining

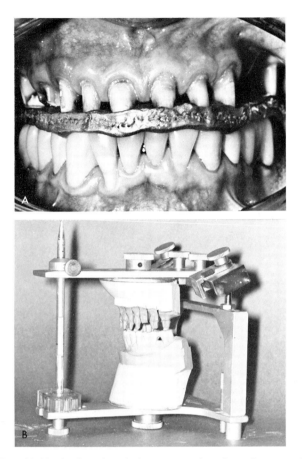

FIG. 29-22. *A. Centric relation wax registration of prepared maxillary teeth and mandibular provisional restoration. B. Maxillary master cast of prepared abutment teeth opposing the mandibular cast of the provisional restoration.*

accurate centric relation registrations. The manner in which this is done for jaws that have all the remaining teeth prepared as abutments is slightly different from that described in Chapter 12. Because there has been considerable occlusal reduction of both the upper and the lower teeth, the interocclusal wafer should be thicker to compensate for the occlusal reduction. Centric relation registration should be obtained at exactly the same vertical dimension as is desired for the reconstruction. This is especially important if an arbitrary face-bow transfer rather than a kinematic transfer has been used. Variation in vertical dimension tends to introduce error. Thus several wafers of wax (up to four) may be required to make a wafer of sufficient thickness. The center wafers may be of Moyco° hard baseplate wax and the surface wafers the usual Aluwax† cloth form wafers. The hard wax helps to reinforce the wafer. Additional reinforcement can be gained by the use of Ash's No.7 relief metal,‡ which is

° J. Bird Moyer, Philadelphia, Pa.
†Aluwax Dental Products, Grand Rapids, Mich.
‡Claudius Ash & Sons, Inc., Niagara Falls, N.Y.

applied in a similar manner to that described in Chapter 12 (Fig. 29-23A–D).

Obtain the centric relation imprints of the abutment teeth in the usual manner (Chapter 12). Chill the registration and check for warping and correct if necessary. The imprints of all mobile abutment teeth should be relieved by scraping, and the wafer should be rechecked to make certain that these teeth do not contact the wax.

Mix a sufficient amount of quick-setting zinc oxide-eugenol paste, and apply a small amount to each imprint in the wafer. Paint the occlusal surfaces of the prepared teeth with a thin film of petroleum jelly, and carefully replace the wafer over the maxillary abutment. Guide the lower jaw to its correct centric relation position, and hold gently until the paste has set. Carefully remove the wafer, chill, and recheck for warpage.

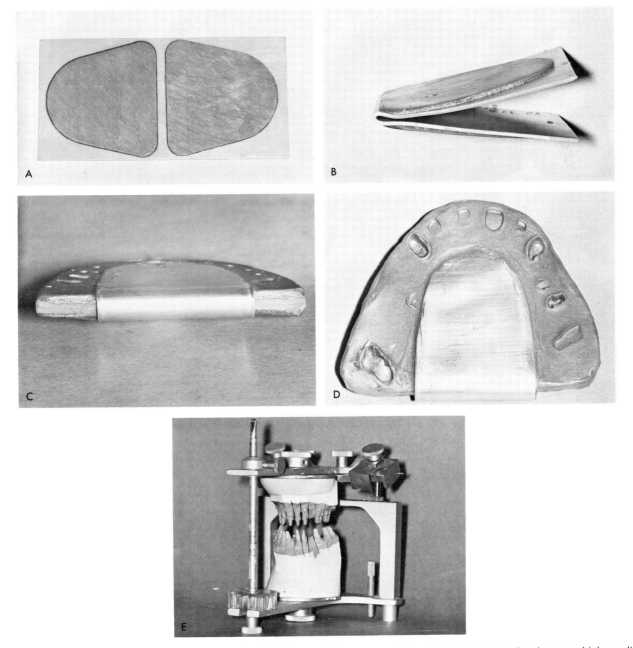

FIG. 29-23. *Fabrication of centric-relation wafer that is thick enough to compensate for increased interocclusal space which results from coronal reduction. A. Aluwax wafers luted to sheet of hard baseplate wax. B. Hard baseplate wax folded. C. View showing four-layered wafer further supported by Ash's #7 relief metal. D. Centric relation registration wafer showing depth of imprints. E. Mandibular master cast secured to lower member of articulator.*

With the aid of this wafer (Fig. 29-23D), secure the mandibular master working cast to the lower member of the articulator (Fig. 29-23E). Check the accuracy of the mounting by comparing the point(s) of initial contact in the mouth and on the articulated master working casts. If these points coincide, set the articulator to the correct vertical dimension and incisal guidance.

Determination of Vertical Dimension and Incisal Guidance

For most patients, the vertical dimension and incisal guidance have been decided during the diagnostic waxing and provisional splinting phase. For various reasons, however, these may have been altered by adjusting the acrylic provisional splint and it will be necessary to correct the settings for the articulated master working casts.

PROCEDURE

Remove the master working casts and replace with the casts of the provisional restorations. Set the incisal pin to this dimension. Re-articulate the master working casts and examine to see if there is sufficient clearance for waxing procedures. If more clearance is required, the articulator can be opened slightly (approximately 1 to 2 mm) to the necessary amount. Keep in mind that the free-way space must not be violated by excessive increase of vertical dimension. Any increase in vertical dimension should usually be tested for tolerance by allowing the patient to wear the altered provisional splint for a sufficient period of time.

If any adjustments of the acrylic provisional splints have affected the original incisal guidance as determined from the diagnostic waxing, this will have to be altered accordingly. Make certain that the incisal guidance pattern is satisfactory by examining all excursive movements of the articulated stone casts of the provisional restoration. If it is not, adjust as necessary by scraping all areas of interference on the stone casts. Alter or customize the incisal guidance table to the corrected pattern of excursive movements. Remove the casts of the provisional restorations and re-articulate the master working casts of the prepared abutment teeth. These may now be prepared for the waxing procedures.

DESIGNING AND FABRICATING THE PROSTHESIS

At this time the design of the prosthesis is determined. Decisions must be made with regard to the extent of splinting required and the manner in which this is to be accomplished. If the waxing and casting phases of the prosthesis are to be carried out by a technician, the prescription of the design must be carefully outlined. If individual copings are planned for all or some of the abutment teeth, their fabrication will be the next phase of the reconstructive procedure.

Copings as Substructures in Periodontal Prosthetics

The use of copings overcomes several of the many problems encountered in reconstructive procedures. Copings are especially advantageous when oral rehabilitative procedures include the rebuilding and long-term splinting of all or most of the teeth in an arch, as is often necessary in periodontal prosthetics. In such cases, copings are used as substructures for some or all of the abutment teeth, over which a splint or superstructure is constructed. This is often referred to as "the telescopic principle"[9] or "telescope reconstruction."[4]

The advantages of telescoping in periodontal prosthetics are numerous. The modern application of this concept allows the periodontist to accomplish the following:

1. Severely malposed teeth that would otherwise have to be realigned orthodontically or reduced to the degree where the pulp must be extirpated can readily be made parallel.
2. Abutment preparations of excessively long clinical crowns, which are often encountered after periodontal treatment, can be kept parallel. For dentitions that require extensive splinting, it is often impossible to achieve composite parallelism by tooth movement and maximum coronal reduction, except by removing the pulps of many teeth. A better alternative is to use properly designed individual copings as substructures to achieve parallelism of the entire arch or segments of the arch (Fig. 29-24).
3. By selectively joining copings, telescopic full-arch splints can be constructed in two or three segments and still provide cross-arch stabilization by cross-linkage of the segments (Fig. 29-25A, B, C). This principle overcomes the many disadvantages of a full-arch, one-piece prosthesis. It allows for single segments to be removed for reasons of repair or additional therapy without disturbing the remaining segments (Fig. 29-25C). An additional advantage is that different veneering material can be used for different segments: for example, porcelain fused to gold for the anterior segment and acrylic veneer for the posterior.
4. Future additional splinting of teeth or segments

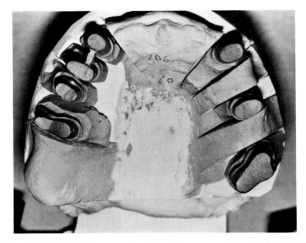

FIG. 29-24. *Maxillary cast of dentition requiring periodontal prosthodontic reconstruction, showing composite parallelism achieved by using copings as substructures.*

of the arch is provided for. This is accomplished by using a specially designed coping that is soldered to a single-segment fixed splint (Fig. 29-2). An individual superstructure crown is fabricated

and temporarily set. If the need to gain cross-arch stabilization arises, the remaining teeth may be splinted and joined to the existing splint without the need to disturb or remake it.

5. The coronal portions of the abutment teeth are better protected against caries by precise permanent cementation of the individual copings. It is virtually impossible to permanently cement a large segment or a full-arch splint with the accuracy that is possible for single units, especially if the abutments are mobile as is often the case following periodontal therapy.

6. The telescopic prosthesis can safely be cemented onto the coping with temporary cement, since each coping is set with a permanent type of cement. The superstructure can then be removed if trouble appears, and remedial measures can be taken without undue difficulty.

In most cases, a cement is required to stabilize a fixed periodontal prosthesis. For a variety of reasons, it is often necessary to remove splints of this kind, and

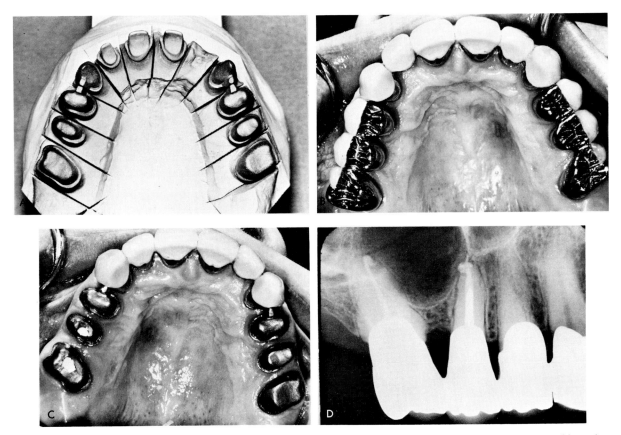

FIG. 29-25. *Copings designed to interlock telescoped segments of splint for cross-arch stabilization. A. Master cast with copings on all teeth except incisors. Note design of cuspid and premolar copings to allow for soldering. B. Telescoped segments of reconstruction cemented with temporary cement. Segments extend from molar to first premolar on both sides and from cuspid to cuspid. C. Posterior telescoped segments removed for endodontic therapy of right molar and premolar and for repair of porcelain veneer of the left segment. Note occlusal perforations of copings which were later repaired with gold foil. D. Radiograph of right quadrant to show telescoped splint in place over treated teeth. (Courtesy Dr. C. Filipchuck.)*

when a permanent type of cement is used it is usually impossible to remove the splint without mutilation of the splint or damage to the abutment teeth. A temporary cement will solve the problem. However, along with many advantages, temporary cements have one serious disadvantage. Invariably, the temporary cement dissolves, and some or all of the retainers become loose, often without the knowledge of the patient or the dentist. If this happens and copings have not been used, the risk of caries and pulpal involvement is extremely high, and the destruction may reach the point where the entire crown of the abutment tooth becomes desensitized and slowly becomes totally destroyed through carious involvement. If, however, each abutment tooth has first been covered with a permanently set coping, the underlying tooth structure is protected. The superstructure can thus be stabilized with temporary cement and left in place with little or no risk of caries.

Abutment teeth showing signs of pulpal degeneration can be tested for vitality through a small occlusal or buccal perforation in the coping. If root-canal therapy is necessary, it can be accomplished through the small occlusal perforation (Fig. 29-25C, D). The perforation can then be filled with either amalgam or gold foil, and the splint can be reset. Thus, endodontic therapy is accomplished without perforating the telescoped superstructure crown.

Abutment teeth that have a doubtful periodontal prognosis can be preserved until they are no longer useful and must be extracted. The telescopic splint can then again be removed, the teeth can be extracted, and the retainer can be converted easily into a pontic.

Further periodontal therapy such as examination procedures, probing, curettage, and surgery can be more easily and accurately performed if the splint can be removed. If gingival irritations due to improper coronal contours, lack of interproximal embrasure space, faulty margins, or improper pontic adaptation develop, the splint can be readily removed, modified, and reset. Any renovations or repairs to worn acrylic veneers, broken porcelain facings, additions to pontics, broken solder joints, or additional splinting of approximate segments on teeth are also more easily managed.

Coping Fabrication

As stated earlier in the chapter, among the many factors that determine success in oral rehabilitative procedures, proper tooth preparation is one of the most critical. This becomes more evident if copings are to be used. The single most prevalent fault in full-coverage tooth preparation is insufficient reduction. Insufficient reduction will result in excessively over-

contoured crowns that will seriously affect the health of the supporting tissues. In successful telescope reconstruction, the following qualities in full-coverage tooth preparation are necessary if both the coping and the telescoped retainer are to be accommodated within the limits of physiologic contour:

1. Adequate occlusal or incisal reduction (allow at least 0.5 mm for the coping and 2 mm for the retainer of the splint)
2. Adequate facial reduction to allow for veneering
3. Adequate interproximal reduction to allow for proper embrasures
4. Adequate reduction of the occlusal third of the facial and lingual surfaces to allow proper width of the functional occlusal table

All of these qualities are necessary for any full-coverage crown preparation, but it is evident that the overall reduction must be slightly greater if the use of copings is planned. In addition, the preparation must be as parallel as possible to give maximum retention and afford resistance to dislodging forces. Retention can often be improved by placing well-designed axial grooves in any axial surface of the preparation. Axial grooves are not limited to mesial and distal surfaces but can be placed facially and lingually as well (Fig. 29-19B). It is evident from the above that if copings are to be used in the reconstruction this must be decided before or at the time of tooth reduction, so that enough tooth structure can be removed to allow for the extra thickness of the coping.

Wax is applied to each die to an overall thickness of 0.5 to 1.0 mm before the gingival collar and margins are formed. For this step, some prefer to use the new resins that are vacuum-adapted to the dies because the thickness can be more easily controlled and the coping is structurally sturdier and resists warping during investment and casting procedures (Fig. 29-26A). If the resins are used, the thimble should be trimmed approximately 1 mm short of the gingival finish line of the die. The gingival collar and margin of each coping can then be individually waxed (Fig. 29-26B).

Interproximally and lingually, and in many cases facially, the gingival collar is waxed to an estimated position relative to the die that would place it slightly coronal to the free gingival margin when the casting is set in place in the mouth. This is done so that the gingival collar of the telescoped retainer remains coronal to the gingiva wherever esthetics will allow. If esthetics are of primary concern, as on the labial surfaces of anterior and, in some cases, premolar teeth, the width of this collar may be reduced accordingly (Fig. 29-27A)

For posterior abutments with long fluted preparations, the gingival collar may have to be extended more coronally, in order to eliminate many undercuts that would normally interfere in gaining composite taper relative to all the other copings in the arch (Fig. 29-27B). Interproximally, the collar should always be extended coronally to the free gingival margin. The embrasures should never be constricted by improperly designed copings.

The shoulder of the collar is made sufficiently thick to accommodate an adequately structured telescoped retainer, constructed so that its facial, lingual, and mesiodistal dimensions in no way exceed those of the original tooth. The shoulder is waxed to approximately a 45° taper (Fig. 29-28A, B). Some prefer to wax this to a chamfer (Fig. 29-28C) rather than to a sharp-angled shoulder. Others groove the shoulder internally on its interproximal and lingual aspects for increased retention and to reduce the risk of temporary-cement washout[1,9] (Fig. 29-28D). In both methods there is only a 10° to 15° taper of the axial walls of the copings.

When all the copings have been waxed, the overall

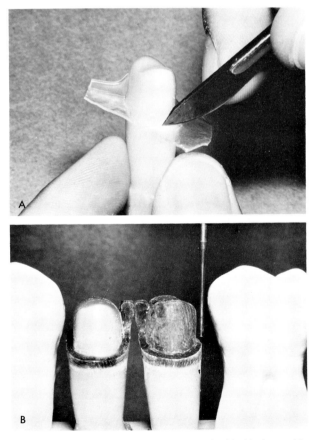

FIG. 29-26. *Fabrication of copings. A. Resin thimble formed by Vacuform method to fit die. B. Resin and wax copings with gingival collars waxed and designed for interproximal soldering checked for proper taper with a surveyor.*

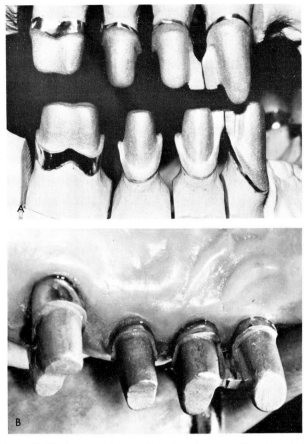

FIG. 29-27. *A. Buccal view of cast copings on dies, showing progressive reduction in width of the gingival collars posteroanteriorly. Esthetics here are of primary concern. B. Lingual view to show increased width of collar. Esthetics here are of no concern. Width of collar must usually be increased when preparations are long and fluted as in the case of the molar which had mesiobuccal root amputation.*

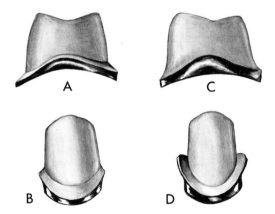

FIG. 29-28. *Mechanical forms of gingival third of copings. A. Interproximal view showing beveled gingival shoulder and increased occlusogingival width of collar both interproximally and lingually. B. Buccal view of A. C. Interproximal view showing chamfered gingival shoulder. D. Buccal view of C showing internal bevel of shoulder in interproximal region designed to increase the retention of the superstructure.*

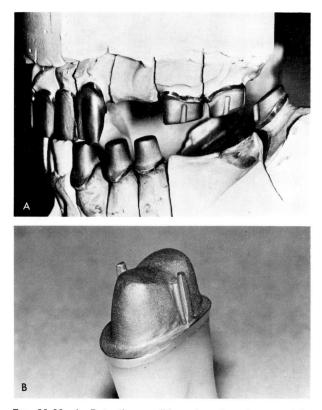

FIG. 29-29. A. Retentive qualities of copings increased by strategically placed grooves (buccal aspects of maxillary molars and mesiobuccal aspect of mandibular molar). B. Extracoronally placed pins as another means of increasing retention of superstructure.

taper of each coping is checked with the aid of a surveyor (Fig. 29-26B), and any wax additions or subtractions are made, as necessary. It is imperative that the gingival third of each coping remain fairly parallel, with only a slight taper (approximately 10° to 15° to the line of draw). This is necessary to ensure adequate retention of the splinted segments. In some instances, tapered internal grooves (Fig. 29-29A) or extracoronally placed pins (Fig. 29-29B) will greatly increase the retention of the telescoped retainer. Either technique is recommended for abutments that are relatively short occlusogingivally.

When it is planned to solder adjacent copings, the interproximal design of the copings is altered, as seen in Figure 29-30A. The mechanical form of the interproximal extensions will allow for an adequate solder joint and will improve the retention of the retainer that is fabricated to fit such a coping. The design of these interproximal extensions should allow for adequate clearance for the interproximal papilla (Fig. 29-30B). This is to ensure that the solder joint will not encroach on this vulnerable area. Occlusogingivally, the facial

and lingual walls of the proximal extensions are designed with a slight taper and act in a similar manner as grooves (Fig. 29-30C, D). The base of the solder joint should be shaped and refined in a manner that does not encourage microbial plaque retention and allows for easy plaque removal (Fig. 29-30E).

Prior to investing the waxed copings, the gingival margins are carefully checked for accuracy. The copings are cast, cleaned, sandblasted, and checked for fit on their respective dies. Electrochemical stripping may be necessary for castings that cannot be seated completely. The stripping creates internal surface relief and facilitates the fitting of the casting to the die. When all the castings are adequately adapted, they are refined, polished, and sandblasted both internally and externally, and the patient is scheduled for trying in the copings (Fig. 29-30B).

Cast Coping Try-in

The provisional splints are removed, teeth are cleaned of all traces of temporary cement, stain, and plaque, and all the copings are tested for accuracy of fit. The margins are carefully tested for overextensions or underextensions. Overextensions and bulky margins are carefully reduced. Underextensions may be due to incomplete seating of the casting on the tooth. This can be verified with the aid of disclosing waxes prepared specially for this purpose. Internal interferences are judiciously relieved either with stones, if the interference is localized, or by additional electrochemical stripping. If marginal deficiencies still exist after complete seating, the coping should be rewaxed and cast from a new die of the tooth.

The gingival collar of each coping is checked for its relation to the sulcus and the free margins of the gingiva. Overcontoured regions of the coping's gingival collar are reduced until, on try-in, there is no blanching of the gingival tissues when the copings are completely seated. The proximal aspects of each collar are especially carefully contoured to accommodate the interproximal papillae adequately.

Interproximal extensions of copings that are to be soldered are contoured so as not to impinge on the soft tissues. Such copings are then joined with Duralay,° and an index is taken with impression plaster. The copings are invested, soldered, refined, and checked to verify accuracy of fit. If the fit of all copings is satisfactory in every respect, they are transferred back to the articulated master working casts and prepared for waxing of the superstructure.

° Reliance Dental Mfg. Co., Chicago, Ill.

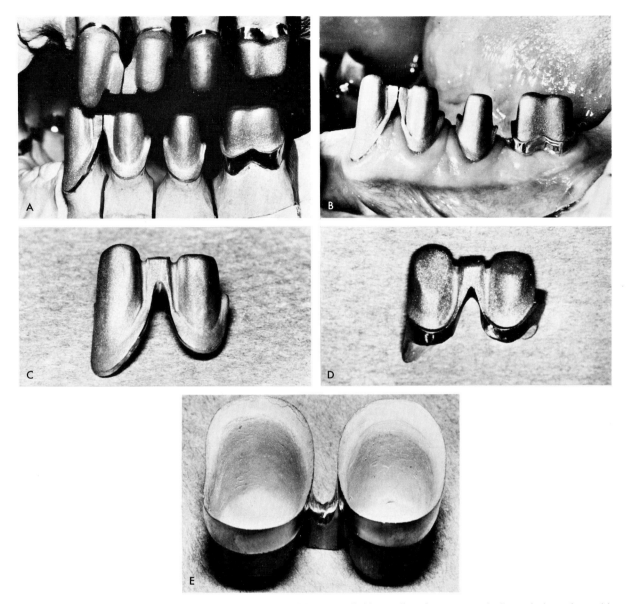

FIG. 29-30. *Interproximal design for copings to be soldered for cross-linking splinted segments. A. Buccal view of cuspid and premolar copings showing such design. B. Copings tried for fit and contour prior to soldering. Note that interproximal contour of cuspid and premolar coping allows for adequate embrasure space. C. Buccal view of soldered copings, showing refined grooves for increased retention of the superstructure. D. Lingual view of grooves and rounded gingival aspect of solder joint designed for ease of plaque removal. E. Gingival view showing rounded and polished interproximal surface of soldered copings.*

Waxing the Superstructure

Of the many technical phases of oral rehabilitation, most dentists who are capable of undertaking this technical aspect of dentistry agree that the most difficult is the waxing of the functional form of the prosthesis. This phase requires much skill if it is to be correctly performed. In full-mouth rehabilitation, the waxing of the coronal morphology with respect to its axial contours and functional occlusion must be correct from all aspects, so that these forms do not contribute to further deterioration of the hard and soft tissues. The occlusal and incisal morphology must be formed in such a manner that the teeth not only occlude accurately in centric relation but also function in harmony throughout all excursive mandibular movements. For these reasons, attempts to perform this phase without the necessary skill and training usually end in failure.

The current trend in waxing is toward functional waxing techniques. Functional waxing creates functional occlusion in a precise step-by-step fashion that is controlled from start to finish. This method coupled with the use of an accurately programmed adjustable articulator permits the occlusal morphology to be harmonious with the patient's condylar influences.

Functional waxing was originally developed to incorporate the tooth-to-tooth, cusp-fossa relationship with mutual protection rather than the tooth-to-two-tooth cusp-to-embrasure fully balanced principle of occlusion.[14,15] It is beyond the scope of this book to outline and describe in detail all the intricate steps necessary to complete such a waxing.

Essentially our technique incorporates most of the principles taught by Thomas in his add-on, functional waxing technique. The slight variations were found advantageous when applying these principles to periodontal prosthodontics.

1. *Maximum intercuspation in the centric relation occlusal position* (Fig. 29-38). However, if the remounting and milling procedures of the completed prosthesis result in slight freedom in CRO (i.e., long centric), there is no objection, as long as the vertical dimension is the same throughout the range.

2. *Cusp-to-fossa relationship rather than cusp-to-marginal ridge relationship* (Fig. 17-4). This principle is important in occlusal reconstruction, especially where splinting is not required, since it eliminates "plunger cusp" effects. A cusp-to-fossa relationship also results in greater stability, since it is possible to wax the occlusal surfaces so that functional forces are contained more within the long axis of the teeth.

3. *Tripodism.* Wherever possible, the cusp contact with a fossa is a three-point contact rather than a one-point contact (Fig. 29-38). Authorities in gnathology believe that this is a more stable type of relationship as compared with a single point of contact. There is no scientific evidence to show that one is better than the other. In striving to attain tripodism, the dentist need not be overly concerned if this is changed to cusp-tip-to-fossa contact after remounting and milling procedures, as long as the cusp tip contacts a flat-based fossa (Fig. 17-20) rather than unreciprocated inclined planes (Fig. 17-19).

4. *Simultaneous contact.* All posterior centric holding cusps should contact simultaneously and with uniform precision. This type of contact also tends to keep the forces within the long axis of the teeth.

5. *Protection of anterior teeth.* The anterior teeth in CRO should be such that they are just out of contact. This is especially important if the anterior teeth are not included in the splint. It is impossible to maintain anterior contact relationships in CRO so that the forces are axially inclined, since these contacts are usually on inclined planes. Therefore, the posterior occlusion should take the load and protect the anterior teeth.

6. *Mutual protection by the principle of disclusion, whenever possible.* According to theory, the immediate disclusion of the posterior teeth by the anterior teeth during any excursive movement of the mandible protects the posterior teeth from deflective contact relationships on the working and balancing sides. It also tends to protect them from excessive wear of the posterior cusps, since there is no contact of these cusps during functional or parafunctional activities. Therefore, adequate overjet and overbite relationships of the anterior teeth and especially of the cuspids are created according to the dictates of esthetics and the programmed articulator.

A slight modification of this principle as it relates to cuspid function in lateral excursion of the mandible is recommended. The posterior occlusion is waxed in such a manner as to provide for group function on the working side, and then the lingual concavities of the maxillary cuspids are waxed so as to disclude the posterior teeth during lateral excursions. This waxing is advantageous in the event that the cuspid wears or migrates or the "cuspid rise" is not tolerated. It can be readily adjusted so that the working side will immediately assume group function. However, the manner of waxing should always ensure that cross-arch and cross-tooth balancing interferences do not appear even if the cuspid wears or is reduced.

7. *Shallower occlusal form, progressing backwards from the premolars.* There is no need for deep intercuspation, even though the articulator programming would allow for this. A shallow posterior occlusion ensures rapid disclusion of the occlusal surfaces during excursive movements and lessens the risk of balancing contacts arising if the cuspid wears or migrates.

8. *Narrowed occlusal tables.* Narrowing occlusal tables allows for better control of contact relationships during excursive movements.

9. *Physiologic morphologic characteristics of all embrasures, axial contours, and marginal ridges.* All the principles of good contours as outlined in Chapter 26 should be adhered to.

It is recommended that either the stone duplicates of the diagnostic waxings (Fig. 28-3) or the stone duplicates of the provisional restorations (Fig. 29-32B, C), whichever is better, be used for guidance to facilitate the waxing of the superstructure. In either case the waxing technique is the same, but the stone casts of the provisional restorations are the ones that are described here. If the casts of the provisional restorations are to be used, it is essential that the provisional restorations be carefully fabricated, adapted to the prepared teeth, corrected, and evaluated over a considerable period of time for proper function, esthetics, and phonetics.

bles of the maxillary posterior copings and pontic regions, and the morphologic characteristics are formed in keeping with the axial contours and occlusal dimensions of the posterior teeth. No attempt should

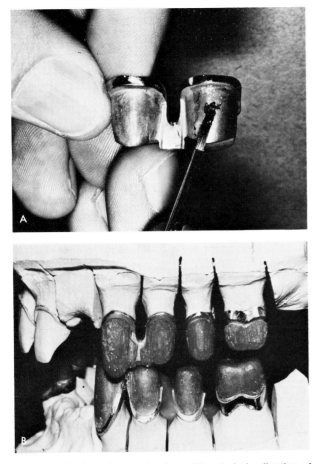

FIG. 29-31. *Waxing of superstructure—Step 1. A. Application of resin onto lubricated coping to fabricate a thimble (one for each coping) prior to waxing of superstructure. The thimble will greatly increase the strength of the waxed crowns. B. Resin thimbles refined to uniform 0.05 to 1.0 mm thickness and trimmed 2 mm short of the gingival margin of the copings.*

1. Each coping is lubricated, and a thin layer of a resin such as Duralay (0.5 mm in thickness) is shaped to form a thimble for each coping or for each die if copings are not being used. Each thimble is trimmed approximately 2 mm short of the gingival margin and all excessively thick regions are reduced so that all are uniformly 0.5 to 1 mm thick (Fig. 29-31A, B).

2. The articulated mandibular master working cast is replaced with the stone duplicate cast of the provisional restoration (Fig. 29-32A). Molten inlay wax is flowed over the resin thimbles of the maxillary anterior copings or dies and, using the maxillary stone cast of the provisional restorations as a reference, the morphologic characteristics of the six maxillary anterior teeth are formed. Any necessary additions or subtractions are made so that they function with the lower teeth according to all the dictates of the programmed articulator (Fig. 29-32B).

3. Molten inlay wax is flowed over the resin thim-

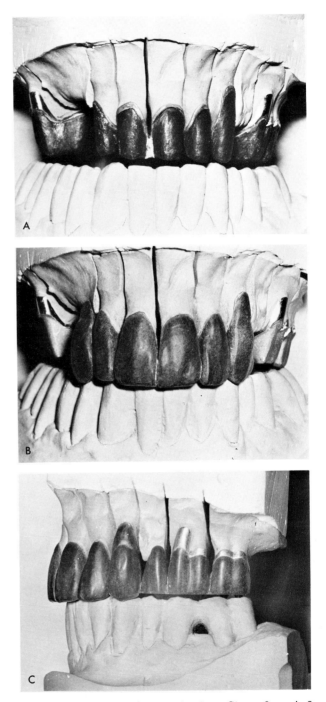

FIG. 29-32. *Waxing of superstructure—Steps 2 and 3. A. Maxillary master cast articulated with mandibular casts of provisional restoration. B. Maxillary anterior teeth waxed to function with mandibular anterior teeth of the stone duplicate of the provisional restoration. C. Axial contours of maxillary posterior teeth waxed leaving sufficient space for structure of occlusal surface.*

be made at this time to establish the functional occlusion, but the wax should be reduced so that there is 2 to 3 mm clearance between the maxillary wax occlusal surface and the mandibular stone occlusal surface (Fig. 29-32C).

4. The maxillary master working cast is replaced with the cast of the provisional restoration. The mandibular cast of the provisional restoration is replaced with the mandibular master working cast, with care to maintain the same vertical dimension (Fig. 29-33A). Using the maxillary cast of the provisional restorations as a guide, the morphologic characteristics of the lower anterior teeth are formed so that they function with the maxillary cast of the provisional restoration, according to the dictates of the programmed articulator (Fig. 29-33B).

5. The morphologic characteristics of the mandibular posterior teeth are formed, and the wax of the occlusal surfaces is reduced to provide a clearance of 2 to 3 mm between the maxillary stone occlusal surfaces and the mandibular wax occlusal surfaces (Fig. 29-33C).

6. The maxillary cast of the provisional restoration is replaced with the master working cast, and the functional characteristics of the maxillary and mandibular anterior waxing are precisely refined, according to the functional dictates of the programmed articulator and esthetic requirements (Fig. 29-33D). Zinc stearate powder is dusted over the functioning wax surfaces to mark any uneven contact or deflective interferences during excursive movements of the articulator. A check is made to see that there is adequate clearance (approximately 4 mm) between the posterior occlusal surfaces in CRO and throughout all excursive movements.

7. The mandibular master working cast is replaced

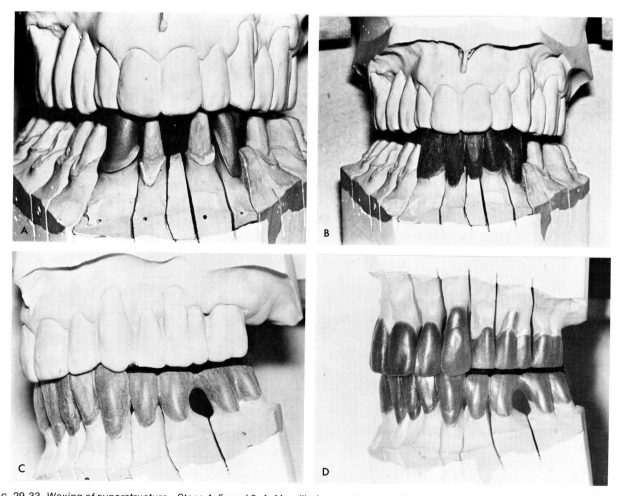

FIG. 29-33. *Waxing of superstructure—Steps 4, 5, and 6. A. Mandibular master cast articulated to the correct vertical dimension with maxillary cast of the provisional restoration. B. Mandibular anterior teeth waxed to function with maxillary anterior teeth of the stone duplicate of the provisional restoration. C. Axial contour of the mandibular posterior teeth waxed, leaving sufficient space for structure of occlusal surface. D. Maxillary cast of the provisional restoration replaced with the maxillary waxings. The functional qualities of the anterior teeth are perfected accordingly.*

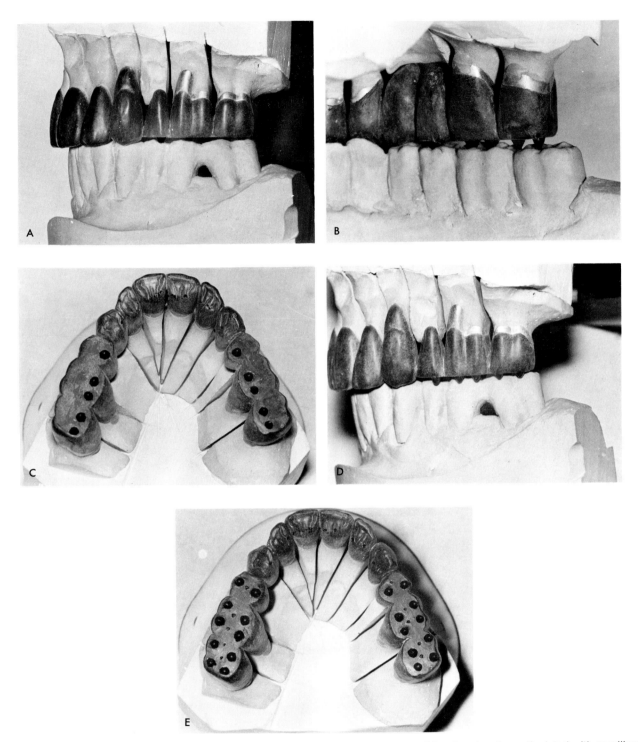

FIG. 29-34. *Waxing of superstructure—Steps 7 and 8. A. Mandibular cast of the provisional restoration articulated with maxillary waxings (buccal view). B. Maxillary centric-holding lingual cones formed to articulate with respective fossae of the mandibular cast of the provisional restoration (lingual view). C. Occlusal view of maxillary lingual cones. D. Maxillary buccal cones formed. E. Occlusal view of maxillary waxings.*

with the cast of the provisional restorations (Fig. 29-34A), and the wax cones that will locate the centric holding cusps of the maxillary posterior teeth are formed (Fig. 29-34B, C). The most suitable mandibular

fossae to receive these are determined, and the tips are projected to contact the base of each respective fossa. A check is made to see that each cone tip clears the opposing occlusal surface during all excursive movements of the articulator. Contact should occur only in the CRO position, and the maxillary anterior teeth should effect an immediate disclusion throughout excursive movements.

8. The maxillary buccal cones are formed so that all the maxillary buccal cusps are located according to the estimated cusp height and occlusal position and so that they effect the correct width of the occlusal table (Fig. 29-34D, E).

9. The maxillary master working cast is replaced

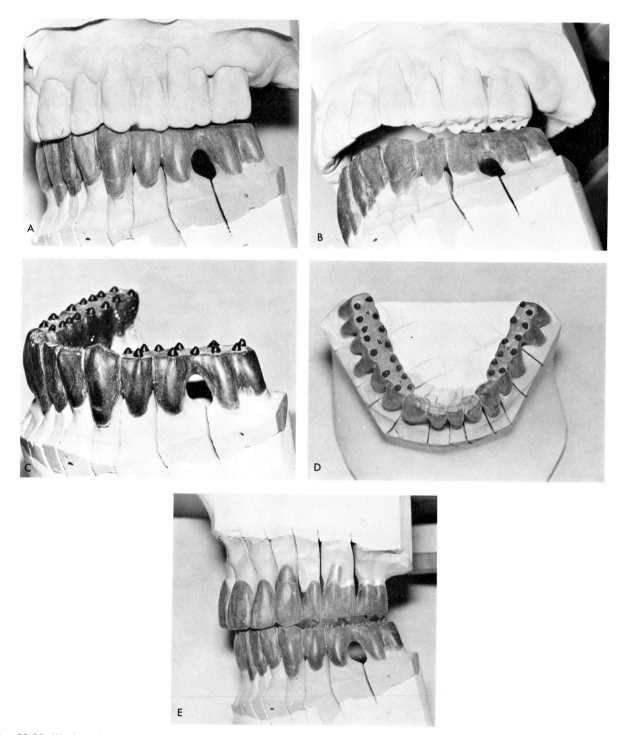

FIG. 29-35. *Waxing of superstructure—Steps 9 and 10. A. Mandibular waxings articulated with maxillary cast of the provisional restoration. B. Mandibular centric-holding buccal cones formed to articulate with respective fossae of the maxillary occlusal surface. C. Mandibular lingual cones formed. D. Occlusal view of mandibular cones. E. Maxillary and mandibular waxings articulated for refinement of cone height and positions in centric relation and all excursive movements.*

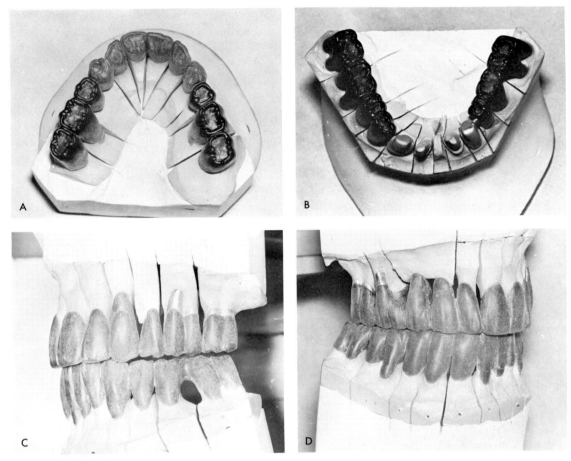

FIG. 29-36. *Waxing of superstructure—Steps 11 and 12. A. Maxillary cones connected to form marginal ridges and perimeter of occlusal surfaces. B. Occlusal view of waxed mandibular marginal ridges. C. Buccal view of left side, showing disclusion of buccal cusps during lateral excursion. D. Buccal view of right side, showing group function during lateral excursion after cuspid rise is reduced.*

with the cast of the provisional restoration (Fig. 29-35A) and the mandibular buccal cones are formed so that the tips of the mandibular centric holding cusps are located in the respective fossae of the maxillary occlusal surfaces (Fig. 29-35B). The mandibular lingual cusp cones are then formed (Fig. 29-35C, D).

10. The maxillary cast of the provisional restoration is replaced with the master working cast and all cusp cones are examined for proper height, position, and function (Fig. 29-35E).

11. The maxillary cones are connected to form the marginal ridges and the perimeter of the occlusal surfaces (Fig. 29-36A). The same is done with the mandibular cones (Fig. 29-36B). At this stage there should be immediate disclusion of the cusp tips during all excursive movements of the articulated models (Fig. 29-36C).

12. The degree of cuspid rise is reduced by carving the lingual sides of the maxillary cuspids, and the cusp tips and marginal ridges of the maxillary buccal cusps and mandibular buccal cusps are adjusted to effect group function on the working side (Fig. 29-36D). Any

balancing contacts on the nonfunctioning side or during protrusive excursion are checked for with zinc stearate powder and, if present, are eliminated.

13. The triangular and oblique or transverse ridges

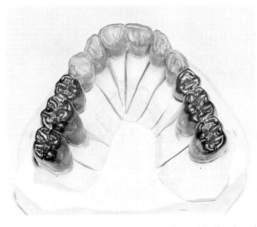

FIG. 29-37. *Waxing of superstructure—Step 13. Occlusal view of waxed maxillary triangular and oblique ridges. Some of the centric contact points are developed during this step.*

are formed. A number of centric relation contacts are established at this time in addition to contact relationships on the working side (Fig. 29-37). Any balancing contacts on the nonfunctioning side or in protrusive excursion are eliminated.

14. The developmental grooves are formed by filling in the remaining occlusal voids, one at a time and, while the wax is soft, closing the articulator in CRO to register the relationship of the centric holding cusp tips to the fossae. The developmental grooves are es-

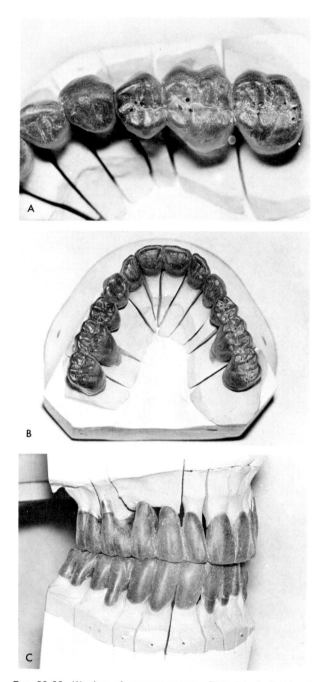

FIG. 29-38. *Waxing of superstructure—Step 14. A. Occlusal view of completed waxings of maxillary quadrant, showing detail of supplemental grooves and three-point contact for each centric holding cusp. Cusp tip does not touch opposing occlusal surface. B. Occlusal view of completed waxings of superstructure. C. Buccal view, showing posterior group function on working side.*

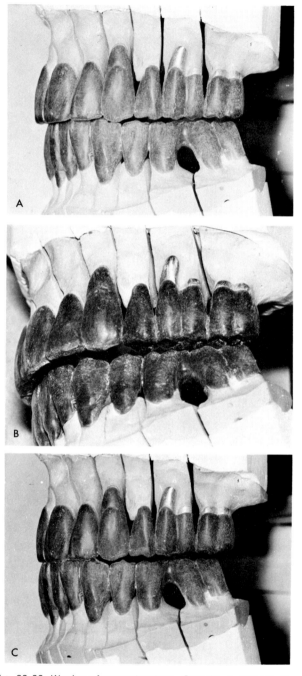

FIG. 29-39. *Waxing of superstructure—Step 15. A. Buccal view showing disclusion of all posterior cusps during excursive lateral movement after cuspid rise is rewaxed. B. Buccal view, showing disclusion of occlusal surfaces on the nonfunctioning side. C. Buccal view showing disclusion during protrusive movement.*

tablished by breaking up the large contact area of the fossa and removing the contact mark of the cusp tips, so that contact is at three points on the perimeter of each centric holding cusp (Fig. 29-38A, B). If this tripod principle is not desired, a single contact can be established between each centric holding cusp tip and the base of its respective fossa. The contact relationship in CRO is carefully checked with the aid of zinc stearate powder and is refined to ensure that all centric holding cusps contact simultaneously and with uniform pressure.

15. Before creating the cuspid rise, posterior group function should be reestablished, and balancing contacts again should be checked for and eliminated. (Fig. 29-38C).

The lingual aspects of the cuspids are then rewaxed according to their original functional characteristics, so that they effect the necessary disclusion during the lateral (Fig. 29-39A, B) and protrusive (Fig. 29-39C)

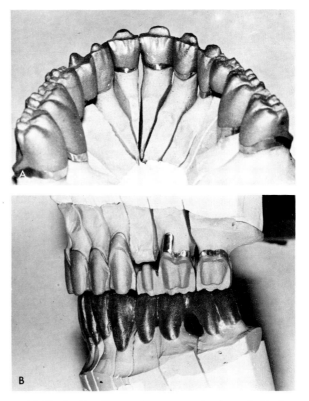

FIG. 29-41. *Casting the maxillary superstructure. A. Occlusolingual view of castings. B. Buccal view of articulated castings.*

excursive movements of the articulated waxings. A careful check is made in all excursive movements to see whether the posterior cusp tips make any contacts. All such contacts must be eliminated. Posterior contact should occur only in CRO.

The facial surfaces of the maxillary waxings are cut back as desired (Fig. 29-40), and the axial contours, proximal contact relationships, and lastly the margins are perfected. The maxillary wax patterns are sprued, invested, and cast (Fig. 29-41). The mandibular waxings should not be cast at this time. Each casting is examined for imperfections, and the fit is tested on each respective die. The patient is then scheduled to try all the castings for fit.

Cementation of Maxillary Copings and Superstructure Soldering

Prior to the try-in and cementation of the maxillary copings, a wire-reinforced acrylic rim is fabricated to act as a remount impression matrix. The copings and superstructure castings are reassembled on the master working cast, and heavy-gauged wire (coat-hanger wire) is bent to conform to the arch (Fig. 29-42A). The occlusal surfaces of the castings are lubricated, the wire is placed in position, and acrylic resin is adapted

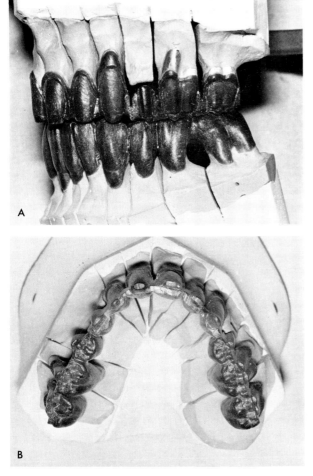

FIG. 29-40. *Preparation of maxillary waxing for casting. A. Buccal view of maxillary waxings cut back to allow for porcelain veneering. B. Occlusal view of maxillary waxings cut back.*

to form a rim containing the imprints of the occlusal surfaces (Fig. 29-42B). This is then trimmed and set aside to be used for the remount procedure (Fig. 29-42C).

The maxillary provisional restorations are removed, and the temporary cement is thoroughly cleaned from all abutment surfaces. Each coping with its respective

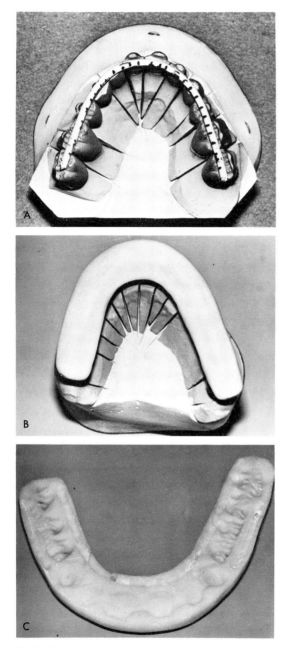

FIG. 29-42. *Remounting the maxillary superstructure—fabrication of the remount plastic matrix. A. Occlusal view of coathanger wire, bent to conform to the occlusal surfaces of the castings. B. Acrylic resin adapted over wire and occlusal surfaces. C. Completed matrix, showing occlusal imprints of castings.*

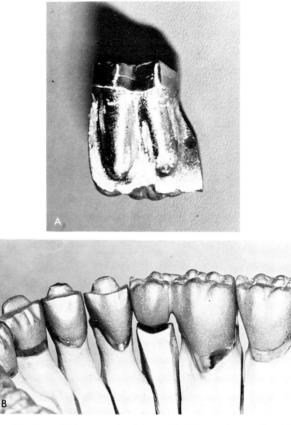

FIG. 29-43. *A. Telescoped retainer fitted to coping and gold-to-gold margins polished. B. Lingual view of refined polished and sandblasted gold-to-gold margins of the telescoped retainers and polished margins of copings. This step is completed prior to permanent cementation of the copings.*

telescoped retainer is examined for marginal fit, coronal and embrasure contour, and degree of proximal contact, and the pontics are examined for ridge relationship. Corrections are made as necessary, and the margin of the telescoped retainer and the gingival collar of the coping are definitively polished (Fig. 29-43).

The coronal surfaces of the abutment teeth are flooded with Metimyd and glazed with a cavity varnish, and the maxillary copings are set with a permanent type of cement (Fig. 29-44). After the initial set, the excess cement is thoroughly removed. The cast superstructure is precisely seated into place over the copings, each joint is luted with Duralay, and sectioned plaster core index impressions are made in order to make the solder joints. The soldered segments are tested for accuracy of fit. If satisfactory, a maxillary remount cast is made in order to rearticulate the soldered superstructure to the waxed mandibular superstructure (Fig. 29-45).

The maxillary master working cast cannot be used for this purpose, because the copings are now perma-

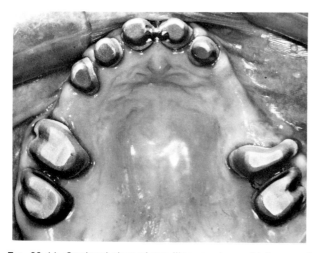

FIG. 29-44. *Occlusal view of maxillary copings which are set with a permanent type of cement prior to making plaster occlusal cores of superstructure for soldering procedure.*

nently seated and the superstructure will not fit the dies. Conversely, the provisional splint will no longer fit the maxillary arch, now that the copings are seated, and it will have to be readapted to the copings or in some instances even remade.

Remounting of Maxillary Superstructure

In most cases, the main objective of remounting is to refine the functional occlusion. At this stage of the rehabilitation, however, the first remounting procedure is solely for the purpose of rearticulating the soldered maxillary framework to facilitate the veneering process. A second precise remount may be performed upon completion of the veneering of the maxillary superstructure for the purpose of refining the functional occlusion of the mandibular waxing, and a third to refine the occlusion of the completed maxillary and mandibular prostheses.

The first remount is especially necessary when the buccal cusps and incisal thirds of the teeth are to be veneered in porcelain, since there is no way other than by rearticulation to determine the morphology of what will be the functional surfaces.

A centric relation registration is now taken of the maxillary telescopic superstructure and the mandibular tooth preparations.

The acrylic rim that was previously made for the remount procedure (Fig. 29-42) is now used as a matrix for a zinc oxide-eugenol impression of the soldered segments of the maxillary superstructure now in place (Fig. 29-45A). The zinc oxide-eugenol paste is allowed to set, and an alginate impression is made of the entire maxillary assembly (Fig. 29-45B). Upon removal of this impression, the soldered superstructure will usually

remain within the impression. If not, it should be carefully replaced. All undercuts are eliminated with wax or hydrocolloid (Fig. 29-45C), the internal surfaces of the retainers are lubricated with Mucolube° (Fig. 29-45D), and molten low-fusing metal is poured into the occlusal portion of the impression. While the metal is solidifying, metal washers or paper clips are partially inserted into selected regions to provide retention for the second pouring of stone mix that will form the base of the model (Fig. 29-45E). This remount cast is related in CRO to the waxed mandibular superstructure and is secured to the upper member of the articulator (Fig. 29-45F).

Provisional Splint Readaptation

Because the copings are now permanently attached to the abutment teeth, the provisional splint has to be readapted to fit the copings. The internal surface and gingival margin of each acrylic retainer are reduced to a shell stage with a large round carbide bur. It is tested for fit and, if found satisfactory, relined with acrylic, trimmed, polished, and reseated with temporary cement. Some find it more expedient to remake the provisional splint entirely by the Vacuform† process. A thin resin matrix is vacuum-adapted to fit the cast of the provisional restoration, is then trimmed, and used in the same manner as a shell in fabricating a new provisional splint (Fig. 29-46).

Completion of Maxillary Superstructure

The soldered segments are refined and prepared as necessary to accept the veneer. The veneer of choice is applied and finished to the degree that is necessary for trial in the patient's mouth (Fig. 29-47). If the veneer is of porcelain, it should not be glazed or stained prior to trial in the mouth. The patient is rescheduled for this trial, and all necessary corrections in contour and surface features are made to satisfy the cosmetic requirements. Stains are applied as necessary, and the veneer is glazed. The superstructure is polished and reseated on the copings but not cemented to them.

Refinement of Waxed Mandibular Superstructure

The mandibular provisional restorations are removed, and a new centric relation registration of the seated, completed maxillary superstructure and the mandibular abutment teeth is taken at the correct

° Cosmos Dental Products, Inc., New York
† Omnivac V Vacuum Adapter, Omnidental Corp., Harrisburg, Pa.

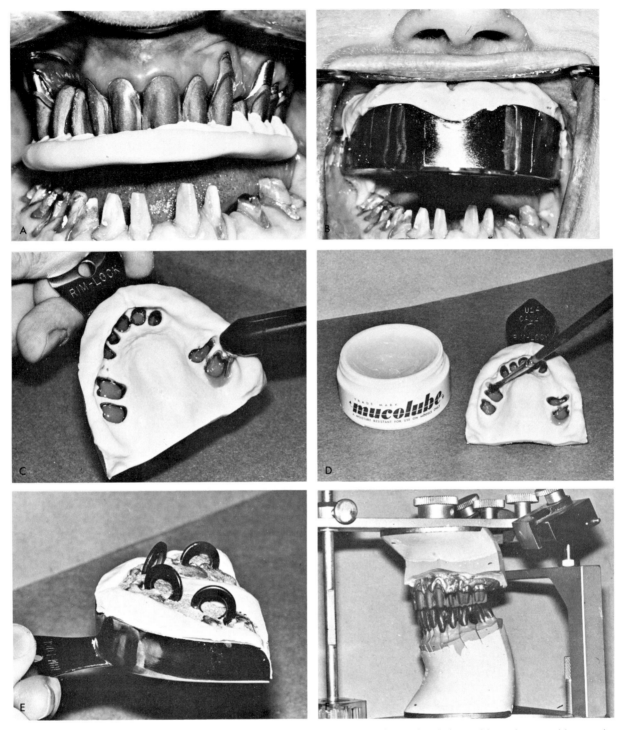

FIG. 29-45. *Impression for remounting procedure. A. Acrylic matrix used to make occlusal zinc-oxide-and-eugenol impression of soldered segments of superstructure. B. Alginate impression being made of the remount matrix in position. C. Alginate impression containing acrylic matrix, with splint segments in place. D. All undercuts are filled with hydrocolloid impression material and the castings are lubricated. E. Low-fusing metal poured into impression and metal washers inserted to provide retention for a second pouring of stone to form the base. F. Maxillary remount cast secured to upper member of articulator.*

vertical dimension. The mandibular waxings and their respective copings are removed from the dies of the master working cast. A new centric relation registration and mounting are made of the mandibular master working cast to the maxillary remount cast containing the complete maxillary superstructure. The mandibular copings with their waxed superstructures are reassembled on the dies of the master working cast and then checked with zinc stearate powder in CRO and all excursions of the articulator. Almost all restorations will require some refinement of the occlusal waxing and the gold occlusal surfaces to satisfy the principles of occlusion as outlined earlier in the chapter (Fig. 29-48). After this is completed, the facial aspects of the wax patterns are cut back and contoured, and their margins are refined. The retainers and the pontics of the superstructure are cast, cleaned, and sandblasted (Fig. 29-49), and the patient is rescheduled for trial of the castings.

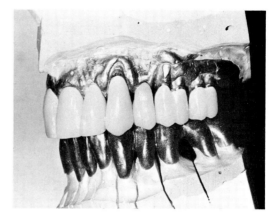

FIG. 29-47. *Veneering of the maxillary superstructure.*

Cementation of Mandibular Copings and Completion of the Mandibular Superstructure

The try-in of the mandibular copings with superstructure, cementation of the mandibular copings, and soldering of the mandibular superstructure are carried out in a manner similar to that described for the maxil-

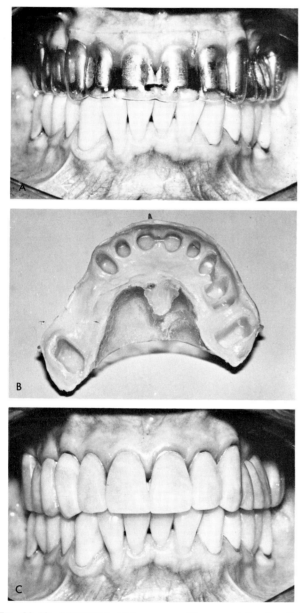

FIG. 29-46. *Adaptation of a new maxillary provisional splint using the Vacuform process. A. Trial of the trimmed Vacuform shell. B. Shell filled with tooth-colored autopolymerizing acrylic resin and precisely repositioned over the lubricated copings. C. New provisional splint trimmed, polished, and set with temporary cement.*

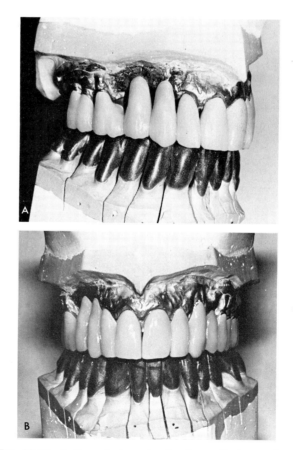

FIG. 29-48. *A. Buccal view of refined mandibular waxings. B. Anterior view of mandibular waxings refined to function accurately with the maxillary superstructure.*

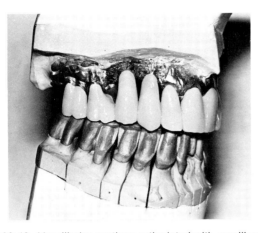

FIG. 29-49. *Mandibular castings articulated with maxillary superstructure.*

lary prosthesis. After completion of the soldering, the segments are checked for accuracy of fit. If the fit is found to be satisfactory, the maxillary provisional restorations are removed, the copings are thoroughly cleaned, and the completed superstructure is precisely seated in place. A new centric-relation registration is made. A remount cast containing the soldered segments of the mandibular superstructure is made in a similar manner to that described earlier in the chapter and is re-articulated to the maxillary cast containing the completed superstructure. The mandibular provisional splint is relined to fit the copings.

The occlusion of the re-articulated prosthesis is precisely refined to correct all discrepancies that may have appeared during the soldering procedures or for other reasons. Only after this is completed should the mandibular superstructure be veneered (Fig. 29-50). The patient is rescheduled to test accuracy of fit, functional occlusion, correction of contours, characterization staining, and glazing of the mandibular super-

structure. Any modifications to the procelain of the maxillary superstructure will require reglazing.

CEMENTATION OF THE PROSTHESIS AND CASE MAINTENANCE

If all aspects of the prosthesis are satisfactory, a decision is made as to what type of cementation is best for the patient. For most patients with complex problems it is best to set the superstructures in place (Fig. 29-51) with petroleum jelly or with a mix of temporary zinc oxide-eugenol cement considerably weakened by incorporating petroleum jelly into the mix. This will allow for easy removal of the superstructure, which will be necessary within 2 to 4 weeks. Prior to dismissal of the patient, oral-hygiene methods must be thoroughly reviewed.

As with periodontal therapy, the success or failure of any restorations, regardless of how expertly fabricated, will greatly depend upon the patient's capabilities in oral-hygiene management. It is impossible to design restorations that are entirely self-cleansing; they must be cleaned by the patient. Often the reason for lack of adequate oral hygiene after placement of restorations stems from the fact that the patient was not sufficiently motivated prior to restorative therapy. It is imperative that the patient comprehend the need for, and be able to demonstrate expertness in, plaque control before and during the period of rehabilitation. If this goal can be realized prior to completion of therapy, then the slight modifications required after cementation of the prosthesis are easily learned. Under no circumstances must the construction of the prosthesis be continued if the patient is not effective in plaque control. Patients who are rehabilitated without adequate instruction and supervision in plaque control or information regarding their responsibility in maintaining the restoration are

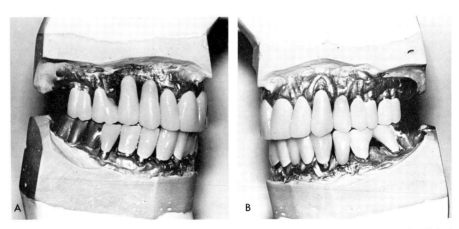

FIG. 29-50. *Mandibular superstructure veneered and articulated with the maxillary superstructure. A. Right buccal view. B. Left buccal view.*

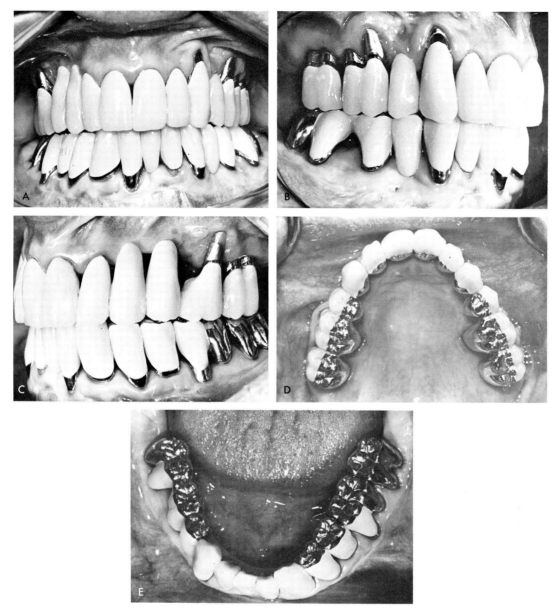

FIG. 29-51. *Cementation of the maxillary and mandibular superstructures with temporary cement. A. Anterior view. B. Right lateral view. C. Left lateral view. D. Occlusal view of maxillary prosthesis. E. Occlusal view of mandibular prosthesis.*

victimized, since the time, effort, and money spent will be for naught.

The method of debridement of plaque and particulate matter for the rehabilitated patient is similar to that described for any patient undergoing other periodontal treatment. The only exception is in the use of dental floss or nylon yarn (Fig. 29-52), since the teeth are splinted and the solder joints prevent the use of floss or yarn in a conventional manner. The patient must also be instructed in the cleaning of the gingival aspects of the pontics. Any oral irrigation device is an extremely useful adjunct. The patient must be informed, however, that these devices are useful in flushing out the plaque and other particulate matter only after it has been loosened by brushing and flossing.

All areas of the patient's mouth that may be potentially problematic are discussed with the patient, and any specialized hygiene and physiotherapeutic procedures for the maintenance of such areas are reiterated. It behooves the dentist to explain that the prognosis of such localized situations may be beyond control, in spite of meticulous care, and the prosthesis may need modification if key abutment teeth are lost.

The regimen of oral hygiene and physiotherapy for patients who have received extensive therapy is described in detail in Chapters 15 and 30.

The patient is rescheduled for an appointment approximately 2 to 4 weeks after initial cementation of the prosthesis. At this time the occlusion is carefully examined, and necessary adjustments are made. The effectiveness of the patient's oral hygiene and his physiotherapeutic efforts is discussed. In the majority of cases, improvements are usually found necessary. Accumulations of microbial plaque are demonstrated with disclosing solutions. It is wise to tap out a splinted segment prior to removal of the plaque, so that the patient can clearly visualize where the plaque commonly accumulates. Procedures for plaque debridement should be reinforced and carefully supervised.

All segments of the prosthesis are now removed, and any necessary modifications in the contour of gold and acrylic surfaces are carried out, and the surfaces are repolished. If porcelain axial surfaces are modified, these will require reglazing.

At this time a decision should be made as to the type of cementation that should be used. Temporary cementation is usually indicated for restorations that have copings as substructures for all the abutment teeth of the splinted segment. The advantages of temporary cementation for such restorations have been discussed earlier in the chapter. In addition, the removal of the telescopic superstructure at prescribed intervals greatly facilitates curettage and root-planing procedures (Fig. 29-53).

Temporary cementation can also be used for abutment teeth when the health of the pulp or surrounding periodontium is questionable. Temporary cementation for such cases is advisable until there is more certainty of their ultimate disposition. It should be realized, however, that if the abutments are not protected by permanently cemented copings, temporary cementation of splinted segments more often than not requires a rigidly adhered-to recall schedule. Such splints should be routinely tapped off, and the abutment teeth should be checked for recurring caries every 6 months or sooner. Except in cases where each abutment is protected by a coping as a substructure, it is inadvisable to use temporary cementation indefinitely, since it is usually only a matter of time until the temporary cement will at least partially dissolve, exposing the tooth to the dangers of caries and gingival inflammation.

Following any cementation procedure, whether of a temporary or permanent type, the occlusion requires

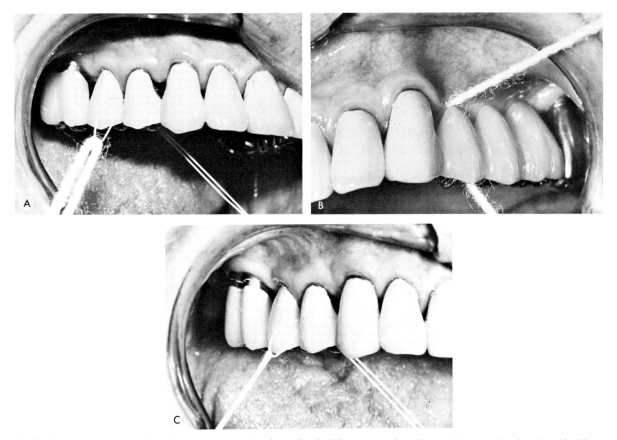

FIG. 29-52. *Oral hygiene procedure for plaque control, using nylon knitting yarn and/or floss. A. Appropriate length of knitting yarn being pulled through embrasure with the aid of a monofilament loop (Butler). B. Nylon yarn passing under pontic. C. Floss being introduced through embrasure with the aid of a monofilament loop.*

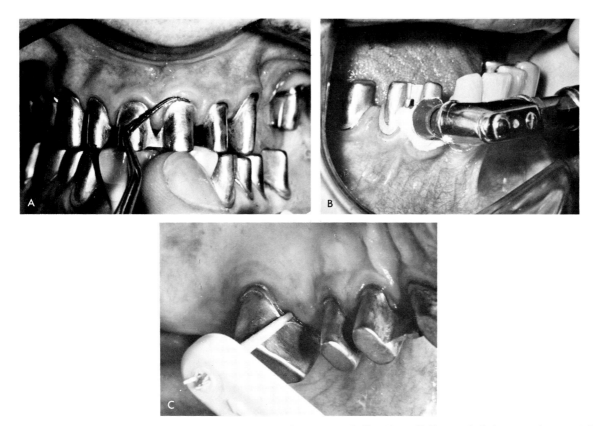

FIG. 29-53. *Temporarily set superstructure removed for ease of curettage. A. Curettage. B. Removal of plaque and cement debris. C. Burnishing of root with fluoride.*

rechecking. All cement debris should be carefully and completely removed.

Recall intervals vary with each patient and will depend greatly on the type of cementation used, the capability of the patient to perform adequate oral hygiene, and the number of potential problems that the patient may have. Some patients may have to be recalled every 3 to 4 months. Each should be recalled at least every 6 months, at which time the mouth should be examined completely and any necessary therapy provided.

References

1. Amsterdam, M., and Abrams, L.: Periodontal prosthesis. *In* Periodontal Therapy, 4th ed. H. M. Goldman and D. W. Cohen, Eds. St. Louis, C. V. Mosby Co., 1968.
2. Amsterdam, M., and Rossman, S.: Technique of hemisection of multi-rooted teeth. Alpha Omegan, 53:4, 1960.
3. Bohannan, H., and Abrams, L.: Intentional vital pulp extirpation in periodontal prosthesis. J. Prosthet. Dent., 11:781, 1961.
4. Gordon, T.: Telescope reconstruction an approach to oral rehabilitation. J. Am. Dent. Assoc., 72:95, 1966.
5. Ingraham, R., Bassett, R., and Koser, J.: An Atlas of Cast Gold Procedures, 2nd ed. Buena Park, California, Uni-Tro College Press, 1964.
6. Johnston, J., Phillips, R., and Dykema, R.: Modern Practice in Crown and Bridge Prosthodontics, 3rd ed. Philadelphia, W. B. Saunders Co., 1971.
7. Kornfeld, M.: Mouth Rehabilitation, vols. I and II. St. Louis, C. V. Mosby Co., 1967.
8. Mann, S. W., and Pankey, L. O.: Oral rehabilitation, Parts I and II. J. Prosthet. Dent., 10:135, 1960.
9. Prichard, J., and Feder, M.: A modern adaptation of the telescopic principle in periodontal prosthesis. J. Periodontol., 33:360, 1962.
10. Rosen, H., and Gitnick, P. J.: Integrating restorative procedures into the treatment of periodontal disease. J. Prosthet. Dent., 14:343, 1964.
11. Schyler, C.: Factors of occlusion applicable to restorative dentistry. J. Prosthet. Dent., 3:772, 1953.
12. Stallard, H., and Stuart, C.: What kind of occlusion should recusped teeth be given? Dent. Clin. North Am., Nov., 1963, p. 591.
13. Stuart, C. E.: Why dental restorations should have cusps. J. So. Cal. Dent. Assoc., 27:198, 1959.
14. Stuart, C. E., and Stallard, H.: A Syllabus on Oral Rehabilitation and Occlusion. School of Dentistry, University of California.
15. Thomas, P. K.: Syllabus on Full Mouth Waxing, Technique for Rehabilitation, Tooth-to-Tooth, Cusp Fossa Concept of Organic Occlusion, 2nd ed. School of Dentistry, Post-graduate Education, University of California, 1967.

Section IV

Maintenance

30

Maintenance of the Periodontal Patient

30

Maintenance
of
the
Periodontal
Patient

ALFRED L. OGILVIE

Each year increasing numbers of people throughout the world receive the benefits of periodontal treatment. At the same time, more of these individuals are living for extended periods after treatment. Awareness of what treatment can offer is being increasingly linked with a recognition that beneficial results are fleeting if not maintained; thus, the prospects are that the interest in and demand for maintenance therapy will continue to increase.

Relatively few authors have discussed maintenance therapy in practice.[1,5,20,21,26,28,32,34] It stands to reason that there is a growing need to analyze the whole field of periodontal maintenance and to decide the extent to which each patient requires it, who shall perform it, and how it can be most effectively carried out.

In the long-term sense, there are some encouraging prospects. A number of studies have already demonstrated what can be expected from an intensive program of preventive recall.[2,3,6,16-18,33] Knowles has shown that plaque scores for patients can be reduced to lower levels and held there over several years in the course of periodontal maintenance care.[13]

From another point of view the picture may be changing even now. Because the emphasis upon plaque control and the early treatment of periodontitis is so substantial within the preventively oriented practices of our time, dentists can expect that fewer incipient lesions of young adults will progress to advanced periodontitis. To this extent at least, the proportion of the total population with severe periodontal disease should eventually diminish.

In the public health sense, of course, the control of periodontal disease is a vast problem. Professional intervention remains so time-consuming and costly that for many it is beyond reach. From the point of view of many patients, plaque control demands so much in personal resolve and manual dexterity that it is unattainable. It seems likely, therefore, that only when gingival inflammation can be controlled by means other than minimal personal oral hygiene and professional treatment, i.e., by some means entirely removed from the individual, through measures analogous to caries control by fluoridation of drinking water, will the problem become truly manageable.

This chapter is written from the perspective of the periodontist. Particular influences bear upon the periodontal specialist, and it can only be helpful to bring these to light. However, concentration upon such a viewpoint should not be taken as an argument against the effective maintenance therapy carried out by many general practitioners. The usual approaches of the generalist and the specialist and the essential cooperation that each must sustain will be discussed.

PSYCHOLOGIC ASPECTS OF MAINTENANCE THERAPY

Successful long-term maintenance after treatment is, more than anything else, an attitude of mind, both of the therapist and the patient. We all realize that a short-term therapeutic improvement, essential though it is, can be only a beginning. By itself, it means little. Ahead is the far more elusive goal of preserving the dentition in a state of health for the longest possible time. To attain this goal, the therapist must generate resolve within the patient, and this resolve must stem from an even firmer resolve within himself. His own conviction comes first. The periodontist must believe that maintenance procedures count a great deal and must show that he cares. To one degree or another, he must participate in the maintenance. Repeated personal contacts with the patient over the years give the periodontist a chance each time to rekindle the sense of mutual challenge that existed at the beginning of treatment. Without such reinforcement, it seems that most patients are unable to continue making the sacrifices that are required of them—namely, the continued plaque removal at home, the keeping of periodic office appointments, and the payment of the substantial recall fee.

Barriers in the Mind of the Therapist

Most periodontists find within themselves more than enough psychologic barriers to carrying out long-term therapy, barriers that are surely just as important as those built up in the patient. What are the factors within the periodontist that work to prevent him from continuing adequate maintenance of the treated patient? Possibly, the most important factor is the appeal of what is new, to the exclusion of the old and therefore dull. Periodontal training has been oriented toward marshaling facts about new patients and treating the complexities so brought to light. After these problems have been recognized and treated, however, the picture changes. We become insensitive to what is known. It is much more difficult to give one's full concentration to familiar surroundings.

Recall care also requires the practitioner to "police" his own results. To a considerable degree, it means keeping alert to changes more subtle than those in new patients with full-blown disease. The periodontist, returning to the patient he has treated, finds himself in much the same position as the general medical practitioner viewing a patient who has been healthy for a long time. His guard is down, so to speak, at the very time when the level of suspicion needs to be kept high.

In the same sense, a new dental patient may appear so healthy in all respects to the general dentist that he omits a thorough examination. It is understandable, therefore, that familiarity with the treated patient as a "healthy" person makes it doubly difficult for the periodontist to see that patient as anything other than healthy, particularly when he himself has "created" the health.

This personal block is encountered by all dentists at one time or another. There is a natural reluctance to face treatment that has not turned out well. Yet what completed case is perfect? Which case does not contain an area that could have been treated more satisfactorily?

Once the periodontist admits to the presence of adverse changes in a mouth that he has treated, he faces several other psychologic barriers before he can take effective action. Assume that the patient has been conscientious about plaque control and keenly interested in preserving the improvement which he knows was obtained as a result of active treatment. Now it appears that an area is going downhill or, worse, that the whole mouth is deteriorating, in spite of good oral hygiene. In these circumstances the dentist may be reluctant to explain to the patient the full extent of the deterioration that has taken place. For one thing, the change may prove reversible. By intervening, the dentist may be able to bring back a state of health. And this does often happen. On the other hand, if breakdown has resumed and the periodontist points it out, he risks disheartening the patient. The patient may then give up on intensive plaque control efforts and routine recall visits. This dilemma of telling or not telling places a considerable burden on the therapist, for he knows that by imparting somewhat less than the whole truth to a certain type of patient he can elicit continued cooperation and can hold ground for a good time to come.

Unfortunately, the periodontist is often required to continue treatment of patients whose dentitions are failing. He experiences only too often the psychologic pain of seeing a mouth deteriorate. When he can attribute this to an unavoidable resumption of active disease or to the patient's neglect, that is one thing; when he can see that his own oversight or inadequate treatment has contributed to the deterioration, it is another matter. He may realize, for example, that the area has been handled too aggressively. In retrospect, it would have been better to have treated in a less complex fashion, perhaps through root curettage, selective grinding, provisional wire-and-acrylic splints, and bite guards. Perhaps an earlier reluctance to remove a maxillary molar with a poor prognosis has resulted in furcation involvement of a neighboring tooth. Whatever the reason, the dentist needs to keep in mind that hindsight is easy and foresight difficult. His treatment represented his best judgment and effort at the time.

The positive approach for the periodontist lies in learning from disappointments and in modifying his behavior so that he can better cope with similar situations later on. The tendency in the presence of personal error is to rationalize in one way or another. A patient's neglect of plaque control can be magnified to assume key importance, or the blame can be placed upon the patient's failure to adhere to the exact recall appointment schedule. Realistically, there is seldom a single cause, and in periodontal disease the patient's omissions do not explain everything.

The periodontist needs to recognize that loss of tooth support is to be expected during the maintenance of a great many patients. Often, patients enter treatment beyond the stage when total arrest of the disease process can be expected. Chronic systemic disease does lower resistance, and patients do age. Many people experience a decline in their capacity to control plaque. Arthritis limits manual dexterity, and senility puts an end to complex motor performance. Just as often, it is neither arthritis nor senility, but merely a diminution in the patient's zest for living that stops the hands from carrying out their essential work. It is at this time that the encouragement of the periodontist can be the deciding factor between maintenance and deterioration.

Other psychologic determinants intrude. For the periodontist, sheer monotony is one. The search for signs of gingival inflammation, for calculus deposits and roughened surfaces, for root caries and for pathologic sulcus depth may be thought of as boring and without interest. In reality, it is a challenge. Unless performed with close concentration, the search is almost sure to be incomplete. Dentists may grow tired of seeing the same patient, but the satisfaction of helping to maintain a treated patient is considerable. One should remember that the odds against long-term success are quite high. Consequently, it is legitimate to derive satisfaction from the knowledge that health has been sustained in the face of what once was and could again be caries susceptibility, heavy plaque deposit, a significant rate of calculus formation, and/or heavy occlusal stress.

Therapists encounter still another block within themselves at recall, namely, the reluctance to confront the patient when surgical retreatment is indicated. They observe a change in the patient's dentition, such as a 6-millimeter pocket where only a few months earlier there was one half of that depth at the end of treatment. They know that the recent treatment placed heavy demands on the patient and that the surgical phase in particular may have been barely tolerated. The patient has since come to look upon all periodontal surgery as being behind him. Yet, now the dentist is faced with a significant new lesion. Should another surgical effort be mentioned so soon after active treatment? Would it not be better to treat with a curet for a time, observe, and then move again toward surgery only when and if there are multiple areas of concern? To do or not to do? These are valid questions. Often it is better to wait than to turn immediately to surgical procedures. This principle applies as much to recall decision-making as to the original treatment planning, but there are occasions when additional surgery can abort the recurrent disease. If a key multirooted abutment tooth is involved, for instance, there is little time to wait.

Fees can become another barrier to maintenance therapy. Financial compensation for services is surely essential, and the level of that compensation is a compelling factor in day-to-day practice. There is no question that the hourly fee customarily received for recall treatment is discouraging when compared with that earned for surgical and restorative services. Recurrent battles of conscience become inevitable. Should one meet the recall needs of patients and suffer a relative monetary loss, or should one let maintenance supervision suffer and engage almost totally in the active treatment of new patients? There seems to be no certain solution. On the one hand the periodontist faces the needs to forego (immediate) maximum income and to realize that, over the long term, considerable recall management will be essential to his own satisfaction and to his reputation; on the other hand, the periodontist must eventually release many patients from recall in his office, or the maintenance care of treated patients will come to occupy a disproportionate amount of his practice time. If he is to remain a qualified specialist, he must maintain numerous skills, some of which can only be brought into play during the treatment of new patients. He also has the obligation to treat new patients in the community. Finally, it is obvious that a specialist's livelihood depends upon a continued willingness to accept new patients from referring dentists. Few periodontists appear to have solved all aspects of this dilemma underlying recall and maintenance.

Links between the Periodontist and Other Dentists

The relationships between general dental practitioners and periodontists constitute another entire segment of interpersonal psychology. At least three studies attest to the strength of the proprietary interest in the patient that is felt by many referring general dentists.[4,35,37] A sense of ownership within human relationships is universal. "My patient" and "my dentist" are commonplace terms, after all. The difficulty arises when the dentist's sense of possession is exaggerated.

There should be a definite tie between the referring dentist and the specialist. When this link is absent, when the patient is viewed by the generalist as "belonging" to him and is sent to the specialist only for the completion of a predetermined aspect of treatment, then the patient is denied the maximum contributions that the specialist can make. Periodontal matters that have a direct bearing on the restorative plan, and vice versa, receive too little consideration at too late a time. Consequently, the periodontist gains less than sufficient satisfaction from treating the patient.

It is only natural that specialists in periodontics seek to draw their patients from generalists and other specialists who demonstrate an interest in closely integrated treatment. The survey of Brustein and Rauschart makes clear that the major stumbling block is the restorative treatment plan.[4] It is often the critical area of treatment. Some generalists feel that the restorative plan is theirs to establish. The periodontist, realizing the impact of restorative measures upon the long-term health of the complex case, feels that he must have the last word, at least in general restorative terms. Many an impasse has developed on this issue, the generalist ending his referrals to the periodontist because of it or the periodontist finding himself too busy thereafter to treat the patients of the particular general dentist. Both generalist and specialist must learn to use the common language of periodontics with one another. Otherwise seeds of anger and hostility are planted, and the professional relationship cannot grow. When both the generalist and the specialist can acknowledge the unique qualities of each other, and can express this mutual confidence openly, then the joint professional efforts of the two are greatly enhanced. Furthermore, the intangible day-by-day satisfactions of both are increased a great deal.

Consequences of the Patient's Moving Away

In the urban practices of our time, patients and dentists share another problem that has striking psychologic overtones. This is the mobility of the North American population and the feelings of deprivation and impermanence that are engendered by patients moving away. The patient who moves is deprived of ties that have often become surprisingly strong. He must add to his other losses the person who has been the center of knowledge about his periodontal condition in all its detail. He is faced with the need to find a replacement and realizes rather keenly that it will take time to replace the person he has so comfortably taken for granted. One definite contribution the periodontist can make to this patient is to give him or her a firm referral to one specific periodontist in the new location. The specialist can promise to forward all pertinent case records as soon as he learns from either the patient or the new periodontist that an appointment has been made. And he can follow through on the promise.

The periodontist, of course, also experiences a comparable loss when a patient moves away. He may say to himself that the departure of a single patient represents little in the way of subtraction. However, the important point to remember is that the effect is cumulative. Over the years, an awareness of the dozens of patients who have moved away, combined with thoughts about those who have died and about those who have chosen not to persist with maintenance, can produce a sense of futility and true loss in the therapist. The saving grace lies in accepting the inevitability of change and in assisting those patients who do move away with their transfers to other periodontists.

Change, of course, can mean substitution as often as it means loss. The departure of one long-term patient is softened by the arrival of another who has been referred by a periodontist or other specialist beyond one's own geographic area. The responsibilities in caring for the newly arrived maintenance patient help the periodontist to accept the departure of a patient he has treated for years and has come to look upon almost as a friend.

Actually, patients referred for continued maintenance care from other periodontists are our own former patients in reverse. The more quickly one helps them meet their need for identification with a therapist and the more evident to them the sense of caring becomes, the less they will tend to neglect their part of the joint patient-periodontist maintenance agreement. By the same token, the less one criticizes the treatment that went before, whether by open comment or by implication, the more smoothly the transition seems to take place. There is time enough later to erase what one perceives as errors or omissions in the treatment of the referring therapist.

Cooperation, mutual recognition, and mutual support are the keys to adequate recall care. Periodontists, hygienists, and general practitioners alike are very much one another's keepers, the sustainers of each other's good name. When there is regression, as so often happens with periodontal therapy, it is easy to turn one's disappointment toward the shortcomings of the patient's last dentist or to decide that the former periodontist should not have done such and so. Stainbrook has indicated how essential it is that the dentist retain a strongly positive image of himself.[31] Surely, though, there is no need for that image to be maintained at the expense of others.

CONCEPTUAL ASPECTS OF MAINTENANCE THERAPY

Periodontitis is a chronic inflammatory disease with a predilection to return and to localize at the sites of previous occurrence and treatment.[9] Like diabetes, it is difficult to keep under control. Ultimately, of course, in most periodontal disease and in most examples of diabetes it is our patients who control their own conditions. However, the patient's control of periodontitis is dependent upon the simultaneous help of others and, most of all, upon the help of the dentist and the dental hygienist.

Why Recall Is Necessary

The realization that periodontal breakdown tends to recur and with speed in the susceptible patient should be enough to keep the dentist committed to frequent recall visits. Even when he is conscientious in recall, there are numerous occasions when he must give ground to periodontitis. Having made the effort, however, the dentist is in a far better position to accept a compromise. For one thing he can then take honest comfort from the realization that other methods of treatment evolve in time. The dentist has no alternative but to employ today's mode of therapy, although he can remain ready to apply improved techniques to today's unmanageable situations when these improvements become available.

Like it or not, at the present stage of knowledge both the dentist and the periodontally susceptible patient are committed to a maintenance regime. Recall continues to be the price paid for the successful management of chronic periodontal disease in the face of the ever present initiators of the disease.[14] The dentist who finds himself wrestling with the maintenance of his treated patients will have less of a problem if he recognizes that maintenance is simply treatment continued. It is treatment that requires cerebration, treatment that can and does vary considerably rather than being a routine which one is obliged to follow out.

Responsibility for Office Phase of Maintenance Care

In today's scheme of things, the maintenance of a periodontal patient involves the activities of at least six persons—namely, the referring dentist, the periodontist, the dental hygienist in the periodontist's office, the office receptionists of both referring dentist and periodontist, and, most important of all, the patient. Who is responsible for the recall evaluation and the actual performance of recall treatment? Definite understandings about the recall interval, the individual who is to be responsible for the recall, and the communication of findings must be reached by both referring dentist and periodontist. From working with the referring dentist again and again, the periodontist more often than not comes to know the dentist's preference in dealing with long-term maintenance. However, there is a better way than trial and error to establish the roles. Generalist and periodontist can meet beforehand and establish policy on the management of the several categories of recall patient. A far more comfortable situation will then exist when patients enter into the relationship.[10] Sometimes, of course, a specific agreement on recall will be required for a particular patient, even though a general protocol has been established.

A good suggestion bordering on a rule of thumb can be made with respect to three types of patients: (1) those who are highly susceptible to periodontal disease, (2) those whose treatment has been initiated after breakdown has become well advanced, and (3) those with a complex periodontal prosthesis. Individuals in the above categories should have their periodontal reviews in the periodontist's office. Otherwise, the planning and performance of maintenance treatment tend to be given short shrift. Another risk encountered in the referring dentist's office is that there will be neglect of important signs of breakdown for too long an interval. Such oversights as these are usually traceable to the failure of the dentist to spend sufficient time on an inspection of the patient's mouth for evidence of change.

Thus it remains the responsibility of the periodontist to determine which patients should be maintained by the referring dentist. The decision rests upon an assessment of the severity of existing breakdown, the patient's age relative to the extent of destruction, the presence or absence of a periodontal prosthesis, the caries susceptibility of the patient, and the patient's demonstrated level of plaque control. It must also be based on a knowledge of the temperament and periodontal experience of the referring dentist. Every periodontist is aware of at least one outstanding, periodontally oriented general dentist who refers the surgical aspects of periodontal treatment because he thinks it best to do so. This dentist is seeing his patients on a regular basis for maintenance care. He is more than capable of supervising all aspects of a complex case. Obviously, the patients of this dentist are exceptions to the premise that periodontal recall should take place in the periodontist's office.[29] By and large, however, patients who have been seen by a periodontist for major periodontal treatment, or have had extensive periodontal restorative care, should continue to be seen by the periodontist. These patients form a minority, but a sizeable minority of any periodontist's case load. They tend to constitute a larger and larger part of the practice as time goes by.

Sandrew studied the attitudes of patients who had completed active periodontal therapy.[27] Among other things, he questioned them regarding their views on whether a general dentist or a periodontist should do their recall treatments. He found that confidence in the therapist was a major factor with these patients. They looked upon the ability of the periodontist to detect recurrent periodontal disease in its early stages as important. Most patients felt that this diagnostic experience of the periodontist had a bearing upon recall effectiveness and that the periodontist was therefore the one whom they wished to have in charge of the recall.

Surely, a case can be made for the more careful training of the pre-doctoral student in periodontal maintenance and for the upgrading of the practicing dentist in this respect.[22] It is hoped that at a later time the majority of generalists will exhibit sensitive diagnostic acumen in the periodontal area. At present, patients with only moderate involvement are often returned to their referring dentists, only to receive a quality of recall supervision that is not consistent with their active periodontal therapy. When most dentists do demonstrate a strong periodontal understanding, the recall picture will undoubtedly change, and patients will be far better off. Furthermore, at this future time, the periodontist will no longer experience the dilemma of an excessive recall load. He will concentrate his recall efforts upon the truly complex cases and feel confident about returning the less involved patients to the referring dentist for all care.

The Origins of Sound Recall Treatment

Since the periodontist's recall treatment and the patient's maintenance prove to be at least as significant as the active multi-appointment office treatment, they ought to loom large in the thinking of the therapist from the beginning. Maintenance and primary active treatment must be introduced conceptually at the same time. It is essential that the patient have realistic expectations of each. The patient must be advised against the folly of relying on short-term gain (via active primary treatment and brief plaque control) when long-term retention of the teeth in function (via extended professional recall treatment and extended personal plaque control) is the only sensible goal.

Effective maintenance care begins during the earliest appointments with the patient. The concept of future office appointments devoted only to maintenance is presented at the same time that the forthcoming "active" therapy is discussed. The patient is made aware of his vulnerability to recurrent disease. He is advised of the usual frequency of maintenance treatment, the features of such treatment, and the amount of the average recall fee in the practice.

The periodontist discusses with the patient the responsibilities that each of them will carry. He makes clear that the referring dentist, whether general practitioner, specialist in restorative dentistry, or prosthodontist, will also carry certain clear and recurring responsibilities. The patient is assured that should several dental professionals become involved, their actions will be coordinated. The point is made that each will probably require of him recall visits. Recall by the periodontist may be the most frequent, however, and the most critical, because the underlying susceptibility to periodontal breakdown will remain. The significant role of the dental hygienist is explained as well, particularly now that this co-professional performs increasing amounts of both initial therapy and maintenance therapy.

Maintenance During Active Therapy

Active treatment of a periodontal patient, by its very nature, has always spanned months of time. The sequence of active treatment, observation, and more active treatment is well accepted in periodontics. Presently, however, patients are being treated in ways that extend the total time of active involvement beyond months and into years. The patient with a multiphase surgical prosthesis and the one with combined periodontal-orthodontic-restorative intervention are examples enough of the greater time that is implicit in current therapy.

There is a real danger of periodontal neglect once initial treatment has been provided and while other forms of treatment are undertaken. One can meet that danger, however, by thinking and acting in terms of maintenance during the active treatment of the patient.

DURING SURGICAL TREATMENT

Maintenance of the surgically treated patient begins as soon as the final dressing is removed from the first surgical area or, if no dressing is employed, at the end of the first postsurgical week. During the surgical phase of treatment it is all too easy to concentrate upon the region of immediate surgical interest and neglect the other areas of completed surgery. Thus, if the left upper and lower segments are treated surgically and several weeks later the right segments are too, the teeth on the left must not be neglected while attention is focused on those on the right. All the teeth in each surgically treated area require periodic curettage and polishing, most critically in the zone of tooth structure adjacent to the new gingival margin. Gentle curetting and polishing in that zone is beneficial from the third week onward to remove accumulated plaque and to slow the establishment of new inflammatory lesions.[19]

Needless to say, oral hygiene must be employed concurrently. Curettage and polishing should be repeated in each area no later than 3 months after surgery when the tissues have healed and become partially stabilized. To paraphrase Chace, if the knife and the chisel cure, then the curet preserves the cure.[5] The time involved is slight; the benefit, in conjunction with good oral hygiene, great.

Patients in the middle of surgical periodontal treatment also require a review of their occlusion at frequent intervals. Surgically treated teeth remain looser than normal for a long time, as the recent investigation of Selipsky makes clear.[30] By selective grinding one should be able to reduce the secondary traumatism. Usually this is done on the teeth opposing the surgically treated segment because then the patient will experience less discomfort.

DURING COMBINED PERIODONTAL-ORTHODONTIC THERAPY

Curettage maintenance is also essential for the patient receiving combined periodontal-orthodontic treatment. One must presume, of course, that before orthodontic treatment is undertaken, initial therapy has already included oral hygiene and definitive curettage to bring the periodontal inflammation under control. Despite curettage, some patients for whom orthodontic treatment is planned will continue to show a high plaque level, localized deep pockets, and extensive gingival inflammation. It is the deeper pockets in such patients that need curettage most of all. Ideally, a curet should be used lightly every week in those deeper pockets. The emphasis must be on light instrumentation, frequently employed. Frequent light curettage is also needed (every 2 to 3 weeks) when a lower molar with a potential furcation involvement is being uprighted. When a relatively passive maxillary removable appliance is in use and eruption of the posterior teeth is anticipated, the curet ought to be used with particular care and lightness. In these instances, curettage can be less frequent (every 2 months) unless there is deep pocket involvement. In the case of

the adult with banded teeth, yet with controlled periodontal disease, the maintenance and curettage interval should approach that of the periodontal patient who is not receiving orthodontic treatment; i.e., every 3 months.

The ultrasonic scaling instrument is of great help in the periodic debridement of a mouth burdened by fixed appliances. The Cavitron apparatus can be brought into use each time an arch wire is removed. Of course it is no panacea. Its vibrating tip can loosen or separate a band from a tooth if the tip is not used carefully and there are bound to be interproximal regions into which only a curet will reach. Nonetheless, in periodic maintenance one ought to use whatever instruments will accomplish debridement and curettage at minimal cost to the attachment apparatus of the teeth.

Repeated selective grinding is another and often essential part of maintenance during combined periodontal-orthodontic treatment. The most obvious example of this is during the uprighting of mesially inclined lower molars. A molar being moved to a more upright position will require a check on its possible interference, at frequent intervals. Selective grinding must be done repeatedly before the movement is complete.

The Role of Dental Personnel

Under present-day circumstances both the dental hygienist and the dental practitioner should contribute to maintenance treatment. Although the dentist retains the overall responsibility, the hygienist ought to be responsible for more and more of the documentation at recall and for more and more of the actual recall therapy. In fact, generalists and periodontists alike who hope to maintain any degree of balance between their treated patients and their new patients must delegate duties extensively. The hygienist can determine and document facts about the patient and when appropriately trained and experienced, can be relied upon to complete most of the therapeutic procedures required at recall.

Logic aside, however, experience proves that there can be no blanket delegation of maintenance therapy to the hygienist. In any periodontal practice some patients will object to a dividing of recall care between the hygienist and periodontist. Usually these patients will fall into two categories. The first consists entirely of patients who have received all their previous periodontal treatment from a periodontist. Some of them may refuse to be treated at recall by anyone other than a periodontist—for example, patients of the specialist who at one time practiced without a hygienist or certain transfer patients from another periodontist whose hygienist has not been involved in their initial therapy or recall. The second group may object to treatment by the periodontist's hygienist on quite different grounds. Interestingly enough, their protest will be made not to the periodontist, but to the referring dentist. They may phrase their objection somewhat as follows: "When I go to Dr. X's (the periodontist's) office, his hygienist does the treatment anyway, so why can't your (the referring dentist's) hygienist do it?" If periodontists are meeting their responsibility, neither they nor referring dentists have reason to feel ill at ease when addressed with this question. The answer to the question is, of course, that the hygienist associated with the referring dentist could do the therapy. In practice the periodontist discourages the move because of the better control of the patient and the improvement in the attention to critical detail that result when the patient is seen by a hygienist more familiar with the periodontist's recall procedures and likewise more conversant with the periodontal background of the patient. The hygienist in the periodontist's office, after all, has access to the patient's chart, can review promptly any point in question with the periodontist, and usually has the additional advantage of her association with the patient during the whole active treatment span.

The fact is that the periodontist's hygienist performs a share of the maintenance treatment of each patient according to a "prescription" developed by the periodontist for that patient.[7] When the division of duties is legitimate, the hygienist gathers and records facts and reports them to the periodontist before maintenance treatment is begun. At this point they examine the patient together. Drawing on the current observations, and earlier experiences with the patient, the periodontist then decides on the treatment. He may designate certain areas of the mouth to receive special emphasis in oral hygiene and others in curettage. The hygienist proceeds according to this prescription. Once the steps have been completed, the periodontist sees the patient again. Plans for further treatment are developed where necessary, and usually the periodontist will perform this additional treatment.

Thus, when the periodontist can demonstrate that he sustains a personal interest in the patient and himself participates in the maintenance treatment of his patients, the picture changes. The referring dentist who has a hygienist in his own office appreciates only too well what it means to be associated with a hygienist trained and willing to render particular forms of treatment efficiently. Appreciating that point, and assured of the periodontist's personal control, he can meet the patient's objection. If the patient then becomes a willing partner in periodontal office maintenance over the long term, so much the better. If not, just as the patient insists, the hygienist in the referring office is enlisted, and the maximum possible communication is established with her.

To still another small yet even more adamant group of recall patients no hygienist is acceptable, whether as the associate of the periodontist or of the referring dentist. It is the rare periodontist who does not himself perform all recall treatment for the occasional patient in this category.

The selection of who is to perform recall treatment is made by the periodontal patient in another way more often than either the periodontist or the general dentist may realize. An informed patient who has known the comfort and the sense of well-being that can follow regular, careful recall treatment is equally aware of their absence. When such a patient moves to another city and enters a practice where recall root curettage, for example, is less than adequate, he or she is often able to sense the fact. Sometimes nothing is said or done; sometimes the patient will speak up. Obtaining no satisfaction, the patient will seek out another office wherein the time and attention given to recall treatment match those in the practice of the original periodontist.

Finally, there will always be a few patients in any practice who exhibit particular emotional needs in treatment or whose maintenance involves special technical skill. These patients also remain the periodontist's responsibility alone when it comes to actual treatment.

A consideration of recall care must include the general dentists who refer periodontally involved patients yet who wish to assume total supervision, once the active phase of periodontal treatment has been completed. In assuming total responsibility, these practitioners may act against the suggestion of the periodontist. Should it happen that they do not or cannot maintain the necessary periodontal follow-through, the patient suffers. One approach that has proven helpful in this circumstance is to suggest that the hygienist of the referring dentist see the patient at the time of the dentist's own twice-annual recall. Shortly afterward and by mutual agreement, the periodontist himself has an appointment with the patient. By this time coronal scaling, polishing, oral hygiene review, and much or all of the needed root planing have been completed. During his appointment, the periodontist is able to reexamine the patient carefully, to complete what root instrumentation may be required, and to project any necessary additional treatment. This form of joint recall does enable the referring dentist to keep the patient under review, yet meets the exacting needs of patient and periodontist.

Alternating the recall visits between general practitioner and periodontist appears on the surface to have distinct merit. The busy periodontist in particular may see it as a means of coping more effectively with an ever-increasing number of treated patients. Unfortunately, the arrangement tends to break down in practice. Delays in communication between the offices and between both offices and the patient have the effect of lengthening the recall interval. Oversights occur also in the relaying of important information about the patient. In short, the patient tends to be left too long without close attention to areas of concern. It is for this reason that one finds the alternative recall plan abandoned so often.

The question of who should perform recall treatment grows increasingly important. The very availability of specialist care comes to be influenced by the views which generalists and specialists develop toward this question. Many periodontists, in the early phase of practice, accept virtually all patients referred to them. Sooner or later, most decide that they can achieve reasonable peace of mind only when they are free to direct the periodontal maintenance of the involved patient. Translated into the language of referral, this means that periodontists come to accept patients from certain dentists only. In effect, they restrict themselves to the patients of dentists who approve of continued periodontal supervision in the periodontal office.[15,24]

Frequency of Maintenance Treatment

Obviously, office maintenance procedures should be performed when necessary, but no more frequently than that. A person's circumstances and health fluctuate and with them both the oral environment and the attention to hygiene. The level of periodontal disease activity also changes. For these reasons, there must be flexibility in the setting of the recall interval. Nonetheless, some useful generalizations apply. A more frequent recall (every 2 to 6 months) is needed by patients whose plaque formation is inherently heavy, whose maintenance is poor, or whose periodontium can be best described as thick. On the other hand, patients whose plaque formation was light even at the outset of treatment, whose oral hygiene has become excellent and has remained so, or who have a thin periodontium usually require less frequent office attention. For them, recall every 9 months or even every year makes good sense.

Some patients susceptible to periodontal disease cannot or will not perform oral hygiene, but are willing to receive and pay for office care. A number of patients in this category have been treated with some success by frequent coronal scaling and root curettage over many years. Office treatment of these individuals must be scheduled at the highest practical frequency,

e.g., every 6 weeks to 2 months. It is interesting to note the growing evidence of periodontal disease containment associated with frequent tooth "cleaning" by trained therapists, with or without personal oral hygiene efforts by the patient.[2,6,17]

PROCEDURAL ASPECTS OF MAINTENANCE THERAPY

A casual and impromptu approach to maintenance therapy invites unpleasant surprise. Unless a rather formal procedural approach is taken, unwelcome contingencies will almost certainly follow.

Prerequisites to Effective Periodontal Maintenance

The allotment of sufficient time is the most important single prerequisite to effective recall. There must be time for the hygienist to perform the essential steps. Time must be allotted to enable the periodontist to phase in with the hygienist and to decide how much further he must go himself. Whatever additional treatment steps are needed, time must be set aside for them. Finally, there has to be a time for correspondence and telephone communication with the general practitioner, the patient's physician, and any other dental specialists who may be involved.

One cannot treat a patient rationally until there is knowledge of that patient. Every therapist involved in recall treatment, whether hygienist, general dentist, or periodontist needs enough time to tune in—in other words, to derive, to organize, and to apply information. Certainly the periodontist must have time at regular intervals to compare present findings with similar objective data from the past. In addition, one needs time to develop present subjective impressions of the patient through observation and conversation. The overview of the patient, derived by the combining of subjective impressions with objective data, is so valuable that it must be obtained periodically if one is to do the patient justice year by year.

Recall attention to the patient with periodontal disease takes longer than one anticipates. In some respects the recall can be looked upon as a capsulized total treatment regimen. The therapist derives information, develops a plan based upon it, acts on that plan, and then observes the response.

The grouping of maintenance appointments on a given day has much to commend it.[15] A therapist who follows this practice is able to assume and retain the mind-set of the detective for a half day or even a full day at a time, as the case may be. He is not required nearly as often to break away from, say, a surgical appointment or a demanding occlusal adjustment to make an all-too-brief review of a recall patient. He is not tempted to indulge in wishful thinking and to say to the patient that everything is fine when the time available is not sufficient for the careful scrutiny that should precede such a statement.

Recording observations of significance made at any time during recall examination and treatment should become part of the procedure. This means the dictation or actual writing of notes as an appointment proceeds. Often the close observation given to gingiva and teeth during curettage brings much to light (e.g., a floss cut, an area of food retention, an isolated facet, or recurring caries). The hygienist and periodontist must record such minutiae promptly or they will be forgotten.

Functioning of the Office Force

The established periodontal office today has a work force consisting of at least a dental hygienist, a dental assistant, and a receptionist. In a large practice there are often two or more of each. A secretary-typist and a plaque control therapist may round out the force. Just how the members of the group should handle all office situations is obviously beyond the scope of the present review; nonetheless, the members have their collective and individual places in the maintenance of the periodontal patient.

All the personnel share the basic assignments of (1) ensuring appointments at the necessary time intervals, (2) establishing necessary amounts of time when an appointment is needed, and (3) keeping appropriate records that are understandable to all. As a rule, only the periodontist and the hygienist are directly involved in treatment. Of course, when a plaque-control therapist is on the staff, she assumes most of the initial responsibility for educating the patient in oral hygiene.

The *dental hygienist* today is being assigned an increasingly large part of periodontal maintenance therapy. After all, the ties of the dental hygiene profession to the prevention of periodontal disease and to periodontology have been so close over the years that it is difficult to imagine the situation evolving otherwise. However, maximum contributions can be made by the hygienist only when the periodontist stays closely identified with the hygienist's activity and with the patients under the hygienist's care.

Today as always it is the periodontist who determines to a large degree the sense of accomplishment the hygienist derives from being in the office and the thoroughness of the recall treatment that the patients receive. The conscientious periodontist will have set out a recall plan at the end of active therapy. It re-

mains for him to reinforce and modify that plan as time goes by. He must encourage the hygienist's careful examination and instrumentation and not be too busy with treatment of new patients, leaving the hygienist too much on her own. He must help the hygienist to recognize the danger signals in the patients that should trigger her concern and attention. He should then take early action based upon the hygienist's findings and advise her of that action. He must provide the hygienist with enough time to render her own professional treatment. This is achieved by letting the hygienist schedule the return visits of maintenance patients whose recall is incomplete. Certainly the receptionist should not be the one to determine the length of the hygienist's appointments. The hygienist needs freedom to do this according to her requirements. Finally, the periodontist should try to make himself available to her for review of her record taking and/or treatment when she requests it. If he finds this impossible, he has the obligation to do his review at an early subsequent appointment and thereafter to report promptly to her.

The *receptionist* plays the invaluable role of bringing together the periodontist, the hygienist, and the patient. She does this through (1) her management of a single master appointment book for the office and (2) her contact with the patients at the time of their arrival, at their departure, and over the telephone between appointments. In doing all this, she functions as an intermediary for, but not as the manager of, the dental hygienist and the periodontist.

The *secretary-typist* (or the receptionist in her absence) is the compiler of information and the person who supervises the transfer of information from the periodontist to the referring dentist and vice versa. This is a basic and critical function in the office. Many patients suffer delay in their follow-up treatment because letters or radiographs are held up as a result of office inefficiencies.

The *dental assistant* is an indispensable co-worker of the periodontist and the hygienist. This individual, once trained, can record data dictated by the hygienist during the recall examination and can chart specifics that come to light during treatment (caries, functional tooth mobility, special root sensitivities). Her services at the chair enable the therapist to move swiftly into treatment with appropriate instruments at hand. Yet to perform efficiently, she must already have been well trained and the periodontist must already have established the plan of treatment. No assistant should be required to guess the next step in treatment. Instead, the therapist should dictate directly to the assistant a brief verbal summary at the end of each appointment. This information is written directly onto the treatment page of the chart, establishing the treatment just completed, giving the steps in treatment to be rendered at the next recall visit, and stating what correspondence or telephone call, if any, is now required. In this way, the assistant establishes an accurate record before the therapist's train of thought is interrupted. She also leaves herself and the therapist invaluable written signals that may be needed in preparing for the next appointment with that patient.

Management of Particular Types of Recall Patients

The patients who continue with the periodontist on a recall basis are a most varied cross section. The majority, of course, have been referred from a local general practitioner. They enjoy reasonable health, have completed a standard periodontal treatment regimen, and do their best to uphold their part of the maintenance. On the other hand, there are numerous patients who do not fit this mold. Most of these exceptions can be grouped into ten categories. Suggestions for management of patients within each category are included in the following list.

1. The patient who won't cooperate in oral hygiene but will pay for office care.
   Management: Frequent, thorough curettage (see page 712).

2. The patient who has refused surgical treatment.
   Management: The recall interval must be shorter than for patients who have received surgical therapy. The curettage phase will involve more time and will be relatively more difficult to do properly.

3. The patient who, for one of a variety of reasons other than personal refusal, is not a surgical candidate—for example, the alcoholic and the patient with high caries susceptibility.
   Management: The same as for category 1.

4. The patient who is hospitalized and has been for several weeks.
   Management: The patient's condition permitting, there should be periodic scaling and review of oral hygiene by the hygienist in the hospital dental clinic. This patient will do best if given daily encouragement and assistance with oral hygiene by the nursing staff.

5. The patient who has been bedridden for a time and is now ambulatory.
   Management: Short appointments, major emphasis on renewal of oral hygiene, thorough caries examination, curettage, and a display of honest concern.

6. The patient who has been fully and "success-fully" treated, yet who now shows distinct breakdown in localized areas.
   Management: A general health review. If this is favorable, then aggressive surgical retreatment of involved areas. Control of occlusal forces.

7. The patient referred to the periodontist from another specialist, such as an orthodontist or a prosthodontist. The referral is often made with a particular surgical end result in mind, the other specialist having realized that he should wait until periodontal evaluation and/or treatment has been completed. Frequently a patient in this group will not require periodontal maintenance as such.
   Management: Surgery and/or other therapy, if required, with maintenance therapy. If no therapy is indicated, return the patient to the referring specialist.

8. The patient whose original periodontist has retired from practice.
   Management: If possible, obtain complete information about the patient's present condition and past treatment from the original therapist. Review these data. If past data are not available, take a detailed history of past dental treatment. During the first 6 months at least continue basic maintenance care. This is preferable to repeating surgical treatment in the same areas or embarking on a new periodontal-restorative or orthodontic approach.

9. The patient who has just moved into the area having been referred to you for continued maintenance by a periodontist in another part of the country.
   Management: Obtain all possible information from the original specialist. Communicate directly with the referring therapist by telephone, in addition to sending a letter of inquiry. A letter from the referring office may bring only the most basic information. Why? Because it may well have been prepared by an assistant who has had access to the patient's record but has no direct recollection or personal knowledge of the patient at all. Comments from the referring dentist should be taken to heart, particularly when they relate to the patient's temperament and response to treatment. Proceed cautiously with forms of treatment other than those used by the referring specialist in his maintenance of the case.[32]

10. The patient who is moving away. The growing mobility of modern society gives rise to a surprising turnover of patients in any periodontal practice. The periodontist can take it for

granted that he will remain in the community while a great many of his patients will move away. Axiomatically, he must be prepared to pass on useful data and records to the periodontist or generalist who is to continue therapy. *Management:* Select a specific periodontist or generalist in the patient's new community and give his name to the patient. Select and photocopy essential records and address a covering letter to the specialist or generalist selected. However, before sending any records, wait to hear that the patient has made contact. Patients do act capriciously. A patient whom you judged to be well briefed may decide to go to an entirely different practitioner, who will not therefore receive the useful data you have developed over the years unless some attempt at recovery is made.

Instead of going to a different specialist, the patient who moves away may reach the recommended periodontist later than anticipated. Many patients need to spend some time adjusting to their new environments before they are willing to resume dental treatment—a tendency that can result in delayed maintenance. Again, when a patient has adjusted and is ready to call for an appointment, the periodontist's name may have been misplaced, causing more delay.

A useful means of reducing such problems is to send a follow-up letter to all patients being referred elsewhere. The letter simply prompts needed maintenance attention by again offering the name and address of the periodontist in the new community. The periodontist can remind himself to send the letter by entering the patient's name and the words *reminder of referral* in the office memo book under the appropriate future date.

Maintenance Therapy Proper

Orderly procedure is the rule in all aspects of periodontal therapy. Neither the generalist nor the periodontist can dispense with careful treatment planning and constant reevaluation of effort.

THE BASIC ROUTINE

Although it is folly to do the same thing for each patient at recall, the efficient performance of maintenance therapy requires a basic routine. The pattern must vary, but usually it should take the following form:

1. Brief review of the patient's chart, especially the medical history, the original diagnosis, and the outline of active treatment.
2. Determination of significant events between the last periodontal appointment and the present date, recorded under the headings of "interim medical history" and "interim dental history."
3. Brief clinical examination and partial recording of the present dental status. At least the occlusion and the level of oral hygiene should be evaluated at this early stage in the recall appointment. Radiographs are taken now if the time interval calls for it.
4. Occlusal adjustment (selective grinding), as required.
5. Oral hygiene instruction and review, as required.
6. Instrumentation of the teeth concurrent with further periodontal examination. (Instrumentation is used in the broad sense to include removal of all deposit, root planing, polishing of the clinical crowns, application of fluoride, if indicated.)
7. Further notes recorded, under the heading of "present dental status" during the course of root instrumentation.
8. Determination of the additional treatment needed: New periodontal treatment? Periodontal retreatment? Restorative treatment?
9. Reappointment for the next maintenance visit.
10. Communication with the dentist(s) who will be performing the needed additional treatment (usually restorative care).

COMMUNICATION WITH THE PATIENT

Any effective recall appointment requires some forethought in planning and coordination. First, one must plan to bring the patient back at a certain future date. The patient is told at the end of one recall visit when the next will take place. If that future appointment is to be less than 3 months away, a definite appointment time is entered. If the interval is 3 months or more, the patient is told the month of the next appointment and assured that a specific date will be established by telephone approximately one month prior to the appointment. Where possible, appointments are made for a time before rather than beyond the desired interval; e.g., if the patient is on a 4-month recall schedule and will be away on the 4-month date, it is preferable to make an appointment for $3\frac{1}{2}$ months rather than 5. Second, any unduplicated records (be they photographs, models, or records) that have been sent to any other dentist in the interval should be retrieved. So often, when they are not on hand is the time when they could be examined to advantage. Third, there is the need to make sure that the patient brings to the appointment all removable dental appliances. Patients should be reminded of this requirement when the recall appointment is made (the receptionist having noted the appliance alert on the chart folder). Of course, a final telephone prompting needs to be given on the day prior to the visit.

The periodontist will do well to have his office staff, if not himself, review the charts of those who are appearing at recall at least 3 days ahead of time. If this suggestion is not followed, all too often one is facing the patient before the absence of a reply from another dentist to an important question is noticed. Usually, it is too late to obtain the information then, another appointment must be made, and valuable time is lost.

COMMUNICATION WITH OTHER DENTISTS

The periodontist must also keep up a useful working relationship with the general practitioner as to the status of each long-term maintenance patient. Unless he does this, the patient ceases to be under control and drifts into a disconcerting gray zone. Every periodontist who has been at all long in practice is bound to have reflected on the problem. He cannot avoid asking himself the reason for the one-way nature of the communication between himself and the generalist. Put another way, why is it so difficult to obtain firm confirmation in writing of a treatment plan both should agree upon? Similarly, in a matter even more basic to their joint care of the patient, why does the referring dentist so seldom confirm in writing what restorative and other treatment he has done for the patient?

The absence of two-way communication leads to the unfolding of a story such as the one which follows: The periodontist, after seeing the patient on recall and noting root caries, advises the general practitioner in writing of this finding. He also advises the generalist that he has asked the patient to contact his dentist. Months pass without word from the referring dentist. The time of the next periodontal maintenance appointment arrives, and the patient is seen. "Did you visit Dr. X after our last appointment?" "Oh yes, and he filled those teeth where you found decay. On examining the mouth the periodontist finds that, while some of the carious teeth have been restored, others have not. The periodontist naturally wonders why the interim restorative treatment took the turn it did. However, until he takes the initiative himself and speaks directly to the general dentist on the telephone, he will never know. Even then, he may not learn the reasons behind the decisions taken because the generalist may be a person who records little on a pa-

tient's chart. To expect him to recall from memory the reasons for a decision made months ago with respect to one area in one mouth among hundreds is indeed asking the impossible.

Fortunately, improvements in communication already are noticeable. Between numerous practitioners there is definite two-way communication. The greatest frustration arises when all messages seem to go one way. The tendency of many generalists to telephone their views and to reach decisions purely on the strength of a two-way verbal exchange without making detailed written notes also complicates the picture. At the least, decisions made on the telephone should be dated and recorded on the chart. When both parties to the decision follow this rule, there is little room for misunderstanding. When they do not, the door to vagueness and unintentional delay is opened.

Ideally, then, the most effective and satisfying communication between professionals combines writing with speaking. There is no substitute for a written plan that has been agreed upon and that can be referred to at any time by both parties to the agreement. For this reason, the first letter to the referring dentist should be mailed when the periodontist is beginning active periodontal treatment.

Usually the second occasion for a letter comes when active periodontal treatment has been completed and restorative moves are to follow or when a summary of the results of periodontal treatment is needed. Sometimes a telephone conversation may be preferable to a letter at this stage. Most dentists would choose to telephone rather than to write. There is the saving of precious time involved when one can speak instead of writing or dictating. An even greater advantage, of course, is that during telephone conversation one can rapidly exchange details and impressions about a patient. This voice exchange often culminates in a decision about the patient that would have taken much longer to reach, or simply could not have been reached at all, through writing alone.

Many periodontists employ a printed three-copy recall report page or simply an office no-carbon-required (NCR) form to communicate with the referring dentist after maintenance appointments.[26] The NCR three-part reply form, sent on to the referring dentist, is of tremendous value also in recording and confirming the essence of a telephone conversation. The periodontist retains one copy, and the referring dentist receives two, one to keep and another on which to send his reply to any question.[24]

Each letter or form sent or received and each telephone communication should be noted by date on the chart. The treatment record page is the logical area for this. When films are mailed to another dentist or a duplicate charting is sent along, this transmission is likewise entered either on the treatment record page or on the inside of the chart folder, after the date.

Good communication between the office and the patient has a great deal to do with the return of the patient after the maintenance interval. Again, the telephone seems to add a certainty and warmth of persuasion to these contacts that no reminder note or appointment card alone can match. At the completion of one recall visit, the patient is handed an appointment card giving only the month of the next appointment. The recall file card is updated and then filed, so that 4 weeks before the time of the next recall visit the receptionist is alerted and telephones the patient. Only then do receptionist and patient agree upon a specific date and appointment time. One day prior to this time, the receptionist calls again to impart a sense of genuine interest and to confirm the arrangement in a business-like way. Surprisingly few patients are remiss after two telephone contacts.

THE USE OF RADIOGRAPHS

Radiographs should be part of periodontal maintenance therapy. They have great value in that they afford a comparison of bone levels at different stages. Unfortunately, they cannot offer any true indication of the amount of soft-tissue reattachment that has occurred. They should be taken at sensible intervals as nearly identically as possible, using the long-cone paralleling technique or period-identical devices.[25] They offer a unique means of assessing the alveolar bone crest and any change therein from year to year. The following outline lists several categories of maintenance patient, a suggested type of radiographic survey for each, and the advisable intervals between surveys:

1. Originally, severe marginal periodontitis with or without prosthesis: full-mouth periapical series; every 3 years.
2. Originally, slight-to-moderate periodontitis: full-mouth periapical series; every 5 years.
3. Standard maintenance patient in categories (1) and (2): posterior bite-wing films; every year.
4. Any patient with a known high susceptibility to caries: posterior bite-wing films; every 6 months.
5. Areas of particular concern in any patient, e.g., a surgical area treated by means of an osseous graft or the intrabony technique:[23] individual periapical films of the areas; annually at least, often every 6 months.

Some have advocated that the first posttreatment films be taken when active treatment actually ends.

Others point out that the first recall (usually 3 months after treatment) is a more appropriate time, because then the alveolar bone has had sufficient time to demonstrate a response to the therapy employed.[12] The Fixott-Everett grid offers another supplemental means of evaluating bone loss over the long term.[8]

It is essential, of course, that films be mounted and preserved for later use in the assessment of change. All films should be placed in mounts and arranged chronologically, the most recent on top. If all radiographs are held within a large envelope securely attached to the inside of the patient's folder, they will remain readily accessible.

SPECIFIC TECHNICAL PROBLEMS IN MAINTENANCE TREATMENT

The effectiveness of maintenance treatment is improved when periodontist and hygienist are alert to the various technical problems that may appear. More often than not, these problems have to do with the completion of curettage and the handling of persistent pockets in an otherwise healthy periodontium. Typical challenges and instruments that can be useful in meeting them include the following:

1. The proximal surfaces of two very closely placed anterior teeth
   Suggested instruments: anterior Jacquette scaler rendered very slender by repeated sharpening, or the Ransom and Randolph D-6 scaler
2. The curved facial and lingual surfaces of lower anterior teeth
   Suggested instruments: Columbia 13/14 curet, Hirschfeld files 3 and 7, or small curets such as the Hutchinson 1 and 2
3. The pocket localized to one surface of a tooth and approachable only through a narrow orifice
   Suggested instruments: Hirschfeld files 3 and 7
4. The furcation area that is difficult to instrument, even though it can be probed
   Suggested instruments: Hirschfeld files, McCall 4R/4L curet with narrowed blade, Gracey 7/8 curet
5. The distal surfaces of the most distal teeth in the mouth
   Suggested instruments: McCall 4R/4L curet, Gracey 13/14 curet

One is no sooner applying the level of scrutiny and detailed attention to the teeth that goes with maintenance root planing than other needs often become apparent. New carious surfaces come to light. These are recorded when discovered, and their locations are communicated to the restorative dentist. Unfortunately, one finds the occasional carious area still untreated long after the mention of it in the recall summary sent to the referring dentist. When caries of root dentin has been detected in a fluting or in a furcation area, there is concern; when the root caries has been left untreated for any length of time, there is urgency. At this point, a follow-through to the referring dentist by note or telephone call is obviously indicated because of the speed with which root caries can progress toward the nearby pulp.

Persistent and generalized tooth sensitivity is another challenge. It is usually related to fairly recent surgical exposure or to overly vigorous curetting of tooth roots near the cementoenamel junction.[11]

Sensitivity of one tooth can also be a problem when the patient returns on a maintenance visit. Frequently in the periodontal patient, it is a feature of occlusal traumatism and is closely associated with parafunctional stress.[36] Vitality testing may be indicated. In fact, a more general use of the electric pulp tester during maintenance treatment is advised.

The most difficult decisions to make in long-term maintenance involve unmistakable evidence of progressive breakdown since the time of the original treatment. Assume for the moment that the dentition has been maintained for a long time. If the deterioration relates to a single terminal tooth that stands isolated and does not support a prosthesis, the decisions can be fairly straightforward. Extraction of that tooth is sometimes the best step, especially when bite guards are already in use or when a fixed prosthesis is already present in the opposing segment. Either of these appliances prevents the eruption of the opposing teeth.

When several posterior teeth in the continuous arch, are almost equally affected, one is required to resolve a more complex problem.[14] Should one or more of the teeth with furcation involvements receive endodontic treatment and subsequent root amputation? Should one of them be extracted? The periodontist must weigh not only the new clinical findings, but also his knowledge of the patient's oral hygiene and the skill of the associated dentist. He must consult with that dentist and of course reach an understanding with the patient on cost and prognosis. Maintenance treatment becomes once again active treatment. Perhaps this having to resume multidisciplinary treatment, the expense of it, and the reminders offered to all concerned that periodontitis is a tenacious, chronic disease are what make the examples of continued breakdown, in spite of maintenance, so disturbing to all concerned.

DOCUMENTATION

There is a great need for documentation at the end of active or primary treatment. Without such documentation, an essential baseline for evaluation during maintenance treatment is lost (another baseline, of course, is the pretreatment record). Fortunately, this need is met by most periodontists today.

The documentation that should appear in one form or another in the posttreatment record includes (1) a full charting, (2) written notes (or a check-off review) on the soft-tissue response to treatment, the oral hygiene status, and the areas of concern, and (3) alerts.

Areas of concern are specific areas that will bear careful watching in the future. They may be ones that had and still have only a fair prognosis or areas where the response to treatment was disappointing, e.g., where less than one millimeter of true attached gingiva remains over the buccal aspect of a lower first bicuspid. The value of a note about an area of concern is increased if one adds the reason for accepting the given result in that area despite treatment.

Alerts are warning signals to the periodontist and to all who will be dealing with the patient. The need for some alerts is determined at the outset of treatment. They are added or removed as circumstances change during the maintenance years. Colored adhesive tape makes an excellent signal because it is both visible and adherent. Tape markers should be applied to the top right-hand corner of the chart folder and the current treatment record page, e.g.:

1. Red tab, denoting danger—sensitivity to an antibiotic, local anesthetic or other drug; a history of diabetes, hypertension, hepatitis, coronary disease, or rheumatic fever.
2. Green tab for the patient with root sensitivity and therefore a need for infiltration or block anesthesia, or supplemental nitrous oxide-oxygen analgesia during root instrumentation.
3. Orange tab for the patient with a very active gag reflex.
4. Yellow tab for the patient who uses bite guards, a Hawley appliance or a power brush and who, prior to the recall appointment, should receive a telephone-call reminder to bring in the device(s) for review. This alert is of greatest value when it is attached to the recall card and accompanied by an appropriate memo.

The records kept during the maintenance phase of treatment should be to a large extent an extension of those that have already been developed for the patient. If they are not and are casual, insufficient, or lacking in pattern, they will not serve the periodontist or the patient satisfactorily. It is helpful to remember that the most useful information about the patient is the information that is quickly found. Another point to keep in mind is that much of the data collected at any one maintenance visit has more significance when compared with earlier data than when considered alone. For this reason, it is worthwhile developing a chart containing several pages, each given over to a particular type of data. The reverse side of each page is left blank. Over the months and years following primary therapy, additional pages are added one upon the other so that the most recently developed pages and their data lie on top. It then becomes a simple matter to compare the present with the past by turning back the successive pages. In this way, one quickly gains an impression of the status of the patient's periodontal disease. Soon, if one follows this idea through, the several separate pages of the original chart become separate packages of data pages, with the most recent entry sheet on the top of each packet.

Periodontal charts will always vary according to individual preference. Despite this, a trend toward more uniform periodontal documentation is evident. There is now invariably a separate treatment record page. For good reason, this page is often placed in the first position, so that it is immediately apparent when the chart folder is opened. There is frequently occasion to inspect this page because it offers important clues to the staff and the therapist. Next in the folder, most periodontists use a separate page for some form of pictorial chart. To have that as the second page, after the treatment record, makes good sense. When a patient is entering upon treatment for the first time, many dentists employ still a third page to record such important basics as the summary of etiologic factors, the diagnoses, the prognosis (of individual teeth and of the dentition), and the treatment plan. A fourth page, usually present in one form or another, provides the essential background data gained at the pretreatment history taking and examination.

During the lifelong maintenance of a periodontal patient one must obviously continue to listen, question, examine, plan, treat, and record. The essentials of any treatment rendered are placed on the treatment record (page 1). Examination results, such as pocket depths, recessions, furcation involvements, and tooth mobility, go onto a page 2. Lastly, a modified page 3 receives other data about the patient under such headings as:

1. Interim medical history
2. Interim dental history
3. Present dental status
   Oral mucosa
   Gingiva
     Bleeding
     Color changes
   Teeth
     Plaque
     Stain
     Calculus
     Caries
     Bite guards
     Prosthesis
4. Areas of concern
5. Recall treatment plan

The volume of paper that accumulates is not as great as one might imagine. For example, each charting page will carry at least two separate series of charting entries. One usually re-charts at yearly intervals. Accordingly, a new page 2 is added every 2 or 3 years. If the charting records on a patient do show signs of becoming too bulky, they can be grouped into manageable 10-year packages.

A small but important consideration in record keeping nowadays is the use of a black-ink pen with medium-thickness point. A bold black ink record duplicates clearly, whereas a fine black line or a blue one, fine or otherwise, can prove almost illegible once it has been duplicated. In view of the current amount of duplicating of patient records this is significant.

Documentation of treatment is too important to be left to chance. Many of the activities associated with maintenance ought to be recorded on the treatment record (page 1) when and as they occur, e.g., (1) treatment rendered, (2) examination and charting performed, (3) radiographs taken, (4) radiographs ordered from another office, (5) radiographs received from the patient or from another office, (6) models received, (7) photographs taken, (8) oral hygiene procedures demonstrated or reviewed, (9) oral hygiene aids issued to the patient, (10) notes sent and received, (11) telephone conversations with the patient, a physician, or another dentist, (12) the next recall date (month and year and by whom the recall treatment will be performed, e.g., A.O., periodontist only, or D.H., dental hygienist, + A.O.). The date of the recall should be written out at the end of the treatment entry and circled in red. When another appointment is required to complete the treatment the word *next* is used. It is circled to catch the eye and a short note is added, indicating the specific treatment to follow, e.g., (1) oral hygiene review—lingual lower molars, (2) bite guard check, (3) root planing, UL, LL.

Periodic recording of specific data on the graphic chart (page 2) is also fundamental to good maintenance. How often is this necessary? The nature of the patient's involvement will dictate the frequency. A stable, well-maintained patient should have a complete probing only once a year. In other patients, areas of concern ought to be probed gently at each recall interval. This is particularly true for an area where progressive deterioration is feared. Furcation involvements, gingival recessions, tooth mobilities, and the occlusion all require a similar application of good judgment as to when they should be re-charted. A review and re-charting of these features every 12 months has much to recommend it.

Gingival recession is another feature deserving consistent attention during the maintenance years. Women patients in particular express concern over this. They will often ask about one particular area of root exposure. "Isn't there more root exposed there now than a year ago?" Only by measuring and recording on the pictorial chart the distance from the cementoenamel junction to the gingival margin in a recession area, and doing this annually, can one answer such a question.

Photographs, like radiographs, have their place in the long-term documentation process. If taken periodically, they make a considerable difference to the sense of control the therapist ought to have. Usually recall photographs are confined to areas of concern and are taken at intervals of a year or more. The plastic slide storage pages now available with their pouches for individual 2 × 2 slides have simplified the storage and comparison of serial views.

Maintenance of homeostasis in the periodontal patient has as its objectives the preservation of the beneficial results of treatment and the early discovery and treatment of new lesions. The periodontist exerts a critical influence on this long-term therapy because his conviction is what sustains the demanding effort. Success in this venture is never won. When it is glimpsed, and glimpsed it is increasingly, that is encouragement enough for patient and therapist alike.

References

1. Adams, F.: What is periodontal maintenance care and whose responsibility is it? J. West. Soc. Periodont., 11:12, 1963.
2. Axelsson, P., and Lindhe, J.: The effect of a preventive programme on dental plaque, gingivitis and caries in schoolchildren. Results after one and two years. J. Clin. Periodontol., 1:126, 1974.
3. Brandtzaeg, P., and Jamison, H. C.: The effect of controlled cleansing of teeth on periodontal health and oral hygiene in Norwegian Army recruits. J. Periodontol., 35:302, 1964.
4. Brustein, D. D., and Rauschart, E. A.: A comparative study on the relationship between the specialist and the referring dentist. J. Periodontol., 42:306, 1971.
4a. Chace, R.: The maintenance phase of periodontal therapy. J. Periodontol., 22:23, 1951.
5. Chace, R.: Subgingival curettage in periodontal therapy. J. Periodontol., 45:107, 1974.
6. Chawla, T. N., Nanda, R. S., and Kapoor, K. K.: Dental prophylaxis procedures in control of periodontal disease in Lucknow (rural) India. J. Periodontol., 46:498, 1975.
7. Drennan, G. A.: Personal communication, 1975.
8. Fixott, H. C., Everett, F. G., and Watkins, R. F.: Refinements in diagnostic x-ray technique with the use of wire grids, J. Am. Dent. Assoc., 78:122, 1969.
9. Friedman, N.: Etiology of marginal gingivitis and periodontitis, Alpha Omegan, 55:2, 1962.
10. Heins, P. H.: The generalist and the specialist. Module 1 in Periodontal Surgery for the General Practitioner. Dept. of Periodontics, School of Dentistry, University of Washington, 1974.
11. Hirschfeld, L.: Subgingival curettage in periodontal treatment. J. Am. Dent. Assoc., 44:301, 1952.
12. Hornbuckle, C.: Washington State Society of Periodontists, Seattle, Washington, March 5, 1975.
13. Knowles, J.: Oral hygiene related to long term effects of periodontal therapy. J. Mich. Dent. Assoc., 44:147, 1973.
14. Kramer, G.: Dental failures associated with periodontal surgery. Dent. Clin. North Am., 16:13, 1972.
15. Kramer, G.: Washington State Society of Periodontists, Seattle, February 3, 1975.
16. Lightner, M. L.: Preventive periodontal treatment procedures: results over 46 months. J. Periodontol., 42:555, 1971.
17. Lovdal, A., et al.: Combined effect of subgingival scaling and controlled oral hygiene on the incidence of gingivitis. Acta Odontol. Scand., 19:537, 1961.
18. Lovdal, A., Arno, A., and Waerhaug, J.: Incidence of clinical manifestations of periodontal disease in light of oral hygiene and calculus formation. J. Am. Dent. Assoc., 56:21, 1958.
19. Nyman, S., Rosling, B., and Lindhe, J.: Effect of professional tooth cleaning on healing after periodontal surgery. J. Clin. Periodontol., 2:80, 1975.
20. Ogilvie, A. L.: Recall and maintenance of the periodontal patient. Periodontics, 5:198, 1967.
21. Parr, R. W.: Periodontal Maintenance Therapy. Berkeley, Calif., Praxis Publishing Co., 1974.
22. Parr, R. W.: The approach to undergraduate periodontics at the School of Dentistry, University of California, San Francisco. Am. Assoc. Dental Schools, Section on Periodontics, San Francisco, Calif., March, 1975.
23. Prichard, J. F.: Advanced Periodontal Disease, 2nd ed. Philadelphia, W. B. Saunders Co., 1972, p. 782.
24. Prichard, J. F.: Periodontist-patient-referring dentist interrelationships. Am. Acad. Periodont., Atlanta, Oct. 1974.
25. Ramfjord, S. P.: Design of studies or clinical trials to evaluate the effectiveness of agents or procedures for the prevention, or treatment, of loss of the periodontium. J. Periodont. Res., 9 (Suppl. 14):78, 1974.
26. Robinson, R. E.: Maintenance of the periodontally treated patient. In Periodontal Therapy, 5th ed. H. M. Goldman and D. W. Cohen, Eds. St. Louis, C. V. Mosby Co., 1973, Ch. 35.
27. Sandrew, S. H.: Summary of patient interpretation after experiencing periodontal therapy. J. Periodontol., 43:237, 1972.
28. Schaffer, E. M.: What is periodontal maintenance care

and whose responsibility is it? J. West. Soc. Periodont., *11:*9, March, 1963.

29. Schluger, S.: Personal communication, 1975.
30. Selipsky, H. S.: A longitudinal study of osseous surgery and plaque control in periodontal therapy, and their effects upon tooth mobility. M.S.D. thesis, University of Washington, 1973.
31. Stainbrook, E.: The practice of dentistry and the behaviour of people. Fifth Annual Dean Jones Lecture, University of Washington, Seattle, March 31, 1975.
32. Sternlicht, H. C.: Evaluating long-term periodontal therapy. J. Prevent. Dent., *2:*4, 1975.
33. Suomi, J. D., et al.: The effect of controlled oral hygiene procedures on the progression of periodontal disease in adults: results after third and final year. J. Periodontol., *42:*152, 1971.
34. Thomas, B. O. A.: What is periodontal maintenance care and whose responsibility is it?, J. West. Soc. Periodont., *11:*8, 1963.
35. Weiner, L.: The relationship between the specialist and the referring dentist, Periodont. Abstr., *16:*6, 1968.
36. Yuodelis, R.: Personal communication, 1975.
37. Zaki, H. A., and Stallard, R. E.: The role of the dental hygienist in preventive periodontics, J. Periodontol., *42:*233, 1971.

Suggested Reading

Chace, R.: The role of the dental hygienist in periodontal practice. J. Periodontol., *30:*47, 1959.

Cimasoni, G.: L'hygiéniste dentaire (The right girl in the right place?) Rev. Mens. Suisse Odontostomatol., *84:*329, 1974.
Fisk, A. R.: The future role of the dental hygienist in oral health. Dent. Clin. North Am., March, 1966, p. 219.
Grant, D., Stern, I. B., and Everett, F. G.: Orban's Periodontics, 4th ed. St. Louis, C. V. Mosby Co., 1972, pp. 685–687.
Hamp, S. E., Nyman, S., and Lindhe, J.: Periodontal treatment of multirooted teeth. Results after 5 years. J. Clin. Periodontol., *2:*126, 1975.
Lobene, R. R.: Periodontics and dental hygiene, J. Dent. Educ., *30:*221, 1966.
Lobene, R. R.: What is the future role of auxiliaries in periodontics? Periodont. Abstr., *20:*157, 1972.
McFall, W. R., Jr.: Periodontics—an old challenge revisited. J. Tenn. Dent. Assoc., *45:*28, 1963.
Miller, O. A.: Psychological considerations in dentistry. J. Am. Dent. Assoc., *81:*941, 1970.
Oliver, R. C.: Tooth loss with and without periodontal therapy, Periodont. Abstr., *17:*8, 1969.
Ramfjord, S. P., et al.: Longitudinal study of periodontal therapy. J. Periodontol., *44:*66, 1973.
Robinson, R. E.: Practice management problems with the referred patient. J. West. Soc. Periodont., *8:*8, 1960.

Index

Page numbers in *italics* refer to illustrations. Page numbers followed by the letter "t" refer to tables.